Volume 1

ABDOMINAL OPERATIONS

sixth edition

APPLETON-CENTURY-CROFTS / New York
A Publishing Division of Prentice-Hall, Inc.

Volume 1

ABDOMINAL OPERATIONS

sixth edition

RODNEY MAINGOT

and
British and American Contributors

Library of Congress Catalog Card Number:
73-12963

Library of Congress Cataloging in Publication Data

Maingot, Rodney, 1893
Abdominal Operations, 6th ed.

Includes bibliographical references.
1. Abdomen-Surgery. I. Title.
[DNLM: 1. Abdomen-Surgery. WI900   M225a]
RD540.M24 1974 617'.55 73-12963
ISBN 0-8385-0042-0

DEDICATED
TO
MY WIFE
EVELYN

CONTRIBUTORS

JOHN ALEXANDER-WILLIAMS, M.D., Ch.M., F.R.C.S. (Eng.)
Consultant Surgeon, United Birmingham Hospital; External Scientific Staff, Medical Research Council; Hunterian Professor, Royal College of Surgeons of England 1963 and 1972; Fellow of the Royal Society of Medicine; Association of Surgeons of Great Britain and Ireland

GARNET WALTER AULT, M.D., F.A.C.S.
Diplomate, American Board of Surgery (Proctology); Diplomate, American Board Colon and Rectal Surgery; Honorary Member, Royal Society of Medicine; Surgeon, The Clinic for Intestinal and Rectal Surgery, Washington, D.C.; Clinical Professor of Surgery, Georgetown University School of Medicine; Chairman, Department of Proctology, Washington Hospital Center; Consultant, Walter Reed Army Hospital, Washington, D.C.

J. PEYTON BARNES, M.D., F.A.C.S
Diplomate of American Board of Surgery; Clinical Professor of Surgery, Baylor University College of Medicine; Chief, Department of Surgery, St. Joseph Hospital, Houston, Texas

B. MARDEN BLACK, M.D., M.D. (Surgery), F.A.C.S.
Consultant, Department of Surgery, Mayo Clinic and Mayo Foundation; Professor of Surgery, Mayo Graduate School of Medicine, University of Minnesota, Rochester, Minnesota

LESLIE HAROLD BLUMGART, B.D.S., M.D., F.R.C.S. (Eng.)
St. Mungo Professor of Surgery, University of Glasgow; Honorary consultant Surgeon, Glasgow Royal Infirmary; Moynihan Fellow of the Association of Surgeons of Great Britain and Ireland, 1972; Former Senior Lecturer and Deputy Director, University Department of Surgery, Welsh National School of Medicine, and Honorary Consultant Surgeon, Cardiff Royal Infirmary and the University Hospital of Wales

SCOTT J. BOLEY, M.D.
Director of Pediatric Surgery, Montefiore Hospital and Medical Center; Professor of Surgery, Albert Einstein College of Medicine, Bronx, New York

JOHN BORRIE, M.B.E., E.D., Ch.M., F.R.C.S. (Eng.), F.R.A.C.S.
Surgeon in Charge, Southern Regional Thoracic Surgical Unit, Dunedin and Wakari Hospitals, Dunedin; Associate Professor of Thoracic Surgery, University of Otago Medical School, New Zealand; Formerly Hunterian Professor and Jacksonian Prizeman, Royal College of Surgeons of England; Assistant Thoracic Surgeon, Newcastle-upon-Tyne, England; Thoracic Surgeon, Green Lane Hospital, Auckland, New Zealand; New Zealand Nuffield Surgical Fellow

IAN ARTHUR DENNIS BOUCHIER, M.D., F.R.C.P.
Professor, Department of Medicine, Dundee University, Dundee, Scotland; Formerly, Reader in Medicine, The University of London; Honorary Consultant Physician, The Royal Free Hospital, London, England

THE RT. HON. LORD BROCK, M.S., F.R.C.S. (Eng.)
Director, Department of Surgical Sciences, Royal College of Surgeons of England; Consultant Surgeon Emeritus, Guy's Hospital and The Brompton Hospital, London; President of the Royal College of Surgeons, 1963–1966

ALEXANDER CAMERON, M. B., Ch.B., F.R.C.S. (Edin.), F.R.C.S. (Eng.)
Senior Lecturer and Deputy Director, Department of Surgical Studies, The Middlesex Hospital, London, England

WARREN H. COLE, M.D., F.A.C.S. (Hon.), F.R.C.S. (Eng.), F.R.C.S. (Hon. Edin.)
Professor Emeritus, Department of Surgery, University of Illinois, College of Medicine, Chicago, Illinois

SIR ZACHARY COPE, B.A., M.D., M.S. (London), F.R.C.S. (Eng.)
Consulting Surgeon, St. Mary's Hospital, London; The Bolingbroke Hospital, London, England

JOHN GEOFFREY SANDISON CRABBE, M.R.C.S., L.R.C.P., F.I.A.C.
Consultant Cytologist, I.C.I. Ltd.; Honorary Consultant Cytologist, Royal Free Hospital; Formerly Director, Royal Free Hospital Cytology Training Centre, London, England

ROBERT E. CROZIER, M.D.
Physician, Department of Gastroenterology, Lahey Clinic Foundation, Boston, Massachusetts; Physician, New England Baptist Hospital and New England Deaconess Hospital

ANTHONY MICHAEL DAWSON, M.D., F.R.C.P.
Physician, St. Bartholomew's Hospital; King Edward VII Hospital for Officers, London, England

MICHAEL E. DE BAKEY, M.D.
President, Baylor College of Medicine; Distinguished Service Professor, Chairman, Cora and Webb Mading Department of Surgery, Baylor College of Medicine; Director, Cardiovascular Research and Training Center, Methodist Hospital, Houston, Texas

ANDREW MORE DESMOND, M.B., B.S. (London), F.R.C.S. (Eng.)
Senior Consultant-Surgeon, Surgeon-in-charge, Gastro-enterological Unit, St. James, Hospital, London, England; Formerly, Examiner and Chairman, Court of Examiners, Royal College of Surgeons of England; Examiner in Surgery, Oxford University, Oxford; External Examiner, Mastership of Surgery, Bagdad University; External Examiner, Mastership of Medicine in Surgery, Singapore University; Member of Council of the Association of Surgeons of Great Britain and Ireland; Surgical Tutor to the South West Metropolitan Regional Hospital Board; Member, Executive Committee of the Committee for Higher Surgical Training

EDWARD B. DIETHRICH, M.D.
Instructor in Surgery, Baylor University College of Medicine, Houston, Texas

LESTER R. DRAGSTEDT, Ph.D., M.D., DsC. O.H.S.
Research Professor of Surgery, Professor of Physiology, University of Florida, Gainesville, Florida

HAROLD ELLIS, M.A., D.M., M.Ch., F.R.C.S. (Eng.)
Professor of Surgery, Westminster Medical School (University of London); Member of Council and Vice-President, Clinical Section, Royal Society of Medicine, London; Fellow, Associate of Surgeons of Great Britain and Ireland; Hallett Prize, Royal College of Surgeons, 1950; Member, Surgical Research Society, British Society of Gastroenterologists

HORST S. FILTZER, M.D.
Clinical Instructor in Surgery, Harvard Medical School; Assistant Director, Department of Surgery, Cambridge Hospital, Cambridge, Massachusetts

JOHN ADRIAN FOX, M.B., B.S., F.R.C.S. (Eng.)
Consultant Surgeon, Edgware General Hospital, Middlesex; Honorary Consultant Surgeon, St. Andrew's Hospital, Dollis Hill, London; Fellow, Royal Society of Medicine; Member, Hunterian Society

JOHN CEDRIC GOLIGHER, Ch.M. (Edin.), F.R.C.S. (Edin. & Eng.)
Professor of Surgery, University of Leeds; Surgeon, General Infirmary, Leeds, Scotland

LIONEL GRACEY, M.A., M.Chir., F.R.C.S. (Eng.)
Consultant Surgeon to the Royal Free Hospital, Hampstead General Hospital and New End Hospital, London. Fellow of the Royal Society of Medicine and of the Association of Surgeons of Great Britain and Ireland.

CHARLES A. GRIFFITH, M.D., M.Sc., F.A.C.S.
Clinical Professor of Surgery, University of Washington, Seattle, Washington

JOHN GRIFFITHS, M.S., F.R.C.S. (Eng.)
Consultant Surgeon, St. Bartholomew's Hospital; Consultant Surgeon, Royal Marsden Hospital and Chester Beatty Cancer Institute, London, England

JOHN WILLIAM PETER GUMMER, M.S. (London), F.R.C.S. (Eng.)
Consultant Surgeon, Central Middlesex Hospital, London, England

GEORGE D. HADLEY, M.D, F.R.C.P.
Physician, The Middlesex Hospital, London, England

RICHARD SAMPSON HANDLEY, O.B.E., F.R.C.S. (Eng.)
Senior Surgeon, The Middlesex Hospital, London; Former Chairman, Court of Examiners, Royal College of Surgeons of England; Member of Council, Royal College of Surgeons of England; Honorary Secretary, Royal Society of Medicine; Former President, Section of Surgery, Royal Society of Medicine; Former Honorary Secretary, Association of Surgeons of Great Britain and Ireland

HUGH ROXBOROUGH SWANZY HARLEY, M.S., F.R.C.S. (Eng.)
Consultant, Cardio-Thoracic Surgeon, United Cardiff Hospitals, Welsh Hospital Board, Wales

PETER ROBERT HAWLEY, M.S., F.R.C.S. (Eng.)
Consultant Surgeon, St. Mark's Hospital, London; Senior Lecturer, University College Hospital Medical School, London, England

J. LYNWOOD HERRINGTON, JR., M.D.
Private practice of Surgery; Member, Edwards-Eve Clinic Association, Nashville, Tennessee; Associate Clinical Professor of Surgery, Vanderbilt University Hospital; Attending Surgeon, St. Thomas Hospital, Vanderbilt University Hospital, Tennessee

BASIL ISAAC HIRSCHOWITZ, B.Sc. (Witwatersand), M.D., B.Ch., M.D. (Witwatersand), M.R.C.P. (London), F.R.C.P. (Edin.) F.A.C.P.
Professor of Medicine and Physiology; Director, Division of Gastroenterology, University of Alabama School of Medicine, Birmingham, Alabama; Attending Physician, University of Alabama Hospitals and Clinics; Consultant in Gastroenterology, Birmingham Veterans Administration Hospital, Alabama

ALAN HENDERSON HUNT, D.M., M.Ch., F.R.C.S. (Deceased)
Senior Surgeon, St. Bartholomew's Hospital; Surgeon, The Royal Marsden Hospital, London, England

DAVID GERAINT JAMES, M.A., M.D. (Cantab.), F.R.C.P. (London)
Physician and Dean, Royal Northern Hospital, London; Lecturer, Department of Medicine, Royal Postgraduate Medical School; Consultant Physician, Royal Eye Hospital and St. Charles' Hospital, London; Honorary Consultant Physician to Sydney Hospital, Australia; Consultant Physician to the Royal Navy

SIR FRANCIS AVERY JONES, C.B.E., M.D. (London), Hon. M.D. (Melb.), F.R.C.P. (London)
Physician, Department of Gastroenterology, Central Middlesex Hospital, London; Consulting Gastroenterologist, St. Mark's Hospital, London, and to the Royal Navy.

PETER F. JONES, M.A., M.Ch., F.R.C.S. (Eng.), F.R.C.S.E.
Consultant Surgeon, Royal Aberdeen Hospital for Sick Children, Aberdeen General Hospitals; Honorary Reader, Surgical Paediatrics, University of Aberdeen, Scotland

S. AUSTIN JONES, M.D., F.A.C.S.
Clinical Professor of Surgery, University of California, Irvine; Clinical Professor of Surgery, University of Southern California, Los Angeles, California

GEORGE L. JORDAN, JR., B.S., M.S., M.D.
Professor of Surgery, Baylor College of Medicine, Houston, Texas; Chief of Staff, Harris County Hospital District; Senior Attending Physician, The Methodist Hospital; Consulting Staff, Veterans Administration, St. Luke's Episcopal, and Texas Children's Hospitals, Houston, Texas

SOUHEL, KANDALAFT, M.D.
Department of Surgery, St. Clare's Hospital and Health Center, New York, New York

KEITH A. KELLY, M.D., M.S. (Surgery), F.A.C.S.
Consultant, Department of Surgery, Mayo Clinic; Assistant Professor of Surgery, Mayo Medical School, University of Minnesota, Rochester, Minnesota

RAYMOND MAURICE KIRK, M.S., F.R.C.S. (Eng.)
Consultant Surgeon, Hampstead General Hospital, London Royal Free Hospital Group, Willesden General Hospital, London, England

SYLVAIN KLEINHAUS, M.D.
Assistant Professor of Surgery, Albert Einstein College of Medicine; Assistant Attending, Pediatric Surgery, Montefiore Hospital and Medical Center, New York, New York

BASILE G. KOURIAS, M.D., F.A.C.S. (Hon.)
Associate Professor, University of Athens; Surgeon-in-Chief, The Red Cross Hospital, Athens, Greece; Member, Academie de Chirurgie, Paris; Honorary Member, The German Surgical Society

LOUIS KREEL, M.D., F.R.C.P., F.F.R.
Consultant Radiologist, Northwick Park Hospital; Head, Radiology, Clinical Research Centre, Northwick Park, Middlesex; Chairman, Medical Executive Committee, Northwick Park Hospital, Middlesex; Honorary Consultant Radiologist, Royal Free Hospital, London; Honorary Consultant Radiologist, St. James's Hospital, Leeds, England

KENNETH KYLE, M.D.
Department of Colon and Rectal Surgery, The Cleveland Clinic Foundation, Cleveland, Ohio

LESLIE PHILIP LEQUESNE, D.M., M.Ch., F.R.C.S. (Eng.)
Professor of Surgery, The Middlesex Hospital Medical School, London University; Surgeon, The Middlesex Hospital; President, The Surgical Research Society; Chairman, The British Journal of Surgery; Member, Court of Examiners, The Royal College of Surgeons of England; Formerly Chairman, Association of Professors of Surgery; Arris and Gale Lecturer, The Royal College of Surgeons of England

OSWALD VAUGHAN LLOYD-DAVIES, M.S. (London), F.R.C.S. (Eng.)
Emeritus Surgeon, The Middlesex Hospital; Emeritus Surgeon, St. Mark's Hospital, London; Former President, Section of Proctology, Royal Society of Medicine, London, England

H. LOCKHART-MUMMERY, M.D., Chir., F.R.C.S. (Eng.)
Surgeon, St. Thomas's Hospital, St. Mark's Hospital, King Edward VII Hospital for Officers; Surgeon to H.M. Household; Former President, Section of Proctology, Royal Society of Medicine, London, England

JOHN L. MADDEN, M.D., F.A.C.S.
Chairman, Department of Surgery, St. Clare's Hospital and Health Center; Professor, Clinical Surgery, New York Medical College, New York City; Consulting Surgeon, Department of Surgery, Veterans Administration Hospital, Castle Point, New York

RODNEY MAINGOT, F.R.C.S. (Eng.)
Honorary Consultant Surgeon, Royal Free Hospital, Royal Waterloo Hospital, London; Southend General Hospital, Essex; Sydney Body Gold Medallist; Former Member, Council and President, Section of Surgery, Royal Society of Medicine; Editor-in-Chief, British Journal of Clinical Practice; Fellow of the Association of Surgeons of Great Britain and Ireland; Formerly Visiting Guest Professor in Surgery: Mount Sinai Hospital, Miami, Florida; University Hospital, Colombus, Ohio; Maadi Hospital, Cairo, Egypt; The American Hospital, Beirut, Lebanon, and The Royal Prince Alfred Hospital, Sydney, Australia

CHARLES VICTOR MANN, M.A., B.M., B.Ch., M.Ch., F.R.C.S. (Eng.)
Consultant Surgeon, London Hospital, and St. Mark's Hospital for Diseases of the Rectum and Colon, London; Postgraduate Dean, St. Mark's Hospital, London, England

JEFFREY ADRIAN PRIESTLEY MARSTON, M.A., D.M., M.Ch. (Oxon), F.R.C.S. (Eng.)
Surgeon, The Middlesex Hospital, and The Royal Northern Hospital; Senior Lecturer in Surgery, University of London, London, England

JAMES H. MASON, M.D.
Chief of Surgery, Department of Surgery, St. Francis Hospital, Evanston, Illinois; Clinical Professor of Surgery, Loyola University Stritch School of Medicine, Maywood, Illinois

THEODORE R. MILLER, M.D., F.A.C.S.
Attending Surgeon, Memorial Hospital for Cancer and Allied Diseases; Clinical Professor of Surgery, Cornell University Medical College; Attending Surgeon, Pack Medical Group, New York, New York

ANDREW KILLEY MONRO, M.A., M.D. (Cambridge), F.R.C.S. (Eng.)
Member, Court of Examiners, Royal College of Surgeons of England; Hunterian Professor, Royal College of Surgeons of England, 1946; Senior Lecturer, Royal Postgraduate Medical School, Hammersmith Hospital, London; Surgeon, Southend General Hospital, Essex, England

SIR CLIFFORD NAUNTON MORGAN, M.S., F.R.C.S., F.R.C.O.G., (Hon.) F.R.C.S.I., F.A.C.S. (Hon.)
Honorary Fellow American Surgical Association; Honorary Fellow American Proctologic Society; Commander, Star of the North, Sweden; Consulting Surgeon, St. Bartholomew's Hospital, St. Mark's Hospital, Hospital for Tropical Diseases, London; Civilian Consultant, Royal Navy and Royal Air Force; Former Vice-President, Royal College of Surgeons of England; Former President, Section of Proctology, Royal Society of Medicine, London, England

GEORGE COOPER MORRIS, JR., M.D.
Associate Professor of Surgery, Baylor University College of Medicine, Houston, Texas

BASIL C. MORSON, V.R.D., M.A., D.M., F.R.C.S. (Eng.), F.R.C.Path.
Consultant Pathologist and Director, Research Department, St. Mark's Hospital; Honorary Senior Lecturer in Pathology, Royal Postgraduate Medical School, London, England

RUDOLPH G. MRAZEK, M.D., F.A.C.S.
Director of Medical Education, Academic Director of Surgery, MacNeal Memorial Hospital, Berwyn, Illinois

WILLIAM V. NICK, A.B., J.D., M.Sc., M.D., F.A.C.S.
Associate Professor of Surgery, The Ohio State University College of Medicine, Columbus, Ohio

HAROLD HOMEWOOD NIXON, M.A., M.B., B.Hir., F.R.C.S. (Eng.)
Consultant Paediatric Surgeon, Hospital for Sick Children, Great Ormond Street, Paddington Green Children's Hospital, London; Hunterian Professor; Honorary Fellow American Academy of Paediatricians

M. J. NOTARAS, F.R.C.S., F.R.C.S. (Ed.)
Senior Lecturer in Surgery, University College Hospital; Consultant Surgeon, Barnet General Hospital; Honorary Consultant Surgeon, Italian Hospital, London, England

ALTON OCHSNER, M.D., LL.D. (Hon), F.A.C.S., F.R.C.S. (Hon., Eng. & Ireland)
Senior Consultant, Department of General Surgery, Ochsner Clinic and Ochsner Foundation Hospital; Emeritus Professor of Surgery, Tulane University School of Medicine, New Orleans, Louisiana

MILTON PORTER, M.D.
Professor of Clinical Surgery, Columbia-Presbyterian Medical Center, New York, New York

JAMES T. PRIESTLEY, M.D., M.S. (Exper. Surg.), Ph.D., F.A.C.S.
Emeritus Consultant, Department of Surgery, Mayo Clinic and Mayo Foundation; Emeritus Professor of Surgery, Mayo Graduate School of Medicine, University of Minnesota, Rochester, Minnesota

CHARLES BERNARD PUESTOW, B.S., M.D., M.S., Ph.D., F.A.C.S. (Deceased)
Clinical Professor of Surgery, Emeritus, University of Illinois College of Medicine; Medical Director-Director of Medical Education, Henrotin Hospital, Chicago, Illinois; Distinguished Physician, Veterans Administration, Washington, D.C.

CHARLES V. PUTNAM, M.D.
Instructor in Surgery, University of Colorado School of Medicine, Denver, Colorado

ANTHONY JOHN HARDING RAINS, M.S. (London), F.R.C.S. (Eng.)
Professor of Surgery, Charing Cross Hospital Medical School (University of London); Honorary Consultant Surgeon, Charing Cross Hospital, London, England

WILLIAM H. ReMINE, M.D., M.Sc. (Surg.), F.A.C.S.
Consultant, Department of Surgery, Mayo Clinic and Mayo Foundation; Professor of Surgery, Mayo Medical School, Rochester, Minnesota

JOHN RICHMOND, M.D. (Edin.), F.R.C.P. (London), F.R.C.P. (Edin.)
Reader in Medicine, University of Edinburgh; Honorary Consultant Physician, Royal Infirmary of Edinburgh; Professor of Medicine, University of Sheffield, Edinburgh

GRANT V. RODKEY, M.D.
Assistant Clinical Professor of Surgery, Harvard Medical School and Associate Visiting Surgeon, Massachusetts General Hospital, Boston, Massachusetts

ROBERT JAMES RYALL, M.B., M.Ch., F.R.C.S. (Eng.)
Consultant Surgeon, Edgware General Hospital; Honorary Consultant Surgeon, St. Andrew's Hospital, and Hospital of St. John and Elizabeth, London, England

LARRY J. SANZENBACHER, A.B., M.D.
Instructor in Surgery, The Ohio State University College of Medicine, Columbus, Ohio

SIR RONALD BODLEY SCOTT, K.C.V.O., M.A., D.M. (Oxon.), F.R.C.P. (London)
Physician to H.M. the Queen; Consulting Physician, St. Bartholomew's Hospital, and King Edward VII Hospital for Officers, London, England

CORNELIUS E. SEDGWICK, M.D.
Department of Surgery, Lahey Clinic Foundation; Surgeon-in-Chief, New England Deaconess Hospital; Assistant Clinical Professor of Surgery, Harvard Medical School, Boston, Massachusetts

R. A. SHOOTER, M. A., M.D., F.R.C.P., F.R.C.Path.
Bacteriologist, St. Bartholomew's Hospital; Professor of Bacteriology, University of London, London, England

DAVID B. L. SKEGGS, M.A., B.Ch., F.F.R., D.M.R.T.
Director of Radiotherapy, Royal Free Hospital; Honorary Consultant Radiotherapist, Royal Northern Hospital; Member of the Court of Examiners for the F.F.R. and D.M.R.T., London, England

FRANCES HAYWARD SMITH, M.D.
Gastroenterologist, Lahey Clinic Foundation, New England Baptist Hospital and New England Deaconess Hospital, Boston, Massachusetts

RODNEY SMITH, M.S., F.R.C.S. (Eng.)
Senior Surgeon and Chairman, Department of Surgery, St. George's Hospital; Hunterian Professor Arris and Gale Lecture; Jacksonian Prize Winner, Royal College of Surgeons of England; Dean, Institute of Basic Medical Sciences; Member of Council, Royal College of Surgeons of England; Former President, Harverian Society, London, England

JOHN S. SPRATT, JR., M.S.P.H., M.D., F.A.C.S.
Chief Surgeon, Ellis Fischel State Cancer Hospital; Director, Cancer Research Center, Columbia, Missouri; Professor of Surgery, University of Missouri, Columbia; Lecturer in Surgery, Washington University School of Medicine, St. Louis, Missouri

THOMAS E. STARZL, M.D., Ph.D.
Professor and Chairman, Department of Surgery, University of Colorado School of Medicine, Denver, Colorado

FRANCIS EDGAR STOCK, O.B.E., M.B., B.S. (London), F.R.C.S. (Eng.), F.A.C.S.
Principal and Vice-Chancellor of the University of Natal, Durban, South Africa; Formerly Professor of Surgery, University of Liverpool, and Consulting Surgeon, Liverpool Royal Infirmary and Royal Navy

SAMUEL LOCKINGTON STRANGE, M.B., Ch.B., F.R.C.S. (Edin.), D.T.M.
Assistant Surgeon, Whittington Hospital, London, England

NORMAN CECIL TANNER, M.D., F.R.C.S. (Eng.), F.I.C.S. (Hon.), F.A.C.S. (Hon.), F.R.C.S.I. (Hon.)

Honorary Consultant Surgeon, Charing Cross Hospital, St. James' Hospital, London; Markham-Skerritt Prize, Bristol, 1946; Jacksonian Prize, Royal College of Surgeons of England, 1948; Grand Cross of the Patriarchal Order of St. Mark; Examiner in Surgery, Universities of Cambridge and London; Vice-Chairman and Member Editorial Committee, British Journal of Surgery; Hunterian Professor, Royal College of Surgeons of England, 1960; Member (Former President) British Society of Gastroenterology; Fellow, Royal Society of Medicine (Formerly President Clinical and Surgical Sections); Former Member, Council of the Royal College of Surgeons of England; Guest Professor, Ein Shams University, Cairo, 1954, Royal North Shore Hospital, Sydney, 1960, Universities of Saskatchewan & Alberta, 1965, and Singapore 1971; Honorary Fellow Association of Surgeons of East Africa

HENRY REYNOLDS THOMPSON, F.R.C.S. (Eng.)

Senior Surgeon, St. Mark's Hospital, London, England

IAN PELHAM TODD, M.D. (Tor.), M.S., F.R.C.S., D.C.H.

Consultant Surgeon, St. Bartholomew's Hospital, St. Mark's Hospital for Diseases of the Colon and Rectum; Civilian Consultant in Proctology to the Royal Navy; Honorary Surgeon to Royal Scottish Corporation; Examiner in Surgery, University of London; Hunterian Professor, Royal College of Surgeons of England, 1953; Arris and Gale Lecturer, 1957–58; Fellow of the Association of Surgeons of Great Britain and Ireland; Former President, Section of Proctology, Royal Society of Medicine, London; Honorary Consultant Member various foreign proctological societies

RUPERT B. TURNBULL, JR., M.D.

Head, Department of Colon and Rectal Surgery, The Cleveland Clinic Foundation, Cleveland, Ohio

MALCOLM CHARLES VEIDENHEIMER, M.D.

Chairman, Department of General Surgery, Section on Colon and Rectal Surgery, Lahey Clinic Foundation, Lahey Clinic Division, Boston, Massachusetts; Clinical Assistant in Surgery, Harvard Medical School; Chief of Surgery, Brooks Hospital, New England Baptist Hospital

SIR CECIL WAKELEY, Bt., K.B.E., C.B., K.St.J., LL.D., F.P.R.C.S. (Eng.), F.R.S.E.

Consulting Surgeon, King's College Hospital, Royal Masonic Hospital, Belgrave Hospital for Children, and the Royal Navy, London; Formerly President of the Royal College of Surgeons of England; Editor-in-Chief, British Journal of Surgery

J. GEOFFREY WALKER, M.D., M.R.C.P.

Consultant Gastroenterologist, Department of Gastroenterology, St. Mary's Hospital, London, England

KENNETH W. WARREN, M.D., F.A.C.S.

Chief Consultant in Surgery, Lahey Clinic Foundation; Surgeon-in-Chief, New England Baptist Hospital; Surgeon, New England Deaconess Hospital, Boston, Massachusetts

FRANCIS R. WATSON, Ph.D.

Chairman, Department of Biomathematics, Cancer Research Center, Columbia, Missouri; Associate Director, University of Missouri Medical Center Computer Center, Columbia, Missouri; Associate Professor, Department of Community Health & Medical Practice, University of Missouri

JOSEPH A. WEINBERG, M.Sc., M.D., F.A.C.S.

Retired Clinical Professor of Surgery, University of California at Los Angeles; Retired Chief of Surgery at the Veterans Administration Hospital, Long Beach, California

CLAUDE E. WELCH, M.D.

Clinical Professor of Surgery, Harvard Medical School; Visiting Surgeon, Massachusetts General Hospital, Boston, Massachusetts

ALAN CAMPBELL YOUNG, M.B., B.S., D.M.R.D.

Director Radiodiagnostic Department, Dean of Postgraduate Studies, St. Mark's Hospital for Diseases of the Rectum and Colon; Member of the Radiodiagnostic Department, London Clinic, London, England

ROBERT M. ZOLLINGER, B.S., M.D., F.A.C.S. (Hon.), F.R.C.S. (Eng.), (Hon.), F.R.C.S. (Edin.)

Regents Professor and Chairman, Department of Surgery, The Ohio State University College of Medicine, Columbus, Ohio

PREFACE

Owing to the great reception this book has been accorded by surgeons throughout the world and also owing to the recent advances that have been made in Abdominal Surgery since the publication of the fifth edition of *Abdominal Operations* in 1969, it has been necessary to bring this edition up to date, to revise the whole work thoroughly and completely, to delete a number of out-dated chapters and many old illustrations, to enlarge and to reset it entirely into new Sections, Chapters and Parts, and to design a new format. *Revision for this Sixth Edition has been so extensive that it really represents a completely new book.*

To ensure that certain specialized subjects in this vast field should receive expert consideration the aid of 97 eminent contributors has been invoked, with the addition of 26 new Chapters and Parts and 604 illustrations, the majority being drawn by well known medical artists.

This work by a combined team of distinguished Anglo-American authors is intended to present *a complete and explicit account of the technique of all of the approved abdominal operations* as are practised today in the Teaching Hospitals, large General Hospitals, and Surgical Clinics in Great Britain and the United States.

It also deals with the choice of operations; the preoperative preparation and the postoperative care of the patient; the immediate and remote results of the various procedures described; the difficulties and dangers which sometimes arise during the conduct of operations; the consequences of altered physiology (metabolic disorders) which follow many abdominal procedures; *recent progress in abdominal surgery,* as well as the importance of decision in the time of emergency.

Throughout these two volumes my prime object has been to provide top priority and especial emphasis to the numerous technical steps of abdominal operations. This will be appreciated by realizing that fully 80 percent of the illustrations and contents are devoted to the minutiae of present-day technique.

However, brief and relevant accounts have also been submitted on modern diagnostic procedures including radiological, endoscopic, biochemical and other laboratory investigations, as well as on the clinical and pathological aspects of many lesions of the abdominal viscera.

In a work of this nature dealing as it does with a large number of subjects, many of which are closely related, it is impossible to avoid a certain degree of repetition, overlapping, difference of opinion and controversy. According to Moynihan * "Controversy in surgery may often tend to be coarsening, but we cannot gainsay it has occasional advantages. It serves to challenge opinions which might be too readily accepted; to oppose reason to authority; to destroy prejudices, or to support a truth which otherwise might long pass unnoticed. . . . Controversy is the very soul of scholarship."

As all literature is personal, the contributors have been given a free hand with their individual sections. A certain latitude in style and expression is stimulating to the thoughtful reader.

The occasional diversity of opinion expressed may be helpful by encouraging a closer study of such subjects to enable the reader to form his own conclusions. I also believe that a certain degree of repetition in order to emphasize a point in teaching, to enforce a precept, or to offer an illustration cannot well be avoided.

It is hoped that this new edition will gain even further favour and will continue to appeal, as it has done in the past 33 years, to abdominal surgeons, to chief assistants on surgical units, to surgical registrars, to resident surgical officers, to general surgeons, to

* *The Spleen and Some of Its Diseases,* John Wright & Sons Ltd., Bristol, 1921.

postgraduates studying for higher degrees in surgery and to all those who are interested in the present-day progress of abdominal surgery.

I tender my most cordial, appreciative and grateful thanks to the following: (1) to the contributors for their ready and loyal cooperation, and also for the excellence of their articles and illustrations which have played such an important part in enhancing the value of this work; (2) to many distinguished authorities (some of whom are contributing authors) who have supplied me with statistical data, drawings, and concise accounts of the techniques they employ for certain operations, or who have submitted other data. These include among many others: Dr. Henry L. Bockus; Dr. Bentley Colcock; Dr. George Crile, Jr.; Dr. Loyal Davis; Dr. Cuthbert Dukes; Professor Harold Ellis; Dr. W. L. Estes, Jr.; Dr. Frank Glenn; Professor J. C. Goligher; Dr. Robert E. Gross; Sir Charles Illingworth; Dr. Edward S. Judd; Dr. Lucien Leger; Dr. John L. Madden; Dr. C. B. McVay; Dr. R. W. ReMine; Mr. George Qvist; Professor Sheila Sherlock; Mr. Rodney Smith; Dr. Richard Warren; and Professor Robert Zollinger; (3) to the numerous editors, publishers of Journals and monographs, and authors who have generously allowed me to quote important passages from their works, to abstract valuable statistical data, to borrow tables and sketches, or to reproduce, adapt, or modify their illustrations, the full recognition of which is made under Acknowledgments or under the captions; (4) to the surgeons at home and abroad, who have so kindly extended me the privilege of witnessing their work and of attending their lectures, sessions, ward rounds or conferences; (5) to those who have readily assisted me with the loan of radiographs; (6) to those surgeons and reviewers who have tendered me their suggestions, advice and helpful criticisms (and these were indeed many!) and who have done so much to stimulate and encourage me in this most difficult and highly responsible task; and, finally, (7) to the publishers, Appleton-Century-Crofts, to Mr. David Stires, their highly efficient Director and his able associates, Miss Joan Donovan, Marketing Director, and Mrs. Berta Steiner Rosenberg, Managing Editor, for their great help in arrangement of this book, for their readiness to adopt my suggestions, for their cooperation and hospitality and, above all, for overcoming every obstacle so that success might be achieved.

The illustrations constitute one of the outstanding features of this edition. Believing, as I do, in the great potentialities of good illustrations, I have introduced as many as 604 new pictures in the text, making a grand total of 1727 illustrations. The majority of the time-honoured illustrations of the previous editions have been eliminated but I have retained a few of the original, vivid, artistic and instructive pictures which were drawn by that talented artist, Miss Pauline Larivière, who was a pupil of Max Brodel, the greatest medical artist of all time.

I have been fortunate in having the valuable aid of Mr. Robert Lane, who has drawn many illustrations for me and for British Contributors. His pictures are, in my opinion, masterpieces in that the technical details of the various operative procedures which are so faithfully reproduced are, after careful study, vigorously and indelibly impressed upon the mind. I am indebted to him and also to a number of other British artists for their fine craftsmanship, artistic skill and accuracy, and for the great pains they have taken to make their contributions a success.

The very high standard of illustration is also well maintained in the superbly drawn pictures which have been so generously supplied by the American authors.

I should like now to express sincere gratitude to my wife for her forbearance and I sincerely hope that the wives of the contributors have been as tolerant as mine has been.

To my secretaries, Miss E. Margaret Thomas and Mrs. B. K. Mason, I owe a great debt of gratitude for helping me with every step of the work, for typing and retyping numerous manuscripts, for reading and editing the galley and page proofs with me after consulting hours, and for their encouragement and perseverance during our joint labours.

Rodney Maingot

25 Wimpole Street
London, W1M 7AD
England

ACKNOWLEDGMENTS

The publishers and editor wish to express their thanks and acknowledgments to the following:

1. MEDICAL PUBLISHERS AND JOURNALS

E. Arnold Company; Annals of the Royal College of Surgeons of England; Australian and New Zealand Journal of Surgery; Appleton-Century-Crofts; Annals of Surgery; American Journal of Diseases of Children; American Journal of Radiology; American Journal of Roentenology & Radiotherapy; American Journal of Digestive Diseases; American Journal of Gastroenterology; American Journal of Surgery; American Surgeon; Archives of Surgery; British Journal of Surgery; British Journal of Radiology; British Journal of Clinical Practice; Bulletin of the Johns Hopkins Hospital; Bulletin American College of Surgeons; British Medical Journal; Blackwell Scientific Publications, Ltd., Oxford; Ballière, Tindal and Cassell; Butterworths, London; Blakiston Company, Toronto; Cleveland Clinic Quarterly Journal; Canadian Medical Association Journal; Cancer; J. & A. Churchill Ltd.; Churchill-Livingstone; Cassell & Co. Ltd.; Edinburgh Medical Journal; Gut; Guy's Hospital Reports; Gastroenterology; Harper & Row, Inc., Medical Department; Wm. Heineman Medical Books; Harvey & Blythe, Ltd., Sussex, England; International Abstracts of Surgery; Journal of the American Medical Association; Journal of the Royal College of Surgeons, Edinburgh; Journal-Lancet; Henry Kimpton, London; Lancet, London; H. K. Lewis & Co. Ltd.; E. & S. Livingstone, Edinburgh & London; Lloyd-Luke, London; Lahey Clinic Foundation Bulletin; Lea & Febiger; J. B. Lippincott Company; Little, Brown & Company; McGraw-Hill Book Company; Humphrey Milford; Simpkin Marshall, Ltd., London; The C. V. Mosby Company; Methuen Medical Publications; The Medical Clinics of North America; New England Journal of Medicine; Oxford University Press; Max Parrish, London; Pitman Medical Publishing Company; Practitioner, London; Proceedings of the Royal Society of Medicine; Postgraduate Medical Journal, London; W. F. Prior Company; Proceedings of the Mayo Clinic; Proceedings Royal Society of Edinburgh; Postgraduate Medical Journal; Postgraduate Medicine; Royal Free Hospital Medical Journal; St. Thomas's Hospital Gazette; W. B. Saunders Company; Surgery, Gynecology & Obstetrics; Surgery; Southern Surgeon; St. Thomas's Hospital Reports; The London Clinic Medical Journal; The Williams & Wilkins Company; The University of Chicago Press; The Surgical Clinics of North America; Charles C. Thomas, Publisher; Transactions of the Medical Society of London; John Wright & Sons, Ltd., Year Book Medical Publishers, Chicago.

.   .   .   .

Acta chirurgica scandinavica; Archiv für klinische Chirurgie; Annels de Chirurgie; Bordeaux Chirurgie; Chirurgie (Swiss); Clinical Proceedings, Cape Town, South Africa; Chirurgia (Milan); Deutsche medizinische Wochenschrift; Deutsche Zeitschrift für Chirurgie; Gazette medica Italiana; Indian Journal of Surgery; Journal de Chirurgie; Journal of the Medical Association of Eire; Journal of Surgery, Athens; Klinische Wochenschrift; La presse medicale; Masson et Cie, Paris; Munchener medizinische Wochenschrift; Revista de gastro-enterologia de Mexico; Schweizerische medizinische Wochenschrift; Wiener klinische Wochenschrift; Zentralbatt für die gesamte Chirurgie und ihre Grenzgebiete.

2. AUTHORS AND EDITORS OF TEXTBOOKS, MONOGRAPHS AND BOOKS OF REFERENCE

a. Anaesthetics
Lee (J. A.) & Atkinson (R. S.), *A Synopsis of Anaesthesia*, 7th ed., 1972; Wylie (W. D.) & Churchill-Davidson (H. C.), *A Practice of Anaesthesia*, 3d ed., 1972.

b. Anatomy
Cunningham's *Textbook of Anatomy* (Abdominal Section), Revised by G. J. Romances, 11th ed., 1971; Grant (J. C. B.), *An Atlas of Anatomy*, 6th ed., 1972; *Gray's Anatomy* (Abdomen), edited by D. V. Davies, 34th ed., 1967; Hollingshead (W. H.), *Textbook of Anatomy* (Abdomen and Pelvis), 2d ed., 1967; Anson (B. J.) & McVay (C. B.), *Surgical Anatomy*, 5th ed., 1971.

c. Physiology

Davenport (H. W.), *Physiology of the Digestive Tract*, 3d ed., 1971; Starling and Lovatt Evans, edited by H. Davson & M. C. Eggleton; *The Principles of Human Physiology*, 4th ed., 1968; Wright's *Applied Physiology*, Revised by C. A. Keele & F. Neil, 12th ed., 1971; Jamieson (R. A.) & Lay (A. W.), *A Textbook of Surgical Physiology*, 3d ed., 1972.

d. Pathology

Boyd (W.), Revised by W. Anderson, *Pathology for the Surgeon*, 8th ed., 1967; Illingworth (Sir Charles) & Dick (B. M.), *A Textbook of Surgical Pathology*, 10th ed., 1968; *Muir's Textbook of Pathology*, Revised by D. F. Chappell, 9th ed., 1971; Willis (R. A.), *Pathology of Tumours*, 5th ed., 1972.

e. Diagnosis and Laboratory Methods

Conn (H. F.) et al. *Current Progress*, 1970–1972; *French's Index of Differential Diagnosis*, by A. H. Douthwaite, 10th ed., 1972; Hunter (H.) & Bomford (R. R.), Hutchinson's *Clinical Methods*, 15th ed., 1968.

f. Diagnostic Radiology

Abrams (H. L.) edited by, *Angiography*, 2d ed., 1971; Cummack (D. H.), *Gastrointestinal X-ray Diagnosis: A Descriptive Atlas*, 1969; Gough (M. H.) & Gear (M. W. W.), *The Plain X-ray in the Diagnsois of the Acute Abdomen*, 1971; Prior (C.) & Valente (J.), *Scintiography of the Pancreas*, 1971; Shanks (S. C.) & Kerley (P.), edited by, *A Textbook of X-ray Diagnosis by British Authors, The Abdomen*, 4th ed., 1970.

g. Monographs

Ariel (I. M.) & Kazarian (K. K.), *Diagnosis and Treatment of Abdominal Abscesses*, 1971; Cantor (M. D.), Abdominal Trauma, 1970; Colcock (B. P.), *Diverticular Diseases of the Colon* (Major Problems in Clinical Surgery) Vol. II, 1971; Dowdy (G. S.), *The Biliary Tract*, 1968; Goligher (J. C.) et al., *Ulcerative Colitis*, 1968; Ladd (W. E.) & Gross (R. E.), *Abdominal Surgery of Infancy and Childhood*, 1941; Madding (G. F.) & Kennedy (P. A.), *Trauma to the Liver*, 2d ed., 1971; Jackman (R. J.) & Beahrs (O. A.), *Tumours of the Large Bowel*, 1968; Welch (C. E.), *Polypoid Lesions of the Gastrointestinal Tract*, 1964.

h. Gastroenterology

Boley (S. J.) et al. edited by, *Vascular Disorders of the Intestine*, 1971; Badenoch (J.) & Brooke (B.), edited by, *Recent Advances in Gastroenterology*, 2d ed., 1972; Cope (Sir Zachary), *The Early Diagnosis of the Acute Abdomen*, 13th ed., 1968; Jones (Sir Francis Avery) & Lennard-Jones (J. E.), *Clinical Gastroenterology*, 2d ed., 1969; Morson (B. C.) & Dawson (I. M. P.), *Gastrointestinal Pathology*, 1972; Smith (R.), Strictures of the Bile Ducts, in *Proc. Roy. Soc. Med.* 62: 138, 1969; Thompson (T. L.) & Gillespie (L. E.), edited by, *Postgraduate Gastroenterology*, 1966; Truelove (S. C.) & Reynell (P. C.), *Diseases of the Digestive System*, 2d ed., 1971.

i. Medicine

Price's Textbook of Medicine, edited by Sir Ronald Bodley Scott, 11th ed., 1972; *Cecil-Loeb Textbook of Medicine*, edited by P. B. Beeson and W. McDermott, 13th ed., 1971; Davidson (Sir Stanley) & MacLeod (J.), edited by, *The Principles and Practice of Medicine*, 10th ed., 1971.

j. Abdominal Surgery: Abdominal Operations

Harding Rains (A. J.), Bailey & Love's *A Short Practice of Surgery*, 15th ed., 1971; Bailey (Hamilton) *Emergency Surgery*, by T. J. McNair, 9th ed., 1972; Cooper (P.), edited by, *Surgery Annual* Vol. III, 1971; Cooper (P.), edited by, *The Craft of Surgery*, 2d ed., 1971; Christopher's *Textbook of Surgery*, edited by Loyal Davis, 9th ed., 1969; Goligher (J. C.), *Surgery of the Anus, Rectum and Colon*, (in print) 3d ed., 1974; Gross (R. E.), *An Atlas of Children's Surgery*, 1970; Harkins (H. N.) & Nyhus (L. M.), edited by, *Surgery of the Stomach and Duodenum*, 1969; Madden (J. L.), *Atlas of Technics in Surgery*, 2d ed., 1964; Morson (B. C.), edited by, *Diseases of the Colon, Rectum and Anus*, 1969; Netter (F. H.), *Ciba Collection of Medical Illustrations*, Vol. 3, Part III; Nixon (H. H.) & O'Donnell (B.), *The Essentials of Pediatric Surgery*, 3d ed., 1973; Nora (P.), edited by, *Operative Surgery*, 1972; Patel (J.) & Leger (L.), edited by, *Nouveau Traite de Technique Chirurgical*, Tomes X, XI, XII, 1969; Puestow (C. B.), *Surgery of the Biliary Tract*, 4th ed., 1970; Rhoads et al. *Surgery: Principles and Practice*, 4th ed., 1970; Rob (C.) & Smith (R.), et al. edited by, *Operative Surgery*, 2d ed., Vols. IV and V, 1969; Schwartz (S.), *Principles of Surgery*, 1969; Smith (R.), edited by, *Progress in Clinical Surgery*, Vol. III, 1969; *Surgical Clinics of North America* (published quarterly), W. B. Saunders Company, 1970–1973; Taylor (S.), edited by, *Recent Advances in Surgery*, 7th ed., 1969; Welch (C. E.), edited by, *Advances in Surgery*, Vol. 4, 1970; Welch (C. E.), *Surgery of the Stomach and Duodenum*, 5th ed., 1972; *Year Book of Surgery*, 1970–1973.

k. Consultant Radiologists to the Following Hospitals:

Charing Cross Hospital, London; Mayo Clinic Foundation; Middlesex Hospital, London; Northwick Park Hospital, Middlesex, England; Royal Free Hospital, London; St. Bartholomew's Hospital, London; St. David's Hospital, Cardiff; St. Mark's Hospital, London; St. Mary's Hospital, London; Southend General Hospital, Essex; The London Clinic; The London Hospital; The Lahey Clinic Foundation; University College Hospital, London; Western University, Glasgow.

CONTENTS

Section Three SPLEEN

Section Four **PANCREAS**

Section Thirteen   **TUMOURS OF THE RECTOSIGMOID,**
RECTUM AND ANAL CANAL

Section Fourteen SOME NONMALIGNANT LESIONS OF THE ANO-RECTAL REGION

Section Fifteen SPECIAL SUBJECTS

Frontis Figures

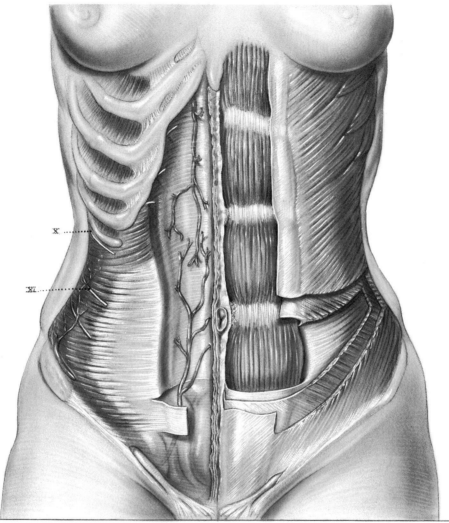

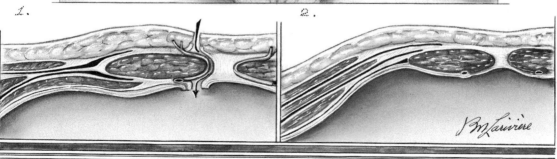

FIG. 1. Anatomical study depicting the muscular and aponeurotic distribution and the nerve and blood supply of the anterior abdominal wall. 1. Illustration of a transverse section of the anterior abdominal wall above the umbilicus. 2. Illustration of a transverse section of the anterior abdominal wall below the semilunar fold of Douglas. *Note* the direction of the dorsal nerves, the position of the superior and inferior epigastric arteries and of the fibrous inter-sections of the rectus muscle.

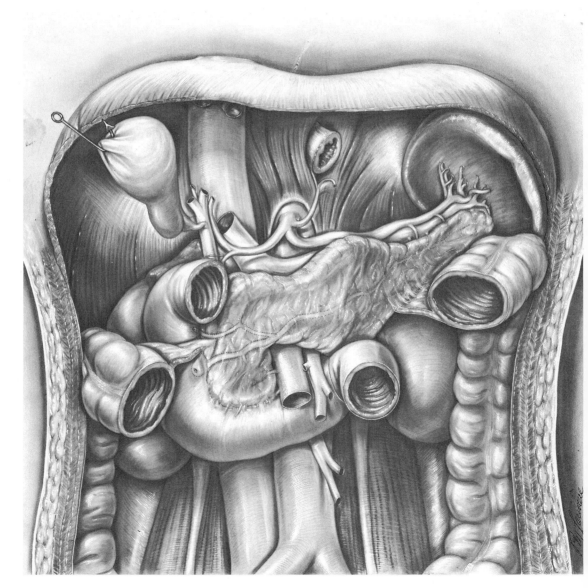

FIG. 2.   The anatomy of the pancreas.

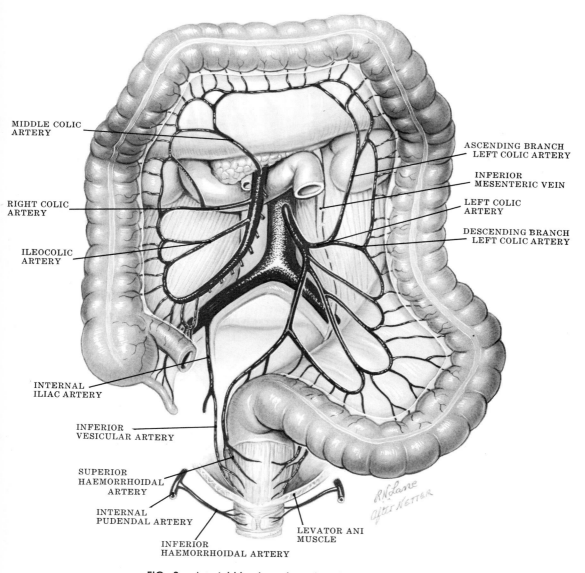

MIDDLE COLIC
ARTERY

ASCENDING BRANCH
LEFT COLIC ARTERY

INFERIOR
MESENTERIC VEIN

RIGHT COLIC
ARTERY

LEFT COLIC
ARTERY

DESCENDING BRANCH
LEFT COLIC ARTERY

ILEOCOLIC
ARTERY

INTERNAL
ILIAC ARTERY

INFERIOR
VESICULAR ARTERY

SUPERIOR
HAEMORRHOIDAL
ARTERY

INTERNAL
PUDENDAL ARTERY

LEVATOR ANI
MUSCLE

INFERIOR
HAEMORRHOIDAL ARTERY

RNLane
after NETTER

FIG. 3.   Arterial blood supply to the colon and rectum.

Volume 1

ABDOMINAL OPERATIONS
sixth edition

Abdominal Incisions

1

GENERAL REMARKS AND PRINCIPLES
A. DESCRIPTION OF INDIVIDUAL INCISIONS; SUTURE MATERIAL; CLOSURE OF ABDOMINAL WALL

RODNEY MAINGOT

Never judge the surgeon until you have seen him close the wound—MOYNIHAN

It is probably no exaggeration to state that in abdominal surgery wisely chosen incisions and correct methods of making and closing such wounds are factors of paramount importance. Any mistakes here, such as a badly placed incision, a careless disregard of the motor nerves that supply the abdominal muscles, inept methods of suturing, an ill-judged selection of suture material, or omitting to protect the wound from contamination during the conduct of operation, may result in serious immediate or later complications such as haematoma formation, infection by pyogenic organisms, disruption of the wound, stitch abscess, a weakened scar, an ugly raised keloid, or a tell-tale rupture.

It should be the surgeon's aim to employ the type of incision that he considers to be the most suitable for the particular case with which he is dealing, and in doing so he must achieve the three essentials: (1) *accessibility,* (2) *extensibility, and* (3) *security.* He should therefore, in my opinion, not only make the correct incision but he should also suture the wound efficiently *himself,* except when assisted by one of his own junior colleagues, who is not only able but who has made a special study of the techniques of abdominal operations. Some assistants, capable though they may be, may not possess the knowledge that the expert surgeon has acquired by experience. For example, in certain types of patients, such as the aged, obese, and cachectic, and those suffering from the destructive lesions of the gastrointestinal tract—including cancer of the stomach and colon, acute peritonitis, congenital lesions of the intestines in infancy, etc.—the recognized routine methods of incision and closure of the abdominal wall may not be applicable, and the success of the particular operation will in no small measure depend upon the length and the judicious placing of the incision and upon a wise selection of suture material and of the method of closure to be adopted. This advice should be given serious consideration in view of the fact that many of the postoperative complications of the wound already mentioned frequently follow in the wake of abdominal operations. Ronald Reid states:

It is not uncommon to see a surgeon cutting his way briskly through the abdominal parietes to perform some internal operation meticulously, and finally leaving the closure to an assistant of limited experience. In consequence, the most brilliantly devised and executed operation may be marred by complication in the abdominal wound and the patient's safety, and maybe his life, thereby risked unnecessarily.

GENERAL PRINCIPLES

The principles that govern all abdominal incisions can be briefly enumerated as follows:

1. The incision must give ready and direct access to the part to be investi-

gated and must also provide sufficient room for the required procedure to be performed. A satisfactory operative field, however, is obtained not only by means of a well-made adequate incision but also by means of the apt use of retractors, forceps, and packs, the correct posture of the patient on the operating table, efficient illumination, and a well-administered anaesthetic.

2. The incision should be extensible in a direction that will allow for any probable enlargement of the scope of the operation. It should also interfere as little as possible with the functions of the abdominal wall, both in the immediate postoperative phase and later on when the patient's normal activities are resumed.

3. The closure of the wound must be reliable and should leave the abdominal wall as strong after the operation as before. The third essential, therefore, is security.

4. A good cosmetic result should be aimed at, when time and circumstances permit, by employing the methods adopted by the plastic surgeon.

5. Strict measures must be enforced to avoid contamination of the wound (see Chap. 3).

Types of Abdominal Incisions

The incisions chiefly used for exploring the abdominal cavity may be described under the following headings:

Vertical. These are supraumbilical or infraumbilical and may be median, paramedian, or muscle-splitting incisions. Some of these vertical incisions are often extended well below or above the umbilicus, e.g., resections for colonic cancers.

Transverse and oblique. The best examples of these are McBurney's gridiron incision for appendectomy, Kocher's subcostal incision for displaying the gallbladder and bile ducts, Pfannenstiel's infraumbilical curved incision in the interspinous wrinkle for certain gynaecological operations, and the transverse or oblique epigastric incisions fot operations upon the stomach, pancreas, and colon.

Alphabetical. These incisions for the most part assume the distorted form of certain alphabetical characters. They include S (Bevan), ⌐ (Czerny), ⌐ (Bardenheuer), 人 (Sloan), ⊏ (Mixter), ⋁ (Sprengel), ⌣ (Maingot), and the T incisions. With the exception of the T incisions, the alphabetical incisions are now rarely employed.
   Cherney
   Abdominothoracic

Choice of Incision

The choice of incision depends upon so many factors (e.g., the organ to be investigated, whether the disease is acute or chronic, whether speed is an essential consideration, the build of the patient, the thickness of the abdominal wall, the degree of relaxation obtainable, the accuracy of the diagnosis, the presence of multiple lesions or of unforeseen complications) that it would be impossible to lay down any hard and fast rules; but in subsequent descriptions of the individual incisions an attempt will be made to guide the surgeon in his choice.

In a general way, however, it may be stated that operations upon the *stomach and duodenum* are best conducted through a vertical midline epigastric incision, an upper right or left paramedian incision, a vertical rectus muscle-splitting incision, a transverse incision, an oblique incision, or an inverted U subcostal incision.

If the patient is thin and has a narrow subcostal angle, a vertical incision is preferable to a transverse one, while, on the other hand, if the patient is obese or the subcostal angle is unduly wide or there is one or more vertically placed scars of previous gastric operations, the surgeon would be well advised to explore the stomach and duodenum through a transverse incision or through an oblique one that stretches from the tip of the left eighth costal cartilage across the epigastrium toward the tip of the ninth right costal cartilage.

As a rule, a right paramedian incision affords the best access to the duodenum and the head of the pancreas, while a left paramedian incision is commonly employed for operations upon the stomach and for truncal and selective vagotomy.

The *spleen* is usually approached through a left upper paramedian incision, although some surgeons prefer a left oblique subcostal incision. A transverse incision may be called for in some cases of familial haemolytic anaemia when splenectomy may be followed by cholecystectomy (combined with choledochostomy) for pigment gallstones. When the spleen is enlarged and firmly adherent to the diaphragm, a left abdominothoracic incision may be employed with advantage (see Chap. 31).

For operations upon the *pancreas,* while the exposure afforded by a transverse incision is adequate, most surgeons prefer a lengthy vertical epigastric incision, usually a paramedian or a vertical rectus muscle-splitting incision.

For operations upon the *gallbladder and biliary passages,* the incision of choice is a right upper paramedian or a Kocher oblique paracostal. The latter incision is usually reserved for obese patients or for those who have an unduly wide costal angle. For secondary operations upon the bile ducts, a vertical right epigastric rectus muscle-splitting incision affords the best access to the part to be attacked. Previous closely placed vertical scars should, of course, be excised in making this incision.

Complicated flap incisions or those that vertically traverse the danger zone of the outer border of the rectus muscle (the so-called pararectal incisions) should be condemned, as postoperative hernia is a common sequel.

For exploration of the *pelvic organs,* the lower paramedian is superior to the midline incision, although in certain instances Pfannenstiel's transverse incision in the interspinous wrinkle possesses distinct advantages, as will be shown later. Pfannenstiel's incision has never been popular in Britain, although it is frequently used on the continent of Europe. *Cherney's incision* can be employed with advantage in pelvic exenteration procedures and is often indicated in extensive urological operations such as total cystectomy for cancer of the bladder.

In cases of *chronic appendicitis* in children and young adults, if the diagnosis is amply supported by good clinical and radiological evidence, the appendix should in most instances be removed through a McBurney incision. In cases in which it is difficult to support a diagnosis of "grumbling appendix," and chronic or intermittent low right-sided abdominal pain is associated with the possibility of lesions in the pelvic organs, however, the safest course is to examine through a generous right infraumbilical paramedian incision, by sight and touch, the caecum, the appendix, the lower coils of the ileum, the sigmoid loop and rectum, and in women the uterus and adnexa in addition.

In all cases of *acute appendicitis* in which the diseased organ is known to be lying low in the right iliac fossa or in the pelvis, or, again, if the patient is obese, this method of approach cannot be bettered.

In infants suffering from acute appendicitis, I prefer a right low vertical muscle-splitting incision to the gridiron incision for gaining access to the inflamed organ, although a limited transverse incision has many adherents.

Lengthy paramedian incisions have much to recommend them for resection with primary anastomosis in cases of *carcinoma of the colon.* In cases of cancer of the left colon and where primary resection and anastomosis are indicated for cases of diverticulitis of the sigmoid loop, good exposure is afforded by a left subumbilical paramedian incision combined with an oblique incision that extends from the umbilicus to the tip of the ninth costal cartilage, and that follows the course of the ninth dorsal nerve. This incision does not divide any of the intercostal nerves and readily displays the complicated anatomy around the splenic flexure of the colon. When performing right hemicolectomy for malignant lesions of the caecum and ascending colon, Peyton Barnes prefers a low epigastric transverse incision (see Chap. 89). When performing an *abdominoperineal operation* for cancer of the rectum, I often make use of a long left paramedian incision that extends from the symphysis pubis to 2 to 3 inches (5 to 8 cm) above the umbilicus.

In *upper abdominal catastrophes,* the abdomen is best investigated through a vertical midline epigastric incision or a right paramedian incision, while in acute diseases involving the lower abdomen the right lower paramedian incision is chosen.

When it is known that an acute intra-abdominal lesion exists but its exact situation cannot be determined by any means available, the rectus muscle should be drawn aside through a right paramedian incision, 5 inches (12.7 cm) in length and placed half above and half below the umbilicus, thereby securing adequate access to every recess in the abdominal cavity for exploratory purposes.

Vertical rectus muscle-splitting incisions, in fact any vertical incisions that are not strictly median or paramedian, are popular in many clinics in America. I frequently make use of these incisions as they afford good exposure and are easy to make and to close. The rectus muscle should be split longitudinally in its *inner third.* If, however, the incision is placed more laterally, the medial fibres of the rectus muscle tend to atrophy and leave a weakened abdominal wall.

Lengthy pararectal incisions through the linea semilunaris are particularly maleficent, as the cut passes at right angles to the course of the motor nerves supplying the rectus muscle, inevitably severing many of them with the result that the rectus, and in certain cases even adjacent portions of the large flat abdominal muscles, become partially or wholly paralysed, then waste, thin out, and bulge, often resulting in a hernia of varying proportions.

Battle's pararectal oblique incision is still widely used for exposing the appendix; it is made a little to the outer side of the lower portion of the right rectus muscle. The wound is deepened and the anterior sheath of the rectus muscle is opened for the full length of the incision. The lateral edge of the sheath is clipped with forceps and the muscle mobilised medially, after which the assistant retracts the muscle toward the middle line. After the nerves that enter the deep aspect of the rectus muscle have been retracted, the peritoneum is opened. This incision has many drawbacks. The epigastric vessels may be injured when the belly of the muscle is being dissected free from the rectus sheath, during retraction, or while the peritoneum is being sutured. The wound cannot be extended for any great length without seriously injuring the motor nerves, two or three of which will have to be retracted out of harm's way while the peritoneum is being opened. If considerable retraction of the wound proves to be necessary, some of these nerves may be unduly stretched or damaged, or they may even snap and lead to partial atrophy of the lower portion of the rectus muscle. The exposure, too, cannot be compared to that which is obtained through the lower paramedian incision; in fact it is, to my mind, one of the most unphysiological of all abdominal incisions in common use today.

Abdominothoracic or thoracoabdominal incisions are employed for cases of: (a) cancer of the upper reaches of the stomach and of the cardia; (b) benign and malignant strictures of the oesophagus; (c) right hepatic lobectomy; (d) marked splenomegaly, more especially when the spleen is firmly tethered to the diaphragm; (e) large cystic benign or malignant tumours of the tail of the pancreas; (f) certain types of diaphragmatic hernia; and (g) penetrating and nonpenetrating wounds of the upper abdomen associated with injuries of the diaphragm and/or thoracic viscera.

Technique of Making and Closing Abdominal Incisions

When the patient is fully anaesthetised and has been placed upon the operating table, the preliminary dressings are removed, and an area extending from the nipples to the upper third of the thighs and including the flanks is fully exposed and lavishly washed with cetrimide and then painted with chlorhexidine (Hibitane).

It is impossible to render the skin sterile without damaging it. Skin antiseptics are therefore always something of a compromise because they must cause the greatest possible destruction among the huge bacterial population of the skin while doing the least possible damage to the skin itself:

Probably the skin antiseptic which most efficiently destroys bacteria is 2 percent iodine in 70 percent alcohol. Unfortunately iodine may cause skin irritation, and this has been reported even when the iodine was removed with spirit within five minutes of application. Owing to the risk of skin reactions many surgeons prefer not to use iodine for routine skin preparation.[1]

However, povidone-iodine (Betadine, Napp Laboratories), which contains 7.5 percent povidone—iodine releasing 0.75 percent available iodine—has proved popular as a skin antiseptic in England during the past few years.

Every surgeon knows that the number of antiseptic solutions that have been used for skin preparation are legion, but at one time or another I have relied mainly upon Cetrimide, chlorhexidine, povidone-iodine or thimerosal (tincture of Merthiolate), used singly but more often in combination.

For this painting, it is most important to hold the swab, or Rondic surgical sponges, already soaked in the solution, on a long swab holder or ring forceps so that no portion of the surgeon's gloves or sleeves comes in contact with the patient's skin while the operative field is being prepared. Waterproof sheeting and towels (or drapes) are next applied in such a way that only the small area of skin through which the incision is to be made can be seen. It is essential that neither the surgeon's hands nor those of his assistants touch the skin of the abdominal wall while the incision is being made, or indeed during any stage of the operation.

Before making the incision, a series of transverse markings can be painted with some sterile indelible ink, Bonney's blue, or special sterilised coloured pencils, parallel to one another and about 1 inch (2.5 cm) apart, across the proposed line of incision in order to ensure that when the skin edges are approximated with interrupted sutures these are inserted symmetrically at regular intervals and with mathematical precision.

Transverse scratches made with a straight needle or with a scalpel are to be deprecated, as there is a tendency for such scratches to become keloid when the wound heals.

When the skin is *dry*, a Steri-Drape (3M) of suitable size is stretched tight and applied to the exposed area of skin and adjacent sterile towels. This avoids the use of towel clips and "fixation" sutures. The Steri-Drape is, of course, sterile, self-adhering, impermeable, transparent, and prevents any bacteria in the surrounding area of skin from gaining access to the incision.

The incision itself is made with a clean firm sweep of the knife. There must be no bungling, or a jagged, irregular cut will result which will afterwards appear unsightly. The knife that has been used to make the incision in the skin should be discarded

and another one employed for completing the dissection. This prevents the possibility of carrying infection from the skin surface to the depths of the wound. Similarly, all instruments that are used in making the incision should be laid aside as "contaminated" and not be employed again during the operation.

I always use three sets of *freshly sterilised* instruments during the performance of any major abdominal operation. The first is used for making the incision, the second for the intra-abdominal procedure itself, and the third set for the closure of the wound. All too frequently I have seen blood-stained scissors, artery forceps, and other instruments that have been employed in the initial stages of making the incision, washed and cleansed in saline solution or some antiseptic preparation and returned to the surgeon for use during the all-important intra-abdominal stage. One contaminated instrument is capable of spreading sepsis in the cleansing solution employed and thus to all the other instruments, to the gloves of the operating team, and to the ligature and suture material.

The points, and only the points, of all bleeding blood vessels in the subcutaneous tissues should be picked up with the tips of Halsted or Dunhill artery forceps and immediately tied with the finest silk, Dexon, or 000 plain catgut. The smaller the amount of tissue clipped with the blood vessels, the less sloughing there will be and the less likelihood also of stitch abscess and such complications.

Haemostasis must be complete and final before the peritoneal cavity is opened. If the surgeon prefers, small bleeding points can be held with haemostats and then coagulated with a diathermy needle; but sizeable vessels are best ligated or underrun and tied off, the ends being cut as close to the knot as possible. This electrocoagulation method of dealing with bleeding points in the subcutaneous and muscular tissues must not be overdone, as charred areas in the wound provide a ready-cooked meal for the ubiquitous bacteria, particularly those of the *Staphylococcus aureus* type.

In vertical epigastric incisions, the peritoneum should be opened at the bottom end of the incision to avoid the falciform ligament of the liver, while in subumbilical vertical incisions, the peritoneum should be incised in the upper part to avoid injury to the bladder, which may be distended. The peritoneum should always be opened with the greatest care, particularly if the patient is taking the anaesthetic badly and is straining or if there is any abdominal distention, as it is then easy to puncture the intestine, which may be lying hard and fast up against the peritoneum. A safe method is to pick up a fold of peritoneum with dissecting forceps, shake it to ensure that no other structure has been caught up with it, clip it with two haemostats placed slightly apart, and then divide this raised fold with the utmost care, using a knife with its blade held on the slant. This small opening is then enlarged to admit two fingers, which are used to protect the underlying viscera while the peritoneum is being divided throughout the whole length of the wound. Pains must be taken during intra-abdominal manipulations, when retracting the edges of the wound and when introducing packs into the abdominal cavity, not to injure the delicate endothelial lining of the peritoneum, as this would predispose to postoperative adhesions. Furthermore, the wound, the peritoneum, and the viscera should be shielded as far as possible from all kinds of injury, whether physical or chemical.

SUTURES AND LIGATURES

Historical Note

The story of sutures and ligatures is, in some respects, the story of surgery itself from its earliest, crude beginnings. Neither the date of the first surgical operation nor the origin of sutures is known.

The oldest medical writings to be found to date are those recorded over 4,000 years ago by the Egyptians, who made many references to the use of sinews and strings for ligating and suturing. Prior to the development of ligatures, attempts were made to control bleeding by cautery, boiling oil, tourniquets, and in the case of dismemberment, by amputation through the upper limit of the gangrenous segment.

The Greeks were leaders in the field of medicine, and their techniques were later adopted by the Romans. In Homer's *Iliad* and in his *Odyssey*, 140 wounds sustained in battle are described in some detail, for which the extraction of arrowheads, the control of haemorrhage and the appli-

cation of compresses, and the use of bandages were undertaken.

> A wise physician, skilled in wounds to heal,
> Is more than armies to the public weal.
> —Virgil's *Aeneid*

Hippocrates, the father of medicine, wrote of the use of sutures and ligatures in his works.

In the pre-Christian era, surgery was practised by the Chinese, Hindus, Japanese, and also by the Aztecs of South America. Celsus, in the reign of the Emperor Augustus, mentioned the use of sutures in his treatise, *De Medicina*, but his manuscripts were not discovered until 1443 in the Church of St. Ambrose at Milan by Thomas Sezanne, afterwards Pope Nicholas V. An unknown Greek surgeon who practised in Rome about the time of the Emperor Trajan was one of the first to describe the technique of ligating blood vessels.

Claudius Galen, a Mycenean physician in Rome, in the second century, used silk and hemp cord for ligating. He also used strands of animal intestine to close the wounds of Roman gladiators. Of Galen's life and character we know much, for he was vain and ambitious, garrulous and verbose. Nevertheless, his claim to honour is an imperishable one, as he was the first physician to bring experiment to medicine.

The Arabs and Moors, at the time of Avicenna (*c.* 950 A.D.), were perhaps the most proficient of early medical practitioners. The Arab surgeon Rhazes (*c.* 860 to *c.* 932 A.D.) is credited with being the first to stitch abdominal wounds with harp strings made from spun strands cut from animal intestine.

During the Middle Ages surgery regressed and sutures were forgotten until revived by Ambroise Paré (1510–1590). Paré reformed the treatment of wounds, substituting the ligation of blood vessels for cauterization.

John Hunter (1728–1793) was the first English-speaking exponent of scientific medical research. Hunter did much to demonstrate that the cause of disease is important in relation to surgery. He advocated the practise of arterial ligation for the cure of aneurysm. Dr. Wright Post, of New York, ligated the external iliac artery in 1796. Dr. Philip Syng Physick (1768–1837), first Professor of Surgery at the University of Pennsylvania, is credited with the development, in 1806, of absorbable ligatures using kid and buckskin. In 1820, Dr. Horatio Gates Jameson used buried sutures from animal sources.

During the period preceding Joseph Lister (1827–1912), infection and pus seemed an inevitable condition of the process of wound healing due to the suture material itself. Except for isolated instances, such as those mentioned above, sutures, particularly absorbable suture materials, fell into general disuse until Lister applied the discoveries of Pasteur to surgery.

Modern aseptic surgery began in 1865 with Lister's development of antiseptics which helped to reduce postoperative wound infection and made possible the widespread use of suture materials. Lister discovered that it was the bacteria present in the suture strand and not the suture itself that caused wound infection. He obtained good results in wound healing by disinfecting ligatures with carbolic acid. He also found that chromic acid made ligatures more resistant to digestion by the tissues. Lister's principle of using only sterile sutures made possible the use of buried sutures in a clean wound without infection.

It is only since Lister's discoveries that the use of sutures has become safe, and only since Lister have the sutures themselves, and the technique of suturing, been brought to a high state of development.

Many kinds of suture material have been used through the centuries. These have included gold, silver, and iron wire; linen and cotton cord; ox, kangaroo, whale, and rat tendons; and camel-hair and horsehair. Many of these materials were treated with various chemicals such as iodine, mercury, silver, and dyes. Catgut was also treated with such substances as alcohol, turpentine, ether, and volatile oils.

As late as 1909, vast areas in the art of suture manufacturing still remained to be explored and perfected. The last 50 years have seen the evolution of a highly technical and specialized manufacturing process—backed by continuous research to advance the art and science of surgery. American Cyanamid Company has played a vital role in the pioneer research necessary to solve the many problems encountered in the development of modern sutures.

One of the most difficult problems in abdominal surgery concerns the *choice of suture and ligature material* and the satisfactory closure of abdominal wounds. Every surgeon has his individual preference insofar as suture material is concerned.

The various recognised methods of closing vertical, oblique, and transverse incisions will be given in detail presently. In clean cases, I prefer to close the pertitoneum and posterior sheath of the rectus muscle with a continuous suture of 0 or 1 chromic catgut, while the anterior sheath of the rectus muscle is approximated with interrupted sutures of 0 chromic catgut, medium silk, or with monofilament nylon. In septic cases, it is advisable to use Flexon stainless steel multistrand on 26-mm, 37-mm, or 48-mm half-circle atraumatic needles in sizes of 000 or 0 (Davis and Geck) or Ethilon (Ethicon), 00, 0, or 1 mounted on 40-mm half-circle Mayo (1 or 2) trocar pointed needles.

The subcutaneous tissues are drawn together with interrupted sutures or a con-

tinuous suture of fine plain catgut, as illustrated in Figure 1 (1) (inset), while the skin edges themselves are evenly united with interrupted vertical mattress sutures of 000, 0, or 1 black serum-proof silk, Deknatel, Mersilk, or Dexon, as is well shown in Figure 1 (3) and inset. The skin edges of small incisions can be approximated with Michel clips, and in some instances a subcuticular stitch can be used, as depicted in Figure 1 (5). (*Sutureless skin closure* technique is discussed later in this chapter.)

When the last suture has been introduced, the wound is again freely painted with the selected antiseptic solution and a gauze dressing is applied and kept in position with a series of strips of Micropore tape.

An attempt should be made to obliterate all dead spaces. Drains and tubes should be introduced through stab incisions rather than through the wound itself.

When large skin flaps have been created, as for example in operations for incisional hernia, *suction catheters* are always used to remove accumulations of blood and serum as well as to obliterate the wound space.

Polyethylene tubes of different sizes are used, either as a prepared apparatus, for example, Redi-Vac Bottle (Zimmer Orthopaedic Limited) (Figs. 2 and 3) or by using the modern and silent Genito-Urinary Mfg. Co. Roberts (portable suction) pump (Fig. 4). These suction catheters or Redi-Vac plastic tubes are similarly led to the exterior through lateral "trocar" stab incisions, and are usually removed after 48 to 72 hours. Gentle suction by negative pressure with the Snyder Hemovac (Zimmer) or Porto-Vac (Howmedica) have also proved invaluable.

If the wound was grossly contaminated at the time of operation, a 1 percent solution of neomycin is used to irrigate the wound before "spraying it" with Polybactrin antibiotic spray, which contains zinc bacitracin, neomycin sulphate, and polymyxin B sulphate (Calmic Ltd.). Other antibiotic sprays include Cicatrin aerosol (Calmic Ltd.), Rikospray (Ricker Laboratories), and Disbiotic powder spray (Pigot and Smith, Ltd.). In my opinion, spraying open abdominal incisions with the bacitracin-polymyxin-neomycin spray has had an effect in reducing infection following operations for suppura-

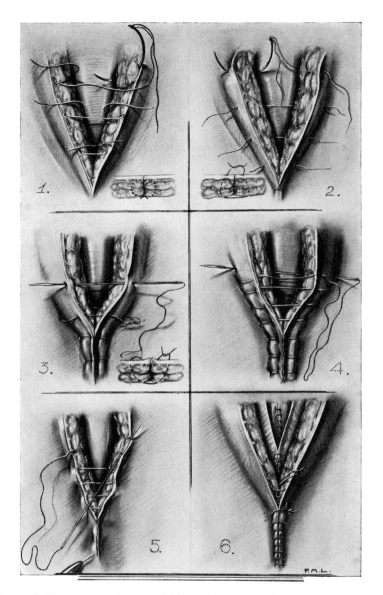

FIG. 1. Types of skin sutures and others. (1) Inverted interrupted sutures for approximating sub-cutaneous tissues. (2) Simple interrupted sutures for approximating subcutaneous tissues and skin edges. (3) Interrupted vertical mattress sutures. (4) Continuous vertical mattress suture. (5) Subcuticular suture. (6) Method of closing all layers of abdominal wall with closely applied interrupted sutures of fine silk in clean cases—Halsted's silk technique.

tive appendicitis, diverticulitis, and cancer of the stomach and colon. However, Jackson, Pollock, and Tindal,[4] in a recent article on The Effect of an Antibiotic Spray in the Prevention of Wound Infection, state: "In a random controlled series of 704 operation wounds the use of an antibiotic spray such as bacitracin-polymyxin-neomycin was not found to cause a *statistically significant improvement* in the overall wound infection-rate." The causes of wound infection are discussed in Chapter 3.

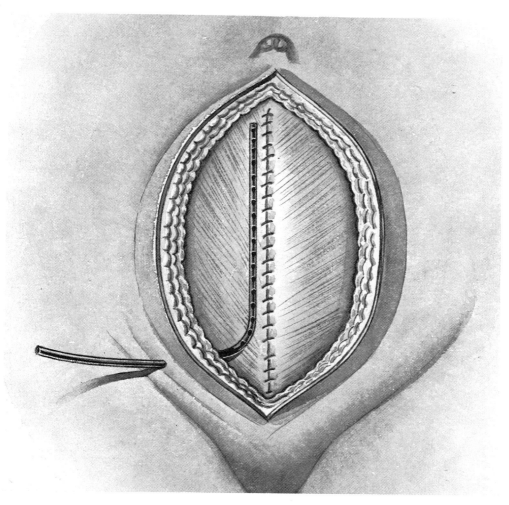

FIG. 2. Redi-Vac plastic tube in position.

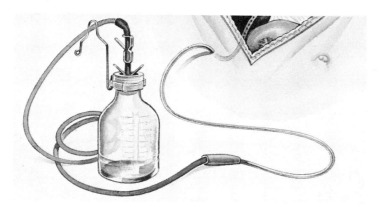

FIG. 3. Redi-Vac apparatus. (Courtesy of Zimmer Orthopaedic Limited.)

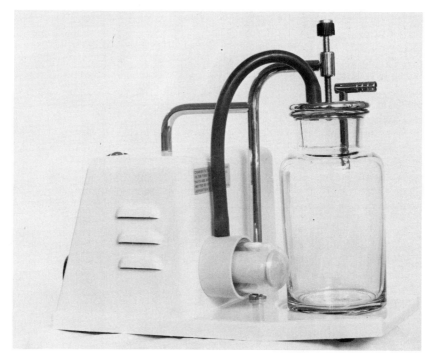

FIG. 4.   Genito-Urinary Mfg. Co. portable suction pump. (Roberts Pump).

DESCRIPTION OF INDIVIDUAL INCISIONS

VERTICAL INCISIONS

Midline epigastric incision.   Many operations upon the stomach, duodenum, gallbladder, and pancreas can be performed through this incision, which possesses certain advantages in that it is almost bloodless, no muscle fibres are divided, no nerves are injured, and it affords good access to both sides of the upper abdomen. It is very quick to make and to close, and is therefore unsurpassed when speed is essential. Its main disadvantage is that there is a tendency for the scar to stretch, as here the *cleavage lines of Langer* run transversely and there is considerable lateral pull in the epigastrium (Fig. 5). Ventral hernia occurs more frequently with this incision than with the upper right or left paramedian, and this is

probably true as the former is more often used for emergency operations, e.g., suture of a perforated peptic ulcer.

This incision does not afford satisfactory exposure of the stomach, duodenum, and gallbladder in patients who are obese or where the distance from the tip of the

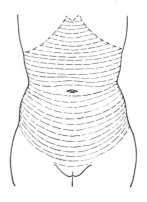

FIG. 5.   Langer's cleavage lines.

xiphisternum to the umbilicus is unduly short. In these types of patients, better exposure is afforded by a lengthy paramedian incision, a highly placed oblique epigastric incision, or an inverted U subcostal incision.

The incision is placed exactly in the midline, and extends from the tip of the xiphisternum to about ½ inch (1.3 cm) above the umbilical cicatrix, dividing the skin, subcutaneous tissues, linea alba, extraperitoneal fat, and peritoneum. The extraperitoneal fat is abundant and vascular in the upper half of the incision, and the suspensory ligament of the liver is best avoided by opening the peritoneal cavity well to the left, or preferably to the right, of the midline under the belly of the rectus muscle, as shown in Figure 6 (2). If this ligament interferes with the exposure of the stomach or duodenum, or cramps the surgeon's movements in any way, it should be clamped in two places, divided, ligated, and completely excised. The wound can be closed in a variety of ways, five of which will now be described.

First method. By this method, which was frequently used by Stiles and by Wilkie, additional security can be obtained by making a vertical incision into each anterior rectus sheath, about ½ inch (1.3 cm) from the midline, and dissecting these inner portions of the sheath away from the underlying muscle. The edges of the peritoneum and linea alba are approximated by a continuous suture of 0 medium chromic catgut threaded on a cutting needle, after which figure-of-eight sutures of stout Dexon, Deknatel, or nylon are inserted at regular intervals, picking up the rectus sheath in the manner depicted in Figure 6 (3). The inner margins of the sheaths of the rectus muscles are sutured together with a continuous stitch of 00 chromic catgut. The skin edges are then stitched together, after which the figure-of-eight tension sutures are threaded through short lengths of fine rubber tubing and snugly tied. The suture line is in this way protected from any lateral pull, thus guarding against ventral hernia.

Second method. Special wound hooks, as illustrated in Figure 6 (4), are placed one at each end of the incision and forcibly lifted upward by an assistant so as to draw the edges of the wound as far away as possible from the underlying viscera. A series of strong 0 or 1 Ethilon or No. 2 Mersilk sutures, mounted on half-circle 40-mm Mayo needles are then inserted through *all* the layers of the abdominal wall, about ¾ inch (1.9 cm) apart and about the same distance away from the margin of the skin on either side. As each is introduced, its ends are clipped and drawn taut. The edges of the peritoneum and linea alba are seized with artery forceps and stitched with a continuous suture of strong chromic catgut, again using a cutting needle as shown in Figure 6 (4). When this layer has been inserted, the through-and-through sutures are threaded through small pieces of rubber tubing and tied, the assistant meanwhile maintaining the upward traction on the wound hooks. When the last suture has been tied, the hooks are removed, and the skin edges between the tension sutures are brought together with Michel clips or interrupted sutures of fine black silk. This method has not proved popular in practise, although it was often performed by Hamilton Bailey and illustrated in his textbooks on operative surgery.

The writer's usual procedure is to close the peritoneum with a continuous stitch of 0 or 1 chromic catgut; to draw the edges of the linea alba snugly together with a series of interrupted sutures of 0 Dexon, 0 monofilament nylon; to obliterate all dead spaces in the subcutaneous tissues with a few sutures of plain catgut; and to stitch the margins of the skin evenly and precisely with interrupted vertical mattress sutures of fine black silk, Deknatel, or Mersilk. "Tension" sutures are used when indicated. The skin sutures are removed on the sixth postoperative day.

Third method. The incision may be securely closed by a series of figure-of-eight sutures of strong nylon or wire which embrace all the layers of the abdominal wall, as shown in Figure 6 (5). McNeill Love's rubber guard (Fig. 7, upper inset) can be inserted between the viscera and the abdominal wall to facilitate the introduction of these figure-of-eight sutures.

Fourth method. The method of closure of abdominal wounds by means of German-silver wire alone (as sponsored by Pauchet and Reid) has been used for many years, and would appear to be *particularly* indi-

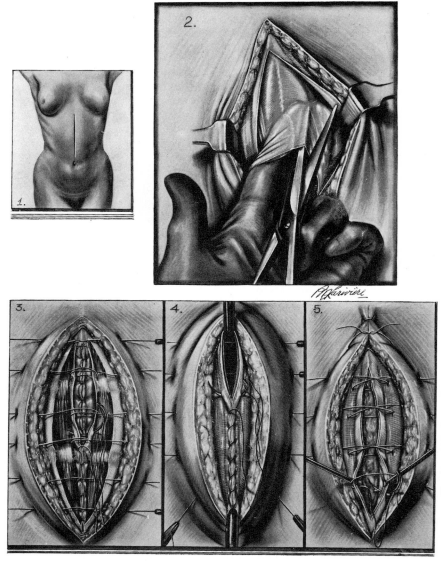

FIG. 6.   Midline vertical epigastric incision. (1) Line of incision extends from xiphisternum to umbilicus. (2) One method of opening peritoneal cavity. (3) Wilkie's method of closing wound. (4) Closure of wound with through-and-through interrupted tension sutures and continuous suture for uniting edges of linea alba and peritoneum. Hook retractors are in position. (5) Incision is here closed with series of interrupted figure-of-eight sutures of wire or nylon.

cated for wounds in which evisceration is prone to occur (e.g., in cases of advanced visceral cancer or when the patient is very debilitated), for those cases in which it is necessary to close the wound under a moderate degree of tension (e.g., general peritonitis and acute intestinal obstruction), and in cases in which a generalised infection of the wound is likely to occur (e.g., perforated diverticulitis associated with a severe degree of peritonitis).

Different types of wire of varying gauges have been used at various times, and these include German-silver wire, phosphor-bronze

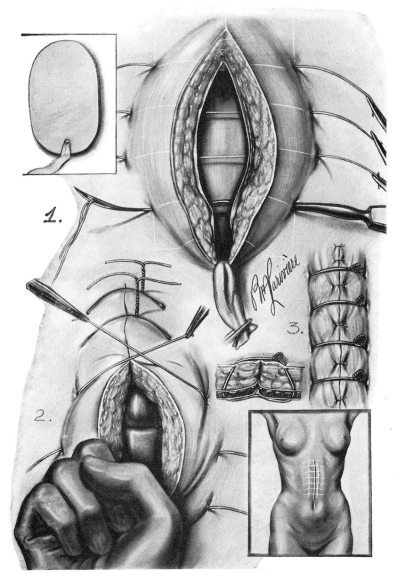

FIG. 7. Steps of suturing abdominal incision by wire method of Pauchet and Reid. (1) Shows how wire sutures are inserted with aid of Pauchet's "aiguille sabre." (2) Method of drawing ends of wire together and twisting. Note that assistant's index finger is inserted beneath edges of rectus muscles to ensure that no appreciable gaps remain after wire sutures have been twisted to desired degree. (3) Final closure. *Top Inset:* McNeill Love's rubber guard. This may be used to protect underlying viscera while wire sutures are being introduced.

wire, Pilling wire, bronze wire, and Nickeline (Minine and Voskrensenski), while Babcock favoured rustless alloy of stainless steel wire (noble metal). In Okkel's opinion, the most suitable alloys are chrome steel and duralu-min. My preference, at the present time, is for German-silver wire.

The method of inserting lengths of *German-silver wire* and using them as through-and-through stay sutures is simple, and any incision can be closed in as short a time as 10 minutes, especially when the technique has been mastered. Reference to Figure 7 will enable the surgeon who is interested in this method, which was popularised by Reid, Zinninger, and Merrell,[9] to appreciate the salient points in the technique employed in closing abdominal incisions with a series of through-and-through sutures of pliable metal.

The following *objections* have been raised against the above through-and-through (all layers of the abdominal wall) wire method of closure of abdominal wounds:

1. That more pain is experienced when wires are used than when ordinary methods of closure are employed.
2. That infection is very prone to occur around the wires.
3. That since the wires are inserted under tension they cut into the skin and leave an ugly crosshatching of the wound.
4. That as the peritoneum is not sutured, incisional hernia, intestinal obstruction, or crippling intraperitoneal adhesions *may* follow.
5. That a block slough of the abdominal wall is a possibility.

The proponents of this method claim that it has certain advantages, which they enumerate as follows:

1. The closure is most secure, in fact so secure that even cachectic and decrepit patients may be allowed to get out of bed at a very early stage after operation.
2. The abdominal wall can be closed very rapidly and under tension, which is a great advantage in cases of wound disruption or intestinal obstruction, or when other methods of suture have failed.
3. The wound can be rapidly reopened by untwisting or cutting the wires if a second laparotomy is necessary shortly after the original one.
4. In cases of peritonitis, drainage tubes are not required, as there is a free discharge between the wires.
5. The absence of any suture material,

such as catgut, in the line of closure of a contaminated incision favours more kindly healing and renders infection less likely.
6. Disruption of the abdominal wound is unlikely to occur.

Fifth method. A series of interrupted sutures of floss nylon or floss silk (impregnated with penicillin) are inserted through all the layers of the abdominal wall except the skin and subcutaneous tissues and are tied securely, after which the skin edges are approximated with silk sutures (Fig. 8). By this method the abdominal wound can be closed rapidly and securely, and the possibility of ventral hernia is remote. If a stitch sinus develops later on during convalescence, as occurs in about 2 percent of cases, it is an easy matter to extract the offending suture. About 1 yard of floss nylon or floss silk is required for the closure. The floss nylon or floss silk is supplied in hermetically sealed glass tubes filled with Bard-Parker antiseptic solution (Bell and Croyden).

Upper paramedian incision. This incision can be made on the right or left side of the midline in the epigastrium. It is employed on the right side for operations upon the stomach, duodenum, gallbladder and biliary passages, and pancreas, and on the left for cases of cancer of the stomach, gastric ulcer, vagotomy, and splenectomy. The incision is a vertical one, starting at the costal margin and finishing about 1 to 3 inches (2.5 to 7.6 cm) below the umbilicus, being placed 1 to 2 inches (2.5 to 5 cm) from the midline.

When the anterior sheath of the rectus muscle has been exposed, it is incised for the whole length of the wound, after which the inner portion of the rectus sheath is carefully dissected from the linneae tranversae to permit the belly of the muscle to be drawn outward, as shown in Figure 9 (*I*). The posterior sheath of the rectus muscle, and the peritoneum, are then incised vertically, again for the whole length of, and in a line with, the skin incision. In this way a trapdoor incision is made.

It is essential to start the incision at the costal margin just to one side of the xiphisternum, as efficient access to the gallbladder

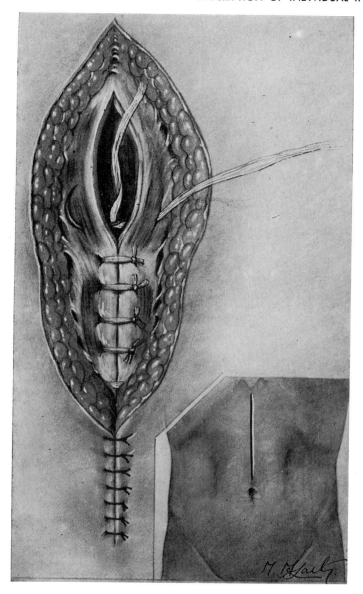

FIG. 8.   Floss-nylon or floss-silk method of closure of midline epigastric incision. Series of closely applied interrupted sutures of floss silk are made to embrace all layers of abdominal wall except skin and subcutaneous tissues. Skin edges are drawn together with fine sutures of black silk. Method is simple, quick, and secure, and leaves a strong abdominal wall. Chief drawback is stitch sinus, which occurs in about 2 percent of cases.

cannot be obtained unless the upper portion of the muscle is dislocated. This incision fulfills all anatomical and physiological requirements, as it gives direct access to the organ to be investigated, e.g., the stomach; no muscles or nerves are divided; *it can be enlarged to the pubis if required;* and, if efficiently sutured, it is not followed by any weakness.

There are many methods employed for suturing the peritoneum. It may be closed with a continuous through-and-through su-

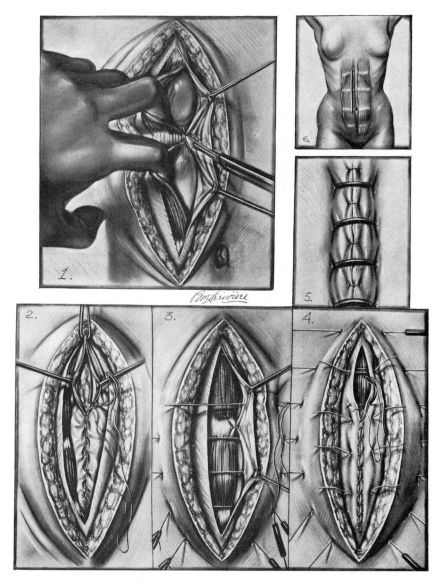

FIG. 9.   Upper right paramedian incision. (1) Dissecting rectus muscle at the middle linea transversa. (2) Peritoneum and posterior sheath of rectus muscle are being approximated by a continuous suture of 0 or 1 chromic catgut. (3) and (4) Process of suturing anterior sheath of rectus
muscle. Note insertion of tension sutures. (5) Final closure.

ture plus a few interrupted sutures of 0 or 1
chromic catgut, with a continuous mattress
suture, or with a baseball suture, as shown
in Figure 9 (2). Sundry suture materials have
also been used, varying with the practise of
the individual surgeon. For instance, some
will use interrupted sutures of fine silk or
chromic catgut, the usual practise being to

suture this important layer with 0 medium
chromic catgut, used either as a single or a
double strand, a few interrupted mattress
sutures also being inserted in order to relieve
strain on the suture line.

It is best to use interrupted sutures of
nylon for closing the anterior aponeurosis,
and here the sutures can be introduced to

make the edges of the aponeurosis overlap if this is deemed necessary. The subcutaneous tissues should be brought together with fine interrupted sutures, so inserted and tied that their knots lie in the depths of the wound facing the rectus sheath and not near the surface of the skin (see Fig. 1). The skin edges can be closed according to individual preference, a reliable method and one which yields pleasing results being the insertion of fine sutures of Dexon or of Deknatel introduced as vertical mattress sutures. Tension sutures are frequently employed, as is well depicted in Figure 9 (*3*).

Lower paramedian incision. This incision is, of course, used for exploring the pelvic organs, the caecal region, and the lower reaches of the large intestine. It is by far the best subumbilical incision and is infinitely preferable to the midline incision, which is prone to be followed by ventral hernia.

As already stated, it is important to open the peritoneum at the upper end of the incision rather than at the lower end in order to avoid wounding the bladder. This incision is very speedily closed, but it is important to remember that as the posterior layer of the rectus sheath is absent below the semilunar fold of Douglas, it is advisable to include a little muscle when inserting the peritoneal stitches. A few supporting Ethilon sutures are passed through the anterior sheath of the rectus muscle to give added security, while the anterior sheath itself is closed with a series of interrupted or mattress sutures and the skin approximated in the usual manner. As this scar is very likely to stretch, the fatty layer should be stitched with the finest suture material (Figs. 10 and 11).

Vertical muscle-splitting incision. Here the rectus muscle, in its upper or lower half, is split longitudinally in its medial one-third, after which the posterior sheath of the rectus muscle and peritoneum is opened in the same line. This incision can be quickly made and closed, and it affords good access. Although some degree of paralysis of the medial portion of the rectus muscle *may* occur following its use, this incision is nevertheless popular in many clinics. The wound can be closed with interrupted sutures of 0 chromic catgut or medium silk, as is well

illustrated in Figures 12 and 13. The margins of the posterior sheath of the rectus muscle and peritoneum are *usually* approximated with a continuous suture of 1 medium chromic catgut and a few evenly placed mattress sutures, which are inserted to relieve the strain on the suture line, after which the apposing edges of the anterior sheath of the rectus muscle are united with a series of closely applied interrupted medium sutures of silk or of 0 or 1 monofilament nylon.

TRANSVERSE ABDOMINAL INCISIONS

These are excellent incisions, and are, in my opinion, all too infrequently employed. This is probably because of the fact that they entail considerably more time and care in planning and execution than do vertical incisions.

There are two main types. In the *first,* all the layers of the abdominal wall are cut across transversely in line with the incision. In the *second* type, after the transverse skin incison has been made, the anterior aponeurotic sheaths are separated from the underlying muscular mass in an upward and downward direction, and the muscles are widely retracted outward, permitting transverse division of the posterior sheaths and of the peritoneum.

Sanders rightly considered that by this conservation of the continuity of the muscle fibres the anatomical and physiological relations of the abdominal wall are not destroyed and the wall's integrity is maintained. The main drawback to this incision is that it is not easy to separate the aponeurosis at the tendinous intersections without buttonholing or injuring the rectus muscles, although with care, patience, and practise this difficulty can be overcome. It should, nevertheless, be remembered that the rectus muscle can be cut across transversely; however, provided its aponeurotic sheaths are accurately closed, no serious weakening of the abdominal muscles results, as such a cut passes between adjacent nerves without injuring them. The rectus muscle has a segmental nerve supply, so that there is no risk of a transverse incision's depriving the distal part of the muscle of its nerve supply as there would be if a divided muscle were dependent upon a single nerve,

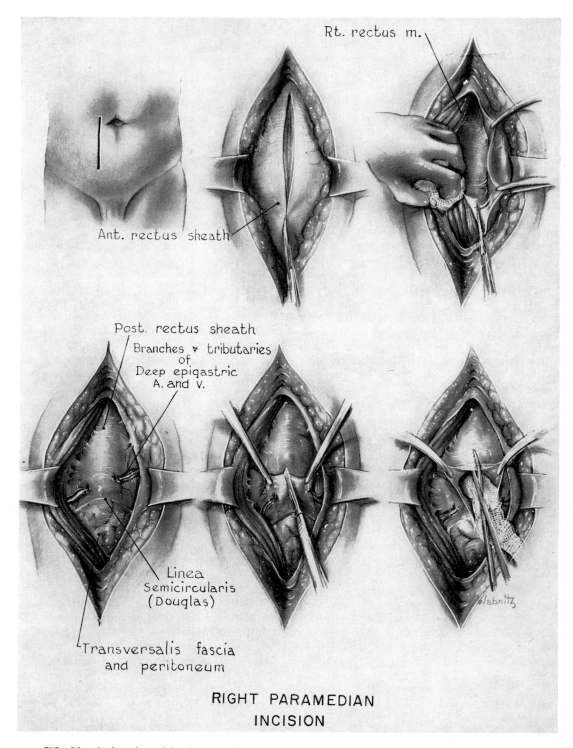

RIGHT PARAMEDIAN
INCISION

FIG. 10.   Right infraumbilical paramedian incision. (From Madden, *Atlas of Technics in Surgery*, 2d ed. Courtesy of Appleton-Century-Crofts, New York, 1964.)

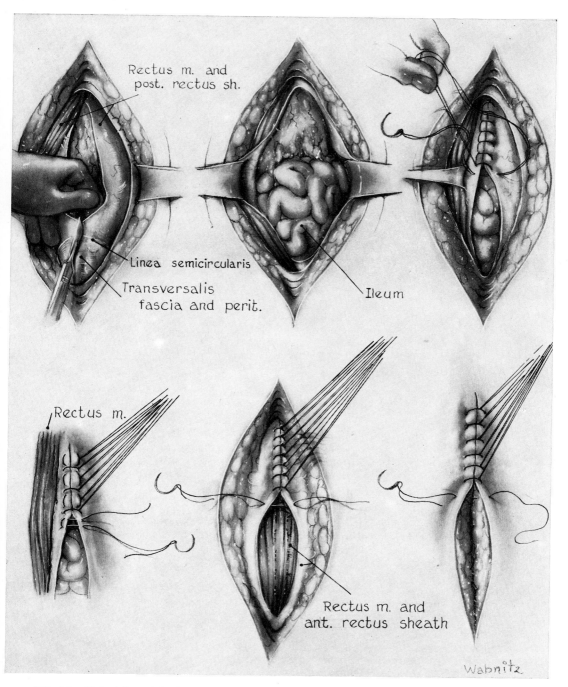

Rectus m. and
post. rectus sh.

Linea semicircularis

Transversalis
fascia and perit.

Ileum

Rectus m.

Rectus m. and
ant. rectus sheath

Wabnitz

FIG. 11.   Right infraumbilical incision. (From Madden, *Atlas of Technics in Surgery*, 2d ed. Courtesy of Appleton-Century-Crofts, New York, 1964.)

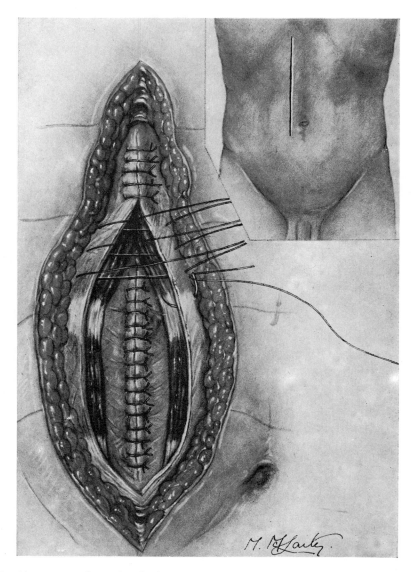

FIG. 12.   Upper vertical muscle-splitting incision. Wound may be closed in manner depicted, with series of closely applied interrupted sutures. There is no need to insert any special sutures to draw muscle edges themselves together, as when anterior sheath of rectus muscle is approximated muscle margins fall together.

e.g., a muscle of the leg. To those surgeons who have rarely employed the Sanders incision it may seem cumbersome and awkward; it may also seem to require that much time be spent on opening and closing the abdomen. Repetition of and familiarity with the procedure should overcome all such difficulties, however.

Sanders' technique.   In Sanders' tech-

nique of the transverse epigastric incision with separation rather than division of the rectus muscles, the skin incision is made transversely, to extend from one costal margin to the other, although when the costal angle is wide a shorter incision can be made according to the requirements of the operation. Again, the exact site of the incision is determined by the width of the

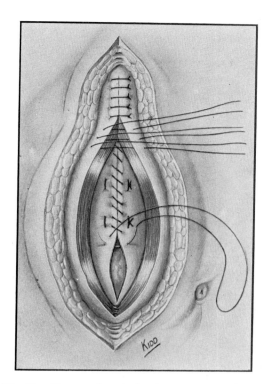

FIG. 13. Closure of vertical epigastric rectus-splitting incision. Peritoneum is closed with continuous sutures of 1 chromic catgut. Note insertion of mattress sutures to relieve strain on suture line. Anterior sheath of rectus muscle is approximated with interrupted sutures of 1 chromic catgut, silk, cotton, or nylon, according to the surgeon's preference.

at the tendinous intersections, the sheaths must be raised carefully and dissected off the muscles with scissors for a distance of 2 or 3 inches (5 to 7.6 cm) upward and downward. During this dissection, haemorrhage occurring from the muscle may be tediously troublesome to control. Bleeding points should not, however, be picked up with haemostats but should rather be underrun with small round-bodied needles, threaded with plain catgut and gently tied. If they are too tightly ligated, the muscle fibers will be cut across; if they are grasped with haemostats, the muscle is likely to be lacerated in the process of ligature and more troublesome bleeding will occur. The utmost caution must also be exercised in freeing the sheaths from the lineae transversae; otherwise the muscles may be weakened and their fibres be more easily torn by retraction. On the posterior aspect of the rectus muscles, the sheaths can be freed quite simply, as adherence here is only minimal.

Both rectus muscles are then firmly retracted laterally, and the posterior sheaths and peritoneum are divided transversely in line with the original skin incision. While the peritoneum is being opened, the ligamentum teres should be clamped and divided between ligatures. Suitable retractors are then placed in position and the wound is opened wide for exploration, as shown in Figure 14 (*3*). Drainage tubes are best brought out through the right side of the wound, lateral to the rectus muscle, as shown in Figure 14 (*7*).

The wound is sutured in layers, starting from the left side. The peritoneum and posterior sheaths of the rectus muscles are adherent and are best approximated with a continuous suture of 0 chromic catgut, the divided ends of the ligamentum teres being brought together by including them in this suture. The rectus muscles now fall back into their normal position, and their anterior sheaths are closed with interrupted or continuous sutures. It will be seen that, although the patient may be straining, there is no tension on the wound side and its edges can be approximated with the greatest ease. When the anterior sheath has been closed, three interrupted sutures of 0 Ethilon wire should be placed in the linea alba as an additional measure of safety. As an alternative,

costal angle; the wider the angle, the higher above the umbilicus the incision should be placed. In the average case, the incision should cross at the junction of the middle and lower two-thirds of an imaginary line drawn between the xiphisternum and the umbilicus. In actual practise, the incision usually crosses the midline at a point about three fingers' breadth above the umbilicus.

After the skin incision has been made, the anterior sheaths of the rectus muscles are displayed, but the subcutaneous tissues are not dissected away from these sheaths in a longitudinal direction, not, at least, for any appreciable distance. The aponeurosis is then divided transversely and is separated in an upward and downward direction from the underlying muscles.

Since the rectus muscles are firmly adherent anteriorly to the sheaths, especially

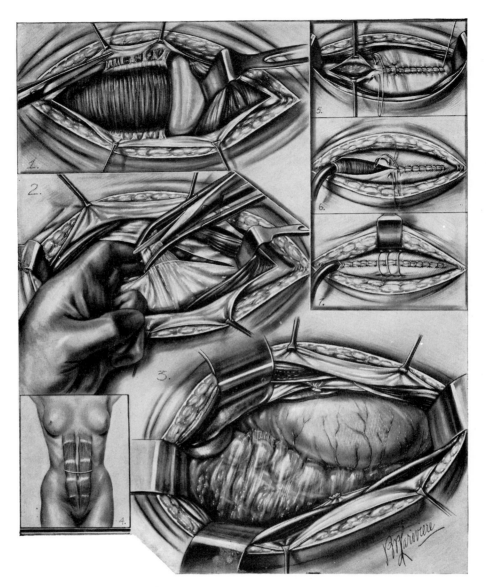

FIG. 14.   Transverse epigastric incision *without* division of rectus muscles—Sanders' technique.

a figure-of-eight suture of stainless steel can be inserted to strengthen this weak spot. The wound edges are closed with Michel clips, interrupted silk sutures, or a subcuticular stitch. The final cosmetic results leave very little to be desired.

Epigastric. A transverse epigastric incision with division of the rectus muscles is placed about three fingers' breadth above the umbilicus and passes transversely across the upper abdomen, reaching to the costal margins (Figs. 15 and 16). The incision is made through the skin and superficial fascia down to the sheaths of the rectus muscles at the level indicated. The skin and subcutaneous tissues that overlie the upper portion of the rectus muscles are mobilised with scissors dissection. The second tendinous intersection is then identified and the sheaths of the rectus muscles are opened transversely

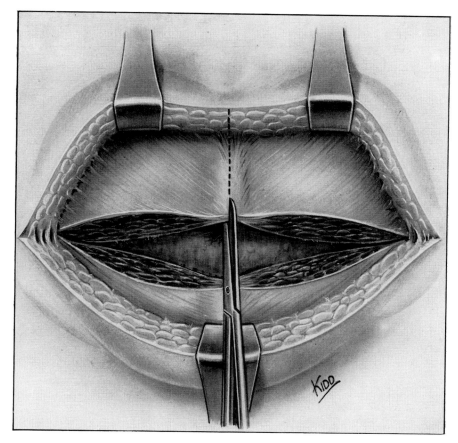

FIG. 15. Transverse epigastric incision *with* division of rectus muscles. After the rectus muscles have been completely divided and the peritoneum opened, the upper flap of skin is mobilised and retracted, and the linea alba is divided with scissors up to the tip of the xiphisternum.

about 1 to 2 inches (2.5 to 5 cm) below (or through) this linea transversa. Both rectus muscles are divided down to the posterior sheaths, the peritoneum then being cut for the full length of the incision. The falciform ligament will need to be freed and completely excised.

The skin flap is retracted as shown in Figure 15, and the linea alba and peritoneum are divided vertically to the tip of the xiphisternum.

The wound is closed as shown in Figure 16. The peritoneum and posterior rectus sheath are sutured with a continuous suture of 1 chromic catgut; the edges of the linea alba are approximated with a figure-of-eight suture of nylon, after which the margins of the anterior sheaths of the muscles are drawn together with interrupted vertical mattress sutures of chromic catgut or silk.

Note that a figure-of-eight stitch is inserted at the point where the vertical incision meets the transverse incision (Fig. 16).

Noordenbos considered that transverse incisions offered the following advantages as compared with vertical incisions:

1. The scars are less visible as they are made in Langer fissure lines.
2. Exposure and drainage (when required) are both better, and less retraction is necessary.
3. Closure of the wound is easier and more secure.
4. Chest complications are rare; owing to the comparative absence of pain with such wounds, the patients are not afraid to cough and are able to get out of bed early after major operations.
5. Ventral hernia is seldom encountered.

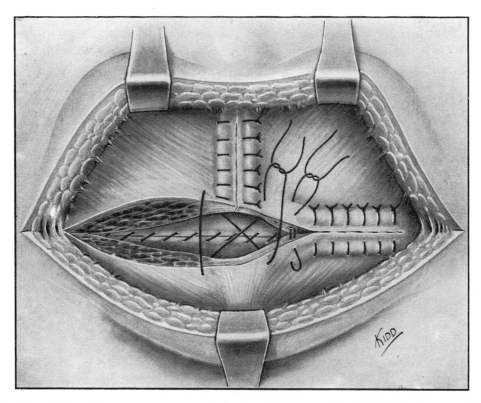

FIG. 16. T-shaped epigastric incision *with* division of rectus muscles. Method of closure is depicted. Note insertion of figure-of-eight suture.

It is nevertheless true that transverse incisions through the abdominal wall take longer to make and to close and that bleeding is more troublesome than with vertical incisions. There is, however, no truth in the statement that sectioning of one or both rectus muscles is followed by some anatomical or physiological impairment of the abdominal musculature; I have been able to satisfy myself that the muscles when healed simply present an extratendinous intersection without any functional disablement.

The criticism that should infection follow the use of a transverse or oblique incision such complications as dehiscence of the wound, evisceration, and ventral hernia are relatively common events is certainly not substantiated by a careful follow-up of my own cases or by a study of the published figures.

Epigastric _/-shaped incision. This incision may be indicated for obese broad-chested patients and those with an unduly wide costal angle, as it affords good access to the upper abdominal organs. It is placed transversely about 3 inches (7.62 cm) above in the umbilicus in Langer's lines and is deepened to expose the middle linea transversa, which is then divided to display the underlying posterior sheaths of the rectus muscles and peritoneum.

After opening the peritoneum, the incision is extended, through all the layers of the lateral abdominal wall, towards the tips of the ninth right and left ribs. The lateral and upward incisions follow the course of the ninth dorsal nerves. The wound is closed in three layers, as already described (Fig. 17).

The *T incisions* are illustrated in Figure 18.

Pfannenstiel's incision. This incision can be used for certain gynaecological operations, such as ventrosuspension of the uterus, removal of a solitary uterine fibroid or

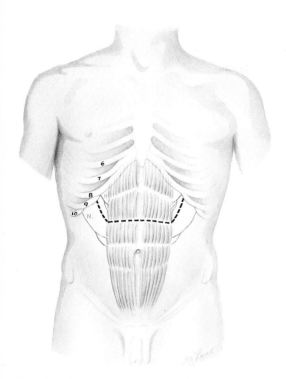

FIG. 17.   The epigastric ___/ -shaped incision.

ovarian cyst, or for appendectomy when it is desired to explore the pelvis. Incidentally, it is the incision of choice for retropubic prostatectomy.

This incision is usually about 5 inches (12.7 cm) long and is placed in the curving interspinous crease, its central point being approximately 2 inches (5 cm) above the symphysis pubis, as shown in Figure 19 (*1*). It is deepened, and the aponeurosis is exposed and divided for the whole length of the wound, i.e., transversely. Haemostats are clipped to the upper and lower edges of the rectus sheath, which is then widely separated above and below from the underlying rectus muscles. It is necessary to separate the aponeurosis in an upward direction almost to the umbilicus and downward to the pubic arch. The rectus muscles are then retracted laterally, and the peritoneum is opened vertically in the midline, care being taken not to injure the bladder at the lower end of the wound; see Figure 19 (*3*), (*4*), and (*5*).

When it is intended to employ this incision, it is advisable to catheterise the patient prior to operation, as a full bladder may lend itself to injury and will also limit the exposure of the pelvic organs. The exposure afforded is somewhat limited, but is nevertheless adequate for the purpose for which it is usually employed, especially if retraction is good; see Figure 19 (*6*).

In those cases in which, after having dealt with some pelvic condition, it is desired to remove the appendix, but the caecum lies tethered far afield in the right iliac fossa and cannot be drawn into the wound, it is an easy matter to approach the appendix by firmly retracting the belly of the right rectus muscle inward toward the midline and cutting across the peritoneum and lateral abdominal muscles in line with the right outer portion of the curved incision. In this way no nerves are divided, but the inferior epigastric vessels will require ligation.

After dealing with the appendix, the outer portion of the wound is sutured in layers, the rectus muscles fall back into position, and after suturing the peritoneum the aponeurosis is approximated with a series of closely applied interrupted mattress sutures, as shown in Figure 19 (*7*). The subcutaneous tissues and the skin are then brought together in the usual manner.

Pfannenstiel's incision leaves an imperceptible scar as it is placed in one of the natural creases of the body and consequently the major part of the wound is hidden by pubic hair.

Inverted U.   The inverted U subcostal muscle-cutting incision may be indicated in broad-chested, muscular or obese patients in whom a small hypertonic stomach is tucked away beneath the liver. It affords good access to the cardia, the duodenum, the biliary tract, and to the liver. Figure 20 depicts the more important steps in the making and the closing of this incision. The margins of the linea alba are best approximated with three interrupted sutures, 0 or 1 Ethilon or 2 Mersilk mounted on atraumatic Mayo (No. 1) trocar-pointed needles.

Kocher's subcostal incision.   This is used frequently in surgery of the gallbladder and biliary passages, and is the incision of choice in unduly obese and muscular patients. For the majority of operations upon the gallbladder and biliary passages, the right

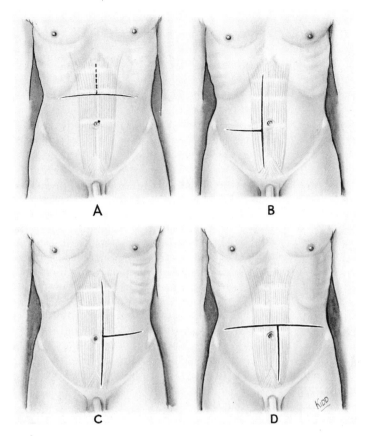

FIG. 18.   The T incisions.

paramedian or vertical muscle-splitting incision cannot be bettered and is the one favoured by the writer (Fig. 21).

Kocher's subcostal incision commences exactly at the midline, about 1 to 2 inches (2.5 to 5 cm) below the xiphisternum, and extends for 5 inches (12.7 cm) downward and outward about 1 inch (2.5 cm) or so below the costal margin (Fig. 21). It should not be extended as far round as the flank, or too many nerves will be severed. The rectus muscle should be completely divided, after which the lateral abdominal muscles are cut in an outward direction *for a short distance.* This complete division of the rectus muscle, preferably between the upper and middle tendinous intersections, must be emphasised, because to leave some of the inner fibres of the muscle intact would restrict the surgeon's manipulations and thereby prevent adequate access to the gallbladder and biliary passages. The nerves will be seen entering the rectus muscle at its outer border, and although the small eighth dorsal nerve will almost invariably be cut, the large ninth nerve must be seen, dissected free for an inch or so, and drawn out of harm's way. Under no condition is it permissible to divide this important nerve.

The incision is very easily closed by using a continuous suture of 0 or 1 chromic catgut for the peritoneum and posterior rectus sheath, and at the same time picking up some of the lateral abdominal muscles. The edges of the anterior rectus sheath and the external oblique muscle are brought together by a series of interrupted sutures of 0 silk or nylon, and the skin edges are approximated in the usual manner. Drainage tubes and/or suction tubes are made to emerge

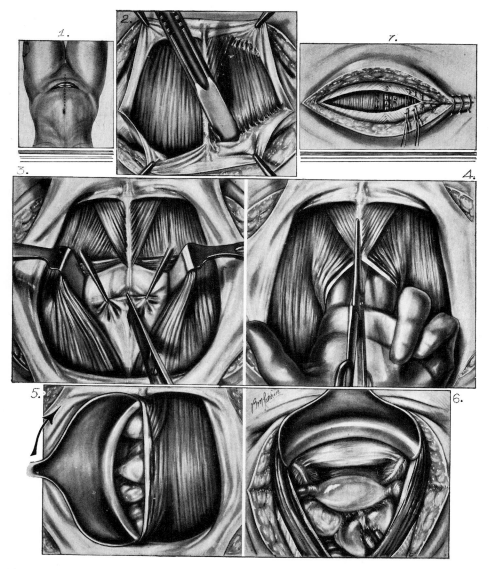

FIG. 19. Pfannenstiel's infraumbilical curved incision in interspinous wrinkle. Details of making and closing incision are depicted.

through a stab incision placed lateral to the lower end of the incision.

McBurney's gridiron incision. This is the incision of choice for appendectomy in most cases of acute appendicitis, although in certain instances already indicated, the right lower paramedian incision is preferable. The level and length of the McBurney incision will vary according to the position of the appendix and the thickness of the abdominal wall. Whenever possible, it is advisable to employ a transverse or oblique incision and to place this in one of Langer's lines in order to ensure a good cosmetic result.

In cases of acute appendicitis, when the patient is fully anesthetised it is advisable to palpate the abdomen carefully in order to determine, as far as possible, the exact position of the appendix so that the incision

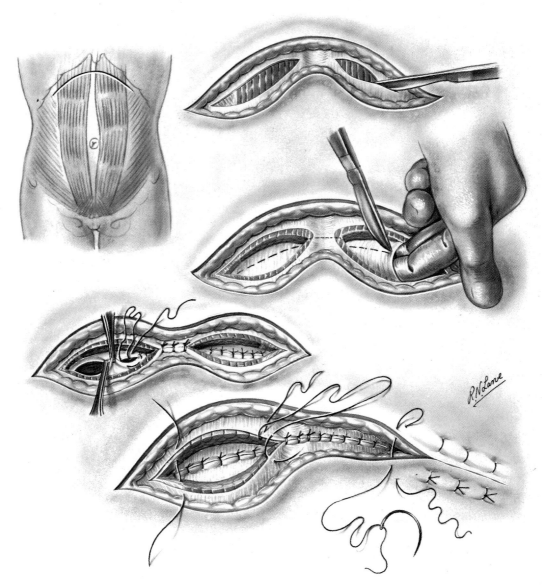

FIG. 20.   The inverted U subcostal incision. The more important steps of making and closing this incision are well depicted by the artist.

can be placed directly over the diseased organ. In certain cases, for instance in children in whom the diagnosis is unequivocal, and in athletes when the minimum amount of damage to the abdominal wall is essential, the incision can be made very small—2 inches (5 cm)—"buttonhole" and transverse.

After the skin incision has been made, the external oblique aponeurosis is divided in the direction of its fibres as shown in Figure 22 (1), each edge being picked up with haemostats and retracted widely, after which the internal oblique muscle will be seen with its fibres running transversely toward the outer border of the rectus muscle; see Figure 22 (2). A small incision is then made in this

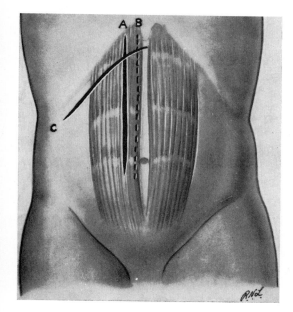

FIG. 21.   Incisions employed in biliary tract surgery: (A) vertical rectus muscle-splitting incision; (B) paramedian; (C) subcostal or Kocher incision.

muscle near the outer border of the rectus muscle, and this is enlarged with the handle of the knife or the points of a pair of Mayo scissors to permit the introduction of the two index fingers between the muscle fibres so that this muscle can be retracted with a minimal amount of damage; see Figure 22 (3). A fold of peritoneum is then picked up and nicked with a knife, after which this little incision is enlarged so that it can be fully stretched with the index fingers. This tends to produce a circular hole in the peritoneum which, at the completion of the operation, is easy to close with a purse-string suture; see Figure 22 (6). As the separated edges of the internal oblique and transversus muscles tend to fall together, they need only be united with a few sutures, but these should not be tied too tightly, as this would lead to strangulation of the muscles and an outpouring of serum. The aponeurosis is stitched with interrupted sutures and the skin is closed as already described, although at times it may be advisable to insert a subcuticular stitch in order to attain a perfect cosmetic result; see Figure 1 (8).

If, during the course of the operation, the appendix is found to be somewhat in-

accessible, the wound can be very easily enlarged by employing the Fowler-Weir extension, whereby the anterior sheath of the rectus muscle is divided in line with the incision and the belly of the rectus muscle retracted inward, after which the opening in the peritoneum can be suitably widened to afford the necessary access. This will provide adequate exposure not only of the whole caecal region and of the lower coils of the ileum, but also of the uterus and its adnexa.

In a small proportion of cases, which has so far not been accurately assessed, inguinal hernias is found to follow the use of the gridiron incision. A consideration of the anatomy of this incision explains this unfortunate complication. The iliohypogastric and ilioinguinal nerves play a large part in supplying those portions of the internal oblique and transverse muscles that constitute the conjoined tendon. This muscle mass is certainly a most important constituent of the inguinal canal and is responsible for the shutter action by which the muscle descends, protecting the posterior wall of the canal during straining or coughing. If these nerves are injured, this important muscle will atrophy, predisposing to the development of an inguinal hernia. The iliohypogastric and ilioinguinal nerves lie between the internal oblique and the transversus abdominis muscles at or near the site of the gridiron incision, and when the wound is enlarged may be damaged by retraction that is too firm, by strangulation with sutures, or in the case of sepsis, by constriction due to scar tissue.

Cherney incision. This may be indicated when a wide exposure of the pelvic organs is imperative in order to simplify certain extensive urological operations or pelvic exenteration procedures.

Culp and DeWeerd [2] give an admirable account of the Cherney incision, including the technique, applications, and complications of this particular suprapubic transverse incision. The illustrations (Figs. 23 to 29) are by that excellent artist, R. Drake, and are depicted here by the courtesy of Dr. Ormond Culp and Dr. James H. DeWeerd, of the Mayo Clinic. They write:

We have been impressed by several commendable features of the Cherney incision. Magnificent exposure has been obtained in obese as well as thin patients. Scars from previous suprapubic opera-

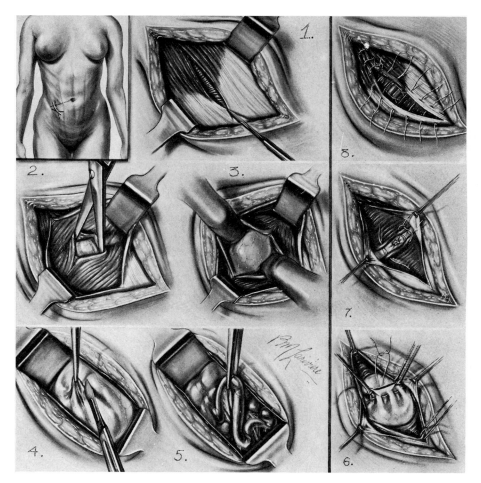

FIG. 22. McBurney or gridiron incision for appendectomy. Note the purse-string method of closing peritoneum.

tions have not made this type of exposure more difficult. It not only has been ideal for procedures on the bladder and adjacent structures, but has afforded ample visibility for transplantation of the ureters and exploration of the peritoneal cavity. Furthermore, lateral extension of the conventional Cherney incision has permitted simultaneous operations on the upper part of the urinary tract, including complete nephroureterectomy. Our patients have been astonishingly comfortable during the immediate postoperative period and so far there have been no hernias or eviscerations after employment of the following type of exposure.

All the important technical features of making and closing this incision are clearly portrayed in Figures 23 to 29.

SUTURELESS SKIN CLOSURE

This technique of closure of abdominal and other incisions appears to be gaining in popularity. For detailed information on this subject, the reader is referred to the following contributions by Golden et al.,[3] Skoog,[13] Rothine and Taylor,[11] Nova,[6] Peterson,[7] and Shepherd.[12]

Skoog, reporting on the use of porous tape for wound closure, refers to a "dry suture" technique used by Ambroise Paré, in the sixteenth century, for closure of facial

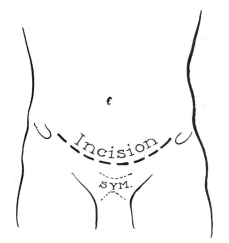

FIG. 23. Cherney incision. Note position of incision—in interspinous crease to afford full exposure of underlying muscles and yield good cosmetic result.

wounds" . . . lest that the scar should become deformed."

However, until the development of microporous surgical tape and unique chemically inert adhesives, the effective use of tape strips for skin closure was impracticable.

Golden [3] reported:

An entirely new type of surgical tape, namely, 3M Micropore Tape, renewed interest in the application of strips for wound healing, and its clinical investigation over a period of 33 months provided impressive facts indicating that the technique with this special tape is feasible, and dependable.

Nova [6] enumerated the advantages of this sutureless skin closure method:

1. Elimination of tissue contraction;
2. elimination of foreign body reaction and introduction of skin micro-organisms;
3. complete closure of dead spaces; and,
4. excellent cosmetic results.

Nova reported a series of 150 cases of which 123 were judged to be excellent; 24 good; and 3 unsatisfactory.

Rothine and Taylor,[11] in recording their experiences of sutureless skin closure in 281 cases, write:

All wounds were prepared for closure by accomplishing hemostasis to keep the surrounding skin dry and free of ooze, and also applying tincture of benzoin to the surrounding skin. Although the over-all results were good and usually more satisfactory than closure by sutures, a few failures occurred. Inadequate hemostasis with oozing from the wound resulted in loss of adhesion with loosening of the adhesive tape and subsequent gaping of the wound. Failure to apply an adequate number of strips of tape close enough together resulted in insufficient tension along the wound edges, which in turn resulted in gaping of the wound.

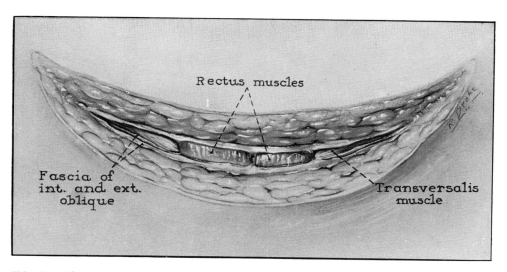

FIG. 24. Cherney incision. Incision of anterior sheath of rectus muscles and aponeuroses of external and internal oblique muscles.

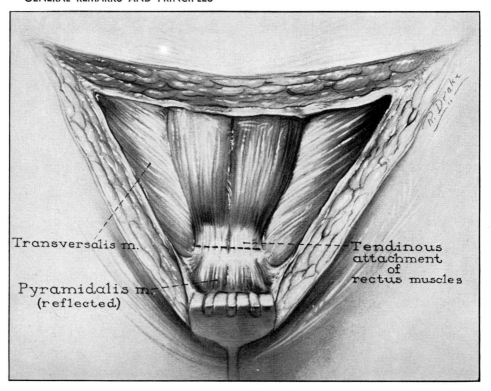

FIG. 25.   Cherney incision. Exposure of tendinous insertion of rectus muscles on symphysis and proposed level for division of tendons.

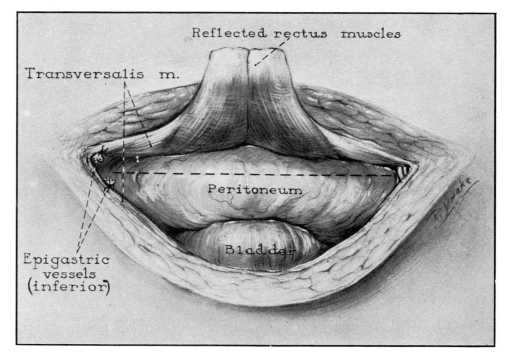

FIG. 26.   Cherney incision. Recti reflected upward, exposing bladder, peritoneum, and proposed position of peritoneal incision.

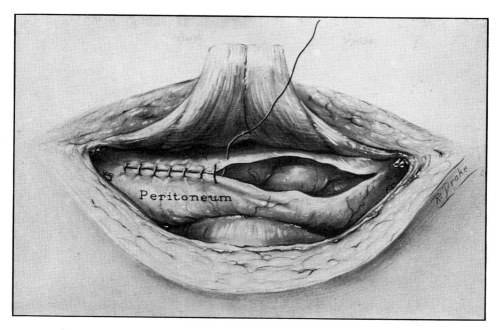

FIG. 27.   Cherney incision. Closure of peritoneum.

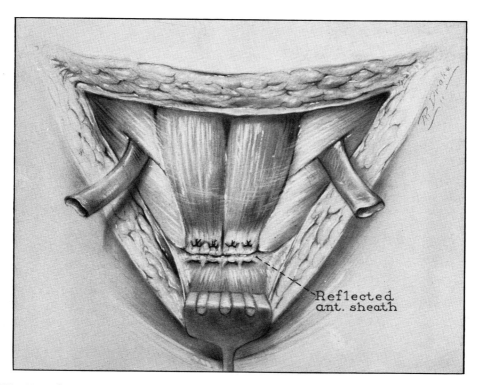

FIG. 28.   Cherney incision. Reattachment of rectus tendons. Note position of drainage tubes.

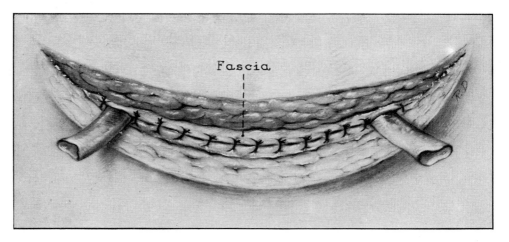

FIG. 29. Cherney incision. Closure of anterior sheath of rectus and aponeuroses of oblique muscles.

Peterson [7] describes his technique as follows:

The tape was applied in ¼ in. widths at ¼ in. intervals and was allowed to remain in place for 8 to 14 days. Then a 2 in. wide strip of microporous tape was placed directly over the incision along the axis of the wound in an attempt to achieve a finer cosmetic result. There was one failure of tape closure when persistent oozing from the wound prevented adequate skin-tape contact and suture closure was required. Postoperative wound complications included 6 wound infections. Cosmetic results have been evaluated in 54 patients followed up for 1 to 3 years, and these results have been universally good. Patient acceptance is high, and the final cosmetic result is adjudged superior to that of suture or clip closure.

No study of this subject would be complete without reference to Miss Mary P. Shepherd's article in the *British Journal of Surgery* (1966).

The following are some excerpts from this paper; the technique is based on use of 3M Steri-Strip Closures on 507 thoracic and abdominothoracic surgical cases:

1. The skin preparation used was cetrimide and Hibitane.

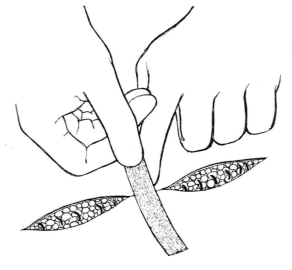

FIG. 30. Sutureless skin closure.

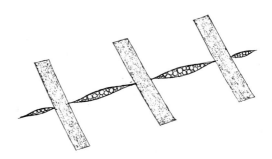

FIG. 31. Sutureless skin closure.

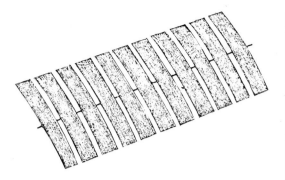

FIG. 32. Sutureless skin closure.

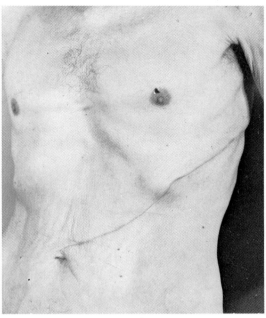

FIG. 33. Sutureless skin closure. Scar 7 months after oesophagogastrectomy. (Courtesy of Miss Mary P. Shepherd, F.R.C.S., and the *British Journal of Surgery.*)

2. 3M "Steri-Drape" was applied to the operative area.

3. In all cases the subcutaneous tissues were closed carefully using a continuous suture of 0 or 00 plain catgut inserted with a curved cutting needle, making sure all knots were buried. If there was an abundance of subcutaneous fat, deep subcutaneous and subcuticular stitches were put in. Particular attention was paid to the level at which the most superficial suture emerged near the skin edge. It was important that this site should be through the dermis, so that the superficial portion of each stitch approximated the skin edges at this level and the subcutaneous fat was buried.

Suture of the subcutaneous layers therefore not only approximated the skin edges, but also produced haemostasis, thus contributing to the dryness of the final wound.

4. The wound and surrounding skin were then washed with cetrimide and Hibitane and carefully dried. The skin was painted with simple tincture of benzoin, care being taken to apply it right to the skin edges.

5. The adhesive tapes were then applied. One end of each tape was stuck carefully to one skin edge, the wound drawn together, and any bulging subcutaneous fat being replaced, the epidermis accurately approximated, and application of the tape completed.

6. To close the average thoracotomy wound, about twelve tapes of ½ in. width and twelve ¼ in. tapes were required. In this way, tension necessary to close the skin was distributed along the wound (Figs. 30 to 32).

The taped incision was covered with a light dressing, using 1 in. width 3M Micropore Surgical Tape to prevent early curling of the ends of the skin tapes and to soiling of linen. The outer dressing was removed in 36 to 48 hours and the wound sealed with transparent dressing, which was sprayed on.

7. The skin tapes were removed on the tenth day in most cases.

8. Of the 507 cases, results were satisfactory in 478. The ages of the patients ranged from 1 day to 90 years.

9. Adhesive-tape skin closure was found to have several advantages over skin sutures, confirming the finding of others.

The incidence of wound infection was reduced and the final cosmetic result of the scar was invariably superior to that produced by skin stitches (Fig. 33).

REFERENCES

1. Annotation, Lancet 2:1164, 1958.
2. Culp and DeWeerd, Proc. Mayo Clin. 43:144, 1951.
3. Golden et al., Am. J. Surg. 104:603, 1962.
4. Jackson, Pollock, and Tindal, Br. J. Surg. 58:340, 1971.
5. Jackson, Pollock, and Tindal, Br. J. Surg. 58:565, 1971.
6. Nova, Milit. Med. 129:349, 1964.
7. Peterson, Obstet. Gynecol. 26:520, 1965.
8. Reid, R., in The Management of Abdominal Operations, R. Maingot, ed., 2d ed., 1957.
9. Reid, Zinninger, and Merrell, Ann. Surg. 98:890, 1933.
10. Rickett and Jackson, Br. Med. J. 4:206, 1969.
11. Rothine and Taylor, Br. Med. J. 2:1027, 1963.
12. Shepherd, Br. J. Surg. 53:445, 1966.
13. Skoog, Svensk Lakartidn, 59:3386, 1962.

B. STAINLESS STEEL WIRE FOR CLOSING ABDOMINAL INCISIONS

ALAN HUNT

Stainless steel wire was first used systematically in abdominal surgery by Babcock.[1] It has certain advantages over other suture materials: (1) It is very strong.[2] Standard wire gauge 33 is satisfactory for most purposes in abdominal surgery. (2) It is inert and induces no inflammatory or foreign body response.[4] In this respect it is preferable to nylon.[3] Its smooth surface does not harbour infection. Almost invariably granulating wounds close over the steel sutures without the formation of residual sinuses. Tension sutures are unnecessary for wounds closed with steel.

It has two disadvantages: a tendency to kink (which can be overcome by appreciating the fact that it requires to be handled in a manner different from other suture materials) and a tendency to fragment (which usually occurs some months or years after it has been sewn into the tissues). A thin person may then become conscious of its presence and a troublesome fragment may need to be removed. This occurs in about 1 case in 50. These disadvantages are those of inconvenience; whereas, to its credit, the material gives the greatest possible security of abdominal closure. The risk of disruption is virtually eliminated.

INDICATIONS

Stainless steel wire is at present the material of choice in the following circumstances:

1. When there is likely to be delay in the biological processes of wound healing:
   a. In nutritional deficiencies, or when the diet has been restricted, or when the absorption of food is in any way impaired.
   b. In all cases of abdominal malignant disease.
   c. In patients with jaundice, cirrhosis, or other liver disease.
2. When the abdominal wall is weak or may be submitted to any undue disruptive force such as distention, coughing, vomiting, or hiccoughing.
3. When infection is present or when an intestinal, biliary, or pancreatic fistula may be expected to form—circumstances which not only delay healing but also accelerate the dissolution of catgut sutures and render healing wounds particularly likely to disrupt.

The value of stainless steel has been demonstrated by the author in a series of more than 800 major operations on patients suffering from diseases of the liver and spleen.

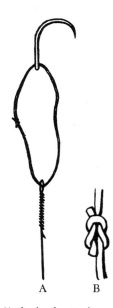

FIG. 34. (A) Method of attaching needle to wire with intervening loop of thread. Needle (Symonds') is suitable type for inguinal and femoral hernia repair. (B) Tight square-lying reef knot, ends of which are cut short.

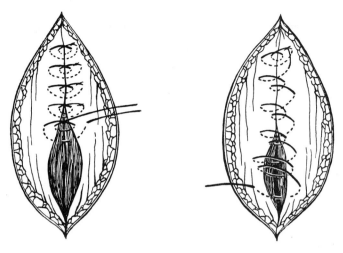

FIG. 35.   Closure of paramedian incision by far-and-near sutures: (A), interrupted and (B), continuous.

Ascites and portal hypertension are well known to cause enormous abdominal distention and render the wounds particularly prone to indolent and sometimes prolonged infection. All except seven incisions were closed with stainless steel wire, and in none did the wound give cause for anxiety. Four were closed with nylon, and in three of these the sutures had to be removed because of persistent infected sinuses. Three were closed with catgut, and in two the wounds disrupted.

METHODS OF USE

The wire is best affixed to the needle by an intervening 2-inch (5-cm) loop of 40 or 60 thread (Fig. 34). This allows manipulation of the needle without bunching of the wire at the eye of the needle, and without fracture, as happens when the wire is affixed to an atraumatic needle. Any needle can be used. I am fully aware that many surgeons are successfully using single or multistrand stainless steel sutures with atraumatic (eyeless) needles, in the closure of abdominal incisions.

However, as I am fully satisfied with the immediate and late results of the technique I have employed for many years, I can see no reason for employing atraumatic needles, as they are very prone to fracture when grasped by needle-holders.

Knots. Knots should be tied with forceps. To be secure, they should always be in the form of a true-close-tied reef (Figs. 34–37). The loose end or ends should be cut flush with the knot. A special pair of scissors, preferably curved on the flat, should be reserved for cutting wire.

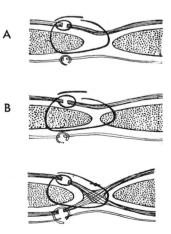

FIG. 36.   Paramedian incision. A and B show relationship of wire to rectus sheath and muscles; below is shown the fold of Douglas.

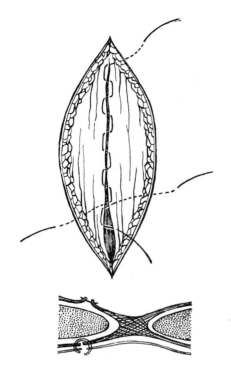

FIG. 37. Method of inserting steel stitch for early removal.

The handling of the wire. This is important. It should be unwound and not twisted off the reel. During the process of sewing it into the tissues the assistant should hold the wire in a loose open loop, using both hands for this purpose only. He must allow the wire to follow the needle without tension and without slack. If this is not done, the wire will kink and soon break.

The peritoneum. The peritoneum is first closed in the usual manner with a con-tinuous catgut stitch. The fibromuscular layers are then approximated with stainless steel. The sutures, whether continuous or interrupted, should never be drawn up tighter than necessary to produce accurate approximation of the tissues. Strangulation of muscle and fascia must be avoided.

Midline incisions. These are closed with a simple over-and-over interrupted or continuous suture.

Paramedian, oblique, and transverse incisions. The far-and-near stitch, whether interrupted or continuous (Fig. 35), gives approximation both deeply and superficially (Fig. 36).

Reopening of abdominal incisions closed with wire. The previous skin scar is excised down to the anterior rectus sheath or external oblique. The cutting diathermy needle is then used lightly to divide the fibrous scar. Contact of the needle with the wire will cause a momentary spark. The loop of wire is pulled up and divided between artery forceps. A succession of such breaks enables the wire to be removed rapidly. If it is certain that a wound will require to be reopened in the near future, the flat back-and-forth stitch illustrated in Figure 37 may be used. Short lengths of a thicker wire (standard wire gauge 31) allow easy removal on the twelfth or fourteenth day, though a brief anaesthetic or an opiate may be required for this purpose.

REFERENCES

1. Babcock, J.A.M.A. 102:1756, 1934.
2. Douglas, Lancet 2:497, 1949.
3. Large, Am. J. Surg. 60:415, 1943.
4. Nelson and Dennis, Surg. Gynecol. Obstet. 93: 461, 1951.

C. THE THORACOABDOMINAL INCISION

JOHN L. MADDEN

The thoracoabdominal incision, both right and left, is of proved value if used for specific indications. Its primary advantage is the conversion of the pleural and peritoneal cavities into one large cavity by which excellent exposure of the operative area is obtained. The closure of the wound, however, is time-consuming, which may predispose to a higher incidence of complications postoperatively. Furthermore, it is believed that the thoracoabdominal incision is used all too frequently as a routine when either an abdominal or a thoracic incision alone would suffice for the operation that is contemplated. It has been observed repeatedly that the greater the experience of the surgeon in operations upon the upper abdominal viscera, the less is the use of thoracoabdominal incision.

The right thoracoabdominal incision, which is illustrated, may be particularly useful in reconstructive operations upon the common duct, lobar resections of the liver, and the performance of portacaval shunt procedures. The association of ascites in patients with portal hypertension, however, is considered a contraindication to the thoracoabdominal approach because pleural effusion as a postoperative complication invariably occurs. This is the result of leakage of the ascitic fluid through the line of closure in the diaphragm.

On the left side, this incision may be used effectively in resections of the lower end of the esophagus and cardia of the stomach, for total gastrectomy, for the removal of large and adherent spleens, and in the performance of splenorenal shunt operations. It must be stated again for emphasis, however, that the thoracoabdominal incision is one that should be used selectively and never routinely.

(See Fig. 38, A to O.)

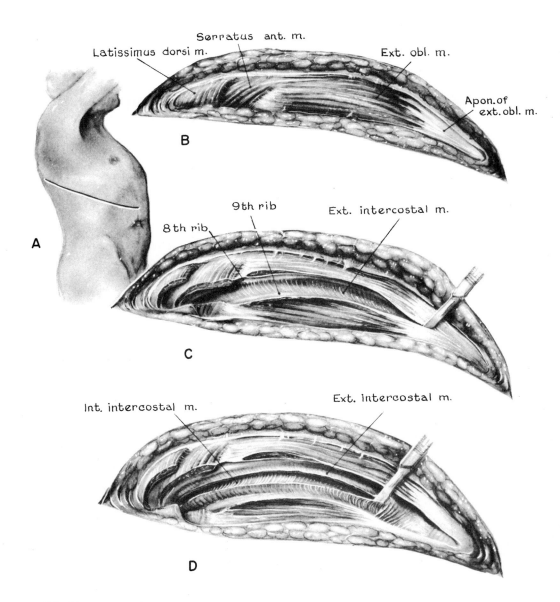

FIG. 38.
- A. The incision overlying the eighth interspace and extending across the right costal margin onto the anterior abdominal wall is shown.
- B. The incision is deepened through the skin and the subcutaneous fatty tissue layers to expose the underlying musculature of the anterolateral thoracic and the anterior abdominal walls.
- C. The exposed muscles—the latissimus dorsi, the serratus magnus, and the external oblique muscle and its aponeurosis—are severed with a scalpel to expose the eighth and ninth ribs and the intervening external intercostal muscle.
- D. The incision is continued through the external intercostal muscle layer, and the fibers of the internal intercostal muscle, which course in a different plane, are depicted.

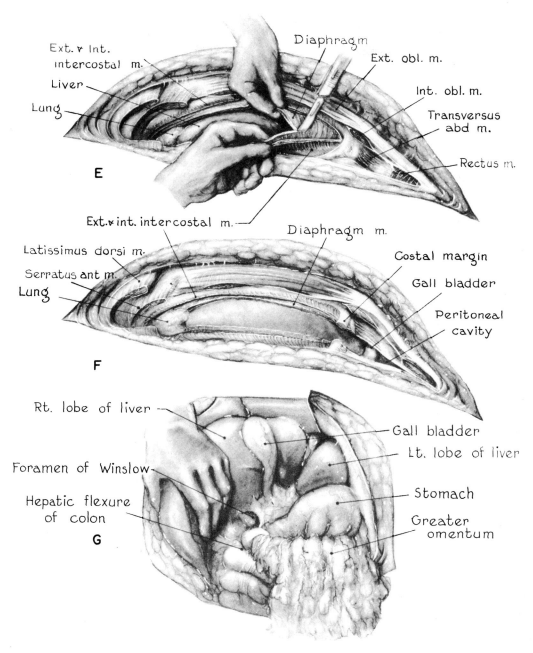

FIG. 38. (cont.)

E. The incision is deepened posteriorly through the internal intercostal muscle, the endothoracic fascia, and the parietal pleura to enter the right pleural cavity. This incision is then extended anteriorly to the costal arch severing the fibers of the internal intercostal muscle and the underlying fibers of the right leaflet of the diaphragm.

F. The incision is continued across the costal arch and through the musculature of the anterior abdominal wall to enter the peritoneal cavity.

G. The incision is completed, and the adequacy of the exposure of the operative field obtained by the conversion of the pleural and peritoneal cavities into a common cavity is shown.

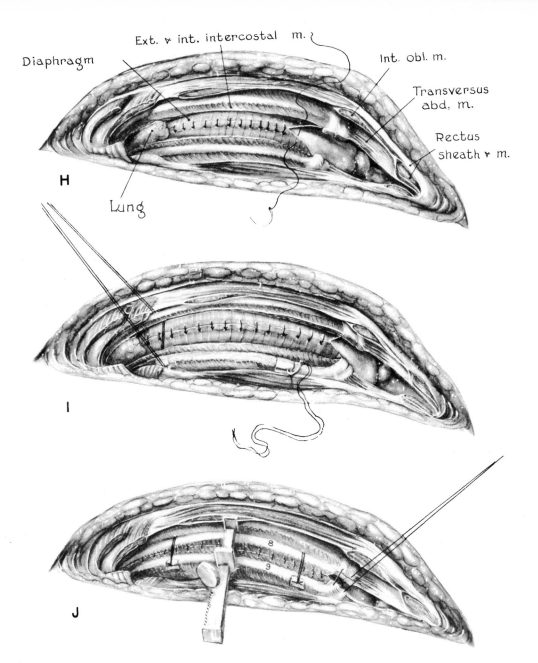

Ext. & int. intercostal m.

Diaphragm

Int. obl. m.

Transversus
abd. m.

Rectus
sheath & m.

H

Lung

I

J

FIG. 38.(cont.)

H. The closure of the incision is begun by the approximation of the cut margins of the diaphragm with interrupted sutures of silk (00). The surrounding related structures are indicated.

I. Two pericostal sutures of double strands of No. 2 chromic catgut are inserted preliminary
to the approximation of the eighth and ninth ribs. Prior to the insertion of these sutures,
periosteal "windows" are made along the inferior border of the lower or ninth rib. This
is done to prevent the impingement of the sutures upon the periosteum and thereby possibly
lessen both the incidence and/or the severity of postthoracotomy pain.

J. The rib cage is approximated with a self-retaining Bailey-Gibbons rib approximator, and
the pericostal sutures are tied and cut. The sutures of silk (000) in the intercostal muscle
layers are first inserted and, after approximation of the ribs, they are tied and cut. A
figure-of-8 mattress suture of No. 1 braided silk is inserted to unite the cut margins of the
costal arch.

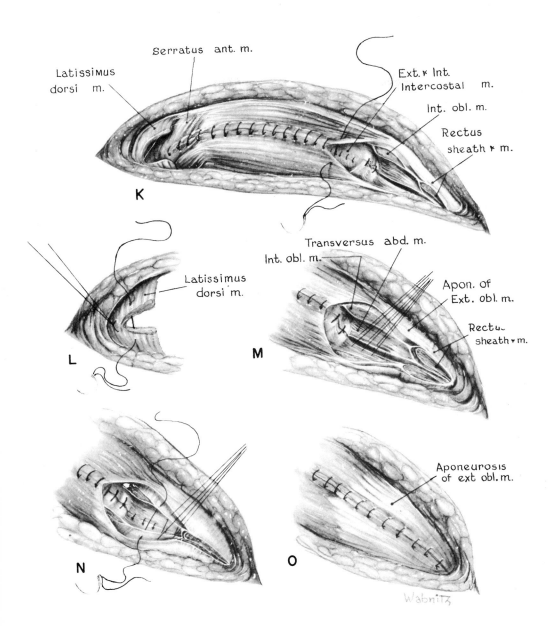

FIG. 38. (cont.)

K. The closure of the rib cage is completed, and the cut margins of the serratus anterior and the external oblique muscles are sutured with interrupted sutures of silk (00).

L. Close-up showing the approximation of the severed fibers of the latissimus dorsi muscle with the interrupted silk (00) sutures.

M. The transversus abdominis muscle layer is approximated with a series of interrupted sutures of silk (000), which are shown inserted but not tied.

N. The closure of the transversus abdominis muscle is completed, and the suturing of the internal oblique muscle is begun, using sutures of silk (000).

O. The closure of the muscle layers is completed by suturing the aponeurosis of the external oblique muscle and the anterior rectus sheath. Although not illustrated in the drawings, water-seal drainage of the pleural cavity is routinely employed.

(From Madden, *Atlas of Technics in Surgery* 2d ed., Courtesy of Appleton-Century-Crofts, New York, 1964.)

2
MANAGEMENT OF THE WOUND

RODNEY MAINGOT

The management of the wound is best discussed under the following classifications:

CLEAN CASES

The dressing that has been applied to the wound in so-called clean cases that have been sutured under ideal sterile conditions should not, as a rule, be disturbed until the skin sutures are due to be removed. The following circumstances would, however, call for an earlier inspection of the wound: (1) when there are signs of infection; (2) when the dressing has been displaced; (3) when there is soiling of the dressing with blood or serum; and (4) when drains have been inserted, either into the abdominal cavity or between the various layers of the wound to give vent to the oozing of blood, serum, or purulent exudates.

Infection of the wound, however trivial, occurring in a series of clean cases, should always be a matter of concern and is frequently a reflection upon the technique employed by the surgeon and his team. It calls for a complete revision of the methods that have been adopted by the surgeon or his personnel in the operating room or his management of the wound in the postoperative period (see Chapter 3).

If the dressing becomes displaced or blood-stained, the wound should be promptly re-dressed and thereafter inspected daily for the next 2 or 3 days to make sure that progress is satisfactory. In clean cases in which drains have been inserted, it is best in many instances to remove the dressing and withdraw the drains at the end of 48 hours. These wounds will also require daily dressing until the skin sutures are removed; they should, in fact, always be suspect until they are firmly healed.

Since reading an article by Herman et al.,[20]

I have tried their methods, in a selected group of clean cases, with good results.

At the completion of the abdominal operation, the incision and an area of skin around it is cleansed with solvent ether and then sprayed with Nobecutane (which is a transparent plastic dressing containing acrylic resin in acetic esters, with inert propellant gases, and made by Evans Medical Ltd.), after which a small gauze dressing is applied and strapped in position with strips of Micropore, or Ethistrip (Ethicon) tapes. After 48 hours the tapes and dressing are removed and the wound is inspected. If the edges of the wound appear to be evenly united and sealed off, the area is once again sprayed with Nobecutane.

No further dressings are applied. Herman et al.[20] write:

What then is the explanation of our observations that postoperative dressings may be removed from a wound healing *per primam* after the second day, without increasing the incidence of infection? The answer must lie in the fact that wound edges, carefully approximated, are sufficiently sealed by coagulum and overlying epithelial regrowth to resist contamination. Of additional importance, it would seem, is the fact that an exposed wound is a dry wound, and few bacteria retain their vitality on a dry surface. These studies have shown that clean, surgically closed wounds, managed by a technique of early exposure, do not have an increased incidence of infection. Our infection rates of 1.4 percent in clean wounds and 5 percent in contaminated wounds are comparable to the incidence of infection in clean wounds of from 1 to 5 percent generally reported.

Thus the major potential disadvantage to this type of wound care, namely increased risk of infection, has not materialized.

The advantages to early wound exposure appear to outweigh the possible disadvantages. These *advantages* are: the healing wound remains clean and dry with less surface moisture or evidence of minor inflammation than the wound dressed with occlusive bandages; daily inspection or palpation of the wound is possible; and the patient does not have the annoyance of tape and bandages to contend with. We have been most gratified by the acceptance by patients of this technique of wound care.

It should be emphasized, that this technique of early wound exposure is being reported on wounds that are clean and are surgically closed. It is not being used on grossly infected wounds or on granulating wounds.

Howells and Young,[21] MacLaren,[30] John Madden,[28] and a number of surgeons throughout the world have gone one step further, and in their articles dealing with *completely undressed surgical wounds,* maintain that there are two fundamental conditions that must be satisfied before dressings can be omitted with safety. First, the wound must be kept dry. This is accomplished by elimination of dead spaces, careful haemostasis, and accurate approximation of the margins of incision with Michel clips, closely applied interrupted sutures of fine serum-proof silk, 000 Deknatel, etc. Secondly, *Staphylococcus aureus* of phage group I must be kept away from the edges of the wound at least until the coagulum has formed.

Attempts to achieve this are made by strict adherence to aseptic principles with careful bacteriological control of sterilisation and theatre cleansing.

If the wound could be kept free of microorganisms until the coagulum has formed, subsequent infection would be unlikely and any additional artificial covering unnecessary. No dressings are required in drained wounds if suction drainage is employed.

The absence of dressings brought great benefits to the patients and staff, and an all-around reduction in expenditure.

Superficial interrupted skin sutures of silk, Dexon, Ethilon, Deknatel, fine wire, or nylon are as a rule removed between the fifth and seventh days, while continuous sutures are allowed to remain a day or two longer. If Michel or Kifa clips have been used to approximate the skin edges, the majority of them should be removed on the third postoperative day, and the remainder on the fifth day. Subcuticular sutures should not be withdrawn too early; they are best left in position for eight days, while tension or supporting sutures inserted through the outer margins of the anterior sheaths of the rectus muscles are generally removed on the tenth day. Through-and-through wire, nylon, or silk sutures are withdrawn between the twelfth and eighteenth postoperative days.

Should there be any gaping at the edges of the wound after extraction of the sutures, it is wise to apply a few sterile Ethicon Steri-Strip skin closure strips across the wound at intervals to hold the edges together.

No hard and fast rules with regard to the *time for removal of drainage tubes* can be laid down, as this will, of necessity, vary with the purpose for which they have been inserted. But in a general way it may be stated that drains that have been introduced to give vent to oozing of blood or serum should be withdrawn at the end of 24 to 48 hours. Again, in cases of general peritonitis or when there is gross contamination of the abdominal cavity during operation, the drains that have been inserted should not be allowed to remain in situ for more than 3 days; but where a localised abscess, e.g., appendix abscess, has been drained, the tube or tubes will have to remain in position for a longer period. After a few days they should be rotated and shortened, until eventually they are replaced by tubes of smaller caliber. In cases of cholecystectomy, a drain is usually inserted in the region of the gallbladder fossa to allow for the escape of serum or possibly bile. When there is little or no discharge from such tubes, it is well to remove them on or about the third postoperative day; however, if there is a discharge of bile, it would be unwise to remove these tubes until the discharge has ceased or is minimal.

When dealing with the various operations in which drainage is called for, I will attempt to indicate to the surgeon where the tubes should be placed and for how long they should remain in position. One thing is certain: that some antiseptic solution, such as tincture of thimerosal (Merthiolate), should be applied to the dressing around Penrose drains, T tubes, etc. It is interesting to see how the skin surrounding the emerging tubes usually remains normal when antiseptics are applied, whereas when they are not applied there is often some redness or discharge about the tube hole. The value of the Hemovac or the Redi-vac drainage apparatus is discussed in Chapters 1 and 9.

INCISIONS WITH COMPLICATIONS

Stitch abscesses. These are usually seen about the tenth postoperative day, but they may occur earlier than this before any of the skin stitches have been removed or even some days or weeks after the wound has apparently healed quite soundly. Stitch abscesses may be superficial or deep. When deep, they may be felt as rounded, indurated masses in the depths of the wound and are painful to the touch. When superficial, they may appear as brown or mauve-coloured, fluctuating, circumscribed blisters more or less in line with the incision. They produce a certain amount of uneasiness and pain in the wound, and although some of the more deeply situated ones may become absorbed and disappear, the superficial ones are best evacuated by incising the blistered area and expressing the contents, which very often include a knot of catgut or silk with some blood-stained pus. Cultures should now be taken, and the responsible organisms identified and appropriate tests for sensitivity carried out. Such sinuses heal rapidly as soon as the offending stitch is removed, leaving only a slight scar.

Cellulitis. In cases of cellulitis of the wound, the appearances are usually quite typical. As a result of the surrounding inflammatory oedema, the stitches appear to be buried deeply in the skin; the edges of the wound are covered here and there with inspissated pus or blood; there may be some oozing of serum between the sutures; and a faint red blush will be discernible in the region of the line of incision or stitch holes, extending outward for a variable distance.

The haemolytic streptococcus is sometimes the infecting agent, although the haemolytic *S. aureus* is commonly responsible.

The condition becomes evident a few days after operation and is generally associated with raised temperature and constitutional symptoms such as headache, anorexia, and malaise. By removing a few skin stitches to relieve tension, by applying heat to the affected area, and by the wise use of antibiotics, these wounds can often be induced to heal without further complications.

The *intelligent use* of antibiotics depends upon: (1) a knowledge of the organisms involved; (2) their sensitivity to the various antibiotic agents now available; (3) the maintenance of an adequate concentration of the drug; and (4) a decision as to whether the substance should be used locally, systemically, or both.

At times a *localised abscess* may form or suppuration may be extensive and involve some of the deeper layers of the abdominal wall. In such an instance, an incision should be made over the abscess and the contents be evacuated, after which a small tube should be inserted to afford drainage and to permit instillations of the selected antibiotics into the depths of the wound. Intramuscular injections or the oral administration of the selected antibiotics is indicated until the acute phase has subsided.

When there is a large collection of blood and/or pus under the skin or when there is much fat in the abdominal wall which has become infected during the process of operation (e.g., appendectomy for perforated gangrenous appendicitis), infection with *Escherichia coli* is very prone to occur with the formation of an extensive abscess. Such wounds have a dusky, mottled appearance, being boggy and tender, the tenderness rendering it impossible at times to elicit the signs of fluctuation; but the appearance should guide the surgeon to remove a stitch or two and to probe the depths of the wound for deep-seated pus which, when located, is often found to be brown, oily and foul-smelling, and, being under great pressure, it will gush from the depths of the wound with considerable force and soon flood the surrounding area. In such cases it is best to open up the wound in part and to irrigate it with hydrogen peroxide followed by warm normal saline solution, and to provide adequate drainage. Subsequently hot compresses are applied and antibiotic therapy is instituted (see Chap. 107).

Prior to drainage, however, much serious damage may have been inflicted upon the muscles and their sheaths, and upon other structures. Considerable necrosis may also have occurred, and if this involves a large blood vessel in the abdominal wall, there may be signs of copious haemorrhage which even packing or firm compression of the wound may fail to control effectively. These cases of *secondary haemorrhage caused by suppurative myositis* are best dealt with by completely opening up the superficial portion of the wound under a general anaesthetic and, after locating the bleeding area, applying ligatures a short distance above and below the oozing surface in the muscle. This is no light task, for as the tissues are cheesy with inflammation, the sutures may readily cut out when applied, and the vessels responsible for the haemorrhage may almost defy detection and isolation. When proximal and distal ligature of the responsible vessels proves impossible, a fresh incision will have to be made in healthy tissue to permit isolation and ligature of the artery that is deemed to be the primary cause of the haemorrhage.

When bleeding has been controlled, the wound should be lightly packed with gauze soaked in zinc peroxide cream and the major portion left unsutured to permit repacking, frequent irrigation, and subsequent healing by granulation tissue. In such cases, a broad-spectrum antibiotic or a combination of two suitable antibiotics, as indicated by bacteriological studies, may be administered, these providing high serum concentrations. Madsen et al.[29] state that topical treatment of abdominal wounds with ampicillin reduces the incidence of wound infection in colon surgery and after appendectomy for perforated appendicitis.

Gas gangrene infection of abdominal wounds. It is surprising that gas gangrene infection of abdominal wounds is so rare when it is realised how often such wounds become contaminated with septic peritoneal fluid and even with colonic contents. About 40 years ago, Orr[38] could collect only twenty-one cases from the literature, although the incidence must undoubtedly be very much higher today than this figure would suggest. During World War II and the Korean conflict, a few cases of gas gangrene infection of the abdominal wall following gunshot and other types of wounds were reported in the medical journals. Findings on this grave infection during World War II have been reported by Cutler and Sandusky,[12] Jeffrey and Thompson,[23] Sachs,[42] and others. A few

cases have been published during the last 10 years, including the recent contributions by McNally, Price, and MacDonald;[33] Willis;[49] Sanders;[43] Duff et al.;[13] and Morgan, Morain, and Eraklis.[37] One of great interest followed resection of a perforated gangrenous portion of the small bowel, reported by Spann and McGill.[44] Apart from gunshot injuries and wounds of the abdominal wall and viscera associated with lacerations or the crushing of a muscle, are cholecystectomy for acute emphysematous cholecystitis caused by anaerobic infections; operation on the bowel for closed-loop obstruction, such as volvulus of the sigmoid colon or small intestine; and caecostomy or colostomy for large gut obstruction. According to Sanders,[43] a few cases of gangrene of the abdominal wall have followed shortly after operations for acute peritonitis and perforation of malignant growths of the large bowel.

The infection is ushered in by severe pain in the wound, usually 12 to 72 hours after operation; the pain is associated with a high temperature (103°F to 106°F), rapid pulse rate (120 to 140), severe shock, and a feeling of apprehension. The patient is gravely ill from the start; the usual malar flush associated with pyogenic infection is replaced by a greyish pallor, weakness, and profuse sweating; and the mental state is often one of apathy and indifference.

McNally and Crile[32] write:

The onset of *shock* ranges from within a few hours to four or more days after operation, but occurs most commonly between the twelfth and seventy-second hours. Tachycardia out of all proportion to the temperature elevation and hypotension are often the earliest signs of the infection. Characteristically, the hypotension does not respond to the usual methods of treatment.

The important features of the diagnosis are:

(a) a high index of suspicion of the diagnosis when the first signs of shock appear, (b) recognition of the characteristic discoloration of the skin, and (c) histological proof from a smear of the discharge. If the smear contains bacteria resembling *Clostridium welchii*, appropriate treatment should be started at once.

When such wounds are examined in the early stages, the edges are found to be oedematous, red, and acutely inflamed, while later on they become dusky, dark brown, and finally black from putrefaction. In some cases the reddened area around the skin incision takes on the yellowish-brown or bronze tint so characteristic of this infection. The wound is crepitant and discharges pus containing gas bubbles and an irritating brownish watery fluid that has a peculiar foul odour. To an experienced observer with a keenly discriminating sense of smell, there is a characteristic acrid or "mousy" odour. Difficulty is often experienced in differentiating between toxigenic infection produced by clostridia in secondary mixed infection in abdominal wounds. It should be remembered that crepitation may result from nonclostridial organisms. Altemeier et al.[2] state that demonstration on x-ray films of gas in the soft tissues may permit an earlier diagnosis than by clinical findings alone. Altemeier remarks that as there are no satisfactory laboratory tests for *early* bacteriological diagnosis of gas gangrene, it is practical to explore surgically and without delay anyone suspected of being infected. Valuable information can, of course, be obtained from microscopic examination of the exudate.

Treatment. As soon as the condition is recognised, the following *treatment* should be carried out:

1. Debridement of wounds and any surrounding area of cellulitis is the most important single therapeutic factor. When gas gangrene is suspected in the immediate postoperative phase after an elective abdominal operation, the patient must be taken to the operating room and given a light anaesthetic, after which the incision should be opened widely and deeply into the muscular layers, and all necrotic tissue removed. Necrotic tissue is, of course, nonviable, noncontracting, and nonbleeding muscle, and requires ablation.

2. The wound should be thoroughly cleaned with hydrogen peroxide (20 volumes) and there is no doubt that this irrigation of the wound at the time of debridement and subsequently is of distinct value.

3. Specific antitoxin is considered by some authorities to be of therapeutic value when used in adequate doses as an adjunct to surgical debridement and

antibiotic therapy. The first dose of equine antitoxin should be strong, that is, 20,000 to 60,000 units or possibly more; it should be given at 4- to 6-hour intervals. The local use of antitoxin in the wound has not been found to be of any value, but, as stated above, irrigations of hydrogen peroxide are more efficient.

4. The antibiotic of choice is penicillin. The average dose of ampicillin (Penbritin, isolated at Beecham Labs.), which should be given intravenously, is 20,000,000 units every 24 hours, combined with 3 g of chloramphenicol every 24 hours, partly intravenously and partly intramuscularly, for about 5 to 6 days.

5. *Hyperbaric oxygenation is considered to be most efficient and highly effective:* 90 to 100 percent oxygen is usually given by mask at a flow rate of 8 to 10 litres per minute under 2 to 3 atmospheres pressure for 1 to 2 hours, 2 to 3 times daily for 2 to 4 days. Reduction of fever is a most welcome symptom.

6. These patients require special continuous nursing and strict isolation; a polyethylene tube should be inserted into a sizeable vein, as blood transfusions will be used freely and several checks will have to be carried out to determine the degree of hydration, anaemia, electrolyte loss, protein loss, etc. Blood volume expanders might be indicated in some cases. Vasoconstrictors have proved to be of little value unless the infection is treated vigourously on the lines already suggested.

7. The use of steroids should be considered individually in each case, but their efficacy is debatable.

The authoritative articles on this subject—by Baffes and Agustsson,[3] Wallyn et al.,[48] Trippel et al.,[46] Willis,[49] and Aldrete and Judd[1]—which emphasize the value of hyperbaric oxygen in the treatment of gas gangrene—are worthy of careful study. Special attention should be given to the review by Aldrete and Judd, who reported five cases from the Mayo Clinic during 1935–64 in which gas gangrene occurred after elective operations.

Postoperative progressive bacterial synergistic gangrene. This is a rare complication of the wound. Cullen,[11] the first surgeon to draw attention to this interesting development and to give an accurate clinical picture of the condition, described vividly the havoc wrought to the abdominal wall in a case of his, which occurred after the drainage of an abdominal abscess. Brewer and Meleney[8] subsequently reported cases with laboratory studies demonstrating the *synergistic origin of this disease*. Stewart-Wallace[45] collected from the literature thirty-seven cases of postoperative progressive gangrene of the skin, and since then additional cases have been reported by a number of surgeons. Behrend and Krouse,[4] after discussing the literature on this subject, described a fatal case following appendectomy for suppurative appendicitis. I saw two cases in 1966 in which the patients were successfully treated by systemic antibiotic therapy with penicillin and erythromycin. But in a recent case (1971), in which synergistic gangrene complicated drainage of a chronic pancreatic abscess, the treatment included radical excision of the ulcerated lesion followed by skin grafting by a plastic surgeon.

The majority of the reported cases of postoperative synergistic gangrene have followed drainage of a lung abscess, a putrid empyema, or a deep-seated peritoneal abscess, such as an appendix abscess; a few have occurred after elective procedures such as partial colectomy for diverticulitis of the sigmoid colon.

The first sign of the inauguration of the gangrenous process occurs during the first or second week after operation, although rare cases have been known in which it has shown itself as early as the second day or as late as the twenty-first day, when the wound and stitch holes take on a carbunculoid appearance and become so exquisitely tender that the application of even the most soothing dressings can hardly be tolerated.

In the early stages, the patient's general condition appears to be satisfactory, although his temperature may be slightly raised; but as the process continues its aggressively relentless course, he gradually becomes worn out with the anxiety that something serious is amiss, with discouragement on seeing the disease spread in spite of constant attention,

and also with intractable pain. The first noticeable change in the wound is that it becomes sore, red, and tender. In the course of a few days, the process very slowly extends, and the central area becomes purple or mauve-colored, while the outer zone is tinted brilliant red or vermilion. Later on, the purplish zone spreads outward and the part first affected shows all the signs of gangrene. The dead, black or mud-brown, leathery, liquefying sloughs of skin, bathed in thin watery pus, undergo a slow but steady disintegration and, on separating, leave a comparatively healthy base covered with pale-pink waterlogged granulation tissue. The purple area creeps outward into the red zone, and as it does so this spreading edge becomes raised and oedematous (Fig. 1). It advances slowly without respite unless checked in its career by surgical measures or antibiotic agents.

If this spreading edge is examined closely, it will be seen that the central portion of the purple zone, i.e., the part that lies close to the gangrenous area, is well defined but irregular, crenated, and here and there slightly undermined, although undermining is not a prominent feature. On the other side, it fades off into the red zone and eventually flattens to the level of the healthy skin (Fig. 1A). In certain places the edges show a tendency to heal and become shelving and nonoedematous, while virile epithelium grows across the base to meet islets of deep epithelium that have sprung from hair follicles or sweat glands that have not been destroyed.

Meleney,[94] *whose work is the most important contribution toward the understanding of the aetiological factors of this condition, concludes that chronic progressive postoperative gangrene of the skin is caused by synergistic activity of a symbiosis of a specific microaerophilic nonhaemolytic streptococcus present in pleural, peritoneal, or intestinal exudates, and a haemolytic* Staphylococcus aureus *introduced from without—usually from the patient's skin, and this opinion has since been confirmed by all workers in this field.*

Treatment. Before 1925 the treatment was unsuccessful, as the lesion progressed with a dogged irresistibility in spite of all kinds of local and systemic therapy. About a year later Brewer and Meleney[8] showed that the spreading gangrenous area could be cured

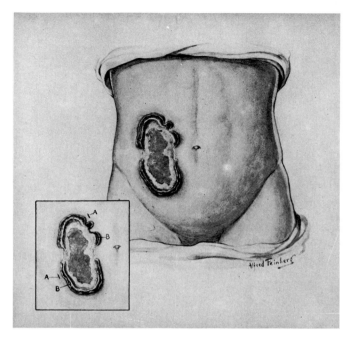

FIG. 1. Postoperative progressive bacterial synergistic gangrene of the abdominal wall. (Courtesy of Dr. Vier.)

by *wide excision*. Afterward many surgeons found that this dread disease could be eradicated by an extensive excision, including the outer zone of redness, performed either with the knife or cautery followed later by skin grafting. Zinc peroxide, suspended in doubly distilled water and applied *after* the excision, helps to prevent a recurrence of the infection. The defect left by this radical operation may, after a few days, be repaired by skin grafting.

The modern treatment consists of giving 20,000,000 to 30,000,000 units of penicillin intravenously every 24 hours and tetracycline 500 mg orally every 6 hours until healing is well advanced. *But sometimes antibiotic therapy is disappointing* because of the production of penicillinase in the wound by one of the secondary contaminants (see Chap. 107).

Better results can be achieved sometimes by treatment of such cases both locally and systemically with large doses of bacitracin combined with Genticin (Nicholas), and sometimes by a combination of neomycin and Ceporex (Glaxo). When antimicrobial agents fail to effect a cure, wide excision of the

diseased area followed by skin grafting should be performed. Similar lesions may be caused by the synergistic action of a microaerophilic streptococcus with other strains of bacteria such as Proteus.

Haematoma. The incidence of haematoma occurring in clean operative wounds is about 2 percent.

Haematomas are, of course, caused by faulty haemostasis of the layers of the abdominal wall but are not serious unless they become infected. They usually give rise to an aching pain in the wound, which is accompanied by a slight rise in temperature. Small haematomas may be difficult to detect, but on careful palpation they may be felt as small, hard, rounded areas, usually underneath the line of the skin incision. Sometimes they may be more deeply placed between the layers of the abdominal wall. When they are near the surface, they may produce a brown or mauve-coloured blister that is tender, soft, and fluctuating. As these small haematomas usually resolve, they may be left alone. If large, and particularly if soft, they should be aspirated with a wide-bore needle, or the edges of the wound which overlie them should be separated with a probe or a sharp-pointed scalpel and the contents evacuated. A small cigarette drain should then be inserted into the cavity to prevent a reaccumulation of serum and to facilitate the process of healing. Haematomas occurring after operations for the repair of hernia, and in which unabsorbable suture material has been employed, are best left alone and allowed to absorb slowly, as drainage of such collections of blood will leave a sinus that may become infected from the organisms that abound in the skin.

If there is a *large extravasation of blood* giving rise to a fluctuating mass, it is best to return the patient to the operating theatre open up the wound, evacuating the clot and ligating or coagulating with a diathermy needle any bleeding vessels that are visible, after which the wound should be closed (with drainage).

If cultures taken from the wound during operation do not yield a growth of microorganisms, no postoperative antibiotic treatment is indicated; but many surgeons, as a precautionary measure against subsequent sepsis, often prescribe treatment with such antimicrobial agents as penicillin, chloramphenicol, or neomycin, either singly or in combination.

Keloid scars. There is no doubt that some persons have a greater tendency to form keloid scars than others.

Crockett [10] discussed the susceptibility of 12 different areas of the body according to the severity and consistency of keloid formation as follows: (1) keloid seen consistently: presternal region and upper back; (2) keloid may be severe or occur in susceptible people: bearded area, ear, deltoid and preaxial region of upper limb, anterior chest wall excluding the midline, and scalp and forehead; (3) keloid change is rarely severe: lower back, abdomen, lower limb, postaxial region of upper limb, central area of face, and genitalia. Tuberculous patients and those who are said to have the "strumous diathesis" are also frequent victims.

King and Salzman [25] submit the following data (Table 1).

The cause of keloid is unknown. It occurs in human scar tissue and is essentially an excessive accumulation of collagen in re-

Table 1. LOCATION OF KELOID SCARS IN 89 PATIENTS

Scar Location	Cause	
	Surgical	Nonsurgical[a]
Head and neck	27	7
Trunk	25	11
Extremities	12	7

Source: King and Salzman, Surg. Clin. N. Am. 50:595, 1970.
[a]Including unknown.

sponse to trauma, which may be (a) surgical, (b) thermal, (c) accidental, (d) infectious, or (e) minimal. Keloid scars may grow progressively, and they are always unsightly and discoloured.

The appearance of keloid is unmistakable. The scar is shiny, pink or red, raised above the level of the surrounding skin, firm and hard, with a surface that may be smooth, rough, or grooved. It has irregular feelers projecting laterally from the parent stem. The various marks made by the needle while suturing the skin are likewise keloid in appearance, being red, shotty, and angry-looking. Although the margins of the keloid may appear sharply defined, they are not actually so, and on palpation the hardened, knotty scar tissue can be felt spreading downward from the surface into the subcutaneous tissues and in some cases even into the deep fascia and muscles. A keloid scar has the microscopical appearance of a soft fibroma and never becomes malignant.

No case of malignant degeneration was reported by Garsb and Stone in 248 keloids observed in the Department of Dermatology of the New York Hospital and in the Skin and Cancer Unit. Although, as previously stated, *the cause of keloid scars is unknown,* some surgeons and pathologists have submitted their "impressions" regarding possible aetiological factors.

They believe it is possible that some keloid scars that disfigure abdominal scars can be traced to errors of operative technique, such as the use of swabs soaked in *hot* saline solution; painting the open wound with skin disinfectants that may contain damaging and irritating mercurials, phenols, or alcohols;

and the use of occlusive dressings that exclude the atmospheric air and promote local sweating. It may be noted, furthermore, that if the patient is allowed to have baths immediately after the skin stitches have been removed or if the wound is inadvertently soaked with water during the process of blanket-bathing, the wound may become soggy, pruritic, and keloid. Age and race show no significant trend. In most recent series on keloids, women predominated in a ratio of 2 to 1. I can find no evidence,. however, that the occurrence of this lesion following abdominal operations is more common in blacks than in whites.

Treatment. As my personal experience of the management of keloids is limited, the reader would be best informed regarding *treatment* by my quoting certain passages contained in a current, valuable, and expert article written by King and Salzman,[25] who state:

Numerous approaches have been employed in the past; some of the popular methods were partial or complete excision alone, kilovolt radiotherapy alone, combination excision and radiotherapy, intralesional steroid infection, and a combination of steroid infections with compression of the keloid. No method of treatment has been predictably satisfactory. The basically attractive combination of keloid excision with conventional radiotherapy has been used sparingly because of the possibility of radiation injury to the skin and underlying structures. This objection to radiation therapy was at least partly resolved in 1951, with the development of the Van de Graaff low megavolt electron accelerator at M.I.T. Capable of delivering monoenergetic electrons in the 1 to 3 million volt range, it permits accurate irradiation of the skin to a thickness of 1 cm. Other advantages are ease of shielding and low accompanying x-ray background.

Patients with keloid scars may be treated (1) with electron beam therapy alone or (2) electron beam therapy after excision of the keloid. In most cases, it is advisable to perform the keloid excisions under local anaesthesia followed by electron beam therapy on the same day.

Ossification in abdominal scars. This complication in abdominal cicatrices has been discussed by Pertl,[41] McCurrick and Millington,[30] and many others.

During the last 20 years, I have seen seven cases in which the ossification occurred in vertical epigastric incisions. In these patients,

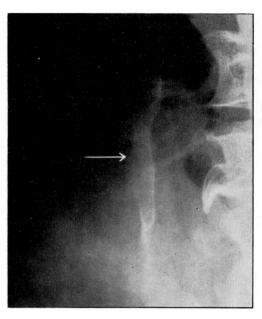

FIG. 2. Ossification in an old vertical right epigastric paramedian incision. The ossified structure was excised over 20 years ago, and when the patient was submitted to a straight x-ray film of the area in 1972 there was no evidence of recurrence. (Author's patient at Royal Free Hospital, London.)

the rock-like masses were widely excised and the resulting abdominal wounds were closed in the usual manner, employing absorbable suture material for the aponeurosis. Figure 2 is a straight x-ray film of the abdomen of one of these patients.

Illingworth and Dick [30a] state:

Heterotopic ossification has been observed quite frequently in the scar of an old abdominal incision, and it may occur in an old haematoma, in tumours, and in many other situations.

. . . In the past, heterotropic ossification was generally attributed to the activity of osteoblasts derived from local or distant sources. Thus, ossification in the abdominal wall was ascribed to injury to the pubis, xiphisternum or the periosteum of the ribs of the costal margins, with consequent liberation of osteoblasts; whereas ossification in other situations was thought to be due to the action of osteoblasts migrating from the blood stream into the injured tissues.

The present-day view is that the presence of specific cells (osteoblasts) is not essential, and that if the requisite conditions of vascularity and calcium supply are present, any primitive mesenchymal cells may assume the osteoblastic function.

The patient may complain that the scar

feels tight and sore; on abdominal palpation the tissues underlying the cicatrix feel densely hard; and straight x-ray pictures of the abdomen show the linear area or areas of heterotopic ossification.

Treatment. The scar and a healthy margin of tissue on either side of the "bone" should be excised, after which the wound is closed in the usual manner. Recurrence is rarely observed.

Desmoid tumours of the abdominal wall. This subject has been most ably and exhaustively dealt with by Pearman and Mayo,[40] Pack and Ehrlich,[39] Booker and Pack.[6]

Desmoid tumours arise in musculo-aponeurotic sheaths, and although they may be found in any part of the body, they usually occur in the anterior abdominal wall. They grow slowly and steadily by expansion from their site of origin and infiltrate all the tissues with which they come in contact. They are benign in character but simulate malignant tumours macroscopically and microscopically. Pack puts it this way:

The borderline between fibroma and fibrosarcoma is well recognised as a zone of histological uncertainty.

Cattell and Wiedman [9] have shown that if surgical excision of the tumour is delayed, it may attain a large size and seriously interfere with function. These tumours present a relatively simple surgical problem if they are diagnosed at an early stage and completely removed. Unfortunately, they are commonly unrecognised as desmoids or are considered as a primary or metastatic lesion. If they are allowed to luxuriate amongst the muscles of the abdomen, they seriously interfere with function and *may* even defy heroic attempts at complete eradication. In addition, local recurrence after excision may complicate further surgical measures.

Macfarlane (1832), in the *Clinical Reports of the Surgical Practice of the Glasgow Royal Infirmary,* was the first to describe these tumours; Müller (1838) applied the name desmona; Sänger (*Arch Gynäk 24*:1, 1884) was first to advocate radical removal; and Pfeiffer (*Beitr Klin Chir 14*:334, 1904) collected 400 cases from the literature for his classic monograph.

Pack and Ehrlich [39] state that desmoids comprise 7 percent of all benign tumours of the abdominal wall. In Pearman and Mayo's series, 71 percent were found in the abdominal wall.

Desmoid tumours are more common in females than in males, as much as 70 to 85 percent occurring in females. Whilst they may be found at any age (Booker and Pack reported 19 cases occurring in childhood), the common age incidences are: for males 40 to 60 years and for females 20 to 40 years. *Pregnancy is undoubtedly the commonest predisposing factor in the development of these tumours;* thus, in Pack's series of 15 female patients, all but one had appeared shortly after delivery; in Pearman and Mayo's series, there was a history of pregnancy in 25 of the 40 women; and in Pfeiffer's series, 94.3 percent of the women had been pregnant. Geschickter and Lewis [17] state:

. . . the predominance of desmoid tumours of the abdominal wall in parous women and the frequent appearance of such tumours following pregnancy, emphasises the connection between these growths and sex physiology.

Cattell and Wiedman [9] write:

This factor is thought to be due to a defect in the organization of small hematomas of the abdominal wall secondary to the trauma of labour. Many desmoids develop in surgical incisions, and at sites of trauma to the abdominal wall. The importance of pregnancy or of abdominal incisions in the production of these tumours is difficult to substantiate in view of the frequency of these factors and the rare development of desmoids. Furthermore, Musgrove and McDonald (*Arch. Path.,* 45:513, 1948), in a careful histologic study of 34 desmoids, were unable to find hemosiderin in 31 of them, which would be an expected finding if they developed as a result of trauma or in an organizing hematoma.

Desmoids are densely hard, fibrous tumours that invade and compress muscle and other structures at their periphery. They tend to be rounded or oval in shape and have a nodular surface.

The usual report on the microscopical sections reads, "Fibroma, or possibly low grade fibrosarcoma." All authorities agree that the differentiation of a cellular desmoid from a low grade fibrosarcoma is very difficult.

Treatment. Desmoids should be diagnosed early, when they are small, and be treated by wide excision. In view of the possibility of local recurrence after operation, generous margins of normal tissue should be excised well beyond the confines of the tumour. This may entail the removal of a large area of the abdominal wall, which may render closure a difficult and exacting problem even to a plastic surgeon. Lundh [27] states that in none of their cases were metastases to regional lymph nodes seen. Twenty-four of these tumours were radically excised and two recurred. Of the seven tumours not excised radically, five recurred at the operative site. Because of the infiltrating nature of this tumour, radical local excision is recommended as the best hope for cure. Early decision relative to the nature of the tumour is, therefore, imperative.

Desmoids are not radiosensitive.

Abdominal wound disruption and evisceration. Disruption of abdominal wounds has been discussed under various titles, such as separation of abdominal wounds, broken-down abdominal incisions, postoperative dehiscence of abdominal wounds, postoperative eventration, and burst abdomen. The title here adopted would appear to be the one most generally accepted.

Disruption of the abdominal wound may be partial or complete. It is *partial* when one or more layers have separated, but either the skin or the peritoneum remains intact. When *complete,* all the layers of the abdominal wall have burst apart, and this may or may not be associated with protrusion of a viscus—evisceration.

Wound disruption is a grave and tragic complication which may follow any abdominal operation in either sex at any age, and when it occurs it presents many serious problems in the management of the case.

Incidence. Estimates of the incidence vary between 0.2 percent and 3 percent. Most surgeons would regard an incidence of 3 percent as being unduly high, and consider a fair estimate for all cases to be in the region of 0.5 percent to 1 percent. Nevertheless, a careful study of the literature dealing with this subject does reveal some discouragingly high figures. Let us study some of the published reports.

Wolff,[50] in a series of 1,700 consecutive abdominal operations, reported 45 cases, an incidence of 2.6 percent. Joergenson and Smith [24] state that in 39,574 laparotomies performed at Los Angeles County General Hospital between the years 1936 and 1946 there were 97 instances of wound disruption abdomen, i.e., an incidence of 0.245 percent. Tweedie and Long [47] state that during a 12-year period (1941 through 1952) 22,311 major operations were performed on the general surgical services and the obstetrical and gynaecological services of the Royal Victoria Hospital in Montreal and that in this large series there were 113 cases of abdominal wound disruption. The incidence of this complication on the general surgical service was 0.47 percent in 15,711 abdominal procedures, while on the obstetrical and gynaecological services the incidence was 0.5 percent in 1,434 caesarean sections and in 5,166 gynaecological procedures. Miles et al.[36] state that during the period from 1947 to 1963, 177 cases of abdominal wound disruption occurred at the Baptist Memorial Hospital, Memphis. The overall incidence was 0.36 percent; the rate for the last 2 years of the series dropped to 0.30 percent. Efron [14] reviewed the cases of *complete* abdominal wound dehiscence at St. George's Hospital, London, during the 5-year period ending December 1964. The overall incidence was 2.2 percent, that is, 128 cases following 5,634 laparotomies.

Mendoza et al.[35] reported a series of 2,988 operations for duodenal ulcer following which wound disruption occurred in 67, or 2.2 percent. Wound disruption occurred more frequently in the older age groups and in those who had emergency operations for haemorrhage (6.2 percent). The death rate in those who had wound disruption was 11.9 percent.

Mortality. The death rate in the reported series varies considerably. It may be as low as 8 percent or again it may be as high as 30 percent, the *average* operative mortality rate of resuture being about 11 to 12 percent. Ferrer [16] states that during a 2-year period 2,058 laparotomies were performed in the local hospitals to which he was attached. In this series, there were 37 wound disruptions, giving an incidence of 1.8 percent. The incidence was greater in aged patients (43 percent were over the age of 50), and the mortality rate was 11 percent. Guiney et al.[19] state that in most cases disruption of the abdominal wound was only one of a number of contributing factors leading to a fatal termination.

If a series of cases were carefully analysed, it would be found that although many patients would eventually have died from the primary disease for which the operation was performed, even had the complication not occurred, the disruption actually precipitated the fatal issue.

Aetiology. Efron [14] writes:

No single cause accounts for all wound disruption, and as a rule a combination of factors is responsible. Basically there are two reasons for abdominal wound disruption (Lythgoe, 1960): the intra-abdominal pressure is too great, or the wound is too weak, or it may be due to both.

AGE AND SEX. Disruption of abdominal wounds is 3 to 6 times more common in patients over the age of 60 than in the younger group.

The sex incidence shows a predominance for males, the ratio being about 4 to 1, but it may be as high as 7 to 1. For instance, Tweedie and Long [47] point out that in their series the overall ratio of wound disruption of males and females was 2.6 to 1; but on the general surgical services alone, which is probably a much more accurate comparison, this ratio was 6.7 to 1.

TYPE OF ANAESTHESIA. It would seem obvious that the type per se of anaesthesia employed for the operation plays an insignificant and unimportant part, as it has been established beyond dispute that disruption occurs with equal frequency after local, spinal, and inhalation anaesthesia (with or without a muscle-relaxing drug given intravenously), specific reports, as well as a study of many cases, seem to bear out this point.

It is, nevertheless, true that a badly administered inhalation anaesthetic associated with straining and struggling of the patient, entailing, as it does, hasty, forcible and perhaps inaccurate suture of the abdominal wall under great tension, is a contributing factor, especially when the suturing is performed by inept hands.

FACTORS IN TECHNIQUE. While it is generally accepted that faulty methods of closure, increased intra-abdominal pressure and other mechanical factors in the immediate postoperative period, operation for malignant disease in patients over the age of 60, aged and poor-risk patients, and diseases associated with malnutrition, hypoproteinaemia, anaemia, and vitamin deficiencies leading to poor and ineffectual healing are the primary preoperative causes of dehiscence of the wound, a number of cases are directly attributable to certain factors in the *operative technique* itself.

The surgeon is responsible for: (1) a sterile technique; (2) the choice and type of incision; (3) damage to the tissues; (4) the control of bleeding; (5) the choice of suture and ligature materials; (6) the type and position of the drainage material employed; and (7) the method of closure of the wound and the use of additional measures to safeguard against undue tension.

It is essential, if the surgeon is to limit to a minimum his incidence of disrupted wounds, for him not only to have an irreproachable sterile technique, to inflict the least possible degree of trauma upon the tissues, and to ensure complete haemostasis and obliteration of all dead spaces, but also to adapt his technique in those cases which are particularly prone to dehiscence, as, for example, in patients who are grossly obese or who are bronchitic, anaemic, cachectic, diabetic, alcoholic, or debilitated from some severe septic form of intoxication, by a careful selection of the methods of suturing and also of the suture material itself, as his experience in such cases may dictate.

INCISIONS. Wound disruption is related to the type of incision employed in the primary operation, and statistics reveal that upper abdominal *vertical* incisions, whether these be epigastric or subumbilical, are more prone to disruption than other types, e.g., transverse or oblique.

Vertical upper abdominal incisions, and more especially *midline ones,* are more likely to disrupt than any other. The McBurney and transverse incisions have always afforded a high degree of protection, and dehiscence following these incisions is rare.

The placing of a viscus in the incision, e.g., colostomy, definitely increases the risk of disruption of the wound, and of the formation of a subsequent ventral hernia.

It is noteworthy that there is a low incidence of disruption following caesarean section. The magnitude and the time consumed by the operative procedure have some bearing on the problem, as has the performance of more than one operative procedure at a time. The longer the operation, the more complicated the procedure, and the performance of two or more procedures at the time of primary operation all increase the risk of this complication.

METHODS OF CLOSURE OF THE WOUND. Do the actual method of closure of the abdominal wound and the type of suture material used affect the question of dehiscence? While it is true that rupture is possible with any type of closure and with any type of suture material, it is the opinion of many surgeons that a wise choice of suture material plays an important part in the matter, although it must be emphasised that no suture material is immune to the accident.

Catgut is extensively used in most clinics throughout the world for suturing abdominal wounds, the usual practice being to employ a continuous suture of 0 or 1 chromic catgut for the posterior rectus sheath and peritoneum, and interrupted sutures of catgut, silk, Dexon, nylon or Ethilon for the anterior sheath, the subcutaneous tissues being closed with interrupted sutures of 000 plain catgut, while the skin edges are brought together with interrupted sutures of fine serumproof silk or with Michel clips.

Tweedie and Long [47] state that it is not possible accurately to assess the relative frequency of disruption in respect of each type or combination of suture materials. In their series, catgut was used in the majority of closures, and they consider that there is no evidence to suggest that the incidence of disruption in such cases is proportionately higher, or that the type per se of suture material used influences the incidence of wound disruption. They state that in the combined usage of catgut with silk or wire, the former was usually employed to close the peritoneum while silk or wire was used to close the fascial layers.

For frankly infected and for *contaminated* cases, Ethilon, silk, wire, or monofilament nylon is almost universally employed; but in *clean* cases, the peritoneum and posterior sheath of the rectus muscle are commonly approximated with a through-and-through continuous-stitch of a single- or double-strand of 0–1 chromic catgut or 0–1 Dexon,

interrupted sutures of chromic catgut—fine silk, nylon, or wire being employed for drawing together the edges of the anterior sheath of the rectus muscle. Wounds sutured solely with fine silk after the Halsted technique are less likely to rupture than those sutured with catgut, and this is attributable largely to the fact that silk is used only in the most favourable types of cases.

The use of tension sutures has undoubtedly reduced the incidence of wound disruption. One-layer closure, with interrupted through-and-through figure-of-8 tension sutures of nylon or wire, is mandatory in gravely ill patients suffering from severe malnutrition or advanced malignant disease (see Chap. 1).

DRAINAGE. Wound disruption is commoner in cases that have been drained, although it is interesting to note that the statistics of certain surgeons show a higher incidence of disruption in undrained than in drained cases. This may be accounted for by the fact that the number of undrained abdominal wounds is considerably higher than the number of drained wounds. It would seem almost self-evident, however, that disruption is likely to occur in a higher percentage of drained cases than of undrained cases, the very necessity for drainage indicating that the patient is suffering from intra-abdominal suppuration with attendant toxaemia, a combination of factors which is well recognised as often being associated with a comparatively high incidence of wound dehiscence.

It is probable that drainage tubes are used too frequently and too long, even in cases of acute peritonitis. Nevertheless, in cases of frank purulent peritonitis there are very few surgeons who would have the temerity to dispense with the use of a drainage tube, however dubious they might be as to its actual benefits. In some 50 percent of "clean" cases, which have undergone disruption of the wound, infection becomes apparent within 24 hours. Mendoza,[35] in 1970, assessed the incidence as high as 65 percent.

Factors responsible for poor healing of the tissues. *The general state of the patient.* Where the patient is obese, emaciated, aged, decrepit, cachectic, toxaemic, jaundiced, diabetic, nephritic, uraemic, anaemic, alcoholic, or suffering from any diseased state associated with prolonged adrenal steroid medication, detectable serum protein deficiencies or vitamin C deficiency, the regenerative powers of the tissues are much diminished, and in such patients extra precautions should be taken to guard against the possibility of disruption of the wound following operation.

The use of vitamins to accelerate healing has been investigated by numerous observers including Hunt,[22] Bourne,[7] and Beattie.[4] Vitamin C is necessary for the formation of collagen in tissue repair, and there seems to be little doubt that the development of tensile strength in wounds is retarded by a partial or complete lack of vitamin C. In the preoperative and postoperative phases, the level of intake of ascorbic acid should be at least 3 times the accepted optimum for adults.

Clinically and experimentally, the association of hypoproteinaemia and dehiscence has often been noted. This subject has received the emphasis it deserves from Elman.[15] Preoperative correction of nutritional deficiencies and restoration of normal fluid and electrolyte balance in dehydrated patients need no further emphasis here. Anaemia as part of a general depletion should be corrected by transfusions of whole blood.

The nature of the primary disease. Although mechanical cause, such as increased intra-abdominal pressure, is one of the primary factors in the production of disruption, there is no doubt that the primary disease is an important aetiological factor. Wound disruption may occur in any disease that affects the peritoneum or its contents, and, as would be expected, it is more common with some diseases than with others. It is well known that illnesses of a protracted nature attended by emaciation, cachexia, and weakness, and those of acute or chronic intoxication associated with long bouts of fever, devitalise the individual sufficiently to interfere with the reparative powers of the tissues and healing of the wound. The condition is therefore most commonly seen after operations for visceral cancer, intraperitoneal suppuration (generalised or localised), acute pancreatitis, jaundice, and ascites. The comparatively high incidence following operations for cancer of the abdominal viscera is due in large measure to the anaemia and debility often present in such cases. For instance, Tweedie and Long [47] state that wound disruption associated with malignant disease is relatively rare below the age of 60 years, but it increases very steadily with advancing age, accounting for 72 percent of all disruptions at the age of 65 and over.

Acute appendicitis associated with spreading or diffuse peritonitis furnishes a number of cases, as suppuration of the wound in such cases is common, peritoneal drainage is frequently required. and other factors, such as septic intoxication and marked debility, are often associated with such mechanical disruptive forces as coughing, vomiting, and distention, which all combine to play an important part in causing the accident.

Increased postoperative abdominal pressure. This is one of the most important underlying causes of disruption of the wound. There can be no doubt that postoperative vomiting, meteorism, hiccough, explosive coughing, violent sneezing, and any undue strain such as might be occasioned by restlessness, by the patient getting out of bed, or by difficulty in defaecation or micturition, as well as the straining associated with gastric lavage, impose upon freshly sutured abdominal wounds stress which is sufficient at times to cause disruption. When, for one reason or another, healing is poor, such as may be the case in the presence of sepsis or malnutrition, or when the suture material used or the method of suturing is unsuitable for the. special needs of the case, disruption is to be anticipated, particularly when the intra-abdominal pressure is of great force or is continuous.

To sum up: The prevention of wound disruption depends upon the anaesthetist, the surgical technique employed, the nature of the disease, and the patient's diet. The anaesthetist by his skill can diminish cough and vomiting and can give the surgeon that relaxation of the abdominal wall that favours gentle handling and ease in suturing the wound. The surgeon must neglect no point of technique that will contribute to firm and secure approximation of the edges of the wound, and he must remember the vitamin C requirements and the demands of his patient for abundant proteins both orally and intravenously.

Clinical picture of wound disruption.

There are many clinical types of wound disruption. There is a type in which the patient's progress appears to be satisfactory, although the temperature may be slightly raised and meteorism may be troublesome. When the stitches are removed on the seventh or eighth day, the wound literally falls apart, or a day or two after the removal of the sutures, the dressings and sometimes even the binder and bedclothes are drenched with a pink serosanguineous discharge. This *pink discharge* is almost pathognomonic of dehiscence, and when it occurs early, i.e., before the seventh day, the wound should be examined, a stitch or two removed, the edges of the wound gently separated with a probe, and the deeper layers inspected to see whether union is satisfactory. Sometimes this pink discharge is associated with a large subcutaneous haematoma or a soft, tympanitic, boggy swelling that distends the wound. Both of these should be investigated in the operating theatre, and if a large haematoma has formed, it should be evacuated and the depths of the wound examined to see if any separation has occurred. The soft tympanitic swelling generally indicates that a knuckle of gut has burst through all the layers of the abdominal wall and lies under the skin incision, but although this may still remain intact, the condition is in itself an indication that immediate repair is imperative.

There is another type in which the wound appears to be soundly healed. There may or may not be the pink discharge I have described, but the patient, following some excessive strain, may feel a sudden "give" in the wound, which when examined is found to be torn asunder and the gut eviscerated. It is surprising how painless this condition may be, and how little if any shock results; shock, in fact, is rarely seen in cases of dehiscence of the wound except when evisceration is extensive. In cases where the edges of the skin incision have separated, the surgeon, after having inspected and probed the depths of the wound, may often lull himself into the belief that what he is seeing is actually rectus sheath or muscle fibres coated with fibrinous clot. More often than not, however, it is the omentum, the transverse colon, or a portion of the small intestine that is protruding into the depths of the wound, and the best way of ascertaining the truth is to explore the wound in the operating room.

In another type, the immediate postoperative course is very stormy, and it should be noted that patients who take anaesthetics badly often have a stormy convalescence. There is usually considerable postoperative vomiting and marked distention, hiccough may be troublesome, respiratory complications are frequent, and suppuration of the wound is common.

When postoperative rupture occurs in a wound that is frankly suppurating, the onset is nearly always gradual. An abscess forms, which is usually drained, and in the discharge, portions of the sloughing aponeurotic sheath or fibres of muscle are carried away, this being followed by separation of the deeper layers. Here the matted omentum and intestine are often adherent to the necrotic muscle.

Extensive evisceration, in which the intestines literally prolapse into the bed, is rarely seen except when large incisions have been made with the object of exploring the abdominal cavity in cases of visceral carcinoma.

Disruption generally follows the removal of the sutures between the seventh and tenth days, but it may occur later (on the fourteenth day) when supporting or stay sutures have been used, or even later than this after the wound appears to be soundly healed, especially in cases of ascites, or when suppuration is a late complication. It is rare for disruption to take place before the skin sutures have been removed, but when it does occur prior to this and is treated promptly, the prognosis is usually hopeful.

PROGNOSIS. As previously stated, the mortality rate of this condition has been computed by different authorities as being between 8 percent and 30 percent, the average being 11 to 12 percent. In Efron's series,[14] the mortality rate was 24 percent, and of the 31 patients who died, only two patients were under 50 years of age. In Guiney's series,[19] the mortality rate was 15 percent. Miles[36] reported that the mortality rate of dehiscence was 14.1 percent. Mendoza[35] recorded the death rate in his large series as being 11.9 percent; while Ferrer[16] reported 37 cases of wound disruption following 2,058 laparotomies. In his series, the mortality rate was 11 percent.

The earlier the accident is recognised and

treated, the better will be the prognosis, and especially in clean cases in which the dehiscence is partial or, if complete, is not associated with prolapse of the intestine.

When there is extensive suppuration of the wound or general peritonitis, the prognosis is very grave.

The most common causes of death are listed in their order of frequency and importance as follows: atelectasis, acute peritonitis, intestinal obstruction, renal failure, or some cardiovascular accident. The primary condition for which the patient was operated upon is more often the exciting cause of death than the rupture itself or the measures required in its treatment.

TREATMENT. There are three methods in common use today:

1. Packing the wound followed by strapping with adhesive plaster.
2. Temporary packing and strapping followed by secondary suture.
3. Immediate resuture.

Packing and strapping the wound is indicated: (a) when the patient's condition is such that any secondary operative procedure would be too hazardous, i.e., he is in a critical state and suffering from shock; (b) when the disrupted wound is very foul and freely suppurating; and (c) when disruption has occurred in a case of frank purulent peritonitis.

Therefore in the severe critical case, strapping is to be preferred to resuturing. In the desperate case, the problem is to get the patient safely through the immediate crisis with the least possible interference. As soon as he has recovered from the early effects of the wound disruption and of the treatment by strapping, and provided there is no evidence of gross infection, *secondary suture* (when indicated) may then be carried out with much less risk.

It is true that *postoperative ventral hernia* is an invariable sequel to this method of treatment, but this can be repaired at a later date with comparative safety and success.

When *strapping* is indicated, the patient should be given an injection of thiopental followed by a general anaesthetic, with a muscle-relaxing drug; the wound edges and any protruding viscera should be freely washed in warm normal saline solution.

After this, the omentum and gut should be gently replaced below the level of the edges of the peritoneum. A long strip of gauze is soaked in a concentrated solution of penicillin-streptomycin cream and is then cautiously placed on top of the reposited viscera, and the skin edges are closely approximated with Ethistrip or Micropore adhesive strips and a firm dressing applied. Free peritoneal drainage is afforded by the gauze, which protrudes through the lowest portion of the wound. If all goes well, the plaster strips and the gauze dressing are removed in a few days, and the process is repeated at intervals until healing is advanced. Secondary suture may be contemplated at this stage, but if this is deemed inadvisable, the wound is allowed to granulate slowly and cleanly.

Resuture of the disrupted wound is recommended for the majority of cases, and especially for those in which the edges of the wound, although these may be frayed and torn, are relatively clean. It may also be advised for those cases in which shock is absent or, if present, is responding readily to treatment; when sepsis is controllable; and when the accident has occurred early in the postoperative phase and is recognised promptly.

As soon as the condition is recognised, an intramuscular injection of sodium phenobarbital, 180 mg, is given, and the wound and protruding viscera are freely bathed with warm normal saline solution and covered with large sterile towels wrung out in the same solution, over which a many-tailed bandage is lightly applied. Atropine and morphine are given in suitable dosage for preoperative medication, and the patient is told that he must not cough or strain.

When the patient has been moved to the operating room, he is given an intravenous injection of thiopental, followed by gas and oxygen, and one of the curare-like drugs to ensure the maximum relaxation. I dislike using a local or spinal anaesthetic for these cases. A nasogastric tube is passed and the gastric contents are aspirated. The patient is then given a blood transfusion and fluid and electrolyte loss is replaced. After the binder and the dressings have been removed, the surrounding skin and prolapsed viscera are again washed with saline solution. The edges of the abdominal wall are then lifted upward and the prolapsed gut is replaced

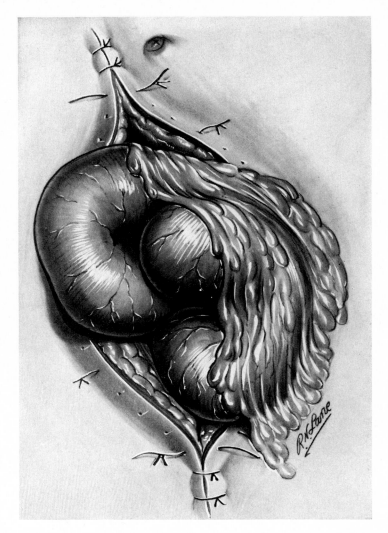

FIG. 3. Wound disruption; prolapse of small intestine and omentum with little evidence of healing in wound margins. (From Maingot, *Management of Abdominal Operations*, 2d ed., 1957. Courtesy of H. K. Lewis & Co., Ltd., London.)

below the level of the peritoneal edges. At this stage, the wound is mopped dry, painted with Cetrimide and Hibitane, disintegrated fragments of catgut or nonabsorbable suture material are extracted, and the edges of the wound are freshened up by clipping away necrotic tissue and oedematous skin tags. It will be noted in many cases that the edges of the wound are very swollen and boggy, and that the peritoneum and posterior sheath of the rectus muscle are glued together and retracted outward, a state of affairs which

immediately suggests that any thought of suturing layer by layer is quite out of the question. Were this attempted, the surgeon would in any case at once realise that the tissues were too friable and cheesy to permit it. If only a very small area of the wound has disrupted, this portion alone should be sutured. If, however, more than half has torn asunder, the correct procedure is to open up the remaining part and suture the whole wound afresh.

Resuture is performed as follows: Hook

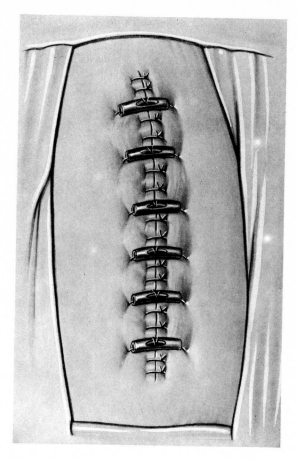

FIG. 4.   Tension sutures tied and held in position and supported by rubber tubing. Note the "eyes" or windows in the tubing with suture-knots in position. (From Maingot, *Management of Abdominal Operations*, 2d ed., 1957. Courtesy of H. K. Lewis & Co., Ltd., London.)

retractors are placed at each extremity of the wound and these are handed to an assistant whose sole duty it is to exert firm upward traction, not only during the introduction of the sutures but until the last through-and-through suture has been tied, at which stage the retractors are removed. The sutures will consist of strong plaited silk, floss silk, strong silkworm gut, nylon, or braided steel wire. They are inserted 1 inch (2.5 cm) from the margin of the wound and about 1 inch (2.5 cm) apart, and are made to transfix *all* the layers of the abdominal wall on both margins of the wound (Figs. 3 and 4). As they are introduced, the free ends are clipped with haemostats. The sutures should be threaded through 2-inch (2.5-cm) rubber tubing and firmly tied. When wire is used, the individual strands are twisted together on one side of the wound until the necessary tension is obtained. They are then clipped fairly short and their spiky ends are blunted by twisting them over. For the reapproximation of the skin edges, interrupted vertical mattress silk sutures are placed between the through-and-through sutures.

Figure-of-eight wire sutures are commonly used for resuturing incisions.

The methods of closure by figure-of-eight sutures are well illustrated in Chapters 1 and 35.

The skin sutures are removed on the eighth postoperative day, the through-and-through sutures being left in until the twelfth or fourteenth day. After the extraction of all the sutures, the wound will require further support by means of a ready-made Abdoplast corset or a Tubi-grip abdominal belt (Seton Products, Ltd.). Active measures should be taken to combat peritonitis, including gastric suction—decompression, intensive antibiotic therapy, parenteral alimentation, etc.

Postoperative ventral hernia. The operative treatment of this complication is discussed in Chapter 71.

REFERENCES

1. Aldrete and Judd, Arch. Surg. 90:745, 1965.
2. Altemeier et al., Arch. Surg. 74:839, 1957.
3. Baffes and Agustsson, Dis. Chest. 49:83, 1966.
4. Beattie, Proc. R. Soc. Med. 39:239, 1946.
5. Behrend and Krouse, J.A.M.A. 149:1122, 1952.
6. Booker and Pack, Cancer 4:1052, 1951.
7. Bourne, Lancet 1:688, 1944.
8. Brewer and Meleney, Ann. Surg. 84:438, 1926.
9. Cattell and Wiedman, Lahey Clin. Bull. 8:2, 1952.
10. Crockett, Br. J. Plast. Surg. 245:17, 1964.
11. Cullen, Surg. Gynecol. Obstet. 38:579, 1924.
12. Cutler and Sandusky, Br. J. Surg. 32:168, 1944.
13. Duff et al., Arch. Surg. 101:314, 1970.
14. Efron, Lancet 1:1287, 1965.
15. Elman, Med. Clin. North Am. 27:303, 1943.
16. Ferrer, Md. State Med. J. 18:57, 1969.
17. Geschickter and Lewis, Am. J. Cancer 25:630, 1935.
18. Given, Khirugiya 23:93, 1970.
19. Guiney et al., Arch. Surg. 92:47, 1966.
20. Herman et al., Surg. Gynecol. Obstet. 120:503, 1965.
21. Howells and Young, Br. J. Surg. 53:436, 1966.
22. Hunt, Br. J. Surg. 28:436, 1941.
23. Jeffrey and Thompson, Br. J. Surg. 32:159, 1944.
24. Joergenson and Smith, Am. J. Surg. 79:282, 1950.
25. King and Salzman, Surg. Clin. North Am. 50:595, 1970.
26. Leading Article, Br. Med. J. 1:447, 1969.
27. Lundh, Acta Chir. Scand. 126:305, 1963.
28. Madden, Personal communication, 1972.
29. Madsen et al., Scand. J. Gastroenterol. 6:237, 1971.
30. McCurrick and Millington, Br. J. Surg. 31:86, 1943.
30a. Illingworth and Dick. Textbook of Surgical Pathology, 10th ed., London, Churchill, 1968.
31. MacLaren, J. R. Coll. Surg. Edinb. 9:61, 1963.
32. McNally and Crile, Surg. Gynecol. Obstet. 118:1046, 1964.
33. McNally, Price, and MacDonald, Am. J. Surg. 116:779, 1968.
34. Meleney, Surgery 18:423, 1945.
35. Mendoza, Postlethwaite, and Johnson, Arch. Surg. 101:396, 1970.
36. Miles et al., Am. Surg. 30:560, 1964.
37. Morgan, Morain, and Eraklis, Ann. Surg. 173:617, 1971.
38. Orr, J.A.M.A. 120:208, 1934.
39. Pack and Ehrlich, Int. Abstr. Surg. 79:177, 1944.
40. Pearman and Mayo, Ann. Surg. 115:114, 1942.
41. Pertl, Minn. Med. 24:338, 1941.
42. Sachs, Surg. Gynecol. Obstet. 80:411, 1945.
43. Sanders, Congress de la Société Internationale de Chirugie, 1963.
44. Spann and McGill, Ann. Surg. 146:98, 1957.
45. Stewart Wallace, Br. J. Surg. 22:642, 1935.
46. Trippel et al., Surg. Clin. North Am. 47:17, 1967.
47. Tweedie and Long, Surg. Gynecol. Obstet. 99:41, 1954.
48. Wallyn et al., Surg. Clin. North Am. 44:107, 1964.
49. Willis, Clostridia of Wound Infection, 1969.
50. Wolff, Ann. Surg. 131:534, 1950.

3

THE SOURCES AND SEQUELAE OF INFECTED ABDOMINAL INCISIONS

R. A. SHOOTER

Twenty years ago staphylococci were generally accepted as the most important organisms in the causation of postoperative wound infection. This may still be true, but an account of wound infection must now in addition pay serious attention to gram-negative bacilli.

The reason for this change is not known. In part it probably represents the increasing ability of surgeons to operate successfully on old or debilitated patients who at one time might have been thought to be beyond operation. It may, too, reflect the success of measures taken to prevent staphylococcal cross-infection and the problem inherent in the treatment of residual infections due to gram-negative organisms, many of which may be resistant to antibiotics.

In part, however, it probably represents a real change in the capacity of staphylococci to cause sepsis. Conclusive evidence in support of this view is difficult to obtain, but there is, of course, no doubt that strains of staphylococci may differ enormously in their capacity to cause infection. For instance up to 70 percent of staphylococci from acute cases of impetigo have been found to belong to phage type 71.[3] In the 1950s staphylococci of phage type 80/81 were notorious causes of infection in many countries. During long-term surveys in surgical wards, strains have been repeatedly isolated from carriers over long periods without any evidence of clinical infection,[33] as compared with other strains that were responsible for sepsis in no less than a third of the patients whose noses were colonised by them.[43]

What we may be seeing now is a relative and probably only a temporary lack of strains of real virulence. In a review of changes of virulence, Williams cites the experience of three hospitals between 1958 and 1968. In all three there was an almost identical drop in the isolation of antibiotic-resistant staphylococci. In one hospital this was attributed to an antibiotic-control policy, and in another to energetic measures to control cross-infection. The third hospital, although carrying out control measures, did not pursue them so rigorously, and it is tempting to conclude that in all three the main factor behind the decline was a change in the nature of the staphylococci themselves.

Many investigations have shown that staphylococcal infection rates for surgical wounds commonly run from 5 to 10 percent, and that these rates may be considerably exceeded from time to time (for a review, see Williams, Blowers, Garrod, and Shooter).[42] Surgical wounds may be infected at the time of operation or subsequently in the ward. It is not always possible to make the distinction, but unless it can be made, investigation of the source of infection becomes more difficult.

STAPHYLOCOCCAL INFECTION

At the Time of Operation

Epidemiological investigations have done nothing to minimise the vital role of the surgeon and his team in preventing sepsis by strict adherence to established surgical practices. Not all practices are of equal value, and in the Report on Aseptic Methods in the Operating Suite [29] they were divided into those for which there was adequate bacteriological and/or clinical evidence, those that needed further evaluation but could be provisionally recommended, those that seemed desirable but could not be evaluated, and those that were traditionally observed but were probably unnecessary and perhaps potentially harmful.

Hand-washing has received much attention, and the conventional scrubbing for 5 to 10 minutes has been shown to be inadequate. A number of methods will give appreciably lower bacterial counts on the skin, and many surgeons advocate the regular use of a short wash or scrub with a hexachlorophene detergent cream or with povidone-iodine. Both preparations have the advantage that, when used repeatedly, their effect becomes cumulative. It is a common finding that up to 30 percent of gloves have tears after operation. These tears may not be discovered by the old-fashioned practice of twirling the gloves around in the air. Testing can be done much more efficiently by blowing up the glove with air and immersing it in water. The use of disposable gloves saves such labour.

Surgical gowns worn by surgeons and nurses protect the patient from direct contamination but do almost nothing to prevent the staphylococcal carriers in the surgical team from shedding staphylococci and other skin organisms to the air. In a well-ventilated operating room, and for most operations, this may not matter. For operations with a high risk of infection, or for operations on patients whose defences are suppressed, consideration should be given to wearing operating suits made of closely woven fabrics that will effectively prevent the dissemination of bacteria. For them to be fully effective, trousers with the legs closed at the ankles must be worn.[5, 6, 7]

A shower bath for members of the surgical team before operation might seem a sensible precaution and has been advocated. Perhaps surprisingly, showers have been shown to *increase* substantially the shedding of skin bacteria into the air for 1 to 1½ hours afterwards; thus showers should be kept for use after operation, or used well before the operation begins.[7, 37]

Surgeons tend to hold strong views about the most suitable preparation for sterilising the patient's skin. Lowbury and his colleagues, who have studied bacteriological aspects of this subject in detail, have found little to choose between single applications of 1 percent iodine, and 0.5 percent chlorhexidine (both of these being dissolved in 70 percent alcohol). Mercurial antiseptics and quaternary ammonium compounds were much less effective.[21]

There remain a number of causes of infection at the time of operation that are perhaps beyond the day-to-day control of the surgeon and deserve separate consideration.

FROM CARRIERS

It can be anticipated that up to half of the surgical and nursing members of the team will carry pathogenic staphylococci in their noses. Fortunately, people who carry staphylococci only in their noses rarely seem to give rise to infection, although there is good evidence that patients have been infected through the unsatisfactory practice of wearing one mask throughout an operating session, lowering it to the neck between cases (Fig. 1).

Hand carriage of staphylococci is another matter. True hand carriage—in which staphylococci grow in the skin of the hand—is rare, but disasters owing to the presence of such carriers in the team have often been recorded.[16, 28, 32] Such people may accumulate pools of sweat in their gloves; this fluid, laden with staphylococci, reaches the patient through tears in the glove. Hand carriage is not appreciably diminished by washing with soap and water, but can be controlled by the regular use of hexachlorophene compounds, and sepsis should be prevented in

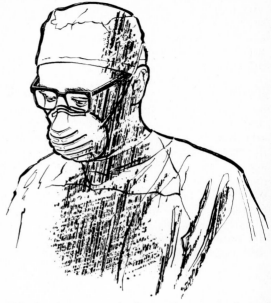

FIG. 1. Aseptex mask. (From Shooter, Smith, and Hunter, *Brit. J. Surg.* 47:246, 1959. Courtesy of 3M Company.)

this way rather than by the employment of uncertain and time-consuming bacteriological searches for staphylococcal carriers.

If sepsis can be caused by a carrier in the operating room, it is not surprising that it may result from the presence of someone with a septic lesion; this possibility has also been well documented.[22, 25, 27] Unless there are very strong overriding reasons, no person with a septic lesion should be present in the operating room.

FROM THE AIR

Bacteria get into the air of the operating room from the patient, from members of the staff, or by being sucked into the room from other parts of the hospital. Suspended in the air they do no harm, but they may settle in the wound or on the much larger sterile field and from there be transferred to the wound. Modern plenum or positive-pressure ventilation greatly reduces this risk (see report of the Medical Research Council's Operating-Theatre Hygiene Sub-Committee [23]). By blowing air under pressure into the operating room, bacteria from the staff and the patient are diluted and blown out, and as air movements through doorways should always be outwards, there should be no opportunity for bacteria from other parts of the hospital to be carried by air into the operating room.

Ventilation, as well as playing a part in preventing infection, is also needed to remove anaesthetic gases, to control humidity, and to provide comfortable and safe conditions for both the staff and the patient. There is some dispute about the way to satisfy the last two requirements, but there is considerable experience that supports the most effective way of providing ventilation to prevent infection. Ventilation rates for operating rooms used to be expressed as air changes per hour, and a figure of 17 changes per hour or more was often quoted as that quantity necessary to give adequate dilution of air in the operating room and a sufficient pressure gradient at its doors. This terminology is being abandoned because the elimination of bacteria in the air depends on the absolute volume of air delivered to the room. It is now usual to specify a delivery of 1,000 to 1,500 cubic feet of air per minute. The filtered air may enter through grilles at high level, producing a turbulent system of air movement, or it may be introduced through symmetrically placed diffusers in the ceiling —with the object of producing a downward displacement of air over the whole area of the room. Although the matter was at one time the subject of controversy, it is now agreed that so long as there is adequate air entry there is nothing to choose between the two systems.

Positive-pressure ventilation has meant extra work for the hospital engineer because the plant must be maintained quite thoroughly and regularly. It is essential that its performance be checked on installation and thereafter at stated intervals.[42] The direction of air flow between various parts of the operating room and movements of air through the doors of the room can be observed by using smoke clouds generated by titanium tetrachloride. This simple procedure should be carried out regularly. Determination of the rate of air flow is usually the task of the ventilation engineer.

Recently there has been interest in the laminar flow techniques that have been developed in industry to provide dust-free air in factories assembling delicate equipment. In this form of ventilation, large volumes of air are used and it may be blown in from all the ceiling or the whole of one wall of a room.[39]

There is little doubt that laminar flow ventilation can produce lower particle and bacterial counts than does conventional positive-pressure ventilation.[14] So far, however, there is no clinical evidence that it will produce lower rates of wound infection.

It is worth remembering that in a well-run and properly ventilated operating room, the rate of staphylococcal sepsis caused by organisms acquired at operation should not normally exceed 1 percent; this figure should be borne in mind when considering some of the more elaborate precautions that have been suggested for the prevention of infection. At this level, additional precautions will not prevent infection in more than one patient in a hundred, and may in fact prevent many fewer.

In the Ward

Patients who return from their operation with the edges of the wound in close and regular contact are unlikely to acquire infection during their subsequent stay in the ward. On the other hand, patients whose wounds are poorly closed or are being drained may suffer a higher incidence of sepsis, although this may not be so true for small-bore suction drains. Considerable time has been spent in trying to trace the source of the infecting staphylococci. Infection may occur from the air while the dressing is being done, but except for burns and perhaps in the case of very large wounds this does not seem to be a common occurrence. Some wounds become infected as a result of poor technique in the course of applying the dressing, staphylococci being transferred to the patient from the dresser.

Recent papers show that an appreciable proportion of ward infections may be caused by organisms carried by the patient himself. Some of these staphylococci may be carried in the nose or on the skin of the patient when he is admitted to hospital. Others may come from other patients in the ward, or, uncommonly, from members of the staff. The acquisition may be the result of physical contact, but is probably more often the outcome of airborne staphylococci being inhaled or settling on the patient's skin or bedding.

Once acquired by the patient, either in the nose or on the skin, staphylococci presumably reach the wound by direct contact or by spreading along the skin to the wound —aided by gravity or movements of clothes or bedding. However the wound is reached, surveys have shown that patients who carry staphylococci during their stay in hospital may be more likely to develop wound sepsis than those who do not.[11, 43] In a few surveys this has been shown not to be the case, and this serves to illustrate the point that sepsis may originate in a variety of ways, not all of which will be working at one time. If most of the infection is occurring at the time of operation, sepsis acquired in the ward will be less evident.

Parker et al.[26] reported that when patients were nursed in single rooms there was very little transfer of staphylococci, and there have been subsequent reports that by nursing patients in wards consisting of a number of small rooms, the spread of staphylococci could be cut down to a degree that significantly reduced the sepsis rate.[17, 20, 40]

For a variety of reasons, hospitals are no longer being designed with large open Nightingale-type wards. The smaller units now being built appear to give greater protection from infection.

INFECTIONS CAUSED BY FAILURE OF STERILISATION

In many papers attention has been drawn to the unsatisfactory methods that have been used to produce sterile instruments and dressings, and recommendations have been made for their improvement.[8, 18, 24] While there may be some doubt as to how often failure to achieve complete sterility causes infections with nonsporing organisms such as the staphylococcus, the ubiquity of the spores responsible for tetanus and gas gangrene makes it absolutely essential that instruments and dressings used for the treatment of patients should be sterile beyond question.

For use in hospital, steam under pressure

in the autoclave remains the best agent for sterilising instruments and dressings. There have been many changes in the design of autoclaves, and for descriptions of these and for a general discussion of steam sterilisation reference can be made to the M.R.C. Reports already cited or to Williams et al.[42]

It is unlikely that plants that sterilise by ionising radiation will become established in hospitals because of the size and cost of such units. It is, however, probable that they will become the usual means by which commercially produced articles are sterilised. Many of these articles are designed to be used once and disposed of, and often, as they are made of plastic, they may be unsuitable for heat sterilisation.

The use of ethylene oxide gas provides another method of sterilising heat-sensitive materials. It may be used commercially or on a small scale in the hospital. With proper safeguards, ethylene oxide will kill sporing and nonsporing bacteria, but it needs constant and detailed supervision, as cleanliness and control of humidity in the process are vital.[19]

Sterilisation by steam at subatmospheric pressure entails holding steam in an autoclave at subatmospheric pressure and at a temperature between 80° and 90°C. When formalin is added, both vegetative bacteria and spores are killed. The method has still to be fully developed, but it shows signs of being the most convenient way of sterilising the increasing number of delicate pieces of equipment used by the surgeon.[1]

Finally, mention should be made of the role of central sterile supply in preventing infection.[2] This system ensures that the hospital's sterilisation is carried out reliably at a place where the machinery is regularly maintained and the process supervised by trained staff. It also frees time previously used in the ward in the preparation of sterile instruments and dressings, allowing the nurse to devote more attention to the proper performance of aseptic procedures.

Theatre instruments may be sterilised in a central sterile supply department (C.S.S.D.), but a more usual development is to attach a Theatre Sterile Supply Unit to each suite of operating rooms. In such a unit it may be decided to make use of the Edinburgh preset tray system, in which a trolley top is laid out before sterilisation with all the instruments, drapes, dressings, etc., required for one operation.[9, 36]

It hardly needs to be said that the value of a central sterile supply department will be largely wasted if steps are not taken to see that its products are used in an aseptic way. The introduction of such a system provides a golden opportunity to reexamine and recast the aseptic techniques on which prevention of infection is so dependent.

INFECTIONS CAUSED BY GRAM-NEGATIVE BACTERIA

In recent years infection by gram-negative bacilli such as *Pseudomonas, Proteus,* and *Escherichia coli* has become of real concern to the surgeon. Why gram-negative organisms have become more prominent is not clear; we do not know if it is because of the increasing age of patients coming into hospital, the different diseases for which they are admitted, or the treatment they receive when they are there.

Some wound infections can be traced to soiling of the wound with bowel contents during the course of the operation, suggesting the need for greater care in handling the tissues and more attention to such things as towelling technique. Some gram-negative bacilli, and *Pseudomonas aeruginosa* in particular, are relatively resistant to many disinfectants, and there are now numerous records of infection arising from disinfectant solutions or medicaments used in the treatment of patients.[4, 35] In addition, the increasing use of respirators for patients has added an additional hazard, as these pieces of apparatus readily become infected and are difficult to clean and disinfect.

Prevention of the infections described so far lies in greater attention to aseptic techniques and in rigorous control of lotions and other articles used in the treatment of patients

The use of typing methods for gram-negative bacilli has opened up new and interesting fields. Epidemiological studies have suggested that as well as spreading in the ways that have been mentioned, infections with *P. aeruginosa* may be autogenous in

that they are caused by the organisms in the patient's own bowel.[15, 34] About 5 percent of normal people carry *P. aeruginosa* in their bowels, but the rate for hospital patients may rise as high as 40 percent. Why this should be is not clear, but one way in which the increase can occur is by contamination of food and medicines with the organism.[30] The elimination of infections with *P. aeruginosa* by better hygiene and the prevention of intestinal carriage is not an impossible target at which to aim.

Similar studies with *E. coli* have shown that hospital food may contain these organisms in large numbers and that strains swallowed in the food may become established in the gut.[10, 13, 31] Until more is known about the differences in pathogenicity between strains of *E. coli,* it is difficult to assess the significance of this finding. It is, however, a matter of concern that strains of *E. coli* in food are apparently derived from animals and poultry and may carry resistance transfer factors against antibiotics as a result of feeding antibiotics to livestock.[13, 38]

REFERENCES

1. Alder, V. G., Brown, A. M., and Gillespie, W. A., J. Clin. Pathol. 19:83, 1966
2. Allen, S. M., et al., Lancet 2:1343, 1965.
3. Anderson, E. S., and Williams, R. E. O., J. Clin. Pathol. 9:94, 1956.
4. Bassett, D. J. C., Proc. Roy. Soc. Med. 64:980, 1971.
5. Bernard, H. R., Speers, R., O'Grady, F. W., and Shooter, R. A., Lancet 2:458, 1965.
6. Bernard, H. R., Speers, R., O'Grady, F. W., and Shooter, R. A., Arch. Surg. 91:530, 1965.
7. Bethune, D. W., Blowers, R., Parker, M., and Pask, E. A., Lancet 1:480, 1965.
8. Bowie, J. H., Pharmacol. J. 174:473, 489, 1955.
9. Bowie, J. H., Gillingham, F. J., Campbell, I. D., and Gordon, A. R., Lancet 2:1322, 1963.
10. Buck, A. C., and Cooke, E. M., J. Med. Microbiol. 2:521, 1969.
11. Colbeck, J. C., Robertson, H. R., Sutherland, W. H., and Hartley, F. C., Med. Serv. J. Canada 15:326, 1959.
12. Cooke, E. M., Breaden, A. L., Shooter, R. A., and O'Farrell, S. M., Lancet 1:8, 1971.
13. Cooke, E. M., Shooter, R. A., Kumar, P. J., Rousseau, S. A., and Foulkes, A. L., Lancet 1:436, 1970.
14. Coriell, L. L., in Proceedings of the International Conference on Nosocomial Infections. American Hospital Association, 1971.
15. Darrell, J. H., and Wahba, A. H., J. Clin. Pathol. 17:236, 1964.

16. Devenish, R. A., and Miles, A. A., Lancet 1:1088, 1939.
17. Edmunds, P. N., J. Hyg. (Camb.) 68:531, 1970.
18. Howie, J. W., and Timbury, M. C., Lancet 2:699, 1956.
19. Kelsey, J. C. J., J. Clin. Pathol. 14:59, 1961.
20. Lidwell, O. M., Polakoff, S., Jevons, M. P., Parker, M. T., Shooter, R. A., French, V. I., and Dunkerley, D. R., J. Hyg. (Camb.) 64:321, 1966.
21. Lowbury, E. J. L., Lilly, H. A., and Bull, J. P., Brit. Med. J. 2:531, 1964.
22. McDonald, S., and Timbury, M. C., Lancet 2:863, 1957.
23. Medical Research Council Operating-Theatre Hygiene Sub-Committee, Lancet 2:945, 1962.
24. Medical Research Council Reports, Lancet 1:425, 1959; 2:1243, 1960; and 2:193, 1964.
25. Mitchell, A. A. B., Timbury, M. C., Pettigrew, J. B., and Hutchinson, J. G. P., Lancet 2:503, 1959.
26. Parker, M. T., John, M., Edmond, R. T. D., and Machacek, K. A., Br. Med. J. 1:1101, 1965.
27. Payne, R. W., Br. Med. J. 2:17, 1967.
28. Penikett, E. J. K., Knox, R., and Liddell, J., Br. Med. J. 1:812, 1958.
29. Report to the Medical Research Council on Aseptic Methods in the Operating Suite, Lancet 1:706, 763, 831; 1968.
30. Shooter, R. A., Cooke, E. M., Gaya, H., Kumar, P., Patel, N., Parker, M. T., Thom, B. T., and France, D. R., Lancet 1:1227, 1969.
31. Shooter, R. A., Cooke, E. M., Rousseau, S. A., and Breaden, A. L., Lancet 2:226, 1970.
32. Shooter, R. A., Griffiths, J. D., Cooke, J., and Williams, R. E. O., Br. Med. J. 1:433, 1957.
33. Shooter, R. A., Smith, M. A., Griffiths, J. D., Brown, M. E. A., Williams, R. E. O., Rippon, J. E., and Jevons, M. P., Br. Med. J. 1:607, 1958.
34. Shooter, R. A., Walker, K. A., Williams, V. R., Horgan, G. M., Parker, M. T., Asheshov, E. H., and Bullimore, J. F., Lancet 2:1331, 1966.
35. Shooter, R. A., in 3d Symposium on Advanced Medicine. A. M. Dawson, ed., London, Pitman, 1967.
36. South Eastern Regional Hospital Board, Scotland: Report of Theatre Service Centre Committee, 1965.
37. Speers, R., Bernard, H. R., O'Grady, F. W., and Shooter, R. A., Lancet 1:478, 1965.
38. Walton, J. R., Lancet 2:501, 1970.
39. Whyte, W., Shaw, B. H., and Barnes, R., Lancet 2:905, 1971.
40. Williams, R. E. O., Bacteriol. Rev. 30:660, 1966.
41. Williams, R. E. O., in Bacterial Infections. *Bayer Symposium III,* Springer-Verlag, Berlin, 1971.
42. Williams, R. E. O., Blowers, R., Garrod, L. P., and Shooter, R. A., Hospital Infection: Causes and Prevention. London, Lloyd Luke, 1966.
43. Williams, R. E. O., Jevons, M. P., Shooter, R. A., Hunter, C. J., Girling, J. A., Griffiths, J. D., and Taylor, G. W., Br. Med. J. 2:658, 1959.

SECTION TWO # Stomach and Duodenum

4
ENDOSCOPY
A. Fibre-Optic Endoscopy

BASIL I. HIRSCHOWITZ

Endoscopy of the upper digestive tract serves not only as a means of resolving or amplifying diagnoses made by indirect means, such as physical examination or radiology, but also as a primary diagnostic procedure for conditions not otherwise diagnosable in the intact patient. As such, its advantages and limitations should be familiar to any surgeon concerned with abdominal surgery who wishes to avoid needless surgery and who would like to have a more precise diagnosis in planning necessary surgery.

INSTRUMENTS

In one form or another, endoscopy of the esophagus and stomach has been practised since 1880. Until recently the instruments used have depended on vision through straight tubes for the oesophagus or on a system of lenses for the gastroscope, limiting the instrument to a virtually straight rod. Because the upper digestive tube is not straight, the passage of those instruments required great skill and subjected the patients to much discomfort and risk of injury. With the invention of the *fibre-optic gastroscope* in 1957,[1, 2] and the rapid evolution of fibrescopes since then,[3] intubation and endoscopy of the oesophagus, stomach, and duodenum has become easy, and the risk of injury less. Because of this, endoscopy of the upper digestive tract is now very widely practised, and its value has been extended by making it possible to obtain biopsy specimens and cytology samples under direct vision. The only indication for use of the rigid *oesophagoscope* is in the removal of large foreign bodies from the oesophagus. Otherwise fibre-optic instruments have completely replaced both the rigid oesophagoscope and the *lens-optic gastroscopes.*

The fibre-optic bundle. The image-transmitting element of the fibrescopes [4] is a bundle of 200,000 or more glass-coated glass fibres, each about 1/1000 inch in diameter, each going from end to end and so arranged that the spatial orientation of the fibres at each end of the bundle is the same. The fibres are permanently bonded to each other at the ends, but are free in between, so that the bundle is completely flexible. There is no distortion of the transmitted image by any degree of bending or flexion between the fixed ends. Each fibre transmits a minute part of the image as a separate spot of light and contains it within the glass core of the fibre by a process known as *total internal reflectance*. The image, or picture, at the other end, is made up of these individual spots of light, so that the quality of the picture depends on the exactness of the orientation of the fibres to each other. Compared with a multiple-lens system of equivalent length, fibre bundles transmit more than 20 times the light. Fibre bundles are also being used to transmit large amounts of light from external high-intensity light sources to supply brilliant, cold illumination, and they have replaced the distally placed incandescent lamp in all types of endoscopes.

The fibrescopes. There has been a profusion of instruments in the last few years, with a strong tendency towards multipurpose instruments.* These instruments are of essentially similar basic design, all using fibre-bundles of 1.5- to 3-mm diameter for illumination, and 2- to 5-mm optical bundles

---

* *The three major manufacturers are American Cystoscope Makers, Inc.; Olympus; and Machida.*

for image transmission. At the distal end, the image is focused on the optical-image fibre bundle by a lens system that has a fixed-focus arrangement in some instruments and a variable, externally controlled focussing system in others. There are essentially two types of instruments distinguished by whether the distal lens looks straight ahead (oesophagoscopes, and oesophago-duodeno-scopes), or sideways (gastroscopes, gastro-duodenoscopes). In all the latest instruments, the distal 7- to 15-cm segment is more flexible than the rest of the instrument and the curvature of that segment controllable in one plane or in all directions from the external end by a single or a pair of controls. The degree of flexion from the longitudinal axis varies from 80 degrees to 170 degrees, the latter forming a J or U configuration.

The diameter of the instruments is from 7 to 12 mm. The instruments may also be distinguished by their working length, varying from 65 cm to 105 cm. The shorter, forward-viewing instrument is useful only for the oesophagus. The 75- to 90-cm side-viewing instruments are essentially gastroscopes and are the best instruments for complete examination of the stomach. The 105-cm instruments are of two types. The end-viewing instrument is being used for examining the oesophagus, stomach, and duodenum. It has a fairly small field and thus does not always provide a thorough view of the whole stomach. The side-viewing instruments of similar length are of use only in the stomach and duodenum. They are the only instruments that allow intubation of the ampulla of Vater, and in certain cases they provide better visualization of the duodenal bulb. The proximal end of the instruments has a lens for enlarging the image from the proximal end of the image bundle, the connections for air and water, the controls for image focussing and control of the distal flexible tip.

Biopsy and cytology. All the instruments incorporate an open channel for air or water to distend the organ and to wash the lens; the same channel can be used for aspiration in most instruments, and in some it is also used as a biopsy channel. The more satisfactory arrangement with the forward-viewing instruments is that in which one channel is used only for insufflation of air or water to wash the lens and a second open channel is provided for aspiration, for biopsy forceps or cytology brushes, for introduction of fluid to wash the mucosa, or for cytological sampling. Biopsy capacity has broadened the scope of the fibrescopes and though small in size (5 to 7 French), they are usually adequate. Some instruments have additional distal controls to make the siting of biopsy specimens more precise. In all cases however, biopsy or jet washing for cytological sampling is under direct vision.

Photography. Light transmission through the optical bundles of the length used is high enough for adequate photography, especially with the ability to introduce much more light using fibre bundles. With optical resolution of the bundles in the range of 40 lines per millimeter, still or moving pictures in color can be taken at normal speeds with standard camera equipment requiring only a built-in light meter for proper exposure and a simple clamp to attach the camera to the eyepiece of the fibrescope. By the same token, there is enough light for television photography in black and white or in color.[4]

By a marriage of the fibrescope and the gastrocamera, some instruments take direct photographs in the stomach under endoscopic visual control. These instruments have a much longer rigid portion and are limited to the stomach.[3]

Teaching fiberscope. This separate device, which can be removably attached to the eyepiece of the instrument being used for normal endoscopy, consists essentially of an image-splitting prism and a 1-meter fibre-optic bundle. Use of this device allows the examiner to make a normal examination and it also allows the student to see the field at the same time.

PROCEDURE

Preparation of the Patient

Most persons gag or retch while swalling tubes, especially when anxious, so that premedication should be used routinely. The patient should have the procedure explained to him and be told why it is to be done. Since the stomach should be as empty as possible, the patient should fast from 8 to 12 hours. It is seldom necessary to empty the stomach by Ewald tube before endoscopy, as most of the normal fasting gastric contents can be aspirated through the fibrescope during examination. Both barium sulfate and aluminum gel antacids cling to the surface of the stomach in patches, making it difficult to exclude discrete lesions such as ulcers. Thus these antacids should not be given within 10 hours of examination and barium within 18 to 24 hours of endoscopy.

The patient should generally be sedated, though cautiously if he has been bleeding and is hypotensive. Meperidine, 50 to 100 mg I.M. or 25 to 50 mg I.V., and diazepam (Valium), 5 to 10 mg I.M., are the drugs most commonly used today, either alone or in combination. A surface-active anesthetic is applied to the throat either by gargling or by a spray-nebulizer. We have used 0.5 percent dyclonine hydrochloride (Dyclone) for almost 5,000 examinations without a single reaction. The amount used by spray is very little; onset of anaesthesia is within 30 seconds and lasts about 1 hour—all advantageous for endoscopy.

Passing the Fibrescope

With this preparation the fibrescope may be passed with the patient sitting and the neck slightly flexed, or he may be lying either supine or on the left side. The instrument is guided over the back of the tongue by the left index finger and the patient asked to swallow. When the tip is in the oesophagus, it is steadily pushed into the stomach. If there is undue resistance, pain, difficulty in breathing, coughing, or marked patient agitation during the initial part of the intubation, the instrument should be withdrawn and a fresh start made. (See Fig. 1.)

For oesophagoscopy, the instrument is passed into the stomach, if there is no obstruction, and gradually withdrawn while the oesophagus is being distended with air. The lumen is kept in constant view by control of the distal end. The major landmarks are the diaphragm, which can be identified by a sharp movement caused by sniffing; the squamocolumnar oesophagogastric mucosal junction; and the lower oesophageal

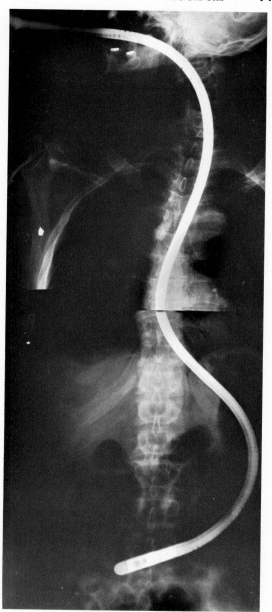

FIG. 1. Composite x-ray of patient with fibrescope in place, showing instrument's curvature in one plane. Upper and lower halves were taken separately at same examination.

sphincter. The major oesophageal lesions amenable to endoscopic diagnosis are tumors, oesophagitis, and ulcer, all of which can be confirmed by biopsy specimen; stenosis and achalasia; diverticula; hiatal hernia; and varices.

In gastroscopy, the major landmark is the angulus. With the newer instruments, in which the distal end is both very flexible and controllable, it is essential to develop a routine for the systematic examination of the entire surface of the mucosa, including a view of the fundus obtained by retroflexion of the instrument into the U or J shape. If the stomach is being examined with the duodenoscope, the small field of view makes it even more imperative to be systematic. Passing this instrument into the duodenum is easily accomplished under direct vision. Because the diameter of the duodenum is relatively small, it is difficult to obtain much perspective in the first part, and thus difficult to be certain about the absence of a lesion. The valuable technique of cannulation of the ampulla is dealt with in a later section.

INDICATIONS FOR ENDOSCOPY

Since intubation with the flexible fibre-optic instruments is not subject to such contraindications as a short fixed neck, small mouth, obesity, or kyphosis, the indications for endoscopy are based on the ability of the endoscopy to make or clarify a diagnosis. The only definite contraindications are a totally uncooperative patient (where necessary, general anaesthesia may be used), recent ulcer perforation, and the acute phase after corrosive ingestion.

Except in emergency situations, such as bleeding, it is always preferable to x-ray the oesophagus, stomach, and duodenum first. Radiography serves to focus attention on particular lesions or areas, and it also may give warning of potentially troublesome anatomical problems such as oesophageal diverticulum or obstruction, para-oesophageal hernia, and any unusual configuration of the stomach. Though this may sound like a counsel of perfection, any lesion of the upper gastrointestinal tract shown by x-ray should be directly visualized by endoscopy, and, if indicated, further clarified by a biopsy specimen or cytological sample. Furthermore, symptoms such as dysphagia, x-ray negative dyspepsia, persistent vomiting, upper gastrointestinal bleeding, and any symptoms after

gastric surgery provide clear indication for endoscopy. Gastroscopy is recommended as a screening procedure in patients with high risk of gastric cancer, such as pernicious anemia; in the follow-up to healing of gastric ulcer; and late after gastric surgery to determine the state of the gastric mucosa.

RISKS OF ENDOSCOPY

The major risk of intubation is perforation of the oesophagus, which may occur in the neck or at the site of stricture; severe oesophagitis; or diverticulum. This occurs about once every thousand examinations and carries a mortality rate of about 20 to 25 percent. An oesophageal varix may be torn, especially if suction is applied, though in the vast majority varices are not greatly at risk from endoscopy. Inhalation of regurgitated gastric contents may occur if too much surface anaesthetic has been used, if the patient has been oversedated, if inadequate suction is applied to keep the mouth clear, and especially if the patient is vomiting large amounts of blood. This can cause troublesome pneumonia, particularly if blood has been inhaled.

SPECIFIC APPLICATIONS OF FIBRE-OPTIC ENDOSCOPY

Upper gastrointestinal bleeding. Any patient who presents with acute gastrointestinal bleeding is a potential candidate for emergency operation. Should surgical intervention be necessary, it is self-evident that foreknowledge of the lesion to be dealt with offers the surgeon, and consequently the patient, a considerable advantage. The commonest lesions responsible for significant bleeding are chronic or acute gastric or duodenal ulcers, while other lesions such as oesophageal or gastric varices, tears at the cardio-oesophageal junction (Mallory-Weiss syndrome), benign or malignant tumors, and diffuse hemorrhagic gastritis together are responsible for about 15 to 20 percent of cases, thus forming a significant fraction of the differential diagnoses.

The value of endoscopy rests principally

upon its ability to localize the source and nature of bleeding early in the course and thus to determine in part subsequent treatment. As soon as resuscitative measures have been instituted—securing an intravenous line for infusion and measurement of central venous pressure, blood sampling for typing and cross-matching and for blood count and chemistry, and institution of intake-output measurement—the stomach is gently aspirated with an Ewald tube to free it of as much of its bloody contents as possible. With appropriate sedation, the fibrescope is passed without moving the patient. It is unusual not to obtain an adequate endoscopic view except in instances of massive bleeding.

Since the endoscopist has only the history to guide his examination, he should systematically examine as much of the oesophagus, stomach, and duodenum as possible.

It is thus a matter of choice which instrument to use. In most cases, it is preferable to start with a long forward-viewing fibrescope (e.g., ACMI panendoscope), with which it is possible to make a comprehensive examination of the oesophagus, antrum, and duodenum. Because of the direction of view and the relatively small field, the body and fundus of the stomach are less certainly fully examined, and if the diagnosis is not clearly established by this instrument, a gastroscope, i.e., a lateral-viewing fibrescope, is then used. A minimal amount of air should be used as massive air distention of the intestine may make closure of the abdomen in subsequent operation more difficult. The first objective is to determine how much, if any, blood is in the stomach and then to attempt to localise the anatomical site of origin of any fresh blood. Bleeding at the cardia is most often caused by varices (which should be suspected from the prior history and physical examination) or by a Mallory-Weiss tear, which can usually be positively diagnosed by endoscopy but rarely by x-ray study. In fact, many cases of haematemesis after heavy drinking are due to this lesion rather than to so-called alcoholic gastritis. The Mallory-Weiss lesion may also occur in other instances when vomiting has preceded bleeding.

In the body of the stomach, diffuse mucosal bleeding can be readily appreciated and, although an infrequent cause of massive bleeding, it occurs in uremia, in blood

dyscrasias, and occasionally with no antecedent cause. The commonest source of bleeding in the stomach are chronic and acute ulcers (i.e., acute gastric erosions), the latter accounting for almost 30 percent of all cases of upper gastrointestinal bleeding, including patients with coexisting chronic ulcers in the stomach or duodenum. In the greatest majority of cases, bleeding from acute ulceration is self-limiting.

Gastric tube suction may produce lesions of the mucosa often indistinguishable from acute ulcers or erosions. They are usually multiple, however, occurring in rows of three or four, and on careful inspection are seen to be small hematomas. Twenty-four to 48 hours later, however, they may slough, leaving small ulcers. It is highly desirable therefore to examine the stomach before vigorous suction is applied.

Tumours of the stomach that may bleed include leiomyoma or leiomyosarcoma and carcinoma, both of which can be readily distinguished from other lesions by endoscopic examination. Together they account for between 2 and 3 percent of massive haematemesis.

Duodenal ulcers account for about 30 to 50 percent of massive upper gastrointestinal bleeding. With the new fibrescopes, it is now possible to examine the duodenum much more easily and comprehensively than before. Even if the duodenum can not be entered, the sight of fresh blood returning through the pylorus is usually a sufficient indication of duodenal ulcer. The mere presence of a duodenal ulcer or deformity on x-ray does not automatically implicate duodenal ulcer as a source of bleeding—30 percent of our bleeding patients who had duodenal deformity on x-ray were found to be bleeding from other lesions, especially acute erosions in the stomach.[5] It is thus important to make a positive diagnosis of the site of bleeding by direct inspection.

If surgical intervention is not immediately necessary and the patient can be moved safely, *x-ray examination* of the upper tract should logically follow endoscopy. In many cases, however, the site and source of bleeding are so clearly identified by endoscopy that x-ray can be delayed until the acute problem has subsided.

Although chronic persistent occult bleeding from the gastrointestinal tract is generally caused by the presence of a malignant lesion, especially of the colon (now also amenable to fibre-optic endoscopy), the stomach occasionally is the seat of the responsible lesion. These lesions include leiomyoma, carcinoma, and vascular anomalies such as hereditary telangiectasia and hemangioma and unsuspected aspirin-induced erosive gastritis. The postgastrectomy stomach is also quite commonly responsible for persistent or repetitive occult bleeding. In our experience hiatal hernia is not a source of such bleeding. The finding of a number of stools containing blood should ultimately be an indication for gastroscopy if other sites, especially the colon, have been exonerated.

Cancer and ulcers. Although the diagnosis of gastric cancer is generally quite clear-cut from x-ray findings, especially since most tumors present as a mass rather than as a crater, it is always possible that any ulcer crater, regardless of size, may actually represent a cancer. Consequently, gastroscopy is essential in the differential diagnosis of every gastric ulcer shown by x-ray. It is only rarely that the diagnosis still remains in doubt after adequate gastroscopy and the examination of a biopsy specimen. Furthermore, gastroscopy tells whether the ulcer is healing or not, whether it is bleeding, and how it distorts the contraction pattern or the pyloric orifice. Associated abnormalities such as the state of the mucosa, the evidence for duodenal ulcer disease, acute ulceration, and the like, can also be determined by gastroscopy.

Healing of gastric ulcer should also be followed gastroscopically, at least after the last apparently normal x-ray, since the ulcer may be present for as long as from 6 to 8 weeks after it no longer shows on x-ray, and it may be present even longer after the disappearance of symptoms. In gastric cancer, gastroscopy not only identifies the principal lesion but defines it and detects the presence of mucosal seeding at a distance, indicating local metastases. Other tumours, such as adenomatous polyps, leiomyomas, lymphomas, and ectopic pancreas, generally have a characteristic appearance.

Deformity of the antrum presents a special diagnostic problem. It is usually first recognized by x-ray in a patient with chronic peptic ulcer disease, and it often raises the possibility of malignancy. By endoscopy it is usually possible to resolve the problem, but if the issue is still in doubt after both endoscopic and cytological examinations, operation should be considered.

Diffuse mucosal lesions. For the most part, diffuse superficial lesions of the gastric or duodenal mucosa are not detectable by x-ray. The most important of these lesions are gastric mucosal atrophy of varying degree up to the total atrophy of pernicious anemia and vascular anomalies such as telangiectasia and hemorrhagic gastritis.

Duodenal ulcer. Endoscopy of the duodenum has been made routine by the addition of about 25 cm to the length of the fibrescope used for oesophagus or stomach, and it has been made more reliable by the controllable tip movement. In endoscopy there is no clear superiority of forward-viewing instruments, which are used by most, over lateral-viewing instruments, though most find it easier to penetrate the pylorus with the former. The ulcers located in the duodenal cap fornix, however, are especially difficult to see with the forward-viewing instrument.[6]

In addition to visualizing the duodenal ulcer itself, endoscopy also reveals associated lesions such as edema, deformity or stenosis of the pylorus, antral gastritis or ulceration, hyperplastic gastric mucosa, hiatal hernia, and oesophagitis. These all help in formulating management of the patient with duodenal ulcer.

THE POSTGASTRECTOMY STOMACH

It is in the patient who has undergone gastric surgery that endoscopy provides information not obtainable by any other means.[7] In a period of 10 years, we have examined over 600 patients complaining of one or more of the following symptoms: pain, dyspepsia, bleeding and anemia, dumping, weight loss, and diarrhea. Most had undergone surgery for duodenal ulcer, and about one-third of these for bleeding. All types of surgery in vogue over the past 30 years were represented in this group, and no particular symptom or abnormality occurred

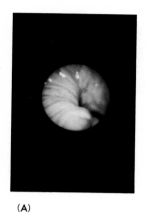

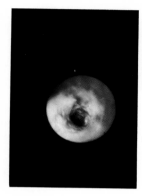

(A)

(B)

Endoscopic photographs.
(A) Hiatal hernia showing normal gastric mucosa "gathered" at the level of the diaphragm.
(B) Severe oesophagitis with stricture in a 27-year-old man with long-standing hiatal hernia with reflux.

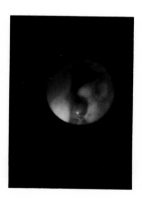

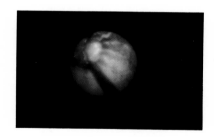

(C)

(D)

(C) Granulating Mallory-Weiss tear of the lower oesophagus approximately 1 week after acute episode.
(D) Retroflexed gastroscopic view of the fundus showing a tumour next to the shaft of the gastroscope as it emerges from the oesophagus.

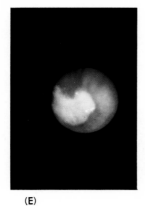

(E)

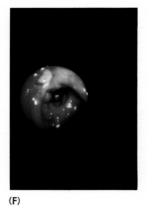

(F)

(E) Gastroscopic picture of a benign gastric ulcer.
(F) Chronic duodenal ulcer somewhat above the ampulla.

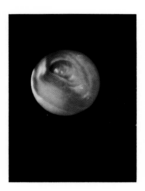

(G)

(G) Descending duodenum with the ampulla on the top left perimeter.

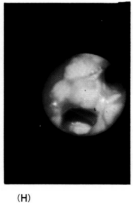

(H)

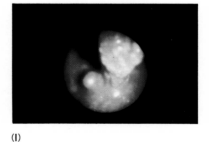

(I)

(H) Double-barrel Billroth II stoma showing afferent and efferent loop orifices separated by a bridge of jejunal mucosa, superficially ulcerated.
(I) Gastric adenomatous polyps developing 2 years after partial gastrectomy for gastric ulcer in a 34-year-old man.

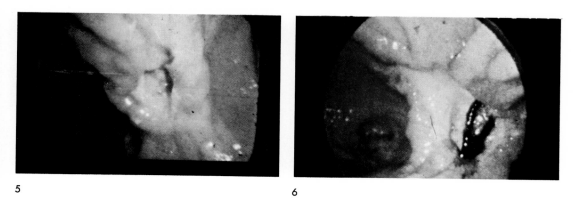

5

6

FIG. 5. Ulcerating carcinoma of angulus. Note broadening and infiltration of angulus round the ulcer.

FIG. 6. Ulcerating carcinoma of lesser curve. Fresh blood clot is seen in the base of the crater.

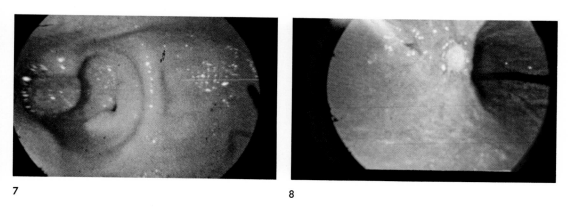

7

8

FIG. 7. Benign antral polyp. Clinical presentation with unexplained anaemia.

FIG. 8. Benign lesser curve ulcer. Clinical suspicion of malignancy.

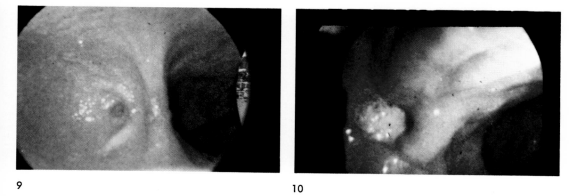

9

10

FIG. 9. The same ulcer after 3 weeks of medical treatment. The ulcer is virtually healed.

FIG. 10. A deep lesser-curve benign ulcer. Note surrounding oedema which at x-ray was sufficient to arouse suspicion of a filling defect.

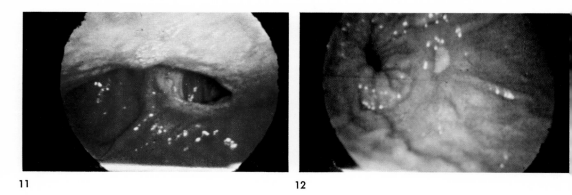

11   12

FIG. 11. Gastroenterostomy. A small superficial marginal ulcer is seen on the bridge between the two loops.

   FIG. 12. Benign antral ulcer in an active phase. Note surrounding oedema.

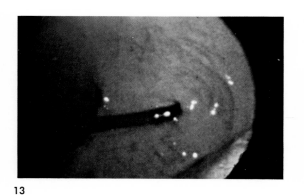

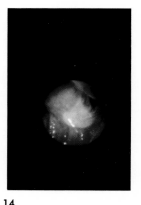

13

                 14

FIG. 13. The "reverse loop" (Olympus G.T.V Camera). The shaft of the instrument emerges from a normal cardia.

   FIG. 14. Large anastomotic ulcer. (A.C.M.I. fibrescope.)

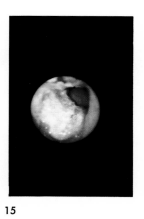

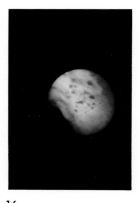

15   16

FIG. 15. Lymphadenoma of stomach. A flat ulcerated plaque not typical of carcinoma. Histological confirmation. (A.C.M.I. fibrescope.)

FIG. 16. Multiple haemorrhagic erosions. Emergency gastroscopy for unexplained melaena. (A.C.M.I. fibrescope).

predominantly with any one operation.

The lesions diagnosable by endoscopy * can be conveniently grouped under anatomical headings as follows:

The gastric stump. *Gastritis* of moderate to marked degree is present in about two-thirds of patients after gastric resection. No consistent symptom complex can be ascribed to this gastritis, although some have pain after eating and some bleed from hemorrhagic gastritis. In addition, about 20 percent have atrophic gastric mucosa, in some cases advanced enough to have lost intrinsic factor secretion and in all cases indicating the need for vitamin B_{12} therapy. Atrophy may be the end-stage of gastritis. In contrast with the gastritis usually seen, the Zollinger-Ellison stomach mucosa is very healthy looking, and may be seen to be actively secreting gastric juice.

Other mucosal lesions include vascular anomalies such as hereditary telangiectasia, which may be responsible for chronic bleeding.

Disorders of the stoma. *Chronic marginal ulcer.* This lesion was found in 30 percent of the symptomatic patients and could be visualized by endoscopy in nine out of ten cases, whereas only 50 percent of marginal ulcers were correctly diagnosed radiologically. The difficulty of radiological diagnosis in an area distorted by surgical manipulation is not hard to understand. Many a surgical tuck has been read as a crater, especially since the stoma is relatively inaccessible to palpation, being generally above the costal margin. Consequently an almost equal number of ulcers diagnosed by x-ray were not in fact present. If for no other reason, then, endoscopy is essential in the symptomatic postgastrectomy patient.

Stomal inflammation (stomatitis). Superficial ulceration, redness, and exudation of the stomal margins were seen in 42 percent of patients, and was the only lesion in almost 20 percent. These findings were often associated with pain and were sometimes the only abnormality in patients presenting with

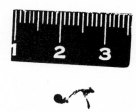

FIG. 2. Suture removed with biopsy forceps from a Billroth II anastomosis of patient presenting with pain and bleeding 2 years after gastrectomy for duodenal ulcer.

bleeding or anemia. Stomatitis may represent a lesser variant or interval stage of chronic marginal ulcer; several of these patients had demonstrated ulcers at other admissions.

While stomal edema is frequent early after surgery, long after surgery this may be the only finding in patients who are complaining of pain or bleeding, and it may thus be hiding small ulcers. It is more commonly seen in Billroth I anastomoses. A late result of stomal inflammation or ulceration is *stomal stenosis*, which may cause persistent vomiting and is easily diagnosed endoscopically.

Foreign body. Not infrequently, suture material is seen at the anastomosis and quite commonly it causes ulceration through which it is extruding into the lumen. It is now possible and advisable to remove these materials with the biopsy forceps under direct endoscopic vision (Fig. 2, and see colorplate). Suture material may also cause localised mucosal hyperplasia, sometimes enough to obstruct the stoma.

Double-barrel stoma. This is a disorder of stomal anatomy in which both afferent and efferent loops present side by side in the stoma, separated by a bridge of jejunal mucosa at the same level as the gastric margins of the stoma. This abnormality was found in about one gastrojejunostomy in ten. In these patients, several significant difficulties arise: the bridge of mucosa is frequently traumatised and bleeds as a result, and ulceration of the bridge and of either loop occurs in over 50 percent. The afferent loop fills easily from the stomach and often produces afferent loop stasis. Since

---

* *The postgastrectomy lesions are illustrated in a 16-mm motion picture "The Symptomatic Postgastrectomy Patient," 22 min., color, sound; Cat. M1714, National Medical Audiovisual Center, Atlanta, Georgia, from whom it can be borrowed.*

afferent-loop secretions have to enter the stomach first, gastritis and bilious vomiting are frequent. When found, this disorder should be surgically corrected, preferably by conversion to Billroth I.[8]

Size and motility of the stoma. When the stoma is small and the gastric resection 50 percent or less, the stoma generally retains circular contractions on the gastric side. Large stomas (over 3.5 cm) with higher resections usually have abortive or no gastric contractions and never close. Vagotomy reduces or eliminates these contractions. Dumping, when present, is found 5 times more frequently with large nonclosing stomas than with smaller closing stomas.

Jejunal disorders. The jejunum may suffer from jejunitis, jejunal ulceration, stenosis of the efferent limb due to stricture or twist with proximal dilatation, and stasis in the afferent limb. These can all be visualized endoscopically. Also, not only biopsy specimens but material for culture can be obtained under direct vision.

REFERENCES

1. Hirschowitz, B. I., Curtiss, L. E., Peters, C. W., and Pollard, H. M., Gastroenterology 35:50, 1958.
2. Hirschowitz, B. I., Lancet 1:1074, 1961.
3. Morrisey, J. F., Gastroenterology 62:1241, 1972.
4. Hirschowitz, B. I., Med. Biol. Illus. 4:224, 1965.
5. Hirschowitz, B. I., Luketic, G. C., Balint, J. A., and Fulton, W. F., Am. J. Dig. Dis. 8:816, 1962.
6. Belber, J. P., Gastroenterology 61:55, 1971.
7. Hirschowitz, B. I., The Postgastrectomy Stomach. In L. Berry, ed., Gastrointestinal Endoscopy. Springfield, Ill., Thomas, 1972.
8. Demaret, A., Hirschowitz, B. I., and Luketic, G. C., Scand. J. Gastroenterol. 6:77, 1970.

B. Gastroscopy and Gastrophotography

GEORGE D. HADLEY

The recent innovations in fibre optics and their application to problems of medical diagnosis are the latest developments in the long history of gastric endoscopy. For practical purposes, this work began in the early 1930s, with the introduction of the Wolf-Schindler semiflexible gastroscope. The safety and comparative ease with which this instrument could be used resulted in a considerable number of physicians and a few surgeons devoting much time and care not only to acquiring technique and experience themselves, but also to imparting their results to others, and by 1939 there were, scattered over the country, nuclei of technically competent gastroscopists who were convinced of the intrinsic diagnostic value of the procedure and capable of passing their expertise on to the next generation. Hermon Taylor's modifications considerably increased the technical efficiency of the instrument but at the cost of greater bulk and diminished flexibility. This instrument became for the next 20 years, however, the standard gastroscope in England, and probably no better gastroscope of this type was ever built.

The remarkable flexibility and optical efficiency of fibre-optic endoscopes inevitably led to the introduction of this system to gastroscopy. The first of these instruments emerged from the U.S.A. almost 20 years ago. It was safe, relatively comfortable for the patient, and was long enough to enter the duodenum. It had, however, a narrow arc of vision and lacked means of controlling the distal end once the instrument had been passed. These were serious defects in an otherwise excellent instrument, and it is perhaps surprising that it should have taken so long to correct them and to produce the far more effective and completely controllable instruments available today. This American fibre gastroscope was, however, the only one available for many years. Its use was limited, and most gastroscopists in this country and in Europe continued to employ up-to-date versions of the Wolf-Schindler and Hermon Taylor semiflexible gastroscopes.

Meanwhile an entirely new technique had been quietly developed in Japan, so quietly, in fact, and with so little publicity, that it was in widespread use all over Japan long before any real knowledge of it reached the Western world. This new technique of blind intragastric photography using colour film had evolved in Japan in response to the challenge set by the formidable incidence of gastric cancer, which is numerically the most common form of malignant disease in that country. The limitations of radiology in the early detection of this disease were obvious, and the physical characteristics of the Japanese race ruled out any possibility of the extensive use of orthodox gastroscopes. Their clinicians urgently needed a method of endoscopy that was safe, easy, rapid, and capable of widespread outpatient use by doctors (and sometimes by nurses) with relatively little training. This range of "blind" gastrocameras, culminating in the Olympus Co. GTV and GTVa models, used 5-mm Anscochrome film, each examination taking 32 photographs which, after processing, could be inspected and reported very quickly by experts. These simple yet sophisticated little cameras with their safety, reliability, and speed in use gave magnificent service. They were introduced into this country in 1963 and have been described in detail elsewhere.[1, 2, 5, 6] They must now, however, be regarded as obsolete. Fibre-optic gastroscopes with optional photography have replaced them completely. It is better to look first and photograph later.

FIBRE OPTICS— TECHNIQUES

Once the difficulties of constructing sufficiently fine glass fibres had been surmounted and—an even more serious problem—their accurate laying together so that each fibre emerges at the proximal end in precisely the same position that it occupies at the distal end, a most valuable means had been achieved of inspecting any kind of interior surface. Human endoscopy is by no means the only application of this technique.

Extreme fine-ness of the glass fibres is important not only in resolution and clear definition of the transmitted image but also in longevity. One fractured fibre in the bundle implies one tiny black spot in the image, and too many of these render the image valueless. The finer the fibres the more flex-

ible they are and the less liable to fracture in normal use.

There is no theoretical limit to the length of these fibre bundles. In endoscopic terms, this means not only that instruments can readily be made long enough to pass down the duodenum but also that the light source can now be outside the patient and transmitted down the bundle. This is a great improvement, as the light can now be far more powerful (and is of course, intragastrically, a "cold" light). Furthermore, previous difficulties with burnt-out filament bulbs are eliminated.

The range of fibre-optic gastroscopes and gastroduodenoscopes now available is bewildering. They may be grouped approximately as follows:

Side-viewing gastroscopes. These instruments are equipped with a built-in distal camera and distal light source. An example is the Olympus Co., Model G.T.F.A. This is

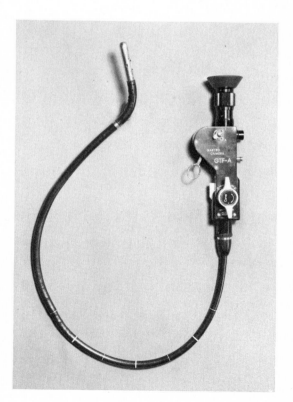

FIG. 3. The Olympus GFTA fibre gastroscope with built-in distal camera.

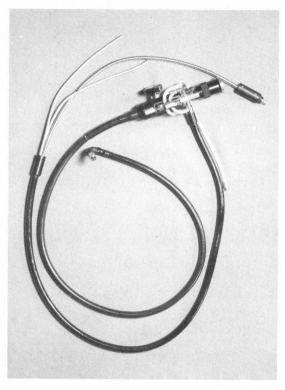

FIG. 4.   The ACMI end-viewing fibrescope with biopsy channel. (Optional photography using a proximal ½-frame 35-mm camera.)

an admirable gastroscope for general use (Fig. 3).

Other versions of this instrument omit the distal camera, which is replaced by arrangements for performing gastric biopsy under direct vision or for brush cytology.

End-viewing fibrescopes. These instruments are equipped with optional proximal camera and external light source. They are effective oesophagoscopes and give excellent coverage of the distal stomach, but they are less reliable in the proximal stomach. They can usually be passed into the duodenum, but in the important region of the "duodenal cap" the views obtained are necessarily at close range and are not always easy to interpret. Examination of the postoperative stomach with this type of gastroscope is, however, most rewarding, as the area around the anastomosis can usually be very adequately inspected. An example of this type is the American A.C.M.I. instru-

ment, which also provides arrangements for biopsy, and which possesses a mechanism for distal end directional control that will not easily be bettered (Fig. 4).

Side-viewing duodenoscopes. These instruments are designed for the express purpose of cannulation of the ampulla of Vater, which can then be injected with a radiopaque substance. This examination must, of course, be carried out in an x-ray department, and at present it appears to be uncertain whether the biliary tree or the pancreatic duct systems will be outlined. The author has no personal experience of this instrument but in capable hands its potentiality in the diagnosis of obscure jaundice and also in pancreatic neoplasm is obvious.

INDICATIONS FOR GASTRODUODENOSCOPY

The indications for gastroscopy and gastrophotography have been reviewed previously, but during the past 5 years the list has been increased considerably. They may be summarized as follows:

X-ray negative dyspepsia. The patient presents with a history compatible with peptic ulcer, but the barium meal shows no abnormality. In 119 patients of this group, gastrophotography showed a benign gastric ulcer in 13, multiple polyps in 1, and carcinoma in 1. The majority of these ulcers were shallow; some, however, were deep and obvious enough to occasion surprise that no niche had been demonstrable at x-ray. It is probably generally true that radiological diagnoses of duodenal ulcer occur too frequently and gastric ulcer too seldom, and the results of gastrophotography in this group of cases support the latter half of this contention. The ease and safety of the procedure suggest that it should be employed routinely in patients who fall into this category.

Gastric ulcer—benign or malignant? When all the clinical facts are known, the number of cases in which this issue seriously arises is not large, but the radiological criteria of malignancy in a gastric ulcer niche are uncertain enough to make a proportion of the reports necessarily equivocal, and in these circumstances a direct view of the ulcer crater, in colour, is extremely valuable. (See Figs.

5–16, colorplate.) If good views can be obtained, mistakes are few, and the opinion of the gastrophotographer (or gastroscopist), in the author's experience, compares favourably with that of the surgeon at laparotomy. Because the operation of gastrectomy for cancer is so much more extensive than that of gastrectomy for ulcer, it is important that surgeons be given the fullest possible information before the abdomen is opened, and a series of photographs that can be inspected and discussed together is of greater practical value in this respect than the written report of the gastroscopist.

Though an experienced gastroscopist's visual impression of the nature of an ulcer crater is usually correct, mistakes can be made, and one must also face the fact that very occasionally a malignant ulcer can be seen to heal,[13] though only temporarily, of course. Biopsy of the margin of a suspicious ulcer crater will certainly decrease this error.

Uncertain x-ray findings.

Deformed or apparently rigid gastric mucosal folds. Here there is always suspicion of carcinoma, and direct inspection of the area, if it can be adequately achieved, is diagnostic: Of 40 cases in which x-ray findings were "suspicious of carcinoma," carcinoma was verified in 8; benign gastric ulcer in 6; and benign tumour in 2. The stomach was normal in 15; and in 9, inadequate photographs with the GTV camera were obtained.

"Spastic antrum." Again there is often suspicion of neoplasm, and gastrophotography has been valuable. Under full premedication, many of these antrums prove to be normal. In others, the deformity has been shown to be caused by the presence of an unsuspected benign ulcer or scarring from a healed ulcer. None in our series so far has shown carcinoma.

So-called "hypertrophic gastritis." Genuine examples of Menétrier's disease are rare but the x-ray appearance often simulates extensive carcinoma, and gastroscopic confirmation, preferably with biopsy, is valuable. Apart from this small and reasonably well-defined group, there remain many instances of what appears radiologically to represent an unusually coarse and thickened mucosal pattern, and this is not infrequently reported on in such terms as "evidence of gastritis" or as "gastroduodenitis." Most of these are examples of the hyperrugose and hypertrophic mucosa often associated with duodenal ulcer, but gastric ulcer may occur and radiological mistakes are not infrequent. A genuine gastric ulcer may easily be missed amongst the big tortuous folds, while on the other hand, flecks of held-up barium may give the impression of an ulcer that does not, in fact, exist. We have found gastrophotography extremely useful in this group of cases in both confirming and refuting x-ray diagnosis of ulcer.

Postoperative stomach. Whether because of subsequent pain or bleeding or both, these cases have always posed a difficult diagnostic problem. Radiology is at best uncertain, and gastroscopy and gastrophotography with the older instruments usually missed the anastomotic ulcer situated distal to the rim of the stoma. With modern fibrescopes, accuracy is greatly increased, and for this purpose an end-viewing instrument is more effective. This applies of course to cases in which gastric resection has been carried out, but the same may be said of the increasing numbers of patients appearing with symptoms after vagotomy and pyloroplasty. This operation inevitably results in gross deformity of the pyloric region, and interpretation of barium studies is often quite impossible. Again examination with an end-viewing fibrescope is invaluable. Recurrent ulcers in this situation are often small and superficial: they appear, they heal, and they relapse, and a positive result is not likely to be achieved unless gastroscopy is carried out at a time when symptoms are actually present.

Haematemesis and melaena. Avery Jones,[8] in a planned research project, showed clearly how frequently acute lesions can be visualised at emergency gastroscopy carried out as soon as possible after admission. Modern fibrescopes have brought this procedure now into the category of "routine and necessary." It is less disturbing to the patient than emergency barium studies and usually more informative. It is probably advisable to employ an end-viewing instrument; if oesophageal varices are unexpectedly present, they can not only be seen but can also be safely negotiated, as the tip of the instrument can be steered under direct vision down the oesophageal lumen into the stomach and duodenum.

THE FUTURE

After many years of very limited use, gastroscopy has now entered into a phase of rapid expansion. It is a diagnostic aid that no hospital department concerned with gastroenterology can afford to be without, and this very obvious fact is now becoming increasingly recognised throughout the country. Expansion brings with it implications both personal and financial, for endoscopy of the stomach and duodenum is both expensive and time-consuming. Both of these aspects must be foreseen and planned for not only by the doctors concerned but also by hospital management committees.

At the time of writing, it would not be possible to equip fully a gastroscopic unit with instruments alone for less than £5,000. Replacement of instruments is necessary occasionally, and repairs to damaged instruments can be extremely expensive.

In considering time allotment, it must be realized that while gastroscopy alone with a side-viewing instrument such as the Olympus Co. G.T.F.A. should take no more than 20 minutes, a full examination of oesophagus, stomach, and duodenum with an end-viewing endoscope may take up to 1 hour, and four or five examinations will usually occupy one complete session. Much additional time is spent when teaching, and demonstration must be included, as is nearly always the case. The extra time can be minimised when it is possible to fit a teaching side piece to the instrument in use.

Assistance is also necessary and it is desirable that both Consultant and Registrar become expert. The gastroscopic needs of the average general hospital in the United Kingdom will not be fulfilled by fewer than two operators working without interruption for at least one full session weekly. Expertise attracts and engenders work, and the above outline should be regarded as a current minimum, likely to be expanded as colleagues gain confidence in a fresh and valuable diagnostic approach.

REFERENCES

1. Blendis, L. M., Cameron, A. J., and Hadley, G. D., Gut 8:83, 1967.
2. Blendis, L. M., et al., Br. Med. J. 1:656, 1967.
3. Chrysopathis, P., Surgery 54:292, 1963.
4. Gibbs, D. D., et al., Postgrad. Med. J. 45:577, 1969.
5. Hadley, G. D., Br. Med. J. 2:1209, 1965.
6. Hadley, G. D., Lond. Clin. Med. J. 7:33, 1966.
7. Hara, Y., et al., Ann. Surg. 159:542, 1964.
8. Jones, F. A., Br. Med. J. 2:477, 1947.
9. Jones, F. A., Lond. Clin. Med. J. 2:25, 1963.
10. Lucchini, M. A., et al., Gastrointest. Endosc. 16: 56, 1969.
11. Morrissey, J. F., et al., Gastroenterology 48:711, 1965.
12. Morrissey, J. F., et al., Gastroenterology 53:456, 1967.
13. Sakita, T., et al., Gastroenterology 60:835, 1971.
14. Tagaki, T., et al., Surgery 65:597, 1969.

C. Duodenography

LOUIS KREEL

In spite of significant advances in biochemical, radiological, and scanning techniques in recent years, accurate early diagnosis of pancreatic lesions remains a problem. At times it has appeared that selective arteriography and then isotope scanning would lead to a higher rate of detection of small carcinomatous lesions and consequently to a better prognosis. No real evidence of this has as yet materialised, however. It is therefore imperative that evidence of pancreatic disease must be sought for in the clinical history and examination, and it must be sought for in the routine investigations such as the plain film, barium meal, and follow-through examination as well. In an examination utilising the barium meal, it is essential to pay particular attention to the posterior wall of the stomach, particularly while the patient is in the prone position in

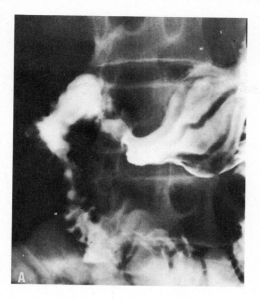

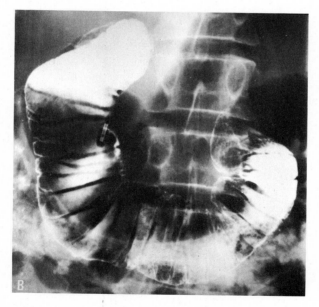

FIG. 17. (A) Coarse mucosal pattern in second part of duodenum. Frequently found in presence of duodenal ulceration and often called "oedema" of the duodenal mucosa. (B) Gas distention duodenography in same patient shortly after previous examination; demonstrates normal duodenal pattern with no evidence of thickening or "oedema" of transverse bars (valvulae conniventes).

deep inspiration. A localised rounded impression with an irregular margin is an important sign. Straightening and fixity of the gastric lesser curve may also occur, and the impression of a dilated common bile duct or markedly enlarged gallbladder on the duodenal bulb or descending limb of the duodenum is also most significant.

In pancreatic disease, special care must be paid to the duodenal loop, but in this respect it must be noted that the examination of the duodenal loop, whether by the conven-

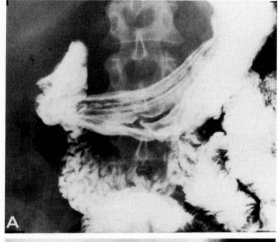

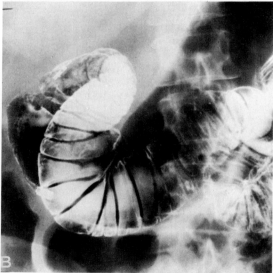

FIG. 18.   (A) Normal feathery mucosal pattern in duodenal loop. Proximal part of duodenal loop is hidden by duodenal bulb and distal part by body of the stomach. (B) Corresponding duodenography film shown by gas-distention technique. Appearances are quite different from those obtained on conventional barium-meal examination.

tional barium meal or as a separate examination, is required for two purposes. Firstly, the loop may be involved because of disease of the duodenum itself; secondly, it may be involved owing to disease of the pancreas. The intimate relationship of the duodenum to the head of the pancreas is such as to make it possible to diagnose pathological lesions of the pancreas by visualisation of the duodenum. During the conventional barium meal, however, there is a constantly

changing pattern caused by the inherent movements of the duodenum. Furthermore, the mucosal pattern is also influenced by the adhesive qualities of the barium and by gastric acidity. The coarse mucosal pattern in the second part (Fig. 17), associated with ulceration in the duodenal bulb, may be due to actual oedema of mucosal folds or merely to changes in the properties of the barium. Another difficulty in using the conventional barium meal to assess changes in the duo-

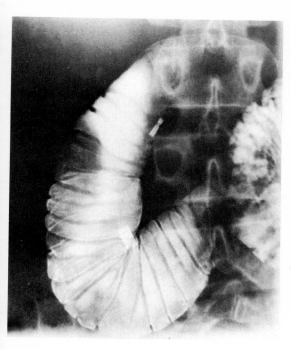

FIG. 19. Duodenography with warm half-strength normal saline producing double-contrast effect. Appearances are similar to gas-distention duodenography, but view is not always so clear. No discomfort whatever is produced by this method, however.

denal loop is that frequently a part of the loop may be hidden either by the duodenal bulb or by the stomach (Fig. 18A). In many cases it therefore becomes desirable to examine the duodenum at a separate examination and in such a way as to obtain constant appearances.

The normal appearance of the duodenal loop during the conventional barium meal is that of a feathery pattern (Fig. 18A) which, as has been mentioned previously, tends to vary from film to film. Transient filling defects that could be interpreted as being caused by extrinsic pressure are not infrequently seen. It is difficult in this situation to know whether the important factor is that the variability indicates the loop is normal, or whether the inherent motility of the duodenum is tending to hide a lesion. The normal pattern of the duodenum on duodenography is, however, quite different (Fig. 18B), with the circular folds of mucous membrane (valvulae conniventes) showing as

transverse bars that reach from margin to margin of the duodenum; between these transverse bars the mucosal margin is convex (Figs. 17B, 18B, 19). The distal half of the second part of the duodenum is usually larger than the proximal part, and there may be slight flattening of the medial margin of the folds in this region (Fig. 19).

TECHNIQUES

Basically, in duodenography there are three separate phases. The first is to introduce the tip of a gastroduodenal tube into the duodenum and inject a small amount of slightly diluted barium; the second is to render the duodenum atonic with oxyphenonium bromide (Antrenyl) given intravenously; and the third is to produce distention of the duodenum and a double-contrast effect.

A double-lumen gastroduodenal tube such as the Scott-Harden tube has been found to be particularly suitable, and recently the "guided" Dotter tube has been recommended. After the pharynx has been anaesthetised with a lozenge and then a spray, the tube is inserted into the stomach. The inner tube is then passed on for about 4 inches (10 cm). Both tubes together can then be pushed on so that they follow the greater curve. When the tip of the inner tube reaches the pyloric canal, it is manipulated into position by palpation (with a lead glove for protection) under fluoroscopic control.

When the tip of the tube is in the second part of the duodenum, the fluoroscopy table is tilted into the horizontal position so that the patient lies supine.

Fifty milliliters of barium of low viscosity but high concentration, such as Baritop, is injected down the tube, and simultaneously 6 mg of Antrenyl is slowly injected intravenously. To allow adequate coating of the duodenal mucosa, some of the barium mixture must be given while the duodenum is still active.

As soon as the duodenum is seen to be atonic, it can be distended and films taken. Distention can be done either with a gas such as carbon dioxide or with warm, half-strength saline. If gas distention is used, the flow should be approximately 4 litres per minute

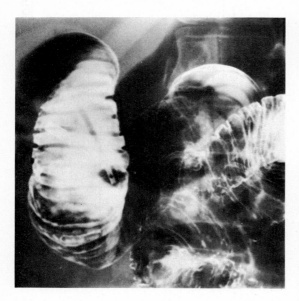

FIG. 20. Steep oblique view of second part of duodenum, showing posterior wall and retro-duodenal space. This can be clearly seen as stomach does not obscure the area, being filled only with gas.

of duodenography a clear view of the posterior margin of the duodenum can be obtained, as it is not obscured by the stomach (Fig. 20).

INDICATIONS FOR DUODENOGRAPHY

Pancreatitis. In acute pancreatitis both the conventional barium meal (Fig. 21) and duodenography demonstrate a marked alteration in the duodenal pattern, particularly in the second part. Not only do the valvulae conniventes appear markedly thickened, but the ridges between appear very pointed. This change usually extends over a long area involving not only the duodenal loop but possibly the proximal jejunum as well. The radiological signs of chronic pancreatitis can usually be detected by the conventional barium-meal technique only in the late stages or in the presence of calcification. In distention duodenography, abnormal signs can frequently be detected. The earliest changes are a definite flattening of the medial margin of the duodenal loop so that the convex bowing between the transverse bars is lost. To be quite sure of this sign, gas distention and not fluid distention must be used. Subsequently the medial aspects of the circular folds are obliterated, giving a smooth bald appearance (Fig. 21A). Later the medial margin becomes quite straight or may even give the inverted "3" sign, and the transverse bars are no longer visible (Fig. 22). An irregular filling defect may even appear on the medial part of the duodenum (Fig. 23).

The straightening of the medial border of the second part of the duodenum may extend to include the upper border of the third part of the duodenum. A real difficulty arises with this sign, however, in the presence of diverticula, as the adjacent border of the inner margin of the duodenal loop may show flattening with a perfectly normal pancreas. Thus minor degrees of flattening of the inner margin of the duodenal loop in the areas adjacent to diverticula must be interpreted with caution. Localised slightly irregular indentations of the inner border of the duodenal loop can also occur in chronic pancreatitis (Fig. 24A and B) and may be mistaken for a carcinoma of the head of the pan-

and the patient should be warned that slight discomfort may occur. Gas distention should be only momentary, just enough to take an exposure, i.e., 1 to 2 seconds, and then be discontinued. This is repeated prior to each exposure. If warm, half-strength saline is used (Fig. 19) it must be injected with a large syringe as rapidly as possible. Gas distention is more effective and produces better quality double-contrast films, but fluid distention produces no discomfort whatsoever. Gas distention must be used if detailed examinations of diverticula are to be carried out; however, for the best demonstration of polypi, fluid is advisable. Thus the particular variation in technique will depend on the lesion to be shown and the general reaction of the patient.

Antrenyl has been used, as it acts rapidly and appears to cause few or no side reactions. The dose may be varied (according to the size of the patient) from 4 to 8 mg. As regards fluid distention, it has been found that tap water and cold fluid cause active contractions in the duodenal loop. Warm half-strength saline is therefore recommended. Another point to be mentioned is that with this type

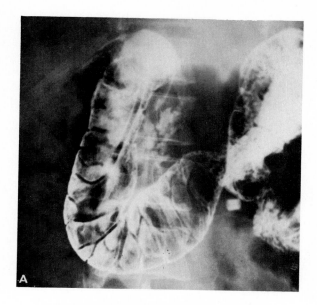

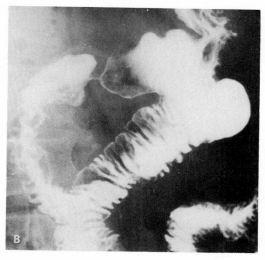

FIG. 21.   (A) Gas-distention duodenography in patient with chronic pancreatitis. Inner margin of duodenum is straightened and there is loss of the transverse folds on inner aspect of second part of duodenum. Pancreatic calcification is also visible. (B) Barium-meal film showing thickened duodenal folds with irregular inner and outer margins in a case of acute pancreatitis.

creas. In this connection it is important to note that a carcinoma in the body of the pancreas, producing oedema or displacement of the head of the pancreas, may cause flattening of the medial margin of the duodenal loop and so be mistaken for chronic pancreatitis.

Carcinoma of the head of the pancreas. There is no doubt that carcinoma of the head of the pancreas produces more definite radiological signs during duodenography than when the conventional barium-meal technique is employed. The late signs of widening of the loop and the inverted "3" sign of Frostberg can be replaced by those of small filling defects (Fig. 25) or areas of constriction (Fig. 26) on the duodenal loop. The filling defect associated with carcinoma of the head of the pancreas differs from that

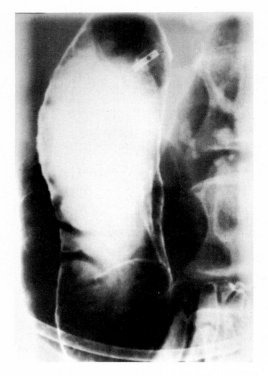

FIG. 22. Marked changes in chronic pancreatitis with early inverted "3" sign. Marked flattening of medial margin and complete loss of transverse folds medially. Slight pancreatic calcification visible.

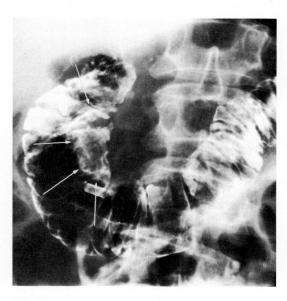

FIG. 23. Late changes in chronic pancreatitis with extrinsic filling defect (*arrows*).

of chronic pancreatitis in that the folds become compressed from side to side, producing a spikiness in pancreatic carcinoma. Often this is only in a very localised region but is constant during duodenography. It shows up best when the patient is placed in the slightly oblique supine position, with the right shoulder raised. These localised filling defects with spiky margins may occur not only on the medial margin of the second part of the duodenum but also on the upper border of the third part.

Carcinoma of the ampulla of Vater. The small smooth localised filling defect in the region of the second part of the duodenum that is associated with a carcinoma of the ampulla of Vater (Fig. 27A) is not caused by the actual growth itself; it is caused by the impression of the associated dilated common bile duct (Fig. 27B). It thus differs in its duodenographic appearance from both chronic pancreatitis and carcinoma of the head of the pancreas. It must be noted, however, that although this smooth localised filling defect is most commonly caused by a carcinoma of the ampulla of Vater, it can also be caused by other lesions that produce distal obstruction of the common bile duct with marked dilatation proximally such as a gallstone impacted at the sphincter of Oddi.

As a further aid in the preoperative differential diagnosis of obstructive jaundice, combined percutaneous cholangiography and duodenography can be used (Fig. 28). In carcinoma of the head of the pancreas, the extent of the lesion will be shown. The lower margin will be demarcated by the filling defect on the duodenal loop, and the upper margin will be shown by the lower end of the obstructed common bile duct; in primary carcinoma of the common bile duct, there will be a perfectly normal duodenal loop and only the obstructed common bile duct will be shown (Fig. 28).

Other lesions impinging on the duodenum. Occasionally other lesions also produce signs caused by extrinsic pressure. Paravertebral lymph node enlargement can produce obliteration, compression, and distortion of duodenal folds with spikiness of their margins (Fig. 29A). This has been seen, for instance, in lymph nodes involved secondarily to a carcinoma of the transverse colon.

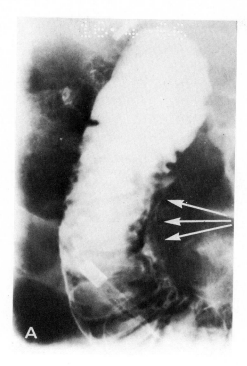

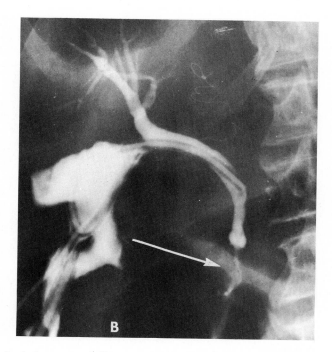

FIG. 24.   (A) Extrinsic pressure effect caused by chronic pancreatitis with smooth inner margin (*arrows*). (B) T tube cholangiogram in same patient shows appearances at distal end of common bile duct (*arrow*), which is markedly narrowed with irregular margins.

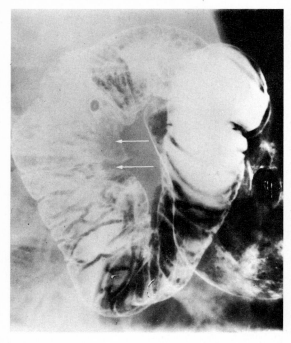

FIG. 25. Extrinsic filling defect owing to pancreatic carcinoma. Inner margin of duodenum has spiky appearance.

Enlarged lymph nodes in the region of the descending limb of the duodenum can produce scalloped smooth impressions often on both the inner and outer margins, as well as half-shadowing filling defects, by pressure on the anterior and posteror duodenal wall (Fig. 29B). A more localised and more linear extrinsic defect can be caused by fibrotic bands (Fig. 30) or associated with arterio-mesenteric ileus.

Intrinsic lesions of the duodenal loop and duodenal diverticula. Intrinsic lesions are not so common in the duodenal loop as in the oesophagus, stomach, or duodenal bulb, but they are more common than in the remainder of the small bowel. Frequently these lesions are overlooked owing to a lack of awareness of their possibility and to difficulties in adequately visualising such lesions. The commonest abnormality is that of the coarse mucosal pattern variously described as "oedema" of the duodenal mucosa, "thickening" of the mucosal folds, and even as the "angry-looking" duodenal pattern. This is commonly associated with peptic ulceration in the duodenal bulb. On duodenographic

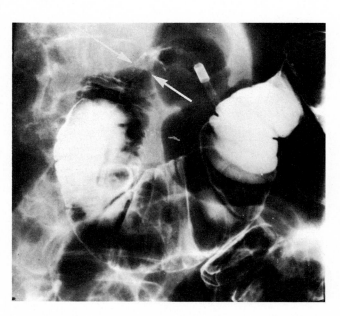

FIG. 26. Constrictive lesion at junction of first and second parts of duodenum, caused by pancreatic carcinoma.

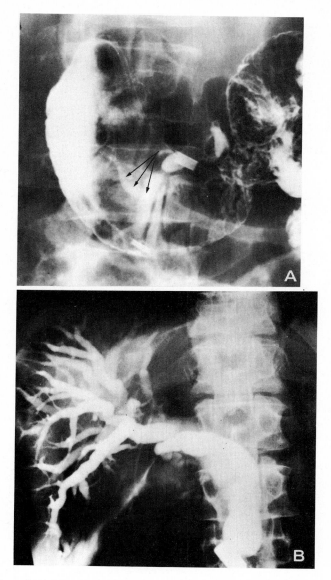

FIG. 27.   (A) Smooth crescentic filling defect at junction of second and third parts of duodenum, owing to markedly dilated common bile duct caused by carcinoma of ampulla of Vater. (B) Pre-operative percutaneous cholangiogram in same patient shows markedly dilated common bile duct responsible for extrinsic impression on duodenography film.

examination, most of these cases have perfectly normal duodenal patterns and it can only be assumed that there is either a definite change in the physical properties of the barium in the presence of high gastric acidity or that there is increased smooth muscle tone or "spasm." On occasion, however, the duodenal pattern may be highly abnormal with large thick transverse bars (Fig. 31), which in one case led to the diagnosis of a Zollinger-Ellison syndrome and the subsequent removal of a pancreatic tumour. Duodenal "atrophy" or a "bald" pattern on duodenography may occur, however, with infestation by the nematode *Strongyloides stercoralis* and also with

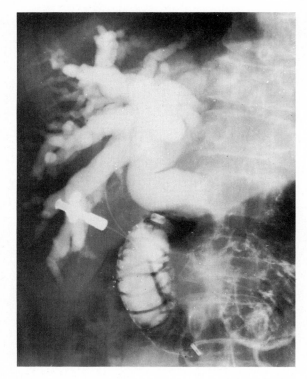

FIG. 28.   Combined duodenography and preoperative percutaneous cholangiography in primary bile duct carcinoma. Duodenal loop is quite normal. If pancreatic carcinoma produced a block at such a high position, duodenal loop would show definite filling defect.

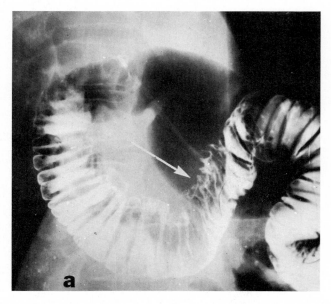

FIG. 29.   (A) Marked compression of duodenal folds of superior margin of ascending limb of duodenal loop (arrow), producing spiky contour. Lesion was metastatic lymph node involvement from carcinoma of the colon.

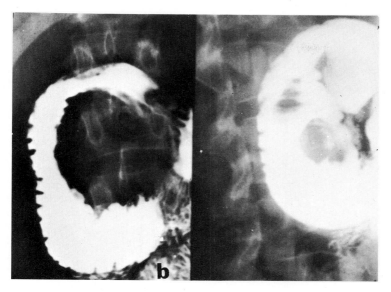

FIG. 29. (B) The medial margin of the descending limb of the duodenum shows impressions producing a scalloped margin, and on the oblique view, with compression, this appears as extrinsic defects. This appearance is caused by enlarged, nonfiltrating lymph nodes, particularly in lymphoma (Hodgkin's disease).

amyloidosis and systemic sclerosis.

A papilla of Vater is present in approximately 80 percent of individuals and can frequently be seen on duodenography with a vertical fold running up into it on the medial side of the duodenum. It produces a smooth semicircular defect on the medial margin which, in the normal way, may be up to 2 cm in diameter.

Papillomas of the duodenum are relatively

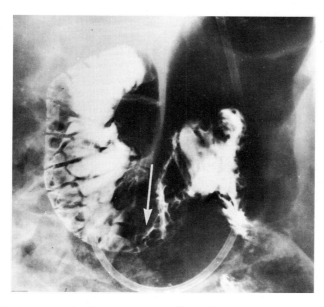

FIG. 30.   Extrinsic compression (arrow) owing to fibrous band across third part of duodenum.

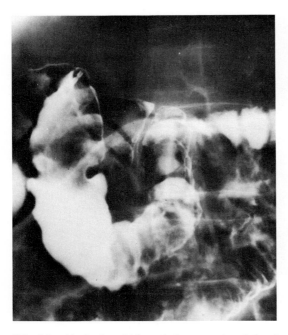

FIG. 31. Markedly thickened but poorly defined valvulae conniventes resulting from prolonged hyperacidity in Ellison-Zollinger syndrome.

rare and are unlikely to be diagnosed during the conventional barium examination. When double-contrast duodenography is employed, especially with warm, half-strength saline, papillomas are clearly visible (Fig. 32). They stand out as rounded filling defects arising from the transverse bars. They may be single or multiple, and may be associated with papillomatosis of the remainder of the small bowel.

Carcinoma of the duodenum is a lesion that will be repeatedly missed unless it is specifically sought for. In any case in which there is evidence of gastric stasis with a marked fasting gastric residue and the cause is not found in the region of the gastric antrum, pyloric canal, or duodenal bulb, the duodenal loop must be clearly shown in its entirety if carcinoma of the duodenum is not to be missed. If there is any question as to the site or nature of such an obstructive lesion, duodenography should be carried out. The site of the obstruction can be clearly

demonstrated (Fig. 33) and usually the differing appearances of carcinoma of the duodenum, infiltration of adjacent metastatic lymph nodes, and extrinsic bands can be distinguished from each other. But primary carcinoma of the duodenum can also produce an intraluminal growth which on duodenography appears as an intrinsic filling defect with irregular margins. Occasionally an infiltrating pancreatic carcinoma may simulate a primary intraluminal duodenal carcinoma. If an extensive lesion with markedly irregular margins and complete obliteration and destruction of duodenal folds is demonstrated, a duodenal sarcoma must be seriously considered. If, on the other hand, there is marked widening of the duodenal loop with the duodenal folds largely intact but showing medial flattening with only a small localised area of spikiness of folds, this would suggest a cystadeno carcinoma of the pancreas. The duodenal sarcoma and pancreatic cystadeno carcinoma are best distinguished on selective arteriography.

Normally there is no difficulty in showing the number and site of duodenal diverticula. The conventional barium meal is more than adequate in this respect. But to demonstrate the intimate details of the appearances of a diverticulum by the conventional barium meal is another matter. This can only be achieved by a double-contrast technique and is quite clearly shown during duodenography. It is thus possible to diagnose the rare complications such as ulceration, food impaction, and carcinomatous transformation. Recently, appearances suggesting prolapse of the duodenal mucosa into the neck of a diverticulum have been demonstrated (Fig. 35) but it is as yet too early to say whether this is a real clinical entity.

The difficulties inherent in examining the afferent loop following gastrectomy are well known. Although this examination is not often required, the afferent loop can be shown with great clarity by a combination of intubation and Antrenyl. As an example of the detail that can become visible, Figure 34 demonstrates the inturned stump of the duodenum showing as a small filling defect.

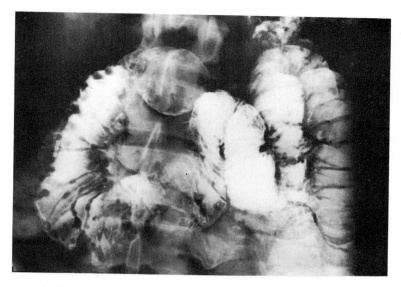

FIG. 32.   Multiple duodenal papillomas in small-bowel papillomatosis. Lesion is best shown by half-strength normal saline rather than gas-distention duodenography.

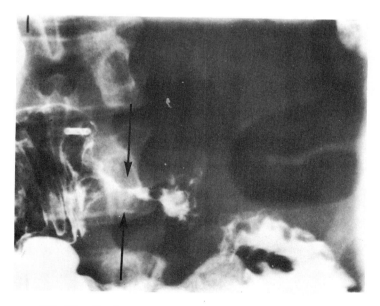

FIG. 33.   Carcinomatous stricture in third part of duodenum.

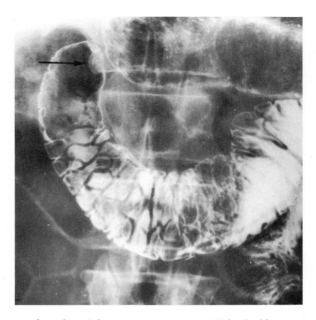

FIG. 34. Duodenography after Polya-type gastrectomy. With double-contrast technique even such a small filling defect as the inturned duodenal stump (*arrow*) becomes visible.

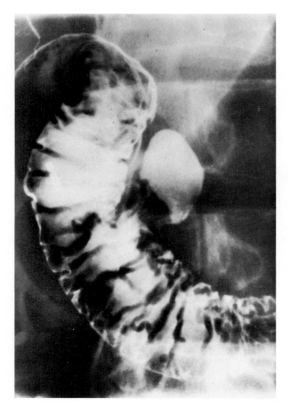

FIG. 35. Duodenal diverticulum with marked mucosal pattern bulging through neck of diverticulum, suggesting presence of mucosal prolapse into diverticulum.

DUODENOGRAPHY DURING CONVENTIONAL BARIUM EXAMINATION

The major objection to duodenography is that it is an examination requiring the insertion of a tube into the duodenum. In order to overcome this objection, the duodenum has been examined during conventional barium-meal examinations by rendering it atonic with 6 mg of Antrenyl administered intravenously. There is no doubt that the appearances after Antrenyl are very similar to those revealed by tube duodenography, although not quite so clear.

A convincing demonstration of the technique's use in pancreatic carcinoma is shown in Figure 36, where it was not really possible to make a diagnosis on the conventional examination. After Antrenyl administration, the filling defect with spikiness of the medial folds of the duodenal margin is shown, indicating the presence of a pancreatic carcinoma. Another example is given in Figure 37 A and B, in which the marked straighten-ing of the medial margin indicates chronic pancreatitis. This was confirmed at operation for the relief of obstructive jaundice when an operative cholangiogram was performed. Although this manoeuvre of giving intravenous Antrenyl during conventional barium-meal examinations greatly enhances the visualisation of the duodenal loop, there are still many cases in which the loop is hidden by the barium in the stomach and in the duodenal cap (Fig. 29B).

The recent introduction of the double-contrast barium meal using gas tablets or powder offers a further refinement in diagnosis of duodenal lesions. In this way, "instant" double-contrast duodenography can then be carried out by giving Antrenyl intravenously once the examination of the stomach and duodenal bulb has been completed. A very important aspect of the use of Antrenyl that must not be forgotten is that the drug subsequently slows the transit of barium through the small bowel, so that a follow-through examination becomes impossible. Thus even when a "no-tube" examination is being contemplated, detailed visualisation of the duodenum and the small

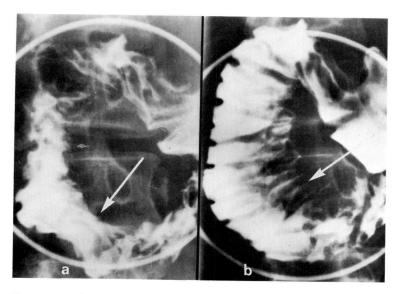

FIG. 36. Conventional barium-meal spot films of duodenal loop. (a) Routine view compared with (b) after I.V. Antrenyl. In (a) there is suggestion of smooth extrinsic filling defect at junction of second and third parts of duodenum. In (b) this is shown more definitely; there is marked compression of inner aspects of duodenal folds producing a spiky margin characteristic of pancreatic carcinoma.

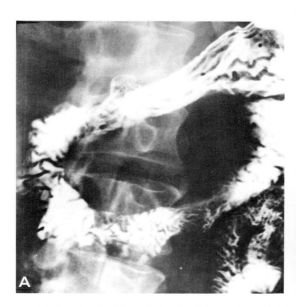 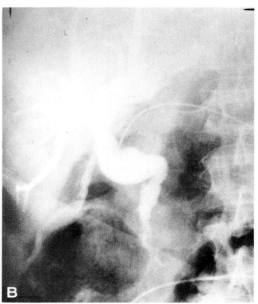

FIG. 37.   (A) View of duodenal loop after I.V. injection of 6 mg Antrenyl shows obvious flattening or "straightening" of medial margin, indicating presence of chronic pancreatitis. (This appearance can, however, also be caused by carcinoma in the body of the pancreas.) (B) Operative cholangiogram. Common bile duct is markedly dilated proximally, but there is marked irregularity at lower end where common bile duct is narrowed. (This was caused by chronic pancreatitis.)

bowel may become mutually exclusive and would in any case require two separate examinations.

SUMMARY AND CONCLUSIONS

The examination of the duodenal loop must become part and parcel of each barium-meal examination. Particular attention must be paid to the duodenal loop in all cases in which the oesophagus, stomach, and duodenal bulb are normal. This is particularly so whenever signs and symptoms point to an upper abdominal lesion in the presence of pain—particularly if this suggests a pancreatic lesion and when there is evidence of gastric outlet obstruction. If in these circumstances the whole of the duodenal loop is not seen, it must be examined by intubation.

Double-contrast distention duodenography

can show lesions such as carcinoma of the head of the pancreas, chronic pancreatitis, and carcinoma of the ampulla of Vater, as well as intrinsic duodenal disease including mucosal thickening, papillomas, and duodenal carcinoma. Duodenal bands and other extrinsic obstructive pathological changes can be accurately localised and duodenal diverticula can be shown with great clarity.

Finally it must be mentioned that "instant duodenography" can be obtained during conventional barium examinations by giving 6 mg of Antrenyl intravenously after the duodenum has been well filled with barium. This, however, usually precludes an adequate follow-through examination at the same session.

The accuracy of duodenography has been shown to be at least as great as that of selective arteriography and greater than isotope scanning. As it is considerably easier to perform, it is now recommended as the examination of choice in lesions of the pancreatic head, and it is imperative in all cases in which intrinsic lesions of the duodenum require delineation.

REFERENCES

Eaton, S. B., Feischli, M. D., Pollard, J. J., Nebesar, R. A., and Potsaid, M. S., New Eng. J. Med. 279: 389, 1968.

Jacquemet, P., Liotta, D., and Mallet-Guy, P., The Early Radiological Diagnosis of Diseases of the Pancreas and Ampulla of Vater. Springfield, Ill., Thomas, 1965.

Kreel, L., Postgrad. Med. J. 43:14, 1967.

Kreel, L., Proc. Roy. Soc. Med. 62:881, 1969.

Kreel, L., Outline of Radiology. London, Heinemann, 1971. Pp. 132–133; 141–148.

Kreel, L., and Mackintosh, C., Gut 9:222, 1968.

Levi, A. J., and Kreel, L., Proc. R. Soc. Med. 56:168, 1963.

Mallett-Guy, P., and Jacquemet, P., J. Radiol. Electrol. 44:249, 1963.

McCarthy, D. M., Kreel, L., Agnew, J. E., and Bouchier, I. A. D., Gut 10:665, 1969.

Mindel, S., and Kreel, L., Br. Med. J. 3:785, 1968.

Poole, G. J., Radiology 97:71, 1970.

Poppel, M. H., Semin. Roentgenol. 3:227, 1968.

Poppel, M. H., Jacobson, H. G., and Smith, R. W., The Roentgen Aspects of the Papilla and Ampulla of Vater. Springfield, Ill., Thomas, 1953.

Raia, S., and Kreel, L., Gut 7:420, 1966.

Rosch, J., Roentgenology of the Spleen and Pancreas. Springfield, Ill., Thomas, 1967.

D. Laparoscopy

RICHARD S. HANDLEY

Laparoscopy (synonyms: peritoneoscopy; coelioscopy) is the technique whereby the peritoneal cavity can be inspected with an instrument closely akin to a cystoscope. First performed in 1901, it has never become popular with surgeons, perhaps because allowances have not been made for its limitations and thus results have been disappointing. Of recent years there has been an upsurge of interest by the gynaecologists, who find that inspection of the female pelvis from within by laparoscopy yields useful results and minor operations can be done through the instrument. The advent of fibre-optic lighting has also greatly improved the laparoscope.

As with all endoscopic instruments, the laparoscope needs "elbow room" for the window of its telescope so that the latter is not in direct contact with what is to be observed. A pneumoperitoneum, either of air or carbon dioxide, must therefore be established as a first step, and the organ to be inspected made to project into this large intraperitoneal bubble; changes in the position of the patient will move the gas bubble and thus allow different areas of the peritoneal cavity to be seen.

In general, therefore, it is only the fixed organs about which useful information can be obtained, and of these the liver is by far the most important for the surgeon. The surface of the parietal peritoneum, the gallbladder, the front of the stomach, and (with a steep Trendelenberg tilt) the female pelvis can also be seen; but the intestines cannot be systematically inspected, and only in the unlikely event of a lesion, free from adhesions, occupying a coil of bowel that happens to lie at the surface of the intraperitoneal air bubble is useful information to be obtained.

INDICATIONS FOR LAPAROSCOPY

From what has been said, the indications are fairly obvious. Hepatomegaly and ascites, of uncertain origin, are the prime indications. Courvoisier's law is much more accurate if the size and colour of the gallbladder are actually seen. Laparoscopy may save a laparotomy in advanced abdominal malignant conditions if it reveals hepatic or peritoneal metastases. Its gynaecological indications are outside the scope of this section.

TECHNIQUE

The patient is prepared for a general anaesthetic, this being much more comfortable for all concerned than attempting the examination under local anaesthesia. Abdominal relaxation greatly facilitates the procedure.

1. After preparation of the skin and towelling, the site for insertion of the pneumoperitoneum needle is chosen. This can be anywhere on the anterior abdominal wall, but the best place is the midline, 1 inch (2.5 cm) below the umbilicus if there is no old operation scar immediately adjacent (Fig. 38). Old scars are likely to have old adhesions behind them, which may lead to perforation of a fixed coil of bowel. An incision is made in the skin, about ¼ inch long. For inducing the pneumoperitoneum, I prefer a fine trocar and cannula (Fig. 39A), though special needles with spring-loaded

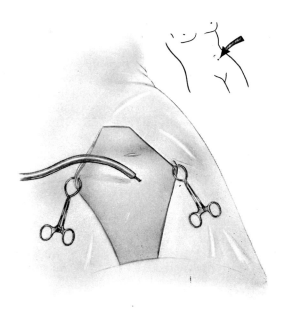

FIG. 38. Induction of pneumoperitoneum. (From Rob, Smith, and Morgan, 1969. *Operative Surgery*, vol. 4. Courtesy of Butterworths, London.)

plungers are available (Fig. 39B). The instrument is pushed through the linea alba in an oblique direction so that the aorta is not punctured by maladroit precipitancy of entry into the peritoneum. When the tip of the instrument is judged to have entered the peritoneal cavity, the trocar is withdrawn and the cannula advanced. The cannula is swung to and fro, and will move easily if its tip lies free in the peritoneum. I like to introduce air into the peritoneal cavity by means of a Maxwell pneumothorax apparatus. Air has been criticised as liable to produce air embolus, and carbon dioxide has been advised as being more soluble. Sudden gross over inflation is possible, however, if the controlling mechanism on the CO_2 cylinder is not correctly used, and this has occurred. A pneumothorax apparatus gives the surgeon more control over the speed, pressure, and volume of air introduced, and the manometer on the instrument indicates whether the air flow is easy and therefore into the peritoneal cavity.

About 1½ litres of gas is then introduced, and the small cannula withdrawn.

2. The large trocar and cannula (Fig. 39C) are then pushed through the abdominal wall into the intraperitoneal gas bubble (Fig. 40), the instrument again being directed obliquely to guard against unduly abrupt and forceful entry damaging the aorta. It is this manoeuvre that the beginner finds most trying because considerable pressure is needed but care is also required to prevent the instrument from entering too suddenly and too far.

3. The trocar is withdrawn, a finger over the end preventing escape of air if the instrument is not valved (Fig. 39D), and the laparoscope (Fig. 39E) is introduced. Inspection can then begin (Figs. 41, 42, and 43), the laparoscope being pushed to and fro, or rotated if nothing can at first be seen; its tip may be covered by a fold of omentum, which can easily be shaken free. Insufficient gas in the intraperitoneal gas

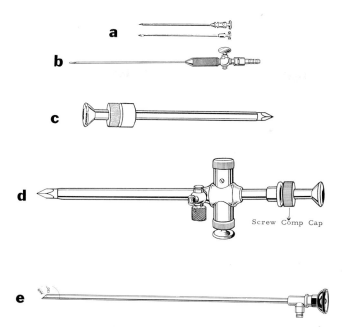

FIG. 39.   The Frangenheim G.U. Co. Laparoscope: (A) small trocar and cannula; (B) Verres Spring-Plunger Pneumoperitoneal Cannula; (C) large plain trocar and cannula; (D) large valved trocar and cannula; and (E) oblique forward fibre-optic telescope. (Courtesy of the Genito-Urinary Manufacturing Co. Ltd.)

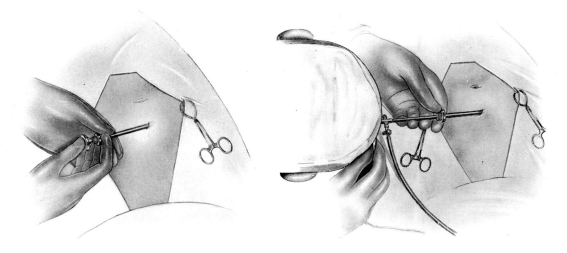

FIG. 40.   Introduction of the large trocar and cannula. (From Rob, Smith, and Morgan, 1969. *Operative Surgery*, vol. 4. Courtesy of Butterworths, London.)

FIG. 41.   Inspection of the peritoneal cavity. (From Rob, Smith, and Morgan, 1969. *Operative Surgery*, vol. 4. Courtesy of Butterworths, London.)

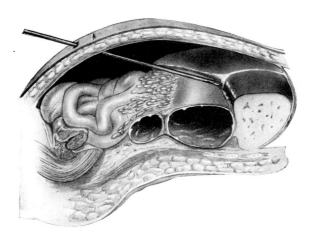

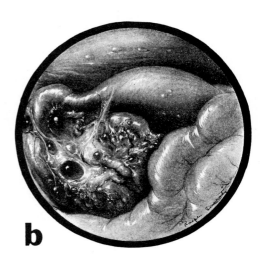

FIG. 42.   Schemiatic section of the abdomen with the laparoscope in position. (From Rob, Smith, and Morgan, 1969. *Operative Surgery*, vol. 4. Courtesy of Butterworths, London.)

FIG. 43.   (B) Papillary cystadenoma of the ovary with peritoneal implantations.

bubble is another common reason for difficulties in visualisation.

4.   Laparoscopic biopsy specimens can be taken. It is best to introduce a second cannula for this, so that biopsy forceps can be introduced; the latter can be insulated and connected to a coagulat-

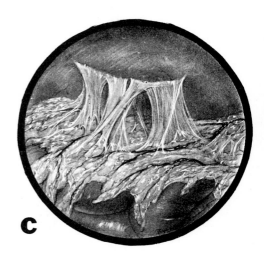

FIG. 43.   (C) Intra-abdominal adhesions. (Courtesy of J. C. Ruddock, M.D., and *Surg. Gynec. Obstet.*)

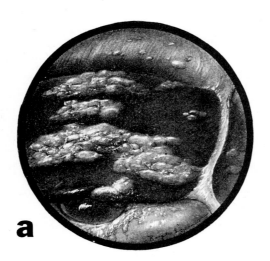

FIG. 43.   Views as obtained through a peritoneoscope: (A) Carcinoma metastases in the liver. Note the metastatic implantation on underside of diaphragm.

ing diathermy so that bleeding can be checked. It must be emphasized, however, that *biopsies introduce a greatly increased hazard to the procedure, owing to the risk of bleeding.* The liver and nodules under the parietal peritoneum are the only lesions that can yield biopsy specimens with reasonable safety, and then only when the operator is quite familiar with the technique of examination. The gynaecologists have perfected a technique for sterilisation by diathermy coagulation of the fallopian tubes, and for dealing with small ovarian cysts and pelvic adhesions.

5. At the end of the inspection, the laparoscope is withdrawn, as much gas as possible is expelled, and the cannula is then withdrawn. A stitch closes the tiny skin incision. If there is no pathological reason to detain him, the patient can be discharged from hospital as soon as he is fully recovered from the anaesthetic.

6. Laparoscopy should be performed only in a fully equipped theatre so that, in the rare event of serious trouble, a laparotomy can speedily be done.

COMPLICATIONS

Most of the very uncommon fatal complications of laparoscopy have been due to *haemorrhage,* and special care must be taken to check prothrombin levels if laparoscopy is performed on jaundiced patients. Liver biopsy has been the main cause of fatal haemorrhage, and it should not, in my opinion, be carried out in jaundiced patients because there is also the added risk of bile leakage from the liver into the peritoneum. Other accidents, due to the introduction of the trocar and cannula, have produced grave and perhaps fatal haemorrhage; the aorta has been punctured, the portal stalk wounded, and the external iliac artery lacerated. Less serious bleeding may be produced by damage to the smaller vessels of the anterior abdominal wall or the omentum.

Damage to the bowel is uncommon and has occurred most often when the bowel is fixed to the anterior abdominal wall by adhesions. It seems almost impossible to damage normal mobile coils of intestine.

Induction of the pneumoperitoneum has given rise to complications, some of them fatal. I have already said that I regard air as safe if it is introduced with care, but fatal pulmonary air emboli have been reported. Gross subcutaneous emphysema from faulty placing of the pneumoperitoneum needle, has occurred, but this appears to be more alarming than serious. Mediastinal emphysema and pneumothorax have also been reported. Carbon dioxide has its disadvantages too; death has resulted from sudden gross overinflation when no metering device has been interposed between the CO_2 cylinder and the cannula. Acidosis from rapid CO_2 absorption is a possible hazard as well.

In *conclusion* it must be emphasised that laparoscopy is much safer than exploratory laparotomy. It is also much less painful for the patient and many times more economical in hospital bed occupancy. Against these advantages must be set the more limited information that it can give. It is contraindicated in patients who are grossly obese, who have extensive intra-abdominal adhesions, or who are unfit for a general anaesthetic, but it may be extremely useful if its indications are remembered and its limitations accepted.

REFERENCES

Cohen, M. R., Laparoscopy, Culdoscopy and Gynecography. Philadelphia, Saunders, 1970.
Handley, R. S., and Nurick, A. W., Br. Med. J. 2:1211, 1956.
Ruddock, J. C., Surg. Clin. North Am. 37:1249, 1957.
Steptoe, P. C., Laparoscopy in Gynaecology. Edinburgh, Livingstone, 1967.

5

FOREIGN BODIES IN THE ESOPHAGUS, STOMACH, AND DUODENUM

MICHAEL E. DeBAKEY and GEORGE L. JORDAN, JR.

A wide variety of foreign bodies in the esophagus, stomach, and duodenum have been encountered. They may be broadly classified into three major categories: (1) swallowed foreign bodies, (2) bezoars, and (3) transmurally introduced foreign bodies.

SWALLOWED FOREIGN BODIES

By far the most frequently encountered foreign bodies in the gastrointestinal tract are those that are either accidentally or deliberately swallowed. Usually accidentally swallowed objects are recovered from the gastrointestinal tracts of children and infants, who have a great tendency to place objects into their mouths. In fact, the highest incidence of swallowed foreign bodies occurs in children from 1 to 3 years old. Adults also inadvertently swallow objects, such as toothpicks, which have been held in their mouths; and even dentures are swallowed by the elderly. The elderly who wear dentures are more prone to swallow foreign bodies because of the lack of tactile sensation in the mouth.[26] Care must be taken not to place objects into the mouths of unconscious or delirious persons; for instance, thermometers have been found in the stomachs of persons after a severe illness as a result of attempts to take oral temperatures in temporarily irresponsible patients. There are two types of patients who deliberately swallow foreign bodies. In mentally unbalanced patients, the swallowing of a wide variety of foreign bodies may represent a compulsive habit, a masochistic tendency, or a suicidal effort. Numerous reports appear in the literature regarding this type of individual, but one of the most remarkable is the case described

by Chalk and Foucar of a manic-depressive patient from whom 2,533 foreign bodies were removed at laparotomy.[4] Numerous other cases of this type have been described in which more than a thousand foreign bodies were removed from the stomach. The other type of person who deliberately swallows foreign bodies is the professional juggler or mountebank whose showmanship prompts him to ingest various apparently dangerous objects, such as broken glass, razor blades, pins, or needles. Inmates of prisons also deliberately swallow foreign bodies at times, in attempts to gain certain privileges or to aid in accomplishing specific objectives. Johnson reports an inmate who ingested razor blades on ten or twelve occasions, and we recently have encountered a prisoner who purposely swallowed safety pins held partially closed, which would open after entrance into the stomach.[14] This has been done on three different occasions. Recently, it has also been suggested that jealous siblings may on occasion purposely feed foreign bodies to small children as a primitive solution to social problems, and it is suspected that mentally ill adults may feed harmful objects to children as a variant of the battered child syndrome.[26]

The nature and types of swallowed foreign bodies are extremely variable. It would appear that almost any object that can be placed in the mouth can be swallowed. The objects encountered most commonly, particularly in infants and children, are pins, coins, small toys, buttons, tacks, nails, and screws. Many unusually large foreign bodies have been swallowed by adults, including full dentures, table forks, and knives.[16] A bolus of food may function as a foreign body in a partially obstructed intestinal tract.

Certain factors influence the fate of foreign

bodies in the gastrointestinal tract. Ordinarily, the size is not in itself an important consideration. The shape or configuration of the object, on the other hand, plays an important role. Coins, buttons, marbles, and other smooth objects will ordinarily pass along without difficulty, whereas long pointed objects may cause considerable concern. Open safety pins are the most difficult and potentially the most dangerous of all foreign bodies. Hairpins, needles, and straight pins may also become impacted in the stomach or duodenum. Even an open safety pin will usually pass along satisfactorily if the spring end of the pin is in the leading point. Other factors, such as the nature and consistency of the foreign body, are relatively unimportant.

There are a number of normal points of relative constriction in the gastrointestinal tract which represent the sites of possible lodgement of a foreign body. After an object passes the cricopharyngeus muscle, there are two areas of narrowing in the esophagus. One is at the bifurcation of the trachea and the area of compression by the aorta. The second is at the diaphragm and the esophagogastric junction. In about 10 percent of patients with esophageal foreign bodies, local disease with stricture formation will serve to produce obstruction. Ordinarily, if a foreign body will pass the cardiac end of the esophagus, it may be expected to pass readily through the entire gastrointestinal tract. In about 5 percent of cases, however, the foreign body may become lodged. This is more likely to occur in the presence of inflammatory or constricting lesions and with relatively long, sharp, pointed objects. Even in the absence of obstructing lesions the pylorus may impede passage, and small foreign bodies may remain indefinitely in the stomach or may pass along after several weeks. Beyond the pylorus the next most common point of obstruction is encountered in the second, and sometimes the third, portion of the duodenum, where relatively long objects are often unable to negotiate the curve. After a foreign body has passed the ligament of Treitz, the ileocecal region is the next point of possible impaction. The area of the peritoneal reflection in the pelvis impedes passage, as does the anus. It is remarkable that such a high percentage of objects of all kinds run this obstacle course without difficulty.

Esophageal Foreign Bodies

CLINICAL MANIFESTATIONS

Gross states that in children approximately 25 percent of foreign bodies lodge in the esophagus.[8] This figure is undoubtedly too high for the general population; in adults there is reason to believe that most foreign bodies that are swallowed never come to the attention of any physician and pass from the gastrointestinal tract without being of concern to the patient.

When lodgement in the esophagus occurs, the symptoms are quite variable. If they are flat, even large objects may occasionally cause no symptoms until some complication develops, food passing into the stomach without difficulty. When symptoms occur, they may direct attention to the esophagus or they may point primarily to the respiratory tract. Choking, dysphagia, and vague discomfort are the most frequent signs. Because of obstruction, however, spillage of ingested liquid or food into the trachea may produce cough, dyspnea, and expectoration of sputum. The presence of a foreign body in the esophagus is one cause of pneumonia and lung abscess. Foreign bodies retained for long periods ultimately erode the esophagus, causing ulceration with perforation or hemorrhage. Although a rare complication, fatal hemorrhage has been reported.[27] If not promptly removed, sharp objects may puncture the esophagus and may perforate surrounding structures. Furthermore, the object may actually migrate completely through the esophagus. Perforation of the trachea, pleura, lung, and even the heart or aorta has been reported, with disastrous consequences. Norman and Cass recently reported a case in which a child was found dead in bed. Autopsy revealed cardiac tamponade due to an open safety pin in the esophagus. It had not perforated the heart but had simply scratched the surface, causing tamponade.[21] Perforation of the carotid artery has also caused death.[20] Perforation into the mediastinum will produce mediastinitis with fever, chest pain, and often crepitation in the neck, as air dissects superiorly.

DIAGNOSIS

Diagnosis is suspected on the basis of history and symptomotalogy. Unless a complication has occurred, there are no significant physical findings. Ultimate diagnosis is by radiological examination. Posterior-anterior and lateral views of the chest are indicated. Fortunately, most objects are radiopaque and easily seen. A nonradiopaque object may be suspected if on the lateral view there is widening of the space between the thoracic vertebrae and the trachea. Ingestion of radiopaque material to aid in determination of location and size will occasionally be necessary. If so, use of water-soluble media is indicated rather than barium. This is safer, as no complications will develop if some aspiration occurs, and it will not coat the object and make it difficult to see through the esophagoscope.

TREATMENT

Although an occasional small, smooth object in the distal esophagus may be observed for a few hours to allow passage into the stomach, most objects—particularly large or sharp ones—should be removed as soon after diagnosis as possible. Removal is an endoscopic procedure, described in detail in the publications of Jackson and Jackson.[13] Foreign bodies have also been removed by more indirect means without anesthesia. Symbas reported 11 cases removed by passage of a Foley catheter under fluoroscopy and careful withdrawal of the object after inflation of the balloon. In the experience of most physicians, however, use of the esophagoscope is preferable, and the introduction of the flexible esophagoscope has made the procedure easier.[24] General anesthesia will be required in most small children and may increase the safety of the procedure in many adults. The foreign body usually is too large to remove through the esophagoscope. Therefore, it is grasped with forceps, brought against the end of the esophagoscope, and the instrument, forceps, and foreign body are removed simultaneously.

Foreign Bodies in the Stomach and Duodenum

CLINICAL MANIFESTATIONS

For the most part, swallowed foreign bodies in the stomach and duodenum cause no symptoms and progress down the alimentary tract to be passed spontaneously without any discomfort. It is of interest in this regard that many of the reported cases of multiple foreign bodies in the stomach of mental patients produced no symptoms. Some patients, however, complain of vague abdominal discomfort, particularly if there is anxiety from the knowledge that the object is in the abdomen. Occasionally, mild abdominal cramps and vomiting may occur if the foreign body is unusually large. Patients with multiple long-standing foreign bodies may have a sense of heaviness and discomfort in the epigastrium as well as anorexia and malnutrition. When an object becomes impacted, severe obstructive symptoms with vomiting and retching may occur. Signs of peritonitis with abdominal pain. tenderness, distension, fever, and leukocytosis are indicative of perforation. Fortunately, this complication is relatively uncommon. In a series of 800 cases reported from the Boston City Hospital by Henderson and Gaston, perforation occurred in only one percent.[9] These observers also found that the stomach and duodenum were the sites of perforation in approximately half of a collected series of 71 perforated cases; the remaining cases were equally divided among the small intestine, the cecum, and the colon. Hematemesis and melena may accompany impaction of a foreign body. A sharp-edged or pointed object may actually lacerate the mucosa and result in brisk hemorrhage. Migration completely through the wall of the stomach or duodenum occasionally occurs with eventual perforation of another organ. Able and associates report the finding of a needle in the liver of an 11-month-old boy in whom there were no symptoms. At operation, a healed tract from the stomach to the liver was found.[1] Baird and Spence have reported ingested foreign bodies migrating to the kidney from the gastrointestinal tract. The right kidney is usually in-

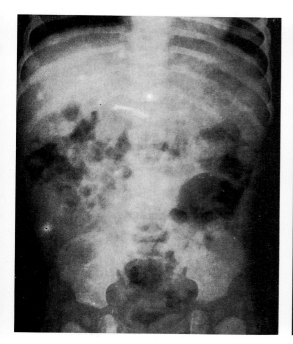
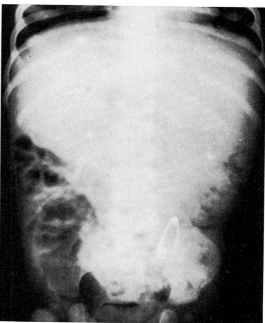
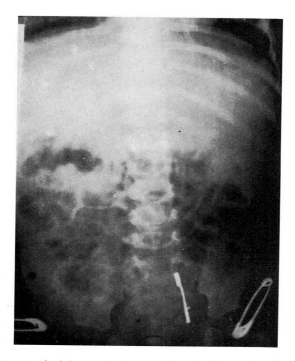

FIG. 1.   Roentgenograms of abdomen in 7-month-old male infant who swallowed open safety
pin. On admission to hospital foreign body was located in stomach (A); on subsequent consecutive
days pin was demonstrated in small bowel (B) and rectum (C). (Diaper pins may be noted on
each side.) Next day the pin was recovered from stool and patient was discharged.

volved, representing presumed perforation of the duodenum. Needles, a pin, and a straw were removed from the kidney in three reported cases.[2]

DIAGNOSIS

The diagnosis can usually be made from the history and from roentgenographic examination. A child's mother can frequently describe the type of object the youngster was holding in his mouth at the time that it disappeared, and an adult will often volunteer the fact that he was holding a nail, screw, or other object in his mouth when some sudden incident caused him to swallow it. In the absence of obstruction or perforation, there are no characteristic physical findings, although a mass of matted foreign bodies may be of such size as to be palpable, particularly in an emaciated patient. Actual diagnosis is usually based upon demonstration of the foreign body by fluoroscopic or roentgenographic examination, as many such objects are radiopaque. Contrast media, such as barium or iodized oil, may be helpful in the roentgenographic demonstration.

TREATMENT

Treatment of ingested foreign bodies depends upon the nature and type of object swallowed and the occurrence of complications. Since spontaneous passage may be expected in most cases, conservative management with close periodic observation of the patients is usually adequate. Thus, Clerf[6] reported spontaneous passage of the foreign bodies in 827 of a series of 834 patients, and Ladd and Gross reported this occurrence in 323 of 337 patients.[17] When objects are relatively small and smooth, such as buttons, coins, and even closed safety pins, observation may be accomplished on an outpatient basis. Careful daily examination of the abdomen and roentgenographic observations should be made to determine the occurrence of any untoward manifestations and to watch the progress of the foreign body through the gastrointestinal tract (Figs. 1 and 2). It is preferable to hospitalize patients who have swallowed open safety pins or relatively sharp, pointed, or irregular jagged objects for closer observation. Although spontaneous

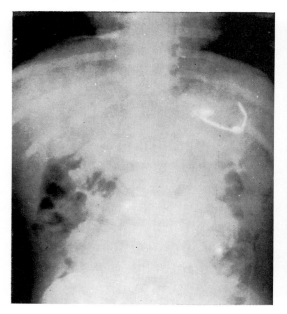 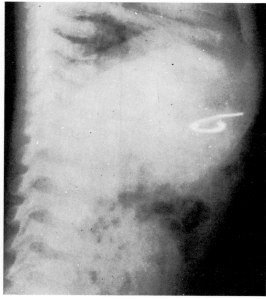

FIG. 2. (A) Roentgenogram of abdomen in male infant of 17 months who swallowed open safety pin and was admitted to hospital. (B) Foreign body's failure to progress after 4 days and apparent impaction prompted early removal by gastrotomy. Patient recovered uneventfully.

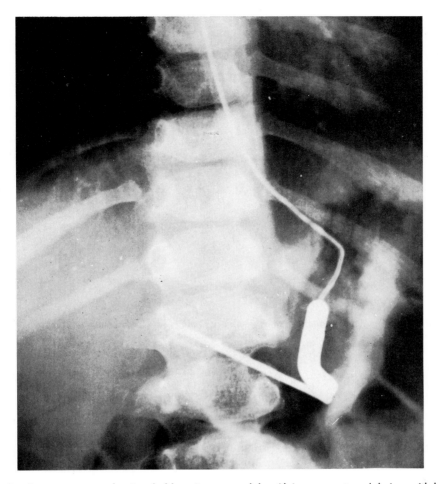

FIG. 3.   Roentgenogram showing bobby pin engaged by Alnico magnet and being withdrawn into esophagus. (From Singleton, *X-ray Diagnosis of the Alimentary Tract in Infants and Children*, 1959. Courtesy of Year Book Medical Publishers, Chicago.)

passage will usually take place in several days to a week, it is well to exercise patience when the object is relatively smooth or rounded, for the risk of complications is comparatively small and passage may take place even as long as 3 or 4 weeks after ingestion. Special diets and cathartics are not recommended. The patient or his relatives should be instructed to examine all stools for the foreign body and to report any untoward symptoms.

Numerous conservative methods of removal have been employed with varying success. Endoscopic removal with the aid of the esophagoscope or rigid gastroscope has been accomplished by some and others have proposed a special forceps for this type of extraction. Currently, the use of the flexible gastroscope has extended the use of this technique. Special forceps have been devised for this type of extraction. Ordinarily these manipulations are done under fluoroscopic control.

Another ingenious technique which has enjoyed some popularity is use of magnets for removal of metallic foreign bodies.[12, 23] Alnico, an alloy of iron, aluminum, nickel, and cobalt that has been magnetized, has been used successfully in many instances in removing foreign bodies from the stomach. An instrument made of this substance is useful for ferrous metallic objects, such as bobby

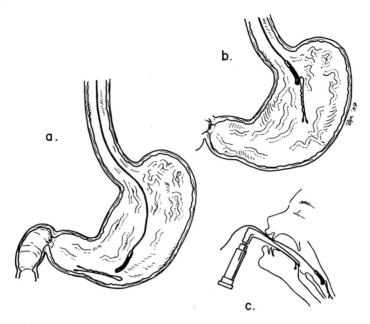

FIG. 4. Use of Alnico magnet to remove object containing ferrous metal. General anesthesia was used; as bobby pin was withdrawn into esophagus, glottis was exposed in order to prevent damage to esophagus and pharynx.

pins and needles, but is not applicable to brass safety pins, coins, etc. Thus, a duplicate of the object should be obtained before insertion of the magnet in order to estimate the magnetic qualities. The patient swallows the magnet or the magnet is introduced with a flexible tube and the foreign body is engaged under fluroscopic control (Fig. 3). The foreign body is then manipulated and drawn into the esophagus. One complication that may occur as the object is withdrawn into the esophagus is perforation, particularly as the object is delivered through the proximal esophagus and cricopharyngeus muscle (Fig. 4). It is advisable, therefore, to administer a general anesthesia and expose this area by elevating the epiglottis with a laryngoscope in order to prevent damage to the esophagus and pharynx if the patient were to strain. This is particularly important in children and uncooperative patients. Complications, such as impaction of the foreign body in the esophagus with perforation, loss of the magnet itself, and others, have limited the acceptance of this method.

In most instances, it is best to employ the conservative method of treatment until there are good indications for surgical intervention. These include: (1) failure of progress or evidence of impaction indicated by constancy of location in repeated roentgenograms taken over a period of 1 or 2 weeks; (2) signs of obstruction, impending penetration, or perforation—such as persistent abdominal pain and tenderness; (3) very long or large, sharp, pointed, or jagged objects; (4) accumulation of a large number of foreign bodies; and (5) excessive gastrointestinal hemorrhage (Fig. 5).

In preparation for surgical removal of a foreign body, a roentgenogram of the abdomen should be made immediately prior to laparotomy to confirm the fact that the foreign body has not changed its position. The stomach should be thoroughly aspirated of its contents by means of a gastric tube. The laparotomy incision is ordinarily placed in the upper part of the abdomen and may be either vertical or transverse, depending upon the preference of the surgeon. If the foreign body is located in the stomach, it may be readily found by palpating the stomach between the fingers. If it has entered the duodenum and become impacted, it is preferable

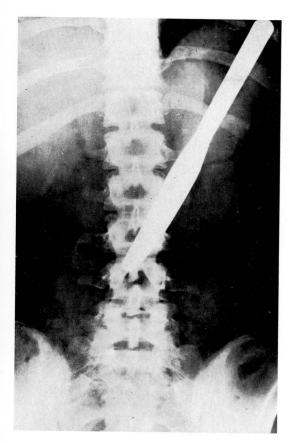

FIG. 5. Roentgenogram showing table knife in stomach of 12-year-old psychopathic girl. Objects of this size and shape should be removed surgically without preliminary trial of conservative management or nonoperative techniques.

to manipulate it into the stomach prior to its removal. Ordinarily, by means of a small gastrotomy incision, the foreign body may be removed with insignificant peritoneal contamination (Fig. 6).

In order to avoid opening the stomach, various methods have been proposed for removal at the time of laparotomy. For example, it has been suggested that an open safety pin may be closed by manipulation through the intact abdominal wall and then allowed to pass spontaneously. Another procedure is to impact or attach the foreign body to the end of an indwelling catheter, which may then be withdrawn along with the foreign body. If surgical intervention is necessary, however, direct removal of the foreign body

through a small gastrotomy is preferable, for such a procedure if properly performed provides no additional risk and is a more reliable and decisive method of removal.

Slender, pointed objects, such as straight pins or needles, are best removed by pushing the sharp end through the wall of the intestine after a Lembert mattress suture has been placed around this point. The protruding end of the object is then grasped with forceps and as it is withdrawn the suture is tightened and tied (Fig. 6).

For multiple foreign bodies, a large gastrotomy as described in the section on bezoars must be employed. In such cases, care should be taken to assure complete removal of all foreign bodies. Roentgenographic examination in the operating room is useful for this purpose.

In addition to removal of the foreign body in the presence of such complications as perforation and peritonitis, appropriate therapy is directed toward control of infection and associated ileus.

BEZOARS

Bezoar, believed to be derived from the Arabic *badzehr* or Persian *padzahr* ("counterpoison"), is applied to concretions of various foreign or intrinsic substances found in the stomach and intestine of both men and animals. The several varieties of bezoars include: (1) trichobezoars (pilobezoar, hairballs), (2) phytobezoar (hortobezoar), and (3) concretions. Although bezoars are encountered relatively infrequently, their occurrence cannot be considered rare. Up to 1938, DeBakey and Ochsner, in a comprehensive review of the literature on this subject, were able to find 303 recorded cases; and Tondreau and Kirklin noted that 100 additional cases were cited during the ensuing 12 years.[7, 25] The trichobezoar is by far the most common type, comprising well over half the reported cases, with the phytobezoar next, representing about 40 percent.

The trichobezoar, as the term implies, consists of a large quantity of hair of varying lengths, firmly matted together, forming when fully developed a perfect cast of the stomach, and even part of the duodenum (Fig. 7). Not infrequently, mixed with this hair may

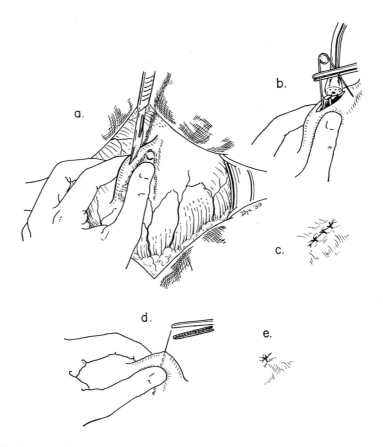

FIG. 6. Technique of gastrotomy for removal of foreign body in stomach. (A) With pin held firmly against anterior wall of stomach midway between greater and lesser curvature, small incision is made in wall of stomach immediately overlying end of pin. (B) As pin is extruded through opening, it is grasped with artery forceps and drawn out. Contamination from intragastric contents is minimized by proper use of suction upon opening the stomach, and gastrotomy is repaired in layers. (C) Pins or needles may be removed by transgastric manipulation and pushed through the gastric wall without incision in stomach. (D) Single suture may be applied over needle hole (E).

be various filamentous substances and other hairs besides the patient's, such as cotton or wool thread, string, bristles, vegetable fibers, and animal hair. Usually it is dark greenish-brown or black in color with a glary, slimy surface and an extremely nauseating odor, presumably caused by the fermentation, decomposition, and putrefaction of the various foods and organic residue intimately interspersed in the hair.

These bezoars are encountered most frequently in young girls. In the series collected by DeBakey and Ochsner, more than 80 percent occurred in persons under the age of 30 years and over 90 percent in females.[7] Although trichobezoars develop primarily from habitual ingestion of hair, the precise etiology and pathogenesis are not clearly understood. Whereas only 9 percent of patients in whom they are found showed overt psychic or mental disturbances, it is generally believed that trichophagy, like other habitual body manipulations such as nail-biting, toe-biting, and thumb-sucking, represents an expression of personality maladjustment.

The phytobezoar, as signified by its Greek prefix phyton ("plant"), may be composed of a variety of vegetable material, including

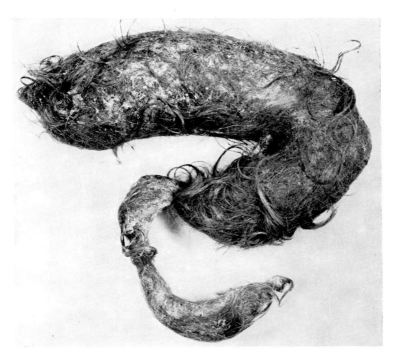

FIG. 7.   Trichobezoar surgically removed from stomach and duodenum of 15-year-old girl with history of trichoplagy and vomiting. Hairball forms perfect cast of stomach and duodenum. (From DeBakey and Ochsner, *Surgery* 4:934, and 5:132, 1939. Courtesy of The C. V. Mosby Company, St. Louis, Missouri.)

fibers, skins, seeds, leaves, roots, and stems of plants moulded together to form a compact mass. The most common form of phytobezoar, comprising about three fourths of the cases, is the one owing to ingestion of persimmons. These masses vary considerably in shape and size, being ovoid, cylindrical, oblong, or pyramidal, and ranging from 2 to 4 inches (5 to 10 cm) in length and 3 to 6 cm in diameter. Usually dark brown or black in color, they may have a smooth and attrite surface or a bosselated and pitted one (Fig. 8). Although firm and compact when freshly removed, they tend to be friable and crumble readily after drying. Upon section they are found to be composed of an amorphous, somewhat gummy material interspersed with cellulose fibers and occasionally seeds and skin.

The most plausible explanation for the mechanism of formation of this form of phytobezoar, for which the more distinctive term, diospyrobezoar, has been proposed (from the Greek etymon, *Diospyron,* the generic name for the wild persimmon), has been presented by Izumi et al.[11] According to their investigations, the mechanism is essentially chemical and depends upon the presence of soluble shibuol, a phlobatannin which, under the influence of gastric juice, becomes transformed into a sticky coagulum cementing into a ball pieces of skin and seeds that may be present. The unripe persimmon contains the greatest amount of soluble shibuol, but traces of it remain in the ripe fruit. Thus, ingestion of slightly unripe persimmons, especially when the stomach contains little or no food matter to interfere with the contact and aggregation of the seeds and fragments of the skin, predisposes to development of this form of bezoar.

Phytobezoars may also be caused by ingestion of vegetable material other than persimmons, such as coconut fibers, heather roots, celery fibers, pumpkin, skins and stems of grapes, prunes, raisins, salsify, leek, mal-

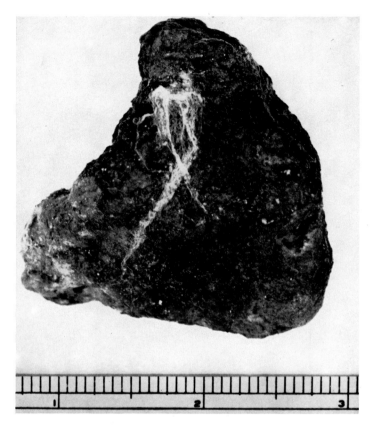

FIG. 8. Diospyrobezoar surgically removed from 44-year-old black female complaining of recurrent bouts of epigastric pain, nausea, and vomiting following ingestion of persimmons.

low, wild beets, and couch grass. Their formation is believed to be essentially mechanical and to depend upon the insoluble and indigestible fiber content.

Concretions are relatively unusual forms of bezoars, representing less than 5 percent of the reported cases. They result most commonly from the imbibition, by painters or furniture workers, of furniture polish, which consists mainly of a strong alcoholic solution of shellac. The drinking of water after its ingestion precipitates the resin into an accumulated mass and the constant repetition of this process produces the amassment of large concretions. More rarely concretions have occurred, presumably from the ingestion of certain medicaments such as bismuth carbonate (in a patient who was given bismuth as a contrast meal for roentgenological examination), salol (taken for the treatment of

cystitis), magnesium and sodium carbonate (for peptic ulcer), and paraffin (derived from a laxative preparation).

CLINICAL MANIFESTATIONS

The clinical manifestations associated with bezoars depend upon several factors including the nature and type of bezoar, the degree of gastric irritation, and the development of certain complications—such as ulceration or obstruction. The characteristic manifestations of trichobezoar are a rather large, firm, freely movable epigastric mass associated with some pain, nausea, vomiting, anorexia, weakness, and loss of weight. Usually the onset of anorexia, dyspepsia, malaise, weakness, loss of weight, and sense of weighty oppression in the epigastrium is insidious. Later there develop attacks of nau-

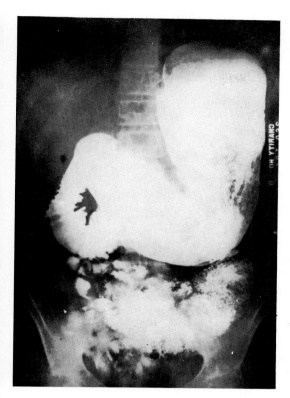

FIG. 9. Roentgenogram of stomach following ingestion of barium in patient referred to in Figure 7;
defect in gastric shadow extends throughout distended stomach with no irregularity in contour, a
feature characteristic of trichobezoar.

sea, vomiting, and epigastric pain which may
be paroxysmal in character. The pain varies
from a slight vague discomfort to severe colic.
About one third of the patients complain of
constipation or diarrhea, often alternating in
character. A foul breath, a furred tongue,
and scanty hair (especially in the frontal and
temporal regions) are often evident. The most
characteristic physical finding is a large,
readily palpable and freely mobile abdominal mass, usually located in the epigastrium
but sometimes occupying lower positions,
with a well-defined, smooth outer surface and
uniform firmness.

Phytobezoars, particularly diospyrobezoars,
have a somewhat different clinical picture.
Careful questioning of the patient usually
elicits the history of an initial attack of nausea, vomiting, cramping epigastric pain, and
diarrhea shortly after ingestion of persim-

mons. This is followed by recurrent attacks
of a milder character between varying intervals of almost complete relief. In some patients, however, the onset is not characteristic,
and the patient may not even recall eating
the fruit. This is especially true in patients
with relatively mild complaints. Occasionally, hematemesis and even melena may occur, especially in the presence of ulceration.
Except for the characteristic initial acute
attack and the history of eating persimmons,
the symptoms of phytobezoars other than
diospyrobezoars are in general similar to
those of the latter. The most constant finding on examination, occurring in slightly
over half the cases, is a freely movable, hard,
palpable mass with well-defined contours,
usually located in the epigastrium and readily displaced to the right or left hypochondrium. Associated tenderness is rarely a
prominent manifestation.

The clinical manifestations of concretions
are generally similar to those of phytobezoars
except for the history of ingestion of persimmons or other plant material. A history
of furniture polish imbibition, particularly
in painters or furniture workers, may be
obtained in cases of shellac concretions. In
other forms of concretions derived from certain medicinal agents, an appropriate history
of such ingestion may be obtained.

LABORATORY STUDIES

Most cases of bezoars are associated
with slight secondary anemia and mild leukocytosis. Gastric analysis and fecal examinations, particularly in trichobezoars, sometimes reveal significant findings, especially
strands of hair. Gastric acidity tends to be
normal or low in trichobezoar and normal
or high in phytobezoar.

The most useful laboratory procedure,
however, is roentgenography, the diagnostic
value of which was first pointed out by
Kampmann,[15] and by Clairmont and Haudek.[5] Later the characteristic fluoroscopic
and roentgenographic appearances of trichobezoars were thoroughly described by Holland [10] and by Ramsbottom and Barclay.[22]
Typically, fluoroscopic examination performed with the patient in the erect position
shows the swallowed barium held up in the
cardiac end of the stomach for a few seconds

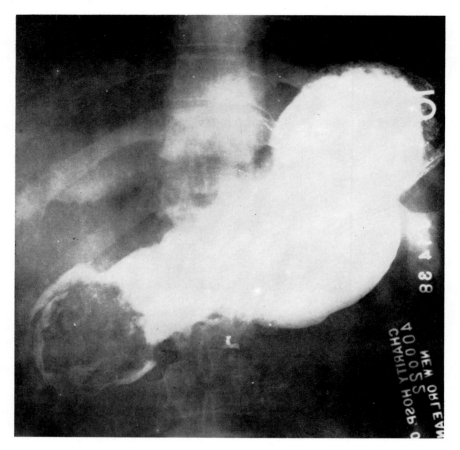

FIG. 10.   Roentgenogram of stomach following ingestion of barium in patient referred to in Figure 8; characteristic mottled transradiant area in prepyloric portion of stomach produced by diospyrobezoar.

as though "forming a cap to something inside the organ," then suddenly diffusing slowly downward on either side of a nonopaque foreign body, following the regular contours of the greater and lesser curvatures to map out the normal contour of the stomach (Fig. 9). At the end of 6 hours, most of the barium has left the stomach, but usually a sufficient amount remains attached to the mass to outline the stomach in a lacelike pattern. Insufflation of the stomach with air may also aid in demonstrating the intragastric character of the foreign body.

Phytobezoars and concretions also have characteristic roentgenologic appearances. With the patient in the erect position, the barium is observed to flow freely into the fundus, and as it enters the pars media it seems to split around a nonopaque body into two columns which join later near the pylorus. As the entire mass becomes coated with barium, it gives a less dense appearance than the barium in the remainder of the stomach (Fig. 10). The free mobility of the mass is readily demonstrated by palpation or by having the patient assume different positions. At the end of 6 to 12 hours, most of the barium has left the stomach, but adherent flecks usually reveal the mass as a reticulated or mottled transradiant area.

DIAGNOSIS

The diagnosis of bezoars can usually be made once the condition is suspected. The diagnosis of trichobezoar is suggested by the characteristic clinical manifestations of a rather large, firm, freely movable epigastric mass accompanied by some pain, nausea, vomiting, anorexia, and loss of weight in girls or young women with a history of trichophagia. The presence of long strands of hair in the stools or gastric contents provides additional evidence. With such a clinical picture, the characteristic fluoroscopic and roentgenological findings should readily indicate the correct diagnosis.

The diagnosis of phytobezoar is based upon the history of the ingestion of persimmons or other plant food and the presence of a freely movable, firm abdominal mass in the epigastrium which is readily displaced beneath the left costal margin, associated with some pain or tenderness and recurrent attacks of nausea and vomiting, loss of weight, and constipation or diarrhea. The characteristic fluoroscopic and roentgenographic findings in the presence of such clinical manifestations should establish the diagnosis. Direct visualization by means of gastroscopy as suggested by Moersch and Walters may be a valuable diagnostic aid, particularly in cases in which the intragastric nature of the mass remains questionable.[19]

COMPLICATIONS

The complications resulting from bezoars include essentially obstruction, ulceration, hemorrhage, perforation, and peritonitis. The most frequent complication is intestinal obstruction, occurring in about 10 percent of patients with trichobezoars and about 25 percent of those with phytobezoars. In the former, it is usually a result of the breaking-off from the main hairball of a small portion which frequently extends through the pylorus into the duodenum and lodges in the terminal ileum. The greater frequency of this complication in phytobezoars is probably caused by the fact that they are more likely to be multiple and of harder consistency. Gastroduodenal ulceration, the next most common complication, occurs only slightly less frequently than intestinal obstruction. Of particular interest is the fact that the characteristics of these ulcers are much the same as those of peptic ulcers. Perforation has occurred in about

one-third of the cases—a particularly serious complication in trichobezoars, as most of these patients died.

TREATMENT

The treatment of large bezoars and concretions is essentially surgical, consisting in operative removal from the stomach and, in cases associated with intestinal obstruction, from the intestines. Although conservative measures directed toward chemical or mechanical disintegration of these foreign bodies may be indicated in certain forms of food boli, they are rarely of any value in true bezoars or concretions and may even be harmful. Small bezoars, however, may occasionally be fragmented through the gastroscope so that the small remaining particles may pass through the gastrointestinal tract.

Certain factors in the surgical management of these cases deserve emphasis. Proper preoperative preparation is important, especially in patients with long-standing bezoars associated with inanition, dehydration, and anemia. The type of abdominal incision may vary and is dependent upon the surgeon's preference. Experience has shown that an upper paramedian or midline incision is quite satisfactory. Special care should be exercised to exclude the abdominal wound and peritoneal cavity by packs placed around the stomach in order to minimize contamination from the intragastric contents. This is particularly important in trichobezoars, which are characterized by an associated slimy, foul, putrid material. Proper use of the suction upon opening the stomach will also aid in carrying out this precaution. The gastrotomy incision should be made on the anterior wall of the stomach at right angles to its longitudinal axis. As the trichobezoar often extends through the pylorus and well into the duodenum, special care should be taken to assure extraction of the entire mass. Similarly, in phytobezoars it is well to bear in mind the frequency of occurrence of more than one mass not only in the stomach but also in the intestines. For this reason, it is important to search the stomach and intestines carefully to assure complete removal of all intragastric and possible intestinal foreign bodies.

In cases associated with simple ulcers, removal of the foreign body is usually sufficient. Experience has shown that following removal of the foreign body most of these ulcers heal satisfactorily and cause no further disturbances. This has been confirmed by Walk, who found good late results in 13 such cases collected from the literature.[28] In the presence of ulcer complications, such as hemorrhage, perforation or penetration, or stenosis, appropriate supportive and surgical measures are indicated, however.

TRANSMURALLY INTRODUCED FOREIGN BODIES

Occasionally foreign bodies enter the stomach or duodenum by passage across the gastrointestinal wall as a result of trauma or ulceration. They may be produced by gunshot wounds or other penetrating injury in which the missile is not removed at the time of the accident and remains in the stomach or duodenum or subsequently migrates across the wall of these organs from adjacent structures. In some instances the foreign body is a surgical instrument, towel, or sponge that was inadvertently overlooked at the time of a previous abdominal operation. Such objects may have been originally placed in the stomach or duodenum or may ulcerate through the wall of these organs from the peritoneal cavity. A number of curious and bizarre cases of this kind have been encountered. Perhaps the most common form of foreign body of this type is produced by migration of gallstones into the stomach or duodenum, usually through the formation of a fistula between these organs and the gallbladder or common bile duct. This occurs more frequently into the duodenum, owing to the closer anatomical relationship of this organ to the biliary tract. In an analysis of 404 collected cases of spontaneous biliary-gastrointestinal fistulas, Lapeyre et al. found that about one half were cholecystoduodenal, almost one fourth choledochoduodenal, about one seventh choledochocolic, and the remainder cholecystogastric or multiple.[18] In most instances, the stones are passed spontaneously through the intestinal tract with few or no symptoms; only about 10 percent or less cause obstruction. In the latter circumstances, the stones may become impacted in the duodenum or at the pylorus, producing obstruction and even perforation; or more commonly they pass beyond this point and tend to become impacted in the terminal ileum.

The clinical manifestations of this type of foreign body in the stomach are variable and depend upon a number of factors including the nature of the object, its method of introduction, and particularly, the development of such complications as ulceration, perforation, peritonitis, and hemorrhage. Roentgenographic examination is the most useful diagnostic procedure.

Treatment consists essentially in operative removal of the foreign body. Additional appropriate measures, such as repair of a constricting pyloric lesion, closure of a perforation, or excision and repair of a fistula, may be necessary in the presence of such complications.

REFERENCES

1. Abel, R. M., Fischer, J. E., and Hendren, W. H., Arch. Surg. 102:227, 1971.
2. Baird, J. M., and Spence, H. M., J. Urol. 99:675, 1968.
3. Barbary, A. S., Foadh, and Fathia, J. Laryngol. Otol. 83:251, 1969.
4. Chalk, S. G., and Foucar, H. O., Arch. Surg. 16:494, 1928.
5. Clairmont, P., and Haudek, M. (Minutes of a case presentation at a meeting) Offizielles Protokoll de K. K. Gesellschaft de Aerzte in Wien. Sitzung von 5. Mai, 1911.
6. Clerf, L. H., Surg. Clin. North Am. 14:77, 1934.
7. DeBakey, M. E., and Ochsner, A., Surgery 4:934, 1938; and 5:132, 1939.
8. Gross, R. E. Bronchoscopy, Esophagoscopy and Gastroscopy. Philadelphia, Saunders, 1953.
9. Henderson, F. F., and Gaston, A., Arch. Surg. 36:66, 1938.
10. Holland, C. T., Arch. Roentg. Ray. 18:373, 1914.
11. Izumi, S., Isida, K., and Iwamoto, M., Jap. J. Med. Sci. Biol. 2:21, 1933.
12. Jackson, C., Laryngoscope 15:257, 1905.
13. Jackson, C., and Jackson, C. L. Bronchoscopy, Esophagoscopy and Gastroscopy. Philadelphia, Saunders, 1953.
14. Johnson, W. E., J.A.M.A. 208:2163, 1969.
15. Kampmann, E., München Med. Wochenschr. 58:413, 1911.
16. Katsas, A. G., Arch. Surg. 96:929, 1968.
17. Ladd, W. E., and Gross, R. E., Bronchoscopy, Esophagoscopy and Gastroscopy. Philadelphia, Saunders, 1941.
18. Lapeyre, N. C., Joyeux, R., and Carabalona, P., J. Chir. 67:568, 1951.

19. Moersch, H. J., and Walters, W., Am. J. Dig. Dis. Nut. 3:15, 1936.
20. Morris, G., Delayed perforation of the internal carotid artery by an ingested foreign body. Br. J. Surg. 56:711, 1969.
21. Norman, M. G., and Cass, E., Pediatrics 48:832, 1971.
22. Ramsbottom, A., and Barclay, A. E., Arch. Roentg. Ray. 18:167, 1913.
23. Silber, S., Kaplan, C., and Epstein, B., Ann. Otol. Rhinol. Larynol. 53:589, 1944.
24. Symbas, P. N., Ann. Surg. 167:78, 1968.
25. Tondreau, R. L., and Kirklin, B. R., Surg. Clin. North Am. 30:1097, 1950.
26. Tucker, G. F., Mod. Treat. 7:1301, 1970.
27. Vella, E. E., and Booth, P. J., Br. Med. J. 2:1042, 1965.
28. Walk, L., Arch. Intern. Med. 84:824, 1949.

6

INFANTILE PYLORIC STENOSIS
Ramstedt's Pyloromyotomy

RODNEY MAINGOT

Hypertrophic pyloric stenosis is the most common condition calling for surgical measures during the first few weeks of life.

AETIOLOGY

The *incidence* of congenital hypertrophic pyloric stenosis is most difficult to determine with accuracy, owing to the widely diverse reports given by various hospitals, but Downes estimates its occurrence as being 1 in every 200 male births, while others place it at 1 in every 200 births regardless of sex.

According to Cockayne and Penrose [4] this abnormality is caused by transmission of a faulty gene. If this view is correct, with a greater number of affected children now reaching maturity as a result of successful treatment, the incidence may be expected to rise, and the condition therefore may well assume an even greater importance in the future than in the past.

The condition was first accurately described by Maier,[9] shortly before Hirschsprung's clinical account.

The disease is strikingly *more frequent in the male than in the female sex,* as is shown in a total of 1,664 cases reported by 13 different authors. There were 1,462 males (88 percent) against 202 females (12 percent). Ladd et al.[6] stated that males predominate in all reported series. At the Children's Hospital, Boston, approximately 85 percent of the cases occurred in male infants, and this percentage is about the same at the present date.

No one has ever offered a satisfactory explanation of this overwhelming incidence. Romano and McFetridge pointed out that this is out of all proportion to the incidence of male and female births and that it is also entirely beyond any reasonable explanation.

Still was one of the first to remark on the frequency with which *first-born children* are affected, Barrington-Ward placing the incidence in his cases at 60 percent, Malmberg at 64 percent, and Ladd at 55 percent. Wallace and Wevill, by a number of control studies, have shown that this preponderance is real and not merely apparent.

More than one infant in a family may be affected. Bidderback [3] and others reported the condition in twins, and Tribble [16] and David Levi [7] record multiple cases in the same family.

The condition occurs most frequently in breast-fed babies, but it is doubtful that this factor has any aetiological significance.

A large number of *theories* has been brought forward to explain the cause of infantile pyloric stenosis, but at present there does not seem to be any general agreement on the subject, which may be regarded as one of only academic interest. There are three principal views held to explain the condition: (1) that the pyloric hypertrophy is caused by spasm (Thomson); (2) that there is a primary or *congenital* developmental overgrowth of the circular coat of the pylorus with a consequent reduction in the pyloric lumen (Hirschsprung); and (3) work hypertrophy. The views of Lehman (quoted by Szilagyi and McGraw [15]) are interesting in this regard, as he considers that work hypertrophy results as the pyloric muscle attempts to overcome a resistant sphincter; that the development of the neuromuscular plexus has been delayed; and that the pyloric sphincter fails to relax and consequently hypertrophies.

The fact that several cases have been reported in which the tumour has been present from birth and even in premature babies militates against this view. There is no racial disposition to the condition.

PATHOLOGY

The most striking feature is the pyloric tumour, which is due to an abnormal overgrowth of the circular muscle. The tumour is felt as a tensely hard cartilaginous mass which is olive- or barrel-shaped, varying from 1.5 to 2 cm in length and 1 cm in diameter. It is interesting to note that in the early cases the tumour is small and pinkish, while in the later stages it becomes whiter, the peritoneum over it being stretched to the utmost capacity. When the tumour is incised, it will grate to the knife, and it will be found that the circular coat of the pylorus is as much as 3 or 4 times its normal thickness. The tumour terminates very abruptly at the pyloric outlet and projects into the duodenum as the cervix projects into the vagina. When the duodenal mucous membrane is reflected onto the tumour, a definite fornix is formed, and it is at this point that perforation of the duodenum may occur during pyloromyotomy. The thickening of the pylorus, although abrupt at the duodenal end, gradually thins out as it is traced into the antrum (see Fig. 9).

When the stomach is opened at autopsy, it will be found to be dilated, with gastritis a notable feature. In the pyloric region, the mucous membrane is crammed into a very narrow space and thrown into longitudinal folds. Wollstein [17] has shown that after operation healing occurs slowly by contraction of the fibrous tissues of the serous and submucous coats, and that the stomach and pyloric regions return to their normal size in about 3 months. If the pylorus is carefully examined after this time, only the faintest linear scar will be discernible. The duodenum is normal in every respect.

Armitage and Rhind [1] reported a case of stomal ulcer following gastrojejunostomy for congenital hypertrophic pyloric stenosis for which partial gastrectomy was performed. Examination of the excised specimen showed that the pyloric tumour had persisted into adult life.

The writer [10] reported the case of a boy with infantile pyloric stenosis who was treated by posterior gastrojejunostomy at the age of 6 weeks. Thirty-seven years later, partial gastrectomy by the Billroth II method was carried out for gastrojejunocolic fistula. In this case, too, the resected specimen showed that the pyloric tumour had persisted.

CLINICAL PICTURE

In most cases the child is healthy and of normal weight at birth. Occasionally, however, he may be below or above normal weight. The first symptoms usually appear between the first week to 10 days or after 2 to 3 weeks. I treated one infant who commenced vomiting on the second day after birth; at operation 2 days later, a typical tumour was found and this was treated by pyloromyotomy. Gross found from a study of his large series of cases that the majority of the patients were 3 to 4 weeks old at the time of admission to hospital for treatment. In the average case, all appears to be progressing satisfactorily until about the end of the first or second week, when it will be noted that instead of gaining weight the child is actually losing, the bowel actions are somewhat irregular, and there may be an occasional attack of vomiting. From then onward the symptoms daily become worse, and vomiting, which is always the first and most important of all the symptoms, is a most troublesome feature. In the early stages, the vomiting may be described as slight, and occurs after feeding. It will give the mother or the nurse the impression that the child is being overfed or that the wrong diet is being prescribed. With a change in the diet there may be a temporary improvement; but this is soon followed by regurgitation of food, small quantities and mucus-laden opalescent fluid welling up into the mouth from time to time and trickling down the cheeks. Later, larger amounts are vomited at longer intervals, and then the vomiting becomes definitely *projectile*. The child is seized with a sudden spasm, and a large quantity of fluid is forcibly projected a distance through the mouth and nostrils. *This type of explosive vomiting is seen in no other condition, with the possible exception of congenital duodenal atresia.* Projectile vomiting is present in from 90 to 96 percent of the cases. In the final stages, when the stomach becomes flabby and atonic, projectile vomiting ceases, being replaced by the effortless overflow of gastric content. The vomitus is never bile-stained, although it may be tinted yellow because of the type of formula or vitamins being offered the baby. The attacks of vomiting are not usually preceded or accompanied by pain; there is, for instance, no screaming or drawing up of the legs such as is seen in cases of intestinal colic or simple curd indigestion, and the vomiting appears to produce little discomfort. The appetite is always voracious, but seems to diminish just before each attack of vomiting. As soon as the child has voided the contents of the stomach, he will eagerly and keenly take more food.

The bowels, as in most cases of pyloric obstruction, are constipated in fully 80 percent of cases. In the remaining 20 percent, they may be normal or there may even be diarrhoea. Diarrhoea denotes that infection is present, and this type does not differ from other types of infective diarrhoea of infancy. The movements are small and green-brown in colour, there being little faecal matter but large quantities of mucus. Persistent vomiting causes a rapid loss of weight. As a result of this loss of weight and the dehydration produced by vomiting, the skin becomes dry, thrown into folds, and inelastic. In a marked case the face becomes pale, ashen grey, or slightly cyanosed, the brow is furrowed, the nose pinched, and the cheek bones prominent. Wrinkles appear around the eyes and the corners of the mouth and the neck, and the child presents the peculiar wizened, shriv-

elled mien of a very old person. The eyeballs may be soft and the fontanelles sunken. It should be noted here that the greater the loss of weight the worse the prognosis, as this implies that the disease has been present for some considerable time without having been recognised.

Tetany may appear in late cases, while jaundice has been noted in a number of instances.[14]

When the abdomen is examined, it will be seen that the upper half is bulging and domelike, while the lower half is empty and flaccid. *Visible waves of peristalsis* will be observed in every genuine case, sweeping from the left costal margin across the epigastrium to disappear at the outer border of the right rectus muscle. These waves will outline the position of the stomach, and the point where they disappear will indicate the position of the pylorus. It is here therefore that the tumour is to be sought. The visible peristalsis is specially marked after a feeding or after stroking or tickling the skin over the left rectus muscle in its upper half.

The surgeon should have some definite scheme for palpating the abdomen to locate the tumour. The best time to palpate the tumour is immediately after the infant has vomited, which empties the bloated stomach and facilitates examination. The child should be taken from the cot, placed on the nurse's knee, and given a drink of sweetened water. The abdomen is exposed and the knees are slightly drawn up to relax the abdominal wall. The surgeon then places his well-warmed left hand below the right costal margin and gradually presses the fingers in an upward, inward, and backward direction, aiming to press the pylorus against the spinal column. He should particularly note the exact point at which the peristaltic waves stop, and search this region very carefully with the tips of his fingers in order to locate the tumour. It may take a considerable time before the tumour is felt, in fact when the stomach is very full it may be impossible to do so at all. In such cases the stomach should be emptied with a small nasogastric tube and another attempt be made. If this fails, further palpation is advised when the peristaltic waves are more vigourous. A tumour is palpable in 85 to 90 percent of cases, and visible peristalsis is observed in from 75 to

85 percent. The surgeon should be careful not to confuse the lower pole of the right kidney with the tumour.

If all the symptoms point to a diagnosis of infantile pyloric stenosis and if after repeated examinations no tumour is palpable, the child should be anaesthetised and a final examination conducted, after the gastric contents have been evacuated with a nasogastric tube. The value of these repeated examinations in a difficult case cannot be too strongly stressed. The more conversant the surgeon is with this disease the more easily palpable will be the tumour, and the later the case the more readily will the mass be felt. The tumour is often described as being acorn-shaped, the size of a hazelnut or small olive, as hard as a lymph node, like the tip of a finger, and so forth. It is, as I have said, most readily felt after the infant has vomited or during a severe spasm, and it may seem to disappear when the child is quiescent.

In connection with a barium meal x-ray examination as an aid to diagnosis in hypertrophic pyloric stenosis, Ladd [6] makes these important observations:

The more facile one becomes in palpating a pyloric tumor, the fewer will be the indications for roentgen confirmation of the diagnosis. A plain film of the abdomen may be of no value if the baby has just vomited. The administration of a thin barium mixture is therefore desirable in obscure cases, but not without danger owing to the possibilities of aspiration. If examination shows almost complete retention, a tube should be then passed and the barium removed.

The essential roentgen features of diagnosis are (1) gastric dilatation, (2) intermittent hyperperistalsis, (3) a greatly elongated pyloric canal which is only 2 to 3 mm. in width and (4) delayed gastric emptying time. Retention of over 75 percent of a barium meal at the end of three hours indicates definite pyloric obstruction.

DIFFERENTIAL DIAGNOSIS

The diagnosis depends chiefly upon feeling the tumour, as this is found in no other infantile condition.

The projectile vomiting, the visible peristalsis, the marked constipation which is usually present, and the palpable tumour, all afford such a typical picture that the condition should be most readily recognised.

Occasionally *pylorospasm* may be a cause of difficulty in diagnosis, but in such cases there is quick response to treatment and no tumour can be felt. In *congenital duodenal atresia* and in *malrotation of the colon,* the obstructing agent is present at birth and the baby starts vomiting shortly after birth. Bile may be found in the vomitus, and here again, no tumour is palpable.

A barium meal x-ray examination is of considerable help in indicating the site of the obstruction. In *gastritis,* although there may be frequent attacks of vomiting in which large quantities of mucus are brought up, the vomiting is never projectile and there is no visible peristalsis. Other features include diarrhoea, poor appetite, and urine that is loaded with urates and chlorides. *Internal hernia* and *volvulus* and other such rarities may at times cause confusion in diagnosis. *Intracranial injury or haemorrhagic disease* is a cause of vomiting and may have to be considered in the differential diagnosis. It should be noted, however, that in these conditions the surgeon is likely to find other evidence of neurological disorders, such as spasticity, convulsions, bulging fontanelles, or possibly bloodstained fluid following spinal puncture. *Congenital heart disease or other anomalies* may be rarely associated with infantile pyloric stenosis.

TREATMENT

In a diagnosed case, Ramstedt's operation of pyloromyotomy for relief of the obstruction is the accepted method of management.

Dr. Robert E. Gross has collected the data shown in Table 1 from the Children's Hospital, Boston. In recent personal communication (1971), Dr. Gross writes:

Regarding the Ramstedt's procedure, I checked up our statistics and find that from January 1, 1953 through the year 1966 there were 928 operations for pyloromyotomy. During this time there were nine deaths. We like to think of this as an operation which carries practically no mortality and very rare morbidity and of course, things do really go along very well. The fact remains though, that in a hospital such as ours, we do have—along with much excellent material —an occasional youngster who has some pretty complicated problems. Hence, we do have the occasional loss of a pyloric child, from cardiac anomaly, some other intestinal abnormality, or some condition which far overshadows the picture of pyloric obstruction. *For the three years, 1964 through 1966, there were 188 pyloromyotomies, with no fatalities.*

For the 5 years beginning 1967 through 1971 there were 274 pyloromyotomies. There were no deaths. (Table 1.)

Table 1.   SUMMARY OF RESULTS IN 2,097 CASES OF PYLORIC STENOSIS TREATED BY RAMSTEDT OPERATION

Years	Number of Cases	Deaths	Mortality (percent)
1915-22	125	13	10.4
1923-28	150	11	7.3
1929-31	151	3	2.0
1932-35	162	8	4.9
1936-39	177	1	0.6
1940-45	380	4	1.0
1946-50	490	4	0.3
1964-66	188	0	0
1967-71	274	0	0

Source: R.E. Gross, Children's Hospital, Boston, Mass.

FACTORS THAT HAVE REDUCED THE OPERATIVE MORTALITY

1. The recognition that early operation is the treatment of choice. The longer the duration of the symptoms and the lower the weight at the time of operation, the higher the mortality. This is indeed a strong plea for early diagnosis and early operation.

2. The adoption of preoperative treatment. This includes:

   (a) Careful intensive preparation of the patient for a period of at least 2 days before operation is undertaken. These cases should not be regarded as surgical emergencies or be operated upon without due preparation. Isolation of these undernourished babies is an essential feature in management.

   (b) Body fluid loss and chemical deficiency are restored by giving small frequent nourishing feedings of 5 percent glucose in water up to 2 hours before operation, by the administration of intravenous glucose-saline solutions, and, if necessary, by blood transfusions. The small feedings are given every 2 hours and should be rich in sugars, proteins, vitamin C, and salts.

With regard to preoperative preparation of the patient, Benson and Lloyd [2] favour the following routine. I quote from them:

Infants admitted to the hospital with a minimal or moderate degree of dehydration and alkalosis can be prepared by the oral route alone. In our institution, 5 percent dextrose in 0.33 percent normal saline solution in amounts up to 3 ounces is offered every two hours. When a satisfactory state of hydration is reached, 3 to 4 mEq. of potassium chloride is added to every second or third bottle, not to exceed 4 mEq. per kilogram per day. We have used this regimen in a limited number of patients and it has proved quite satisfactory. However, the preoperative preparation of most patients in our series has been managed by the administration of intravenous fluids. The stomach is emptied of curds and barium by careful saline lavage and oral fluids are withheld. Routinely 5 percent dextrose solution in 0.33 percent normal saline solution is administered, usually by a scalp vein. The amount of infusion varies from 60 to 90 cc. per pound of body weight per day, depending on the degree of dehydration. When adequate urinary output has been established, 10 mEq. of *potassium chloride* is added to every 250 cc. of solution. We never exceed a concentration of 40 mEq. per liter unless there is electrocardiographic evidence of a severe potassium deficiency. Laboratory data obtained on admission are usually limited to a complete blood count, urinalysis, serum chloride and carbon dioxide determination.

With breast-fed babies, the mother is instructed to pump her breasts during the preoperative period because the infant will be back on the breast by the afternoon of the day of operation.

   (c) In every case a small nasogastric tube is passed through the nostril into the stomach, and the stomach is aspirated and irrigated with normal saline solution. The lavage should be performed routinely 1 hour before operation. This reduces gaseous distention, thus rendering operation more simple; it rids the stomach of much mucus and decomposing food; and it tends to alleviate the gastritis that is always present. The catheter should be left in situ during the operation to keep the stomach deflated.

(d) Precautions are taken to prevent loss of body heat before, during, and after operation. The operating room should be specially heated to not less than 75°F, and the operating table itself may with advantage be warmed.

(e) Premedication. Morphine should not be administered because of its depressing effects on the respiratory system. Atropine should be given, 0.7 mg intramusculary, about 30 minutes before operation.

(f) *General anaesthesia* is the method of choice, although in a few desperately ill infants local anaesthesia by the infiltration method using a 0.5 percent solution of procaine, may be employed.

3. The universal acceptance of the Ramstedt operation as the technical procedure of choice. The best guarantee of a good and dependable operation for the cure of any condition demanding operative interference is its worldwide acceptance.

The popularity of the Ramstedt operation for infantile hypertrophic pyloric stenosis has remained unchallenged for over half a century. Before the advent of this operation the majority of cases were treated medically with a mortality of about 80 percent. The crude and complicated operations which preceded the Ramstedt method had such a damning mortality that the claims of medical therapy were richly strengthened. All these operations lacked the ease, simplicity, speed and security of Ramstedt's method. Pylorectomy had a mortality of 100 percent, the Heineke-Mikulicz procedure was associated with a death rate of close to 95 percent, gastrojejunostomy certainly not less than 50 percent, while Pietro Loreta's operation of instrumental avulsion of the pyloric tumour was a lethal undertaking except in the very safe and capable hands of Burghard. Fredet obtained better results by longitudinal division of the thickened muscles of the pylorus, but he prolonged and complicated the operation by transverse suture of the margins of the severed friable muscle, which is almost incapable of efficient closure in this way. Ramstedt, in attempting Fredet's operation upon an emaciated infant, was unable to complete the *transverse* suture of the divided pyloric muscular mass owing to the sudden collapse of the patient. He rapidly replaced the stomach in the abdominal cavity and hastily inserted a few through-and-through stitches to close the abdominal wall. The child was then returned to the ward in a moribund condition, but to Ramstedt's surprise and gratification a splendid recovery followed and he had the good sense to appreciate the fact that simple longitudinal division of the tumour, allowing full protrusion of the mucous membrane of the pyloric canal, was all that was necessary to effect a cure, and he had the courage of his convictions to repeat this method in subsequent cases with most satisfactory results.

(As regards the spelling of Ramstedt's name, which, it will be noted, varies in different articles and journals, apparently he originally used the form Rammstedt and that is the one he was using when he published his original article in 1912. Following an investigation he made of family records, in 1920 he changed the spelling of his name to Ramstedt. This accounts for the fact that in modern editions of medical dictionaries the spelling is given with a single m.)

4. A well-planned scheme of postoperative treatment is essential. In Britain most of the cases are handed over to the care of a physician-pediatrician who supervises both the preoperative and postoperative treatment.

Hugh B. Lynn [8] summarises the essential points of postoperative feedings, as follows:

Within two hours of the operation these infants seem to be completely recovered from the effects of the anesthetic and are hungry and making vigorous sucking efforts. Sugar water is safest for the first few feedings. Dextrose in water is given as desired during the day of operation and will prepare the infant for full formula feedings the following morning. Breast feedings are restarted the afternoon of the operation.

About 50 percent of these infants vomit postoperatively. This should stop by the fourth, fifth, or sixth postoperative day and should not recur.

THE RAMSTEDT OPERATION

Procedure

The upper and lower limbs are wrapped in cotton wool and lightly swathed. The child is then bandaged to a wooden

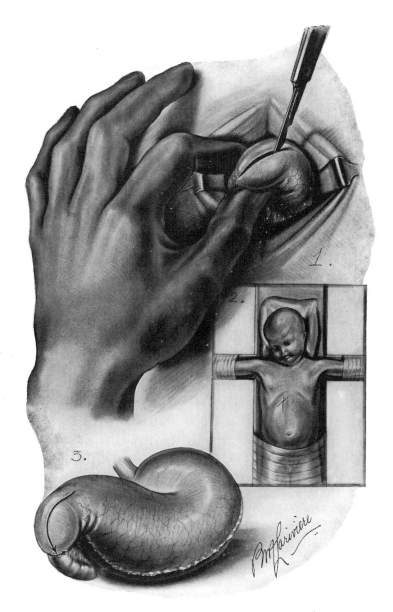

FIG. 1.   Ramstedt's operation of pyloromyotomy. (1) Method of steadying pyloric tumour and of making incision through seromuscular layer. (2) Position of child on operating table and choice of incision—vertical or subcostal. (3) Small *arrow* marks pyloroduodenal junction while large *arrow* indicates position of incision for pyloromyotomy.

cross which is well padded with soft spongy rubber. A small air cushion is placed under the lower ribs to throw the epigastric region forward and to render the pyloric zone more accessible. The abdomen and lower half of the chest are painted with warm Humerosal (tincture of Merthiolate solution), after which the operative field is rapidly draped.

There is a choice of many incisions, some of which are vertical and others transverse. *Vertical incisions* include the midline, the paramedian, and the vertical muscle-splitting (Fig. 1). The *transverse incision* is made just below the costal margin, through the body

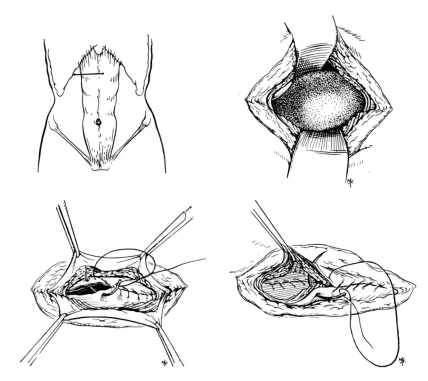

FIG. 2.   Transverse epigastric incision for Ramstedt's operation.

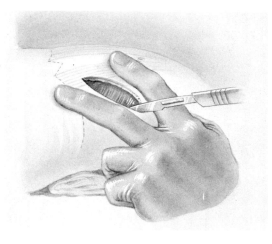

FIG. 3.   The gridiron incision. The incision is made one finger breadth below and parallel to the costal margin. The external oblique fibres are then divided in line of the incision.

of the right rectus muscle. It affords excellent exposure and decreases the likelihood of any extrusion of the omentum, colon, or small intestine if the child strains during the operation. Again, being transversely placed, there is very little tension and the suturing of such an incision is consequently a simple matter (Fig. 2).

Randolph [13] has given an account, The Evolution of an Ideal Surgical Incision for Pyloric Stenosis, in which he discusses the standard right paramedian incision, the McBurney type subcostal incision with muscle-splitting, and the transverse incision with rectus transection.

I have no hesitation in stating that by far the best incision to employ for pyloromyotomy is the gridiron (McBurney) incision placed one finger breadth below the right costal margin, as the grave complication of dehiscence is eliminated. Figures 3 and 4 clearly depict the essential steps of the gridiron incision.

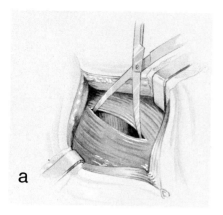

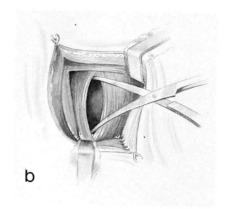

a

b

FIG. 4. (A) Gridiron incision. The internal oblique fibres are divided toward the upper and medial end of the incision.

FIG. 4. (B) Transversus abdominal muscle fibres split, and peritoneum can be seen beneath.

The transversus muscle and peritoneum must be very carefully picked up before incising them transversely, as it is so easy inadvertently to wound the underlying liver. The liver should be hooked upward with a small, malleable, ribbon retractor, and the pyloric region of the stomach grasped with non-toothed dissecting forceps and coaxed into the wound, aided by gentle manipulation with the fingers. The pyloric tumour should then be fixed with the thumb and index finger of the left hand, the tips being placed underneath the tumour and adjacent duodenum to prevent the tumour from slipping

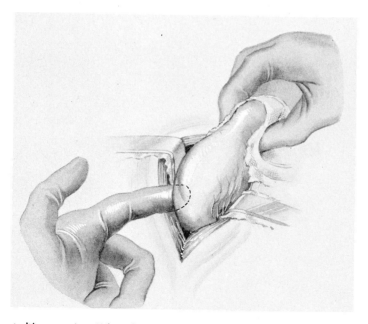

FIG. 5.   Ramstedt's operation. When the pylorus is drawn through the wound and is steadied by the assistant, the surgeon places his left index finger against the tumour, and retractors are not needed.

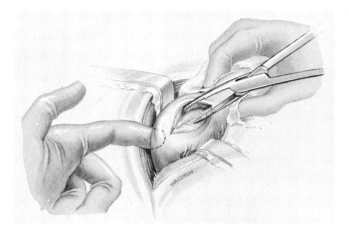

FIG. 6. Ramstedt's operation. Note the surgeon's left index finger supporting the pyloric tumour. When the division is complete, as shown in Figures 8 and 9, the end of the pyloric ring, which the surgeon is pressing in an upward direction, will lose its definite ring and become soft and poorly defined.

back into the abdomen (Fig. 5). It is then firmly gripped and rotated slightly to the left so that the anterior aspect of the tumour, the commencement of the duodenum, and the antrum are clearly visible. *The tip of the surgeon's left forefinger should press against the end of the pylorus to stabilise the tumour and also to point out clearly its termination* (Fig. 6).

A longitudial incision should then be made in the hypertrophied area at the junction of the middle and upper thirds of the anterosuperior aspect where the blood vessels seem to be scarce (Figs. 1 and 6). This incision, which should be ½ to 1 inch (1.3 to 2.5 cm) long, is slightly curved, with its concavity downward, starting just proximal to

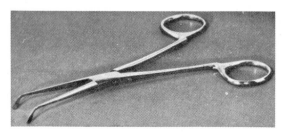

FIG. 7. Pyloric spreader for Ramstedt's operation, as used by Benson and Lloyd.

the pyloric vein of Mayo, which indicates the gastroduodenal junction, and being carried through the serosal and superficial muscular coats over the pyloric tumour and a little beyond it upward into the antrum of the stomach. Using the handle of the knife, or better yet, by employing the so-called pyloric spreader as used by Benson and Lloyd (Fig. 7), one widely separates the muscle fibres throughout the length of the incision until the glistening white mucous membrane is visible and eventually bulges through the gap (Figs. 6 and 8). A little gentle stretching of the fibres with a haemostat or a pyloric spreader, as is well shown in Figure 8 [5], and a little cautious dissection here and there, may be necessary to make absolutely sure that all constricting fibres, particularly those close to the gastroduodenal junction, have been severed and that an efficient patency is ensured. This part of the dissection is simple, as the thickened circular coat rapidly springs apart, producing an oval wound in the pyloric region of the stomach, the base of which is formed by the tough mucous membrane of the pyloric canal. A width of at least ½ inch (1.3 cm) of mucosa must be exposed in the centre of the incision.

As soon as the patency of the pylorus has been assured, a hot compress is firmly applied to the cut surface in the pyloric region to

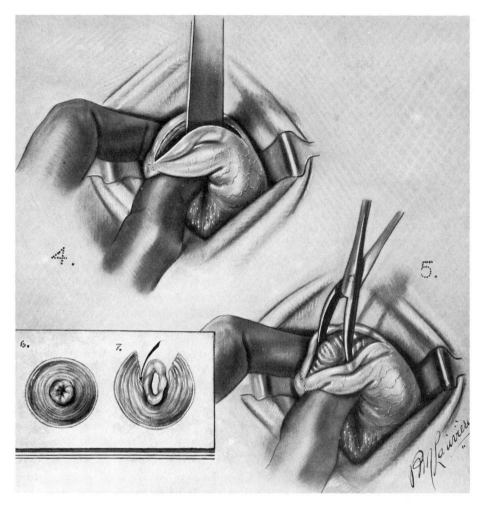

FIG. 8.   The Ramstedt operation of pyloromyotomy. (4) Thickened muscles of the pyloric region are being separated with the handle of a knife. (5) Mucous membrane is made to gape widely into the wound through incision into the pylorus. (6) Transverse section of the pyloric tumour. (7) Dilated pyploric canal after division of muscle fibres.

arrest any oozing, which is usually trivial. No attempt should be made to stop the bleeding, which is usually venous, mild, and temporary.

It is always a wise precaution to make sure that the duodenum has not been punctured at the fornix (Fig. 9). In most cases, such a mishap is immediately recognised by the escape of a few drops of glary, blood-stained fluid. In other cases, by compressing the body of the stomach, air can be forced into the duodenum and if a small perforation exists, this can be detected by the hiss of air through the aperture. Such perforations should be closed immediately with sutures of fine chromic catgut and the area protected with a wisp of omentum. This added precaution does not in any way detract from the completeness of the success of the operation. If the duodenum has been accidentally opened, it is a wise measure to keep the baby on *nasogastric suction* for 72 hours after the operation before starting any feedings. If the puncture is not recognised at the time of the operation, peritonitis will, of course, develop. Therefore, when the surgeon has made quite

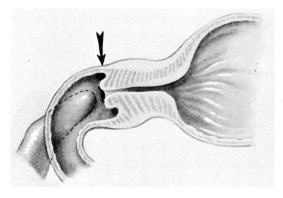

FIG. 9. Ramstedt's operation. Note the critical zone (the fornix). It is at this point (indicated by the arrow) where the protrusion of hypertrophic muscle into the lumen of the duodenum creates a critical zone of folded duodenal muscle.

sure that the pyloric outlet is widely patent, that there is no bleeding, and that no perforation of the duodenal mucous membrane exists, the stomach is returned to the abdominal cavity and the wound closed in layers with a 5–0 running chronic catgut suture to unite the peritoneum and the edges of the transversus muscle together. Several 6–0 Mersiline, interrupted sutures are used to approximate the edges of the internal and external oblique muscles. The skin is closed with a subcuticular stitch of 4–0 Ethilon or with Micropore strips. No dressing is used.

Postoperative Complications

These are best classified into two main groups:
1. Surgical
   a. Wound sepsis
   b. Dehiscence of the wound
   c. Incisional hernia
   d. Incomplete operation
   e. Haemorrhage
   f. Peritonitis
   g. Acute otitis media
2. Medical
   a. Diarrhoea
   b. Pneumonitis
   c. Postoperative collapse of the lung

Wound sepsis, stitch abscess, dehiscence of

the wound, and ventral hernia occur in a small but sufficiently significant number of cases to imply that modern operative technique is not always infallible.

An incomplete operation, which is due to inadequate division of the constricting pyloric muscular fibres, especially near the dangerous fornix, blatantly declares itself by the return of stubborn vomiting after the sixth postoperative day. The surgeon should be quick to realise the true state of affairs and not lull himself into the belief that the vomiting is caused by postanaesthetic sickness. He must act promptly: the abdomen must be reopened, and, after drawing the pylorus through the wound, the constricting fibres concerned must be freely but cautiously severed.

The grave complication of diarrhoea, which is so often caused by bacterial enteritis, is rarely observed in modern pediatric hospitals. Nevertheless sporadic cases are seen and these patients require prompt treatment which includes the correction of dehydration, anaemia, alkalosis, malnutrition, and potassium deficiencies, as well as the cautious administration of such potent antibiotics as neomycin and kanamycin.

Pneumonia and other chest complications do not occur in more than 1 to 2 percent of cases, and can usually be avoided by good nursing.

Acute otitis media occurs in some 2 percent of cases after pyloromyotomy, but this complication does not appear to affect the prognosis in any way. It is probably caused by vomiting, the eustachian tubes becoming blocked by gastric contents or becoming infected through use of a stomach tube.

REFERENCES

1. Armitage and Rhind, Br. J. Surg. 39:39, 1951.
2. Benson and Lloyd, Am. J. Surg. 107:429, 1964.
3. Bilderback, Northwest Med. 27:182, 1928.
4. Cockayne and Penrose, Lancet 1:898, 1934.
5. Fredet, Rev. Chir. Paris 37:208, 1908.
6. Ladd et al., J.A.M.A. 131:647, 1946.
7. Levi, D., Postgrad. Med. 26:24, 1950.
8. Lynn, H. B., Operative Surgery, Rob and Smith, eds., 2d ed., Vol. 4. P. 55. Butterworth
9. Maier, Virchows Arch. Path. Anat. 102:413, 1885.
10. Maingot, Lancet 2:910, 1952.
11. Ramstedt, Med. Klin. 8:1702, 1912.
12. Ramstedt, Zbl. Chir. 39:1741, 1912.

13. Randolph, Arch. Surg. 93:489, 1966.
14. Rhea, Headrick, and Stephenson, Surgery 51: 687, 1962.
15. Szilagyi and McGraw, Surgery 13:764, 1943.
16. Tribble, J.A.M.A. 101:278, 1933.
17. Wollstein, Am. J. Dis. Child. 22:512, 1922.

7

GASTRIC AND DUODENAL DIVERTICULA

RODNEY MAINGOT

Gastric and duodenal diverticula should no longer be regarded as surgical or pathological curiosities. Owing to worldwide improvements in diagnostic methods (especially in radiology), a more scrupulous performance of autopsies, and a more painstaking and searching scrutiny of the viscera as displayed at exploratory operation, it has been proved that diverticula occur more frequently than was formerly supposed and must now be reckoned in the differential diagnosis of upper abdominal diseases.

Feldman [10] stated that in 10,923 cases, barium-meal x-ray examination revealed 328 cases with diverticula involving all portions of the gastrointestinal tract. The oesophagus was involved in 2.8 percent; stomach, 0.9 percent; duodenum, 31.4 percent; jejunum and ileum, 0.9 percent, and colon, 63.5 percent. Diverticula thus occur in different parts of the alimentary canal in the following order of frequency: (1) large bowel, (2) duodenum, (3) oesophagus, and (4) stomach and jejunoileum.

Although gastric and duodenal diverticula have certain features in common, it is here deemed preferable to discuss them separately.

GASTRIC DIVERTICULA

Historical Note

On Voigtel's authority (*Handbuch der pathologische Anatomie*, Halle, 1804, p. 512), it is frequently stated in papers relating to gastric diverticula that Van Helmont was the first to report this condition; but the claim of any individual to priority in recording any known pathological lesion or in performing any surgical procedure is always most difficult to establish and can rarely be placed beyond dispute. For instance, while Van Helmont (1804) is credited with being the first to describe a divetriculum of the stomach, Thomas Baillie (*The Morbid Anatomy of Some of the Most Important Parts of the Human Body*, 1793, Chapter 7, p. 92) gave an accurate account of this very abnormality. He wrote:

"A part of the stomach is occasionally formed into a pouch by mechanical means, although very rarely. I have seen one instance of a pouch being so formed, in which five halfpence had been lodged. The coats of the stomach were thinner at that part, but were not inflamed or ulcerated. The halfpence had remained there for some considerable time, forming a pouch by their pressure, but had not irritated the stomach in such a manner as to produce inflammation or ulceration."

Reich (*Amer J Dig Dis 8*:70, 1941) considers that the credit of the discovery of gastric diverticula as a pathological entity should be given to Fournier (1774), while Moses (*Arch Surg 52*:59, 1946) states that the first case was undoubtedly reported by Moebius in 1661.

Pathology

AETIOLOGY

The aetiology of gastrointestinal diverticulosis is not clearly understood, and this confusion is reflected in the nomenclature and classifications that exist to describe the lesions. Adjectives employed more or less synonymously are *true, primary,* and *congenital*. These describe diverticula, which are usually composed of all layers of the gastric or intestinal wall and are probably present from birth. By way of contrast are the *false, pseudo, secondary,* or *acquired* diverticula, which may be found in a breaking-down neoplasm, a penetrating ulcer, from

129

the traction of adhesions, or the pulsion of mucosa through a weakened muscular wall. Diverticula in the stomach may in fact be false, secondary, or acquired, or contain all the layers of the gastric wall with no obvious underlying cause (true, primary, or congenital). This section is mainly concerned with the so-called true diverticula.

INCIDENCE

The incidence of gastric diverticulum is unknown, but the reported incidence covers a wide range, varying between 0.01 percent and 2.6 percent. Palmer,[25] in a searching review, was able to collect 412 cases from the literature. One hundred and sixty-five of these were diagnosed during 380,099 routine barium-meal x-ray examinations—an incidence of 0.043 percent. Meeroff [19] collected a series of his own of 30 cases from 7,500 radiological examinations, an incidence of 0.4 percent—this is, 10 times higher than that of Palmer. Whatever the true incidence, it is fair to say that gastric diverticula are distinctly rare.

The lesion is more common in women than in men. For instance, 17 of 19 patients reported by Bigg and Judd from the Mayo Clinic [5] were women, and all three of Young's patients were women.[32]

These diverticula have been found at all ages but most of them have been discovered in patients between the ages of 20 and 60. In Palmer's series, 214 out of 267 patients presenting with symptoms during life came within these ages, an incidence of 80 percent. As might be expected with a congenital lesion, however, the condition may be manifest at a much earlier age; Neil Sinclair [27] reported a case of a 4-month-old child upon whom he successfully operated for a diverticulum of the fundus of the stomach.

The most common site for a gastric diverticulum is the cardiac region. Eighty percent of Meeroff's patients and 86 percent of those reported by Bigg and Judd had juxtacardiac diverticula. Juxtapyloric diverticula account for almost all the remainder.

Gastric diverticula vary in size and shape but are usually saccular or tubular in form. They may be as small as a pea or as large as a lemon. The majority of the recorded cases have measured from less than 1 inch to almost 2½ inches (1 to 6 cm) in diameter. The diameter of the opening also varies considerably, and may be large enough to admit one or more fingers, or be so attenuated as to allow the introduction of only the finest probe. The usual size of the ostium was between 2 and 4 cm in the series recorded by Bigg and Judd. The size of the opening is important, because, when it is large, the gastric contents can enter and leave the pouch without producing any stagnation. When small, however, it may easily be missed on x-ray screening owing to the inability of the opaque substance to enter the sac. Again, retention of food with subsequent decomposition and inflammatory change is prone to take place when the stalk is narrow.

COMPLICATIONS

Complications of gastric diverticula are rare: (1) *Acute diverticulitis* with ulceration of the lining mucosa may develop leading to perforation. (2) *Haemorrhage* may also occur and haematemesis result. Should haemorrhage be associated with perforation, a haemoperitoneum may develop (3) Ward, Oca, and Cartz,[29] C. H. Mayo; [18] and Mellon [20] reported cases in which *carcinoma* developed at the base of a gastric diverticulum.

Cases have been reported in which the sac contained enteroliths or foreign bodies.

Diagnosis

Diverticula may cause no symptoms. although, in some instances, failure of the pouch to empty normally during digestion has been responsible for epigastric fulness and uneasiness, flatulent dyspepsia, and gnawing pain. In some cases the local stasis is followed by diverticulitis or peridiverticulitis; when this occurs, the pain is accentuated. According to Meeroff,[19] the diagnosis of gastric diverticulum is usually unsuspected on clinical grounds, and in most patients an associated lesion such as a duodenal ulcer or a hiatal hernia is found and held responsible for the symptoms.

There is, then, no typical picture of gastric diverticula, and the condition can only be diagnosed in the living person by means of radiology, gastroscopy, or at operation. Today the main reliance is placed upon screening after the ingestion of an opaque meal, but even the expert radiologist will on occasion have great difficulty in interpreting his findings. Äkerlund [2] was one of the first to describe the radiological appearances of gastric diverticula, especially the type that occurs near the cardia, as a circumscribed, smooth, evenly rounded projection from the gastric lumen, and in which the barium pools at the bottom of the sac and a bubble appears above it when the patient is placed in the erect position (Figs. 1 to 3). Diverticula arising from the anterior or posterior wall may easily be overlooked if the examination is carried out only with the patient in the erect position and with distended filling of the stomach. By using a mucosal relief technique and by examining the patient in all positions between the extreme Trendelenburg and the erect, the diverticulum can be projected clear of the stomach and its stalk and point of origin determined. The most

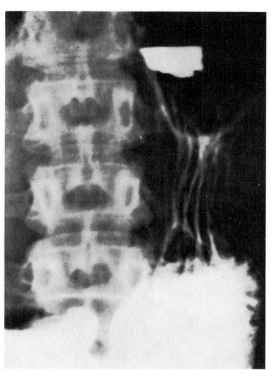

FIG. 2. Gastric diverticulum; the patient is standing erect. Note the "fluid level."

common fault is to mistake a diverticulum for a large penetrating gastric ulcer (Fig. 3). Diverticula usually occur, however, in those portions of the stomach where ulcers are rarely seen, i.e., near the cardia in the posterior wall of the fundus and along the upper end of the greater curvature. Other differential diagnostic factors include carcinoma of the cardia of the stomach with pseudodiverticulum formation, hiatal hernia, diverticulum of the lower oesophagus, and cascade stomach caused by gastric torsion.

Gastroscopy may be of some diagnostic help and may yield valuable information about the orifice of the diverticular sac and adjacent gastric mucosa. Complications may thus be detected and a photographic record made by means of a gastric camera (see Chap. 4. Parts A and B.)

Treatment

The mere proof that a diverticulum exists is not in itself a reason for its im-

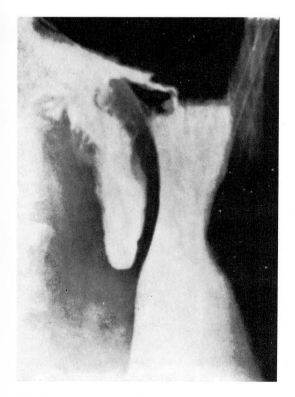

FIG. 1. Large gastric diverticulum. (Courtesy of Dr. E. B. Madden and the Radiological Department, Royal Free Hospital, London.)

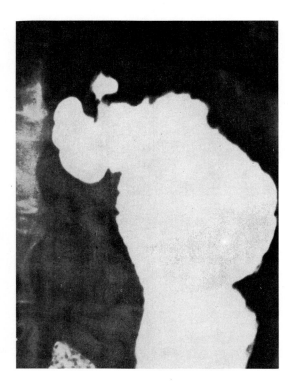

FIG. 3. Gastric diverticulum which in some respects resembled a simple peptic cardial ulcer. Note the large size of the stoma.

mediate excision. If it is causing no distress and is not associated with any concomitant gastric or other abdominal lesion, it is well to leave it alone.

For those patients in whom there are mild symptoms, medical treatment is advised. This consists of giving the patient a bland, nonresidue, peptic ulcer diet as well as alkalis and antispasmodics, and the adoption of postural treatment. It is unlikely, however, that such measures, even when carried out with care and discrimination, are likely to afford the patient much permanent relief. Palmer [25] states that the records show most patients with gastric symptoms were operated upon if a gastric diverticulum could be demonstrated on radiological examination.

Operation is advised under the following conditions:

1. When the symptoms are severe and there is no relief obtained after a careful course of medical treatment.

2. When complications such as diverticulitis and haemorrhage have occurred.

3. When the diagnosis is uncertain and the presence of malignant disease cannot be excluded.

4. When there is an associated lesion present, e.g., gastric ulcer.

5. In cases in which a diverticulum has been demonstrated in the pyloric region of the stomach and is associated with symptoms of obstruction.

6. When the pedicle is narrow but the fundus is unduly wide; in such circumstances, the onset of diverticulitis may be predicted with certainty.

OPERATIVE TECHNIQUE

The actual operative procedure will depend upon: (1) the position of the diverticulum and (2) the presence or absence of associated lesions.

Diverticula near the cardia. The cardia is best approached through the left paramedian, a vertical muscle-splitting, or a left oblique subcostal incision. The diverticulum should be displayed by dividing the left lateral portion of the gastrocolic ligament and the entire gastrosplenic omentum by drawing the liver upward and by rotating the upper third or more of the stomach in such a way that its posterior aspect close to the gastroesophageal orifice is brought into view (Fig. 4). A little careful dissection in this rather inaccessible area, the division of any adhesions that tether the sac to the pancreas or to the stomach wall itself, and a certain amount of traction on the diverticulum will be necessary before the neck of the pouch is clearly identified and then clamped flush with the gastric wall. The diverticulum is next amputated, the stump oversewn with 000 medium chromic catgut, inverted with a continuous suture and reinforced with interrupted sutures of fine silk, after which a portion of the omentum is stitched in place to afford added security.

Operative experience with these diverticula will show that they are very difficult to approach by dividing the gastrohepatic omentum and rotating the posterior wall of the stomach medially. It is well to make sure that the Ryle or Levin tube, which was passed through the nose into the stomach cavity before the operation and which was used for aspiration purposes during the excision, is lying in the stomach, as it will be needed for suction purposes during the first

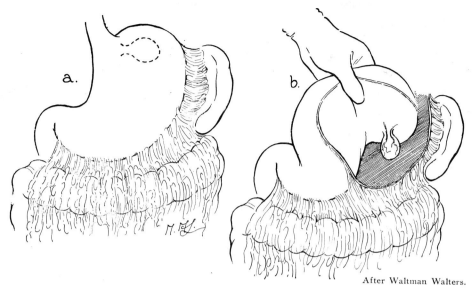

After Waltman Walters.

FIG. 4.   Gastric diverticulum. (a) Position of the diverticulum high up near the cardia and on the posterior wall of the stomach. (b) Exposure of the diverticulum by division of the gastro-splenic omentum and a portion of gastrocolic ligament. The stomach is rotated to bring the diverticulum clearly into view.

few postoperative days to keep the stomach deflated.

Diverticula of the lesser and greater curvatures of the stomach.   These should be excised by an ample V excision and the gap in the gastric wall repaired with a three-tier suture. In some cases, when the stalk of the diverticulum is small, the neck may be dampled and the diverticulum excised. The stump is transfixed and tied, and then invaginated by means of a purse-string suture of 000 silk. This procedure is preferable to inversion of the sac followed by closure of the defect in the gastric wall, although inversion is acceptable as a method in the poor-risk patient, or when technical difficulty prevents excision and suture. Young [32] reported two cases in which complete relief of symptoms followed a simple inversion procedure.

Diverticula of the pyloric region. When the anomaly occurs in the pyloric region or when there is an associated gastric lesion, it is better to perform partial gastrectomy after the Billroth I plan than to rely upon a limited local excision.

In cases in which local excision is indicated, it is imperative to obtain a good inversion of the sutured margins of the gastric wall because to leave any weakness at that point would predispose to recurrence of the condition.

The immediate and late results of excision of gastric diverticula are highly satisfactory. Some 90 percent of cures are reported from various clinics, and the operative mortality is low, being about 0.2 percent.

DUODENAL DIVERTICULA

Historical Note

Chomel (1710) is given credit for recording the first case of duodenal diverticulum. He found in a woman of 80, who died from an apoplectic fit, a duodenal pouch containing 22 gallstones. Odgers (1930) considered that the pouch was probably a dilated ampulla of Vater containing biliary calculi.

Authentic cases were later reported by Morgagni (1765), by Sommering (1794), and by Fleischman (1815). The abnormality was first observed by barium meal x-ray examination by Case (*Amer J Roentgen* 3:314, 1916), while in 1917 Bauer performed a gastrojejunostomy for a duodenal diverticulum which was producing obstructive symptoms. Forssell and Key 1915) were the first to excise a duodenal diverticulum which had been diagnosed by radiography.

Pathology

CLASSIFICATION

As in the case of gastric diverticula, duodenal diverticula are classified into primary and secondary types. The facts that *false or secondary duodenal diverticula* are sometimes composed of submucosal and mucosal layers of the gut, that they occur at the point of entry of blood vessel pedicles or the common bile duct, and that they are found mainly in the elderly suggest that aetiologically they are secondary to *pulsion* through a weakened duodenal wall. The majority of the false diverticula are *secondary* to chronic duodenal ulcer, traction by adhesions, and acute calculous cholecystitis. We are here solely concerned with the *primary types.* More than 30 per cent of patients have concomitant diverticulosis of the colon.

INCIDENCE

About 90 percent of duodenal diverticula are solitary and 70 percent occur in the second portion of the duodenum, mostly on its concavity. It is difficult to assess the incidence of duodenal diverticulum with any accuracy. Harold Edwards [8] found 82 cases in 9,631 x-ray examinations and Whitcomb [31] obtained an incidence of 1.064 percent in one million consecutive barium-meal examinations at the Henry Ford Hospital, Detroit. Autopsy series suggest that the con-

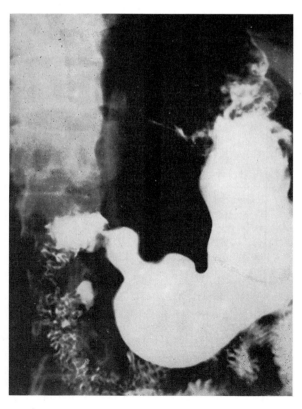

FIG. 5. Small diverticulum of the second part of the duodenum. About 70 percent of duodenal diverticula occur in this area.

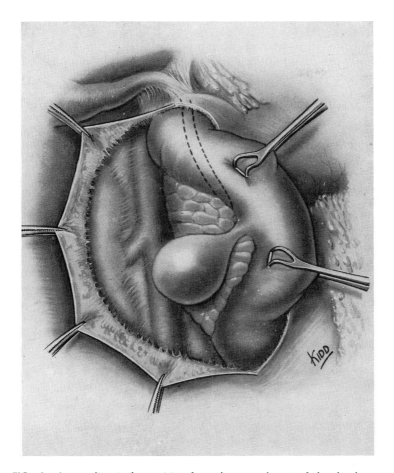

FIG. 6.   Large diverticulum arising from the second part of the duodenum.

dition occurs much more frequently. Grant [12] found an incidence of 11.6 percent and Baldwin [3] one of 14.5 percent. Ackerman,[1] by making plaster-of-paris casts of the duodenum of fifty cadavers selected at random, found eleven specimens with diverticula, an incidence of 22 percent. This discrepancy between radiological and autopsy findings implies that the diverticula may be difficult to demonstrate by conventional barium-meal examination, or that though relatively common, duodenal diverticula rarely produce symptoms.

Duodenal diverticula are rare before the age of 30 and uncommon before 40. The incidence rises rapidly after the age of 60, most cases being diagnosed when the patients are between the ages of 50 and 65. Beals [4] reported a series of 34 patients, their average age being 53.3 years. This conforms to the figures given later by Waugh and Johnston [30] and Cattell and Mudge.[6] The frequency between the sexes is about equal.

MORBID ANATOMY

Studies of the pathological anatomy show that duodenal diverticula may be solitary or multiple. The solitary type is much in preponderance, multiple diverticula being found in only 10 percent of all cases. They very rarely spring from the first portion of the duodenum (this is the prerogative of the prestenotic ulcer type) and while a few are found in the third or fourth portion, from 70 percent are seen in the second part (Fig. 5).

They are retroperitoneal and are situated

on the concave inner aspect near the inferior or mesenteric border of the descending limb of the second portion of the duodenum, usually in proximity to the common bile and pancreatic ducts, with their openings into the gut close to the papilla and with their flask-shaped sacs abutting upon, extending behind, or even penetrating into, the pancreas (Figs. 5, 6, and 10) The common bile duct and the duct of Wirsung may open into the diverticulum itself.

Culver and Pirson[7] reported three cases in which the common bile duct terminated in a duodenal diverticulum.

About 5 percent are located in the convex side of the second part of the duodenum,[14, 24] as shown in Figure 7.

On rather rare occasions, the diverticulum bulges into the lumen of the duodenum. Landau and Norton[16] reported such a case in a 26-year-old woman and Heilbrum and Boyden[13] found eight such cases in the literature and added six more.

COMPLICATIONS

The complications of duodenal diverticula have been well reviewed recently by Neill and Thompson.[22] There are two main groups of complications, namely, those caused by pressure, and those owing to inflammation. *Pressure* may produce jaundice, cholangitis, acute and recurrent pancreatitis, and even duodenal obstruction. *Inflammation* leads on to ulceration and haemorrhage, abscess formation, perforation, and occasionally the formation of an internal fistula. Rhodes and Williams[26] reported three such cases of duodenocolic fistula complicating duodenal diverticulum.

An interesting cause of perforation is stercoral ulceration caused by the presence of a stone in the diverticulum.[21] Such a stone may also pass down the lumen of the intestine before impacting and producing enterolith ileus.[28] Despite the known frequency

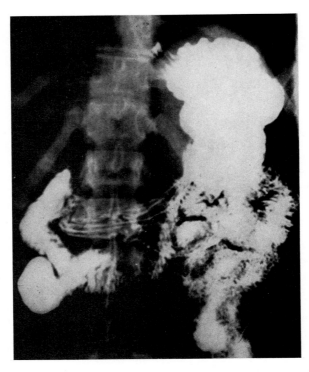

FIG. 7. Duodenal diverticulum. Stalk springing from *convex side* of the third part of the duodenum. This is a rare type, accounting for about 5 percent of cases.

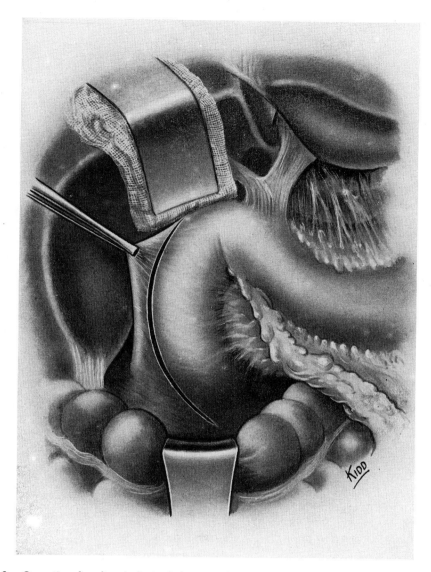

FIG. 8. Operation for diverticulum of the second portion of the duodenum. Kocher's incision is used to facilitate the mobilisation of the second portion of the duodenum.

of duodenal diverticula, the complications described here are decidedly rare. Nevertheless, examples of each have been carefully recorded in the literature.

Diagnosis

There are no pathognomonic signs or symptoms of a duodenal diverticulum, and a diagnosis cannot be made solely upon clinical evidence. A duodenal diverticulum may be present and produce no obvious ill effects.

When symptoms are present for any period of time, they are often indistinguishable from those produced by peptic ulcer, cholecystitis, or pancreatitis and, in all probability, owe to pylorospasm, to distention of the pouch, to pressure effects, or to inflammation of the diverticulum or adjacent structures such as the pancreas or common bile duct.

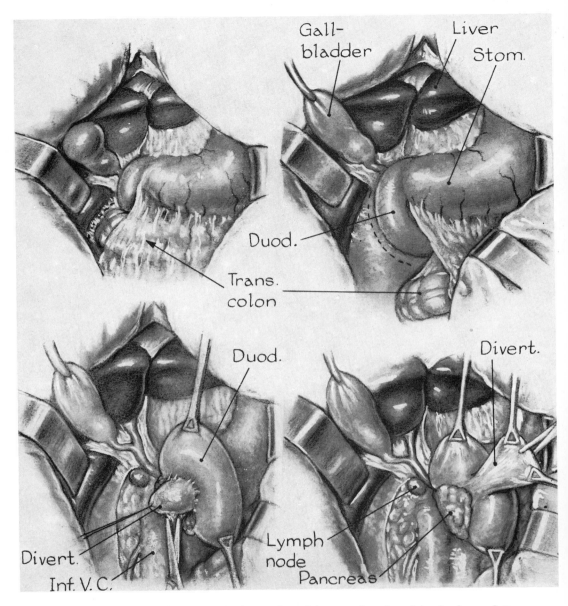

FIGS. 9 and 10. Top, Exposure of the diverticulum of the second portion of the duodenum. Bottom, Operation for diverticulum of the second portion of the duodenum. Note the exposure obtained by the liberal mobilisation of the duodenum and the head of the pancreas. (From Madden, *Atlas of Technics in Surgery*, 2d ed., Courtesy of Appleton-Century-Crofts, New York, 1964.)

In those exceptional instances in which a diverticular process becomes acutely inflamed, the signs and symptoms will resemble those of acute retrocaecal appendicitis, acute cholecystitis, or acute pancreatitis.

Elster and Waugh [9] state that the symptoms are often varied and complex and that many of them are due to functional dyspepsia or to the patient's tendency to complain. They emphasise that a thorough search must be made for associated pathological states.

As already mentioned, the clinical picture is atypical. At times, pain of a deep boring nature or epigastric discomfort is perhaps

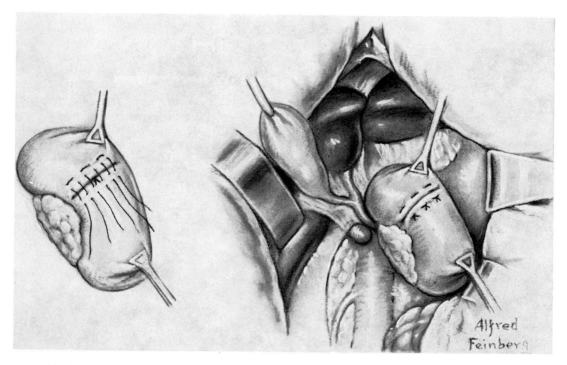

FIG. 11.   Excision of diverticulum of the second portion of the duodenum. After the diverticulectomy, closure of the defect is completed by inserting a few mattress sutures of fine silk. (From Madden, *Atlas of Technics in Surgery*, 2d ed., Courtesy of Appleton-Century-Crofts, New York, 1964.)

a troublesome feature. Tenderness localised to the diverticulum by palpation during fluoroscopy indicates that diverticulitis is present. Preoperative diagnosis is invariably based on an upper gastrointestinal barium meal series. On occasion, duodenography and fibreduodenoscopy may afford valuable information (see Chaps. 4C and 38B). Careful search must always be made for other pathological conditions possibly responsible for the signs and symptoms.

Treatment

Operations for diverticula of the duodenum are best reserved for those cases in which there are complications and incapacitating symptoms. This implies that very few of these diverticula will be submitted to surgical procedures, a fair reckoning being 5 to 6 percent of the total of all cases diagnosed by barium-meal examination. The prognosis is far from being favourable, as less than 50 percent of the patients treated

by operation are entirely relieved of their symptoms. Again, the removal of a diverticulum adjacent to the ampulla of Vater is not an easy undertaking, as injury to the ampulla with interference with the drainage of bile or pancreatic secretions may lead to jaundice, pancreatitis, or even the development of a duodenal fistula. When such postoperative complications ensue, the mortality rate is, judging by modern standards, high, being 5 to 10 percent.

Diverticula that are found in a routine examination of the gastrointestinal tract and that do not appear to produce symptoms are best left alone; their excision may at times be difficult and not free from danger, as mentioned above. Those that are associated with vague upper abdominal symptoms demand a thorough investigation to eliminate other causes. If this investigation should prove negative but symptoms persist, medical measures—a strict ulcer regimen—should be given a trial, and only when these repeatedly fail should surgical intervention be undertaken. In other words, operation is advised only when symptoms persist and when complications have arisen.

OPERATIVE TECHNIQUE

The operative procedure for diverticula of the second portion of the duodenum consists of exploring the abdomen through a right upper paramedian or a muscle-splitting incision; and, after excluding any organic disease by a thorough exploration of the abdomen, the right phrenocolic ligament should be severed prior to mobilising the hepatic flexure of the colon. The duodenum is next mobilised by dividing the peritoneum along its lateral border, as originally described by Kocher. The strong fascia propria, which is exposed after incising the peritoneum, is carefully snipped with scissors, after which the fingers steal under the duodenum and turn it over to the left (medialward) until a small arcade of blood vessels from the pancreaticoduodenal artery can be

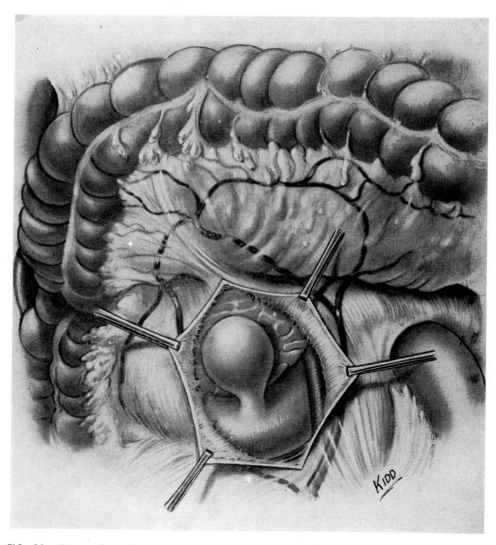

FIG. 12.   Diverticulum of the third portion of the duodenum. Note the method of approach and exposure.

seen entering the concave inner border of the gut. The frail pouch and the yellow lobulated head of the mobilised pancreas now come into view. The diverticulum, which is frequently situated near the termination of the common bile and main pancreatic duct, will be found to be adherent to the pancreas and should be daintily teased away from the compressed connective tissue strands which surround it, using a small swab held in the jaws of a haemostat or fine nontoothed dissecting forceps. The fundus, when freed, should be clipped with two Halsted haemostats to steady it and to facilitate the dissection and isolation of the pedicle (Figs. 8 to 11). A few small blood vessels that will be found supplying the sac should be ligated with fine silk and divided. The liberated sac is drawn medially and split open to obtain a good view of the papilla of Vater, after which the diverticulum is excised flush with the duodenal wall. The opening that results is then sutured transversely with interrupted sutures of fine black silk, the knots of which are placed inside the lumen of the gut. When this row of sutures has been completed, the suture line is reinforced with a series of interrupted mattress sutures (Fig. 11).

In certain instances in which on inspecting the papillary region it would seem likely that the suture line when completed might constrict the bile duct, it is advisable to make a small opening in the supraduodenal portion of the choledochus and to insert one of Maingot's guttered long T tubes into the duct and pass it on well into the duodenum before completing the closure of the defect in the duodenal wall. The intraductal limb of the T tube serves as a useful guide during the dissection, especially when the choledochus opens into the sac. This T tube is left in situ for about 10 days.

In certain cases in which the mouth of the diverticulum is wide, there may be an extensive gap to be sutured in the duodenal wall after the excision of the pouch. Nevertheless, this opening is always capable of being closed securely and in a watertight manner by the careful placement of sutures.

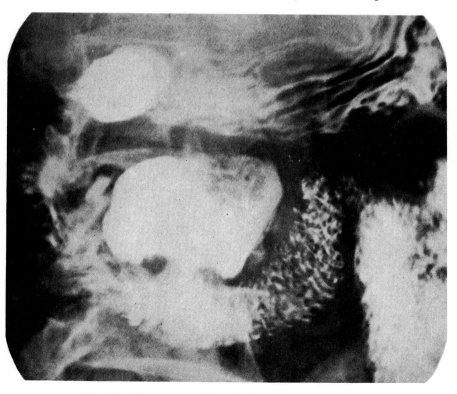

FIG. 13.   Diverticulum of the third part of the duodenum.

Invagination of the sac into the lumen of the duodenum is not advised, as it may lead to obstructive symptoms later. Ferguson and Cameron,[11] however, claim that invagination of the mucosal sac followed by repair of the muscle defect in the gut wall through which the neck of the diverticulum passed is the method of choice. Obstruction of the lumen is thought by them to be a purely theoretical complication. They report that the five patients they treated by this method were cured and did not experience any postoperative complications. Cattell and Mudge [6] voice the opinion held by most surgeons, namely that excision of the diverticulum is the procedure of choice. They report 25 with excellent results in 15, improvement in 4, and failure in 6. There were two deaths in this series. John Madden,[17] states that in his series of 19 patients who were subjected to diverticulectomy, a good result was obtained in each instance, and there were no postoperative complications to report.

Diverticula arising from the third or fourth part of the duodenum may be approached through the posterior peritoneum beneath the mesocolon, and pains should be taken in making this exposure to avoid the vulnerable right colic artery (Fig. 12) and injury to the pancreatic substance; a number of diverticula situated at this point may lie deep to the pancreas or be actually incorporated in pancreatic tissue. Here again, the complete excision of the sac after it has been adequately mobilised is the method preferred by most surgeons. Should complete excision be particularly hazardous, however (e.g., in patients presenting with mainly obstructive symptoms), a short-circuiting operation (side-to-side duodenojejunostomy) is probably preferable. This latter method was successful in the case reported by Lambert, Fitts, and Turk.[15]

REFERENCES

1. Ackerman, Ann. Surg. 117:403, 1943.
2. Äkerlund, Acta Radiol. (Stockh.) 2:470, 1923.
3. Baldwin, Anat. Rec. 5:121, 1911.
4. Beals, South. Med. J., 218, 1937.
5. Bigg and Judd, Am. J. Surg. 105:259, 1963.
6. Cattell and Mudge, N. Engl. J. Med. 246:317, 1952.
7. Culver and Pirson, Am. J. Roentgenol. 96:370, 1966.
8. Edwards, H., Ann. Surg. 103:230, 1936.
9. Elster and Waugh, Surgery 41:674, 1957.
10. Feldman, Clinical Roentgenology of the Digestive Tract, 4th ed. Baltimore, Williams & Wilkins, 1957.
11. Ferguson and Cameron, Surg. Gynecol. Obstet. 84:292, 1947.
12. Grant, Can. Med. Assoc. J. 33:258, 1935.
13. Heilbrum and Boyden, Radiology 82:887, 1964.
14. Holmes and Woodward, Aust. N. Z. J. Surg. 33:227, 1964.
15. Lambert, Fitts, and Turk, Am. J. Surg. 101:808, 1961.
16. Landau and Norton, Am. J. Roentgenol. 90:756, 1963.
17. Madden, Personal Communication on Excision of Duodenal Diverticula, 1972.
18. Mayo, C. H., J.A.M.A. 59:260, 1912.
19. Meeroff, Am. J. Gastroenterol. 47:189, 1967.
20. Mellon, Surg. Gynecol. Obstet. 33:177, 1921.
21. Munnel and Preston, Arch. Surg. 92:152, 1966.
22. Neill and Thompson, Surg. Gynecol. Obstet. 120:1251, 1965.
23. Norton, Am. J. Roentgenol. 90:756, 1964.
24. Norton and Peacock, Br. J. Surg. 40:577, 1963.
25. Palmer, Int. Abstr. Surg. 92:417, 1951.
26. Rhodes and Williams, Surg. Gynecol. Obstet. 123:1017, 1966.
27. Sinclair, Neil, Br. J. Surg. 17:182, 1929.
28. Upson, Culver, and Hermann, Surgery 54:725, 1963.
29. Ward, Oca, and Cartz, J.A.M.A. 196:798, 1966.
30. Waugh and Johnston, Am. Surg. 141:193, 1952.
31. Whitcomb, Arch. Surg. 88:275, 1964.
32. Young, Br. J. Surg. 50:150, 1962.

8

INJURIES OF THE STOMACH AND DUODENUM

CLAUDE E. WELCH and GRANT V. RODKEY

The recent wave of trauma in American cities and on the highways has led to numerous injuries of the stomach and duodenum nearly all of which arise from external force, although a few perforations are iatrogenic, the causative force being applied from within the viscus (e.g., from the gastroscope). The perforations of the stomach and duodenum that are secondary to underlying visceral disease will not be considered in this section; furthermore, the general remarks on abdominal trauma in Chapter 84 are applicable here and will not be repeated.

CAUSES OF INJURY

As is true with all other abdominal injuries, the responsible trauma may be either penetrating or nonpenetrating.

Nonpenetrating trauma is of particular interest in the case of these abdominal viscera —i.e., of the stomach and the duodenum— because of the retroperitoneal rupture of the duodenum that produces a particular syndrome. In addition, the stomach may be ruptured from vomiting when it is full or partially obstructed from some disease. These "emetogenic injuries" include complete perforation of the upper stomach or lower esophagus or laceration of the mucosa alone, as is seen in the Mallory-Weiss syndrome.

Since the incidence of injury to each viscus following penetrating trauma varies directly with the space that the viscus occupies in the abdomen, these wounds of the stomach and duodenum are relatively uncommon, compared with those of other viscera. Thus, Rodkey,[1] in his series of 177 cases, found only three instances of gastric injuries and three of duodenal injuries. Morton et al.[2] observed only two gastric perforations in 120 patients treated for blunt trauma at the University of Rochester Hospital. Harrold[3] observed that rupture of the duodenum oc-

curred in only 9 percent of 717 cases of intestinal rupture caused by nonpenetrating injuries.

Blast injuries have received a great deal of attention as a cause of gastric or duodenal injuries. Cameron et al.[4] believed that there was very little difference whether the pressure was in air or in water. They studied 20 patients who had been subjected to operation and 80 who had recovered without laparotomy. The lesions varied from intramural hemorrhage to complete lacerations of the stomach and intestinal wall; it was of interest that the lungs and colon were the viscera most likely to be damaged. Liebow et al.[5] found that intestinal rupture from air blast was almost unknown following the explosion of atomic bombs in Japan.

Muscular relaxation is an important predisposing factor for duodenal rupture, as Webb et al.[6] have suggested. Compression of the duodenum against the spine with the application of a shearing force is the most important mechanism by which the damage to the duodenum is produced. Although duodenal injuries are much less common than those of the jejunum and ileum, the incidence of injury per unit length is actually considerably greater.

DIAGNOSTIC SIGNS AND SYMPTOMS—GENERAL

While the diagnosis of visceral injury caused by trauma is similar in many respects, regardless of the viscus involved, there are a few important differences in the case of the stomach and duodenum. Thus, the development of pain and tenderness may be very rapid if there is a wide communication of the stomach with the peritoneal cavity. Shock may likewise follow shortly after injury. On the other hand, some of the perforations of the duodenum are retroperitoneal, so that pain and tenderness may be delayed over a period of many hours. The symptoms of these injuries may be obscured by the associated injuries to other viscera that are exceedingly common in wounds of the stomach or duodenum.

While the diagnosis of the exact injuries is usually made by laparotomy, a Levin tube should be inserted prior to operation. The presence of a bloody aspirate will suggest injury to the stomach or duodenum. Vomiting is relatively uncommon following perforating injuries to the stomach, but on the other hand, it is quite common with duodenal injuries. X-ray observations that suggest specific injuries to these two organs include the presence of free gas beneath the diaphragm on erect films, or the demonstration of a perforation by the instillation of Gastrografin. Subcutaneous or submucosal emphysema has also been noted. These findings will be discussed in more detail in later paragraphs.

TYPES OF INJURIES

Gastric Wounds

General characteristics. Wolff [7] studied 416 penetrating wounds of the stomach treated by the Second Auxiliary Surgical Group in World War II. Penetrating wounds were found in 13.2 percent of all abdominal injuries. Wolff concluded that wounds of this organ occurred much more frequently than they heretofore had appeared to, that they were complicated by injury to other viscera in nine out of ten cases, and that the case fatality rate (40.6 percent) was significantly higher than after wounds of the colon, small intestine, liver, or spleen.

Frequency. The frequency of multiple visceral wounds is not surprising when the close relationship of the stomach to other organs is considered. The diaphragm had been traversed by missiles in 47.1 percent of the cases. The liver, spleen, colon, jejunum, kidney, and pancreas, either alone or in combination, were involved in that order of frequency in 90 percent of all the gastric wounds.

The character of the wounds varied with the type of wounding agent. Missiles that

entered in a perpendicular plane usually produced small wounds that soon were blocked by pouting of the mucosa. Those that entered at an acute angle, regardless of size, could produce a large laceration that led rapidly to shock and peritonitis.

Diagnosis. Perforating wounds of the stomach should be suspected whenever a missile track has crossed the left diaphragm. According to Wolff,[7] the only positive preoperative findings that definitely indicate a diagnosis of gastric wounds are emission of undigested food from an abdominal wound or the observation of a laceration in the eviscerated stomach. Subcutaneous emphysema in varying degrees, or gas bubbling from a wound, may also be noted at times when the stomach has been lacerated. The presence of blood in the Levin tube aspirate is of great importance and much more frequent.

Vomiting is not likely to occur following penetrating wounds of the stomach. On the other hand, pain, local tenderness, and shock are exceedingly variable, and, in the presence of large injuries, may be very important almost from the outset. The shock appears to be much more than can be accounted for by blood loss.

Treatment. The stomach may be exposed by an abdominal or transthoracic incision. The latter is preferred if there is damage to the diaphragm as well, as the fundus can be explored adequately at the time the diaphragm is repaired. In Wolff's series,[7] approximately 30 percent of the patients had a thoracic incision alone, while in a few patients it was supplemented by one in the abdomen.

For the laparotomy a *paramedian incision* is preferred. Adequate observation of the stomach will require exposure of both the anterior and posterior surfaces, which means that the gastrocolic omentum must be divided. In a questionable case, the duodenum or pylorus may be occluded by a clamp, and the stomach distended with salt solution containing methylene blue. If the wound is caused by a penetrating shell fragment, and is not tangential, there must be wounds of both entrance and exit in the stomach unless the foreign body is found within the viscus. If a wide defect is found in the anterior wall of the stomach, the posterior wall may be

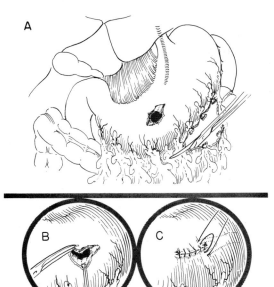

FIG. 1. Treatment of gastric wounds. (A) Penetrating wound of stomach. Division of gastrocolic omentum to observe posterior wall; (B) excision of ragged laceration; (C) (D) closure of incision in two layers.

examined through it. At times a gastrostomy may be necessary for complete observation of the whole internal surface of the stomach.

Perforations of the stomach can be sutured very easily if they are on the anterior wall, but they are difficult to close if they are on the posterior side. Inasmuch as there are large vessels in the mucosa of the stomach, it is well to be most meticulous about hemostasis in order to avoid secondary hemorrhage. It has been found that the best method of closure is to convert the defect by debridement into a linear incision which then can be sutured in two layers. A pursestring closure is more likely to bleed postoperatively because, if the mucosa is not sutured, the margins retract, leaving an open ulcer (Fig. 1).

In a few instances the damage to the stomach may be so great that complete division may require an end-to-end anastomosis or a formal gastric resection. Such extensive injuries have nearly always been fatal.

Postoperative complications. Such complications include shock, peritonitis, secondary hemorrhage, and gastric fistulas. Shock is severe when there is wide disruption of the stomach because of the chemical peritonitis.

The sequel of unsutured lacerations of the stomach is of interest. Wolff [7] found in his series that only two lacerations of the stomach had been overlooked; interestingly enough, at autopsy both were found to have healed spontaneously.

Duodenal Injuries

General characteristics. Penetrating wounds of the duodenum are infrequent. In soldiers of the American Army during World War I, such wounds accounted for 6 percent of the injuries of the small bowel; Wallace [8] reported 16 cases of penetrating wounds of the duodenum in 185 abdominal injuries in British soldiers. Cave [9] found that the Second Auxiliary Surgical group encountered 118 of these injuries, which represented 3.7 percent of all abdominal injuries. Morton and Jordan [10] estimate duodenal wounds occur in 4 to 5 percent of all patients with abdominal injuries. Their report includes 131 patients treated chiefly in Houston.

It is characteristic of penetrating duodenal wounds that nearly always other organs are involved; this occurred in 116 of 118 cases noted above. The pancreas, colon, liver, kidney, ureter, and great vessels are all in close proximity. The high mortality rate of these wounds is, to a great extent, dependent upon this feature.

Mortality. The mortality rate from penetrating wounds in military service is high. In the experience of the Second Auxiliary Surgical group it was 59 percent. In Korea it was estimated to be about 46 percent. In civilian life the rate is lower because many stab wounds are included in this category and the penetrating wounds are likely to be from pistol shots rather than from disrupting shell fragments. Thus, Webb et al.[6] reported on 50 patients from Atlanta and Houston; the mortality rate of the 45 penetrating wounds was 27 percent. The predominant cause of death was shock and hemorrhage, which usually occurred within 48 hours. This series has been extended by Morton and Jordan,[10] who reported a mortality rate of 22 percent for penetrating wounds, 14 percent for blunt wounds, and an overall rate of 18 percent. The death rate is dependent, however, on the wounding agent. In Morton and Jordan's series,[10] it was 23 percent from bullet wounds and 75 percent from shotgun wounds.

Nonpenetrating wounds. Such wounds of the duodenum that are a result of blunt trauma occur even more infrequently, so that most papers have consisted either of single case reports or of collective reviews. While it will not be possible to cite all these references, some of the most pertinent will be discussed here—as adapted from the summary of Webb et al.[6]

The first report available is by Schumaker,[11] who in 1910 collected reports on 91 cases of duodenal rupture caused by nonpenetrating abdominal injuries, of which 24 were retroperitoneal. The mortality rate in the latter group was 93 percent. Subsequently in 1916 Miller and Schumaker [12] recorded 22 additional cases; the death rate continued at almost the same level, but in 14 of the 37 patients who were operated upon the lesion was not found. Other early reports were by Leibowicz [13] in 1931, and by Kellogg [14] in 1933.

By 1944 Johnson [15] was able to collect reports on 52 cases, with cure in 26. It was of interest that by this time the accuracy of diagnosis had improved and in only 7 of these patients was the lesion missed at the time of laparotomy. Many of these early series of statistics were likewise collected and analyzed by Lauritzen.[16] In the past 20 years many more case reports have appeared. One of the largest series is by Webb et al.,[6] who found five retroperitoneal ruptures in a series of 50 wounds of the duodenum. Cohn et al.,[17] in 1952, collected from the literature reports on 25 cases, listing a mortality rate of 20 percent. Cleveland and Waddell [18] found 37 cases of retroperitoneal rupture between 1951 and 1963, with a mortality rate of 16 percent, indicating improvement in therapy. Recent experience has shown that automobile accidents are the cause of the majority of duo-denal injuries, and that most of them are caused by steering-wheel injuries. Traumatic perforations and fracture of the liver are the most commonly associated lesions.

Retroperitoneal ruptures. It is in this small group that the diagnosis is most likely to be missed. Inasmuch as gastrointestinal ruptures occur in the duodenum in less than 10 percent of all cases, and since only one-quarter of duodenal ruptures are retroperitoneal, this group is small. Actually, the most likely areas of rupture are at the two extremities of the duodenum, particularly where the duodenum crosses the spine just proximal to the ligament of Treitz. The dependent portion of the duodenum is protected from the shearing action following blunt force, so that it is not often involved. It should be noted, however, that traumatic hematomas of the duodenum, which will be discussed later, often occur in this area.

The cause of duodenal rupture is usually a severe physical force that is exerted, particularly when the muscles are flaccid. Crushing injuries, severe bruises to the abdomen, kicks, automobile accidents, and severe blows to the back have all been implicated. Steering-wheel injuries have become relatively common, and they are usually found in association with contusion of the pancreas. Blast injuries may also be serious if the pylorus is closed and the duodenojejunal angle is acutely flexed so that the duodenum is full of air at the time of the blast. These causes are summarized by Morton and Jordan [10] as tears, crushes, blowwounds, and penetrations.

Signs and symptoms. The basis for diagnosis of an intraperitoneal rupture is similar to that for a perforated duodenal ulcer; in these instances there is usually a history of a severe blow. A sudden pain may be noted but it usually passes relatively soon, and for a period of a few hours the patient may feel quite well. This is due to the fact that with small injuries there may be pouting of the mucosa, which will block extravasation or secretions for a brief period. Later on, as peritonitis develops, the pain becomes increasingly severe. The period of quiescence is quite variable, depending on the extent of the laceration. Tenderness accompanies the pain. The presence of shock at the outset should lead one to suspect vascular damage as well, although as peritonitis develops the signs of shock will become more pronounced. Shock is not common in the early stages but does occur later. Unless operation is carried out, increasing extravasation will lead to a rapid change in the vital signs. The temperature usually remains near normal but the pulse rises rapidly. Accumulation of fluid in the right side of the peritoneal cavity will produce respiratory embarrassment, shifting dullness, and severe local pain spreading from the flank down to the groin.

The findings on x-ray examination usually are not important in the early stages. As with perforated ulcers, however, gas may appear beneath the diaphragm within a period of a few hours, and in certain instances it may be seen within the tissue planes as well. In questionable cases, confirmation may be obtained by the administration of meglumine diatrizoate (Gastrografin) by mouth. We believe this can be done without any risk. We would not advise the introduction of barium at any time, although some authors have suggested that it can be done with safety. At later stages, air may outline the kidney or extend along the vertebral column. The renal and psoas shadows may be obliterated; these are late and relatively unimportant signs, however, and should not be depended upon for a diagnosis.

Treatment. The stomach is decompressed preoperatively by a Levin tube, which is to be left in for postoperative care. The most important part of the operation is a complete examination of the entire duodenum. Even today, with good anesthesia, it may be possible to overlook these perforations unless a very careful search is made of the entire organ. This will involve the combined use of the Kocher maneuver, the mobilization of the entire right colon, and the freeing of the root of the mesentery from the ligament of Treitz to observe the duodenojejunal flexure. Fatalities still result from the fact that complete exploration has not been carried out; it is imperative that this be done whenever there is cause for suspecting retroperitoneal rupture (Fig. 2).

With retroperitoneal ruptures there may be no intraperitoneal signs of damage whatsoever; on the other hand, free straw-colored fluid, free blood, brownish fluid, right upper quadrant peritonitis, bile extravasation, hematoma formation, or crepitus all may be found at the base of the mesocolon or at the upper portion of the small bowel. Other indications for further exploration include elevation of the peritoneum, with a glossy edema over it, fat necrosis that may be noted even in the absence of any injury to the pancreas, retroperitoneal hematoma about the head of the pancreas or at the base of the mesocolon, or a phlegmon in this area.

The specific treatment of the laceration will vary considerably, depending on the wound's size and location. Small tears can be closed in two layers and the abdomen closed without drainage. In Morton and Jordan's series,[10] this simple method was sufficient in 85 percent of all cases. If the tear is in the second portion of the duodenum, it is wise to carry out a choledochotomy and to leave the T tube in place for at least 2 weeks. If the common duct has been severed, it may be necessary to reimplant it into the jejunum or duodenum. A complete transection may be treated by an end-to-end suture provided there is no great loss of continuity at the posterior wall. If this loss has occurred, it will be almost impossible to secure enough mobility to make an adequate suture, so that some other maneuver will become necessary. At times the surgeon may bring up a loop of proximal jejunum and carry out an anastomosis with it. Some authors have reported closure of both ends of the severed duodenum and the reestablishment of gastrointestinal continuity by gastroenterostomy. In such cases, however, it would seem wiser to carry out a duodenojejunostomy.

A very interesting application of the exclusion principle and its application to traumatic perforations of the duodenum has been made by Donovan and Hagen,[19] who have subjected some patients to closure of the duodenal perforation, antrectomy, vagotomy, duodenostomy, and gastrojejunostomy. This operation was performed on six of 29 patients with traumatic perforations; in four it was primary therapy because of the severity of the injury and in two it was for treatment of a lateral duodenal fistula that developed after closure of the perforation. Five of these patients survived this very extensive operation. The total mortality rate in the 29 patients was only 14 percent. It was noted that in 20 patients without pancreatic injuries

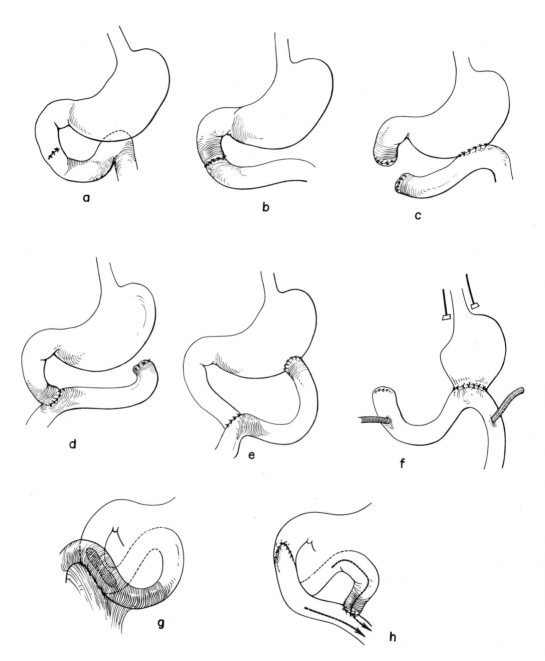

FIG. 2.   Treatment of duodenal wounds. (a) Suture of laceration; (b) end-to-end anastomosis; (c) closure severed duodenum; gastrojejunostomy; (d) closure upper jejunum; duodenojejunostomy; (e) duodenojejunostomy; gastroduodenosotmy; (f) vagotomy, antrectomy, duodenostomy, jejunostomy; (g) duodenojejunostomy, closing an anterior wound, side-to-side; (h) duodenojejunostomy, side-to-end.

the mortality rate was 5 percent, and in nine patients with pancreatic injury, 33 percent. The authors believe that if pancreatic injury is not present, primary closure will be satisfactory, but that otherwise this much more extensive operation is indicated.

There is a very marked hazard if the duodenum is closed more than 12 hours after injury. The chances of dehiscence of the anastomosis are high, and once a wide duodenal fistula occurs, the situation may very well get out of control. If it does occur, consideration should be given to a gastric resection as the primary type of operation, with a Billroth II anastomosis in order to render the duodenal loop functionless, insofar as possible. With the insertion of a catheter duodenostomy and wide drainage, it is possible that the fistula can be controlled.

Very wide drainage is essential to any retroperitoneal injury; the drains are placed close to, but not in apposition with, the line of suture, and they are brought out through a stab wound. Other technical problems arise when there is a wide disruption of the duodenum. Resection and anastomosis may be carried out without difficulty in the jejunum or ileum, but in the duodenum it is difficult because the presence of the pancreas allows only limited mobility of the duodenum, so that an end-to-end suture after resection may be impossible.

In some instances there will be rather wide destruction of the anterior lateral duodenal wall, while the posterior wall is left intact. In these instances it is well to consider closure by the suture of a loop of upper jejunum over the defect. This may be accomplished by suturing the unopened loop of jejunum over the opening. After a few months, the serosa will become covered with a thin layer of mucosa. The strength of the closure has been proved in experimental animals by Kobold and Thal.[20] In other instances it may be possible to bring up a Roux-en-Y loop of jejunum to close the defect so that internal drainage can be provided. Postoperatively the patient is likely to have a complicated course; the chances of pancreatitis are high, and gastric function may be slow to return. Therefore, in many instances, a complementary gastrostomy and jejunostomy at the time of the original operation will be wise.

Early deaths are usually due to hemorrhage and shock. Other than peritonitis, pancreatitis, and external duodenal fistula, late postoperative complications that may occur are subdiaphragmatic abscesses and stenosis of the duodenum secondary to suture. All are extremely serious and contribute to the high mortality.

Of these complications, the most common by far has been sepsis. With heavy doses of antibiotics, the incidence of 11 percent noted by Morton and Jordan[10] should be reduced. Drainage of the subhepatic space also is helpful, but drains should not be placed in direct contact with a suture line.

External fistulas are serious complications. Several methods are available for therapy. Catheter duodenostomy or a Billroth II resection may be chosen. An excellent suggestion made by Tanski and Weismann[21] is to insert a sump drain into the duodenum through a gastrostomy incision. This has led to rapid closure in several cases reported by them.

In most cases a feeding jejunostomy is a good adjunct procedure, since aspirated duodenal contents can be returned to the gastrointestinal tract. Intravenous hyperalimentation, by the technique of Dudrick et al.,[22] is of great value in these cases.

Intramural Hematoma of the Duodenum

Within the past few years an interesting syndrome—the intramural hematoma of the duodenum—has been observed. A series of case reports has been made by Freeark et al.,[23] Mathewson and Morgan,[24] and Bailey and Akers.[25] This hematoma is seen in children who, while riding a bicycle fall and are hit by a handlebar in the right upper quadrant. The patient apparently does well immediately after the accident but in the course of 24 to 48 hours develops mild right upper quadrant tenderness associated with symptoms of duodenal obstruction. X-rays taken at this time may demonstrate a smooth defect in the wall of the duodenum that is producing partial obstruction. The actual pathological condition involves hemorrhage that forms beneath the mucosa; because of lack of penetration, the lesion of the bowel remains localized and produces this defect.

The therapy preferably is conservative because many of these hematomas will gradually absorb and symptoms relent. Should obstruction persist, it will be necessary to operate to establish the diagnosis and evacuate the hematoma. A jejunostomy or a gastrojejunostomy often is necessary.

Iatrogenic Injuries

A gastric perforation may follow several surgical procedures; perhaps the most common one is still that which occurs secondary to gastroscopy. This complication occurs much more frequently when a rigid gastroscope has been used, but it also still occurs occasionally when the fibre-optic scope has been employed). The diagnosis may be evident by observation through the instrument, but in general it is not recognized until a few hours after perforation, when the patient complains of severe abdominal pain and tenderness. Immediate laparotomy is essential.

In the presence of an obstructed or spastic pylorus, the stomach has also been perforated by distension with gas during the administration of anesthesia. The lesser curvature has been torn by the passage of a needle during the repair of a hiatal hernia by the transthoracic route. A perforation of the stomach may be produced by clamps placed too close to the stomach as the vasa brevia were ligated during the performance of a splenectomy.

The duodenum may be damaged during the operation of nephrectomy, cholecystectomy, or colectomy. Such accidents are usually recognized immediately at the time of operation, and repair is carried out. If they are not diagnosed at that time, the normal postoperative pain is likely to obscure the increased pain from this cause, and a lateral duodenal fistula may occur. This is an extremely serious type of injury because it leads to very severe and quite rapid depletion of electrolytes. Furthermore, the operative repair of a duodenal fistula is extremely difficult and carries a high incidence of failure because of a breakdown of the suture line.

SPONTANEOUS RUPTURE OF THE STOMACH

Rupture of the stomach in a newborn infant is a clinical entity that was recognized first in 1825. Vargar et al.[26] collected reports on a total of 55 cases in 1955, and added 11 others. Surgical repair was attempted in 22, and nine of the infants survived operation. The disease is most common in premature infants, and usually occurs within the first 2 weeks of life. Acute gastric ulcers account for the perforation in less than one-half of the cases; a few occur spontaneously, and the remainder are caused by a congenital muscle defect. These defects may be single or multiple; the infant usually presents with abdominal pain and tenderness, and a pneumoperitoneum. The operation may be very difficult because the area of perforation may be quite large. It is important that the sutures be placed in viable muscle or reperforation may occur. Obstruction of the lower intestinal tract must be ruled out by careful observation, as the condition is not uncommon in these cases. A gastrostomy tube is used for decompression.

Spontaneous rupture of the stomach occurs also in adults. Actually the term should not imply that the rupture occurs in the absence of any exciting cause; as a general rule the catastrophe is most likely to follow an attack of vomiting, when the stomach is distended. It is observed in alcoholics, occasionally in those patients who have taken large amounts of sodium bicarbonate, and in some patients whose stomachs have been overdistended with anesthetic gases at the time of anesthesia administration. Probably the most important factors that lead to this rupture are obstruction either at the cardiac or pyloric outlet; the pylorus may be blocked by ulcer or tumor, or the cardia may be blocked by hiatal hernia or by gastric volvulus. A block of the cardia is dangerous if the patient attempts to vomit and is unable to do so.

Probably spontaneous rupture is closely related to the syndrome described by Weiss and Mallory,[27] in which only the mucosa about the cardia has been lacerated. In these instances, the mechanism is exactly the same; the disease is manifested by acute massive hemorrhage.

Case reports by Millar et al.[28] and by Cronin [29] may be consulted for further information on this condition.

REFERENCES

1. Rodkey, G. V., Surg. Clin. North Am. 46:627, 1966.
2. Morton, J. H., Hinshaw, J. R., and Morton, J. J., Ann. Surg. 145:699, 1957.
3. Harrold, A. J., Br. Med. J. 2:949, 1951.
4. Cameron, G. R., Short, R. H. D., and Wakeley, C. P. G., Br. J. Surg. 31:51, 1943.
5. Liebow, A. A., Warren, S., and DeCoursey, E., Am. J. Pathol. 25:853, 1949.
6. Webb, H. W., Howard, J. M., Jordan, G. L., and Vowles, K. D. J., Int. Abstr. Surg. 106:105, 1958.
7. Wolff, L. H., Medical Department, United States Army, Surgery in World War II, Vol. II, Office of the Surgeon General, Department of the Army, Washington, D.C., 1955, pp. 223–233.
8. Wallace, C., War Surgery of the Abdomen. London, Churchill, 1918.
9. Cave, W. H., Medical Department, United States Army, Surgery in World War II, Vol. II, Office of the Surgeon General, Department of the Army, Washington, D.C., 1955, pp. 235–240.
10. Morton, J. R., and Jordan, G. L., J. Trauma 8:127, 1968.
11. Schumaker, E. D., Beitr. Klin. Chir. 71:482, 1910.
12. Miller, R. T., Ann. Surg. 64:550, 1916.
13. Leibowicz, M., Abl. Chir. 58:2205, 1931.
14. Kellogg, E. L., The Duodenum. New York, Hoeber, 1933.
15. Johnson, M. L., Am. J. Surg. 94:251, 1957.
16. Lauritzen, G. R., Acta Chir. Scand. 96:97, 1947.
17. Cohn, I., Jr., Hawthorne, H. R., and Frosbese, A. S., Am. J. Surg. 84:293, 1952.
18. Cleveland, H. C., and Waddell, W. R., Surg. Clin. North Am. 43:313, 1963.
19. Donovan, A. J., and Hagen, W. E., Am. J. Surg. 111:341, 1966.
20. Kobold, E. E, and Thal, A. P., Surg. Gynecol. Obstet. 116:340, 1963.
21. Tanski, E. V., and Weismann, R. E., Am. J. Surg. 121:426, 1971.
22. Dudrick, S. J., Wilmore, D. W., Vars, H. M., and Rhoads, J. E., Surgery 64:134, 1968.
23. Freeark, R. J., Corley, R. D., Norcross, W. J., and Strohl, E. L., Br. Med. J. 2:949, 1951.
24. Mathewson, C., Jr., and Morgan, R., Am. J. Surg. 112:299, 1966.
25. Bailey, W. C., and Akers, D. R., Am. J. Surg. 110:695, 1965.
26. Vargas, L. L., Levin, S. M., and Santulli, T. V., Surg. Gynecol. Obstet. 101:417, 1955.
27. Weiss, S., and Mallory, G. K., J.A.M.A. 98:1353, 1932.
28. Millar, T. McW., Bruce, J., and Patterson, J. R. S., Br. J. Surg. 44:513, 1957.
29. Cronin, K., Br. J. Surg. 47:43, 1959.

9

INTERNAL AND EXTERNAL GASTRIC AND DUODENAL FISTULAS

RODNEY MAINGOT

There are two varieties of gastric fistula, namely: (1) internal gastric fistula communicating with some other hollow viscus, such as the gallbladder, the duodenum, or the colon; and (2) external gastric fistula opening onto the surface of the body.

GASTRIC FISTULAS

Internal

Internal gastric fistulas may be divided into two groups:

1. The spontaneous variety, in which, as a result of a gastric ulcer or carcinoma of the stomach, the viscus opens spontaneously into the duodenum, the colon, the gallbladder, or the jejunum.
2. A gastrojejunocolic fistula that develops following gastric operations, such as partial gastrectomy or gastroenterostomy for duodenal ulcer.

The *gastroduodenal* fistulas may be caused by a chronic penetrating ulcer of the stomach or by malignant disease of the organ. The first case of gastroduodenal fistula secondary to a benign gastric ulcer was described by Deitrich in 1847. The first operation for a **gastro**duodenal fistula caused by cancer of the stomach was reported by Ludin in 1924.

Moran and MacLean [23] recorded an interesting case of gastroduodenal fistula caused by a large penerating posterior wall gastric ulcer, in which the ulcer eroded through the pancreas and the anterior wall of the fourth portion of the duodenum. Prior to the publication of this case, only 12 proved cases had been reported, the majority of them being caused by cancer of the posterior wall of the stomach.

There are two types of gastroduodenal fistulas. In one type, the fistula occurs between the stomach and first part of the duodenum, whereas in the second type, the fistula occurs between the stomach and the third or fourth part of the duodenum. In the first type, it is conceivable that the pylorus is drawn up toward the lesser curvature of the stomach, where the ulcer in contracting draws up the remaining portion of the lesser curvature and the duodenum toward its destructive margin. Eventually the inflammatory process embraces the duodenum and finally perforation occurs between the stomach and the duodenum. Of course *it is possible* that, when there is a gastric ulcer and a duodenal ulcer present at the same time, the lesions may be attracted to each other by scarring and contraction. They first of all become what are called "kissing" ulcers, and then perforation occurs between these hollow viscera, with or without a concomitant abscess.

A number of cases have been reported of *gastrocolic fistula* secondary to benign gastric ulceration, to cancer involving the body of the stomach, ulcerative colitis, localized peritonitis, and stab wounds. In the case of chronic gastric ulcer, this lesion is decidedly rare, whereas in cases of malignant disease it may be encountered as a terminal event. Cases are reported in the literature in which benign or malignant gastric ulcers have become anchored to the jejunum and perforated it, thus producing a *spontaneous gastrojejunostomy;* or again, in rare instances, the ulcerated stomach may become glued to the colon, to the gallbladder, or even to the bile ducts, and eventually perforate them.

Deshpande [9] reported a case of benign gastric ulcer with concomitant gastrocolic and gastrojejunal fistulas.

Gray [12] published a case of benign gastric ulcer penerating the colon and also reviewed the literature. She found only 30 cases of gastrocolic fistulas caused by benign gastric ulcer (see Chap. 24). Arthur and Morris [1] have given an able and interesting account of *renoalimentary fistulas.* They state that Abeshouse (1949) was able to collect only six authentic cases of *renogastric fistula* from the literature, and as far as can be ascertained no further cases have been added since that time. Abeshouse collected nine cases of *renoduodenal fistula* from the literature, and, since that time, at least six other cases have been recorded. In most of the reported cases, the fistula at its renal end has communicated with the pelvis of the kidney.

Gastrojejunocolic fistula caused by peptic ulceration following gastrojejunostomy or partial gastrectomy for duodenal ulcer is discussed in Chapter 24.

SIGNS AND SYMPTOMS

The signs and symptoms of an *internal gastric fistula* due to primary or secondary peptic ulceration or malignant disease are indistinguishable from those of cancer of the stomach, but the diagnosis can often be confirmed preoperatively by means of a barium-meal x-ray examination and by the expert use of the fibrescope. It is true that at operation the surgeon might easily be misled into believing that a nonresectable carcinoma of the stomach was present, but sometimes following a judicious dissection of the parts his endeavors may be rewarded by finding that the lesion is in fact innocent.

TREATMENT

The treatment of gastroduodenal fistula caused by benign gastric ulcer calls for partial gastrectomy of the Billroth II variety, whether the first part of the duodenum or the third or fourth portions are implicated in the fistulous communications. In cases of gastric cancer, resection is rarely feasible owing to the advanced stage of involvement of neighboring viscera and adjacent vital tissues, e.g., abdominal aorta, portal vein.

External

External gastric fistulas are usually man-made, as in the case of *gastrostomies* performed for feeding purposes. But a number may be observed after imperfect closure of a perforated gastric ulcer, after gastric resections or short-circuiting procedures, following the drainage of a perigastric abscess caused by slow leakage from a chronic ulcer of the stomach, or after the receipt of a penetrating wound of the epigastrium such as a stab or gunshot wound.

External gastric fistulas can be divided into two main groups: In the *first* group, the clinical picture is that of a slow leak from a perforation of the stomach, leading to a small area of erosion of the abdominal wall. Such a fistula produces a minimum amount of disturbance and may heal spontaneously, following an intensive course of medical therapy.

The *second* group comprises some of the postoperative catastrophes of a drainage operation for duodenal ulcer, partial or total gastrectomy, or oesophagogastrostomy, in which the suture line partially breaks down, and this is followed by a subphrenic abscess, general peritonitis, or a discharge through a breaking-down abdominal incision. In such cases, where gastric fluids pour through the wound following a gastric operation, the prognosis is grave.

Treatment

Conservative measures may be advised under the following conditions:

After catheter gastrostomy for perforated gastric ulcer. When the perforation has resulted in a hole more than 1 cm wide and the surrounding stomach wall is cheesy with inflammation, Neumann (1909) and Keynes (1934) considered that it was harmful to attempt closure by means of interrupted sutures. A rubber catheter passed through the hole and led downward into the duodenum will serve both as a stopper and also as a means of administering fluid nourishment. When the gastrostomy tube works loose and has to be withdrawn, a gastric fistula results; but if the abdominal wound is protected with aluminum paste or with one of the modern commercial liquid plastic substances, and if the medical treatment instituted for the cure of the ulcer is efficient, the fistulous tract may slowly close. At a later date, when the patient's general condition is satisfactory, the stomach should be examined by means of gastroscopy and barium-meal x-ray examination to ascertain whether the ulcer crater has healed, is healing, or is still active. If medical measures prove ineffectual, as is often the case, partial gastrectomy by the Billroth I or Billroth II method should be carried out.

When a cutaneous fistula develops after suture of a perforated gastric ulcer. This is a serious complication and is caused either by faulty closure of the hole in the stomach or by inadequate plugging of the perforation with an omental pad. If in attempting closure of the perforation the surgeon finds that the sutures persistently tear out, producing a large aperture in the stomach wall, the omentum should be gathered together and sutured over the opening, as practised by Roscoe Graham, or as an alternative method an expeditious partial gastrectomy by the Schoemaker-Billroth I method should be performed. (See Chap. 22.)

Following the Roscoe Graham procedure, the stomach should be kept empty by means of continuous or intermittent suction for at least 7 days. Nothing is allowed by mouth, but glucose-saline solution and blood should be introduced into the circulation in order to maintain the patient's strength. Blood chemistry determination should be carried out frequently so that the necessary parenteral replacements can be accurately prescribed. If after a few days of such therapy there is still an ominous discharge of gastric juice through the incision in the abdominal wall, emergency partial gastrectomy offers the only means of saving the patient's life.

Following the drainage of a subphrenic abscess caused by a leaking gastric ulcer. In such cases the wound and the surrounding skin for a wide area should be thickly smeared with aluminum paste or some other suitable preparation, such as Nobecutane, that protects the skin from coming into contact with the gastric juices. A Chaffin's sump drain should be inserted into the fistulous tract, and attached to a silent

CHAFFIN

SUCTION

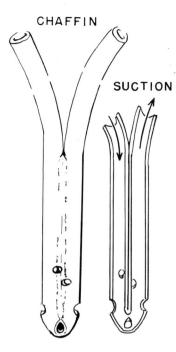

FIG. 1. Chaffin's tube.

electric suction apparatus such as the one illustrated in Figure 2, which is the oil-immersed low-pressure suction pump with overflow valve (No. GU. 2394). This is a most efficient apparatus. (Figs. 1, 2, and 3.)

Chemical tests of the blood are carried out, and dehydration and loss of electrolytes are made good by blood transfusions and intravenous infusions of water, sugar, salt, proteins, and vitamins. No food or fluid nourishment is allowed by mouth, pain is assuaged by intramuscular injections of pethidine (meperidine), and sleep is ensured by giving intramuscular injections of soluble phenobarbital. At some future date, when the general condition of the patient permits, partial gastrectomy should be carried out.

Disruption of the line of anastomosis is rare in comparison with leakage from the duodenal stump. The most serious cause is *ischaemic necrosis* of the gastric remnant. When a fistula due to ischaemia occurs, a fatal outcome is highly likely unless the ischaemic tissue can be expeditiously and boldly excised and alimentary continuity restored. Hardy [15] writes:

In contrast, anastomotic leakage in the absence of serious ischemia of the tissues involved carries only a moderately greater risk than does duodenal stump fistula. Such anastomotic fistula will often close spontaneously with supportive therapy; but if it does not close, it can be repaired by freshening the margins and suture-approximation at a second operation weeks later, once the peritonitis has subsided and a chronic drainage tract established. If a feeding tube can be passed into the distal jejunal loop, the nutrition of the patient can be maintained fairly well over a period of weeks. As an alternative, a jejunostomy for feeding purposes may be performed. . . . For leakage at the anastomotic line, conservative management is usually indicated; *but if ischemic necrosis is suspected,* especially if the splenic and left gastric arteries were sacrificed during the performance of a high subtotal gastrectomy, bold operative intervention and resection of questionably viable tissue may represent the only hope of preventing a fatal issue.

These views also have the support of State,[29] Colcock,[7] and Tanner (1972).

DUODENAL FISTULA

Duodenal fistulas may be external or internal. The majority of the external duodenal fistulas are the result of postoperative complications following procedures upon the duodenum, whereas the majority of the internal variety are of the spontaneous type, of which a good illustration is the cholecystoduodenal fistulas which result from gallstones. (See Fig. 7.)

External

Nearly all the reported cases have followed operations upon the stomach and duodenum, the gallbladder and bile passages, after excision of duodenal diverticula (especially of the second portion), after a difficult right-sided nephrectomy, and in some instances of penetrating or blunt injuries of the epigastrium. This fact was brought out 35 years ago by Kittleson who, in analysing 88 cases of external duodenal fistula, showed that in 30 cases the fistula followed operations upon the gallbladder and bile ducts, in 22 cases operations for perforated duodenal ulcer, in 8 cases nephrectomy, in 8 cases resections of the stomach and the first portion of the duodenum, in 7 cases operations

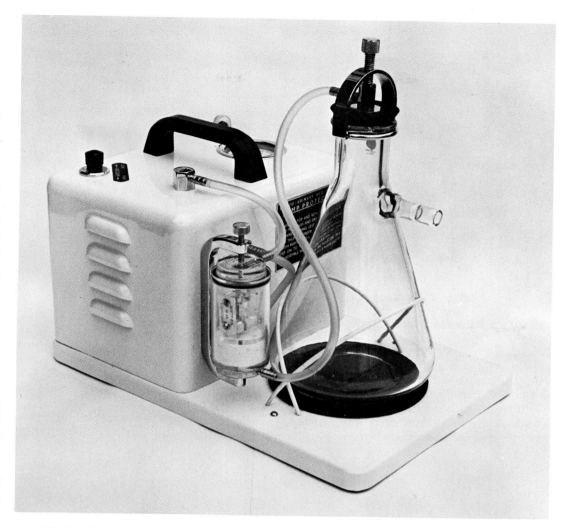

FIG. 2.   Special suction pump as supplied by The Genito-Urinary Manufacturing Company, Ltd. (Courtesy of The Genito-Urinary Manufacturing Company, Ltd., London.)

for acute retrocaecal appendicitis with obstruction, in 6 cases rupture of the duodenum, and in 7 cases as a result of other causes, such as penetrating wounds, e.g., stab or gunshot wounds.

I shall presently attempt to show how in performing operations upon the gallbladder and bile passages the duodenum can be injured, what precautions should be taken to prevent such a mishap, and how during a difficult right nephrectomy a portion of the second part of the duodenal wall may be picked up in a clamp and become crushed or else be ligatured to the vascular pedicle.

It now remains to consider how this complication following operations upon the stomach and duodenum accounts for more than 70 percent of the cases. In the majority of cases in this group, this is caused by inept methods of closing a perforated duodenal ulcer, especially when the hole is very large and the walls of the gut are unduly sodden with inflammatory products, and also to *the "blowing out" of the duodenal stump following the Billroth II types of partial gastrectomy for penetrating duodenal ulcer.* (Fig. 4.)

External duodenal fistula has been known

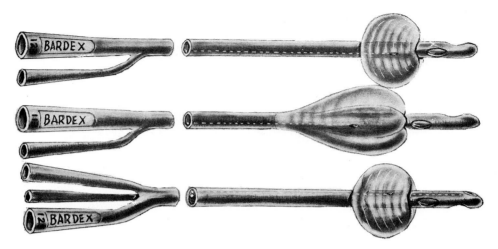

FIG. 3.   Bardex balloon catheters.

to arise after the operation of transduodenal choledocholithotomy for stone impacted in the ampulla of Vater; after transduodenal sphincterotomy or sphincteroplasty for recurrent pancreatitis or residual stones; fibrosis or stenosis of the sphincter of Oddi or for multiple stones in the bile ducts; after cholecystoduodenostomy; and after pyloroplasty or Finney's gastroduodenostomy for duodenal ulcer, particularly when there has been tension on the suture line. Rupture of the duodenum by a penetrating wound accounts for a few cases, as does also the operation of excision of a duodenal diverticulum, more especially when situated in the second portion of the bowel.

The most tragic cases of all are those seen after the Billroth II type of partial gas-

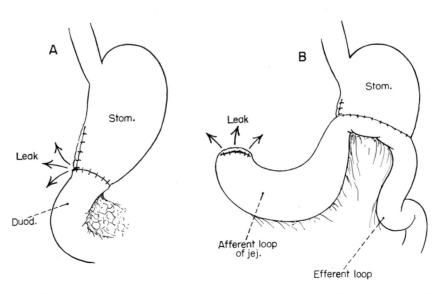

FIG. 4.   Leakage at anastomotic line and blown-out duodenal stump. (Courtesy of Dr. Bentley Colcock and the Lahey Clinic.)

troduodenal resection for peptic ulcer or gastric cancer. Here, owing to afferent loop or stomal obstruction, to imperfect invagination of the duodenal stump, to the use of unsuitable suture material such as plain catgut, to omitting to insert additional sutures of silk after the inversion of the duodenal stump is complete, or to failure to protect the finished suture line in the duodenum with adjacent omentum, a portion or the whole of the duodenal cul-de-sac blows out, with the result that a subphrenic abscess or generalised peritonitis ensues. When the accumulated fluids burst through a portion of the abdominal incision or through an emergency exploratory incision, a grave type of external duodenal fistula results.

It is perhaps surprising to find in the literature several references to this complication following appendectomy for acute retrocaecal appendicitis, but the position of the appendix (high up, retrocaecal and overriding the duodenum), the state of affairs displayed at operation (the appendix large, oedematous, soft with gangrene, and embedded in a mass of adhesions), the technical difficulties associated with its excision, and the necessity for inserting a rubber drainage tube down to the septic oozing area, which may, if left in situ too long, cause pressure necrosis of the duodenal wall, would all at times predispose to fistula formation. More than 40 years ago that wise American surgeon Cameron drew attention to this complication.

An external duodenal fistula may be deliberately constructed by the surgeon in exceptional circumstances when, following gastroduodenal resection for a large, inflamed duodenal ulcer, the closure of the stump has been exceedingly difficult or appears to be insecure.

So excellent an account of this operation of duodenostomy has been given by Priestley and Butler [25] that I cannot do better than quote it here in full:

Occasionally, because of unexpected findings as the operation progresses or for other reasons, one may find that closure of the duodenal stump in a usual manner might result in undesirable encroachment on certain important adjacent structures. Under these circumstances, management of

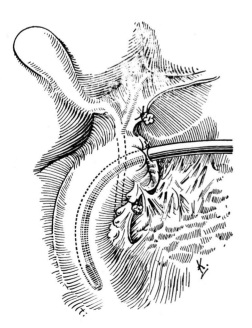

FIG. 5.   Catheter duodenostomy in case of difficult closure of stump following gastroduodenal resection for large penetrating duodenal ulcer.

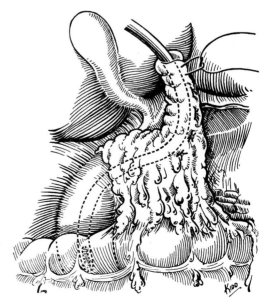

FIG. 6.   Catheter duodenostomy following gastroduodenal resection for penetrating duodenal ulcer. Note that catheter as it emerges from duodenum is encased with omentum.

the duodenal stump by performance of duodenostomy may prove to be quite helpful [Figs. 5 and 6]. This procedure consists simply in closing the open end of the duodenum around an appropriate catheter, perhaps a size 20 F straight latex type. That portion of the duodenum which can be sutured satisfactorily is closed and the catheter is permitted to remain where satisfactory closure is difficult or impossible without endangering adjacent structures or the wall of the duodenum by further mobilization. Purse-string sutures placed around the catheter may be helpful. Nearby fatty tissue may be sutured around the catheter if further protection of the closure appears advisable. The catheter is brought out of the abdominal wall through a stab wound. The catheter is anchored securely to the skin by a sturdy nonabsorbable suture. A Penrose-type drain may be left near the end of the duodenum if one wishes, and brought out by a different tract through the abdominal wall.

The catheter is connected with a bottle at the conclusion of the operation so that fluid which drains from the duodenum may be collected and measured. This, of course, is helpful in judging the need for replacement of fluid and electrolytes. There may be relatively little drainage from the duodenum. Ten or 12 days after operation the catheter may be clamped to observe any untoward effects that might result. In our limited experience with this procedure, no such results have been observed. The catheter may be withdrawn 12 to 14 days after operation. The sinus tract may be expected to heal quite promptly. (Figs. 5 and 6.)

Welch [32] began using this technique as far back as 1946, with excellent results. In 1962 he wrote:

The surgeon may have already accomplished a gastric resection and found himself with a duodenal stump which is most difficult to close, or he may have had to expose the duodenum widely for the control of massive haemorrhage from the gastroduodenal artery.

Particularly in cases of this latter type, it is well to re-emphasize the advantages of *tube duodenostomy* as a method of prevention of death from a duodenal fistula. It was of interest that in 52 instances of tube duodenostomy carried out by the author and his associates, only one death could be ascribed to the procedure.

The mortality of patients with duodenal stump perforations in our hospital is now roughly 50 percent and indicates strongly the great advantages of decompression of the duodenum by catheter wherever closure is unsatisfactory.

Austen and Bane [3] state that the safety of gastric surgery has increased markedly in recent years, but that as long as stomachs are resected, there will be problems with closure of the duodenum.

Difficulty with the duodenal stump remains the largest single cause of death following gastrectomy.

One hundred and sixty-two gastric resections were carried out over a period of two years on a ward service by surgical residents; a mortality rate was 0.6 percent. Catheter duodenostomy was utilized whenever closure of the duodenal stump was not completely satisfactory. This occurred in 24 percent of the resections. There were no duodenal leaks in any of the patients and no cases of pancreatitis in those in whom a catheter was used. In many patients the duodenal closure was either unsatisfactory or impossible, and many of the patients were extremely poor risks. When used properly in such situations, catheter duodenostomy can help reduce the mortality of gastric section to an extremely low level.

SYMPTOMS

The diagnosis of either duodenal or anastomotic leakage should be considered if the patient abruptly experiences abdominal pain, tenderness and rigidity associated with pyrexia, tachycardia, and leukocytosis. It is always wise to insert a small drain down to the closed duodenal stump following the performance of the Billroth II procedures.

The symptoms are dependent upon the character and quantity of the discharge and the size of the fistula itself. When the opening is small and is discharging a little mucus with perhaps only a slight trace of duodenal juice without causing any appreciable irritation of the skin, healing may be rapid. When, however, the fistula is large and great quantities of viscid, bile-stained, acrid fluid constantly gush through the semidigested wound, the patient rapidly becomes emaciated, anaemic, hypochloraemic, profoundly prostrated and dehydrated, and the position is grave, calling for energetic and immediate treatment to prevent a fatal issue.

The patient's chances of survival are endangered when the fistula develops: (1) very soon after operation; (2) after gastrojejunostomy or the Billroth I types of gastroduodenal anastomosis; (3) when the duodenal stump "blows-out" after the Billroth II operation; and (4) when the discharge through the wound is profuse or torrential.

Prognosis

According to Gardner (1951) the fatality rate from duodenal fistula is greater than from fistulas elsewhere in the intestine. Schneider (1944), in reviewing a consecutive series of 33 cases, gave the fatality rate as about 50 percent whether the patients were treated conservatively or by operation.

In 1964, Welch and Hedberg [33] reported a mortality rate for duodenal stump fistula of 50 percent at the Massachusetts General Hospital.

Colcock [7] stated that in a series of 374 patients who had a gastric resection for duodenal ulcer at the Lahey Clinic during the previous 4½ years, a duodenal leak developed in three after operation. Although the incidence of duodenal stump leakage was low (0.8 percent), the mortality rate was 33 percent.

Belding [4] reported the experience of a community hospital in which 512 patients were submitted to gastrectomy over a 10-year period. The incidence of duodenal stump leakage was 5.6 percent, and the mortality rate was 15 percent.

Treatment

Operative measures include: (1) resuture of the aperture at the anastomotic junction and (2) jejunostomy.

In slight cases, for example, in those with a small *chronic fistula* which will not heal with conservative treatment, reopening of the abdomen, excision of the fistula, and resuture of the aperture in the duodenum will often be successful.

In those cases of duodenal fistula caused by the *blowing out of the duodenal stump* following Billroth II operations for chronic duodenal ulcer, gastric ulcer, or pyloric growth, *resuture* is meddlesome and often is doomed to failure owing to the friable and necrotic condition of the bowel wall and to the great pressure within the duodenum during digestive activity. In such cases, conservative treatment, as outlined later, is definitely indicated.

The cases of external duodenal fistula that occur after such operations as Billroth I, Finney's operation, gastrojejunostomy, pyloroplasty or simple suture of a perforated duodenal ulcer, demand prompt decision and action. As soon as the condition is recognised and *closing the hole with interrupted sutures of 00 Mersilk* and protecting the suture line with an omental pad or free omental graft, as would be practised in a case of acute perforation due to peptic ulcer, drainage of the operative field is cogently advocated.

Jejunostomy is the procedure of choice when it is imperative to operate upon a patient who has symptoms of dehydration, malnutrition, alkalaemia, and extreme prostration, as it is a simple and easy procedure and can be carried out under local anaesthesia with comparatively little disturbance. Jejunostomy (by the Stamm or Marwedal method) is the most logical measure, as it permits the ingestion of fluids and foods by the intestine below the fistula and it also permits the introduction of the aspirated duodenal juices into a portion of the gut where it is especially needed for digestive purposes.

It should be emphasized, however, that in cases of "blowing-out" of the duodenal stump, if response to supportive measures proves to be increasingly satisfactory, this procedure is unnecessary.

It is now generally agreed that *conservative measures* offer the best hope of cure when "blowing out" of the duodenal stump follows the Billroth II methods of gastroduodenal resection. Only when this method fails should the surgeon resort to *Fourth Priority*.

Chapman, Foran, and Dunphy [6] maintain that the keys to successful conservative management are: (1) "get control of the fistula"; (2) combat sepsis; and (3) from the very beginning, maintain adequate nutritional support.

They consider the specific priorities of management to be those as summarised in the list below.

First priority (0 to 12 hr)
1. Correct blood volume deficiency.
2. Drain obvious and easily accessible abseses.
3. Control fistula, protect skin by use of sump or bag.

Second priority (0 to 48 hr)
1. Correct electrolyte imbalance.

2. Replace daily fluid and electrolyte losses.
3. Begin intravenous nutritional program.
   Third priority (1 to 6 days)
1. passage of feeding tube beyond fistula.
2. Feeding jejunostomy.
3. Continual search for and drainage of obvious abscesses if they appear.
   Fourth priority (after 8 to 20 days)
Surgical intervention to find occult sepsis and to close or bypass the fistula.

Control of the fistula. The skin must be protected from the searing discharges by kaolin, aluminium paste, a suitable acrylic emulsion such as Octaflex, or by karaya gum powder.

The total output of the fistula is measured and charted every day and the nature of the discharge ascertained by chemical tests.

Local abscesses must be drained and any pocketing of fistulous contents avoided.

Sump drainage tubes, such as the Chaffin (Fig. 1) or Richardson suction tubes, should be inserted into the depths of the wound and then connected to a G-U portable suction apparatus (Fig. 2). It is often advisable to isolate the fistula from the surrounding skin by means of a *disposable ileostomy type of pastic bag,* the mouth of which is firmly affixed around the fistulous opening. Suction by means of sump can be continued through the plastic ileostomy bag.

According to Chapman et al.: [6]

Once a satisfactory tract has been established, the sump should be withdrawn and either suction discontinued or applied only to the bag. The presence of a sump tube may actually impair closure of the fistula by acting as a foreign body. It also may greatly increase the output of the fistula. The use of a plastic collecting bag avoids this difficulty, permits a continued accurate collection of drainage, avoids leakage and often allows only a small portion of the intestinal contents to pass through the fistula. No excess fluid is suctioned from the gastrointestinal tract. . . . The next step in the control of the fistula is delineation of its size and location. This is accomplished by careful x-ray studies using a combination of dilute barium or gastrografin by mouth and by injection of the fistulous tract. *Essential questions to be answered are:* (1) the level of the fistula; (2) its size and whether or not there is bowel continuity; (3) the presence or absence of obstruction distal to the fistula.

Maintenance of nutrition. During the first 10 days, more than 2,000 calories per day can be given by the intravenous route. Proper administration of intravenous electrolytes and blood must be maintained. This entails repeated blood chemistry determinations. The chief losses in gastric and duodenal fistulas will be those of sodium and chloride; but a careful check should be made of calcium, potassium, and *magnesium* loss.

When ileus has abated, early attention must be directed toward passing a nasogastric tube beyond the fistula in order to provide an adequate nutritional regimen. When this cannot be performed, a *feeding jejunostomy* must be considered and should not be postponed beyond the tenth day, unless it is manifest that all infection has been controlled and the fistula shows signs of closing.

Control of infection. One of the first priorities in management is drainage of obvious and easily accessible abscesses.

Continued daily search for potential sites of abscess in the region of the fistulous tract, pelvis, peritoneal cavity, subphrenic spaces, and liver must be carried out.

If the patient remains febrile and is losing ground, exploration of potential sites of infection is in order.

Antibiotic therapy is used freely; the choice of antibiotic is made on sensitivity tests (see Chaps. 106 and 107).

Finally, suction should be maintained for at least 2 days after the discharge of the fluid has ceased. Where haemorrhage through the fistulous tract or haematemesis—a rare complication—occurs, such conservative measures as outlined above, combined with massive blood transfusions, should be persevered. with until all haemorrhage ceases. Haemorrhage is in some instances caused by acute peptic erosions of the stomach pouch. Reopening the abdomen and making a sedulous search for the bleeding point is associated with a prohibitive mortality and should thus not be countenanced.

INTERNAL DUODENAL AND BILIARY FISTULAS

Biliary fistulas can be single or multiple, external or internal. They may be classified as follows: (1) *external or cutaneous:* via elective operations, i.e., cholecystostomy, T tube choledochostomy; and spontaneous,

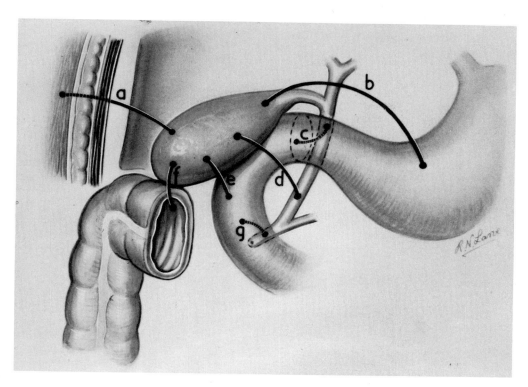

FIG. 7.   Sites of biliary fistulas.

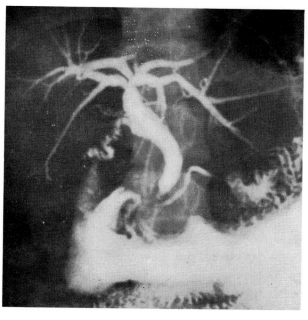

FIG. 8.   Outline of biliary tree, caused by *reflux* of duodenal contents and barium. Patient was young soldier who complained of indigestion. He was admitted to hospital and barium-meal x-ray examination was carried out. Gallbladder, cystic duct, common bile duct, intrahepatic radicals, and pancreatic duct are clearly shown filled with opaque medium. No operation was performed. Patient was subsequently discharged fit and well. (Courtesy of Dr. Edward Holland.)

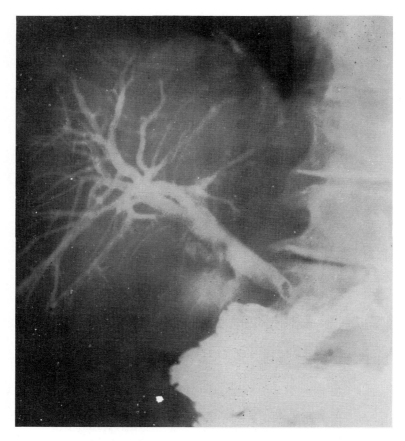

FIG. 9.   Choledochoduodenal fistula caused by stone in common bile duct ulcerating through into duodenum. Picture was taken after a barium-meal x-ray examination.

caused by gallstones or carcinoma of the gall-bladder; or (2) *internal:* after elective operations, i.e., various types of cholecystoenterostomy to relieve obstructive jaundice; and spontaneous, most commonly caused by gall-stones eroding into the duodenum or adjacent colon, to a penetrating duodenal ulcer, etc. (Figs. 7-11.)

Spontaneous internal biliary fistulas, in which the gallbladder communicates with the duodenum, colon, or stomach, are uncommon, being found in 0.4 to 3 percent of all operations on the biliary tract, as has been noted by Noskin et al.[24] Puestow, writing on the subject of biliary fistulas in his *Surgery of the Biliary Tract, Pancreas and Spleen* (4th Ed. 1970), makes these observations: "External biliary fistulas are quite rare, and *spontaneous biliary fistulas* are seldom encountered in modern day medicine.

These usually result from an abscessed gall-bladder pointing through the abdominal wall. Occasionally an abscess of the abdominal wall will form and, when incised, bile, pus and gallstones may be extruded. *Spontaneous internal biliary fistulas are not uncommon.* (See Fig. 7.) I have encountered healed or existing fistulas in 3 percent of patients operated on for biliary tract disease." The majority of internal fistulas are due to gallstones ulcerating from the gallbladder into the duodenum; *only 6 percent are caused by duodenal ulceration.* But in these latter cases, the fistulas nearly always open into the adjacent common bile duct, as has been ably pointed out by Waggoner and LeMone[31] and later by Kyle.[19] Up to the present time about 400 cases of *choledochoduodenal fistula* have been reported in the world literature. (Fig. 11.)

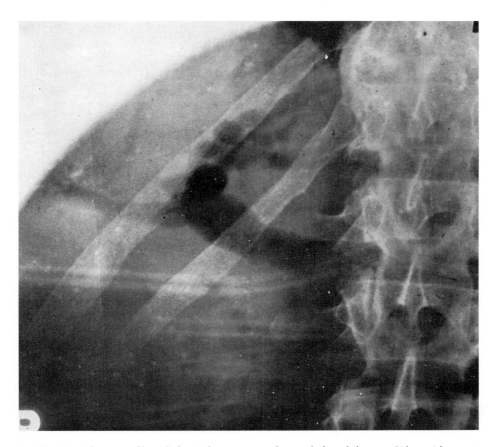

FIG. 10. Straight x-ray film of the right-upper quadrant of the abdomen. Side-to-side anastomosis of greatly dilated common bile duct to first portion of duodenum. Note gas filling biliary tree. (Courtesy of Mr. W. B. Gabriel.)

Hicken and Coray,[17] in a study of 272 gastrointestinal biliary fistulas, found the gallbladder to be involved in 88 percent and the common bile duct in 11 percent, whilst the gastrointestinal component consisted of duodenum in 69 percent, colon in 26 percent, and stomach in 5 percent. Epperman and Walters[10] state that 84 cases of spontaneous internal biliary fistulas were encountered at the Mayo Clinic during the years 1945 to 1950, inclusive. During that period 9,716 operations were performed upon the biliary tract—an incidence of about 1 percent. Haff et al.[14] places the incidence of biliary enteric fistulas as low as 0.4 percent of all biliary tract operations. They reported 24 cases, of which 20 were women and 4 were males. The average age was 71. These were 13 cases of cholecystoduodenal fistulas, 7 cholecys-tocolonic, 1 duodecystogastric, 4 choledoduoduodenal and 2 cholecystocholedochocholedochal.

The fistulous communication can occur as the result of trauma, an operation, or disease between the duodenum on the one hand, and the stomach, colon, gallbladder, or bile ducts on the other hand. As just stated, by far the most common type of internal duodenal fistula seen is that which occurs between the duodenum and gallbladder—cholecystoduodenal—as the result of gallstones (Fig. 12). This is confirmed by the records of many surgeons. For instance, Lasala and Saporta[20] state that of the 51 patients operated upon by them, 49 had fistulas between the gallbladder and duodenum, and in 2 the fistulous tract was caused by a chronic penerating posterior wall ulcer. Caminha and Monteiro [5] write:

The 30 fistulas which were discovered at operation comprised 2 percent of 1,500 cases of biliary tract disease surgically treated in Rio de Janeiro from 1947 to 1957. Of the 30 patients, 27 (90 percent) had calculous cholecystitis, and in 3 there were cholecystoduodenal fistulas secondary to chronic duodenal ulcer. In 16 (59.2 percent) of 27 cases of biliary origin there were cholecystoduodenal fistulas, in 4 (14.8 percent) cholecystocolonic fistulas, in 3 (11.1 percent) cholecystogastric fistulas, and in 2 (7.4 percent) choledochoduodenal fistulas. There were 2 patients with combined fistulas: one had a cholecystohepatic and cholecystoduodenal fistula, and the other had a cholecystocholedochoduodenal fistula.

Glenn and Mannix,[11] in reporting 40 cases of biliary enteric fistula, write:

Cholecystoduodenal fistulas were encountered in 32 cases (76 percent of the total); cholecystocolic in 3; choledochoduodenal in 2; and there were single cases of cholecystogastric, cholecystoduodenocolic and cholecystocholedochoduodenal fistulas.

Marshall and Polk [21] reviewed 41 cases of internal biliary fistulas that had occurred in patients who had not previously had surgical procedures on or near the biliary tract. Of the 41 patients studied, 26 were females and 15 males. They state that fistulas occur approximately *twice as frequently in females as in males.* The majority of fistulas in their series had occurred in the sixth and seventh decades of life, with the fifth decade ranking next in frequency. The *age* of the patients who had spontaneous internal biliary fistulas correlates closely with that of patients who have calculous cholecystitis. Cholesystoduodenal fistula was the most common type; it was found in 73 percent of the cases they studied. Although cholecystocolic and choledochoduodenal fistulas had been regarded as the next most common types, in their series cholecystocholedochal fistulas were more common. Twenty-eight of the 30 cases of cholecystoduodenal fistulas could be attributed directly to chronic gallbladder dis-

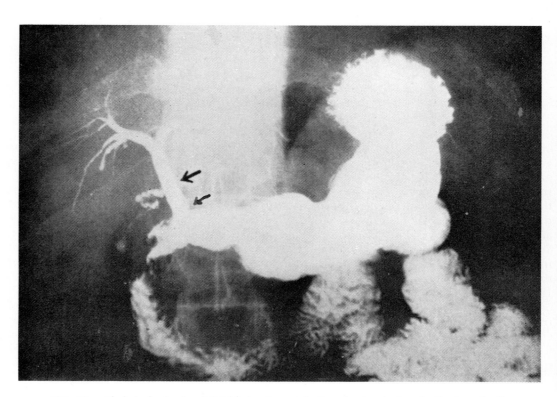

FIG. 11.   Choledochoduodenal fistula due to penetrating duodenal ulcer (author's patient).

ease, although 2 of the 30 were the result of a penetrating duodenal ulcer. They found the *operative mortality* rate to be much higher in cases of internal biliary fistulas than in cases of uncomplicated cholelithiasis. Five of their 40 patients who were operated upon died in hospital, a mortality rate of 12.5 percent. This should be contrasted with their mortality rate for operations upon the gallbladder and biliary tract for cholecystitis and cholelithiasis, which is only 1.1 percent. The final outcome in their 41 cases was "good" in 31.

An adherent gallbladder favours the pressure of calculi against the duodenum, leading to slow necrosis and eventually to the discharge of the stones into the bowel. When this complication arises, it is assumed by some authorities that a permanent communication exists between the duodenum and gallbladder. This is by no means the case, as although most of these fistulous tracts between the gallbladder and duodenum bear evidences of the ravages of past disease, in some instances the fistulous tract may heal without any gross detectable traces. This statement is supported by Hicken and Corby[17] who write:

There is abundant evidence indicating that these fistulas can and do heal voluntarily. Numerous cases have been reported wherein all biliary symptoms subsided after the gallstones had eroded into the duodenum and escaped with the faeces. . . .
We have seen cholecystoduodenal fistulas close spontaneously as soon as the provocative duodenal ulcer has become quiescent under strict medical management.

It can be reiterated here that 6 percent of these spontaneous fistulas between the common bile duct (or hepatic ducts) and the duodenum are produced by perforating duodenal ulcer. If the ulcer is situated posteriorly it usually perforates the choledochus, but if it is situated laterally or superiorly, it may erode the gallbladder itself; such fistulas (caused by chronic peptic ulceration) are rare, however, as are also instances of benign gastric ulcerative lesions forming an attachment to the gallbladder and perforating it.

An impacted calculus in the lower end of the common bile duct may ulcerate through the walls of the duct and then into the duodenum, thus producing another variety of choledochal fistula, but this variety is less commonly encountered than those due to duodental ulceration. The rarity of *spontaneous choledochoduodenal fistulas* seems to me to be a little surprising in view of the frequency of duodenal ulceration and of the proximity of the common bile duct to the first portion of the duodenum. The fistulous tract in such cases is usually quite short, being only 2 to 3 mm long. Interesting cases of *cholecystocolic fistulas* have been reported by Augur and Gracie,[2] Clarence Schein,[28] Grossman,[13] Sherill Rife,[27] and Maingot (see Figs. 12 and 13). When operating on cases of cholecystocolic fistulas, preliminary operative cholangiograms supply useful information regarding the presence or absence of calculi in the biliary tree. A barium enema may display the fistula. The operative procedures include cholecystectomy, closure of the hole in the hepatic flexure of the colon, exploration of the bile ducts, and T tube choledochostomy. The subject of *gallstone ileus*

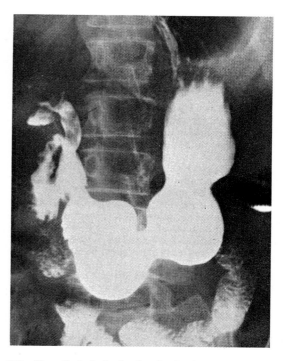

FIG. 12. Choledochoduodenal fistula caused by stones in common bile duct. Such fistulas are rarely encountered (author's patient).

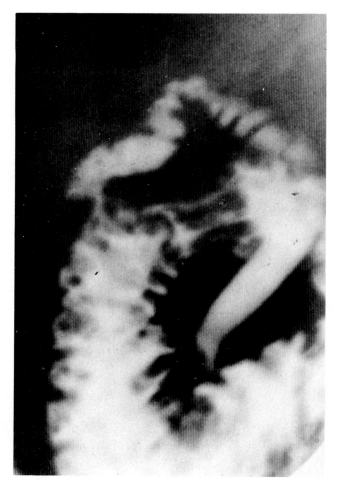

FIG. 13. Cholecystocolic fistula (author's patient). There is a stone in the lower end of the bile duct.

or obturation is discussed by Harold Ellis in Chapter 86.

The *symptoms* are in many respects similar to those associated with disease of the biliary system. Dyspepsia, flatulence, nausea, diarrhoea, vomiting, uneasiness after fatty meals, occasional chills, and bouts of pyrexia usually precede the intense spasms of right-sided colic, the sullen pain of hepatitis, cholangitis, and the onset of deepening jaundice. I say *usually* because the clinical picture may be very confusing; it may simulate that of a stenosing duodenal ulcer, a carcinoma of the stomach, or calculi impacted in the choledochus; or again the preexisting symptoms may abruptly cease concomitantly with the formation of the fistula.

The *diagnosis* can in many instances be confirmed by means of radiographic examination after administration of an opaque meal. The barium will be seen passing through the superior aspect of the duodenal cap into the gallbladder or bile ducts, which will be clearly outlined.

Heron [16] has discussed the radiological features of the condition; these, briefly, are:

1. Direct signs: (a) Gas or barium, or both, in the gallbladder or biliary tree. (b) mucous membrane at the stoma of the fistula.
2. Indirect sign: nonfunctioning gallbladder, as revealed at cholecystography.

A revealing x-ray sign is the presence of *gas in the gallbladder or bile duct*. This may result from one of three conditions:

1. Spontaneous or operative fistulous connection between some part of the biliary system and the gastrointestinal tract.
2. Regurgitation through the sphincter of Oddi via the ampulla of Vater (see Fig. 8).
3. Emphysema from bacterial origin— emphysematous gangrenous cholecystitis (Cottam,[8] and Swalm and Manges.[30]

McCorkle and Fong [22] emphasise the fact that in emphysematous cholecystitis the gas derived from the action of bacteria is usually confined within the gallbladder itself. Rees [26] asserts that the reflex regurgitation of the duodenal gases through an atonic sphincter of Oddi is a very rare event. Intravenous cholangiography employing Biligrafin has proved helpful in diagnosis.

Other rare instances of internal duodenal fistulas include those cases in which a duodenal ulcer has eroded into the stomach, into the small intestine, the colon or even into the pelvis of the right kidney, or the portal vein.

TREATMENT

When the fistula is caused by gallstones—*cholecystoduodenal fistula*—the two viscera should be carefully separated and the aperture in the duodenum closed in such a way that narrowing of the gut does not result. After exploring the common duct and dilating the ampulla with Bakes' or other dilators to make sure that it is amply patent, the gallbladder is removed and the common duct is drained by means of a T tube.

When acute intestinal obstruction is due to the impaction of a large gallstone in the lower reaches of the ileum in the presence of calculous cholecystitis, the correct treatment is first to deal with the emergency, i.e., to relieve the gallstone obturation by enterotomy, to extract the stone, and to carry out transverse closure of the wound in the bowel, this being followed some weeks later by excision of the fistulous tract between the gallbladder and duodenum, and then chole-cystectomy combined with T tube choledochostomy.

The surgical treatment of *choledochoduodenal fistula* caused by an impacted common duct stone entails cholecystectomy, exploration of the biliary passages, the removal of any calculi which are present in the ducts, transduodenal sphincterotomy with T tube choledochostomy, and closure of the duodenotomy incision, followed by control cholangiograms to make sure that the biliary passages are clear and fully patent before closing the abdominal incision. Drainage in these cases is essential.

Good results have followed the treatment of *choledochoduodenal fistulas caused by a penetrating duodenal ulcer by partial gastrectomy based on the Bancroft-Plenk plan*, as Kourias [18] has emphasised.

REFERENCES

1. Arthur and Morris, Br. J. Surg. 53:396, 1966.
2. Augur and Gracie, Am. J. Gastroenterol. 53:558, 1970.
3. Austen and Bane, Ann. Surg. 160:781, 1964.
4. Belding, Surg. Gynecol. Obstet. 117:578, 1963.
5. Caminha and Monteiro, Rev. Brasil. Cir. 34:5, 1957.
6. Chapman, Foran, and Dunphy, Am. J. Surg. 108:157, 1964.
7. Colcock, Lahey Foundation Clin. Bull. 13:190, 1964.
8. Cottam, Surg. Gynecol. Obstet. 25:192, 1917.
9. Deshpande, Br. J. Surg. 51:389, 1964.
10. Epperman and Walters, Proc. Mayo Clin. 28:353, 1953.
11. Glenn and Mannix, Surg. Gynecol. Obstet. 105:693, 1957.
12. Gray, Surgery 40:408, 1956.
13. Grossman, Am. J. Surg. 55:277, 1971.
14. Haff et al., Surg. Gynecol. Obstet. 133:84, 1971.
15. Hardy, Am. J. Surg. 108:699, 1964.
16. Heron, Br. J. Radiol. 31:50, 1958.
17. Hicken and Coray, Surg. Gynecol. Obstet. 82:723, 1946.
18. Kourias, Surg. Gynecol. Obstet. 119:103, 1964.
19. Kyle, Br. J. Surg. 46:124, 1958.
20. Lasala and Saporta, Prensa Méd. Argent. 44:1657, 1957.
21. Marshall and Polk, Surg. Clin. North Am. 6:679, 1958.
22. McCorkle and Fong, Surgery 11:851, 1942.
23. Moran and MacLean, Ann. Surg. 146:937, 1957.
24. Noskin et al., Ann. Surg. 130:270, 1949.
25. Priestley and Butler, Am. J. Surg. 82:163, 1951.
26. Rees, Am. J. Surg. 100:496, 1941.
27. Rife, Arch. Surg. 62:876, 1951.
28. Schein, Acute Cholecystitis, New York, Harper & Row, 1972.
29. State, Surg. Clin. North Am. 44:371, 1964.

30. Swalm and Manges, Amer. J. Surg. 7:52, 1929.
31. Waggoner and LeMone, Radiology 53:31, 1949.
32. Welch, Surg. Clin. North Am. 42:1313, 1962.
33. Welch and Hadberg, J.A.M.A. 187:432, 1964.

10

EXPLORATORY LAPAROTOMY: BEFORE AND AFTER OPERATIONS UPON THE STOMACH AND DUODENUM

RODNEY MAINGOT

Exploratory laparotomy is rarely required in order to establish a diagnosis of destructive organic disease of the stomach or duodenum. Pyloric stenosis, extension of an ulcer to a size which precludes the likelihood of permanent healing, early cancerous change, and the presence of innocent tumours can be detected with certainty by means of clinical methods, radiography, biochemical and other tests, and gastroscopy.

But in spite of the great advances that have been made in diagnosing gastric and duodenal disorders, there are still a few baffling cases of organic disease which defy detection by these means but which, nevertheless, on account of the symptoms present, call for surgical measures. I refer particularly to certain cases of cancer of the stomach which present suspicious symptoms but in which on x-ray examination no abnormality is detected; to some ulcerating lesions of the antrum; to the elusive anastomotic ulcer; and to chronic duodenal ulcers situated in the descending limb of the duodenum proximal to the ampulla of Vater.

Again, some *unusual lesions of the duodenum* such as: inflammatory and stenoic lesions of the ampulla of Vater, diverticulitis, cicatrising enteritis (Crohn's disease), tuberculosis, polypi, adenomas, carcinoid tumours, and melanomas are rarely diagnosed preoperatively, in spite of the fact that they may display symptoms of partial obstruction, unexplained melaena, and radiological evidence of a deformity. During recent years, however, the increasing use of and experience with the fibreduodenoscope has played a significant part in the elucidation of such lesions (see Chap. 34B, by Louis Kreel).

When an elective operation is advised for chronic gastric or duodenal ulcer or for malignant disease of the stomach, it is often wise to conduct a very thorough routine examination not only of the stomach and duodenum but also of the remaining abdominal viscera.

These are best investigated in the following order: stomach and duodenum; liver, gallbladder, and bile passages; pancreas and spleen; duodenojejunal flexure and small intestine; appendix and caecum; and colon and pelvic organs. A search should always be made for diaphragmatic hernia. I have found that a hiatus that admits the tips of only two examining fingers is normal. The cardiac portion of the stomach, which is sometimes difficult to examine adequately on barium-meal x-ray examination, can be inspected and palpated with ease after the left lobe of the liver has been mobilised by division of the left lateral ligament. I agree with Strokl and Diffenbaugh [20] that a diverticulum of the proximal one-third of the stomach is particularly difficult to demonstrate by x-ray examination. These lesions are usually located on the posterior wall of the fundus, adjacent to the cardiac orifice (see Chap. 7).

The whole of the stomach and duodenum must be methodically examined; the anterior surface, the greater and lesser curvatures, the omenta with their lymph nodes, and the cardiac and pyloric regions are palpated and visualised by good retraction, after which the posterior surface of the stomach and the stomach bed itself are explored through an incision made in the gastrohepatic omentum and also by detaching the gastrocolic ligament from the greater curvature of the stomach. When the stomach is elevated, an excellent view of the posterior wall of the stomach, a limited area of the posterior wall of the first portion of the duodenum, the pancreas, and the spleen is obtained. At this stage, it is advisable to inspect and palpate the neck, body, and tail of the pancreas methodically in order to exclude the possibility of a cryptic adenoma (see Chap. 13) (Fig. 1).

The four parts of the duodenum are examined seriatim, particular care being taken in palpating the bulb, testing the patency of the pyloric outlet and the tone of the sphincter, searching for the bed of a hidden posterior ulcer, and noting scarring, distortion, narrowing, and thickening of the bowel if these are present, as well as the condition of the surrounding parts. Kocher's manoeuvre of mobilising the first and descending portions of the duodenum will be necessary as a preliminary step to a number of gastroduodenal operations, and also when a lesion is detected or suspected to be in this portion of the gut (Fig. 2).

The retroperitoneal space is opened and the sweep of the duodenum and the head of the pancreas are firmly rotated medially, exposing the ureter, inferior vena cava, a con-

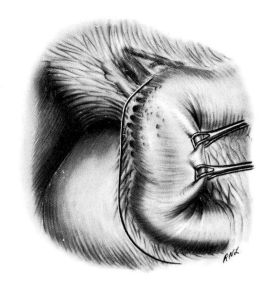

FIG. 2.   Incision for Kocher's mobilisation of first three portions of duodenum. In this illustration the stump of cystic duct is visible following previous cholecystectomy.

siderable portion of the head of the pancreas, the liberated parts of the duodenum, the lower reaches of the choledochus, and the "common duct gland." Many times it is difficult to determine whether the lesion arises in the duodenum or the head of the pancreas or in the periampullary area. If duodenotomy is indicated, the bowel should be opened obliquely, and later closed in this direction, in one layer, by means of a series of closely applied Gambee sutures of fine silk.

The technique for the exposure of the third and fourth portions of the duodenum, the lower half of the head of the pancreas, and the root of the superior mesenteric vessels is less well known and more difficult to accomplish. Here is Sedgwick's account [19] of Cattell's approach to this area:

By reversing the embryologic rotation of the colon and small intestine, the third and fourth portions of the duodenum can be made completely extraperitoneal. To expose the third and fourth portions of the duodenum, this process is reversed first, by freeing the attachments to the cecum and right half of the colon and then by incising the avascular peritoneal attachment to the mesentery of the small bowel from the right lower quadrant up to and including the ligament of Treitz. The right portion of the colon and small intestine are displaced onto the chest wall and direct exposure to the third and fourth parts of the duodenum is obtained [Fig. 3].

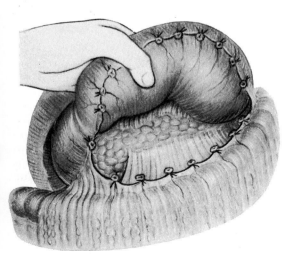

FIG. 1.   Exposure of the pancreas. (From Rob, Smith, and Morgan, 1969. *Operative Surgery*, vol. 4. Courtesy of Butterworths, London.)

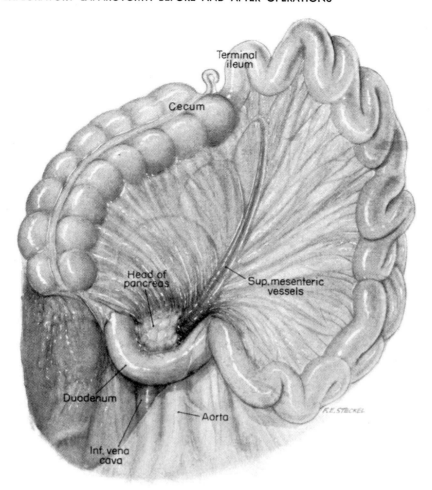

FIG. 3.   Cattell's method of obtaining good exposure of third and fourth portions of duodenum, the ligament of Treitz, the superior mesenteric vessels, and the head of the pancreas. (Reproduced by kind permission of the Lahey Clinic and *Surgery, Gynecology and Obstetrics*.)

The first loop of jejunum is picked up and drawn through the wound to allow inspection of the duodenojejunal flexure (and ligament of Treitz) in order to ascertain whether any congenital or inflammatory bands bind it to the mesocolon and also to find out whether the large mesenteric blood vessels have in their upward course produced any constriction of the third part of the duodenum which they override.

The transverse colon should next be drawn bodily upward to display the mesocolon and the arrangements of the vascular arches therein. If this supporting structure is fat-laden, short, or fixed to the upper coils of jejunum by inflammation or by congenital membranes, or if the blood vessels in it assume an eccentric distribution, it is unwise to incise it in order to draw the stomach or the uppermost jejunal coil through it for the purpose of making an anastomosis.

The liver is easily explored by slipping the hand over its exposed surface and palpating it to test its consistency. Small haemangiomas and subserous cysts of the liver are frequently observed at laparotomy. The superficial cysts of the liver can be readily dispersed by compression.

The healthy gallbladder is sea-green in colour and can be emptied of its viscid contents by gentle compression with the fingers, when its walls will be found to be thin and elastic. It is sometimes impossible to detect a few elusive, small, shotlike calculi in a normal-looking gallbladder, which is tense with bile unless the viscus is first milked dry or aspirated by means of a Mayo-Ochsner trocar and cannula. The signs of chronic cholecystitis are unmistakable: the walls of the gallbladder are found to be thicker and firmer than normal, the sea-green colour is toned down by shades of grey, the subserous fatty tissue is augmented, the cystic lymph node feels prominently enlarged and firm, and inflammatory adhesions drag up the colon with its omenta and shut off the area in preparation for a future crisis.

The common bile duct is next noted, and palpation is carried out with a finger thrust into the foramen of Winslow, while the thumb compresses the structures which lie in the free outer border of the gastrohepatic omentum. The index finger and the thumb sweep upward and downward in their search for stones and enlarged lymph nodes, and an attempt is also made to gauge the calibre of the main ducts. A normal common bile duct is the size of a lead pencil, approximately 7 mm. A common bile duct is judged to be dilated if it measures 1 cm or more in diameter.

The jejunoileum, the caecum, and the everguilty appendix are examined. The last three feet or so of the ileum should be carefully inspected to exclude the presence of a Meckel's diverticulum or the inaugural stages of regional ileitis.

The colon is palpated for growth, polypi, diverticulitis, or other lesions, after which the pelvic organs and the pelvic shelf are systematically and deftly explored with the fingers.

It would be wrong to assume that such a searching investigation of the viscera is required in every case, and under the following conditions it would be even meddlesome and injurious:

1. In cases of infantile pyloric stenosis. Here only the pyloric tumour is sought for and dealt with by Ramstedt's operation.
2. In cases of perforated peptic ulcer. Here, after the perforation has been located and sutured, a rapid examination of the entire stomach and duodenum is carried out, as on rare occa-sions coincidental multiple perforations are encountered.
3. In those cases in which operation is advised on account of severe bleeding from a chronic peptic ulcer, as here exploration of all the abdominal viscera would unduly protract the operation and increase shock.
4. In aged and feeble patients suffering from pyloric obstruction caused by a cicatrising duodenal ulcer. Here an expeditious short-circuit operation (with vagotomy) is performed with the minimal amount of disturbance of the viscera.
5. In cases of acute cholecystitis. Here the gallbladder and extrahepatic bile passages, the liver, the first and second parts of the duodenum, and the head of the pancreas are displayed before the gallbladder is drained or excised.

BEFORE AND AFTER GASTRIC OPERATIONS

Surgery has been made safe for the patient; we must now make the patient safe for surgery.
— MOYNIHAN

All patients with chronic gastric or duodenal ulcer who are admitted to hospital under the care of the surgeon for operative treatment must undergo a course of preoperative medication, the length and nature of which will vary with individual cases. No patient should be refused the benefit of operation because he is deemed a bad surgical risk.

In the *average case* of chronic peptic ulcer without marked gastric retention, when the patient's condition is good, it is best to admit him to hospital and to allow 2 or 3 days prior to operation in order to conduct further investigations, if they are deemed advisable, and to accustom him to his surroundings while the routine preoperative ritual is being carried out. He should not be kept constantly in bed; in fact it is better for him to be up and about for a part of the day in order to maintain muscular and circulatory tone and pulmonary ventilation and to prevent his mind from dwelling unduly upon the thoughts of his pending operation.

A nutritious semisolid and nonresidue diet and a liberal supply of vitamins A, B, and C are prescribed, together with the usual medicines which are employed in the treatment of chronic peptic ulceration. In addition to this, large quantities of fluids and glucose are given to stimulate renal excretion, to guard against dehydration, and to ensure an adequate supply of glycogen in the liver and muscles (see Chap. 12D).

The night before operation a light meal is ordered, and at the hour of retiring a barbiturate drug such as sodium amytal 200 mg, butobarbital 180 mg, Mogadon (Roche) 5 mg, or the like is given. This will usually ensure peaceful sleep, and the patient will wake in the morning fresh, rested, and ready to face all that has to be done in the 2 hours or so which remain before the operation is due to start.

The abdominal field should be closely shaved and thoroughly cleansed with soap and water; the teeth and gums should be cleansed and dentures (if any) removed; the lower bowel should be emptied by means of Dulcolax or glycerine suppositories or enemas; a Ryle tube should be passed through the nose, and the stomach should be irrigated with normal saline solution, and its contents evacuated by aspiration; the patient should be instructed to urinate and if unable to do so must be catheterised. He should also be visited by the anaesthetist, who should conduct a thorough examination of the patient the night before or on the morning of the operation. He should give instructions to the nurse as to the exact time for the intramuscular injection of the preanaesthetic drug or drugs. The Ryle tube is strapped to the cheek and kept in position for use during and after the operation.

It should be routine practise to pass a small stomach tube and aspirate the gastric contents of all patients shortly after admission and again 2 hours before operation.

When *gastritis* is marked or when *obstruction* is present, frequent gastric lavage with normal saline solution is essential. In cases of gastric ulcer, a certain degree of gastritis is always present; in cases of long-standing pyloric obstruction due to a stenosing duodenal ulcer, gastritis and dilatation go hand in hand—the greater the degree of dilatation the more pronounced the gastritis—and here it is not uncommon to find complete absence or a marked reduction of hydrochloric acid in the gastric juice. When the tenacious mucus is removed from the stomach by irrigation and aspiration, when the inflamed mucosa is afforded the rest that it needs, and when it is protected and soothed by drugs,

the return of acid is a token of successful therapy.

In the immediate preoperative stage, purgation, like starvation, is a potent factor in producing acidosis, dehydration, and gaseous distress. If the patient is in the habit of having a normal daily evacuation of the bowels, no purgatives are indicated, but it is usual to give him a rectal wash-out some hours before he is removed to the operating room. When constipation is a marked feature, however, an attempt should be made to clear the bowel thoroughly 2 days before operation by means of a full dose of liquid cascara evacuant or by the aperient the patient is in the habit of taking, plus a glycerine enema; but he is in no sense of the word freely "purged." Repeated enemas are to be deprecated, as they are responsible for a great deal of the intestinal distention seen both during and after operation.

When the patient has a *large penetrating lesion*—one which has breached all the coats of the stomach or duodenum and has deeply pitted the pancreas or liver—when he is exhausted from pain and loss of sleep, and when he shows evidence of dehydration and emaciation through his abstention from food and fluids, a much longer course of preoperative treatment is required, extending in some cases over several days or possibly weeks. He must be confined to bed altogether with complete rest and quiet, sleep being ensured by the administration of sedative drugs. Pain must be relieved by giving either pethidine, physeptone, or morphine, together with alkalis and Pro-Banthine, and a strict ulcer diet is ordered. The stomach should be thoroughly washed out once or twice a day with warm physiological saline in order to remove mucus or any decomposing gastric contents. The reservoirs of the tissues should also be flushed with fluids introduced orally or intravenously. The milk-drip treatment, as popularised by Winkelstein, may be given a trial and will prove invaluable in the management of patients with chronic gastric ulcer in which pain is a marked feature.

Frequent examinations of the blood, of the aspirated gastric juices, and of the stools will be necessary during this period to gauge the efficacy of the treatment instituted. It is common to find that a marked general and local improvement has accrued, even after only a few days of the treatment detailed above. Considerable absorption of the inflammatory products in the vicinity of the ulcer will usually take place, gastritis will be diminished, and even a large, previously fixed and apparently irremovable ulcer may be rendered readily resectable by these measures.

If there is a marked *anaemia* from continued loss of blood, blood transfusion will be necessary, and in such cases, operation should be deferred until the patient is in a fit condition to withstand it. Blood should be given to patients who have lost blood. Blood transfusions, however, are contraindicated in those patients who have a normal blood picture.

Obstruction and retention from organic lesions is one of the most important preoperative considerations. When there is prolonged organic obstruction, the stomach slowly becomes dilated and atonic, and there is in addition a diffuse gastritis accompanied by a decrease in the units of free hydrochloric acid. Vomiting of large quantities of putrid, semidigested food and evil-smelling fluid soon ensues, and the patient becomes dehydrated, emaciated, and alkalaemic.

Brown et al.[2] were among the first to describe accurately the syndrome and blood chemical changes in such cases, and McVicar,[12] in an article which may be read with profit even today, has shown how the blood chemical factors run parallel with the clinical condition of the patient.

It is very important to examine the blood in all cases in which there is the least degree of retention in the stomach to determine the content of chlorides, potassium levels, the nonprotein nitrogen, the CO_2-combining power of the plasma, the serum protein levels, and prothrombin time. In this way, cases of alkalaemia, anaemia, protein deficiency, and malnutrition can frequently be discovered before the symptoms have become definitely established.

The unfortunate effects of *hypoproteinaemia* are well recognised and have been demonstrated experimentally by Thompson, Ravdin, and Frank;[21] Canham;[3] and Rhoads.[18] It has been shown both experimentally and clinically that hypoproteinaemia has a marked influence on gastric emptying and gastrointestinal motility (Barden et al.[1] and Mecray et al.[13]).

After gastrojejunostomy combined with vagotomy and after partial gastrectomy, the oedema associated with hypoproteinaemia may, according to Ravdin et al.,[16] be a decisive factor in preventing normal function of the stoma. Lund[11] states that there is no form of tissue repair in which protein metabolism is not concerned.

I have found Aminosol solutions (Paines & Byrne Ltd.), especially Aminosol—glucose solution or Aminosol—fructose—ethanol solution, given intravenously, to be very helpful in patients suffering from protein-deficiency states.

The size of the stomach should be determined by radiography, both at the start of the preoperative treatment and also at the end of 5 or 6 days, when the maximum degree of improvement is to be anticipated. Shrinkage of the viscus would indicate a return to healthy muscular tone, that obstruction has been successfully overcome, and that the propitious moment for surgical intervention has arrived. Thus the objects of preoperative treatment are: to reduce the size of the dilated stomach and to correct the bad effects of malnutrition, dehydration, hypoproteinaemia, avitaminosis, and electrolyte loss occasioned by the obstruction. The former is achieved by gastric aspiration and lavage, either by passing a nasogastric tube once or twice a day, as may be indicated, or by means of continuous or intermittent suction. The patient should be urged to drink as much fluid as possible to aid in the lavage and cleansing of the stomach, but such treatment should, of course, not be carried to dangerous extremes, as prolonged aspiration causes a further depletion of blood chlorides and potassium through loss of gastric secretion. This loss should be compensated for by means of intravenous injections of 4.3 percent glucose in 0.18 percent saline solution, about 3,000 ml being introduced daily by the slow-drip method, or by feeding the patient by the continuous milk-drip method through an indwelling tube when it has been employed. Blood transfusions often have a remarkably beneficial effect and are advised for all severe cases.

The most rapid and satisfactory method of correcting hypoproteinaemia is by means of transfusions of blood or plasma substitutes. The popular modern commercial protein digests fed into the stomach or duodenum are also of value the moment pyloric patency is established.

It is thought by Lund [11] that patients with gastric lesions commonly have *ascorbic acid deficiency,* rather because of an insufficient dietary intake of vitamin C than because of any metabolic effect caused by the disease. Lund has attempted to estimate as closely as possible the tissue reserves of vitamin C in relation to the healing of gastric lesions. In a study of 45 patients who underwent operations for gastric and duodenal ulcer, few had a normal ascorbic acid intake, plasma level, leukocyte level, or reserve, the operative death rate and complications being considerably higher in those patients who had low reserves of vitamin C. Vitamin B complex in adequate doses should be given intramuscularly or intravenously for a few days prior to operation as well as in the postoperative phase.

Tetany is always associated with severe alkalaemia and is an indication of marked disturbance in the acid-base mechanism. McVicar stated that tetany might be anticipated when the CO_2-combining power exceeded 100 percent by volume. The painful muscular spasms that occur can be partially relieved by intravenous injections of 10 ml of calcium chloride or of calcium gluconogalactogluconate (Sandoz), 10 ml given intramuscularly twice daily combined with occasional intramuscular injections of morphine and atropine.

The *optimal time for operation* in such patients is thus decided by the return of laboratory findings to normal, an all-round improvement in the general condition, and by the degree of reduction in the size of the stomach. It is rarely necessary to prolong the preoperative treatment as outlined above for more than 2 weeks.

It should be noted here that for patients with chronic peptic ulceration the eradication of all *accessible foci of infection* constitutes an important part of the preoperative treatment. The nose, accessory sinuses, tonsils, teeth, and gums should always be carefully examined, and if any septic focus is found it should be dealt with. No gastric operation should be performed shortly after the enucleation of tonsils or after the wholesale extraction of teeth; ample time should be allowed for healing to take place. If, however, the patient is

suffering from an operable cancer of the stomach or, through lack of response to medical treatment, his condition is desperate and the obstruction demands immediate relief, the removal of such foci must be deferred until he is convalescent from his operation.

It should be remembered that there are at least two other likely sources of infection: the appendix and the gallbladder. Therefore during the performance of an operation for peptic ulcer a crippled appendix (when present) should be removed, and the gallbladder, if found to be diseased, should also be excised whenever circumstances permit.

If infection is likely to be encountered or if a carcinoma of the stomach is present, it is advisable to begin antibiotic therapy 48 hours before operation. For this purpose, 500,000 units of penicillin and 0.25 g of streptomycin are given intramuscularly every 6 hours.

When operating for malignant lesions of the stomach, gastric ulcers of the greater curvature, spontaneous gastrocolic fistulas or gastrojejunocolic fistulas caused by recurrent peptic ulceration, it is well to give special care to the preparation of the large bowel. The administration of sulfathalidine or sulfasuxidine orally, 8 g daily for 5 days, and/or of neomycin, 2 g four times daily for 2 days, and adequate preoperative enemas are essential to such preparation.[22]

Finally, deep breathing exercises, supervised by a physiotherapist, should commence a day or two before operation and continue for a variable period postoperatively.

POSTOPERATIVE TREATMENT

Many schemes have been adopted by surgeons in their management of cases after the performance of operations for gastric and duodenal ulcer. The main principles of such treatment, however, are much the same in each and may be briefly outlined as follows:

Pain

On full recovery from the anaesthetic, morphine 10 to 15 mg, omnopon 10 to 20 mg, heroin 10 mg, or pethidine (meperidine, i.e., Demerol) 75 to 100 mg is injected intramuscularly and one or the other of these drugs is given as required, although not more than two or three injections during the first 24 hours is usually necessary. On the second postoperative day omnopon 10 mg or pethidine 75 to 100 mg is injected in the morning and at night if pain is a troublesome feature. After this time, no further injections of these drugs will as a rule be required. The injections should, on the whole, be given sparingly but not too much so. Large doses of narcotic drugs given during the early hours after operation are dangerous, as they encourage pulmonary complications such as atelectasis, while small doses given at lengthening intervals may be wholly ineffective.

Sleep

The following drugs are commonly prescribed: butobarbital, cyclobarbital, quinalbarbital, and syrup of chloral hydrate.

During the first 24 to 72 hours following operation restlessness, anxiety, tension, chronic psychosis as well as nausea and vomiting can best be overcome by intramuscular injections of soluble sodium phenobarbital 180 to 240 mg or Fentazin (A and H), 5 mg per milliliter two or three times daily.

Position in Bed and Early Ambulation

When the patient returns to bed following operation, he is placed in a slight Trendelenburg position so as to prevent aspiration of any regurgitated gastric fluid and in order to facilitate the removal of all bronchial secretion. The position is effectual also in combating threatened hypotension. I used to enforce this position for 24 hours, but I do not now consider this prolonged time to be necessary; in fact, as soon as the patient has regained consciousness, he should be placed in a half-sitting posture. The patient himself, however, usually selects automatically the best and most comfortable position in bed.

Breathing exercises and active and passive movements of the legs and arms are encouraged within a few hours of the patient's full recovery from anaesthesia.

Many-tailed bandages, abdominal binders, "pressure dressings" with their broad strips of flexible adhesive plaster, and tight bedclothes that restrict movements of the belly and legs are to be avoided. One should have faith and confidence in the methods now employed of securely closing abdominal incisions!

A popular method of dressing epigastric incisions is to spray the suture line and a small area around it with a transparent liquid plastic material (such as Nobecutane) and then to apply a small gauze pad over the incision, this being kept in place with a few strips of Micropore tape. In selected cases, the dressings are removed after 48 hours, when the edges of the wound are "sealed off."

I allow my patients to get out of bed *early,* i.e., on the second day after operation. They are helped out of bed, stand erect for a few minutes, breathe deeply, walk around the bed, and give their legs and arms a good stretching. The excursions are increased daily, sometimes in spite of protestations. Nelson [15] states that early ambulation following abdominal operations was first recommended in 1899 by Ries,[17] and that good results depend on the strict observance of contraindications as well as of indications.

The *advantages* of the plan include: (a) the lower incidence of postoperative complications, particularly pulmonary and vascular; (b) the lower incidence of nausea, vomiting, and abdominal distention; (c) the earlier return of normal function of the bladder and bowel; (d) the maintenance of normal muscle tone; (e) the psychological effect on the patient's morale and mental state; (f) the acceleration of convalescence and an earlier return of working ability; and (g) the economic saving to patient and hospital.

Leithauser [9] maintains that the plan of early postoperative ambulation presents a sound surgical advance and its more general employment in properly selected cases is strongly recommended.

D'Ingianni [5] states that the chief *contraindication* to early ambulation after abdominal operation is pulmonary embolism. There are, of course, other contraindications —such as the presence of peritonitis, myocardial disease, shock, exhaustion, and pneumonitis. My aim after a gastric operation is to have the patient up and about as soon as possible. An important contribution to the study of *Early Movement, Early Rising, and Early Discharge* will be found in the *Lancet,* I:95, 1951, while no consideration of early ambulation after surgery would be complete without reference to Leithauser's masterful contribution [10] to the subject.

Elastic stockings are applied regularly before and immediately after operation. These are worn for about 2 weeks unless contraindicated by inadequate arterial circulation in the legs.

Nasogastric Suction

Since 1965, I have been reluctant to employ nasogastric suction in aged and feeble patients, in infants, in those suffering from chronic bronchitis, emphysema or myocardial damage, and also in "high-strung" and agitated patients who cannot or will not tolerate the presence of an inlying tube. In these circumstances, *no fluids are given by mouth for 3 to 4 days after operation;* dehydration, electrolyte and vitamin deficiencies, and protein loss are corrected by the administration of continuous intravenous solutions containing glucose 5 percent and saline 0.18 percent, Parentrovite (B complex with vitamin C), protein (plasma and/or blood), and potassium, when indicated. After 36 to 48 hours, routine blood investigations are carried out and if any deficiencies are brought to light, e.g., chloride loss, they are rectified as soon as possible. If progress is satisfactory, the intravenous polyethylene tube is removed on the third or fourth postoperative day and small amounts of liquid nourishment are given by mouth—intermittently and cautiously. If there is no vomiting or sign of ileus, the feedings can be increased daily until about the seventh postoperative day, when the patient is ordered a light non-residue diet.

Herrington et al,[7] in their instructive paper "Elimination of Routine Use of Gastric Decompression Following Operation for Gastroduodenal Ulcer," state that the routine use of postoperative suction is unnecessary and

definite indications, such as postoperative gastric atony, vomiting, etc., should determine its employment. It is Herrington's practise to pass a nasogastric tube before operation and to leave it in situ during operation and for 6 to 8 hours postoperatively. The tube is then removed and nothing is given by mouth for 72 hours. After that period, for the next 3 or 4 days, only water and clear fluids are permitted by mouth.

During the last 15 years, there has been an increase in the use of *temporary gastrostomy* for decompression of the stomach and proximal small intestine. Advantages of this method have been reported by Farris and Smith,[6] Holder and Gross,[8] McDonald,[14] and others.

A brief account of gastrostomy following operations upon the stomach and duodenum is given in Chapter 28. LeQuesne and Cameron give a detailed account of fluid, electrolyte, and nutritional problems in Chapter 106, and nutritional and metabolic are described by Alexander-Williams in Chapter 27.

REFERENCES

1. Barden et al., Am. J. Roentgenol. 38:196, 1937.
2. Brown et al., Arch. Intern. Med. 32:425, 1923.
3. Canham, Surgery 37:683, 1955.
4. Cattell, Surg. Gynecol. Obstet. 111:378, 1960.
5. D'Ingianni, Arch. Surg. 50:214, 1945.
6. Farris and Smith, Am. J. Surg. 102:168, 1961.
7. Herrington et al., Ann. Surg. 159:807, 1964.
8. Holder and Gross, Pediatrics 26:36, 1960.
9. Leithauser, Arch. Surg. 47:203, 1943.
10. Leithauser, Surg. Gynecol. Obstet. 105:100, 1958.
11. Lund, Surg. Gynecol. Obstet. 83:259, 1946.
12. McVicar, Minnesota Med. 8:429, 1925.
13. Mecray et al., Surgery 1:53, 1939.
14. McDonald, Surg. Clin. North Am. 44:273, 1964.
15. Nelson, Arch. Surg. 49:1, 1944.
16. Ravdin et al., Arch. Surg. 46:871, 1943.
17. Reis, J.A.M.A. 33:454, 1899.
18. Rhoads, Surg. Gynecol. Obstet. 94:417, 1952.
19. Sedgwick, Surg. Clin. North Am. 44:665, 1964.
20. Strokl and Diffenbaugh, Surg. Clin. North Am. 41:15, 1961.
21. Thompson, Ravdin, and Frank, Arch. Surg. 36:500, 1938.
22. Welch, The Surgery of the Stomach and Duodenum, 4th ed., Chicago, Year Book, 1966.

11

A. THE AETIOLOGY AND PATHOGENESIS OF PEPTIC ULCER

Factors Influencing the Choice of Operations

CHARLES V. MANN

Until comparatively recently, gastric and duodenal ulcer were regarded as manifestations of an identical tendency—the "peptic ulcer diathesis." The results of experiments into the aetiology of gastric ulcer were assumed to apply with equal force to duodenal ulcer, and the surgical management of peptic ulcer did not distinguish between the two forms. This situation was made more complicated by the dramatic changes in the epidemiology of peptic ulcer that have occurred in the last 50 years; in the classic writings of Billroth,[22] Finsterer,[92] and others, treatment was primarily directed toward cure for gastric ulcer, and duodental ulcer was a comparative rarity. Nowadays duodenal ulcer is estimated to be between 3 and 8 times more common than gastric ulcer,[85, 86, 137, 138] and these proportions are reflected in the numbers of patients presenting for operation. It was soon apparent that when operations devised primarily for the treatment of gastric ulcer were applied to the treatment of duodenal ulcer, the results were often disastrous, and this realisation coincided with evidence, both clinical and experimental, of sharp differences between the two types of ulcer.[14] A clear understanding of this evidence is essential to the correct handling of peptic ulcer patients presenting for surgery.

THE PEPTIC ULCER DIATHESIS

Illingworth [132] has stated that there is more in common between gastric and duodenal ulcer than otherwise, and it is helpful both historically and in practise to review the evidence underlying this point of view.[236] First, and most important of all, peptic ulcers develop only in mucosa exposed to the influences of gastric juice, of which the most important components are hydrochloric acid and pepsin; consequently, it has always been assumed that peptic ulcers can occur only as a result of an abnormal secretion of gastric juice or from failure of mechanisms that normally protect against the actions of acid or pepsin, or a combination of both. Secondly, gastric and duodenal ulcer are similar in their histopathology and behaviour, and, with the exception of malignant change, which is common in gastric ulcer but very rare in duodenal ulcer,[165] they are subject to the same complications if allowed to persist without treatment. Finally, both types of ulcer when acute heal readily in the first instance with treatment based on rest and antacids, and will just as readily recur under circumstances of stress.[221]

There are also many important differences, however, between the two types of ulcer. Duodenal ulcer is common in Western society, while gastric ulcer is much more rare,[13, 140] and these figures are the reverse of the situation in the past. Duodenal ulcer is much more common in men, whereas with gastric ulcer the sex ratio is almost evenly balanced. Duodenal ulcer afflicts younger subjects than gastric ulcers,[97, 138] and gastric ulcer is associated with a significant incidence of pulmonary disease.[10, 137, 167] Duodenal ulcer is associated with a higher than normal acid production, whereas in gastric ulcer, acid production is usually normal and often diminished.[13, 16, 21, 142, 163, 227] Gastric emptying times appear to be normal or increased in duodenal ulcer subjects,[227] whereas gastric retention appears to be an important factor in the aetiology of gastric ulcer.[31, 32, 33, 39, 69, 74, 121, 130, 133, 140] Patients with duodenal ulcer commonly have a strong family history or are sometimes associated with endocrine abnormalities, which does not seem to happen in instances of gastric ulceration. The relation between gastric ulcer and blood group O, except possibly with prepyloric ulcers, is not as significant as it is with duodenal ulcers.[141, 142, 272]

For these reasons, as well as the experimental work to be discussed, it is usual nowadays to consider the so-called peptic ulcer as representative of different diseases when it occurs in the stomach or in the duodenum. Considerable overlap may occur, however, and it is informative in this respect that the nearer to the pylorus the gastric ulcer occurs, the closer it resembles a duodenal ulcer in behaviour, acid production, and genetic background.[11, 16, 95, 142]

GASTRIC ULCER

Aetiology and Pathogenesis

Focal ischaemia. In work prior to 1930 there were attempts to explain the occurrence of gastric ulcer by local factors at the site of the ulcer that would make the mucosa more vulnerable to acid/pepsin digestion. As far back as 1853, Virchow[252] suggested that the cause was local mucosal ischaemia due to thrombosis. This theory of mucosal infarction was later supported by work showing that microemboli artificially introduced into the gastric circulation of dogs[20, 47, 138, 206] or interference with the blood supply by ligation of vessels or omental stripping[194] would cause gastric erosions and ulcers to develop; more recently Barclay and Bentley[15] have described arteriovenous shunts in the submucosa of the stomach under the control of the sympathetic system. While it is true that nervous influences can certainly cause rapid changes in the blood supply of the mucosa of the stomach (as witnessed by the blanching and reddening of the stomach mucosa observed by Wolf and Wolff in Tom[271] and by Beaumont in Alexis St. Martin[17] under the influence of strong emotional stimuli), there is no evidence that chronic gastric ulcer in man is related to ischaemia; there is no evidence of a persistent change in autonomic control of the blood vessels of the stomach, and none

to suggest that significant vascular shunting is occurring in gastric ulcer subjects. The blood supply to the stomach is characteristically enormous, and Somervell[233, 234] has even advocated an operation (for duodenal ulcer) based on deliberate division of main vessels supplying the stomach. Many operations for curing chronic gastric ulcer actually involve ligation of all the main arteries supplying the stomach, and de Busscher[62] has shown that there is often increased blood supply in the stomach wall in relation to the gastritis associated with chronic gastric ulcer, which does not support an ischaemic basis for the disease. There is some evidence, however, to show that the arteries supplying the lesser curve of the stomach are end-arteries, and this may be a factor in the ulcers occurring at this site, and it may explain why so many of them do, in fact, occur along the lesser curve.

Mucosal trauma. Eighty-five percent of gastric ulcers occur along the lesser curve aspect of the stomach, and 60 percent are within 6 cm proximal to the pyloroduodenal junction.[211] These facts, taken with the observation that food and fluid tend to cling to the lesser curve of the stomach—*The Magenstrasse*—suggested that a mechanical factor might be involved. Although gastric ulcers can be produced by trauma,[99, 111, 138, 270] chemical agents, and irritant drugs (of which aspirin is now probably the most important),[113, 184, 225, 240, 264] heat, and other physical agents,[63] they heal readily,[237] and even if these physical agents are factors in initiating a gastric ulcer, there must be some other equally vital process involved that prevents the normally rapid healing process from taking place, of which the end-arteries, referred to above, are probably the most convincing.

Bacteria. Rosenow[221] postulated that bacteria deposited in the wall of the stomach (principally the streptococcus) were responsible for destroying local resistance to ulceration and predisposing to ulcer formation. While it is certainly true that subjects suffering from septicaemia or bacteraemia may develop a gastric ulcer, subjects debilitated or dying from a wide variety of causes, including severe trauma such as a major surgical operation, also have an ulcerogenic tendency. When attempts were made, in experimental animals, to cause chronic gastric ulcer by injecting suitable organisms into vessels supplying the stomach wall, only transient changes were observed. If infection plays any part in causing chronic gastric ulcer, it is likely that this is achieved through a nonspecific lowering of bodily resistance rather than by a special effect upon the gastric wall.

Diminished mucosal resistance. Amongst other causes of a general lowering of the ability to resist the effects of acid/pepsin digestion may be listed nutritional disturbances, and especially lack of vitamin C,[236] and auto-immune deficiency.[2, 46, 170, 231, 248] It would not seem unreasonable that in certain individuals such abnormalities could play a significant role, but it does not seem to the author that these causes could explain the occurrence of chronic gastric ulcer in most cases; and it would not be possible to reconcile them with the rapid healing tendencies that most gastric ulcers exhibit under favourable circumstances without any need to correct these factors.

Antral stasis. Ever since Dragstedt [68-79] began his brilliant work in Chicago, in much of the experimental work there has been an attempt to explain gastric ulceration by abnormalities of gastric secretory function. Although, in general terms, the evidence that has been uncovered has helped to distinguish between gastric and duodenal ulceration, it has assisted more in the development of treatment than it has revealed of original causes. When vagotomy was first used in attempts to cure duodenal ulcer, it was found that gastric retention occurred; in many cases, the patient learnt to live with his symptoms and in these cases gastric ulcers often developed. Since these patients had low levels of acid production (as a result of vagotomy), it was realised that it was the stasis that was responsible for the appearance of the gastric ulcer. Although Dragstedt has attempted to explain gastric ulceration as a result of such antral stasis in terms of increased acid/pepsin output in response to antral stimulation, it is now known that gastric ulcer patients on the whole have low acid figures, although the nearer the ulcer is situated to the pylorus the higher the acid levels become.[16, 142] The evidence is not nearly so well documented, but

there is no evidence of increased output of pepsin in gastric ulcer subjects either.

Pyloric channel obstruction. Antral stasis from pyloric stenosis—either due to chronic duodenal ulcer, mucosal folds, or muscular hypertrophy have all been shown capable of causing stomach ulcers to develop,[32, 64, 121, 165, 251] and Burge [32, 33] has collected these various causes into a syndrome of "pyloric channel obstruction associated with gastritis and benign gastric ulcer." Dragstedt strongly supports this view, emphasizing that pyloric holdup causes great increase in acid/pepsin secretion.[73, 77]

Gastritis. It is likely that the gastritis that precedes and invariably accompanies benign gastric ulcer [161, 171] is the link between the gastric retention and the development of ulcer. Any cause of gastric retention, especially if associated with gastritis, is liable to lead to the formation of gastric ulcers, and measures designed to alleviate the mucosal inflammation, especially if they abolish gastric stasis, will promote healing of the ulcer.

Pyloroduodenal reflux of bile. Spira [235] has stated categorically that he believes regurgitated bile is the prime cause of preulcerative superficial hypertrophic gastritis. Similar views have been expressed by du Plessis [80] and by Lawson.[160, 161] It was not, however, until this hypothesis was taken up by the Bristol School of Surgery, under the vigorous prompting of Capper,[38] that there was much concrete experimental evidence to support this suggestion.

Bile is known to be an extremely corrosive chemical when put into contact with the oesophageal mucosa, and it is capable of penetrating mucus. It is only rarely found in other than very small quantities in the stomachs of patients with healthy gastrointestinal tracts. One can, therefore, readily accept the opinion that regurgitation of bile in significant quantities into the stomach would cause a stomach ulcer to develop, although Dragstedt's experiments seem to belie this.[73, 79]

This being said, the evidence is still incomplete, however, and much of it can be given more than one interpretation. If one accepts the theory as offered, there is still the problem of why the bile regurgitated in the first place, and why was it not immediately expelled again by the forceful peristalsis of the stomach. It is equally convincing to claim that the gastric ulcer, by causing an inflammation of the gastric wall, prevents the proper motor action of the stomach, and, therefore, bile that is regurgitating is not expelled as it would be in the normal individual. In this case, the bile found in the stomach of gastric ulcer subjects is a *consequence* rather than a prime cause of the ulcer.

Whether it is the prime cause or not, however, biliary regurgitation would seem likely to prolong or accentuate a gastric ulcer, and is probably an important factor in what is most likely to be a complex process. Certainly, not all gastric ulcers are associated with bile reflux. In gastric ulcers developing above a severe pyloric stenosis, bile is frequently absent from the stomach; some gastric ulcers develop in the fundus or at the gastrooesophageal junction, where bile corrosion would seem least active; the preference for lesser-curve sites seems difficult to equate with the tendency of fluid to bathe all parts equally below its surface level. Finally, many gastric ulcers are healed by operations that accentuate the likelihood of biliary reflux.

If one reverts to Burge's hypothesis that pyloric holdup is the most significant *single* cause of gastric ulceration, one could dovetail this with the presence of normally regurgitated bile (which then remains in abnormally prolonged contact with the gastric mucosa) to produce an attractive "combination theory." Since nicotine is known to interfere with the normal motor action of smooth muscle by its poisonous action on nerve ganglia, the well-known clinical observation that smoking will cause or aggravate gastric ulceration can be fitted as yet another factor interfering with normal pyloroduodenal function and enhancing the tendency to retain corrosive bile and peptic juices in the stomach.

Deficient mucus barrier. In a few patients with gastric ulcer, mucosal inflammation may be caused by auto-immune antibodies,[2] but a definite relationship between this form of gastritis and gastric ulcer has not been proved. Cases of auto-immune gastritis tend to develop macrocytic anaemia,[170] but this type of blood picture is not found frequently in patients undergoing surgery for gastric ulcer. Hollander [125] has postulated a different cause of mucosal susceptibility, namely, deficiency of the mucus barrier; by this theory, the parietal cell is protected normally from the digestive effect of hydrochloric acid by a surface layer of mucus: this postulate has been supported by others.[7, 58] It has not been possible to show convincing evidence to support this hypothesis in human beings, however,[104] and it is a matter of common clinical observation that in many cases of gastric ulcer the stomach produces large quantities of mucus.

Biochemical cellular dysfunction. Davenport [58-60] has shown that the production of acid is dependent upon the integrity of the surface epithelial layer. Since many cases of gastric ulcer are associated with low acid production, he has suggested that this is a reflection of the breaching of the surface layer. Marks and Shay [179] have suggested that a gastric ulcer starts at a point of diminished mucosal resistance, that from the ulcer point spreading areas of gastritis develop, which then cause further functional impairment and destruction of mucosal cells. It may be that any cause of prolonged mucosal inflammation, of which pyloric dysfunction with antral retention or bile reflux is an example, is capable of initiating a vicious circle of ulcer formation, further physical and biochemical trauma to the mucosa, interference with ulcer healing, and more ulcer formation. The speed with which gastric ulcers come and go, and the ease with which experimentally produced ulcers heal in otherwise healthy stomachs, strongly suggest that this mechanism, or one very like it, may well be present.

SUMMARY

Many aetiological agents have been postulated for peptic ulcer, including mucosal ischaemia, foci of infection, mechanical trauma, chemical agents, and nutritional disturbance. None of these has been shown to cause a chronic peptic ulcer of the type that surgeons are asked to treat, although all may cause acute gastric ulcer, and some may delay healing processes if they are left uncorrected.

Attention has been focussed recently on

the pylorus as a prime agent in causing gastric ulcer. Pyloric stenosis or duodenal regurgitation, or a combination of both, may underlie many cases of gastric ulcer, and correction of the pyloric abnormality can lead to permanent healing. Gastritis probably plays an important intermediary role and, in some cases of auto-immune disease or biliary reflux, the gastritis may be the sole cause of the ulcer.

Many gastric ulcers are not associated with high levels of acid secretion, and surgical efforts to correct hypersecretion of acid are usually unnecessary. Likewise, there is no evidence of abnormal pepsin or mucus production in human gastric ulcer subjects.

Choice of Operation for Gastric Ulcer

Experimental work on the aetiology of gastric ulcer has failed to disclose a precise cause for the disease at the ulcer site itself. Clinical experience has amply confirmed that local excision operations (based on a hypothesis that local factors at the ulcer site might be responsible for the lesion) are inevitably followed by recurrence of the ulcer.[88, 151] Local excision accompanied by gastrojejunostomy too has disappointing long-term results,[24, 148, 205, 245] particularly if the antrum is not adequately drained. Pyloroplasty alone also gives poor results. If any lesson can be drawn from the results of local procedures, it is that the cause of gastric ulceration does not lie at the site of the ulcer itself.

Partial gastrectomy combines the advantages of removing at the same time the ulcer itself as well as the antrum and pyloroduodenal junction. By this one procedure, the lesion itself, as well as the sites of many of the possible aetiological factors is removed. As might be expected, the long-term results of partial gastrectomy for gastric ulcer are very gratifying. With all types of gastric resection, however, a price must be paid for the benefit conferred of subsequent freedom from disease. In addition to the mortality attached to a major operation, there is a substantial amount of morbidity from loss or derangement of many stomach functions. Gastric storage capacity is reduced, the acid

barrier to organisms is lost, antral production of intrinsic factor is ended, and many of the fine regulators controlling acid production and gastric emptying are abolished. In most patients, excellent adjustment is made to these upsets, but in a few cases, severe disturbance persists. The judgment, personality, and skill of the surgeon can do a great deal to prevent or minimise the effects of gastric resection, but every busy surgeon has one or two disappointing gastric "cripples" amongst the great mass of his satisfied customers. It is fair to state that after Billroth I gastrectomy for gastric ulcer there will be very few dissatisfied patients, and that most poor results after gastrectomy will occur in the duodenal ulcer subjects.

After partial gastrectomy for gastric ulcer, the surgeon has a choice of rejoining the gastric remnant to duodenum or jejunum. In most cases of gastric ulcer, the duodenum is healthy, a normal or subnormal level of acid production is present, and there is no need to remove an excessive amount of stomach. Under these conditions a gastroduodenal join-up of the Billroth I type is to be preferred, since this retains the advantages of normal mixing of the food leaving the stomach with bile and pancreatic juice, and it also preserves duodenal inhibition to acid secretion by fat and acids in the duodenum.[136] In addition, the normal fluxes of electrolytes can take place across the duodenal mucosa (which eliminates one possible source of postgastrectomy disturbance) and the dangers associated with a gastrojejunal loop (afferent loop obstruction, volvulus or herniation) are avoided.[178]

While a gastroduodenal linkup is to be preferred, however, there are certain circumstances in which a gastrojejunal anastomosis has advantages. If the duodenum has been badly scarred or narrowed (for example, by an accompanying duodenal ulcer), it is wiser to use healthy jejunum for the anastomosis. In all cases of gastric ulcer, where an accompanying duodenal ulcer is known or suspected (and Aagard[1] has claimed that a duodenal ulcer is present in one-third of gastric ulcer cases), it is imperative to use a gastrojejunal anastomosis, since the Billroth I type gastrectomy has been shown to have a high incidence of recurrence when used in the presence of a duodenal ulcer.[105, 127, 128, 196, 257]

In a few cases of high gastric ulcer, when a severe gastrectomy has to be performed for technical reasons to enable the ulcer to be resected, such a small remnant will remain that a gastrojejunal hookup is advisable in order to avoid tension on the anastomosis.

Before attention was drawn to the frequent association between stasis and gastric ulcer, for those ulcers situated at or just below the oesophagogastric junction, where resection would carry high risks, removal of the stomach below the ulcer (which is itself not disturbed) was found to be followed by healing of the ulcer.[92, 164] It is now realised that this procedure—the so-called Kelling-Madlener manoeuvre [164]—removes the causes of antral stasis and acid/pepsin production, but the clinical observation was made long before a theoretical justification was available. The operation can still be very useful in a difficult, high ulcer that is penetrating onto the surface of the pancreas. Pauchet and Tanner described other methods [174, 243] for dealing with this problem of the high ulcer by rotating the stomach, but these demand a high degree of technical skill.

Since the demonstration by Harkins,[114] Burge,[31-36] and others,[88, 117] that a drainage procedure combined with vagotomy will heal a gastric ulcer, it would seem that difficult and dangerous operations to remove the ulcer are probably unjustified. But in most cases it is possible to resect the ulcer without undue difficulty, and the Billroth I gastrectomy is a safe and satisfying operation giving excellent results in good surgical hands. In addition, fear of missing an early malignant ulcer [21, 180] has prevented many surgeons from adopting an operation that does not actually remove the ulcer itself. This fear is soundly based; Marshall and Jensen [180] have estimated that 13.2 percent of gastric ulcers are malignant, and others [97, 150, 168, 192] have also found a high rate of carcinomatous change. There have been recent reports of mistaking a malignant gastric ulcer for a benign one, and neither gastroscopy,[198, 224, 246] gastrocamera, acid secretory studies,[21, 200, 249] nor radiological follow-up can be relied upon to prevent mistakes.[21, 94, 210] Nor can four-quadrant biopsy [88] be regarded as a foolproof method of picking up early cancer occurring at one small point of an ulcer margin, although Bachrach [8] feels these fears are exaggerated.

Since the introduction of modern fibre-optic gastroscopes with their capacity to take multiple biopsy specimens, however, it is very unlikely that a malignant gastric ulcer will be overlooked. I believe that vagotomy plus a drainage procedure will be used increasingly in the treatment of gastric ulcer, and especially for those situated in the upper half of the stomach, as an alternative to the Kelling-Madlener manoeuvre. For those ulcers situated lower down in the antrum or pyloric channel, a Billroth I gastrectomy would still seem to be the operation of choice.

Results of Elective Operations for Gastric Ulcer

When considering the results of elective surgery for gastric ulcer, it must be remembered that many patients are poorly nourished individuals, often with significant associated pulmonary disease.[10, 162, 214] For this reason, much of the mortality and morbidity associated with operations for gastric ulcer arises from the general complications of major surgery, especially chest complications.[191, 217] It is likely that significant reduction in the mortality figures will be accomplished, not by switching from partial gastrectomy to vagotomy with a drainage procedure, but through the development of better anaesthetic methods and improvement in treatment of cardiorespiratory complications and the prevention and cure of pulmonary embolism.

Billroth I gastrectomy is presently the most widely used operation for the treatment of chronic gastric ulcer. Most series report a mortality rate of less than 5 percent from Billroth I gastrectomy,[21, 199, 212, 254, 256, 259, 264] of which approximately half arises from complications outside the operative field. These series, however, usually include the results of emergency operations, and when the risks of elective surgery are considered separately, the mortality figures fall sharply. Several series have been reported of gastric ulcer treated by partial gastrectomy with an overall mortality rate between them of 3.4 percent [21, 212, 254, 264]: a figure of 2.7 percent was reported by Walters and ReMine,[259] and Priestley et al.[212] had the astonishingly low figure of 2.0 percent. In 1957, Pearce, Jordan, and DeBakey [207] published a series of 406 cases of benign gastroduodenal ulcer treated by distal subtotal gastrectomy with an operative mortality rate of 0.3 percent. It would appear that when a high degree of technical skill is available, mortality figures for elective gastrectomy of the Billroth I type of around 1.0 percent may be expected, and in the elective case it is hard to support a switch from partial gastrectomy on grounds of operative mortality risks.[219] The incidence of recurrent ulcer after partial gastrectomy for gastric ulcer is also very low; Tanner [243, 244] has reported on 1,000 gastrectomies for gastric ulcer before meeting a recurrent ulcer.

The advocates of vagotomy with a drainage procedure for the treatment of gastric ulcer claim that however low the mortality rate from partial gastrectomy, it will still exceed that from vagotomy. Burge [32, 33] has reported a series of gastric ulcers treated by vagotomy and pyloroplasty with a mortality rate of less than 1 percent, and similar figures have been recorded by others.[88] These series, however, are still comparatively small, and have been compiled by enthusiastic experts, and it is only when the postoperative sequelae are considered that vagotomy with drainage appears to be strongly favoured, although even this has been questioned. Although the Billroth I type gastrectomy has fewer and less severe aftereffects than a Polya-type procedure,[127] weight loss, anaemia, and dumping syndrome occur; [134, 155, 189, 208, 255] in addition, stomal obstruction can develop at the gastroduodenal anastomosis, and some patients suffer aggravation of latent or established pulmonary tuberculosis. Although dumping can occur after vagotomy with gastric drainage (probably as a result of the drainage procedure), weight loss and anaemia do not seem to develop. The only postvagotomy complication of importance is diarrhoea. Although the incidence of postvagotomy diarrhoea in severe form has been reported in as many as 8 percent of cases,[33] this has not been the experience of most surgeons; in many cases, patients are not aware of diarrhoea unless they are questioned, and are frequently glad to exchange their previous costive habits for a more frequent bowel action.[106] Not more than 1 or 2 percent of patients suffer serious disability from diarrhoea, and the adoption of selective instead of truncal vagotomy [35, 266] will prob-

ably further reduce this small number.

The high incidence of recurrent ulceration [88, 117, 151, 245, 264] has made the procedure of wedge excision with or without a drainage procedure unacceptable for the treatment by election of gastric ulcer, unless a situation of extreme urgency should arise to prohibit other procedures. Similarly, since the development of vagotomy with gastric drainage as an alternative to partial gastrectomy for handling a difficult gastric ulcer, the necessity for a Kelling-Madlener-type procedure has largely disappeared. Although the recurrence rate after a Madlener operation is very low,[92] the patient will also suffer the disabilities associated with gastric resection. Occasionally, after distal gastric resection for gastric ulcer, a gastroduodenal linkup is unwise; where a Polya-type gastrojejunal anastomosis is employed after a gastric resection for gastric ulcer, ulcer recurrence is virtually unknown.

Having noted that acid production in most cases of gastric ulcer is normal or on the low side, some surgeons have attempted a gastric drainage procedure alone (pyloroplasty), without the accompanying vagotomy. The early results of this operation, however logical it might appear on the aetiological assumption of pyloric holdup, have been very bad indeed, and it is unlikely that this procedure will remain in the surgical curriculum.

In conclusion, I should like to stress the recent report by Duthie,[81] who compared the results of Billroth I gastrectomy with vagotomy and pyloroplasty, in which the results showed that the gastric resection was much superior: the incidence of recurrent ulcer was 2 percent after the gastrectomy and 15 percent after vagotomy.

DUODENAL ULCER

Pathogenesis

Acid hypersecretion. The problem of duodenal ulceration is seemingly simplified at first sight by a clear relationship to overproduction of hydrochloric acid by the stomach.[11, 16, 72, 179, 228] The question, however, is only pushed one stage back because the problem then becomes—what is the cause of the overproduction of the acid? Until recently, surgery was solely concerned with the most efficient methods of curing acid hypersecretion, because it was known that if acid production was effectively restrained, the duodenal ulcer would heal. This attitude led to the development of more and more radical types of gastric resection. Recently, after ways were developed for testing the physiological background to the increased acid formation, these methods have been adopted for clinical use and in some cases may determine the type of operation employed in the individual case.[40] The most important effect of the increase in physiological knowledge has been the development of vagotomy as an adjunct to and replacement of gastrectomy. Although many surgeons still rely heavily upon a single type of procedure for the treatment of their duodenal ulcer patients, others advocate a more physiological approach, in which the nature of the hypersecretion is investigated and the appropriate procedure is employed.[40, 152, 153, 195] There is agreement by all surgeons that whatever the operation used, it should be based upon a clear understanding of recent knowledge concerned with the production of acid by the stomach.

Hollander has postulated that the gastric parietal cell produces hydrochloric acid of fixed concentration.[124, 175] If this is so, then it follows that acid in greater quantities than normal can only be put out by a greater than normal number of parietal cells, or by a normal number of cells working for an increased proportion of the time; it is probable that in many cases of duodenal ulcer, both mechanisms are active. Histological studies of the stomachs of duodenal ulcer cases have shown a greater than normal area populated by parietal cells (an "increased parietal cell mass"),[27, 53] and comparisons with normal subjects have shown greatly increased volumes of acid produced by many duodenal ulcer subjects per given time (sometimes when the number of parietal cells present has not been shown to be significantly larger).[41, 226]

It is known that acid production depends both upon a neural ("nervous secretion") and a hormonal ("chemical secretion") mechanism, and that the efficiency of the hormonal output depends greatly upon an intact nerve supply to the antrum.[101, 209] The secretory nerve is the vagus, and it has been shown that stimulation of the vagus nerve causes increased acid production[5] and, conversely, vagotomy substantially reduces acid formation by up to 70 percent.[18, 23, 98, 101, 102, 103] The hormone is gastrin, and it is formed by the antral mucosa in response to digestive processes; if the vagus nerves are divided, less gastrin is produced.[93, 209] It is likely that the hyperacidity responsible for a duodenal ulcer is caused either by increased vagal activity or by overproduction of gastrin; in many instances there is both experimental and clinical evidence to support this hypothesis of nervous or hormonal "drive."[29] In a certain number of duodenal ulcer subjects, an enlarged parietal cell mass cannot be demonstrated by the response to maximal stimulation by histamine, and yet in these patients both the hourly unstimulated ("basal") volume and the twelve-hourly collection are greater than normal values; this is generally regarded as resulting from excessive vagal activity, and both figures usually return to normal or subnormal values after vagectomy. Cases of Zollinger-Ellison syndrome[84, 129, 273] are classic examples of wildly excessive acid production in response to a gastrin-like hormone arising from the nonbeta cells forming the pancreatic tumour.[110]

While increased vagal excitation is assumed to underlie the duodenal ulcer diathesis in many if not all cases where a direct cause of gastrin overproduction cannot be demonstrated, the agent responsible for the vagal stimulation itself has not been pinpointed. There is some evidence that the region of the hypothalamus may be the origin of the impulses, but duodenal ulcers have been caused by brain damage in other situations.[28, 57, 138] It is the continued inability to account satisfactorily for the increased vagal activity that has sustained the search in other directions for the cause of duodenal ulcer.

Mucosal susceptibility and genetic factors. It has always been assumed that the "forces of aggression," e.g., hydrochloric acid, are counterbalanced by the "forces of resistance," i.e., the ability of the mucosa to heal, and that in the normal person the balance is maintained in favour of the defence. Although in many duodenal ulcer patients there is ample evidence of excessive acid production, in a great number of instances the acid production is within the normal range; these cases would seem to support a concept of diminished powers of resistance rather than increased acid aggression. This speculation concerning mucosal susceptibility was unsupported by evidence until Aird, et al.[4] drew attention to the significant relationship between certain blood groups and a tendency to develop ulcers; their observations have been extended by others [95] and have shown a significant relationship between blood group O and the development of duodenal ulcer,[227] and that those persons of blood group O who do not possess ABH antigen are peculiarly liable to develop duodenal ulcers of a refractory nature that require more than usually severe measures to cure.[42, 159, 219] It is possible that these cases represent a group of duodenal ulcer patients in which diminished mucosal resistance plays a significant part in the ulcer process. A similar reduction in healing powers may lie behind the known tendency of the corticosteroids to cause or aggravate duodenal ulcers [223] and the known tendency of stress to be associated with peptic ulcers.[216] This aspect is more fully discussed by Kelly in the second section of this chapter. At the present time, although it is recognised that in some cases a duodenal ulcer results from an inability to resist acid digestion rather than an augmentation of the level of acid formation, the surgeon still relies upon reducing acid production for cure of the ulcer: the practical consequence of this is that if the surgeon operates on a duodenal ulcer patient of blood group O, who is a nonsecretor of ABH antigent, an operation of greater-than-normal magnitude is often required if ulcer recurrence is to be avoided.

Endocrine organ dysfunction. In addition to the Zollinger-Ellison syndrome, in which there is overproduction of gastrin by pancreatic tumour tissue with consequent hyperacidity and ulcer formation, other endocrine adenomata may be associated with duodenal ulcer; such ulcer-associated adenomata have been described from the pituitary, the parathyroid, and adrenal glands, and may all be present occasionally in a single subject.[3, 249, 250, 265] Such cases are now commonly referred to as examples of the "pluriglandular syndrome." In the Zollinger-Ellison syndrome, the source of the hyperacidity was uncovered by the demonstration by Gregory et al.[110] of the gastrin-like hormone present in the pancreatic tumour. In Cushing's syndrome, the high level of endogenous steroids may be responsible for the duodenal ulcer. Where a parathyroid tumour is present, there is frequently, but not invariably, hypersecretion of acid.[83] Although hypercalcaemia has been shown by Donegan and Spiro [67] to cause high levels of acid secretion,[260] this had been challenged as the cause of the ulcer by other observers.[108, 172] At present it must be accepted that in a large number of patients suffering from ulcer-associated endocrine organ dysfunction, the links between the adenomata and the ulcer have not been elucidated. In a few cases of the Zollinger-Ellison syndrome, hypersecretion of acid is not present.[51, 182]

Liver disease. An association exists between ulceration of both stomach and duodenum and diseases of the liver, principally cirrhosis.[197, 242, 261] Good summaries of the evidence have been published by Irvine [135] and Frederick.[96] In some cases, increased production of acid has been found, but the nature of the secretagogue has not been established.[197] It is thought that the agent responsible for the hyperacidity is produced by the intestines, but in the presence of liver disease the normal processes of detoxification do not take place. At first it was thought that the agent might be histamine itself, but Livingston and Code [166] have shown that histamine is unaffected by passage through the liver. A recent suggestion by Code [45] has again implicated histamine; this hypothesis postulates that in response to an unknown stimulus, possibly connected with an increase in the blood supply to the gastric mucosa, overproduction of histamine occurs in the stomach wall in close relation to the parietal cell, which is caused to secrete acid. This suggestion takes into account the possibility that the secretagogue does not involve either the neural or the hormonal mechanisms but affects the parietal cell directly; this is of great surgical importance, as it accounts for the failure of operations aimed at interrupting the vagal or the gastrin pathway and seems to be borne out by both experiment and sad clinical experience.

SUMMARY

At present, duodenal ulcer is known to be closely related to hypersecretion of hydrochloric acid. In most cases, vagal or gastric activity is responsible for the parietal cell stimulation, although in many cases both mechanisms may be implicated.[29] It is not known what causes the increased vagal activity underlying the duodenal ulcer. A strong family history can be obtained in some patients, but in general terms duodenal ulcer appears to be a "disease of civilisation" affecting men rather than women;[6] the disease seems to be maximal in the third and fourth decades (younger than gastric ulcer subjects,[90, 97, 149, 156] and the victims are usually otherwise healthy. A factor of increased mucosal susceptibility may also be involved, and there is a tendency for persons of blood group O to develop duodenal ulcer;[4, 159] failure to secrete ABH antigen aggravates this trend.[213] In rare cases, endocrine organ dysfunction or liver disease may be a prime cause of the ulcer, but the secretagogue in these cases is mostly unidentified. Surgical cure of duodenal ulcer still relies upon effective reduction of acid formation, and the standard operations aim to interrupt the physiological mechanisms involved in acid secretion; if vagal dependence is predominant, vagectomy is effective, while antrectomy may be used to prevent gastrin formation. Vagectomy also substantially reduces gastrin production by the antrum. Where factors other than hypersecretion of acid are present, such as a genetic susceptibility implied by blood group O and absence of ABH antigen, additional surgical manoeuvres may be necessary to circumvent ulcer recurrence.

Choice of Operation for Duodenal Ulcer

The aim of any operation for duodenal ulcer is threefold—to reduce the acid secretory level effectively; to achieve this acid reduction as safely as possible; and to sacrifice the minimum of other normal functions of the stomach and duodenum. I believe that these aims have been stated in the order of their importance, and each deserves separate consideration, although all must be borne in mind when a decision has to be made on the operation of choice in the individual case.

Surgical methods of reducing acid secretory potential are vagal nerve section, or antrectomy or resection of parietal cell mass by gastrectomy. Vagotomy will abolish pure nervous secretion, and will also reduce antral release of gastrin.[12, 93, 101] Antrectomy (or a limited gastrectomy) will stop gastrin-dependent acid production, but will not limit acid production by remaining parietal cells that are responding to nervous stimulation. Partial gastrectomy will combine the advantages of removing the antrum with ablation of an additional number of parietal cells proportional to the extent of the gastrectomy.

If acid production in a case of duodenal ulcer has been shown to depend substantially upon the vagus, it would seem unnecessary to perform any larger operation than vagotomy with a drainage procedure, and since the brilliant pioneer work of Dragstedt, this has been widely adopted for the treatment of duodenal ulcer. Since reductions of acid secretion of up to 70 percent of maximal[23, 101] may result from vagotomy, this operation should suffice to reduce acid production in most duodenal ulcer subjects to below the normal mean of around 18 mEq per hour. Since the procedure is also extremely safe, and sacrifices no gastric or duodenal tissue, it is no surprise that the operation of vagotomy with a drainage procedure has been advocated as the best operation currently available for all cases of duodenal ulcer.[34] Unfortunately, the decision is not quite so simple as these arguments would suggest. The operation of vagotomy is associated with a high recurrence rate[255]: in a recent review by a group experienced in both vagotomy and gastrectomy, Goligher, Pulvertaft, and Franz[106] found that the incidence of recurrent ulcer after vagotomy was approximately twice that following partial gastrectomy (five cases in 120 operations as compared with two in 108 operations, respectively), and recurrence rates as high as 13 percent were recorded by Rhea et al.[218] Feggetter and Pringle[89] reported a 5 percent incidence of stomal ulcer after vagotomy and gastrojejunostomy and quoted various other authors with recurrence rates varying between 1 and 5 percent. This problem of recurrent ulcer can be related to several causes. First, some cases of duodenal ulcer have such a high level of acid production (over 50 mEq per hour) that even complete vagotomy effecting 70 percent reduction in acid production would still leave the patient with an abnormally high level of acid secretion; such cases are often examples of extremely severe duodenal ulcer, and it has been shown that they are more than usually likely to relapse after surgery.[30] Second, some cases of duodenal ulcer are not due to excess vagal activity, but to undue gastrin output by the antrum and will be only partially affected by vagotomy. Third, there is a high incidence of "incomplete" vagotomy after attempted truncal division.[115, 205] Lythgoe,[167] in 1961, reported 12 percent of incomplete vagotomies (as measured by a positive insulin test), and in 1964 Ross and Kay [222] recorded a figure of 38 percent. Although the number of incomplete vagotomies performed may be expected to decline with increasing experience of the procedure, it is clear that even in skilled hands incomplete vagotomy with all the consequent risks of recurrence will still occur.

More recently, attempts have been made to gain all the benefits of gastric vagal denervation without the need to suffer the disadvantages of gastric drainage, or to sacrifice vagal nerve supply to other organs such as the gallbladder. One of the disadvantages of gastric drainage is a small number of patients with clinical dumping and a larger number of occult or manifest examples of steatorrhoea. The major side-effect of truncal vagotomy is diarrhoea, but biliary stasis and gallstones seem to be among other more minor defects. The operation of *selective vagotomy* was designed to pick out for division only those branches going to the stomach itself—so avoiding the unpleasant side-effects due to widespread denervation of organs other than the stomach. Complete gastric denervation still led to gastric paralysis, however, in addition to gastric acid hyposecretion, and the operation of *highly selective vagotomy* [144] has been developed to save the normal gastric emptying mechanisms; in this procedure, the pyloric nerve branch of the anterior vagus is deliberately preserved, and a gastric drainage procedure is not used; apart from the pyloric nerve, the other branches of the vagus nerves going to the

stomach alone are divided along the same lines as in the operation of selective vagotomy. The operation of selective vagotomy (with a drainage procedure) seems to be as safe as truncal vagotomy, although much more difficult to perform. Special techniques have been described by Burge, Tanner, and Harkins. Although the operation is still new, it is steadily gaining acceptance. One reason for its adoption has not only been the sound logic lying behind the operation, but the demonstration by carefully recorded trials that the incidence of unpleasant diarrhoea is substantially reduced; an additional, welcome—if somewhat surprising—benefit is that selective vagotomy appears to result in a lower incidence of "incomplete" vagotomies.[154] The operation of highly selective vagotomy is too new for appraisal at this moment, but early reports have disclosed a disquietingly high rate of early and late positive insulin tests.[145] Experience in the past has shown that positive insulin tests are associated with a high risk of recurrent ulcers.

It is similarly too early to evaluate another variant on the attempts to avoid a gastric decompression accompanying vagotomy in which a pyloroplasty is not performed in those patients who show a rapid rate of gastric emptying preoperatively. The author himself is sceptical whether preoperative tests of gastric emptying can be taken as a valid guide to the effects of vagotomy on gastroduodenal motility.

When a gastric drainage procedure is performed with vagotomy, it is usual to prefer one of the varieties of pyloroplasty [32, 91, 116, 186, 262] to gastroenterostomy. A pyloroplasty has the theoretical advantages of preserving the normal direction of the food leaving the stomach, and also it conserves duodenal acid inhibitory mechanisms.[143] Occasionally a pylorus may be so narrowed or inflamed that even one of the special varieties of pyloroplasty designed for these situations [139] would be too dangerous to perform. A gastroenterostomy is then a satisfactory alternative procedure. Although Tanner prefers an anterior juxtopyloric position for the stoma, the classic form is still that perfected by the Mayo brothers [183]— horizontal, retrocolic, and designed to lie at the most dependent portion of the antrum.

Occasionally an antrum is so baggy and flaccid that even a well-designed pyloroplasty will not drain it effectively, and a gastroenterostomy is to be preferred. Although the theoretical basis for favouring pyloroplasty to gastroenterostomy is very strong, in practise, there is little to choose between the results of the two procedures used in conjunction with vagotomy,[106, 126] but it does appear that the problems associated with all gastrojejunal loops are best avoided when possible.

Even if satisfactory vagotomy could be achieved in every case, however, it is clear that some types of duodenal ulcer are not suited to the procedure. In addition to those patients with massive hypersecretion or those who have hormonal-dependent rather than neural-dependent acid secretion, patients who are unsuited to vagotomy will include a certain number who, for technical reasons, must be treated by other methods. In a few cases, the region of the hiatus may be obliterated by adhesions (for example, after a previous ulcer perforation, especially if followed by a subphrenic collection); pyloric stenosis may render a pyloroplasty dangerous to achieve, and yet the bag-like dependent antrum may be difficult to drain efficiently by the alternative procedure of gastroenterostomy. In these examples, a different operation is required, and many surgeons would recommend a partial gastrectomy as the best procedure.

If a partial gastrectomy is to be used in the treatment of duodenal ulcer, it should be one employing a gastrojejunal (Polya-type) anastomosis, as the Billroth I operation has been shown by Orr[196] to have a 15 percent recurrence rate when used for the treatment of duodenal ulcer (compared to a less than 1 percent recurrence rate when used for gastric ulcer) and it has been shown by the Mayo Clinic and by others[264] to have a recurrence rate of between 7 and 14 percent. The Polya-type partial gastrectomy is extremely effective in controlling the duodenal ulcer diathesis; in McKeown's[185] report of 716 cases of duodenal ulcer treated by partial gastrectomy with a gastrojejunal anastomosis, the recurrence rate was 1.5 percent; in the Mimpriss and Birts[187] series of 248 peptic ulcer cases treated mainly by Polya-type gastrectomy (and which included 125 duodenal ulcer patients treated by this method), no case

of ulcer recurrence was recorded: in the report by Pulvertaft,[215] only two recurrences in over 400 cases were found. Although the mortality from "cold" gastrectomy was less than 1 percent in McKeown's group,[185] and other series are reported with a similar very low mortality from elective partial gastrectomy less than 3 percent overall, Fegetter and Pringle[89] have reported on 248 cases of duodenal ulcer treated by vagotomy and gastroenterostomy with no mortality, and the series of Burge and Pick[34] had no death (but a recurrence rate of over 4 percent). Crile[54] and Hoerr[123] have also treated large numbers by vagotomy combined with gastric drainage with virtually no deaths. It appears that in expert hands there is a very low mortality rate from partial gastrectomy. The operation of vagal nerve section with gastric drainage has a still, however, lower mortality rate, and it would be preferred normally to partial gastrectomy in spite of a higher recurrence rate. It remains to be shown, that if the vagotomy and drainage procedure is reserved for those cases of difficult duodenal ulceration where partial gastrectomy would carry high risk from duodenal stump dissection or subsequent breakdown, the operation of Polya-type gastrectomy could not be made as safe as the vagotomy procedures. A recent trial from Leeds has confirmed the astonishing safety of partial gastrectomy in good hands when consideration is given to such technical matters.[107]

Even if Polya partial gastrectomy were to have comparable operative risk to vagotomy with gastric drainage, it has been shown that it is followed by formidable sequelae: these include anaemia,[66, 147, 188, 215, 268] weight loss,[87, 146, 215] protein deficiency,[25] dumping and afferent loop syndromes,[134, 155, 238, 239] as well as osteoporosis and osteomalacia.[65, 267] By comparison, the operation of vagotomy and pyloroplasty appears to be relatively free from side-effects apart from the incidence of diarrhoea already discussed. It would seem to the author that, at present, the higher mortality and greatly increased morbidity of partial gastrectomy would favour truncal or selective vagotomy with gastric drainage as the operation of choice for the usual case of duodenal ulcer, reserving Polya partial gastrectomy for special cases unsuitable for vagotomy; such cases would include hiata obliteration, pyloric stenosis, massive hyper-secretion of acid (especially if vagal dependence had not been shown by the presence of a substantially increased volume of resting juice), combined gastric and duodenal ulcers, and possibly recurrent ulceration after a previous attempt at vagotomy.

Vagotomy combined with antrectomy [52, 82, 118, 119, 202, 203, 232] (or with limited partial gastrectomy) probably gives the most complete control of acid formation, since it not only interrupts both the nervous and the hormonal acid secretory pathways,[20] but it also includes direct resection of parietal cells as part of the procedure. There is evidence that many patients are achlorhydric after this procedure, and that the percentage of achlorhydric cases increases with the passage of time after the operation.[202, 232] Although the mortality rate has been low (2.7 percent in Herrington's series,[118] the addition of gastric resection to the vagotomy must give this procedure a mortality rate akin to Polya partial gastrectomy, while at the same time compounding the rate of morbidity figures associated with removal of gastric tissue with those known to result from vagal nerve division. Since vagotomy is known to reduce antral production of gastrin as well as interrupting nervous secretion of acid, it does not appear that the theoretical basis of the combined procedure is unduly strong. Nor do the mortality or morbidity figures justify preferring this operation to vagotomy or Polya-type partial gastrectomy as an elective procedure for the ordinary case. Vagotomy with antrectomy is possibly best indicated for the extreme hypersecretor of blood group O who is a nonsecretor of ABH antigen; such patients are known to respond badly to either vagotomy or Polya partial gastrectomy.[213] If vagotomy with antrectomy is performed, it would not appear that a gastroduodenal anastomosis carries high risk of recurrence and is to be preferred, since the problems associated with the gastrojejunal loop are avoided.

In summary, then, the three well-tried operations currently available for the elective treatment of duodenal ulcer all have particular advantages and drawbacks, and the best results will be achieved by judicious use of each according to the circumstances. Vagotomy with gastric drainage is probably the safest operation and is associated with the least sacrifice of stomach functions; at present it appears to have a higher rate of recurrent ulceration than the other two operations. Selective vagotomy seems to be the technique that has the lowest rate of incomplete nerve sections plus the advantage of avoiding unnecessary side-effects (such as diarrhoea) resulting from unwanted denervation of organs other than the stomach.[154] Partial gastrectomy of the Polya type is not as safe as vagotomy, but it gives more effective control of the ulcer-forming tendency at an increased price in terms of postoperative disabilities, some of which may be serious; this operation may be used in cases unsuitable for vagotomy, which would include those patients whose parietal cell mass is known to be greatly increased. Vagotomy combined with antrectomy (or limited partial gastrectomy) gives almost complete control of the ulcer diathesis but has many of the dangers and risks of morbidity of both vagotomy and gastrectomy; this operation should probably be reserved for quite exceptional cases in which either the level of acid production or the genetic background is known to carry high risks of recurrent ulceration if vagotomy or Polya partial gastrectomy were to be employed. Whatever views a surgeon may form as a result of studying the available evidence as to the best operation to employ for the usual case of duodenal ulcer presenting to him for surgical cure, circumstances will frequently arise where, in the interests of safety, alternative methods must be used; only when there is willingness to tailor the operation to the patient's needs, of which survival is the most important, will the mortality and morbidity of duodenal ulcer surgery be further reduced. If present efforts to increase both the effectiveness and the specificity of vagotomy (e.g., by changing to selective nerve division) are successful, it is likely that this operation will occupy a permanent position in the elective surgical control of duodenal ulceration.

Tests Used to Measure Acid Secretory Levels

In the previous material, it has been shown that the results of elective operations for duodenal ulcer depend in part upon the nature and degree of acid secretory capacity. While no attempt will be made by the author to supplant more detailed reviews of tests of acid secretion published elsewhere,[56] a brief outline of some of the more important methods and views on their significance in relation to surgical management of duodenal ulcer are relevant here.

Tests of unstimulated (basal) acid secretion. In practise, basal secretion is measured on the fasted stomach with the patient isolated as far as possible from psychic stimuli. Since the hormonal mechanisms dependent upon digestion are assumed to be largely inactive in the fasted subject, the acid collected from the stomach in these tests is assumed to represent mainly nervous (vagal) activity. In most tests, acid is collected by tube aspiration from the stomach, and it has been shown that if the tube is correctly positioned and the aspiration performed with care and skill, the collection is virtually complete.[143] Two frequently used tests of unstimulated acid secretion are the basal 1-hour collection and the 12-hour (overnight) collection.

The basal 1-hour acid collection often forms the preliminary to a test of stimulated acid.production. The volumes obtained are small and there is often some lack of conviction of the reliability of the results for this reason. In control subjects, basal secretion of hydrochloric acid is in the range of 2 to 3 mEq per hour, while in duodenal ulcer subjects this figure is more than doubled. There is wide individual variation, however, and nonulcer subjects can occasionally secrete as much as 13 mEq per hour and more.

Because of this wide scatter, most people favour the *12-hour acid collection,* and for convenience this is often done overnight. In normal subjects, the average collection is 18 mEq, but it is usually much higher in duodenal ulcer patients, often 61 mEq or more.[136]

Tests of stimulated acid production. If the blood sugar falls below 45 mg per 100 ml, intense vagal stimulation occurs, with consequent increased acid formation by the stomach. This forms the basis of the *insulin (Hollander) test,*[9] in which insulin is used to drop the blood sugar to excitatory levels. The test is rather drastic and can be dangerous in the presence of cardiovascular disease.

It is usually employed to test for the completeness of vagotomy if there is suspicion of ulcer recurrence after this operation. The method, however, can give evidence on the amount of vagal-dependent acid formation; the acid collection is usually continued for 3 to 4 hours, as there are two peaks of acid produced after insulin, an early and a late or delayed response; the latter is often thought to represent an effect of vagal release of gastrin.

Histamine appears to stimulate the parietal cell directly, and if given in a sufficiently high dose will cause all the parietal cells of the stomach to secrete. If Hollander's hypothesis is true, that each parietal cell produces acid of the same fixed concentration,[124, 175] the maximal response to histamine will provide a measure of both the parietal cell mass and the total acid secretory potential of the stomach.[40] This argument forms the basis of the *augumented histamine test,*[55, 152, 241] and its later development like the *histology test.* In response to histamine in sufficient dose, control subjects secrete slightly more than 20 mEq of acid per hour, but in duodenal ulcer patients the figure becomes 37 to 40 mEq per hour; in 40 percent of male duodenal ulcer subjects the figure is over 40 mEq per hour.[136]

Since the purification of gastrin II by Gregory and Tracy,[109] it has become possible to measure the effect of direct hormonal stimulation. The amount of acid produced after a *gastrin* (pentagastrin) *test* closely corresponds to the quantities produced after a maximal histamine response.[175, 176, 190]

It can be seen that by applying these methods of measuring acid formation by the stomach, not only is the quantity of acid determined but also in part the excitatory mechanisms responsible for its secretion. Although no absolute rules can be made, if the levels of unstimulated acid are high, and the results of the stimulation tests do not disclose an unduly large parietal cell mass, e.g., less than 50 mEq per hour in response to maximal histamine stimulation, vagotomy and gastric drainage can be expected to give a satisfactory result. If the parietal cell mass is much enlarged, e.g., more than 50 mEq per hour after histamine, a high Polya gastrectomy will give better control of the ulcer diathesis than vagotomy, and if blood group

O and absence of ABH antigen are also present, vagotomy plus antral resection should be considered. It has been shown by Bruce et al.[30] that those patients developing recurrent ulcer after surgery for duodenal ulcer had greatly increased levels of acid secretion in response to histamine; if these patients had been selected for more effective surgical control by vagotomy and antrectomy, it is probable that many of these recurrences could have been prevented. An excellent review of recent views on gastric secretory tests has been provided by Cox.[51]

Results of Elective Operations

Some of the results of cold surgery for duodenal ulcer have already been referred to when considering the choice of operation. Although it is customary to consider the results of all operations under the two principal headings of mortality and morbidity, a hidden factor is present that is frequently overlooked but is often all-important, namely, the skill of the individual surgeon. Many important papers are published by surgeons of exceptional gifts, and operations that appear straightforward in their hands prove disappointing when applied by surgeons of less ability. For this reason, surgical practise changes slowly as it follows the efforts of the pioneers. This attitude of cautious appraisal is especially valuable when consideration is given to the results of procedures for duodenal ulcer, for many of the aftereffects become apparent only with time.

The operations of gastroenterostomy and Billroth I gastrectomy for duodenal ulcer have been abandoned because of their high recurrence rate.[19, 119, 193, 196] Occasionally an elderly enfeebled patient presents with pyloric stenosis, and a gastroenterostomy is performed as the safest and simplest method of relieving the obstruction, but it would be difficult to justify the operation under other circumstances. The author has operated upon several such patients who had been regarded as unsuitable for a "proper operation"—often when they have bled or perforated years afterwards. They have usually survived these much more hazardous emergency operations without any difficulty. Somervell's operation [233, 234] of division of arteries supplying the stomach has not been used extensively,

as the special circumstances lying behind its use in India are not met in Western countries and long-term follow-up studies are not available.

Until the past decade, partial gastrectomy with gastrojejunal anastomosis was the most common operation performed for duodenal ulcer. In most large reported series, the incidence of ulcer recurrence has been low—less than 3 percent.[157, 201, 258] Most Polya-type gastrectomies resect about two-thirds of the stomach, and the greater the amount of stomach removed the smaller the incidence of stomal ulceration; Visick [253] has described an exceptionally high "measured" gastrectomy in which the incidence of stomal ulceration was nil. Such high gastric resections, however, call for an unusual measure of surgical skill to be performed safely, and Perman [208] has shown that the greater the amount of stomach removed, the greater the ensuing morbidity. The Polya operation is followed by a wide variety of aftereffects, and only 60 to 70 percent of patients are virtually symptom-free after the operation, although most patients are so delighted to be rid of their ulcer that they make light of their subsequent disabilities. The best results from partial gastrectomy are achieved in middle-aged men with a long history of ulcer pain; the shorter the history, the more likely the patient is to resent the difficulties experienced after surgery, and women tolerate the operation less well than men. Patients who have associated disease, especially pulmonary disease, do badly after this operation, and patients with quiescent tuberculosis often have a recrudescence after partial gastrectomy. If there is a history of ulcer complications, however, or a long period of painful suffering, most surgeons consider operative intervention justified, and Hadley [112] opined "it can be stated dogmatically that a duodenal ulcer that has been relapsing for 10 years or more has next to no chance of ever becoming permanently healed by *any* medical regime and an ulcer case seen first at this stage should, generally speaking, be offered gastrectomy forthwith."

Although the immediate mortality of partial gastrectomy in skilled hands is very low, Maingot [173] has estimated his mortality rate at 2 percent, and Pennet [204] recorded figures of less than 1 percent for elective operations); and although strict selection of cases **can be** of great benefit in avoiding misguided zeal in recommending surgery, Polya partial gastrectomy may be followed by weight loss, dumping syndrome, anaemia, and bone disease. The weight loss may be as great as one or two stones. The cause of postoperative dumping is not entirely understood, but it is partly due to a smaller gastric reservoir, and Brain and Stammers [26] have shown that a residual stomach of less than 250-ml capacity is associated with increased "small stomach" symptoms; other symptoms may be due to afferent loop mechanical kinking or overdistention, or possibly bacterial fermentation in a stagnant intestinal pool; [48, 247] yet other suggestions have included too rapid gastric emptying,[86, 131] too rapid efferent loop filling,[169] pancreatic-cibal asynchromism,[118] shifts in circulatory plasma volume,[220] electrolyte disturbances,[229] and abnormal peripheral carbohydrate metabolism.[100, 122] It has been shown that a misplaced stoma is more liable to produce postoperative discomfort, and that a short retrocolic gastrojejunal anastomosis is associated with the fewest postoperative disabilities. A recent publication by Taylor and Eadie [247] has shown how a retrocolic "no-loop" anastomosis may virtually eliminate postoperative dumping. The incidence of anaemia may be very high after gastrectomy, and increases with time; both iron-deficient and macrocytic anaemia may occur, and the incidence of the former may reach as high as 70 percent or more; [158] fortunately both types of anaemia are easily treated. Osteoporosis and osteomalacia have been reported after partial gastrectomy, although estimates of its frequency vary greatly.[120, 269] It should be stressed that several recent reports appear to show that the morbidity following gastrectomy has been greatly exaggerated; they also show that it compares not unfavourably with vagotomy.[49, 107]

Insofar as there is virtually no mortality attached to vagotomy,[34, 89] and it is free of most of the above complications, it is preferred by many surgeons for the treatment of duodenal ulcer. Although the reported incidence of recurrent ulcer has been put as high as 15 percent, the advocates of vagotomy would claim that if a complete vagotomy is performed, the incidence of ulcer recurrence is probably less than 5 percent; they would also claim that with increasing experience this figure will fall lower still. Burge and

Vane [36] have devised an instrument to test for the completeness of vagotomy at the time of operation, although Lythgoe [167] has disputed its usefulness. The series reported by Hedenstedt and Lundquist,[115] and others,[18] however, lends hope that the adoption of selective instead of truncal vagotomy will assist in the achievement of complete gastric denervation.

Vagotomy is followed by one serious sequel —diarrhoea. The incidence of this has been estimated between 15 percent [7] and 50 percent,[115] but in the series reported by Williams and Irvine,[266] it occurred in almost 10 percent, and it occurred only in those patients having total vagotomy; they did not find diarrhoea in a comparable group of patients after selective vagotomy. Their results appear to support the claim that selective vagotomy will avoid the problem of postvagotomy diarrhoea without sacrifice of efficiency of the control of acid secretion. Even in those cases where total truncal division is performed, when the incidence appears to be potentially as high as 50 percent, the number of patients who are sufficiently inconvenienced to question the value of the operation is very small. It is the author's view that postvagotomy diarrhoea does not in itself constitute a reason for not using this procedure. The only question that is still to be answered is the long-term effects of vagal nerve division; it has taken nearly 40 years for some of the results of partial gastrectomy to become apparent, and it would be wise to reserve final judgment on vagotomy for a similar period.

When the long-term studies of the results of vagotomy and antrectomy currently available are studied, the operation appears to have a very low mortality, and to be almost free from problems of ulcer recurrence.[61, 82, 118, 202, 232] Theoretically, it should cause all the postvagotomy sequelae with additional aftereffects from the removal of part of the stomach. This possibility is sufficiently strong that it cannot be recommended except for the control of exceptionally difficult ulcer cases.

SUMMARY

The best results from ulcer surgery are achieved through an understanding of present views of their cause.

Motor and biochemical abnormalities at the pyloroduodenal junction appear to play a leading part in causing gastric ulcers, and the operation should endeavour to correct these. Although vagotomy and gastric drainage appear to do this, and benign gastric ulcers heal as a result, fear of malignancy causes many surgeons to favour an operation that removes the ulcer. The Billroth I gastrectomy removes both the ulcer and any causes residing at the pylorus; the operation is safe and has few sequelae.

The cause of duodenal ulcers is intimately related to overproduction of hydrochloric acid by the stomach. Both the vagus nerves and antral gastrin play a major role in acid secretion, and in most cases of duodenal ulcer one or other of these mechanisms is dominant. Preoperative testing can help in determining both the amount and the nature of the acid forming potential of the stomach. Vagal nerve section with drainage appears to be the safest operation for duodenal ulcer and attended by the fewest aftereffects, but it has the highest rate of recurrent ulceration. Selective vagotomy appears the best type of nerve division, with the highest success rate in reducing acid production and the lowest incidence of incomplete vagotomy. Partial gastrectomy of the Polya type is not so safe, although the mortality rate in the best hands is less than 3 percent; the recurrence rate is approximately half that after vagotomy but between 4 and 10 percent of postoperative patients suffer from symptoms due to the operation, some of which are serious. Vagotomy plus antrectomy is almost without risk of recurrent ulceration, but it combines both the dangers and the aftereffects of vagotomy and gastric resection. At the moment, it is probably wiser to choose one of these three operations by a shrewd assessment of both the patient and the acid secretory levels, and to be prepared to sacrifice theoretical advantages in the interests of safety. Certain technical and physiological reasons favour pyloroplasty over gastroenterostomy, and posterior short loop-gastrojejunal anastomoses over antecolic longer loops.

A long history, a male patient, and a highly skilled surgeon are conducive to a favorable outcome; whenever possible, partial gastrectomy should be avoided in women and children.

In a patient with blood group O and a lack of ABH antigen, the likelihood of ulcer recurrence may justify sterner operative measures. Likewise, operations for peptic ulcer in the presence of cirrhosis of the liver or endocrine dysfunction must be treated on an empiric basis of experience of these special categories, as the former group appear to be independent of the usual acid secretory relationships, and in the Zollinger-Ellison syndrome it would seem that total gastrectomy gives the best overall results.

REFERENCES

1. Aagard, P., Andreassen, M., and Kurz, L., Lancet 1:1111, 1959.
2. Adams, J. F., Glen, A. I. M., Kennedy, E. H., MacKenzie, J. L., Morrow, J. M., Anderson, J. R., Gray, K. G., and Middleton, D. G., Lancet 1:401, 1964.
3. Adesola, A. O., Ward, J. T., McGeown, M. G., and Welbourn, R. B. Br. J. Surg. 49:112, 1961.
4. Aird, I., Bentall, H. H., Mehigen, J. A., and Roberts, J. A. F., Br. Med. J. 2:315, 1954.
5. Alley, A., Trans. R. Soc. Can. 27:71, 1933.
6. Alsted, G., Incidence of Peptic Ulcer in Denmark. Copenhagen, Danish Science Press, 1953.
7. Austen, W. G., and Edwards, H. C., Gut 2:158, 1961.
8. Bachrach, W. H., in Proceedings of the World Congress of Gastroenterology, Vol. 1, Baltimore, Williams & Wilkins, 1959, pp. 430–433.
9. Bachrach, W. H., and Bachrach, L. B., Ann. N.Y. Acad. Sci. 140:915, 1967.
10. Balint, J. A., Gastroenterologia 90:65, 1958.
11. Ball. P. A. J., Lancet 1:1363, 1961.
12. Barabas, A. P., Payne, R. A., Johnston, I. D. A., and Burns, G. P., Lancet 1:118, 1966.
13. Barborka, C., and Texter, E. C., Peptic Ulcer, Boston, Little, Brown, 1955, p. 29.
14. Barborka, C., and Texter, E. C., Peptic Ulcer, Boston, Little, Brown, 1955, p. 245.
15. Barclay, A. E., and Bentley, E. H., Br. J. Radiol. 22:62, 1949.
16. Baron, J. H., Gut 4:243, 1963.
17. Beaumont, W., Experiments and Observations on the Gastric Juice and the Physiology of Digestion, Plattsburg, F. P. Allen, 1833.
18. Bell, P. R. F., Gastroenterology 46:387, 1964.
19. Berg, A. A., Ann. Surg. 92:340, 1930.
20. Bergh, B. N., Arch. Surg. 54:58, 1947.
21. Bernardo, J. R., Soderberg, C. G., and Migliaccio, A. V., Surgery 44:804, 1958.
22. Billroth, T., Arch. Klin. Chir. 39:785, 1889.
23. Bitsch, V., Christensen, P. M., Faver, V., and Rodbro, P., Lancet 1:1288, 1966.
24. Bland-Sutton, J., Br. Med. J. 1:272, 1916.
25. Booth, C. C., Brain, M. C., and Jeejeebhoy, K. N., Proc. R. Soc. Med. 57:582, 1964.
26. Brain, R. H. F., and Stammers, F. A. R., Lancet 1:1137, 1951.

27. Bralow, M. D., in The Stomach, New York, Grune & Stratton, 1967, pp. 132–140.
28. Brooks, F. P., in The Stomach, New York, Grune & Stratton, 1967. Pp. 119–123.
29. Broome, A., Bergstrom, H., and Olbe, L., Gastroenterology 52:952, 1967.
30. Bruce, J., Card, W. I., Marks, I. N., and Sircus, W., J. R. Coll. Surg. Edin. 4:85, 1959.
31. Burge, H. W., Postgrad. Med. J. 36:76049, 1960.
32. Burge, H. W., Vagotomy, London, Arnold, 1964.
33. Burge, H. W., Gill, A. M., and Lewis, R. H., Lancet 1:73, 1963.
34. Burge, H. W., and Pick, E. J., Br. Med. J. 1:613, 1958.
35. Burge, H. W., Rizk, A. R., Tompkin, A. M. B., Barth, C. E., Hutchinson, J. S. F., Longland, C. J., McLennan, I., and Miln, D. C., Lancet 2:897, 1961.
36. Burge, H. W., and Vane, J. R., Br. Med. J. 1:615, 1958.
37. Capper, W. M., Hosp. Med. 1:1054, 1957.
38. Capper, W. M., Ann. R. Coll. Eng. 40:21, 1967.
39. Capper, W. M., Butler, T. J., Buckler, K. G., and Hallett, C. P., Ann. Surg. 163:281, 1966.
40. Card, W. I., in World Congress of Gastroenterology, Vol. 1, Baltimore, Williams & Wilkins, 1959, pp. 88–89.
41. Card, W. I., and Marks, I. N., Clin. Sci. 19:147, 1960.
42. Clarke, C. A., Progress in Medical Genetics. New York, Grune & Stratton, 1961, pp. 81–119.
43. Clarke, J. S., McKissock, P. K., and Cruze, K., Surgery 45:48, 1959.
44. Clarke, J. S., Ozeran, J. S., Hart, J. C., Cruze, K., and Reevling, V., Ann. Surg. 148:551, 1958.
45. Code, C. F., Gastroenterology 51:272, 1966.
46. Coghill, N. F., Doniach, D., Roitt, I. M., Mollin, D. L., and Williams, A. W., Gut 6:48, 1965.
47. Cohnheim, J., Vorlesungen über allgemeine Pathologie, 2d ed., Vol. 2, Berlin, Hirschwald, 1882.
48. Coldstein, F., Wirts, C. W., and Kramer, S., Gastroenterology 40:47, 1961.
49. Cox, A. G., Br. Med. J. 2:288, 1968.
50. Cox, A. G., Prog. Surg. 8:45, 1970.
51. Cox, A. G., Modern Trends in Surgery (3), London, Butterworth, 1971. Chap. 4.
52. Cox, A. G., Spencer, J., and Tinker, J., After Vagotomy, London, Butterworth, 1969. Chap. 9.
53. Cox, A. J., Arch. Path. 54:407, 1952.
54. Crile, G., Jr., Ann. Surg. 136:752, 1952.
55. Cummins, A. J., The Stomach, New York, Grune & Stratton, 1967, pp. 189–196.
56. Cummins, H. J., in The Stomach, New York, Grune & Stratton, 1967, p. 192–194.
57. Dalgaard, J. B., in Proceedings of the World Congress on Gastroenterology, Vol. 1, Baltimore, Williams & Wilkins, 1958. P. 387.
58. Davenport, H. W., Gut 6:513, 1965.
59. Davenport, H. W., Gastroenterology 49:189, 1965.
60. Davenport, H. W., Gastroenterology 49:238, 1965.
61. Dean, A. C. B., Edwards, H. C., and Munro, A. I., Gut 7:677, 1966.
62. De Busscher, G., Gastroenterologia 72:154, 1947.
63. Decker, J., Beitr. Klin. Wschr. 24:369, 1887.
64. De La Rosa, C., Linares, C. A., Woodward, E. C., and Dragstedt, L. R., Arch. Surg. 88:927, 1964.
65. Deller, D. J., Begley, M. D., Edwards, R. G., and Addison, M., Gut 5:218, 1965.
66. Deller, D. J., Ibbotson, R. N., and Crompton, B., Gut 5:225, 1964.
67. Donegan, W. L., and Spiro, H. M., Gastroenterology 38:750, 1960.
68. Dragstedt, L. R., Peptic Ulcer, Philadelphia, Saunders, 1951, pp. 490–497.
69. Dragstedt, L. R., Amer. J. Roentgen. 75:219, 1956.
70. Dragstedt, L. R., Maryland Med. J. 8:98, 1959.
71. Dragstedt, L. R., J.A.M.A. 169:203, 1959.
72. Dragstedt, L. R., in Current Gastroenterology, New York, Hoeber, 1962, p. 336–340.
73. Dragstedt, L. R., J. Roy. Coll. Edin. 16:251, 1971.
74. Dragstedt, L. R., Oberhelman, H. A., and Evans, S. O., Ann. Surg. 134:332, 1951.
75. Dragstedt, L. R., Oberhelman, H. A., Evans, S. O., and Rigler, J. P., Ann. Surg. 140:396, 1954.
76. Dragstedt, L. R., Oberhelman, H. A., and Woodward, E. R., Gastroenterology 24:71, 1953.
77. Dragstedt, L. R., Woodward, E. R., Scand. J. Gastroent. 6 (Suppl.) :243, 1970.
78. Dragstedt, L. R., Woodward, E. R., Storer, E. H., Oberhelman, H. A., and Smith, C. A., Ann. Surg. 132:626, 1950.
79. Dragstedt, L. R., Woodward, E. R., Takashi Setto, Jaime Isaza, Rodriguez, J. R., and Resa Samiian, Ann. Surg. 174:548, 1971.
80. Du Plessis, D. J., Lancet 1:974, 1965.
81. Duthie, H. L., Annual Meeting, Association of Surgeons of Great Britain and Northern Ireland, 1970.
82. Edwards, L. W., and Herrington, J. L., Surgery 41:346, 1957.
83. Elliott, D. W., in The Stomach, New York, Grune & Stratton, 1967, pp. 311–312.
84. Ellison, E. H., and Wilson, S. D., Ann. Surg. 160:512, 1964.
85. Emery, E. S., Jr., and Munroe, R. T., Arch. Intern. Med. 55:271, 1935.
86. Eustermann, G. B., and Balfour, D. C., The Stomach and Duodenum, Philadelphia, Saunders, 1935.
87. Everson, T. C., Surgery 36:525, 1954.
88. Farris, J. M., and Smith, G. K., Ann. Surg. 158:461, 1963.
89. Fegetter, G. Y., and Pringle, R., Surg. Gynecol. Obstet. 116:175, 1963.
90. Feldman, M., J.A.M.A. 136:736, 1948.
91. Finney, J. M. T., and Hanrahan, E. M., Jr., in Practice of Surgery, Hagerstown, Md., Prior, 1929, Chap. 6.
92. Finsterer, H., Wien Klin. Wschr. 66:659, 1954.
93. Forrest, A. P. M., in International Congress of Physiology, Vol. 20, Brussels, St. Catherine Press, 1956, p. 299. (Abstract)
94. Fox, N. M., and Remine, W. H., Surg. Clin.

North Am. 41:907, 1961.

95. Fraser-Roberts, J. A., Br. J. Prev. Soc. Med. 11:107, 1957.
96. Frederick, P. L., Surg. Gynecol. Obstet. 118:1093, 1964.
97. Friedenwald, J., Am. J. Med. Sci. 144:157, 1912.
98. Gelb, A., Baronofsky, I. D., and Janowitz, H. D., Gut 2:240, 1961.
99. Gibelli, C., Arch. Int. Chir. 4:127, 1908–9.
100. Gilbert, J. A. L., and Dunlop, D. M., Br. Med. J. 2:330, 1947.
101. Gillespie, I. E., in Postgraduate Gastroenterology, London, Balliere, Tindall and Cassell, 1966, pp. 223–232.
102. Gillespie, E. E., Clark, D. H., Kay, A. W., and Tankel, H. E., Gastroenterology 38:361, 1960.
103. Gillespie, I. E., and Kay, A. W., Brit. Med. J. 1:1557, 1961.
104. Glass, C. B. J., and Boyd, L. J., Gastroenterology 16:697, 1950.
105. Goligher, J. C., Moir, P. B., and Wrigley, J. H., Lancet 1:220, 1956.
106. Goligher, J. C., Pulvertaft, C. N., and Franz, R. C., in Postgraduate Gastroenterology, London, Balliere, Tindall and Cassell, 1966, pp. 246–259.
107. Goligher, J. C., Pulvertaft, C. N., de Dombal, F. T., Conyers, J. H., Duthie, H. L., Feather, D. B., Latchmore, A. J. C., Shoesmith, J. H., Smiddy, F. G., and Wilson-Pepper, J., Br. Med. J. 2:781, 1968.
108. Grant, R., Am. J. Physiol. 132:460, 1941.
109. Gregory, R. A., and Tracy, H. J., Gut 5:103, 1964.
110. Gregory, R. A., Tracy, H. J., French, J. M., and Sircus, W., Lancet 1:1045, 1960.
111. Gross, A., Mitt Grenzgeb Med. Chir. 10:713, 1902.
112. Hadley, G. D., Practitioner 170:18, 1953.
113. Hanzlick, J. P., Actions and Uses of the Salicylates and Cincophen in Medicine. Baltimore, Williams & Wilkins, 1927.
114. Harkins, H. N., Stavney, S. L., Griffith, C. A., Savage, L. E., Kato, T., and Nyhus, L. M., Ann. Surg. 158:448, 1963.
115. Hedenstedt, S., and Lundquist, G., Acta Chir. Scand. 131:448, 1966.
116. Hendry, W. G., Postgrad. Med. J. 37:137, 1961.
117. Herrington, J. L., Surgery 58:619, 1965.
118. Herrington, J. L., Edwards, L. W., Classen, K. L., Carlson, R. I., Edwards, W. H., and Scott, H. W., Ann. Surg. 150:499, 1959.
119. Herrington, J. L., Edwards, W. H., and Edwards, L. W., Surgery 49:540, 1961.
120. Higgins, P. McR., and Pridie, R. B., Br. J. Surg. 53:881, 1966.
121. Hildebrand, H., and Thomson, F. B., Can. Med. Assoc. J. 90:915, 1964.
122. Hobsley, M., and LeQuesne, L. P., Br. Med. J. 1:147, 1960.
123. Hoerr, S. O., Surgery 38:149, 1955.
124. Hollander, F., Fed. Proc. 11:706, 1952.
125. Hollander, F., Arch. Intern. Med. 93:107, 1954.
126. Hopkinson, B. R., Br. J. Surg. 53:1046, 1966.
127. Horsburgh, A. G., and Cox, R., Gastroenterology 49:381, 1965.
128. Horsley, G. W., and Barnes, W. C., Ann. Surg. 145:758, 1959.
129. Howe, C. T., in Postgraduate Gastroenterology, London, Balliere, Tindall and Cassell, 1966, p. 167.
130. Huber, F., and Huntington, C. G., Am. J. Roentgenol. 60:80, 1948.
131. Hurst, A. F., Ann. Surg. 58:466, 1913.
132. Illingworth, C. F. W., in Peptic Ulcer, Edinburgh, Livingstone, 1953.
133. Illingworth, C. F. W., J. R. Coll. Edin. 2:14, 1956.
134. Illingworth, C. F. W., Gut 1:183, 1960.
135. Irvine, W. T., Gastroenterology 42:337, 1962.
136. Irvine, W. T., The Scientic Basis of Surgery. London, Churchill, 1965.
137. Ivy, A. C., Nebr. Med. J. 14:137, 1929.
138. Ivy, A. C., Grossman, M. I., and Bachrach, W. A., in Peptic Ulcer, London, Churchill, 1951.
139. Jaboulay, M., Arch. Prov. Chir. 1:1, 1892.
140. Johnson, H. D., Surg. Gynecol. Obstet. 102:287, 1956.
141. Johnson, H. D., Ann. Surg. 162:996, 1965.
142. Johnson, H. D., Love, A. H. G., Rogers, N. C., and Wyatt, A. P., Gut 5:402, 1964.
143. Johnstone, D., and Duthie, H. L., Gut 7:58, 1966.
144. Johnstone, D., and Wilkinson, A. R., Br. J. Surg. 57:289, 1970.
145. Johnston, D., Humphrey, C. S., and Wilkinson, A. R., Annual Meeting, Association of Surgeons of Great Britain and Northern Ireland, 1970.
146. Johnston, I. D., Welbourn, R., and Acheson, K., Lancet 1:1242, 1958.
147. Jones, C. T., Williams, J. A., Cox, E. V., Meynell, M. J., Cook, W. T., and Stammers, F. A. R., Lancet 2:425, 1962.
148. Jones, T. W., Devito, R. V., Nyhus, L. M., and Harkins, H. D., Surgery 43:781, 1958.
149. Jordan, S. M., in Proceedings of the World Congress of Gastroenterology, Vol. 1, Baltimore, Williams & Wilkins, 1959, pp. 25–29.
150. Judd, E. S., and Priestley, J. T., Surg. Gynecol. Obstet. 77:21, 1943.
151. Judd, E. S., and Rankin, F. W., Surg. Gynecol. Obstet. 37:216, 1923.
152. Kay, A. W., Br. Med. J. 2:77, 1953.
153. Kay, A. W., Gastroenterology 42:501, 1962.
154. Kennedy, T., and Connell, A. M., Lancet 1:675, 1970.
155. Kinsella, V. J., and Hennessy, W. B., Lancet 2:1205, 1960.
156. Klein, N. M., and Bradley, R. L., Am. J. Roentgenol. 77:25, 1957.
157. Klossner, O., Acta Chir. Scand. 131:127, 1966.
158. Krause, U., Acta Chir. Scand. 132:186, 1966.
159. Langman, M. J. S., and Doll, R., Gut 6:270, 1965.
160. Lawson, H. H., Lancet 1:469, 1964.
161. Lawson, H. H., Br. J. Surg. 53:493, 1966.
162. Levij, I. S., and De Fa Fuente, A. A., Gut 4:349, 1963.
163. Levin, E., Kirsner, J. B., and Palmer, W. L., Gastroenterology 12:561, 1949.

164. Lewisohn, R. J. J., Mt. Sinai Hosp., N.Y. 14: 470, 1947.
165. Linares, C. A., De La Rosa, C., Woodward, E. C., and Dragstedt, L. R., Arch. Surg. 88:932, 1964.
166. Livingston, R. H., and Code, C. F., Am. J. Physiol. 181:428, 1955.
167. Lythgoe, J. P., Br. Med. J. 1:1196, 1961.
168. MacCarty, W. C., in The Stomach and Duodenum, Philadelphia, Saunders, 1935, pp. 73 and 87.
169. Machella, T. E., Gastroenterology 14:237, 1950.
170. Mackay, I. R., Gut 5:23, 1964.
171. Mackay, I. R., and Hislop, I. G., Gut 7:228, 1966.
172. Mahfouz, M., and Koskowski, W., Arch. Intern. Pharmacodyn. 118:1, 1959.
173. Maingot, R., in Abdominal Operations, 4th ed., London, Lewis, 1961, p. 156.
174. Maingot, R., in Abdominal Operations, 4th ed., London, Lewis, 1961, pp. 249–250.
175. Maklouf, G. M., McManus, J. P. A., and Card, W. I., Gut 5:379, 1964.
176. Maklouf, G. M., McManus, J. P. A., and Card, W. I., Gut 51:149, 1966.
177. Maklouf, G. M., McManus, J. P. A., and Card, W. I., Gastroenterology 52:787, 1967.
178. Markowitz, A. M., Surgery 49:185, 1961.
179. Marks, I. N., and Shay, H., Lancet 1:1107, 1959.
180. Marshall, S. F., Jensen, A., and Davison, C. M., Am. J. Surg. 101:273, 1961.
181. Mason, M. C., Graham, N. G., Clark, C. G., and Goligher, J. C., Br. J. Surg. 55:677, 1968.
182. Matsumoto, K. K., Peter, J. B., Scholtze, R. G., Hakim, A. A., and Franck, P. T., Gastroenterology 50:231, 1966.
183. Mayo, W. J., Ann. Surg. 43:537, 1906.
184. McCarrison, R., Indian J. Med. Res. 19:61, 1931.
185. McKeown, K. C., Br. J. Surg. 50:131, 1962.
186. Mikulicz, J., Arch. Klin. Chir. 37:79, 1888.
187. Mimpriss, T. W., and Birt, St. J. M. C., Br. Med. J. 2:1095, 1948.
188. Mollins, D. L., and Hines, J. D., Proc. R. Soc. Med. 57:575, 1964.
189. Moore, H. G., and Harkins, H. N., Surgery 32:408, 1952.
190. Multicentre Study, Lancet 1:341, 1969.
191. Nash, T., and Fleming, J., Med. J. Aust. 1:663, 1964.
192. Ogilvie, H., Br. Med. J. 2:405, 1947.
193. Ogilvie, W. H., Lancet 2:295, 1938.
194. Omata, T., Arch. Pathol. Anat. 269:797, 1928.
195. Orr, I., Gut 3:97, 1962.
196. Orr, I., Ann. R. Coll. Surg. Eng. 34:314, 1964.
197. Ostrow, J. D., Timmerman, R. J., and Gray, S. J., Gastroenterology 38:303, 1960.
198. Oyen, O., Acta Chir. Scand. 131:454, 1966.
199. Paine, J. R., Surgery 51:561, 1962.
200. Palmer, W. L., Ann. Intern. Med. 13:317, 1939.
201. Palumbo, L. T., and Sharpe, W. S., Surgery 48:658, 1960.
202. Palumbo, L. T., Sharpe, W. S., Lulu, D. J., Vespa, R., and Colon-Bonet, J., Surgery 46:1005, 1959.
203. Palumbo, L. T., Sharpe, W. S., Lulu, D. J., Bloom, M. H., and Porter, H. R., Surgery 51:289, 1962.
204. Pannett, C. A., Surg. Gynecol. Obstet. 67:485, 1938.
205. Paterson, H. J., Ann. Surg. 1:367, 1909.
206. Payr, E., Verh. Dtsch. Ges. Chir. 36:636, 1907.
207. Pearce, C. W., Jordan, G. L., and De Bakey, M. E., Surgery 42:447, 1957.
208. Perman, E., Acta Med. Scand. 196 (Suppl.) :361, 1947.
209. Pe Thein, M., and Schofield, B., J. Physiol. (Lond.) 148:291, 1959.
210. Plenk, A., and Zeckmann, A., Int. Abst. Surg. 88:409, 1949.
211. Portis, S. A., and Jaffe, R. H., J.A.M.A. 110:6, 1938.
212. Priestley, J. T., Walters, W., Gray, H. K., Waugh, J. M., and Judd, E. S., Proc. Staff Meet. Mayo Clin. 31:62, 1956.
213. Pringle, R., Wort, A. J., and Green, C. A., Br. J. Surg. 51:341, 1964.
214. Pulvertaft, C. N., Br. J. Prev. Soc. Med. 13:131, 1959.
215. Pulvertaft, C. N., Br. J. Surg. 51:44, 1964.
216. Ragins, H., Dragstedt, L. R., II, Landor, J. H., Lyons, E. S., and Dragstedt, L. R., Surgery 40:886, 1956.
217. Ransom, H. K., Ann. Surg. 126:633, 1947.
218. Rhea, W. G., Jr., Killen, D. A., and Scott, H. W., Surg. Gynecol. Obstet. 120:970, 1965.
219. Roberts, J. A. F., Br. J. Prev. Soc. Med. 11:107, 1957.
220. Roberts, K. E., Randall, H. T., and Farr, A. W., Surg. Forum 4:301, 1954.
221. Rosenow, E. C., J.A.M.A. 61:1947, 1913.
222. Ross, B., and Kay, A. W., Gastroenterology 46:379, 1964.
223. Sandweiss, D. J., Gastroenterology 27:604, 1954.
224. Schindler, R., Gastroenterology 10:234, 1948.
225. Schnedorf, J. G., Bradley, W. B., and Ivy, A. C., Am. J. Dig. Dis. 3:239, 1936.
226. Shay, H., Amer. J. Dig. Dis. 4:846, 1959.
227. Shay, H., Amer. J. Dig. Dis. 6:29, 1961.
228. Shay, H., in Current Gastroenterology, New York, Hoeber, 1962, pp. 276–296.
229. Smith, W. H., Lancet 2:745, 1951.
230. Smith, H. W., Texter, E. C., Stickley, J. H., and Barborka, C. J., Gastroenterology 32:1025, 1957.
231. Smith, W. O., Duval, M. K., Joel, W., and Wolf, S., Surgery 46:76, 1959.
232. Smithwick, H. R., Surgery 41:344, 1957.
233. Somervell, T. H., in The Surgery of the Stomach and Duodenum, London, Arnold, 1948.
234. Somerwell, T. H., Br. J. Surg. 30:113, 1942.
235. Spira, J. J., Gastroduodenal Ulcer, London, Butterworth, 1956, Chap. 14.
236. Spira, J. J., Gastroduodenal Ulcer, London, Butterworth, 1956, p. 146.
237. Spira, J. J., Gastroduodenal Ulcer, London, Butterworth, 1956, pp. 145–146.
238. Stammers, F. A. R., Br. J. Surg. 49:28, 1961.
239. Stammers, F. A. R., Partial Gastrectomy Complications and Metabolic Consequences. London, Butterworth, 1963.
240. Sternberg, C., Z Heikl 28 (Suppl.) :280, 1908.
241. Sunn, D. H. C., Ryan, M. L., Chang, P. L., and Keogh, R., Ann. N.Y. Acad. Sci. 140:875, 1967.
242. Swisher, W. P., Baker, L. A., and Bennett, H. D.,

Am. J. Dig. Dis. 22:291, 1955.

243. Tanner, N. C., Ann. R. Coll. Surg. Eng. 10:45, 1952.

244. Tanner, N. C., in Surgery of the Stomach and Duodenum, Boston, Little, Brown, 1962, p. 430.

245. Tanner, N. C., Br. J. Surg. 51:5, 1964.

246. Taylor, H., Br. J. Surg. 24:469, 1936-7.

247. Taylor, H., and Eadie, D. G. A., Br. Med. J., 1:15, 1967.

248. Te Velde, K., Hoedemaker, P. J., Anders, G. J. P. A., Arends, A., and Nieweg, H. O., Gastroenterology 51:138, 1966.

249. Turner, J. C., Dockerty, M. B., Priestley, J. T., and Comfort, M. W., Surg. Gynecol. Obstet. 104:746, 1957.

250. Underdahl, L. O., Woolner, L. B., and Black, B. M., J. Clin. Endocrinol. 13:20, 1953.

251. Van Yzeren, W. Z., Klin. Med. (Mosk.) 43:181, 1901.

252. Virchow, R., Arch. Pathol. Anat. 5:361, 1853.

253. Visick, A. H., Lancet 1:505, 1948.

254. Wallensten, S., and Cothman, L., Surgery 33:1, 1953.

255. Walters, W., Surg. Clin. North Am. 37:921, 1957.

256. Walters, W., Gray, H. K., and Priestley, J. T., Proc. Staff Meet. Mayo Clin. 23:29, 1948.

257. Walters, W., and Lynn, T. E., Ann. Surg. 144: 464, 1956.

258. Walters, W., Lynn, T. E., and Mobley, J. E., Gastroenterology 33:685, 1957.

259. Walters, W., and Remine, W. H., Surgery 55: 585, 1964.

260. Ward, J. T., Adesola, A. O., and Welbourn, R. B., Gut 5:173, 1964.

261. Watkinson, G., Gut 1:14, 1960.

262. Weinberg, J. A., Stempien, S. J., Movius, H. J., and Dagradi, A. E., Am. J. Surg. 92:202, 1956.

263. Weiss, A., Pitman, E. R., and Graham, E. C., Am. J. Med. 31:266, 1961.

264. Welch, C. E., and Burke, J. F., Surgery 44:943, 1958.

265. Werner, P., Am. J. Med. 16:363, 1954.

266. Williams, E. J., and Irvine, W. T., Lancet 1: 1053, 1966.

267. Williams, J. A., Br. J. Surg. 51:125, 1964.

268. Williams, J. A., Baume, P. E., and Meynell, M. J., Lancet 1:342, 1966.

269. Williams, J. A., Nicholson, G. I., and Cooke. W. T., Gut 5:281, 1964.

270. Wittneben, R., Inaugural Dissertation, Wurzburg, 1886.

271. Wolf, S., and Wolff, H. G., Human Gastric Function, New York, Oxford University Press, 1943.

272. Wright, J. T., Grant, A., and Jennings, D., Lancet 2:1314, 1955.

273. Zollinger, R. M., and Ellison, E. H., Ann. Surg. 142:709, 1955.

B. Stress Ulcer

KEITH A. KELLY

Stress ulcer is a life-threatening complication that develops in patients who are already desperately ill from another disease. The sudden onset and devastating effects of the lesion demand prompt attention and effective therapy. Knowledge of stress ulcer is especially important today, since continuing advancements in medical care have resulted in greater numbers of severely ill patients surviving long enough for these lesions to develop.

Stress ulcers are acute erosions or ulcerations of the stomach and duodenum that appear in patients under severe stress. The lesions have also been called *acute peptic ulcers, acute hemorrhagic gastritis, acute erosive gastritis, Curling's ulcer,* and *Cushing's ulcer.*

Several types of stress can lead to the development of stress ulcers. Thus, the pathogenesis of the ulcers may vary, depending on the inciting cause. Until more is known about their pathogenesis, and because of similarities in the acute onset, clinical course, and lethal nature of all types of stress ulcers, however, there is some justification for considering them together.

Stress ulcers should be clearly distinguished from chronic peptic ulcers that exacerbate acutely under stress; chronic peptic ulceration is a different disease and it may continue to produce difficulty after the stress precipitating the acute exacerbation is removed; whereas, the gastrointestinal tract in patients with stress ulcer returns to normal when the patients recover from their primary illness.[1]

HISTORY

Stress ulcerations have been known for at least 150 years. Swan,[2] in 1823, described bleeding stress ulcerations in a burned patient, an association verified and brought into prominence by Curling[3] in 1842. In the 1860s, Billroth[4] noted stress ulcers after operation and with sepsis, while Cushing,[5] in 1932, described alimentary ulceration with lesions of the central nervous system and after neurosurgical operations. In 1966, Harjola and Sivula[6] showed that hemorrhagic shock could result in stress ulcers in animals. More recently, Skillman and colleagues[7] documented increased rates of back diffusion of hydrogen ion, that is, diffusion from the gastric lumen back across the mucosa in patients with stress ulcer; Guilbert and co-workers[8] demonstrated the damaging effect of duodenal content on the gastric mucosa of animals under stress, while DenBesten and Hamza[9,10] demonstrated that bile salts had a similar effect.

INCIDENCE

Stress ulceration is common in severely stressed patients, but the lesions are usually not clinically manifest. Of 42 patients under severe stress, all were found to have lesions in the gastric mucosa when gastroscopy was performed routinely, although most had no clinical signs of stress ulcers.[11] More than half of 85 burn patients had guaiac-positive stools or evidence of abnormalities on x-ray examination of the upper gastrointestinal tract, whether clinical signs of stress ulcer were present or not;[12] however, clinically evident stress ulcers developed in only about 12 percent of burn patients.[13] Only 8 of 150 severely injured patients in a surgical intensive care unit had clinical signs of stress ulcers.[14] Also, stress ulcers developed after only 1 of 2,000 operations at the Mayo Clinic, although these ulcers were four times more likely to follow cardiovascular, thoracic, neurosurgical, or abdominal operations than less extensive procedures.[15]

CLINICAL SETTING

Stress ulcers can result from shock, trauma, operations, infections, burns, hepatic, renal, or pulmonary failure, lesions or injuries of the central nervous system, and ulcerogenic drugs. The disease can occur in anyone undergoing severe stress and appears in patients of all ages.[15] Males predominate over females in most series.[16]

ETIOLOGY AND PATHOGENESIS

The exact cause of stress ulcers is unknown. In fact, different causes may be operative in different patients. In every case, however, stress in some way damages the gastroduodenal mucosa.

A promising hypothesis is that the inciting stress results in poor vascular perfusion of the alimentary mucosa.[11, 17, 18] The resulting ischemia and anoxia damage the integrity of the mucosal capillaries and result in capillary dilatation and extravasation of fluid, plasma, and blood cells. Mucosal necrosis ensues and extends, erosions appear, and hemorrhage begins at erosive sites.

Hydrochloric acid plays a key role in the genesis of stress ulcer, for if there is no acid bathing the ischemic gastroduodenal mucosa of the stressed subject, stress ulcers do not appear.[7, 19] The amount of hydrochloric acid present need not be great. In fact, only small amounts of hydrochloric acid can be aspirated from the stomach of patients with stress ulcer,[20] with the possible exception of those with lesions of the central nervous system.[21] It should be emphasized, however, that the amount of acid aspirated may not represent the total amount secreted by the gastric mucosa.

The quantity of acid aspirated from the gastric lumen is the net result of secretion of HCl by the oxyntic cells and of diffusion of HCl from the gastric lumen back into the blood. In healthy patients, only small amounts of hydrogen ion diffuse from the lumen into the blood, and almost all the secreted hydrogen ion can be aspirated.[22] In patients with stress ulcer, however, the damaged mucosa is no longer an effective barrier to back diffusion of hydrogen ion, and loss of hydrogen ion from the lumen to the blood occurs at an increased rate.[7]

Back diffusion of hydrogen ion enhances the development of stress ulcers. As hydrogen ion reenters the gastric wall, it results in the release of histamine and other vasoactive amines.[17, 22] The released vasoactive amines further augment mucosal capillary dilatation, edema, and ischemia, abetting the development of the ulcers. In addition, the hydrogen ion may act directly on enteric neurons, which in turn stimulate gastric contractions via local reflexes and enhance mucosal congestion, aggravating the mucosal ischemia.[22]

The back diffusion of hydrogen ion also results in the secretion of pepsinogen from chief cells.[23] The released pepsinogen, if activated, could augment the damage to the mucosa.

Damage to the mucosa caused by stress also is worsened by the presence in the gastric lumen of bile salts, proteolytic enzymes and urea, and of drugs such as aspirin and phenacetin, which, except for proteolytic enzymes, have been shown to break the mucosal barrier and increase back diffusion of hydrogen ion.[22]

Sepsis leads to stress ulceration, causing septic shock and poor perfusion in some cases, and capillary damage from bacterial endotoxins in other cases. Also, decreased platelet adhesiveness and prolongation of prothrombin time can result from sepsis and can augment bleeding from stress ulcers.[24]

Menguy and co-workers[25] hypothesized that the secretion of mucus is defective in patients with stress ulcer, especially those receiving corticoids, and that the lack of a protective mucous coat over the mucosa leads to stress ulcers. Davenport[22] stated, however, that mucus does not normally provide such a protective barrier, since hydrogen ion and other agents that break the mucosal barrier can readily diffuse through the mucous layer. Silen and Skillman[18] suggested that changes in mucus production may be secondary to mucosal injury rather than primary causes of stress ulcers.

PATHOLOGICAL FINDINGS

Stress ulcers are more often gastric than duodenal, more often in the oxyntic than in the antral mucosa, and more often multiple than single.[15, 18, 26] They are frequently less than 5 mm in diameter, but their greatest dimension can be up to 10 cm. They may be round or linear. These ulcers characteristically are soft, nonindurated, and

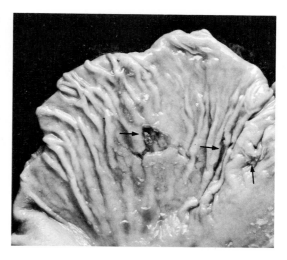

FIG. 1. Gastric corpus from a 45-year-old man who died of gastric bleeding 9 days after a severe burn. Multiple superficial, shallow ulcers are present (arrows), the largest of which is about 1.5 cm in greatest dimension.

superficial, and they usually penetrate only to the muscularis mucosa (Figs. 1, 2). On occasion, however, they penetrate deep into the wall of the viscus and even perforate into the peritoneal cavity.[27, 28]

Microscopically, an early finding is capillary dilatation with edema in the lamina propria and extravasation of erythrocytes. Necrosis of the overlying epithelium occurs with ensuing hemorrhage and ulceration (Fig. 2). The lesions characteristically do not show evidence of chronic inflammation, which is the hallmark of chronic peptic ulcers.

SYMPTOMS AND SIGNS

The clinical onset of stress ulcer usually occurs between 5 and 10 days after the onset of the inciting stress (Fig. 3).

Stress ulcers generally do not produce recognizable symptoms, perhaps because they are masked by the overwhelming distress most patients experience from their primary illness. Pain is characteristically absent.

In about 9 of 10 patients, stress ulcers present with acute gastrointestinal bleeding; in the remainder, they perforate.[16] The onset

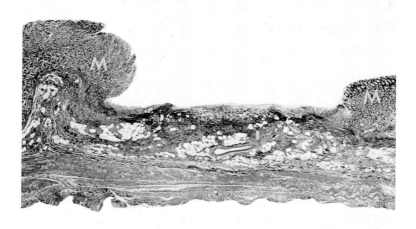

FIG. 2.   Large stress ulcer from specimen shown in Figure 1. The ulcer penetrates mucosa (M) down to but not through the muscularis mucosa. An acute inflammatory reaction is present at the base of the ulcer, but there is no evidence of chronic inflammation. H&E; ×10.

of bleeding is usually heralded by hematemesis, the appearance of blood in nasogastric aspirate, or the passage of blood via the rectum. An increase in pulse or a decrease in blood pressure, however, may be the first sign of a bleeding stress ulcer. The amount of blood lost can range from a few flecks, or just enough to cause a brownish discoloration in the gastric juice, to liters per hour. Once brisk bleeding begins, it usually continues, and the patients may need multiple blood transfusions to maintain their circulating blood volume.[27]

Patients with perforated stress ulcers may have abdominal pain and tenderness,[27] but many cases of "silent" perforation have been reported.[28]

DIAGNOSIS

Bleeding from the gastrointestinal tract in a patient under stress suggests the diagnosis of stress ulcer. The single best diagnostic aid is endoscopy. The superficial, bleeding erosions or ulcerations can almost always be identified with the gastroscope or the duodenoscope.[15] Endoscopy should be done early, however, preferably while the patient is still bleeding, for then the endoscopist has the best chance of detecting the lesion.

Radiology has not been as useful as endoscopy in diagnosis. Plain roentgenograms of the abdomen usually do not show any abnor-

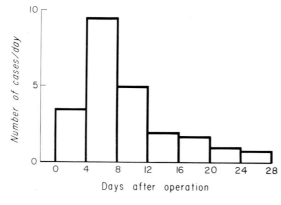

FIG. 3.   Distribution of onset of symptoms in 95 cases of acute postoperative stress ulceration. (From David and Kelly. *Surg. Clin. N. Amer.* 49:1111, 1969. Courtesy of W. B. Saunders Company, Philadelphia.)

mality, although they may show evidence of free air if perforation has occurred. Barium examination of the upper part of the gastrointestinal tract usually is not helpful in diagnosing the lesions, because stress ulcers are so superficial that the radiologist has great difficulty in identifying them. Also, the presence of blood in the stomach and duodenum hinders the examination. Arteriography can be employed, but it is usually not necessary because a diagnosis can be obtained by endoscopy.

In some cases, the patients are bleeding so briskly and are so unresponsive to medical treatment that the diagnosis must be made at operation by direct inspection.

TREATMENT

Prophylaxis

Surgeons must recognize that stress ulcers are likely to develop in patients under severe stress. Vigorous treatment of primary conditions that could result in stress ulcer should be pursued. Medications that damage the gastric mucosa and those leading to bleeding, such as heparin, should not be used unless absoluetly indicated.

Antacids are the mainstay of prophylactic therapy. Neutralization of the hydrogen ion prevents its back diffusion with related consequences, and it also inactivates pepsin. Antacids should be given in amounts large enough and at intervals frequent enough to maintain the intraluminal gastric pH near neutrality at all times. If gastric retention or ileus develops, the patient should be given nothing by mouth, and a nasogastric tube should be positioned in the stomach to remove hydrogen ion, pepsin, and any refluxed duodenal juice. Antacids can then be administered intermittently through the tube.

Medical Management

Once signs of stress ulcer appear, vigorous medical management is indicated initially. When the ulcers present with bleeding, a central venous pressure catheter is inserted and a sample is withdrawn for typing and cross-matching of six units of blood for possible transfusion, and to assess hematocrit, leukocyte count, platelet count, prothrombin time, and other bleeding and clotting parameters. A nasogastric tube is inserted to remove gastric content and to monitor and quantitate the extent of bleeding.

The stomach should be lavaged with iced, isotonic sodium chloride via the nasogastric tube if active bleeding continues. Antacids also can be administered through the tube during periods when suction is not employed. Ulcerogenic drugs and factors promoting bleeding, such as heparin, are withdrawn.

The pulse and the arterial and central venous pressure are carefully monitored. Lactated Ringer's solution and blood are given intravenously to maintain the pulse and the central venous and arterial pressures at normal levels for the patient and to ensure a urine output of more than 30 ml per hour. If poor perfusion of tissue results in acidosis, sodium bicarbonate should be administered. Vitamin K should be given for a prolonged prothrombin time, and transfusion of fresh frozen plasma or fresh platelets for underlying platelet abnormalities.

Surgical Treatment

INDICATIONS

Some patients continue to bleed in spite of vigorous medical therapy. Operation, therefore, must be considered. The decision to operate must be made on an individual basis, according to the surgeon's assessment of the likelihood of continued bleeding or distress from the stress ulcer versus the patient's ability to withstand operation. Patients who can tolerate bleeding the least should be operated on the soonest; but often these patients are the least likely to withstand an operation. Nevertheless, persistence with medical therapy carries an exceedingly high mortality rate. Early operation offers the patient a better chance of survival.

Chong and Kelly [27] found that not one of eight patients who underwent operation died within 3 days of the onset of bleeding and after an average of 5.5 units of blood had been transfused. In contrast, all nine patients who underwent operation after an average delay of 5 days subsequent to onset of bleeding and after an average of 16 units of blood was transfused died.

OPERATIVE TECHNIQUES

A vertical, upper midline abdominal incision should be made to expose the stomach and duodenum. The initial objective is to identify the site of bleeding and to control it quickly. If the stomach is filled with blood, a longitudinal gastrotomy 10 cm in length should be performed through the midportion of the anterior wall of the stomach. The clots should be evacuated from the lumen and the mucosa inspected from cardia to pylorus to determine the source of the bleeding. Sites of bleeding are quickly ligated with sutures. A more leisurely inspection of the entire gastric and adjacent esophageal and duodenal mucosa can then be performed and additional bleeding sites sought.

If no active bleeding is encountered in the stomach, a second longitudinal incision about 7 cm in length should be centered over the pylorus. Bleeding sites in the duodenum can then be identified and ligated.

What else should be done at operation is unclear. The reported series of patients treated surgically are small, and no random, unbiased application of one procedure versus another has been made. Also, most surgeons have not defined the exact type, location, and extent of ulceration in their reports, so that assessment of results is difficult.

Multiple bleeding gastric stress ulcers have been treated successfully by subtotal distal gastric resection. Bleeding was controlled by subtotal gastrectomy in three of three cases reported by Gilchrist and dePeyster [29] and in four of five cases reported by Chong and Kelly.[27] In recent years, however, most surgeons favor the use of truncal vagotomy with the gastrectomy.[11, 17, 18, 30-32] The incidence of recurrent bleeding after the combined operations has usually been less than after subtotal gastrectomy alone.

Menguy et al.[25] recommended total gastrectomy in critically ill patients with bleeding gastric stress ulcers, reporting no rebleeding and only two deaths among ten such patients. But Drapanas et al.[17] cautioned against the use of total gastrectomy because of the likelihood of high morbidity and mortality rates and the adverse long-term

sequelae accompanying the operation. They employ it only if lesser procedures fail to control the bleeding.

Although some have found vagotomy and pyloroplasty satisfactory procedures for bleeding gastric stress ulcer,[33, 34] rebleeding occurred in four of four patients so treated by Bryant and Griffen,[35] in five of nine patients treated by Goodman and Frey,[36] and in two of four patients treated by Chong and Kelly.[27] Also eight of 22 patients treated by Kirtley et al.[37] died after vagotomy and pyloroplasty for bleeding stress ulcer. Menguy et al.[25] and Drapanas et al.[17] did not advise these procedures.

In contrast, vagotomy and pyloroplasty have been used successfully for bleeding duodenal stress ulcer by Kirtley and associates[37] in four patients, and by Chong and Kelly,[27] who effectively controlled bleeding in four of five patients. The modified Heineke-Mikulicz pyloroplasty (Chap. 17) is preferred, since it allows fast, safe closure of the longitudinal, transpyloric incision described previously and used for exploration of the duodenum.

Patients with perforated gastric or duodenal stress ulcers have been treated as well by simple closure (Chap. 22) as by more extensive operations.[27, 31, 38]

RESULTS OF TREATMENT

The results of treatment for stress ulceration have been poor, partially due to the lethal nature of stress ulcer and partially because many patients die from their primary illness even though their stress ulcer is brought under control. Reported mortality rates for medical therapy have ranged from 50 to 80 percent. Patients undergoing operations for stress ulcers have had somewhat better survival rates (10 to 50 percent), but no unbiased, controlled trial of medical versus surgical treatment has been carried out. It seems likely that only patients well enough to tolerate operations have undergone operation, as the most seriously ill patients are often refused operation by surgeons because of the unlikely possibility that they will survive the operation.

The need for controlled trials of medical versus surgical therapy and of various types of surgical therapy for stress ulcer is apparent.

REFERENCES

1. Roth, H., Schweiz. Med. Wochenschr. 100:1278, 1970.
2. Swan, J., Edinburgh Med. J. 19:344, 1823.
3. Curling, T. B., Roy. Med. Chir. Soc. London (Med.-Chir. Trans.) 25:260, 1842.
4. Billroth, T. R., Wien Med. Wochenschr. 17:705, 1867.
5. Cushing, H., Surg. Gynecol. Obstet. 55:1, 1932.
6. Harjola, P.-T., and Sivula, A., Ann. Surg. 163:21, 1966.
7. Skillman, J. J., Gould, S. A., Chung, R. S. K., and Silen, W., Ann. Surg. 172:564, 1970.
8. Guilbert, J., Bounous, G., and Gurd, F. N., J. Trauma 9:723, 1969.
9. DenBesten, L., and Hamza, K. N., Gastroenterology 62:417, 1972.
10. Hamza, K. N., and DenBesten, L., Surgery 71:161, 1972.
11. Lucas, C. E., Sugawa, C., Riddle, J., Rector, F., Rosenberg, B., and Walt, A. J., Arch. Surg. 102:266, 1971.
12. Day, S. B., MacMillan, B. G., and Altemeier, W. A., Curling's Ulcer: An Experiment of Nature. Springfield, Ill., Thomas, 1972.
13. Pruitt, B. A., Jr., Foley, F. D., and Moncrief, J. A., Ann. Surg. 172:523, 1970.
14. Lev, R., Molot, M. D., McNamara, J., and Stremple, J. F., Lab. Invest. 25:491, 1971.
15. David, E., and Kelly, K. A., Surg. Clin. North Am. 49:1111, 1969.
16. David, E., McIlrath, D. C., and Higgins, J. A., Mayo Clinic Proc. 46:15, 1971.
17. Drapanas, T., Woolverton, W. C., Reeder, J. W., Reed, R. L., and Weichert, R. F., Ann. Surg. 173:628, 1971.
18. Silen, W., and Skillman, J. J., Adv. Intern. Med. (In press.)
19. Moody, F. G., and Aldrete, J. S., Surgery 70:154, 1971.
20. McClelland, R. N., Shires, G. T., and Prager, M., Am. J. Surg. 121:134, 1971.
21. Norton, L., Greer, J., and Eiseman, B., Arch. Surg. 101:200, 1970.
22. Davenport, H. W., N. Engl. J. Med. 276:1307, 1967.
23. Johnson, L. R., Gastroenterology 62:412, 1972.
24. Altemeier, W. A., Fullen, W. D., and McDonough, J. J., Ann. Surg. 175:759, 1972.
25. Menguy, R., Gadacz, T., and Zajtchuk, R., Arch. Surg. 99:198, 1969.
26. Fletcher, D. G., and Harkins, H. N., Surgery 36:212, 1954.
27. Chong, G. C., and Kelly, K. A., Surg. Clin. North Am. 51:863, 1971.
28. Kunzman, J., Am. J. Surg. 119:637, 1970.
29. Gilchrist, R. K., and dePeyster, F. A., Ann. Surg. 147:728, 1958.
30. Crawford, F. A., Hammon, J. W., Jr., and Shingleton, W. W., Am. J. Surg. 121:644, 1971.
31. Girvan, D. P., and Passi, R. B., Arch. Surg. 103:116, 1971.
32. Hinchey, E. J., Hreno, A., Benoit, P. R., Hewson, J. R., and Gurd, F. N., Adv. Surg. 4:325, 1970.
33. Flowers, R. S., Kyle, K., and Hoerr, S. O., Am. J. Surg. 119:632, 1970.
34. Sullivan, R. C., and Waddell, W. R., Am. J. Surg. 116:745, 1968.
35. Bryant, L. R., and Griffen, W. O., Jr., Arch. Surg. 93:161, 1966.
36. Goodman, A. A., and Frey, C. F., Ann. Surg. 167:180, 1968.
37. Kirtley, J. A., Scott, H. W., Jr., Sawyers, J. L., Graves, H. A., Jr., and Lawler, M. R., Ann. Surg. 169:801, 1969.
38. Fogelman, M. J., and Garvey, J. M., Am. J. Surg. 112:651, 1966.

12

A. PATHOLOGY, DIAGNOSIS, AND FACTORS INFLUENCING THE CHOICE OF TREATMENT FOR PEPTIC ULCER

RODNEY MAINGOT

While the term *peptic ulcer* is a convenient one to cover both duodenal and gastric ulcer, it must be understood that these are, in fact, two separate diseases related anatomically rather than aetiologically.

Gastric ulcer is more rare than duodenal ulcer and is more common in males than in females; duodenal ulcer also predominates in the male. Gastric ulcer is usually associated with a long, J-shaped, hypotonic stomach with atrophic mucosal changes, and has a level of acid secretion which is normal or below the average, while in duodenal ulcer it is common to find the stomach high in position, steer-horn in shape, hypertonic, irritable, and hyperchlorhydric, with gastric mucosa thicker and the parietal-cell mass greater than is usual in most people, and emptying its highly acid-pepsin contents rapidly and eagerly.

Duodenal ulcer is distributed evenly throughout the adult population of Great Britain, but gastric ulcer appears to be more common in those who are undernourished and underprivileged. Duodenal ulcer is frequently associated with a certain physical and psychological type, such as the thin, highly strung, conscientious, overworked intellectual who is in a constant state of stress and anxiety. There are, of course, exceptions to this generalisation, although there seems to be little doubt that there is an increased incidence among doctors and among individuals who hold responsible positions in industry, such as foremen, business executives, and skilled engineers.

A gastric ulcer responds to medical treatment more speedily and dramatically than does a duodenal ulcer, but it inexplicably breaks down with equal rapidity, and recurrence is all too frequent. It is so unpredictable in its behaviour and simulates a cancerous lesion with such frequency that it demands surgical enquiry and excision in the majority of cases.

The uncomplicated duodenal ulcer is a medical problem. Surgery should be invoked in the case of duodenal ulcer only when complications have occurred or the lesion has proved *intractable* to intensive and well-applied medical therapy, in other words, when conservative treatment and, possibly, the patient himself have failed. Furthermore, the two conditions vary in many essential details, and it is for this reason in particular that I propose to discuss them separately. The *aetiology and pathogenesis* of duodenal and gastric ulcer are fully described by Mann in Chapter 11, Part A, and Zollinger, Nick, and Sanzenbacher discuss the role played by ulcerogenic tumours of the pancreas in Chapter 13. The reader is also referred to articles by Tanner,[31] Orr,[21] Avery Jones,[14] and Judd,[16] Wirthlin and Malt,[35] and to the Annotation in the British Medical Journal 1:256, 1973.

DUODENAL ULCER

Pathology

Approximately 75 to 80 percent of chronic peptic ulcers are found in the duodenum. More than 90 percent of chronic duodenal ulcers occur in the first portion of the duodenum. Portis and Jaffe,[22] analysing over 9,000 autopsy findings, recorded 158 active ulcers; of these 85 percent were within the first 2 cm of the duodenum, 10 percent were within the next 3 cm, and the remaining 5 percent were beyond the first 5 cm and above the ampulla of Vater.

Though *postbulbar ulcers* are uncommon, the proportion situated in the supra-ampullary region is higher than that in the lower half of the descending limb, as would be expected from the changed conditions below the entry of alkaline juices. Brulé et al.[3] collected 94 cases of ulcer of the second part of the duodenum, of which 84 percent were supra-ampullary.

Crymble[9] reported four cases of ulcer in the second part of the duodenum, and came to the conclusion that when a patient had symptoms of duodenal ulcer but the first part was normal on x-ray examination and on surgical exploration, the palpation and inspection of the second part should not be neglected. Cooke and Hutton[8] state that increasing awareness of this lesion has improved their standards of diagnosis considerably. They diagnosed ten cases during the 5-year period 1949 to 1953 in 9,732 barium-meal x-ray examinations, but 15 cases during the 2 years 1954 to 1955 in 4,016 examinations. The average age in their series was 51, and their 25 patients comprised 23 men and 2 women (Fig. 1).

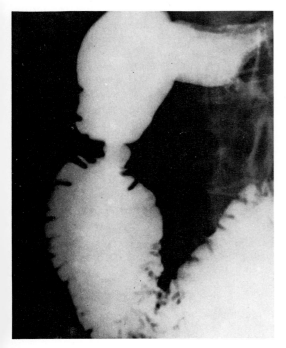

FIG. 1. Postbulbar duodenal ulcer. Patient, a doctor aged 61, was operated upon and Billroth II partial gastrectomy was performed with duodenal occlusion, i.e., first portion of cut end of duodenum was closed and inverted. Patient made good recovery (author's patient).

Certain clinical features of postbulbar duodenal ulcer should be noted: pain is mainly situated in the back, occurs principally late in the day and during the night, and is difficult to relieve by drugs; bleeding is the most common complication; acute perforation is a rare event; and episodes of intermittent duodenal obstruction with sudden pain and vomiting may supervene.

If we exclude the *acute perforations*, which occur most frequently near the superior surface of the lesser curvature of the duodenal bulb, at operation the majority (fully 85 percent) of chronic duodenal ulcers are found to be located on the *posterior wall* or to have extended from the posterior wall to the superior surface of the lesser curve of the duodenum, about 1 cm or so from the pyloric ring, and it is these ulcers that so frequently become attached to or actually penetrate into the substance of the pancreas and that account for most of the technical difficulties associated with partial gastroduodenal resection. I have seen cases at operation where there appeared to be a complete circle of scarring and ulceration.

Multiple duodenal ulcers occur in from 10 to 15 percent of cases. These are usually seen on the anterior and posterior walls, facing one another like contact or "kissing" ulcers, and they produce a considerable amount of scarring and distortion of the bulb.

Combined ulcers, i.e., ulcers in both the stomach and duodenum in the same patient, were reported in 8 percent of cases in Present's series. Wilkie,[33] on the other hand, discovered 51 combined ulcers in 413 peptic ulcer patients, an incidence of 12 percent, while Rivers[24] found a coexistence of 13 percent. Tanner[31] recorded that 20 percent of his gastric ulcer cases were associated with duodenal ulcer. Anthanassiades and Charalambopoupoulou, in a study of the operative notes of the last decade (Jan. 1957 to June 1968), showed that 2,523 operations were performed for gastric and duodenal ulcer; among these were 60 cases of coexistent gastric and duodenal ulcers, an incidence of 2.4 percent. The incidence of duodenal ulcer in patients with gastric ulcer (21 percent) was much higher than gastric ulcer patients with duodenal ulcer (3 percent). The incidence of gastric ulcer is 3 times greater in cases of duodenal ulcer with pyloric stenosis (5.5 percent) than in duodenal ulcer without stenosis (2 percent).

Chronic duodenal ulcers are on the whole smaller than gastric ulcers, the average size being 1 cm, although in rare instances they may measure as much as 5 cm across the crater. They vary considerably in shape and may be circular, crescentic, oval, triangular, or pear-shaped. The ulcer has a punched-out appearance; the margins are overhanging, receding, or terraced; and the granulating base is covered with mucopurulent debris. The depth of the ulcer will depend upon the degree of penetration that has occurred, and at the height of inflammatory activity the muscularis is always breached.

The characteristics of chronic ulcer are: (1) destruction of the muscularis in the centre of the ulcer, (2) dense fibrosis in the base, (3) adhesion of the muscularis mucosae to the muscularis at the margin of the crater, and (4) the presence of periarteritis and endarteritis in the surrounding vessels.

The mucous membrane around the ulcer will, in addition, show the usual proliferative and regenerative changes. As a result of the accompanying fibrosis, the first portion of the duodenum becomes distorted and *shortened*. The normal distance from the pyloric ring to the papilla of Vater is 8 cm, but this may be reduced to 4 cm or even less by contracting fibrous tissue such as is found in long-standing cases of duodenal ulcer—a fact which is well recognised by surgeons who undertake partial gastroduodenal resection for this condition. This marked contraction of the first part of the duodenum consequent upon long-standing ulceration and fibrosis receives but scant notice by radiologists, yet it is of the utmost importance to the surgeon in envisaging the possible technical difficulties that may be encountered in dissection of this scarred zone in the bowel.

Giant duodenal ulcers are rare and at times cause difficulties in diagnosis, as the shape of the ulcer may in some respects simulate a normal cap until close study demonstrates the loss of mucosal pattern.[14]

It is very probable that many chronic ulcers that heal completely break down again many times subsequently. The final result of the cicatrisation of a chronic ulcer will depend upon its situation, size, and chronicity. So far

as duodenal ulcer is concerned, when a severe degree of contraction occurs, pyloric stenosis results, and the commonest cause of occlusion of the outlet of the stomach is a cicatrising duodenal ulcer.

At *operation, chronic duodenal ulcers* are readily recognised, only a very few of the more less visible ones located on the posterior wall of the second or possibly the third part of the duodenum proving difficult to identify.

In ulcer cases, operation is advised for treatment and not for purposes of diagnosis.

With modern methods of investigation, the preoperative diagnosis of duodenal ulcer may be said to be correct in fully 97 percent of cases. At operation, therefore, we expect to find the stigmata of a callous ulcer, i.e., one that has resisted all attempts at cure by medical therapy.

If, on exposing the stomach and duodenum, no evidence of ulceration can be found the position is at once perfectly clear—no operation directed to the cure of a supposed ulcer can be countenanced and we must search elsewhere in the abdomen for lesions that are capable of producing dyspeptic symptoms, e.g., chronic pancreatitis, chronic calculous cholecystitis, etc., and deal with them accordingly. The difficult cases are those in which the patient gives a history of ulcer where a long course of medical treatment has been undertaken without appreciable improvement, when numerous biochemical investigations support the diagnosis of ulcer, and when although a barium-meal examination shows what appears to be an ulcer niche or a deformed cap, at operation no ulcer can be detected and in fact the entire duodenum both on inspection and palpation appears to be normal.

If, on very careful inspection and palpation of the walls of the duodenum, no signs of ulceration are present; if the pylorus is amply patent; and if, after opening the lesser sac and dissecting the posterior wall of the first part of the duodenum free from its pancreatic bed, no lesion can be seen or felt, no useful purpose will be served by opening the anterior wall of the duodenum and extending this incision well into the pyloric region for the purpose of prying into the cavity of the stomach or duodenum. No ulcer will be found if the examination by sight and touch of the viscera concerned has been orderly, purposeful, and fastidious. The surgeon should, nevertheless, be mindful of the rare postbulbar duodenal ulcer which cannot be readily displayed unless the head of the pancreas and the duodenum are mobilised on the lines first suggested by Kocher in 1903.

The presence of a chronic ulcer can be easily verified on exploration. The ulcerated area will be felt as a hard, fibrotic mass or a cartilaginous, button-like tumour; the ulcer bed can often be palpated by the tip of the finger, which invaginates the gut; the portion of the bowel just distal to the vein of Mayo is frequently revealed as distorted, puckered, scarred, narrowed, or pouched; the adjacent gastrocolic and gastrohepatic omenta may be tethered to the pancreas by the penetrating lesion, while the duodenum may be dragged out of position and bound to the undersurface of the liver or to an adjacent structure such as the gallbladder by filmy vascular bands or transparent web-like membranes. The duodenum may be deeply placed and obscured by a sheaf of adhesions, but good retraction and careful dissection will bring it into view, revealing its cicatrised face.

It should be remembered that posterior wall ulcers give rise to unmistakable change on the anterior wall, such as thickening because of oedema, mottling or speckling of the serosa on gentle friction, or superficial scarring. When a healed ulcer is found on the anterior wall, the posterior wall also should be examined for the presence of an active ulcer, as contact or kissing ulcers are by no means infrequent. The crater of a posterior ulcer may be difficult to find, particularly if the anterior wall is sclerosed. On occasion, scarring is very extensive in the region of the pylorus, and it may be almost impossible to say on inspection whether the ulcer that has produced the scarring is pyloric or duodenal; but it can be definitely stated that ulcers that begin at or within 1 inch (2.5 cm) of the gastric aspect of the pylorus are comparatively rare, as examination of specimens removed by partial gastroduodenal resection for pyloric stenosis will readily prove, and that in nearly every case cicatricial stenosis of the pylorus is caused by chronic duodenal ulcer, the scar tissue resulting from which has spread to the left, thus obscuring the exact site of origin of the ulcer. When a duo-

denal ulcer is found at operation, the surgeon should bear in mind the possibility of hiatal hernia and of associated organic lesions in the stomach, appendix, or gallbladder, or even in all three organs simultaneously.

As previously mentioned, *combined gastric and duodenal ulcers* are by no means uncommon.

The development of a duodenal ulcer after healing of a gastric ulcer must be a very unusual event. Both Tanner [30] and Daintree Johnson [12] have noted that the *duodenal lesion always develops first*. Tanner found that the gastric ulcer was active and the duodenal ulcer inactive or healed in 80 percent of these patients, whereas, when in association with an active duodenal ulcer, the gastric ulcer frequently appeared to be an early lesion.

Of 313 patients with gastric ulcer treated by Aagaard and his colleagues,[1] the gastric ulcer was associated with duodenal ulceration in 120, while of 100 duodenal ulcer patients only 2 showed evidence of gastric ulcers.

Among 779 cases of benign gastric ulcer Comfort et al.[7] found 184 that were associated with duodenal ulcer.

Wilkie [34] stressed the frequent combination of cholecystitis, appendicitis, and duodenal ulcer—*the abdominal triad*—and also the association, especially in women, of gallstones with ulcer—the cholecystoduodenal syndrome.

Many writers have discussed the possible relationship between appendiceal disease and peptic ulcer. For instance, Hartman and Rivers [11] reported chronic appendicitis to be present in 35.7 percent of gastric and 44.4 percent of duodenal ulcer patients. Larimore [17] noted that 18 percent of his patients had had their appendices removed, while Somervell and Orr, in their statistics from Southern India, found a concomitance of 73 percent. Many surgeons recommend that on completion of an operation for peptic ulcer the appendix be removed (usually through a small gridiron incision) whether this organ be diseased or not. In 10 percent of my patients with chronic duodenal ulcer subjected to operation, the appendix had been removed previously.

The *complications* of duodenal ulcer—obstruction, perforation, haemorrhage, and duodenocholedochal fistula—are discussed in Chapters 9, 22 and 23.

Diagnosis

The methods commonly employed for the diagnosis of duodenal disorders include the following:

1. History of the case.
2. Physical examination of the patient.
3. Endoscopy employing the modern gastric and duodenal types of fibrescopes (See Chap. 4. Part A, and Chap. 38. Part B).
4. Radiological examination; including duodenography (Chap. 4. Part C).
5. Laboratory investigations. These include:
    (a) Gastric analysis and biochemical investigations (Chap. 12. Part C).
    (b) Tests for occult blood.
    (c) Examination of the urine and tests for renal efficiency.
    (d) Complete examination of the blood, including haemoglobin estimation, leukocyte count, differential leukocyte count, erythrocyte count, colour index, nonprotein nitrogen of the blood serum, the CO_2-combining power of the plasma, the blood chloride, the Wassermann reaction and Kahn test for syphilis, sedimentation rate, blood group, and gastric cytology (Chap. 28. Part E).

I attach the greatest importance to a painstaking history of the case and to a physical examination of the patient—*clinical methods,* and I consider that with our increasing knowledge of the symptomatology of gastrointestinal diseases a correct diagnosis can be arrived at in the majority of cases by these methods alone. Certainly in chronic duodenal ulcer the symptoms are so characteristic that in approximately 85 percent of cases a confident and correct diagnosis can be formed on the history per se. But "seeing is believing," hence the services of the radiologist are required in every case.

No preoperative diagnosis of chronic duodenal ulcer can be upheld unless it receives the joint approval of the radiologist and the surgeon, while at operation no diagnosis of duodenal ulcer can be supported unless the ulcer itself or the consequences of the ulcer can be unequivocally demonstrated.

Symptoms

The cardinal symptoms of *chronic duodenal ulcer* are pain, vomiting, and bleeding, by far the most outstanding being pain. The characteristic story obtained is one of intermittent attacks of epigastric pain extending over a period of months or years with free intervals varying from weeks to months. This periodicity is very typical, at any rate in the early stages of the disease, but at a later date, when obstruction supervenes, the periodicity is lost, and pain, although it may decrease in severity, becomes constant. In young patients, indigestion that persists without interruption from its onset is unlikely to be caused by peptic ulcer. Periodicity is generally more marked in duodenal than in gastric ulcer. Ulcer pain is of a severe nature and may be described as boring, aching, burning, or lancinating. It is felt in the epigastrium, usually a little to the right of the middle line or perhaps further afield below the tip of the right eighth costal cartilage, but it pierces fiercely through to the back when the ulcer erodes the pancreas. It usually starts 2 to $2\frac{1}{2}$ hours after meals, and is often appeased by food (*hunger pain*), alkalis, or by vomiting. It is commonly relieved by rest in bed and by the benison of warmth. The bigger the meal, the greater the interval, but the worse the pain. After breakfast (a small meal), the interval is short, usually less than 2 hours, while after dinner (usually the largest meal of the day), it may be as long as 3 to 4 hours. Certain articles of diet, the intake of alcohol, or smoking will often aggravate the pain, and worry and anxiety will intensify it. A characteristic feature is nocturnal pain, i.e., pain that is bad enough to awaken the patient out of his sleep late at night or in the early hours of the morning. Pain that is sufficiently acute to arouse a patient from sleep is likely to be organic in nature, whereas pain that increases in severity when the patient is in bed or prevents him from sleeping is suggestive rather of functional disorder.

Some patients know to the minute when an attack of pain is due and they will forestall it or at least dull its sharp edge by taking a glass of milk, a biscuit, or some other food.

Any change in the characteristics of the pain, such as increased persistence despite the use of alkaline medicines, denotes that new pathological processes are at work in the ulcer itself. Pain tends to become progressively more severe, and this crescendo characteristic is very marked during an acute attack. The attacks in some patients appear to have a *seasonal occurrence* and to be more common in the autumn and spring. Hunger pain, which was first described by Moynihan,[19a, b] occurs in many other conditions besides peptic ulcer, e.g., carcinoma of the stomach, chronic cholecystitis, hyperchlorhydria, excessive smoking, and in certain nervous disorders. The cause of the pain that occurs in association with ulcer has not been definitely determined, but it is thought by some to be muscular in origin and to be produced either by tension or stretching of the muscular fibres and nerves in the vicinity of the ulcer or else by involvement of the parietal peritoneum. Most gastric symptoms are due to motor disturbances. On the other hand, the ulcer pain is considered by others to be caused by chemical or acid stimulation. Tanner [28] writes:

If acid stimulation be the cause of pain, then the remissions may result from the nerve endings being protected by a thick tenacious plug of mucus or by the new mucosa growing from the edge. Or possibly a little fresh necrosis of the edge or base might cause temporary death of exposed nerve endings, and pain would cease until the slough had separated to expose live tissue again. Symptoms are known to cease abruptly after a haematemesis; in such cases one may at times find the crater filled with blood clot, which would act as a barrier.

The striking and uniform features of ulcer pain, established by clinical methods, are that the pain is frequently relieved by alkaline medicines, by food, and by vomiting. The most probable hypothesis is that pain is due to the action of acid on the ulcer, and that pain comes on when the acidity reaches a certain level, and abates when the acidity falls below that level (Pickering, 1951).

When chronicity is established, the attacks will increase in frequency and will last longer, the interval will shorten, and the symptoms during the attacks will become more exhausting in character.

Vomiting is comparatively rare in uncomplicated duodenal ulcer and is much more frequently seen in association with gastric ulcer. This may be accounted for by the fact that in gastric ulcer spastic occlusion of the pylorus often takes place and nausea is a more prominent feature. When organic pyloric obstruction supervenes, vomiting will occur, but the symptoms will be those of obstruction of the outlet rather than those truly typical of ulcer. Waterbrash is especially frequent in cases of chronic duodenal ulcer, as was observed by Ryle, who considered the abundant production of this watery alkaline saliva to be the natural reaction on the part of the organism to neutralise the excess of acid. In simple cases, the appetite remains good and the patient will often gain weight and appear to be in sound health; but with the onset of stasis, a loss of weight will ensue as a result of vomiting, a distaste for food, dietary restrictions, nocturnal pain, and insomnia. Constipation is common and will be aggravated by the onset of pyloric obstruction. Other symptoms include a fulness or bloating of the epigastrium, belching or eructations, and periodic bouts of nausea, which, however, are more common in gastric ulcer and in calculous cholecystitis than in duodenal ulcer.

Bleeding is so common that it constitutes a symptom rather than a complication. Duodenal ulcer is the most frequent of all causes of gastrointestinal haemorrhage. Bleeding—melaena or haematemesis—mild, moderate, or massive, occurs in from 20 to 30 percent of cases, and peptic ulceration is, at the present time, the most common single cause of haematemesis.

In a small percentage of patients suffering from chronic duodenal ulcer, no pain at all is felt and the ulcer makes its presence known by bleeding or by perforating. Nausea, anorexia, waterbrash, heartburn, and attacks of vomiting, all without pain, may be the only presenting symptoms.

Physical signs. It is often taught that a physical examination of the abdomen will yield a negative result in the majority of ulcer patients, and consequently this method of investigation is likely to be conducted somewhat perfunctorily and carelessly. This is unfortunate, as valuable signs may be present, and in addition physical examination is necessary in order to exclude the possibility of concomitant disease of other organs. In my experience of ulcer cases I have, on deep pressure, usually found a point of tenderness in the epigastrium which may be exquisitely painful even during the period of quiescence. This sensitive area may be quite small, but its discovery is a most valuable piece of evidence. During an acute attack of ulceration, superficial tenderness and muscular guarding can be elicited over the duodenum, but in the reposeful stage, these may be entirely absent. The point of maximal tenderness is situated in the epigastrium, either at the outer border of the right rectus muscle or in the middle line nearer to the xiphisternum than to the umbilicus. It should be remembered in this connection that midline epigastric tenderness may be caused by pressure on the aorta. There may also be a localised area of reflex tenderness at the back close to the right side of the spinal column at the level of the eleventh or twelfth rib. The painful area in the epigastrium is usually constant in position and does not move appreciably on respiration. It may be confused with gallbladder tenderness, but here it is situated more laterally and is intensified by deep palpation during forced respiratory movements (Murphy's sign).

It should be remembered that the earliest sign of response of an ulcer to medical treatment is the disappearance of pain, which is followed successively by loss of tenderness and of muscular rigidity. On rare occasions, a duodenal ulcer may form a palpable tumour. It is difficult, however, to feel such a tumour unless the patient is thin and has a flaccid abdominal wall. Its palpation, too, is more likely when the stomach is empty. It is often most difficult to determine on palpation whether the tumour is a fixed growth or a large inflammatory mass. When detected, it will be found to be tender on pressure and will appear to be fixed to the pancreas, being immobile on respiration.

When dilatation of the stomach results from a stenosing ulcer, there is distention of the epigastrium and splashing gastric sounds. By ordinary physical methods of examination, it is impossible to discriminate between atonic dilatation of the stomach and stasis produced by organic stenosis, and the diagnosis can only be clinched by barium-meal studies.

In the general examination of the patient, particular attention should be paid to any evidence of carious teeth, gingivitis, or enlarged tonsils. Pallor and anaemia may be marked, suggesting haemorrhage, a growth, or some blood dyscrasia. A rectal examination should never be omitted.

Radiological examination. This is indispensable, and no method of enquiry in gastric disorders is complete nor can any diagnosis be accepted as final until this has been undertaken. Not only can the presence of the ulcer often be confirmed, but the severity of the complications that are present can be evaluated, and the efficacy of the treatment that has been instituted as well.

The diagnosis of peptic ulcer by x-ray examination depends upon the demonstration of direct and indirect signs. The *direct sign* is the crater itself, the *indirect signs* being deformity of the bulb and disturbances in the outline and function of the duodenum or stomach.

Diagnostic accuracy is inextricably bound up with technique, and provided this is efficient, there is no portion of the alimentary tract that can be more thoroughly investigated than the duodenal cap.

Excellent accounts of the radiography of the duodenal cap are given in the work of Truelove and Reynell,[32] and Shanks and Kerley,[26] to which the reader is referred for further information on this subject (Figs. 2 to 7).

The use of *gastrophotography* and *cineradiography* will undoubtedly play an important part in the future, in the study of the physiological functions of the stomach and duodenum and in clear demonstrations of the destructive lesions of the upper gastrointestinal tract (see Chap. 4. Part B).

Differential Diagnosis

The differential diagnosis of duodenal ulcer is based upon a careful consideration of the history of the case, a thorough physical examination, a study of the gastric contents and of the blood and stools, endoscopic examination, and radiological studies. Every patient suffering from *chronic indigestion* has a potential ulcer until it is proved otherwise, and in such cases we can only be dogmatic when our investigations have been exhaustive and have followed the lines already suggested.

It is surprising the number of diseases, both functional and organic, which closely simulate chronic duodenal ulcer, e.g.:

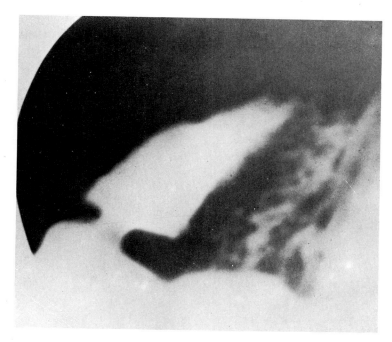

FIG. 2.   Normal duodenal cap.

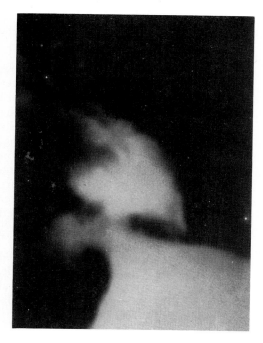

FIG. 3.   Pyloric ulcer.

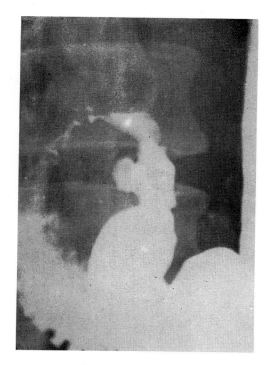

FIG. 4.   Duodenal ulcer.

1. *Nervous Gastric Disorders:* (a) functional; (b) migraine; (c) gastric crises of tabes; (d) psychosomatic disorders and psychoneurotic disturbances.

2. *Reflex Dyspepsias:* (a) appendix dyspepsia; (b) biliary tract disease; (c) dyspepsia from prostatic enlargement; (d) pancreatic disease; (e) carcinoma of the colon and other destructive intestinal lesions; (f) ileocaecal tuberculosis; (g) epigastric hernia; (h) postoperative adhesions; (i) visceroptosis; (j) Crohn's disease; (k) hepatitis.

3. *Hiatal Hernia.*

4. *Other Organic Gastric and Duodenal Disorders:* (a) gastric ulcer; (b) chronic gastritis and duodenitis; (c) cancer of the stomach; (d) innocent new growths of the stomach; (e) syphilis of the stomach; (f) tuberculous ulceration of the stomach; (g) gastric and duodenal diverticula; (h) duodenal bands, adhesions, and duodenal tumours, including periampullary carcinoma, carcinoids, inflammatory lesions and Crohn's disease; (i) acquired hypertrophic pyloric stenosis of adults.

Factors Influencing Choice of Medical or Surgical Treatment

Age. The younger the patient and the shorter the history, the more likely are medical measures to be successful. In the

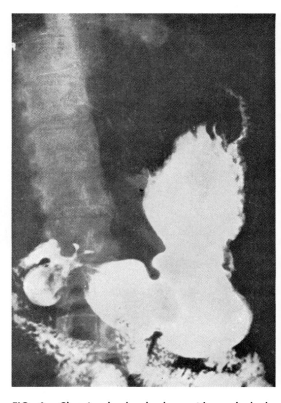

FIG. 6. Chronic duodenal ulcer with marked deformity of cap and prestenotic diverticulum.

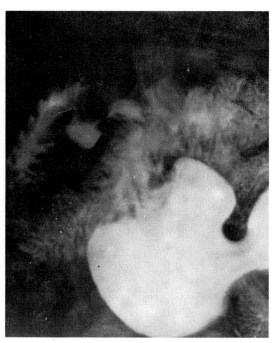

FIG. 5. Large penetrating duodenal ulcer.

absence of complications, operation should not be advised for young patients, i.e., those under 25 years of age, as in most instances the ulcer is of recent date, obstruction and anchorage are rare, and cooperation in the matter of postoperative caution is less easily ensured. It should be noted that in the young, although duodenal ulcers heal rapidly on good medical therapy, they are prone to relapse. Again, as a group, younger people are less likely to follow the details of an ulcer regimen with such enthusiasm as is witnessed in those approaching the midsummer of their lives.

Many cases of duodenal ulcer have been reported in infancy and childhood. As a rule, children do not respond as well to medical therapy as adults, and haemorrhage is a relatively common complication. Ravitch,[23] writing on this subject, reported five children who were operated upon in a 2-year period.

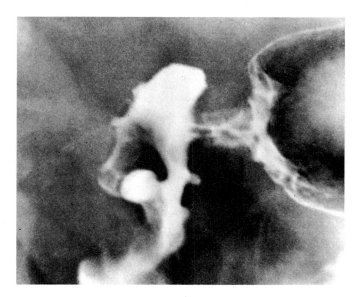

FIG. 7. Large penetrating duodenal ulcer.

All the operations were vagotomy and a drainage procedure. The immediate and late results were good. Nuss and Lynn,[20] writing on *peptic ulceration in childhood* state: "Since January 1960 peptic ulceration of the stomach or duodenum has been demonstrated at the Mayo Clinic in 78 children (15 years old or less). Three children had both gastric and duodenal ulcers, giving a total of 81 lesions. There was no significant increase in numbers between the year 1960 and the year 1970. Related to age, the incidence showed two trends: *acute ulcers* occurred most often in the first 3 years of life, while *chronic ulcers* occurred with progressively increasing frequency from age 10 onward." The majority of patients were treated by means of vagotomy and pyloroplasty, partial gastrectomy employing the Billroth II procedure, or vagotomy with antrectomy.

Operation is called for in patients suffering from duodenal ulcer in whom complications have occurred and the symptoms are undoubtedly intractable.

The best results in gastric surgery for chronic duodenal ulcer are obtained in middle-aged patients, i.e., those between 40 and 55 years of age, and such operations are, in fact, most frequently performed during this 15-year period.

Medical treatment of *elderly patients* is generally much less effective than it is for those who are younger, and this is no doubt in part due to the impaired circulation, diminished recuperative powers, and the presence of associated diseases, such as arteriosclerosis, in the former. On the other hand, surgical measures involve greater risks when undertaken in those of more advanced age. Nevertheless, in spite of this, operation, when unquestionably indicated, should be undertaken.

The mortality rate from the *complications* of peptic ulcer, particularly that from perforation or haemorrhage, markedly increases after the age of 60.

Sex. Sex does not necessarily influence the choice of treatment, although it should be noted that the mortality rate following gastric operations is lower in women than it is in men. This, at least, has been my experience with such patients. Again, stomal ulceration is more rare in women than in men after any type of gastric operation. Women patients, on the other hand, show a greater tendency to develop iron-deficiency anemia following gastric resection.

Type of patient, occupation, and economic status. The following types are all poor candidates for operation: the alcoholic, the nephritic, the drug addict, the obese, the diabetic, the asthmatic, the psychoneurotic, and the visceroptotic, as is also that group so capably classified by Goldthwaite as lean, nervous, anxious-minded individuals who live in a state of perpetual excitement. There is, as I have said, a high incidence of duodenal ulcer associated with hypersecretion, hypermotility, and hyperchlorhydria in the professional classes, whose members comprise doctors, barristers, and accountants, whose mental activities are always at key pitch, and who have to shoulder grave responsibilities. Such patients are, on the whole, unsatisfactory for either medical or surgical treatment, as their work and their habits and mode of life hinder them from paying the necessary attention to the details that are inseparable from the successful management of ulcer cases. On the other hand, the more tranquil patients—farmers and those in certain types of sedentary occupations—often show a good result from treatment whether medical or surgical.

In the medical management of ulcer cases, success may depend not so much upon the type of treatment that is instituted as upon the individuals themselves who are being treated. Cigarette-smoking, continued indulgence in alcohol, and overreating are deterrents to the success of treatment, as already emphasised.

The economic status of the patient is an important factor to be considered when deciding upon the best lines that treatment should take. Expedient circumstances have to be considered in certain cases; for instance, *operation may be needed to save a man's job rather than his life.*

In certain primitive peoples, surgery is the lesser of two evils, and the same applies to ignorant or indigent patients who lack the will or the intelligence to follow out directions to the letter. (See Chap. 12. Part D.)

General condition. Medical treatment should be adhered to for patients who suffer from chronic ill health owing to associated diseases such as phthisis, nephritis, serious cardiac lesions, chronic bronchitis, and emphysema, and operation should be undertaken only in the presence of urgent complications.

Operation, too, is contraindicated during pregnancy and the puerperium except when acute perforation or massive haemorrhage takes place.

Length of ulcer history. The shorter the duration of the disease, the better are the prospects of healing by medical measures. This point at least is undisputed. Therefore, patients giving a short history of duodenal ulcer are not good candidates for operation, and I have no faith in a surgeon who would advise surgical interference in such cases. Patients giving a long history, for example of over 10 years, during which time they have had many courses of medical treatment for a persistent recurrence of symptoms, are best operated upon if no specific contraindications are shown to exist.

There is no doubt that recurrent ulceration or repeated relapse is the prime indication for surgery.

It can be stated dogmatically that a duodenal ulcer that has been relapsing frequently for 10 years or more has next to no chance of ever becoming permanently healed by *any* medical regime, and an ulcer case seen first at this stage should, generally speaking, be offered the benefits of surgery forthwith. A trial of medical treatment at this stage is a waste of time.

Failure of medical treatment. About 65 percent of the cases treated medically relapse within 3 years, and approximately 70 percent within 5 years. The longer the duration of symptoms before medical therapy, the higher is the probability of early relapse.

Thomas Hunt [11a] considers that failure to start treatment at the earliest moment after any return of symptoms is an important point. It is unfortunately a fact that many patients who follow a strict regimen have relapses for no apparent reason, while others who are haphazard with their home treatment and who do not "deserve" a respite may remain symptom-free. About 30 to 40 percent of Hunt's patients with duodenal ulcer develop complications, such as perforation, haemorrhage, or obstruction. About 5 percent of his patients treated medically died as a direct result of ulcer.

Acidity. The significance of hyperchlorhydria is decribed in Part C of this chapter, by Ian Bouchier.

Zollinger-Ellison Syndrome. (See Chapter 13 by Zollinger, Nick, and Sanzenbacher.)

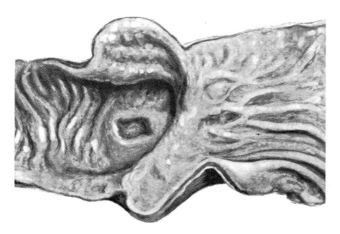

FIG. 8. Chronic penetrating duodenal ulcer. Ulcer has breached all coats of duodenal wall and is anchored to the pancreas. (Museum of the Royal College of Surgeons.)

The site and pathological characteristics of the ulcer. Anchorage denotes chronicity. When a posterior ulcer has breached all the coats of the gut and its base lies deeply embedded in the substance of the pancreas—anchorage—it is unlikely that medical measures will prove of any avail, and surgical intervention will often be required to arrest or to forestall bleeding, to prevent the onset of acute ascending cholangitis owing to perforation of the common bile duct by the ulcer—a rare but grave complication—to overcome stasis, or to rid the patient of an incorrigible and crippling pain that totally incapacitates him (Fig. 8).

Posterior ulcers often produce pyloric obstruction, and it is of the utmost importance for the clinician to distinguish between obstruction caused by scar and obstruction owing to a combination of spasm and oedema. Obstruction by scarring is a long-standing affair; when there is organic obstruction, the dilated, baggy, atonic stomach becomes a receptacle for decomposing, fermenting food, and inert gastric juice, which are voided in enormous quantities towards the close of the day. In such cases, the gastric glands become atrophic and secrete little or no hydrochloric acid. On the other hand, obstruction owing to oedema around a duodenal ulcer is of more sudden onset and is accompanied by severe pain and copious vomiting. The latter patients often respond promptly to medical treatment, but relapse is a common event. Pyloric obstruction caused by a stenosing duodenal ulcer is one of the paramount indications for operative intervention. The wider and deeper an ulcer, the slower it will be in healing and the less likely to heal staunchly. The greater the size of the ulcer, the greater is the risk of acute perforation or haemorrhage.

Prestenotic diverticula of the first part of the duodenum are commonly observed on x-ray examination and at operation. Their presence indicates that the ulcer is *old,* or at least unrelenting, and associated with much scar tissue. (See Fig. 6.)

Indications for Operation for Duodenal Ulcers

Surgical intervention is recommended when the following situations obtain:

1. Acute perforation.
2. Intermittent or continuous haemorrhage arising from the base of a chronic duodenal ulcer that medical therapy is incapable of controlling.
3. Organic stenosis caused by a cicatrising duodenal ulcer.
4. Repeated failure of adequate medical treatment—intractability.
5. Chronic duodenal ulcer associated with chronic gastric ulcer (combined ulcers).
6. Chronic duodenal ulcer associated with chronic arteriomesenteric ileus.
7. Recurrence of ulceration following simple suture of an acute perforation.
8. Postbulbar duodenal ulcer, i.e., ulcer situ-

ated in the second portion of the duodenum above or below the ampulla of Vater, as haemorrhage and obstruction are common complications.

9. Choledochoduodenal fistula.
10. Expedient circumstances and economic reasons *in certain cases*.

Contraindications to Operation

The following groups of patients who have chronic duodenal ulcer should, as a rule, receive medical treatment:

1. All those who have *uncomplicated ulcers,* especially if they have been present for only a short time.
2. Patients under 25 years of age, unless their lesions are complicated.
3. Older patients whose symptoms are mild, the intervals between the attacks are long, and efficiency is not impaired.
4. Any patient whose ulcer is complicated by some medical condition that would render operation hazardous.
5. Psychoneurotic patients who have hyper-irritable gastrointestinal tracts and whose ulcers are not complicated by repeated haemorrhage or pyloric obstruction.

Operations for Duodenal Ulcer

The various operations performed today for chronic duodenal ulcer are as follows:

A. *Vagotomy with a drainage operation*
   1. Pyloroplasty (Chap. 17).
   2. Gastrojejunostomy (Chap. 19).
   3. Finney's gastroduodenostomy (Chap. 18).
   4. Jaboulay's gastroduodenostomy (Chap. 18).
B. Vagotomy with Antrectomy *(or hemigas-*trectomy) followed by
   1. *End-to-end* gastroduodenostomy Billroth I operation (Chaps. 16 and 20).
   2. *End-to-side* gastroduodenostomy.
   3. The Billroth II operation (Chap. 21).
C. *The Schoemaker-Billroth II operation* (Chap. 21).
D. *Operations for the acute complications of duodenal ulcer*
   1. Perforation (Chap. 22).
   2. Haemorrhage (Chap. 23);
   3. Operations for pyloric obstruction; fistula, etc.
E. *Chronic duodenal ulcers associated with ulcerogenic tumours of the Pancreas* (Chap. 13).

F. *Proximal selective vagotomy or parietal ce*[ll] *vagotomy.*

The choice of operation is fully and abl[y] discussed by Judd,[16] Dragstedt (Chap. 14), Mann (Chap. 11), Griffith (Chap. 15), and b[y] Wirthlin and Malt.[35]

GASTRIC ULCER

Avery Jones,[14] in a personal communi[-] cation, writes:

. . . peptic ulcer becomes more frequent as ag[e] advances and, in England, is found in nearly 1[0] per cent of men aged 45–54 years. In lif[e] duodenal ulcer is found four or more times mor[e] often than gastric ulcer under the age of 35 year[s], but after 45 years it is only one or two times a[s] common. Gastric ulcers are two to three time[s] commoner in men than in women, and duodena[l] ulcers are six to 12 times more common, at lea[st] at all ages between 25 and 65 years. At autops[y] the ratio of males to females is 1:1.

It should be noted, however, that whils[t] the incidence of peptic ulcer in patients o[f] the younger age group has declined in recen[t] years, the incidence of acute perforation an[d] severe haemorrhage has significantly i[n]creased.

Pathology

Gastric ulcers may be acute or chronic[.] Approximately 85 percent of chronic gastri[c] ulcers are found on or near the lesser curva[-] ture, the great majority of these being close[r] to the incisura angularis than to the cardia[c] orifice; 12 percent are in the antrum, and o[f] these less than 2 percent are situated in th[e] pyloric canal itself. Whereas 15 percent o[f] cancers arise in the cardia, less than 3 percen[t] of gastric ulcers are found in this region. I[n] the rest of the body of the stomach—i.e., th[e] fundus, the anterior and posterior walls o[f] the body, and along the greater curvature— the incidence of simple ulcer is slight, pos[-] sibly not more than 5 percent. It is rare t[o] find two or more chronic gastric ulcers i[n] a state of activity at the same time (2 pe[r] cent), but combined ulcers, i.e., *a gastri[c] ulcer associated with a duodenal ulcer,* ar[e] encountered in over 5 percent of cases.

Gastric ulcers appear to the naked eye t[o] be similar to duodenal ulcers except tha[t]

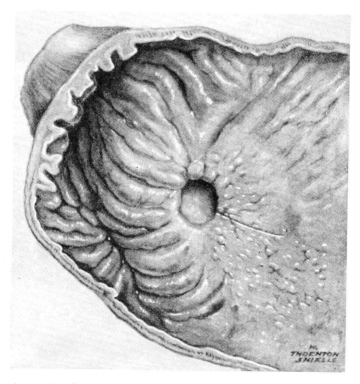

FIG. 9. Chronic gastric ulcer. Gastrectomy specimen. Biopsy proved the ulcer to be benign.

ulcers in the stomach are larger, tend to penetrate more deeply, and are associated with a greater degree of fibrosis.

Gastric ulcers average 1.6 to 1.9 cm in diameter. In the individual cases, the large size of a gastric ulcer is no proof of cancer, since benign ulcers may reach 10 cm or more in diameter, as Cabot[4] has emphasised. The importance of the size of gastric ulcers has perhaps been exaggerated by surgeons.

Small, shallow, flat lesions are easily overlooked at exploratory laparotomy, and in order to locate them it is necessary to mobilise the greater curvature of the stomach; to palpate the whole length of the lesser curvature methodically; to search for inflamed lymph nodes, which are always present; and to examine the pyloric region and cardia with scrupulous care.

The surgeon should also bear in mind the possibility of (1) dual lesions in the stomach, and that when two are present one ulcer may be malignant and the other simple; (2) combined ulcers; and (3) accompanying lesions such as hiatal hernia, calculous cholecystitis, diverticulosis of the sigmoid loop, chronic appendicitis, and so forth.

Marshall et al.[19] found that out of 708 *apparently* innocent gastric ulcer cases treated at the Lahey Clinic, 13.2 percent proved to be malignant. They found no significant difference between the malignant and innocent cases in respect of the patients' age, sex, or length of history. They found their diagnostic error rate to be diminishing with newer diagnostic methods. Clagett[5] writes: "In the past it was generally recognised and accepted that approximately 10 percent of the lesions that appeared to be benign gastric ulcers on radiologic and gastroscopic examination would actually be ulcerating carcinomas. This fact encouraged and supported a policy of early surgical intervention." Today, employing the routine and more recent sophisticated refinements in the techniques of investigating ulcerated lesions in the stomach, I would hazard a guess that the true incidence of carcinoma develop-

CARCINOMA

DUODENUM

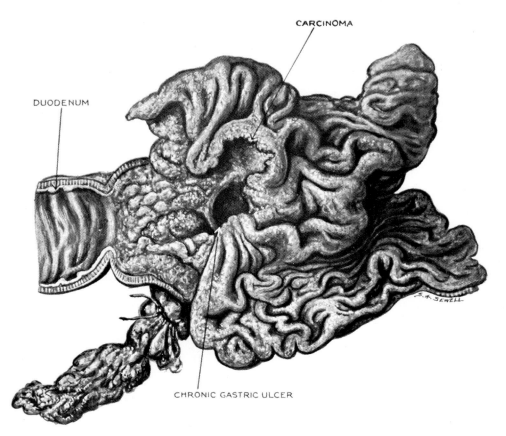

CHRONIC GASTRIC ULCER

FIG. 10.   Carcinoma of pyloric end of stomach involving chiefly the lesser curvature and posterior
wall. Chronic gastric ulcer was found in the proximal portion of the ulcerated zone.

ing in a benign gastric ulcer is about 3 percent, and that the margin of error in differentiating a simple gastric ulcer from an
ulcerating carcinoma is approximately 8 percent (Figs. 9 and 10).

The Clinical Picture

In most cases of gastric ulcer, the
symptoms and *physical signs* are in many respects similar to those found in nonstenosing
duodenal ulcer. As in duodenal ulcer, the
most important symptoms are *pain, vomiting,* and *bleeding.* The pain at first is insidious and slight, amounting to little more than
a sensation of discomfort and fullness in the
epigastrium; but in a well-established case it
becomes severe in character and arises shortly
after the intake of food. The situation of the
ulcer and the onset of certain complications

will cause marked variations in the nature of
the symptoms. For instance, when an ulcer is
situated high up on the lesser curvature near
the cardia, pain will be experienced during
meals or shortly afterwards while, when the
pyloric segment is involved, pain may not
arise for 2 or 3 hours after the ingestion of
food. Pyloric ulcers simulate duodenal ulcers
in that the onset of pain is delayed and food
often affords a measure of relief. On the
other hand, they cause great impairment of
gastric motility and marked spasm of the
pylorus, leading to occasional attacks of
vomiting, nausea, and flatulence, with a
considerable number of visceral disturbances
that demand immediate attention, early investigation, and possibly operation.

Ulcers of the middle third of the lesser
curvature produce symptoms that in some
ways resemble those of duodenal ulcer, but

the pain arises ½ to 1 hour after food intake and slowly disappears before the next meal. Food and alkalis, however, do not alleviate the pain as completely as they do in duodenal ulcer, but belching and vomiting afford instantaneous relief. Small feedings may give relief, but large feedings often cause distress. Patients learn that by taking tablets of malted milk and the like shortly before the pain is due they can almost certainly forestall its onset or mitigate its severity.

Patients with gastric ulcer rarely experience pain during the night, and seldom on an empty stomach in the morning before breakfast. The attacks of pain last a variable time—an hour or two, sometimes less, sometimes more; but when complications ensue, the pain may be continuous and exhausting. The pain radiates to the back or to the left shoulder when the ulcer has penetrated the capsule of the pancreas, the liver, or the crura of the diaphragm. *Backache is therefore a symptom of the greatest importance, denoting anchorage.*

In a typical case, the patient will give a history of recurrent attacks of dyspeptic pain, each lasting for a few days, weeks, or possibly months, with intervals of freedom for a variable period; but as the disease progresses, these remissions become shorter and shorter, pain becomes more intense and incoercible, and the well-tried anodynes are no longer dependable. Vomiting is now more troublesome, and is frequently self-induced. In cases of gastric ulcer, appetite and nutrition are usually good except where the disease has been of long-standing, in which case, owing to the fear of the pain that will follow the intake of food, enforced abstinence often results in loss of weight and a severe degree of malnutrition. With the onset of pyloric obstruction, of hourglass stomach, or of deep penetration of the ulcer, loss of weight may be very marked and the symptom complex becomes irregular, suggesting at times that a primary cancer in the stomach is rapidly advancing. Some patients, especially those in the elderly group, may not complain of pain; and acute perforation or massive bleeding may be the first manifestation of the disease.

On *physical examination* there is often a point of maximum tenderness to be found in the epigastrium, close to the costal margin on the left side, or in the midline below the xiphisternum. Guarding will be marked at the height of the ulcerative activity, but this will be absent when the ulcer is quiescent.

Diagnosis

With our present methods of diagnosis —and these include history of the case, physical examination of the patient, analysis of the gastric contents, exfoliative cytology, complete examination of the blood, occult blood tests, barium-meal x-ray investigations, endoscopic enquiry, and gastrophotography—it is not difficult to arrive at a diagnosis of simple ulcer or ulcerating carcinoma; but to distinguish these two conditions and to divide cases into two groups is on occasion difficult and presents an important problem.

Rivers and Dry [24] suggested that a patient who had a gastric ulcer should be *suspected* of harbouring a malignant lesion if:

1. He is over 60 years of age and gives a brief history of indigestion.
2. The symptoms are of short duration and have persisted *without remission*.
3. There is no relief of symptoms following careful medical treatment, and in addition to this the ulcer crater has not diminished in size after 2 weeks' probationary supervision.
4. Occult blood continues to appear in the stools.
5. The ulcer is situated in the pyloric region, on the anterior or posterior wall of the stomach some distance from the curvatures, or at or near the greater curvature.
6. Gastric analysis shows absence of free hydrochloric acid.

On the other hand, the following criteria would suggest that the lesion is benign:

1. The patient is young or middle-aged.
2. There are long periods during which the ulcer is quiescent.
3. Gastric acidity is normal or high.
4. Symptoms completely disappear under medical treatment, bleeding ceases, pain abates, and the x-ray studies reveal that the breach in the stomach has healed over.

In the differential diagnosis between simple ulcer and ulcerating cancer, some importance is attached to the therapeutic test, although I must emphasise that no preoperative tests or the application of any criteria such as have been enumerated above can be deemed entirely trustworthy. It is significant that a few patients with ulcerating cancers temporarily gain weight, lose all their symptoms, and appear to be progressing satisfactorily while undergoing medical therapy.

Indications for Operation for Gastric Ulcer

The main indications for operative interference may be detailed as follows:

1. Acute perforation (see Chap. 22).
2. Haemorrhage from the base of a chronic ulcer or from multiple acute erosions which threaten the life of the patient. Such bleeding may be continuous or intermittent; or again it may be moderate or massive in degree (see Chap. 23).
3. Anatomical organic deformity of the stomach owing to stenosing ulceration and associated with progressive loss of weight: (a) hourglass stomach; and (b) pyloric obstruction.
4. Failure of the ulcer to heal despite prolonged (e.g., 3 weeks) and well-supervised inpatient medical treatment.
5. Recurrence of ulceration associated with intractable symptoms following: (a) one or more courses of inpatient medical treatment; (b) simple suture of an acute perforation; (c) some inadequate operation such as sleeve resection.
6. Multiple chronic gastric ulcers or *combined* gastric and duodenal ulcer.
7. The suspicion of malignancy that cannot be excluded by combined clinical, biochemical, radiological, cytological, and gastroscopic examination.
8. The patient is 60 years of age or over, having an ulcerating lesion in the stomach and giving a short history of dyspepsia.
9. The ulcer is situated in one of the "danger zones" of the stomach, namely, the pyloric segment, on the greater curvature, high up towards the cardia, or on the anterior or posterior wall of the body of the stomach *some distance away from either curvature.*
10. Large flat ulcers.
11. A gastric ulcer that has penetrated into the substance of the pancreas or liver or some adjacent viscus—anchorage. (Fig. 20.)
12. Expedient circumstances and economic reasons in certain instances, e.g., indigent or mental patients with callous lesions.

Factors Influencing Management

Every patient is subjected to the same routine methods of investigation as already outlined, and if the presence of an ulcer in the stomach has been demonstrated by means of x-rays and gastroscopy, the physician and surgeon should meet in consultation and decide what lines the treatment should take.

The following factors will influence the choice of treatment:

Age.   The patient who is over the age of 60 and gives a short history of indigestion is a candidate for radical surgery. If hypoacidity or anacidity is also present and occult blood is found in the stools, a diagnosis of ulcerating carcinoma should be strongly entertained. Again, operation should be advised in elderly ulcer patients who, in addition to giving a *short* history of indigestion, have *constant* epigastric pain that is unrelieved by bed rest and anodynes. Young patients who have a small ulcer in the region of the incisura may well be given a course or two of medical treatment to see how they respond.

Position of the ulcer.   When the ulcer is situated in one of the "danger zones" of the stomach—the pyloric canal and the antrum, on the greater curvature, high up towards the cardia, or on the anterior or posterior wall of the body of the stomach some distance away from either curvature— partial gastrectomy should be strongly recommended, as the incidence of carcinoma is high when the ulcer occurs in these zones (Figs. 11, 12 and 13).

An ulcer or ulcers occupying any portion of the greater curvature demand subtotal gastrectomy, as some 40 percent of them are cancerous in nature. I have now performed gastrectomy for eight chronic ulcers of the greater curvature of the stomach, and of these, four were benign and four were malignant (Fig. 12).

Presence of multiple ulcers as well as combination of gastric and duodenal ulcer. It is agreed that such combined lesions, when found, are sufficient to warrant surgical measures. I once performed gastric excision upon a patient who had two chronic ulcers in the stomach, one being situated on the lesser curvature about the incisura, and the other directly opposite to it on the greater curvature. The lesser curve ulcer was innocent, but on the greater curve was an ulcerating carcinoma. Multiple chronic ulcers are seen in about 2 to 3 percent of resected stomachs.

Combined ulcers call for surgical measures

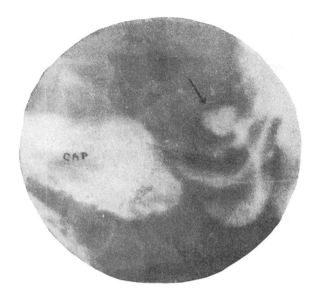

FIG. 11.   Benign prepyloric ulcer.

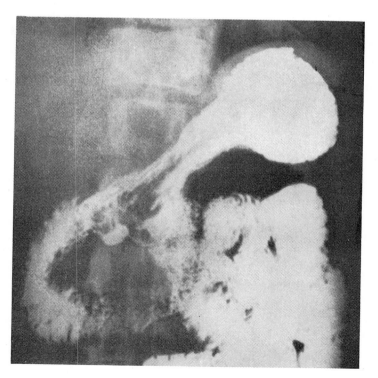

FIG. 12.   Gastric ulcer on the greater curvature of stomach. Partial gastrectomy was performed and the ulcer proved to be benign. (Author's patient.)

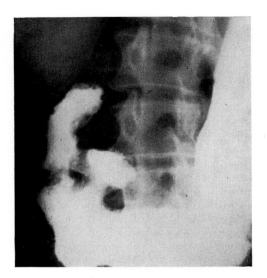

FIG. 13.   Large pyloric ulcer.

as soon as the diagnosis is made, as complications of perforation, haemorrhage, and obstruction are all frequent.

It is interesting to note that with these combined ulcers the duodenal ulcer is almost invariably the primary lesion, the gastric ulcer arising later on when pyloric obstruction has supervened and has led to stasis in the gastric pouch.

The duodenal ulcer retrogresses but leaves a considerable degree of scarring and deformity of the cap, while the gastric ulcer progresses apace and may even attain giant status.

Size of the ulcer.   Scott and Mider [25] wrote:

It was hoped at one time that the size of the ulcer as revealed roentgenologically might be a good index of its character. It is true that many ulcers over 2.5 cm in diameter are malignant, while most of the smaller ulcers (1 to 1.5 cm in diameter) prove to be benign. However, there are so many exceptions to this general rule that it is almost valueless as a guide to therapy in the individual case.

The *size of the ulcer* has often been said to provide a highly significant indication of its nature; the larger the crater the more likely it is to be carcinomatous. This view can no longer be supported, as 50 percent of malignant ulcers are less than 4 cm in size, while

over 10 percent of benign ulcers are larger than this. Fully 20 percent of *small* ulcers are malignant, consequently a small crater offers no guarantee of nonmalignancy.[18]

Personal experience supports the view that many of the so-called *giant gastric ulcers* which, as it were, sprout from the stomach by a narrow stalk, expanding into a bulbous dome, are benign in character. This subject is ably discussed by Strange,[27] who reported a personal series of 73 giant innocent gastric ulcers, the majority of which measured at least 3 cm or more in diameter. There were 47 males and 26 females, giving a ratio of 1.8 to 1. Twenty-five of the patients had severe haemorrhage. During the period in which the 73 cases of giant gastric ulcer presented for treatment, only two giant malignant ulcers of the lesser curve were seen.

Although there is a definite correlation between the size of an ulcer and the likelihood of its being malignant, size alone, no matter how suggestive, is not an absolute criterion of malignancy in the individual case. However, since the incidence of benignancy

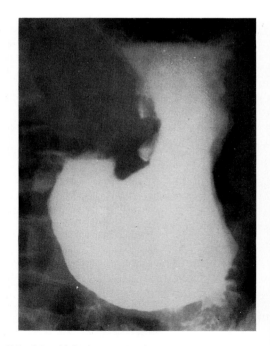

FIG. 14.   Multiple gastric ulcers. Patient was a man, aged 82, with a history of chronic indigestion for over 30 years. Partial gastrectomy was performed and the patient made a good recovery. Microscopical examination proved the ulcers were benign.

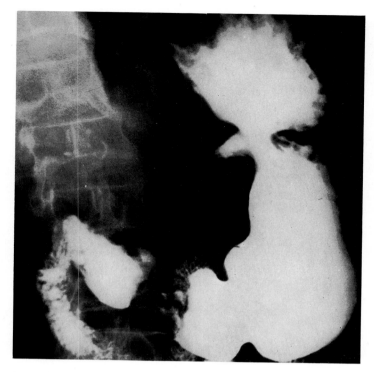

FIG. 15. Radiograph of large chronic penetrating gastric ulcer, with marked spasm of the greater curvature. Partial gastrectomy was performed. The ulcer, which was with difficulty detached fom the pancreas, showed no evidence of malignant degeneration.

among gastric lesions whose longest diameter measures 4.0 cm or more is so low, immediate surgical therapy is advisable. (Figs. 14 to 21.)

Cohn and Sartin [6] wrote:

The theory that a large or giant gastric ulcer is almost certain to be carcinomatous is not supported by our studies, for even the largest ulcers have only a 25 per cent incidence of malignancy in our series.

A review of the literature discloses 613 giant gastric ulcers, 71 percent of which were benign.

Hourglass Deformity

Hourglass deformity may be classified under the following causes:

1. *Intrinsic causes.* These are caused by intrinsic ulcerative processes and include:
   a. Chronic gastric ulcer (over 90 percent.
   b. Gastric cancer.
   c. Gastric syphilis.
   d. Large stomal ulcer, and
   e. Stenosis resulting from corrosive poisoning.
2. *Extrinsic causes.*
   a. Perigastric adhesions.
   b. Pressure from an adherent colon distended with gas, and
   c. Spasmodic hourglass contraction owing to reflex causes.

It is doubtful whether bilocular stomach is ever a congenital condition. This complication is seen in 8 percent of all cases of chronic gastric ulcer occurring in women. The condition is rarely observed in men—in probably 1 percent of all cases of gastric ulcer. The development of hourglass stomach depends upon the size, the position, the form, and the chronicity of the ulcer, the so-called saddle-shaped ulcer of the body of the stomach often being a common precursor (Figs. 22 and 23).

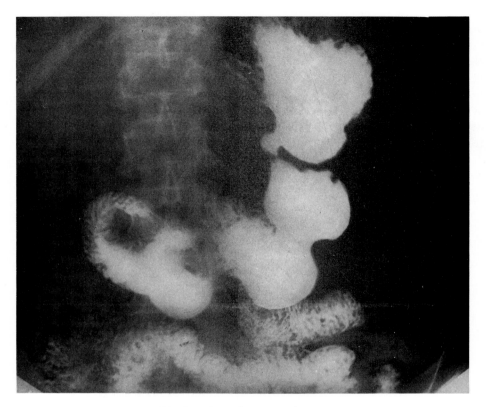

FIG. 16.   Hourglass stomach.

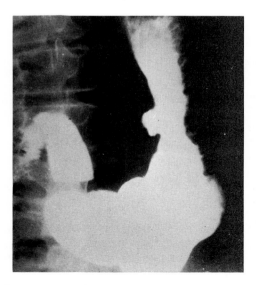

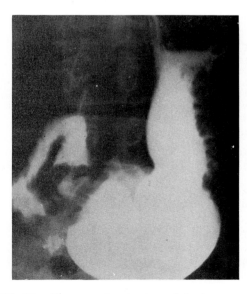

FIG. 17.   Large chronic ulcer of the lesser curvature before milk-drip treatment.

FIG. 18.   The same chronic ulcer of the lesser curvature shown in Figure 17 one month later (after continuous milk-drip treatment) the ulcer has healed.

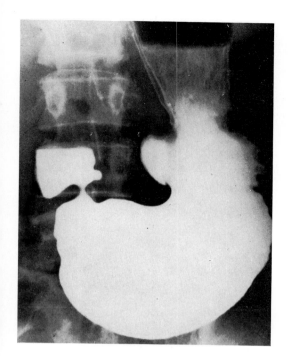

FIG. 19. Large gastric ulcer. Gastrectomy was performed. The ulcer proved to be simple in character.

The complication is nearly always single and is often situated in the region of the incisura, i.e., nearer the pyloric than the cardiac end of the stomach, which is frequently J-shaped. The isthmus is narrow, an ulcer crater may or may not be visible, and the cardiac loculus—which is usually much larger than the pyloric pouch—overhangs and sags across the dilated vestibule. Pyloric obstruction caused by duodenal ulcer is found in 25 percent of cases of hourglass stomach, and when these two complications coexist, the distal pouch may be greatly distended while the proximal pouch may be small. *At operation, in 50 percent of cases the ulcer causing the constriction is healed.* The position and calibre of the isthmus will determine the severity of the symptoms. Perforation and haemorrhage are relatively rare complications.

It is exceptional to find malignant change associated with hourglass deformity of the stomach owing to peptic ulceration. It is conceivable that medical treatment, or, rather, stringent dietetic measures may keep the patient in a moderate state of nutrition when the ulcer, on healing, has left a small but adequate channel for food. But such patients are chronic invalids, and sooner or later operative measures, usually in the form of partial gastrectomy, will be necessary to overcome the effects of obstruction. I would regard hourglass deformity as a definite indication for operative interference at any age.

A series of cases successfully treated by gastrogastrostomy has been reported in the past. In my experience, gastrogastrostomy is doomed to failure if at the time of operation the crater of a chronic gastric ulcer is encountered. Where, however, in elderly, undernourished patients healing is complete and the constriction is situated *high up* in the stomach, this operation offers considerable palliation. As these patients with hourglass constriction withstand resection followed by one of the Billroth procedures very well, this operation should be carried out whenever the local and general conditions permit.

Response to Medical Treatment

It should be remembered that complete disappearance of symptoms with a gain in weight when the patient is subjected to medical treatment is no evidence whatsoever that the ulcer is benign in character; in fact, a cancerous gastric lesion will at times respond in this manner when it presents irrefutable x-ray evidence of its malignancy.

Medical treatment should be persevered with when it has afforded prompt relief of symptoms, when blood disappears from the stools, and when x-ray studies show that there is a progressive decrease in the size of the ulcer crater. But frequent periodical x-ray examinations are necessary to ensure that healing, once established, remains permanent. A return of symptoms while the patient is undergoing medical treatment or failure of the ulcer to decrease appreciably in size immediately suggests to the examiner that the lesion is either a *callous* benign ulcer or a carcinoma and will therefore call for gastric resection after a preliminary course of preoperative treatment. Recurrence spells operation. Clagett[5] puts it this way: "At present, if all diagnostic tests indicate that an ulcerating gastric lesion is benign, a

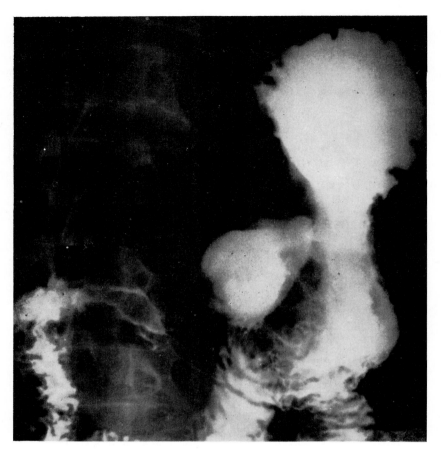

FIG. 20.   Giant gastric ulcer. Note that the ulcer is pear-shaped with a stalk arising from the lesser curvature of the stomach. Partial gastrectomy was carried out successfully. The ulcer proved to be benign.

2-week trial of rigid medical management seems reasonable. And if roentgenologic examination shows the crater is 50 percent smaller at the end of 2 weeks, medical treatment and observation may be continued. Failure to obtain such a response warrants surgical intervention without further delay. Medical treatment of gastric ulcers in general leaves much to be desired." Lasting good results are obtained in only 20 to 25 percent of cases following strict medical therapy. (See Chap. 12. Part D.)

Approximately 8 percent of apparently simple gastric ulcers that are diagnosed by clinical methods, barium-meal x-ray examination, gastroscopy, and cytological studies of gastric material eventually prove to be ulcerating carcinomas. Some authorities place the incidence higher than this.

Tanner [30] states that *gastroscopy* is the most reliable means of differentiation between simple ulcer and carcinoma. He writes:

It is frequently quoted in the North American literature that some 10 percent of ulcers resected in the belief that they are innocent, are, in fact, malignant. With the aid of preoperative gastroscopy we find well under 2 percent of such resected ulcers to be malignant on histological or follow-up investigations. It is reported that an ulcerating carcinoma may appear to heal for a time on x-ray examination. In a series of between 1,000 and 2,000 gastroscopic examinations of gastric ulcers, I have never found a gastric ulcer apparently heal and later turn out to be malignant. Therefore I place considerable value on

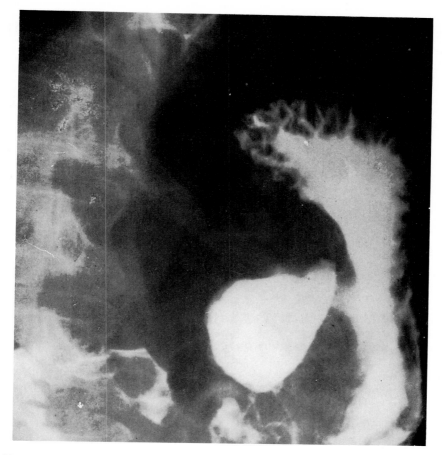

FIG. 21.   Giant gastric ulcer. Note the similarity to the ulcer shown in Figure 20. On subsequent microscopical examination, it proved to be a simple gastric ulcer. The patient made an excellent recovery following Billroth II partial gastrectomy.

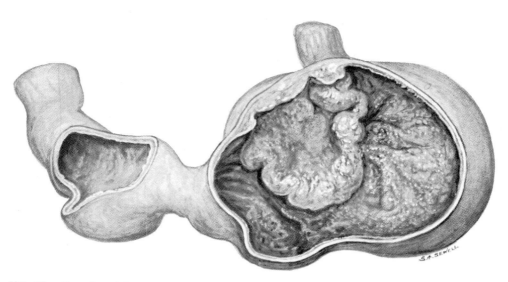

FIG. 22.   Hourglass deformity of the stomach caused by a long-standing gastric ulcer. Ulcerating carcinoma is located in the proximal gastric pouch. (Museum of the Royal College of Surgeons.)

preoperative visualisation of a gastric ulcer. In cases of doubt at laparotomy, I have usually found it safe to trust my preoperative gastroscopic diagnosis. The disadvantage of gastroscopy is the need for very extensive training and an experience of many hundreds of examinations before one is able to interpret the findings.

As has already been mentioned, approximately 70 percent of patients with chronic gastric ulcer investigated by the writer eventually required partial gastrectomy.

Choice of Operation for Gastric Ulcer

In order of preference, the choice of operation may be listed as follows:

1. Schoemaker-Billroth I operation. The ulcer is excised together with 50 percent (hemigastrectomy) or to 65 to 70 percent (partial gastrectomy) of the stomach and a portion of the first part of the duodenum.

2. Schoemaker-Billroth II procedure: antecolic; short jejunal loop used in the anastomosis. This operation is especially indicated in cases of *combined ulcers.*

3. Panchet's operation, for high lesser curve cardial ulcers (Chaps. 20 and 21).

4. Kelling-Madlener operation for paracardial ulcers (Chap. 21).

5. Four-quarter biopsy of high lesser curve ulcers (which are too large or too difficult to resect) followed by vagotomy and a drainage operation.

6. Excision-biopsy of a gastric ulcer combined with vagotomy and pyloroplasty or gastrojejunostomy.

7. Selective proximal vagotomy (Chaps. 11 and 15).

8. Proximal selective vagotomy.

At the present time, it is generally agreed that the Schoemaker-Billroth I operation is the procedure of choice, as the mortality rate is low—below 0.5 percent; the recurrent ulcer

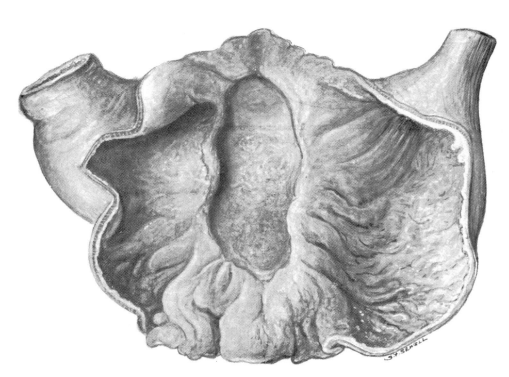

FIG. 23. Hourglass deformity of the stomach caused by a so-called saddle-shaped ulcer of the body of the stomach. (Museum of the Royal College of Surgeons.)

rate is less than 0.5 percent; and the late results are excellent in fully 95 percent of the cases.

Tanner[30] reported only two recurrences after 1,000 Billroth resections for chronic gastric ulcer.

Harkins and his associates,[10] after 140 resections, found only one recurrence.

Daintree Johnson[12] had no recurrence in 140 patients who had undergone Billroth II resection.

In my series of over 300 patients who underwent Billroth I or Billroth II operations for gastric ulcer, there were no instances of recurrent ulceration.

The Billroth I operation for gastric ulcer is one of the best operations in abdominal surgery.

REFERENCES

1. Aagaard et al., Lancet 1:1111, 1959.
2. Anthanassiades and Charalambopoupoulou, Am. J. Surg. 120:381, 1970.
3. Brulé et al., Arch. Mal. Appar. Dig. 29:846, 1936.
4. Cabot, New Engl. J. Med. 235:171, 1946.
5. Clagett, Surg. Clin. N. Am. 51:901, 1971.
6. Cohn and Sartin, Ann. Surg. 147:749, 1958.
7. Comfort et al., Surg. Gynec. Obstet. 105:455, 1957.
8. Cooke and Hutton, Lancet 1:754, 1958.
9. Crymble, Br. J. Surg. 32:500, 1945.
10. Harkins et al., Ann. Surg. 140:405, 1954.
11. Hartman and Rivers, Arch. Int. Med. 44:314, 1929.
11a. Hunt, personal communication, 1972.
12. Johnson, D., Lancet 1:298, 1950.
13. Johnson, D., Gastroenterology 33:121, 1957.
14. Avery Jones, F., Lond. Clin. Med. J. 2:13, 1970.
15. Avery Jones, F., Personal communication, 1972.
16. Judd, Surg. Clin. N. Am. 51:843, 1971.
17. Larimore, Surg. Gynec. Obstet. 50:59, 1930.
18. Lumsden, Gastroenterology 76:89, 1950.
19. Marshall et al., Am. J. Surg. 101:273, 1961.
19a. Moynihan, Lancet 2:1662, 1901.
19b. Moynihan, Br. Med. J. 1:1092, 1908.
20. Nuss and Lynn, Surg. Clin. N. Amer. 51:945, 1971.
21. Orr, Ann. Roy. Coll. Surg. Eng. 34:314, 1964.
22. Portis and Jaffe, J.A.M.A. 110:6, 1938.
23. Ravitch, Ann. Surg. 171:641, 1970.
24. Rivers and Dry, Arch. Surg. 30:702, 1935.
25. Scott and Mider, Am. J. Surg. 40:42, 1938.
26. Shanks and Kerley, A Textbook of X-ray Diagnosis, 4th ed., Parts IV and V, 1970.
27. Strange, Br. Med. J. 1:476, 1959.
28. Tanner, Bristol Medicochir. J. 43:16, 1946.
29. Tanner, Ann. Roy. Coll. Surg. Engl. 10:45, 1952.
30. Tanner, Postgrad Med. J. 30:448, 1954.
31. Tanner, Br. J. Surg. 51:5, 1964.
32. Truelove and Reynell, Diseases of the Digestive System, 2d ed., 1971.
33. Wilkie, Lancet 2:1228, 1927.
34. Wilkie, Br. Med. J. 1:771, 1933.
35. Wirthlin and Malt. Surg. Gynec. Obstet. 135:256, 1972.

B. PYLORIC AND PREPYLORIC MUCOSAL STENOSIS: MUCOSAL DIAPHRAGM

SAMUEL L. STRANGE

In pyloric and prepyloric mucosal stenosis, there is a diaphragm (consisting of a double layer of mucosa with intervening submucosa) present at the pylorus or less commonly in the prepyloric region, and there is an opening in the diaphragm that may be as small as 2 mm in diameter (Fig. 24); it may be eccentrically placed. Sometimes there is superficial ulceration of the margin of the opening, or its previous occurrence may be deduced from the presence of submucosal fibrosis on histological examination. In prepyloric mucosal stenosis, the diaphragm is usually situated 1 to 3 cm proximal to the pylorus, which is normal (Fig. 25). A gastric ulcer is present in about half of the cases of pyloric mucosal stenosis and is probably secondary to the stenosis (Fig. 26). Hypertrophy of the pyloric muscle is sometimes associated with pyloric mucosal stenosis.[1]

INCIDENCE

Pyloric mucosal stenosis is not a rare condition, but an awareness of its existence is necessary for it to be discovered. Prepyloric mucosal stenosis occurs much less frequently than does the pyloric type. In a total of more than 40 cases of mucosal stenosis, Rhind[2]

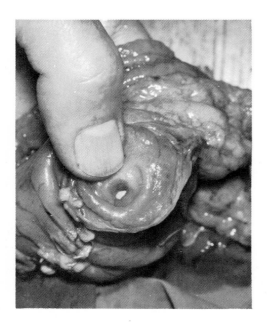

FIG. 24. Pyloric mucosal stenosis viewed from the duodenal aspect. (Aperture, 4 mm in diameter.)

had five that were prepyloric, and the writer has had three out of a series of 34 cases. The sex incidence appears to show a female preponderance. Most of the adult cases present in the sixth and seventh decades, but the condition can occur at all ages. I had a female patient of 91 who required emergency surgery for haemorrhage from a gastric ulcer; she was found to have a pyloric mucosal stenosis with an aperture 6 mm in diameter.

AETIOLOGY

There are two views concerning the cause of pyloric mucosal stenosis: first, that the mucosal diaphragms are congenital in origin, and second that they are the result of the healing of linear annular ulcers, which produce scarring and contraction.[3] This latter view, that peptic ulceration may be responsible, is supported by the presence in some cases of superficial ulceration or of

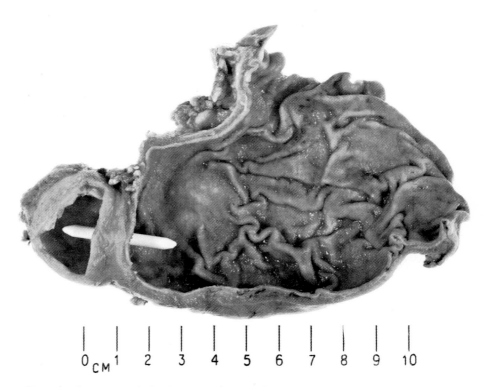

FIG. 25. Prepyloric mucosal diaphragm with a marker in the 5-mm diameter aperture. (From Tanner, Proc. R. Soc. Med. 60:1, 1967.)

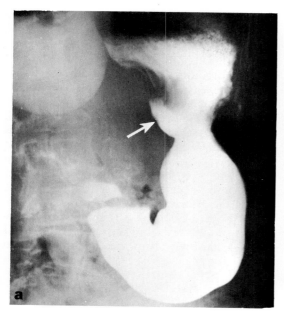

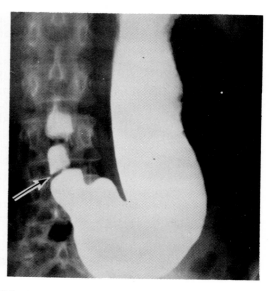

FIG. 27. Radiographic demonstration of prepyloric mucosal diaphragm (arrow) that gives the appearance of two duodenal caps. Partial gastrectomy specimen is shown in Figure 25. (From Tanner, Proc. R. Soc. Med. 60:1, 1967.)

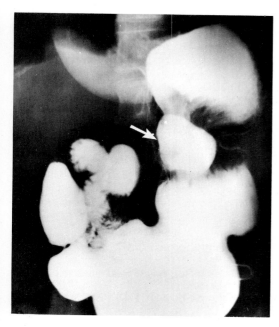

FIG. 26. Radiograms, erect (A) and supine (B), of a giant gastric ulcer 8 cm in diameter, which was associated with a pyloric mucosal diaphragm. (Aperture in the diaphragm was 7 mm in diameter.)

submucosal fibrosis at the margin of the aperture in the diaphragm, and also by the fact that the aperture may be eccentric. In addition, there is some difficulty in understanding why a congenital condition should sometimes commence to give trouble late in adult life. On the other hand, cases of pyloric and prepyloric mucosal stenosis have been found in infants in the first weeks of life, as have cases of imperforate pyloric and prepyloric mucosal diaphragms.[4] Many diaphragms in adults have no evidence of present or past ulcerations, and it is possible that trauma from food could produce superficial ulceration in a congenital diaphragm and perhaps in due course diminish the size of the aperture. Whatever may be the explanation, symptoms often do not commence until after middle age, and there appears to be a parallel with the late onset of symptoms in some cases of the congenital duodenal mucosal diaphragm with a small aperture.

CLINICAL PICTURE

Patients with pyloric mucosal stenosis may give a history of trouble extending from months to many years. One 72-year-old woman had experienced intermittent vomiting from at least the age of 5. The condition may present in one of three ways: with a gastric ulcer, with frank pyloric stenosis, or with symptoms of mild pyloric obstructions. The pain of gastric ulcer may be associated with vomiting of food. In spite of a small aperture in the diaphragm, it is uncommon for patients to present with obvious pyloric stenosis with large "vomits" containing food and a succussion splash present on abdominal examination. More frequently they present with milder symptoms of pyloric obstruction. There may be epigastric discomfort after meals, with occasional vomiting of small amounts of food or even of bile. Discomfort is most marked after large meals and after intake of solid foods; such discomfort is relieved by vomiting, which may be self-induced. As symptoms become more marked, some patients discover that they are more comfortable on a semisolid diet; they may cease eating meat, vegetables, and fruit. Loss of weight may occur. Occasionally vomiting may be completely absent but nausea and heartburn may be troublesome.

DIAGNOSIS

In pyloric mucosal stenosis a barium-meal examination may not show very much abnormality in the absence of a gastric ulcer. The stomach may be somewhat dilated, with evdience of residual fluid, but there may be little or no delay in emptying as the fluid barium passes readily through the small aperture. It is in this group of patients that there may be delay in making the diagnosis, because too much reliance is placed on the largely negative radiological findings, whereas the combination of these findings and the symptoms of some pyloric obstruction should suggest the correct diagnosis. In prepyloric mucosal stenosis, the barium meal may show the condition very clearly (Fig. 27) with the appearance of two duodenal caps—the proximal one being the compartment between the prepyloric diaphragm and the pylorus. Gastroscopy has been performed to confirm clinical and radiological suspicions of the presence of a diaphragm.[5]

At laparotomy it is possible for the lesion to be missed because the pyloric region, as viewed from the outside, looks quite normal. The diaphragm, being only a mucosal fold, is usually not palpable until the stomach is opened and the index finger inserted. The normal pyloric opening allows the passage of an index finger into the duodenum.[3] When performing a partial gastrectomy for gastric ulcer, the associated presence of mucosal stenosis may not be detected if the pyloric region is not examined in the manner indicated or if a crushing clamp has been applied to the region.

TREATMENT

Pyloric mucosal stenosis may be responsible for the development of a gastric ulcer at an earlier age than is usual, and if its presence is suspected, there is little point in treating the ulcer conservatively. If there is clinical evidence of severe stenosis, the stomach is washed out and the patient put on a liquid diet before operation is undertaken. If a gastric ulcer is present a Billroth I partial gastrectomy is advised. In the absence of an ulcer, a low Billroth I partial gastrectomy is favoured,[6] but incision of the diaphragm and pyloroplasty may be performed for pyloric mucosal stenosis and excision of the diaphragm for prepyloric mucosal stenosis.

REFERENCES

1. Desmond, A. M., and Swynnerton, B. F., Br. Med. J. 1:968, 1957.
2. Rhind, J. A., Br. Med. J. 1:1309, 1965.
3. Rhind, J. A., Br. J. Surg. 46:534, 1959.
4. Gerber, B. C., Arch. Surg. 90:472, 1965.
5. Sokol, E. M., Shorofsky, M. A., and Werther, J. L., Gastrointest. Endosc. 12:20, 1965.
6. Tanner, N. C., Proc. R. Soc. Med. 60:1, 1967.

C. THE BIOCHEMICAL INVESTIGATION OF PEPTIC ULCER

IAN A. D. BOUCHIER

The ideal biochemical assessment of a patient with peptic ulcer disease should provide information of diagnostic value, help in the evaluation of the severity of the disease, predict the likely response to therapy, and indicate whether the ulcer is an isolated event or a manifestation of a more general disease process. Insofar as the pathogenesis of this disease is still unknown, tests of gastric function are disappointing in the overall investigation of the ulcer patient, although in certain special circumstances clinically useful information is provided. The aspect of gastric function most commonly assessed in routine clinical practice is acid secretion. Relatively less helpful information is obtained from an examination of the other indices of gastric function: protein secretion, motility, and mucosal resistance.

TESTS OF GASTRIC ACID OUTPUT

An essential feature of any test of gastric acid output is that it should yield consistent results in any one person. A variety of tests have been in use over the years but experience with the augmented histamine test [12] suggests that it remains the most satisfactory method for assessing acid output. The fractional test meal is obsolete: the gruel used is a poor stimulant of gastric acid secretion and stimulates by bulk only. The serial test meal and the 24-hour gastric secretion are of interest mainly to the physiologist. The methods of testing acid output and their value in clinical medicine have been recently summarised by Bouchier [4] and Baron; [3] the latter monograph contains an extensive and valuable bibliography.

Augmented Histamine Test (AHT)

The AHT is a maximal secretory test for any one patient and is generally believed to be an indirect measure of the parietal cell mass. The test and its clinical implications have been discussed in detail by Baron. [2] After an overnight fast, the patient is intubated with a radiopaque Ryle's tube size 12–16 F. Although there has been much debate, most gastroenterologists believe that it is essential to screen the position of the tube so that the holes in the lower end lie at the lowermost part of the body of the stomach. In nearly half the patients, the tube will be shown to be incorrectly placed at the time of screening. The stomach is emptied, the aspirate examined, and the volume recorded. This represents the *early morning volume* of the stomach and is an important guide to the presence of either gastric outflow obstruction or the Zollinger-Ellison syndrome, for in both disorders the volume will be greater than 150 ml. Thereafter, collection of gastric juice is made for 1 hour, using either an electric suction pump or, preferably, frequent hand aspirations with a syringe. This collection is known as the *basal secretion* or *basal acid output*. One hundred milligrams of mepyramine maleate (Anthisan), an antihistamine, is given intramuscularly and gastric secretion collected over the ensuing 30 minutes is discarded. Histamine acid phosphate, 0.04 mg per kilogram of body weight, is then injected subcutaneously and the gastric secretions are collected for the next 60 minutes. This is best done by collecting four samples each of 15 minutes. Each sample is measured for the volume, pH (concentration of hydrogen ions), and millimoles of hydrochloric acid.

In recent years histamine has been superseded as a stimulant by Histalog and Peptavlon. Histalog (Betazole, Ametazole) is an analogue of histamine that can also produce maximal acid output. It has fewer side-effects than histamine and no injection of an antihistamine agent is required. The usual dose is either, 1.5 mg per kilogram of body weight or 1.7 mg per kilogram of body weight; less satisfactorily, a fixed dose of 100 mg has been used. Histalog is administered either intramuscularly or subcutaneously. Peptavlon pentagastrin is an analogue of the C-terminal tetrapeptide sequence of gastrin that possesses all the physiological properties of the natural substance. The usual dose is 6 μg per kilogram of body weight. Adverse effects of pentagastrin are mild and transient and include nausea, faintness, and hypotension. The side-effects of Histalog are similar to those of histamine. Because pentagastrin administration is cheaper than Histalog and has fewer side-effects than any other gastric acid stimulant, it is recommended for general clinical use.

Gastric stimulants may be administered by continuous intravenous infusion with results that are very similar to those obtained using the conventional dosage schemes. Thus equally accurate estimations can be made of acid output using subcutaneous or intravenous administered stimulant.[15]

There is much variation in how the results are expressed because of differences in collecting times, the end-point to which the gastric acid is titrated and the way in which acid output is calculated. Collection of the stimulated samples should be made for one hour and expressed as mmol per hour. Acid output can then be expressed as the *maximum acid output* (MAO), which is the acid output in the first hour following the histamine injection.[6] Baron[2] introduced *peak acid output,* which is the highest output of acid during any two successive 15-minute periods, but the clinical value of this mode of expressive acid output remains to be decided.

The expression *millimoles of hydrochloric acid* should be used. This is readily determined by titrating an aliquot of gastric juice with 0.1 N NaOH in a direct-reading pH meter to a pH of 7.0. Achlorhydria is defined as failure of pH to fall below 6 pH units after a given stimulus. Use of the following terms must be discontinued: *free acid* (titration to about pH 3.5 with Topfer's reagent), *total acid* (titration to pH 8–10 with phenolphthalein), *degrees of acidity, clinical units, ccN/10 NaOH per 100 cc gastric juice,* and *relative achlorhydria.*

Basal acid output. Acid production during a basal period can be measured overnight by collecting the 12-hour nocturnal secretions, or for an hour only on waking, and this is called the basal, 1-hour measurement. The 1-hour measurement is conveniently made as part of the AHT and is generally believed to provide similar information to the 12-hour nocturnal collection. The disadvantages of the longer period of collection include a change in of the position of the tube and the difficulty of collecting samples without disturbing the patient. The nocturnal acid output in normal subjects is 10 to 20 mmol per litre (volume 600 ml); 5 to 10 mmol per litre (volume 600 ml) in patients with gastric ulcer; and 50 to 75 mmol per litre (volume 1 litre) in duodenal ulcer. Dragstedt[9] considers a nocturnal acid output greater than 75 mmol per litre in a patient with duodenal ulcer to indicate severe disease that is unlikely to respond satisfactorily to medical treatment. A nocturnal acid output of 300 mmol per litre (volume 2 to 3 litres) is found in the Zollinger-Ellison syndrome.

Basal gastric secretion is usually assessed on the prestimulant 1-hour collection of the AHT. The overlap between values in normal subjects and those with gastric and duodenal ulcers is too great for the test to have much diagnostic significance (Table 1). Basal acid output and volume are of most value in the diagnosis of the Zollinger-Ellison syndrome and to a lesser extent in gastric outflow obstruction.

Clinical value of the augmented histamine test. The routine clinical assessment of gastric acid output should record the basal acid output (mmol per hour), the basal volume (ml), the maximal acid output (mmol per hour), and the volume during this period. The results to be expected are shown in Table 1.

There is a wide range of acid output in normal subjects and males secrete more than females. A slight reduction occurs with age. Patients with duodenal ulcers have a higher mean rate of acid secretion than do normal subjects, but they do not have "hyperacidity": there are just fewer patients secreting lesser quantities of acid. The overlap between normal subjects and patients with duodenal and gastric ulcers is so great that the augmented histamine test has little diagnostic value. It is of limited value in the diagnosis of x-ray negative dyspepsia. Grossman et al.[11] did not find a benign gastric ulcer in pa-

**Table 1.   GASTRIC ACID OUTPUT IN NORMAL INDIVIDUALS AND PATIENTS
WITH ULCER DISEASE OR CANCER**

Condition	Basal Acid Output (mMol HCl/hr)	Basal Volume (ml/hr)	Maximum Acid Output (mMol/HCl/hr)	Poststimulus Volume (ml/hr)
Normal	2.0 ± 2.0	40	18.0 ± 8.0	250
Duodenal ulcer	4.0 ± 4.0	60	34.0 ± 13.0	330
Gastric ulcer	1.2 ± 1.5	45	14.0 ± 10.0	240
Gastric cancer	0.3 ± 1.0	45	2.5 ± 3.5	240
Zollinger-Ellison syndrome	34.5 ± 30.0	200	47.0 ± 20.0	360

tients who did not secrete acid; failure to produce acid in response to the augmented histamine test is good evidence that a gastric ulcer is malignant. On the other hand, the secretion of acid does not ensure that a gastric ulcer is benign.

Attempts have been made to use the response to the augmented histamine test as a guide to the type of gastric surgery to be used for peptic ulcer disease.[5] This concept has been challenged and the possibility of a stomal ulcer developing cannot be predicted from the preoperative acid output.

Accumulating experience indicates that the augmented histamine test is of limited value in the diagnosis of the Zollinger-Ellison syndrome. In general, the secretion of fluid and acid in patients with the syndrome far exceeds that found in normal subjects or in those with duodenal ulcer. Gastric hypersecretion shows in a variety of ways: a greatly increased basal acid output, a ratio of basal acid output to maximal acid output greater than 0.6, a nocturnal (12-hour) secretion of more than 1 litre, and 100 mmol hydrochloric acid. Aoyagi and Summerskill[1] stressed the value of the basal acid output and suggested that the syndrome should be considered when the basal acid output is greater than 15 mmol per hour, while values above 10 mmol per hour should be regarded with suspicion. In an assessment of basal and maximal acid secretion, Kaye et al.[14] found an overlap between the data obtained in duodenal ulcer patients and the figures usually quoted as indicating the presence of a Zollinger-Ellison syndrome. A basal acid output greater than 15 mmol per hour was found in 10 percent of duodenal ulcer subjects, and 12 percent of these also had a ratio of basal

to stimulated acid concentration greater than 0.6. It is therefore necessary to exercise caution in the interpretation of gastric secretory data in any patient in whom the Zollinger-Ellison syndrome is suspected.

Kay,[13] in an overall assessment of gastric acid secretion tests, concludes that "although its place as a research tool is not in doubt its value in clinical practice is less certain. The measurement is rarely of critical diagnostic value save in excluding the diagnosis of peptic ulcer by the demonstration of total "achlorhydria."

Tubeless gastric analysis. *Dye test.* This test depends on the dissociation of a cation exchange resin by the hydrochloric acid in the stomach. The cation is absorbed and excreted in the urine where it can be measured. The dye commonly used is Diagnex blue (Azuresin). After an overnight fast, the patient empties the bladder and discards the urine. An acid stimulant is given (either 500 ml caffeine orally or 50 mg Histalog by injection) with a glass of water to drink. One hour later the control sample of urine is collected and this is followed by the oral administration of 120 mg of the granules containing the dye; these are taken with a glass of water. The patient is asked to produce a sample of urine 2 hours later. The urine sample is compared to standards supplied by the manufacturers. When necessary, the urine is acidified with a drop of 6N HCl and heated gently to develop the blue colour. The quantity of dye appearing in the urine is not directly proportional to the amount of acid secreted. False positive results occur in 8 percent of patients; false negative results are more frequent and may be recorded in up to 30 percent of patients, but these patients will usually be submitted to gastric intubation.[7]

Radiotelemetry. The Heidelberg capsule contains a pH measuring cell and a miniature radiotransmitter that relays pH measurements continuously. The capsule is 20 x 7 mm and is a simple and rapid method of measuring basal and stimulated acid output. Gastric acid is neutralized by 1 to 2 mmol $KHCO_3$ and measurements are made under basal conditions followed by a maximal acid output. Acid production over 1 hour is measured by the amount of $KHCO_3$ that is required to maintain a continuous intragastric pH of 7.4. If anacidity is found, it is necessary to check radiologically to ensure that the capsule is positioned in the stomach. Potential sources of error with this technique include improper calibration of the capsule, inaccuracies in the administration of the neutralizing solutions, and improper positioning of the capsule (Yarbrough et al., 1969).

All the tubeless tests are unreliable in measuring acid output, both basal and stimulated. The technique can be used in patients who refuse intubation or as a screening procedure for patients with defective gastric secretion and who require further study.

Serum gastrin estimations. The isolation of the gastric acid secretory hormone, gastrin, in 1964, by Gregory and Tracy anticipated the development of a method for measuring serum gastrin levels in man. McGuigan and Trudeau [17] have reported a radioiodine-immunoassay technique for measuring circulating human serum gastrin concentrations. Serum gastrin levels are of much diagnostic value in distinguishing between duodenal ulcers and ulcers in the duodenum and jejunum associated with the Zollinger-Ellison syndrome. Normal fasting serum gastrin values are 165 ± 28.3 (S.E.) pg per milliliter in normal subjects, whereas in the Zollinger-Ellison syndrome fasting values are 3,550 to 21,000 pg per milliliter.[16] Patients with duodenal ulcer disease have normal or slightly reduced fasting levels of gastrin. This probably reflects the inhibition of gastrin secretion that normally occurs when the antral pH is reduced to less than 3.0 units. In the Zollinger-Ellison syndrome, the extragastric secretion of gastrin is autonomous and is obviously unaffected and not suppressed by antral acidification. Thus a fasting serum gastrin level is of no value in distinguishing normal from gastric ulcer or duodenal ulcer but it does differentiate between a patient with duodenal ulcer and one with ulcers accompanying the Zollinger-Ellison syndrome.

OTHER TESTS OF GASTRIC SECRETION

The routine estimation of the chloride content of the gastric aspirate is not helpful. It does not indicate the degree of duodenal reflux nor does it help in making the distinction between benign and malignant gastric ulceration. The analysis of gastric mucus has no direct clinical application. The estimation of blood and urinary pepsinogen values parallels the gastric acid output, as does intrinsic factor secretion. The assessment of gastric proteolytic activity has no direct clinical application.[18]

ABO BLOOD GROUPS AND SECRETOR STATUS

It is known that a high proportion of duodenal ulcer patients are of blood group O. Among these are a significant number who fail to secrete the A, B, and O antigens in the gastrointestinal mucus. Such persons are known as nonsecretors. The earlier suggestion that nonsecretors have a greater tendency to develop stomal ulcer has not been confirmed, and the measurement of secretor status has as yet no clinical value.

MEDICAL VAGOTOMY

Attempts have been made to predict preoperatively the secretion of acid following a surgical vagotomy and drainage procedure. This information might then help to decide which patients with duodenal ulcer would be particularly suited to this form of operation. The test used is known as a medical vagotomy. An AHT is performed before and after-drug induced vagal blockage to determine which patients have only a small reduction in acid output when vagal activity is abolished. Medical vagotomy can be induced either by an intramuscular injection of 1.3 mg of atropine sulphate and 50 mg of hexamethonium bromide or else intravenous injection of 30 mg propantheline bromide in 10 ml of saline. A good correlation will be found between acid output after the medical and surgical vagotomy,[10] but in one-quarter of the tests the prediction for the individual will be misleading. Moreover medical vagotomy, as used at present, is an incomplete vagotomy. The test itself is unpleasant and tedious, and as currently described has no place in the routine preoperative assessment of patients with duodenal ulcer.

ASSOCIATION WITH OTHER DISEASES

No causal factors can be identified in the majority of patients with peptic ulcer disease. There are a few instances in which ulcers are associated with disease elsewhere. The occurrence of peptic ulcers and the Zollinger-Ellison syndrome has been mentioned, but patients with insulinomas show an increased tendency to develop peptic ulcer disease also. An association of interest is that between ulcer disease and parathyroid adenomata.[19] Whether there is a genuine increase of ulcers remains uncertain, but a case can be made for routine screening for parathyroid overactivity in all patients with peptic ulcers. Hyperparathyroidism is associated with hypercalcaemia and hypercalcuria, and the best screening test is the serum calcium, correctly taken: a fasting venous sample obtained without venous constriction. A serum calcium greater than 10.5 mg per 100 ml is abnormal. There is also an increased tendency to peptic ulcer disease in the multiple endocrine adenoma syndrome, and there is an overlap between patients with this syndrome, patients with the Zollinger-Ellison syndrome, and patients hyperparathyroidism or an insulinoma.[8] An increased incidence of peptic ulcer disease is also claimed to occur in chronic pancreatic insufficiency, chronic respiratory disease, and chronic rheumatoid arthritis.

REFERENCES

1. Aoyagi, T., and Summerskill, W. H. J., Arch. Intern. Med. 117:667, 1966.
2. Baron, J. H., Gut 4:136:243, 1963.
3. Baron, J. H., Scand. J. Gastroenterol. 6 (Suppl.):9, 1970.
4. Bouchier, I. A. D., Clinical Investigation of Gastrointestinal Function, Oxford, Blackwell, 1969.
5. Bruce, J., Card, W. I., Marks, I. N., and Sircus, W., J. R. Coll. Surg. Edinb. 4:85, 1959.
6. Card, W. I., and Marks, I. N., Clin. Sci. 19:147, 1960.
7. Christiansen, P. M., Scand. J. Gastroenterol. 1:9, 1966.
8. Condon, R. E., Granville, G. E., Jordan, P. H., Jr., and Helgason, A. H., Ann. Surg. 167:185, 1968.
9. Dragstedt, L. R., Gastroenterology 52:587, 1967.
10. Gillespie, I. E., and Kay, A. W., Br. Med. J. 1:1557, 1961.
11. Grossman, M. I., Kirsner, J. B., and Gillespie, I. E., Gastroenterology 45:14, 1963.
12. Kay, A. W., Br. Med. J. 2:77, 1953.
13. Kay, A. W., Gastroenterology 53:834, 1967.
14. Kaye, M. D., Rhodes, J., and Beck, P., Gastroenterology 58:476, 1970.
15. Makhlouf, G. M., Gastroenterology 55:423, 1968.
16. McGuigan, J. E., and Trudeal, W. L., New Engl. J. Med. 278:1308, 1968.
17. McGuigan, J. E., and Trudeau, W. L., Gastroenterology 58:139, 1970.
18. Turner, M. D., Miller, L. L., and Segal, H. L., Gastroenterology 53:967, 1967.
19. Wilder, W. T., Frame, B., and Haubrick, W. S., Ann. Intern. Med. 55:885, 1961.

D. THE MEDICAL THERAPY OF PEPTIC ULCER DISEASE

IAN A. D. BOUCHIER

The medical management of peptic ulcer is controversial. Widely differing views are strongly held, and it is difficult to tread a sensible path through this forest of controversy. There have been few adequately controlled studies to determine the efficacy of the various therapeutic measures so vigorously promoted. Bedevilling the whole subject is the complete ignorance of the pathogenesis of this disease; any scheme of therapy must of necessity be tentative.

What are the aims of a therapeutic programme? First, to relieve symptoms; second, to heal the ulcer; and third, to prevent a recurrence: relief of pain is not synonomous with ulcer-healing. Pain can be readily controlled, but healing of the ulcer is more uncertain. There is still no understanding of how to prevent either ulcer disease or the relapse of a previously healed ulcer.

In all the confusion of therapeutic measures, it is important that management of the patient as an individual should not be overlooked. Peptic ulcer disease is usually a mild, recurrent, chronic disease. In our therapeutic endeavours, it is not only right but also essential that the patient be permitted to lead a reasonable existence: continue to earn a living, enjoy his family life, and partake of those few pleasures that make modern life bearable. The treatment that converts a patient into a timid, introverted, "stomach conscious" individual fails.

It is proposed here to survey the different measures that have been advocated in the treatment of ulcer disease, giving both the advantages and disadvantages. In a final section, the management that this author currently uses will be given, more as a practical synthesis of the preceding sections than as dogmatic statement of the way to treat peptic ulcers.

Therapeutic measures commonly used include admission to hospital, cessation of smoking, dietary manipulations, antacids, anticholinergic drugs and the use of liquorice derivatives. Only *admission to hospital* and the *stopping of smoking* have been shown to promote the healing of gastric ulcers. No convincing data have been produced that any therapeutic regimen favourably influences the course of duodenal ulcers.

THERAPY

Diet

The aim of effective dietotherapy must be to reduce gastric acid output, improve gastroduodenal mucosal resistance, and suppress pyloroduodenal motility.

Attempts can be made to neutralize acid, but this is rarely achieved or required. It is probably more efficient to prevent acid stimulation. All food stimulates acid secretion, depending on the quantity (causing antral distention) and composition (protein > fat > carbohydrate). Ideally bread, potatoes, and fruit—which have little stimulating effect—might be used, but these fail to provide the protein so necessary for adequate healing. A compromise is generally made: the administration of small, frequent feedings avoiding potent secretagogues such as coffee and alcohol.

Milk would appear to be the ideal nutriment, and milk and milk foods have traditionally held pride-of-place in dietotherapy. The action of milk is, however, peculiar. It is a buffer and will delay gastric emptying, but it is also a most potent stimulant of gastric acid. There are many studies to show that milk causes a slight and only transitory elevation of intragastric pH. In fact, the gastric acidity on a milk-cream diet may be greater than when taking a light diet.

Attempts to maintain or improve mucosal resistance include restriction of hard, bulky, or rough foods and avoidance of mucosal "irritants" such as spices, condiments, and alcohol. The evidence that these do cause mucosal damage, however, is wanting; what burns the tongue does not necessarily harm the stomach.

Strict dietotherapy includes the following regimen. Hourly milk feedings are given for the initial 10 to 14 days and may be administered during the night if there is much pain. Some of the feedings may be substituted by custards and soups, and protein concentrates and carbohydrates (dextrose or lactose) can be added to the milk to improve the caloric value of the diet. Constipation may be a problem on this diet and prune juice can be added.

After the initial period of hourly feedings, the patient is gradually taken through a series of diets in which solid foods are introduced, so that by the eighth or ninth week a normal diet is permitted. Thus, after 2 weeks, the patient receives cereal, creamed soups, soft boiled eggs, butter, cheese, and white bread; later he receives potatoes, rice, and spaghetti. At 5 weeks, fish and chicken are added, and red meats after 9 weeks.

This regimen–complicated, intrusive, and restrictive–undoubtedly relieves pain, but so do the more permissive dietary programmes. Furthermore, such studies as there are do not show any significant improvement in the rate of ulcer-healing with bland foods compared with intake of a more normal diet. Perseverance with this diet may precipitate vitamin deficiencies (vitamin supplements are therefore usually necessary). Because most ulcer diets are "bursting with regulations" many patients find it difficult or are unwilling to hold to them. The patients then relax and cheat, thereby defeating the purpose of the diet.

Antacids

Antacids are drugs that neutralise or reduce the acidity of the gastric contents. Their use is based on the fact that pepsin is active only in an acid medium (optimum pH 1.5 to 3.5), and the belief that gastric acid secretion has a role in the pathogenesis of peptic ulceration. Some form of antacid therapy is generally considered essential for this disease. The ideal antacid should effectively neutralise the acid and has a prolonged action in the stomach without producing unwanted side-effects.

Any scepticism for this form of therapy is because of the many studies demonstrating the short-lived duration of action of antacids, which is somewhere between 20 and 40 minutes. This is probably caused by rapid gastric emptying. Most patients with duodenal ulcers have increased gastroduodenal motility, and doubling the dose of antacids does not increase efficacy. Fordtran and Collyns [3] demonstrated that when antacids were administered 1 hour after a normal meal, the effect (a reduction of gastric acidity to 38 percent of control value) was seen for up to 4 hours. Doubling the dose enhanced the degree and duration of antacidity. When the antacid was given 4 hours after a meal, the effect was short-lived. It would therefore seem more rational to administer antacids soon after a meal rather than at the traditional time of 2 to 3 hours after eating.

Antacids do stop pain but to do so it is *not* necessary for the gastric acid to be neutralized. Indeed, the most completely safe antacids, such as aluminium hydroxide, are virtually incapable of elevating gastric juice pH to any extent. There is doubt whether it is necessary for the acid to be neutralized in order for healing to occur; there is no good evidence that neutralization of the gastric juice hastens the healing of gastric ulcers,[1] and unfortunately there is no good evidence relating to the healing of duodenal ulcers.

Antacids are taken hourly when intensive therapy is being instituted in the hospital, and this should be maintained during the period of hospitalization, which is usually for 3 weeks in the case of a duodenal ulcer and possibly slightly longer for a gastric ulcer. Ambulant therapy is maintained for 1 or 2 months during which time the antacids are taken every hour or two. Placebo doses of antacids (administered 2 or 3 times a day) have no place in ulcer therapy.[10] Antacids should never be dispensed in the same mixture or tablet as anticholinergic drugs or sedatives. Liquid preparations or powders mixed with water are generally more effective than antacids taken in tablet form because of more complete interaction with gastric hydrochloric acid. Nonetheless, the ambulant patient finds that tablets are more convenient to use and a reasonable symptomatic effect can be achieved if the tablets are taken frequently and sucked or chewed thoroughly.

The following is a selection from the extensive number of antacids available. It has been compiled with consideration to the cost of the various agents; this is an important factor in a disease that may affect up to 10 percent of the population and for which treatment is required for a relatively long time.

Calcium carbonate powder: Dose 4 g. Four grams of calcium carbonate is superior to 15 ml aluminium-magnesium hydroxide in lowering the hydrogen ion content of the gastric secretions.
Aluminium hydroxide mixture: Dose 5 ml. Consists of aluminium hydroxide gel B.P.; it contains Al_2O_3 about 4 percent w/w.
Magnesium trisilicate powder: Dose 2 g.
Magnesium trisilicate compound tablets, B.P.C.: Dose 1 or 2 tablets. Consists of magnesium trisilicate 250 mg dried aluminium hydroxide gel 120 mg, with peppermint oil.

A great number of other proprietary and nonproprietary antacid preparations are available (about 50 are catalogued in a current index of ethical preparations) but none offers any particular advantage over those mentioned above.

Unwanted effects. Calcium salts cause *constipation* whereas magnesium induces *diarrhoea,* and it is for this reason that the various compounds are given either as mixtures or in alternating doses. Calcium carbonate in large doses can induce *hypercalcaemia,* and patients receiving this antacid require regular monitoring of the serum levels. *Acid rebound* occurs with potent antacid preparations. This is one of the theoretical disadvantages of sodium bicarbonate (the others being the production of the milk-alkali syndrome and the generation of excess gastric and intestinal gas). It is theoretically possible with calcium carbonate therapy, but it is probable that in the clinical situation any excess acid production is buffered by the antacid remaining in the stomach or by the ingestion of food.[2] The *milk-alkali syndrome* may develop if excess milk and absorbable antacids are administered. It is a real hazard of sodium bicarbonate therapy but may also complicate calcium carbonate administration because a small fraction of the calcium ions may be absorbed. The main signs are hypercalcaemia, hyperphosphataemia, uraemia, and alkalosis with elevated plasma bicarbonate and decreased chloride levels. The syndrome may be conveniently subdivided into "reversible" and "irreversible" forms, the latter being recognised by the occurrence of metastatic calcification and progressive renal failure. Treatment consists of a low calcium diet, high fluid intake, and substitution of the absorbable alkali by nonabsorbable antacids. The hazards of impaired absorption of phosphorus that may accompany long-term use of nonabsorbable antacids containing magnesium and aluminium hydroxides have been reported by Lotz et al.[8] The patients have a syndrome of *phosphorus depletion* in which there is hypophophosphataemia, hypophosphaturia, increased gastrointestinal absorption of calcium, hypercalcuria, debility, weakness, and bone pain. It is not clear how common phosphorus depletion is in clinical practise. Many of the nonabsorbable antacids

that are taken in the form of gels may interfere with the absorption of other pharmacological agents, and this may influence their therapeutic effects.

Anticholinergic Therapy

The place of anticholingeric agents in the management of peptic ulcer disease is highly controversial. They are given to suppress gastric secretion and motility but with the smaller and better tolerated doses it is doubtful whether these objectives are achieved. Piper [10] has suggested that the anticholingeric drugs are given to facilitate the neutralization of gastric acid by antacids and food. The well-recognised side-effects that occur with larger, more effective doses limit the use of such agents. Anticholingeric drugs do suppress basal gastric acid secretion, but there is no evidence that long-term administration reduces the gastric acid output. Furthermore, long-term treatment does not potentiate the short-term antisecretory effect of the anticholingeric agent.[9] A controlled trial of anticholingeric drugs in the management of duodenal ulcer showed that they were no more effective than a placebo.[6]

Anticholingeric drugs are often given with meals in the belief that this will lead to a more even and sustained effect. They are taken with greatest effect at night just before the patient retires. The drugs should never be administered in combination with other agents, for the dose should be carefully adjusted to the individual tolerance of the patient. A variety of preparations are available but there is no conclusive evidence that any one is superior to atropine.

Propantheline tablets, B.P. 15 mg. Dose: up to 45 mg daily in divided doses.
Dicyclomine tablets, B.P. 10 mg. Dose: 30 to 60 mg daily in divided doses.
Poldine methylsulphate tablets 2 mg. Dose: 2 to 6 mg daily in divided doses.

Unwanted effects. The side-effects of the anticholinergic drugs include dryness of the oral and respiratory passages, blurring of vision, and urinary retention. The drugs are contraindicated in glaucoma, prostatic hypertrophy, and oesophageal reflux. They should not be used if there is any gastric outflow obstruction, following a recent gastrointestinal haemorrhage, and if surgery or a barium meal are being undertaken.[5]

Liquorice Derivatives

Two derivatives of liquorice are available and have proven therapeutic value: carbonoxelone sodium and deglycyrrhizinized liquorice. These drugs are of considerable value in the treatment of gastric ulceration, but there is no convincing evidence that either is of benefit in the treatment of duodenal ulcers.

Carbonoxelone sodium ("Biogastrone"). The precise mode of action of this agent is uncertain. It has an anti-inflammatory effect and may also have an influence on the gastric mucus. Carbonoxelone is particularly effective in the outpatient management of gastric ulcers. It is prescribed as 50-mg tablets, which are taken after meals. The recommended dose is 100 mg 3 times daily for the first 1 to 2 weeks of therapy followed by 50 mg 3 times daily for up to 6 weeks. Side-effects are due to the mineralocorticoid effects of the carbonoxelone sodium and include sodium retention, oedema, a gain in weight, hypertension, and a fall in serum potassium levels. These various indices must therefore be monitored very carefully while the patient is under treatment with this drug. Particular care is required in treating elderly or hypertensive patients, and the agent is contraindicated in patients with congestive cardiac failure.

Deglycyrrhizinized Liquorice ("Caved-S"). The active ingredient is taken in tablets that also contain a variety of antacid preparations. The dose is 2 tablets 3 times daily after meals. Caved-S is effective in the healing of gastric ulcers and does not have the side-effects of salt and water retention.

Intragastric Drip Therapy

Some patients continue to have severe abdominal pain despite hospitalization bed rest and careful attention to antacid and anticholinergic regimens. In this situation, an intragastric drip of milk, together with an antacid preparation, is usually of value. One to 2 litres of milk are administered via a nasogastric tube over 24 hours and the programme is maintained for 2 to 3 days. During this period, the patient is kept at strict bed rest. A regular diet and other therapeutic agents may be given as required. If this method is going to be of benefit, the pain will subside within 2 or 3 days; if it does not, either the pain does not arise from peptic ulcer disease or the ulcer is complicated. In either event, there is no value in persisting with the nasogastric drip and some alternate form of treatment must be instituted.

An equally effective technique is continuous gastric suction with intravenous feeding. The pain usually subsides within 36 hours.

Other Forms of Therapy

Because peptic ulcer disease, particularly duodenal ulcer, is regarded by many as a disease of personality and stress, some form of *sedation* is often given. Such evidence as there is suggests that phenobarbitone does not influence the outcome in patients with duodenal ulcers. Many patients give no evidence of undue stress, and moderate sedation causing only minimal blunting of the faculties will often not be tolerated by the tense active "ulcer-prone" individual. Sedation has little to offer in the routine outpatient management of ulcer disease but it may be instituted in the inpatient management of the tense, anxious patient particularly when the abdominal pain persists. Tranquilizers may be used instead of sedatives, but these too have no role in the routine management of peptic ulceration.

Formal *psychotherapy* has been suggested but has not been widely adopted as a method of treating ulcer disease. *Diethylstilbestrol* can be shown to increase the healing of duodenal ulcers in males. The treatment is accompanied by feminization and is clearly of no practical value. *Gastric irradiation* may destroy parietal cells and has been suggested for patients in whom surgery is contraindicated and in patients with the Zollinger-Ellison syndrome. The radiation dose is about 1,650 R total depth dose directed in 10 divided treatments to the fundus and body of the stomach. *Gastric freezing* was introduced in 1962 for the management of duodenal ulcers. Gastric freezing must not be confused with gastric cooling: cooling is used for prolonged periods in the emergency treatment of massive gastrointestinal bleeding; freezing is applied for 1 hour or less as the elective treatment of a nonbleeding duodenal ulcer. There is no evidence that this form causes any significant reduction of pain, suppression of acid secretion, or reduction in the number of recurrences.[4, 11]

There is a risk of patients with peptic ulcer developing complications, particularly bleeding, if they receive anti-inflammatory drugs. Thus aspirin, indomethacin, phenylbutazone, and corticosteroids must be administered under careful surveillance.

AMBULANT VERSUS HOSPITAL MANAGEMENT

Duodenal ulcers are common, and the disease has a marked tendency to spontaneous remission. The majority of patients can and should be managed as outpatients. Inpatient therapy is required if symptoms persist or if complications develop, and is usually for 3 to 4 weeks. Patients with a gastric ulcer may be treated with liquorice derivatives as outpatients initially. If the ulcer fails to heal within 4 to 6 weeks, the patient must be admitted for a period of hospital therapy. Adequate healing of an ulcerative gastric lesion is essential because failure to heal is taken as a sign of malignancy. Barium studies or endoscopy are therefore necessary after the patient has been under adequate medical care for 4 weeks, and if the ulcer has persisted, the patient is submitted to surgery.

PREVENTION OF RELAPSES

The relapse rate of patients treated for symptomatic duodenal ulcer is high; probably less than one-third of patients remain permanently symptom-free.[7] Despite the successful treatment of the active symptomatic ulcer, there is no way to prevent relapse. The patient is generally advised to alter his "way of life," to reduce or stop smoking, to moderate alcohol consumption, and to alter the diet, but with the exception of stopping smoking it is doubtful how effective these measures are. There is no evidence that the prolonged use of antacids prevents recurrences.

FAILURES OF MEDICAL THERAPY

Medical treatment can be considered to have failed if the patient presents with a complication of ulcer disease (haemorrhage, perforation, penetration, or obstruction), and surgical intervention will then be contemplated. Failure to relieve pain, persistent recurrence of pain, or failure of a gastric ulcer to heal despite adequate inpatient therapy is also taken as an indication for surgical intervention. Male sex, long duration of symptoms, and high gastric acid secretion are thought to be factors weighing against the success of medical treatment. There is no evidence to support the concept that the patient should "earn his gastrectomy." Patients who have had a long period of ulcer symptoms do not have any fewer postgastrectomy problems than those patients who have a shorter history at the time of operation.

SUMMARY

In the preceding sections, an attempt has been made to present a broad view of the medical management of peptic ulcer disease. By way of summary, the author's own therapeutic programme will be presented. This produces clinically satisfactory results and has proved acceptable to the majority of patients who appear to cooperate willingly. The author has been influenced particularly by the marked natural tendency of peptic ulcers to heal spontaneously, their uncertain pathogenesis, the need to interfere as little as possible with the patient's way of life, and the avoidance of unpleasant side-effects from therapeutically unproven agents.

The majority of patients are treated as outpatients. After assessment of the patient and his social circumstances, an explanation is given of the nature of the disease and what the treatment will involve. The patient is permitted a normal diet, but restrictions are placed on black coffee or alcohol taken on an empty stomach (small quantities of alcohol are permitted during a meal) and strong condiments. The patient is urged to stop smoking. Regular mealtimes are advised: ideally 6 small meals a day; failing this, 3 meals with midmorning and afternoon snacks and something to eat before going to bed. Two tablets of magnesium trisilicate compound are sucked or well chewed at hourly intervals. The antacid tablet is changed if there is any upset in the bowel actions or if the patient cannot tolerate the flavour. The patient is advised to take a holiday if possible. Patients with a gastric ulcer are started on carbonoxelone sodium, and antacids are added if there is any abdominal pain. These patients are seen twice at weekly intervals and then at two-weekly intervals in order to monitor any side-effects.

Patients usually respond well with relief of pain and radiological evidence that the gastric ulcer is healing. The programme is maintained until the patient has been symptom-free for 1 to 2 months, at which time the antacids are discontinued. Should the patient fail to respond, propantheline is introduced. In the event of this being unsuccessful, the patient admitted to hospital for intensive therapy and for further assessment. Failure of a gastric ulcer to heal radiologically within 4 to 6 weeks is also an indication for hospitalization.

REFERENCES

1. Baume, P. E., and Hunt, J. H., Aust. Ann. Med. 18:113, 1969.
2. Fordtran, J. S., New Engl. J. Med. 279:900, 1968.
3. Fordtran, J. S., and Collyns, J. A. H., New Engl. J. Med. 274:921, 1966.
4. Harrell, W. R., Rose, H., Fordtran, J. S., and Friedman, B., J.A.M.A. 200:290, 1967.
5. Ingelfinger, F. J., New Engl. J. Med. 268:1454, 1963.
6. Kaye, M. D., Rhodes, J., Beck, P., Sweetman, P. M., Davies, G. T., and Evans, K. T. Gut 11:559, 1970.
7. Krag, E., Acta Med. Scand. 180:657, 1966.
8. Lotz, M., Zisman, E., and Bartter, F. C., New Engl. J. Med. 278:409, 1968.
9. Norgaard, R. P., Polter, D. E., Wheeler, J. W., Jr., and Fordtran, J. S., Gastroenterology 58:750, 1970.
10. Piper, D. W., Gastroenterology 52:1009, 1967.
11. Ruffin, J. M., Grizzle, J. E., Hightower, N. C., McHardy, G., Shull, H., and Kirsner, J. B., New Engl. J. Med. 281:16, 1969.

13

ULCEROGENIC TUMORS OF THE PANCREAS

ROBERT M. ZOLLINGER, WILLIAM V. NICK, and LARRY J. SANZENBACHER

A direct relationship between noninsulin-producing islet-cell tumors and a pancreatic phase of gastric hypersecretion, first advanced in 1955,[1] has now been firmly established by experimental and clinical evidence. The original report was based on two cases of severe primary jejunal ulceration, characterized by tremendous hypersecretion and continued ulcer recurrence until total gastrectomy became mandatory. A thought-provoking finding in both cases was the presence of a nonspecific islet-cell tumor of the pancreas, with no clinical or laboratory evidence of increased insulin production. It was suggested that these tumors were producing a potent gastric secretagogue, of islet-cell origin, which caused digestion of the stomach if any acid-secreting surface remained. This clinical syndrome, presented as a triad after the example of Whipple,[2] consisted of (1) the presence of primary peptic ulceration in unusual locations, that is, the second or third portions of the duodenum, upper jejunum, or recurrent stomal ulcers following any gastric surgery short of total gastrectomy; (2) marked gastric hypersecretion despite adequate and even intensive conventional medical or surgical therapy; and (3) the identification of nonspecific islet-cell tumors of the pancreas.

THE CLINICAL SPECTRUM OF ULCEROGENIC TUMORS

Since 1955 hundreds of case reports have documented the islet-cell tumor ulcerogenic syndrome. It is known that these tumors, as well as their metastases, produce 35 times more gastrin than a similar weight of porcine antrum.[3, 4, 5] The diagnosis is often suggested from the history. The onset of a fulminating ulcer diathesis in an elderly individual, in a youngster under 15 years of age, in the immediate postpartum period, or following one or more standard surgical operations for ulcer should suggest the diagnosis.

While the clinical syndrome may be that of severe diarrhea or steatorrhea, the symptoms are ordinarily those of a fulminating ulcer. More than 40 percent of the reported patients have intractability to ulcer treatment as the prime reason for further surgery. Hemorrhage is the principle complication in 33 percent. Perforation was an emergency indication for surgical intervention in 23 percent. A perforated ulcer does not necessarily suggest an ulcerogenic tumor unless a jejunal ulcer perforates just beyond the ligament of Trietz. Eight percent of the patients reported had multiple perforations. Relatively few patients develop pyloric obstruction, which is observed in only 7 percent of the cases. In 16 percent, there was no discernible difference in the symptomatology between the patient with the ulcerogenic tumor and the usual duodenal ulcer patient. All too frequently, the diagnosis is established fortuitously at the time of surgery or is an unexpected finding at postmortem examinations.

Islet-cell tumors have been reported in children under 10 years of age. Nearly 5 percent of the reported cases occurred in patients 10 to 16 years of age. In fifteen recently studied cases of the clinical syndrome in children, all experienced gastrointestinal hemorrhage or perforation prior to surgical intervention.[6] Perforation was the most frequent complication requiring emergency sur-gery. Gastric hypersecretion and characteristic radiographic findings were documented in all children in which these studies were performed. While no associated endocrine abnormalities were evident in any of these 15 young patients, the clinical picture is otherwise virtually identical to that in adults.

The diagnosis can be supported by upper gastrointestinal barium studies that show huge mucosal folds with considerable fluid retention in the stomach.[7] The duodenum tends to be enlarged and irregular in appearance, with one or more ulcers in an unusual location such as the second or third portion of the duodenum. Ulceration just beyond the ligament of Treitz should be considered pathognomonic of an ulcerogenic tumor. Barium studies after previous gastric resection may show multiple deep penetrating ulcers in the mesenteric border of the efferent loop rather than in the usual marginal location.

Accurate gastric analysis studies are helpful. The gastric tube must be carefully placed by fluoroscopy. The typical findings include an output of gastric juice in excess of 100 ml per hour with 10 mEq of hydrochloric acid per hour in an unobstructed stomach. As much as 5 liters of gastric juice with more than 60 mEq per liter of free hydrochloric acid, may be aspirated in 12-hour overnight studies from an obstructed stomach. The stomach is maximally stimulated, producing at least 60 percent or more of the volume obtained following the augmented histamine study.

The diagnosis is currently being made more frequently and with greater accuracy using the gastrin immuno-assay test of McGuigan.[8] High serum gastrin levels are found in the presence of an islet-cell tumor as well as in pernicious anemia. The absence of hydrochloric acid in the latter disease facilitates the differential diagnosis.

Considerable clinical experience has confirmed the possibility of the involvement of secondary glands of internal secretion. An accurate incidence of involvement of these glands in the collected cases cannot be determined since in at least half, an endocrine survey had not been made. Ellison and Wilson have reported an incidence of associated multiple endocrine adenomatosis in about 20 percent of the patients, and an incidence of Wermer's syndrome in approximately 5 percent.[9] Parathyroid adenomas occur in about 20 percent, the parathyroid being the most single endocrine gland involved.

Blood calcium studies must be part of the preoperative evaluation. When the evidence favoring a parathyroid adenoma is definite, it may be advisable to remove the parathyroid adenomas first, to lower the blood calcium and circulating gastrin levels. The decision whether to remove the ulcerogenic islet-cell tumor or the parathyroid adenoma first depends upon the predominant symptoms and the clinical course of the patient. On occasion, the evidence of a parathyroid adenoma is not present for some time after the total gastrectomy.

The clinical problem may be complicated by several factors. Frequently the patient has had one or more previous operative procedures to control the ulcer diathesis. The ulcerogenic syndrome is often suspected when a standard surgical procedure fails to relieve an ulcer diathesis. The most likely cause of this problem is an inadequate or incomplete operation that has not controlled the acid factor. The original operative note must be reviewed in an attempt to determine whether the surgeon had difficulty exposing the vagus nerves, or there was difficulty in closing the duodenal stump. Such a report might suggest that one vagus nerve has not been cut or that a portion of antrum remains. Furthermore, an enteroenterostomy or some other short-circuiting procedure may have been necessary to alleviate an acute problem such as obstruction, but this may predispose the patient to subsequent recurrent ulceration.

The most common cause of recurrent ulceration is an overlooked vagus, particularly the posterior nerve. Secondly, a gastroenterostomy placed too high on the greater curvature with inadequate drainage of the antrum will produce antral distension and continuous overproduction of gastrin. Two common forms of pathologic lesions in the upper adbomen tend to simulate an ulcerogenic tumor: the retained gastric antrum from an inadequate gastric resection and chronic recurrent pancreatitis with severe fibrosis and diffuse calcification. Elliott showed that the severely damaged pancreas is a possible source of continuous gastrin stimulation, producing gastric hypersecretion and further difficulties in controlling the associated pancreatitis in what become a vicious circle, with the pancreas being its own worst enemy.[10]

TUMOR HISTOPATHOLOGY

Tumors of the pancreas have long challenged the pathologist because their identification can be most difficult and the cell of origin of a particular tumor often defies identification. Ulcerogenic tumors of the pancreas often have the microscopic appearance of a carcinoid pattern with the cellular arrangement in ribbons. The rosette configuration about blood vessels is consistent with endocrine activity. Many of the islet-cell tumors cannot be differentiated from carcinoid tumors irrespective of their hormonal activity. The tumors may be single or multiple; they may be very small or as large as an apple. Occasionally only microscopic metastases in the lymph nodes adjacent to the pancreas have been found. Ectopic growth have more rarely been found in the gastric antrum and the splenic hilus.

Approximately 70 percent of the patients with the ulcerogenic syndrome have multiple foci of gastrin-producing tumor due to the high incidence of malignancy. More than 60 percent of these tumors are malignant. Three out of four will have metastasized to either the liver or regional lymph nodes by the time of surgery. Bloodworth and Elliott [11] have emphasized that it is impossible to determine whether the original tumor is benign or malignant unless extension beyond the capsule of the pancreas can be identified. A smaller percentage of patients will have either diffuse islet-cell hyperplasia or multiple benign adenomas. Gross identification is often by palpation, since these tumors may be deep within the gland and do not present any unusual discoloration, which tends to distinguish their borders from normal surrounding pancreas. The tumors are distributed throughout the head, body, and tail of the pancreas.

Of particular importance are small ectopic tumors, which occur in the wall of the duodenum in about 10 percent of the cases. They tend to be overlooked at the time of surgical exploration, since they are usually less than 1 cm in diameter or are found by digital examination of the lumen or following microscopic examination of the entire circumference of the excised duodenal wall.

DIAGNOSTIC METHODS

Gastric Hypersecretion

The patient with an ulcerogenic tumor of the pancreas will usually have tremendous gastric hypersecretion despite previous vagotomy or any ulcer operation other than total gastric resection. The 12-hour overnight gastric aspiration in most cases will measure at least 2 liters with a free hydrochloric acid output content of 100 to 300 mEq per liter, compared to a normal volume of 400 ml and acid output of 18 mEq per liter. There have been reports of patients who secrete as much as 10 or more liters of gastric juice in 24 hours. It is of great importance to avoid marked dehydration and severe electrolyte imbalance when conducting the overnight gastric analysis; careful attention to nocturnal parenteral replacement of these losses will prevent dehydration and imbalance. Caution is warranted in the interpretation of gastric secretory studies in any patient suspected of having an ulcerogenic tumor. Winship and Ellison,[12] and most recently Way, Goldman, and Dunphy,[13] have called attention to the variability of the gastric analysis findings.

The augmented histamine test has been used extensively in evaluating the gastric secretory function of these patients. When performing this test, the tube must be placed in the most dependent portion of the stomach and its location verified by fluoroscopy. An hourly output of 100 mEq per liter of hydrochloric acid is not at all uncommon and should suggest an extragastric cause for the marked hypersecretion in the absence of pyloric obstruction. A fixed acid concentration of more than 100 mEq per liter tends to confirm the presence of an ulcerogenic tumor. Ruppert and others have found that the ratio of basal acid concentration to maximal acid concentration (BAC/MAC) is indicative of an ulcerogenic tumor if it is above 0.6.[14] The anatomical explanation for this tremendous hypersecretion appears to be a

hyperplastic transformation and marked increase in the parietal cell mass resulting from prolonged stimulation of gastric secretion by the gastrin-producing tumor.

DIAGNOSTIC METHODS

Radiography

Often the first clue to the diagnosis of an ulcerogenic tumor may be provided by the upper gastrointestinal series.[7] The tumors themselves are usually so small that indirect signs such as organ displacement, extrinsic compression of the stomach, and changes in the duodenal C-loop are rarely detected. The characteristic signs of marked hypersecretion, however, with large amounts of retained gastric fluid, huge gastric mucosal folds, and a large "shaggy" appearing duodenum with or without an ulcer provide invaluable hints to the alert radiologist who is thoroughly familiar with the clinical history and laboratory results (Fig. 1).

Christoforidis and Nelson [7] emphasized the importance of roentgenological examinations as a means of early diagnosis. They determined that the most significant finding was the markedly hypertrophied gastric mucosal folds. In certain instances, this may be misinterpreted as a protein-losing gastropathy or even lymphoma. There are excessive amounts of retained gastric juice in the fasting state, without evidence of any organic obstruction. While gastric and duodenal ulcers may be present, ulcers distal to the bulb should always raise a suspicion of the ulcerogenic syndrome. The likelihood of ulcerogenic tumor of the pancreas is great with ulcerations of the distal duodenum and, particularly, the jejunum.

Postresection or marginal ulcerations produced by an islet-cell tumor tend to be deep, penetrating, and multiple, and they are almost always located on the mesenteric border of the efferent loop rather than in the usual anastomotic location.

Arteriography may be helpful when the presence of arteriovenous shunts in the gastric mucosa is demonstrated.[15] The extremely early return of contrast media to the venous circulation may have a relationship to the large amount of gastrin produced by the pan-

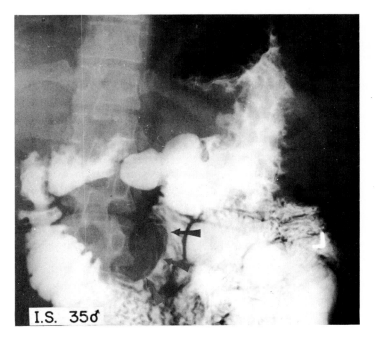

FIG. 1. Barium studies demonstrate large mucosal folds in the stomach and an enlarged and irregular duodenum. Encroachment by tumor on the third portion of the duodenum is indicated by the *arrow.*

creatic islet-cell tumors. Selective arteriography of the pancreas has occasionally demonstrated islet-cell tumors by an increased venous blush that outlines the lesions, though they are relatively small in size. Scanning of the pancreas with selenium 75 rarely demonstrates ulcerogenic tumors of the pancreas.

Radiographic studies may also detect associated endocrine abnormalities. The skull, lamina dura, hands, and clavicles should be x-rayed in an effort to determine secondary signs of pituitary or parathyroid abnormalities.

DIAGNOSTIC METHODS

Immuno-assay Studies

Following the discovery by Gregory that gastrin is the secretagogue present in ulcerogenic tumors, investigators were challenged to develop a diagnostic test that could measure this substance directly.[3, 5] Ghosh and Schild,[16] then Lai,[17] emphasized the value of the isolated rat stomach as a means of studying the effect of gastric secretagogues. Thompson, Cleator, and Sircus affirmed the value of the Lai preparation for the diagnosis of ulcerogenic tumors based on perfusion of the isolated rat stomach and the output of gastric acidity following the intravenous administration of serum, pH-adjusted gastric juice, or urine.[18] Moore and his colleagues reported their experience with this technique in 130 patients, 10 of whom had a positive response.[19] Consistently positive results were obtained in all but one ulcerogenic tumor patient, who had a variable response. Wilson et al. found evidence favoring a potent gastric secretagogue in only 10 of 15 patients with proved ulcerogenic tumors.[20] The bio-assay was negative in 21 control patients and in 22 patients with proved peptic ulcers. They emphasized that a negative bio-assay did not necessarily rule out the presence of an ulcerogenic tumor, since there is a wide range of serum gastrin levels in these patients.

In 1968, McGuigan reported the development of a sensitive radio-immunoassay technique for the measurement of gastrin concentrations in serum and plasma.[8] He utilized this technique to quantitate the excessive amounts of gastrin in the serum of patients with the ulcerogenic syndrome and to document its presence in extracts of the nonbeta islet-cell tumor.

Normal fasting serum gastrin levels have usually been less than 200 $\mu\mu$g per milliliter. While the results from various laboratories vary, the gastrin levels for duodenal ulcer may or may not be slightly elevated above normal. The serum levels in the presence of gastric ulcer may tend to be a little higher than those for duodenal ulcer. Perhaps the latter results are due to lower gastric acidity values in the presence of gastric ulcer. The two conditions thus far associated with high levels of serum gastrin are pernicious anemia and the ulcerogenic syndrome. In both, the serum gastrin levels may be far greater than 1,000 $\mu\mu$g per milliliter.

The increase in serum gastrin levels during the infusion of calcium in patients with ulcerogenic tumor suggests this test may be valuable in the diagnosis of a borderline case.[21] Passaro has reported the use of an intravenous calcium infusion (15 mg per kilogram of body weight per 4 hours) and has shown this produces a gastric acid secretory response at least 75 percent as high as stimulation with Histalog in patients with the ulcerogenic syndrome.[22] Passaro has also advocated the use of a smaller calcium dose (2 mg per kilogram) given intravenously as a bolus over a period of 1 minute, while measuring gastric acid secretion every 15 minutes for 1 hour.[23] These studies indicate that the calcium load may be worthwhile as a screening test for an ulcerogenic tumor when gastrin immuno-assay is not available. The calcium infusion test should be avoided in the presence of high serum calcium levels associated with a parathyroid adenoma.

The gastrin immuno-assay yields quantitative results. As the test becomes more widely available, it should be the most useful test to establish the diagnosis of the ulcerogenic tumor. Markedly elevated gastrin levels in the absence of pernicious anemia will prove very useful to the surgeon in cases where he is unable to find any evidence of tumor at the time of operation. While total gastrectomy has ordinarily not been recommended in the absence of documented tumor, pre-operative high serum levels could change this view and should prove very reassuring as an indication for total gastrectomy.

PREOPERATIVE PREPARATION

Every detail in the preoperative study of the patient must be confirmed, and the evidence for or against the diagnosis of ulcerogenic tumor reviewed, as the overall postoperative mortality in the world literature approximates 35 percent. Irrefutable proof of the tumor, such as a previous biopsy, perforation of a jejunal ulcer, or positive gastrin levels, versus evidence of a prior nonphysiological operation in past operative notes must be carefully weighed, should the tumor not be found. Fortified with such documentation and a carefully prepared and thoroughly informed patient, the surgeon will have the conviction to carry out the proper surgical procedure. Actually, preoperative informed consent should be obtained for a possible total gastrectomy, partial pancreatectomy, and splenectomy in any patient with a severe ulcer diathesis.

The loss of fluids and electrolytes from gastric aspiration or diarrhea must be carefully corrected. Intravenous replacement with cautious monitoring of the patient's weight insures safe preparation for operation and accurate daily laboratory measurements. Measured blood volume and nutritional deficits are replaced. Preoperative antibiotic therapy may be indicated because of the tendency of the ulcers to penetrate the gastrointestinal wall into adjacent tissues and occasionally, the colon. Since steroid therapy may have been given to control the diarrhea, the necessity of additional steroids just prior to and during surgery should not be overlooked to avoid relative adrenal insufficiency.

SURGICAL PROCEDURES

The surgical procedure depends upon a number of factors including the preoperative gastrin levels, gross evidence of a pancreatic tumor, metastasis to the regional lymph nodes or liver, and the nature of the previous surgical procedure. When total gastrectomy is carried out at the initial operation, the mortality rate is reduced to 18 percent. A definite plan of exploration should be reviewed, since the tumor may be difficult to find or indeed defy identification. This tempts the surgeon to follow a conservative course with disastrous results from prompt ulcer recurrence. The major challenge to the surgeon occurs when he can not find either gross or microscopic evidence of a tumor and, second, when an ulcerogenic tumor is found unexpectedly in a patient unprepared or uninformed concerning the possibility of a total gastrectomy.

One or more previous incisions often dictate the placement of the upper abdominal incision. The preferred incision extends from up over the xiphoid process in the midline to below the umbilicus on the left side. The inflammatory appearance of the tissues and the increased vascularity of the stomach will be apparent. This is especially true if the patient has had one or more previous gastric procedures and now may have a marginal ulceration that has perforated and been sealed off by the peritoneum. On occasion, a marked inflammatory mass associated with a gastrojejunocolic fistula is encountered.[24]

The liver is carefully inspected and palpated for evidence of metastatic nodules. If one is found, a biopsy specimen for frozen section confirmation of the diagnosis should be taken. The presence of multiple nodules in the liver is no contraindication for proceeding with a total gastrectomy. Whether the removal of the target organ by total gastrectomy causes regression of the metastasis, as Friesen advocates, requires a longer follow-up study of additional cases. Removal of all acid-secreting surface is important in the presence of multiple metastases, in order to avoid the lethal complications of ulcer, i.e., perforation or hemorrhage. The ulcerogenic islet-cell tumor as well as the metastases grow slowly but both are the source of the potent gastric secretagogue, gastrin.

In the absence of gross metastasis to the

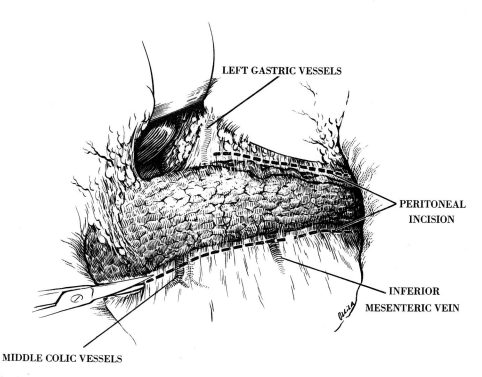

LEFT GASTRIC VESSELS

PERITONEAL INCISION

INFERIOR MESENTERIC VEIN

MIDDLE COLIC VESSELS

FIG. 2. Peritoneum along inferior surface of pancreas is incised, taking care to avoid middle colic vessels and underlying inferior mesenteric vein.

liver or previous proof of an islet-cell tumor, the surgeon is often hard pressed to prove the diagnosis before proceeding with a definitive operation on the stomach. A systematic pattern of exploration should be followed to minimize the chances of overlooking the small and elusive ulcerogenic islet-cell tumor.

The head of the pancreas is first mobilized by the Kocher maneuver to permit direct inspection and palpation between the surgeon's thumb and fingers. The enlarged duodenum should also be carefully palpated in a search of an elusive submucosal adenoma which may occur in one patient out of ten. Any enlarged lymph nodes about the hepatoduodenal ligament or along the superior margin of the pancreas should be removed for frozen section evidence of metastasis. The jejunum just beyond the ligament of Treitz should be examined for evidence of ulceration, since this is such an important diagnostic finding of the islet-cell tumor syndrome. The next step is to open the lesser sac wide for inspection and palpation of the

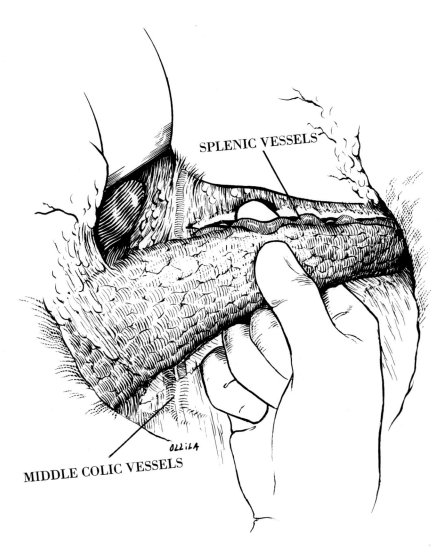

SPLENIC VESSELS

OLLILA

MIDDLE COLIC VESSELS

FIG. 3.   Body and tail of pancreas are mobilized for direct palpation and possible extirpation if tumor is found. Left side of pancreas and splenic vessels can be encircled without mobilizing spleen or compromising blood supply.

body and tail of the pancreas. The greater omentum is reflected upward and traction maintained on the transverse colon as the flimsy omental attachments are divided and all bleeding points ligated. All attachments of the splenic flexure of the colon must be divided in case mobilization of the spleen and tail of the pancreas becomes necessary. Likewise, the greater omentum should be freed on the right side to ensure good visualization of the anterior surface of the head of the pancreas. A large S-shaped retractor is inserted to hold the stomach upward as the body and tail of the pancreas are inspected.

If an obvious tumor is apparent, a biopsy specimen is taken to establish the diagnosis by frozen section. Sometimes little nodules appear to be tumors but they turn out to be localized superficial cysts of the pancreas. Unless a well-circumscribed tumor nodule is visualized or definitely palpated, the pancreas

must be freed up for a more definitive examination. The peritoneum along the inferior border of the pancreas is incised, taking care on the right side to avoid the middle colic vessels, and on the left side the inferior mesenteric vein (Fig. 2). Blunt finger dissection is used to free up the undersurface of the body and tail of the pancreas. Eventually the fingers can be passed up and around the splenic artery to encircle the substance of the left side of the pancreas completely, without mobilizing the spleen or compromising its blood supply (Fig. 3).

Occasionally the islet-cell adenoma will be located very near the end of the tail of the pancreas and can be missed unless the spleen is well mobilized into view. If no tumor is found, the short gastric vessels should be divided as the initial step in further mobilizing the spleen and pancreas. Any ligature of the blood vessels along the greater curva-

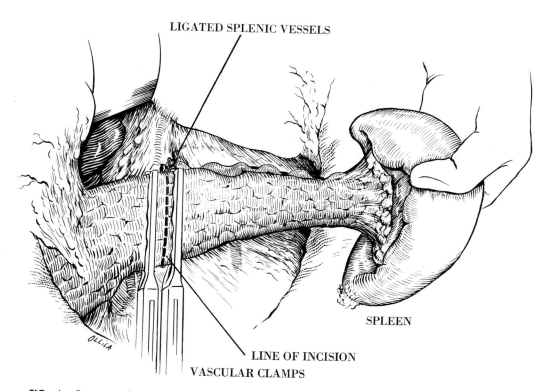

LIGATED SPLENIC VESSELS

SPLEEN

LINE OF INCISION

VASCULAR CLAMPS

FIG. 4.   Presence of microscopic adenomata or hyperplasia of pancreas cannot be excluded by thorough exploration and palpation. Blind resection of body and tail of pancreas is often warranted for microscopic proof of tumor. Mobilization allows spleen and pancreas to be lifted up. Splenic vessels are ligated and divided and distal pancreas and spleen subsequently excised.

ture and fundus of the stomach should include a bit of the gastric wall to make certain there is no slippage of the sutures with subsequent bleeding, should postoperative gastric distension occur. The splenorenal ligament is divided and the spleen delivered outside the wound (Fig. 4). The posterior surface of the body and tail of the pancreas can now be accurately visualized and the gland thoroughly palpated.

If no tumor is found, the surgeon is faced with a dilemma as to how to proceed. The spleen and pancreas can be returned to the abdomen and the pylorus divided to permit introduction of the finger into the lumen of the duodenum in search of a small tumor nodule within its wall. Oberhelman has reported control of the ulcerogenic diathesis following only the local excision of these olive-sized tumors, resection of the duodenal stump, or removal of the head of the pancreas by the Whipple procedure[25] (Fig. 5). The adequacy of the local excision of the tumor in the duodenal wall can be tested by monitoring the output of gastric juice from the gastric tube for 30 or more minutes. If a dramatic decrease occurs, the gastric resection

can be deferred. This location of the tumor is one of the few instances in which local excision of the tumor without removal of all the acid-secreting surface is justified. Should no tumor be found anywhere, it is worthwhile to remove as much of the first part of the duodenum as will permit safe and secure closure without obstructing the lower end of the common bile duct. The pathologist should be urged to study the complete circumference of the duodenal wall in search of microscopic evidence of an aberrant submucosal adenoma.

In general, total gastrectomy has been deferred in the past unless clear-cut evidence of an islet-cell tumor was found. More recently, the widespread availability of the gastrin immuno-assay provides support for total gastrectomy when very high serum gastrin levels have been repeatedly confirmed. On rare occasions, additional support favoring the presence of a hidden tumor can be gained if the output of monitored gastric juice remains high after vagotomy and antrectomy. It is justifiable to delay temporarily total gastrectomy following vagotomy, antrectomy, and removal of the first portion of the duodenum to see if the measured output of gastric juice is altered following these procedures. If the stomach tube continues to yield large volumes of gastric juice, the surgeon may properly proceed with ligation of the left gastric artery and total gastrectomy.

Occasional reports have indicated control of the ulcerogenic syndrome by local excision of tumors of the pancreas other than those occurring in the duodenal wall. The senior author first resected an islet-cell tumor in 1947 with control of the ulcer diathesis for over 4 years by vagotomy and a drainage procedure.[26] The surgeon is loathe to leave behind tumor—especially when it has proved malignant potential—and proceed with total gastrectomy. Either total pancreatectomy or the Whipple procedure can fail because of the high incidence of gastrin-producing metastasis to the liver or lymph nodes, as long as any gastric acid-secreting surface remains. Because of the multicentric location (Fig. 6) of the tumors and the high incidence of malignancy, approaching two out of three cases, it must be realized that an ulcer recurrence rate of approximately 70 percent can be anticipated as long as even a small rim of

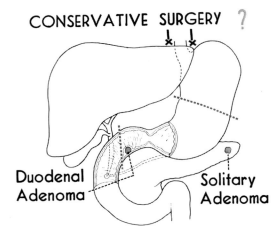

FIG. 5. Total gastrectomy has on occasion been successfully avoided following the local excision of a solitary adenoma within the duodenal wall or the pancreas. The conservative approach may include vagotomy, antrectomy, and removal of the first portion of the duodenum to provide additional insurance against ulcer recurrence.

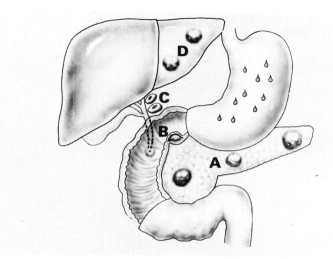

FIG. 6. Multicentric gastrin sources: The very high incidence of multicentric gastrin sources within the pancreas (A), duodenum (B), regional (C) lymph nodes and hepatic metastasis (D) support removal of all acid-secreting surface by total gastrectomy to avoid an extremely high ulcer recurrence rate.

acid-secreting surface remains. Furthermore, it has been suggested by Friesen that the metastases recede or indeed disappear following removal of the target end-organ by total gastrectomy.[27] A much longer period of follow-up will be required to establish this optimistic concept firmly. The patient is indeed exceptionally fortunate who has but one islet-cell tumor that is easily resected. Blind resection of the left side of the pancreas in search of a hidden adenoma or microscopic-size adenomatosis is not difficult, but the yield of tumor is relatively small. A small wedge biopsy of suspicious areas is justifiable as long as the location of the main pancreatic duct is kept in mind and careful hemostasis is maintained.

Once the decision is made to perform total gastrectomy, the surgeon must be certain the abdominal incision is sufficiently large to ensure good exposure. It is helpful to extend the incision up over the lower end of the sternum and remove the xiphoid process. The lower end of the incision should extend to the left and below the umbilicus. The procedure often tends to be complicated, since so many patients have had one, or several previous unsuccessful surgical attempts for ulcer control. Fewer postoperative difficulties can be anticipated if a blind pancreatic resection is not done in search of a hidden adenoma or microscopic evidence of adenomatosis.

A further problem is the difficulty in exposing the esophagogastric junction without potential injury to the musculature of the lower esophagus. This is especially true when the patient has had a previous vagotomy. The usual blind finger dissection carried out in a downward direction after previous vagotomy attempts may result in fraying the esophageal musculature where it is attached to dense adhesions at the hiatus. The diaphragm should be incised just above the hiatus over the lower end of the esophagus to permit blunt finger dissection downward. Sharp dissection under clear vision is used to divide any attachments between the esophagus and the margins of the hiatus. After the left gastric artery has been doubly ligated, and the vagus nerves divided, the esophagus tends to be elongated into the peritoneal cavity for at least 6 to 8 cm. It is advantageous to anchor the esophageal wall to the

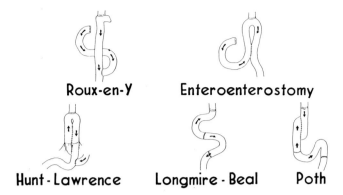

FIG. 7.   Common types of reconstruction after total gastrectomy.

edges of the hiatus with three or four super-ficially placed sutures. Traction on the stomach is maintained to avoid rotation of the esophagus and to provide exposure.

Several 0000 silk sutures are placed in the wall of the esophagus and tied in order to prevent fraying of the lower end of the esophagus as the stomach is divided. These sutures are placed on either side as well as in the anterior and posterior wall of the esophagus just proximal to the point of division. They tend to ensure a firmer cuff of open esophagus for subsequent anastomosis to the jejunum.

Many types of reconstruction have been used after total gastrectomy (Fig. 7). In general, the patient with an islet-cell tumor, for as yet unknown reasons, seems to maintain a better nutritional state than the patient having the same procedure for other causes. The Roux-en-Y has proved to be a satisfactory procedure provided the arm of jejunum is sufficiently long, perhaps 30 cm, to prevent regurgitation. The closed arm of the mobilized jejunum is directed to the left and anchored with interrupted sutures about the hiatus to avoid subsequent tension on the anastomotic suture line. A second layer of sutures anchors the posterior wall of the esophagus to the jejunum before an opening is made into the jejunum. Since a tendency to late stenosis of the esophagojejunal anastomosis has been observed, it appears to be advantageous to pass a large rubber Ewald (20 Fr.) tube after the posterior layer of sutures of the esophagojejunal anastomosis has been placed. The anastomosis is completed with the tube in place, ensuring a larger lumen than could be obtained with the use of the standard Levin tube.

DRAINAGE

After completing the remaining anastomosis of the jejunum to the jejunal limb of the esophageal anastomosis, all openings in the mesentery are carefully tested and closed with interrupted sutures. The large 20 F. tube is replaced by a nasojejunostomy tube, threaded well down into the jejunum beyond the esophageal anastomosis. Some prefer to direct the tube into the duodenum as a precaution against a duodenal stump blow-out. No drainage of the peritoneal cavity is necessary unless the pancreas is resected or a biopsy specimen taken. To ensure external drainage of pancreatic secretions following a left hemipancreatectomy, a small polyethylene tube can be inserted into the pancreatic duct and directed a few centimeters toward the head of the pancreas. This tube, anchored in place by a catgut suture, is brought out through the left upper quadrant with one or more rubber tissue drains.

POSTOPERATIVE CARE

There should be no particular difficulty in the postoperative care of these patients provided the blood volume has been maintained during surgery and the excessive fluid and electrolyte losses from gastric drainage and diarrhea have been corrected. Several liters of gastric juice may have been aspirated before the stomach is removed, which must not be overlooked in calculating the patient's fluid requirement. Antibiotics should be considered, especially in those patients having either a free or walled-off perforation. Fluid collections in the left upper quadrant should be anticipated, especially if a portion of the pancreas has been resected. While leakage at the esophageal suture line can lead to a subphrenic abscess, it is surprising how well the majority of these patients do postoperatively.

Accurate fluid intake and output records, along with daily weights, are essential in monitoring the patient's fluid requirements. Daily serum amylase determinations are made especially if the pancreas has been extensively manipulated or partially resected. Colloid solution, as well as blood, may be required if pancreatitis develops. Within 3 or 4 days, the nasojejunal tube can be removed and oral fluids begun. Within 7 to 10 days, the patient can advance to six small daily feedings. Both the patient and his family should be given dietary instructions, since patients without a stomach tend to be a family curiosity and may unnecessarily become a nutritional problem.

The best results will be obtained if patients are readmitted to the hospital at regular but gradually lengthened intervals.[28] Their weight trends and dietary habits are reviewed. Occasionally additional blood transfusions are helpful in the early postoperative period. The long-term follow-up should include monthly vitamin B12 injections. If difficulty in swallowing occurs or the weight trend is unsatisfactory, the degree of patency of the esophagojejunal anastomosis should be determined by barium studies. Sometimes the area of stenosis responds to dilatation, but a transthoracic approach with revision of the anastomosis is sometimes required. In addition, blood calcium and phosphorus studies should be made over the years

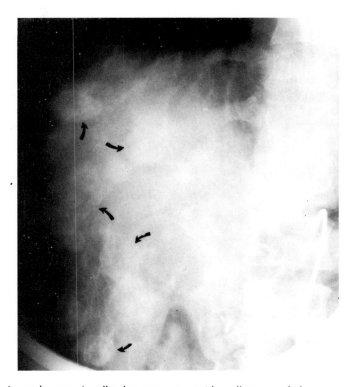

FIG. 8.   Angiography occasionally demonstrates an islet-cell tumor of the pancreas. It is useful in documenting the presence as well as the progress of hepatic metastases. The intrahepatic nodules, shown here, had increased in size 1 year after total gastrectomy.

because of the common association of hyperparathyroidism with the islet-cell ulcerogenic tumor. Many such patients have had a parathyroid adenoma previously resected. Yet in some, the blood calcium will not become elevated until late in the postoperative period.

A clue to the activity of the residual tumor can be gained by serum gastrin determinations. It has been reported by Sanzenbacher, however, that one fasting serum gastrin determination might be normal and therefore not a reliable index of tumor activity. This suggests the additional value of utilizing the calcium gluconate infusion test,[29] which stimulates the release of gastrin. Fifteen mg of calcium gluconate per kilogram of body weight in 500 ml normal saline is given intravenously in a 4-hour test with frequent serum gastrin level determinations. By this test, patients with previously undetected residual tumor may be identified, as serum gastrin levels will be elevated into the ulcerogenic range in patients with residual tumor. Secretin has also been shown to produce a similar gastrin response. Such long-term studies as these may help solve the current riddle of how the metastases of the islet-cell ulcerogenic tumor behave. An aortogram may prove useful not only in demonstrating their presence but also the growth potential after total gastrectomy (Fig. 8).

The morbidity and mortality rates associated with these tumors remain high. As earlier diagnosis can be anticipated from the more widespread availability of the gastrin immuno-assay, the results should improve. A review of the world literature suggests that the overall mortality rate approaches 33 percent. Where total gastrectomy is performed, the mortality rate approximates 18 percent. In a 5-year follow-up of 16 cases having total gastrectomy, there was a mortality rate of 6.5 percent, with 25 percent of the deaths resulting from the persistent growth of the islet-cell tumor. There was an overall 5-year survival rate of 50 percent, which emphasizes that the ulcerogenic islet-cell tumors, although often malignant, have a much better prognosis than other carcinomas of the pancreas.

PALLIATIVE THERAPY

Ordinarily neither chemotherapy nor irradiation therapy is given following total gastrectomy. The growth of the secondary tumor as well as that of the metastases is slow, and the lesions may regress after total gastrectomy. Streptozotocin has been reported to be successful in the treatment of islet-cell carcinomas, especially those of the beta cell type. No doubt new drugs will be available in the future.

DIARRHEOGENIC ISLET-CELL TUMOR SYNDROME

Diarrhea of the steatorrhea type occurs in approximately one-third of the patients with the gastrin-producing islet-cell tumor. Within 2 years of the description of the ulcerogenic islet-cell syndrome, Priest and Alexander reported a patient with an islet-cell tumor; there was an intractable watery diarrhea and extreme potassium depletion, but no ulceration.[30] Verner and Morrison reported two patients, together with more from the literature, who they believed represented a distinct clinical syndrome.[31] Murray, in 1961, documented the presence of achlorhydria in a patient with a watery diarrhea and severe potassium depletion.[32] For a time these rare case reports were considered a variant of the ulcerogenic islet-cell tumor syndrome. The watery diarrhea was so pronounced, however, that the term *pancreatic cholera* was coined to describe the patient's complaints.[33] Marks named this the WDHA syndrome to abbreviate the watery diarrhea, hypokalemia, and achlorhydria typical of these patients.[34] Less than 50 cases have been reported, clearly suggesting that the diagnosis must be frequently overlooked.

The classic syndrome consists of a watery diarrhea of 5 to 6 liters per day.[35] The potassium losses are even more marked than those in patients with a large villous adenoma of the colon. Potassium levels of 2 mEq per liter are not uncommon. Patients are periodically admitted to the hospital in fluid and electrolyte imbalance, often with abnormal abdominal distension from the marked potassium deficiency. These patients may have been hospitalized over a period of months or for several years with signs and symptoms of intestinal obstruction due to low potassium levels. Death has resulted from hypokalemic nephrosis. These patients exhibit achlorhydria or low acid values, which is partially overcome by the augmented histamine test. Hypercalcemia is present in over one-half of the patients, and the incidence of diabetes mellitus approximates 40 percent.

The tumors tend to be much larger than the ulcerogenic type and commonly cause displacement of the stomach or colon as visualized by barium studies. The gallbladder tends to be considerably enlarged and the small bowel filled with a clear fluid due to the physiological effects of the polypeptide produced by these tumors. Evidence has been presented by Zollinger et al. that the hormone produced is secretin.[36] Until an accurate immuno-assay for secretin is developed and sufficient tumor tissue is available for amino-acid sequence studies, a final answer is not available.

Local excision of the tumor is all that is required. No other intestinal procedure is indicated. More than one tumor has been found in the pancreas, which indicates the necessity of a thorough examination of the entire gland. Approximately 50 percent of the tumors are malignant. In this group, the reported survival is about 1 year.

There is no special postoperative care required other than that specifically related to the extent of the resection of the pancreas. If steroid therapy has been given to control the diarrhea, the necessity of continued therapy in the immediate postoperative period should not be overlooked. The diabetes so frequently present requires careful and frequent monitoring. Blood calcium levels may return to normal after removal of the tumor. If the calcium levels remain persistently elevated, the parathyroid glands should be explored.

The diarrhea and potassium loss is immediately corrected after removal of the tumor, and the achlorhydria is replaced by normal or elevated acid values. The latter observation is consistent with removal of the inhibiting effect of secretin. No specific program of chemotherapy or irradiation has been developed because of the limited number of case reports.

REFERENCES

1. Zollinger, R. M., and Ellison, E. H., Ann. Surg. 142:709, 1955.
2. Whipple, A. O., J. Internat. Chir. 3:237, 1938.
3. Gregory, R. A., Tracy, H. J., French, J. M., and Sircus, W., Lancet 1:1045, 1960.
4. Grossman, M. I., Tracy, H. J., and Gregory, R. A., Gastroenterology 41:87, 1961.
5. Gregory, R. A., and Tracy, H. J., Gut 5:103, 1964.
6. Wilson, S. D., Schulte, W. J., and Meade, R. C., Arch. Surg. 103:108, 1971.
7. Christoforidis, A. J., and Nelson, S. W., J.A.M.A. 198:511, 1966.
8. McGuigan, J. E., and Trudeau, W. L., New Engl. J. Med. 278:1308, 1968.
9. Ellison, E. H., and Wilson, S. D., Ann. Surg. 160:512, 1964.
10. Elliott, D. W., Taft, D. A., Passaro, E., Jr., and Zollinger, R. M., Surgery 50:126, 1961.
11. Bloodworth, J. M. B., and Elliott, D. W., J.A.M.A. 183:1011, 1963.
12. Winship, D. H., and Ellison, E. H., Lancet 1:1128, 1967.
13. Way, L., Goldman, L., and Dunphy, J. E., Am. J. Surg. 116:293, 1968.
14. Ruppert, R. D., Greenberger, N. J., Beman, F. M., and McCullough, F. M., Ann. Intern. Med. 67:808, 1967.
15. Alfidi, R. J., Skillern, P. G., and Crile, G., Jr., Cleve. Clin. Q. 36:41, 1969.
16. Ghosh, M. N., and Schild, H. O., Br. J. Pharmacol. 13:54, 1958.
17. Lai, K. S., Gut 5:327, 1964.
18. Thompson, C. G., Cleator, I. G., and Sircus, W., Gut 11:409, 1970.
19. Moore, F. T., Murat, J., Endahl, G. L., Baker, J. L., and Zollinger, R. M., Am. J. Surg. 113:735, 1967.
20. Wilson, S. D., Mathison, J. A., Schulte, W. J., and Ellison, E. H., Arch. Surg. 97:437, 1968.
21. Trudeau, W. L., and McGuigan, J. E., New Engl. J. Med. 281:862, 1969.
22. Passaro, E., Jr., Basso, N., Sanchez, R. E., et al. Am. J. Surg. 120:138, 1970.
23. Passaro, E., Jr., Basso, N., and Walsh, J. H., Calcium challenge in the Zollinger-Ellison syndrome. Surgery 72:60–67, July, 1972.
24. Zollinger, R. M., Vogel, T. T., and Sherman, N., In J. D. Hardy, ed., Critical Surgical Illness, Philadelphia, 1971, p. 15.
25. Oberhelman, H. A., Jr., Arch. Surg. 104:447, 1972.

26. Ellison, E. H., Surgery 40:147, 1956.
27. Friesen, S. R., Ann. Surg. 168:483, 1968.
28. Zollinger, R. M., King, D. R., and Sanzenbacher, L. J., Presented before 9 EME Congres International De L'Association Des Societes National Europeennes Et Mediterraneennes De Gastro-Enterologie, July 8, 1972 (In press.)
29. Sanzenbacher, L. J., King, D. R., and Zollinger, R. M., Am. J. Surg. January 1973.
30. Priest, W. M., and Alexander, M. K., Lancet 2:1145, 1957.
31. Verner, J. V., and Morrison, A. B., Am. J. Med. 25:374, 1958.
32. Murray, J. S., Paton, R. R., and Pope, C. E., New Engl. J. Med. 264:436, 1961.
33. Matsumoto, K. K., Peter, J. B., and Schultze, R. G., et al., Gastroenterology 50:231, 1966.
34. Marks, I. N., Bank, S., and Louw, J. H., Gastroenterology 52:695, 1967.
35. Kraft, A. R., Tompkins, R. K., and Zollinger, R. M., Am. J. Surg. 119:163, 1970.
36. Zollinger, R. M., Tompkins, R. K., Amerson, J. R., Endahl, G. L., Kraft, A. R., and Moore, F. T., Ann. Surg. 168:502, 1968.

14

SECTION OF THE VAGUS NERVES TO THE STOMACH IN THE TREATMENT OF PEPTIC ULCER

LESTER R. DRAGSTEDT

The employment of section of the vagus nerves to the stomach in the treatment of peptic ulcer was based on a long series of experimental and clinical studies on the pathogenesis of peptic ulcer and the physiology of gastric secretion which began in 1924 [1] and has continued to the present time. As a result of these studies, I became persuaded that duodenal ulcers are caused by a hypersecretion of gastric juice of nervous origin brought on in some way by the tensions, strains, and competitive efforts of modern life. It was my view that gastric ulcers, on the other hand, are caused by a hypersecretion of gastric juice of hormonal or gastrin origin brought on by stasis of food in the stomach, due either to pyloric stenosis or to a relative gastric atony. The prolonged contact of food with the mucosa of the antrum causes a continuing release of gastrin with continuing stimulation of gastric secretion, until the gastric content approximates pure gastric juice in its concentration of free hydrochloric acid and pepsin. One of my most significant early experiments on the nature of the ulcer problem was the finding that pure, undiluted gastric juice, as it is secreted by the parietal cells in the body of the stomach, is an exceedingly corrosive fluid and has the capacity to digest away the normal gastric or intestinal mucous membrane.[2] In these early experiments, I drained the gastric juice from Heidenhain pouches into the ileum or jejunum in dogs instead of to the exterior, which is the usual method. Chronic progressive ulcers resembling the clinical lesions regularly appeared in the intestine near the anastomosis with the isolated stomach pouch. In other experiments with isolated whole stomach pouches,[3] I found that the stomach mucosa itself is digested away by pure undiluted gastric juice if the exposure is prolonged. If it be granted that pure gastric juice has this corrosive power, the logical question is: Why then do not all people have chronic, progressive peptic ulcers? The answer seems to lie in the protective effect of the normal mechanism that controls the secretion of gastric juice. In the interval between meals, when the stomach is empty of food, a very meager secretion of gastric juice occurs. The output of free hydrochloric acid in this basal or continuous secretion in normal people averages about 1 mEq per hour. The normal stimulus for gastric secretion is food-taking, and food is the chief agent that dilutes and buffers the acid of the gastric juice and protects the mucous membrane from its corrosive action. Gastric secretion is stimulated initially by impulses in the vagus nerves aroused reflexly by the sight, odor, and taste of food. When food enters the stomach, gastric motility is stimulated and the food comes in contact with the mucous membrane of the gastric antrum. The hormone gastrin is then liberated into the bloodstream and continues the stimulation of gastric secretion until the gastric contents become acid in reaction. At pH 3.5, the release of gastrin from the antrum begins to decrease, and when the acidity of the gastric content reaches pH 1.5, the release of gastrin from the antrum is completely checked. The passage of the acid-gastric content into the duodenum stimulates the secretion of pancreatic juice and bile. This is brought about by the hormone, pancreatic secretin, which is released from the mucous membrane of the duodenum when it comes in contact with acid. Secretin not only stimulates the secretion of pancreatic juice, but also has a profound inhibitory effect on the secretion of gastric juice. There is, thus, a remarkable mechanism that provides for the secretion of gastric juice when there is food in the stomach and provides it in sufficient amounts to digest the food. This mechanism also checks further gastric secretion before the gastric content becomes sufficiently corrosive to break down the mucous membrane. What abnormality in this physiological control of gastric secretion could occur in disease that would provide for a gastric content as corrosive as pure gastric secretion? Two possibilities immediately come to mind: first, if there should occur a stimulation of gastric secretion by agencies other than food, and second, if such a hypersecretion of gastric juice should occur so that the buffering and neutralizing action of the food would be overcome. Both of these factors have been found to be operative in patients with chronic, progressive peptic ulcers, and in my view, they present a sufficient cause for the lesions. This view, of course, does not exclude the possibility that other factors such as impairment of the blood supply to the mucosa, deficiency of mucus secretion, mechanical trauma, or other factors may play an additional role in some patients.

The concept that duodenal ulcers are usually caused by a hypersecretion of gastric juice of nervous origin was stimulated by the report of Henning and Norpoth [4] that patients with duodenal ulcer are often found to contain large amounts of pure gastric juice in the stomach while they are asleep in the hospital at night. We immediately confirmed this observation and began to measure the gastric secretion in the empty stomach of our patients at night when they were shielded from the usual physiological stimuli for gastric secretion. We soon found that duodenal ulcer patients regularly secrete from 3 to 10 times as much gastric juice in the fasting, empty stomach at night as do normal people. The finding of Hay, Varco, Code, and Wangensteen [5] that duodenal ulcers regularly appear in laboratory animals when a continued secretion of gastric juice is induced by the intramuscular injection of pellets of histamine in beeswax indicated that this hypersecretion was probably significant. The occurrence of duodenal ulcers in patients subjected to long, continued mental strains suggested that the hypersecretion was probably of nervous origin and accordingly in 1935 we suggested that division of the vagus nerves to the stomach might well find a definite place in ulcer therapy.[6] We did not perform my first vagotomy, however, until almost 10 years later,[7] when clinical experience with resection of the lower esophagus for carcinoma by Ohsawa's method [8] convinced me that complete division of the vagus nerves in man was compatible with life and good nutrition, as it is in the dog.

In peptic ulcer patients, the therapeutic value of complete division of the vagus nerves to the stomach is due to the marked reduction in gastric secretion produced by the operation and, to a lesser extent, to the reduction of the tonus and motility of the stomach. This is accomplished without causing serious complications or side-effects. The reduction in gastric secretion is effected by abolition of the nervous phase of gastric secretion, abolition of the vagal release of gastrin, and reduction in the sensitivity or responsiveness of the parietal cells to humoral stimuli. The method is relatively new, the first operations of the present type being performed in January and February of 1943. In the succeeding years my associates and I have used these methods in operating upon approximately 2,400 patients with various types of peptic ulcer.

A review of the surgical literature indicates that operations on the vagus nerves to the stomach for the treatment of peptic ulcer, gastric crisis of tabes, and other diseases were performed by surgeons in the past. Stierlin, Bircher, Latarget, and Schiassi, as well as others, have described and illustrated operative procedures on the stomach designed to sever the vagus nerve supply. Brief and incomplete reference has usually been made to the results secured. A study of these reports and inspection of the drawings supplied suggest that the anatomy of the vagus nerves to the stomach was not very well known and that in the operations described a complete vagotomy was not usually obtained. In our own experience, complete division of the vagus nerves to the stomach, when combined with an adequate drainage procedure, has caused such immediate and persistent relief of ulcer distress, together with objective evidence of healing of the lesion, that it seems likely had a similar result been secured by the early workers, the operation would have long since become widely adopted. The fact that vagotomy did not become popular is perhaps the best evidence that the earlier methods were unsuccessful in securing complete interruption of all vagus nerves to the stomach.

CAUSE OF DUODENAL ULCER

The failure of the gastric and duodenal mucosa to be digested away in normal individuals appeared to demand the postulate of a local decrease in resistance if ulceration were to be accounted for on the basis of peptic digestion. This requirement led naturally to the view that peptic ulcers were caused by a local decrease in the resistance of the mucosa brought on by vascular impairment, deficiency of protective mucus, local allergy, anoxia of the cells, or other factors. The prompt recurrence of ulceration after the local excision of peptic ulcers, however, cast grave doubts on this view of a local decrease in resistance as being the causative factor in the disease, and careful examination of resected stomachs has also usually failed to reveal evidence of a pathological vascular condition. It has been possible to produce acute ulcers in the stomachs of experimental laboratory animals by vascular

occlusion, by the local injection of caustic chemicals, or by burning with hot metal discs. These acute ulcers regularly heal in 3 or 4 weeks and rarely display chronicity and progression—cardinal characteristics of the disease seen in man. There is, moreover, good evidence indicating that in human ulcer patients the corrosive and digestive properties of the gastric content are much greater than in normal people. The corrosive properties of the gastric content are a result of the presence of gastric juice secreted by the body and fundus of the stomach. The other material present—mainly food, swallowed saliva, the mucoid secretion from the gastric antrum, and regurgitated duodenal secretions—is largely buffering or protective in effect. When an excessive secretion of gastric juice occurs, the corrosive properties of the gastric content approach that of the pure fundic secretion. The key to the ulcer problem was probably provided by the demonstration that pure, undiluted gastric juice has the capacity to digest all living tissues including the wall of the stomach and duodenum, and that when this digestion occurs ulceration exactly like that encountered in patients is reproduced.[6] The experimental ulcers produced in animals by hypersecretion of gastric juice resembled those seen in man in appearance and in the characteristics of chronicity and progression.

The evidence that duodenal ulcers are caused by a hypersecretion of gastric juice of nervous origin may be summarized as follows: Duodenal ulcer patients usually secrete from 3 to 10 times as much hydrochloric acid in the basal fasting secretion as do normal people. When a hypersecretion of this degree is reproduced in experimental animals, ulcers exactly resembling the clinical lesions usually appear. Complete division of the vagus nerves to the stomach in duodenal ulcer patients abolishes the fasting hypersecretion, indicating that it is of nervous origin and is mediated by the vagus nerves. It seems probable that in some way tensions and strains of modern life produce a secretory hypertonus in the vagus centers and that it is in this way that the central nervous system plays its role in the cause of the disease. When the fasting hypersecretion in duodenal ulcer patients is terminated by vagotomy, the ulcers usually heal, and if an adequate drainage operation has also been performed to prevent stasis of food in the gastric antrum, they remain healed.

THE CAUSE OF GASTRIC ULCERS

The evidence that gastric ulcers are usually caused by a hypersecretion of gastric juice of hormonal origin, while not complete, is nevertheless impressive. Experimental data are now satisfactory to indicate the validity of Edkin's gastric hypothesis, namely, that the gastric phase of secretion is mediated exclusively by the antrum of the stomach, which functions as an endocrine organ, producing and releasing the gastric stimulating hormone, gastrin. Gregory [10] and his associates have isolated gastrin in pure form from the antrum, determined its chemical composition, and synthesized it. Factors causing the release of gastrin from the antrum have been found to be contact of the mucosa with food or the development of tension within the stomach as a result of peristalsis.[9] A hypersecretion of gastric juice of humoral origin with typical peptic ulcer formation in the stomach, duodenum, and jejunum has been reproduced in experimental animals. It is probable that a hypersecretion of gastric juice of hormonal origin occurs in man when prolonged stasis of food in contact with the antrum mucosa occurs. This may be caused either by pyloric stenosis or by deficient gastric peristalsis or atony. We have been able to produce chronic progressive ulcers in dogs and rats by experimental pyloric stenosis. I have also been able to produce typical chronic progressive gastric ulcers in swine and rabbits by producing gastric atony by division of the vagus nerves to the stomach.[11] Delayed emptying of the stomach has been found in a large proportion of gastric ulcer patients, and in approximately 20 percent of these, pyloric stenosis from a previous duodenal ulcer has probably caused hypermotility and increased tension within the antrum as well. Experimental data indicate that stasis of food in the stomach caused by diminished gastric motility and tonus, such as that affected by vagotomy, can produce a hypersecretion of gastric juice of hormonal origin sufficient to produce ulceration in the stomach. These concepts are in harmony with surgical experience. Resection of the antrum exerts a curative effect on gastric ulcers (even those left in situ near the esophagus), and gastrojejunal ulcers rarely or never develop. On the other hand, antrum resection for duodenal ulcer has been followed by a high incidence of recurrent gastrojejunal ulceration, and larger resections or resections combined with vagotomy have been employed.

GASTRIC SECRETORY TESTS IN ULCER PATIENTS

I have become convinced that a measurement of the basal or continuous secretion of gastric juice in the fasting empty stomach is a most important and useful procedure. It has supplanted all other gastric secretion tests in our clinic. The patient is placed on a liquid diet for 24 hours to make sure there is no solid food in the stomach. An intragastric nasal tube is introduced at 9 P.M. and continuous gastric aspiration made for 12 hours (until 9 A.M.). During this time, the patient is shielded from the sight, odor, or taste of food, and he usually sleeps. The volume of the gastric aspirate is then measured, and its free acid concentration determined. If the volume is expressed in liters and the free acid concentration in clinical units, the product of the two gives the amount of free hydrochloric acid in terms of mEq. Normal people put out between 10 and 20 mEq of free hydrochloric acid in the fasting nocturnal secretion in a 12-hour period. Duodenal ulcer patients, in my experience, may put out from 40 to 200 mEq or even more. If the output is 100 mEq or greater, the likelihood of medical management proving successful is remote, and surgical treatment is definitely indicated. In some hospitals the 12-hour basal secretion collection is difficult to obtain and in this case recourse may be had to a 2- or 4-hour test. A 1-hour test is, however, apt to provide inaccurate data. The basal or continuous secretion in the empty stomach of man and animals is almost entirely of nervous origin and is terminated if the vagus nerves to the stomach are completely divided. It provides an index of the importance of the nervous phase of gastric secretion or the secretory tonus of the vagus nerves in the ulcer patient.

The augmented histamine test of Kay is widely employed in the examination of ulcer patients, and I have used it to amplify the information obtained by measurements of the basal secretion. The augmented histamine test provides a rough measurement of the parietal cell mass or the number of acid-secreting cells in the stomach. These are markedly increased in patients with long-standing duodenal ulcers. This increase in the parietal cell mass has been attributed by some investigators to an hereditary defect. I prefer the view that the increase in the parietal cell mass in duodenal ulcer patients is caused by hyperplasia and hypertrophy of the gastric glands as a result of long, continued stimulation by vagus impulses. Indeed, there is experimental evidence now that long, continuous stimulation of gastric secretion produces an increase in the parietal cell mass in animals. The augmented histamine test is reproducible and provides information concerning the amount of gastric juice that is produced when an apppropriate stimulus to gastric secretion is applied. It does not, however, provide information concerning the amount of gastric juice that is secreted in the empty stomach when the patient is asleep, and there is no obvious stimulant for gastric secretion. It is under these conditions, when there is no buffering food in the stomach, that it is important to know how much of the corrosive gastric juice is being produced.

Most gastric ulcer patients put out less acid in the basal fasting secretion than do normal people. This finding has led some observers to doubt that gastric ulcers are produced by a hypersecretion of gastric juice. Here again data from the experimental laboratory have proved helpful. Contact of food with the antrum mucosa evokes a stimulation of gastric secretion through liberation of the hormone, gastrin, and this mechanism persists unabated without evidence of fatigue for at least 24 hours. Hurst [12] was one of the first to point out that the gastric ulcer patient usually has an atonic, slowly emptying stomach, and although at the present time adequate tests to determine the presence or absence of gastric retention in ulcer patients are not usually made, I am persuaded that Hurst was correct in his impressions. Retention of food

in the stomach and contact with antrum mucosa will probably cause a continuing secretion of gastric juice until the gastric content becomes sufficiently acid to prevent the further release of gastrin. Although it is true that most gastric ulcer patients secrete less acid in the basal secretion than do normal people, there are some in which the basal secretion is abnormally great. Many of these patients have had a previous duodenal ulcer that has caused pyloric stenosis and gastric retention. However, my son, L. R. Dragstedt, II,[13] has observed gastric ulcer patients with a high basal secretion but without evidence of a previous duodenal ulcer. It is quite likely that this is the type of gastric ulcer patient who in former times developed a gastro-jejunal ulcer after gastroenterostomy or low gastric resection. If the basal secretion of gastric juice is abnormally high, the probability is that the ulcer is caused by a hypersecretion of gastric juice of nervous origin, whereas if the basal secretion is abnormally low, one must conclude that a hypertonus of the vagus secretory mechanism is not present and the ulcer is therefore probably caused by a hypersecretion of humoral origin. Stimulation of gastric secretion by the gastrin mechanism is absent when there is no food in the stomach except for the relatively rare patients within an associated Zollinger-Ellison tumor. These tumors release gastrin continuously into the bloodstream irrespective of the presence or absence of food in the stomach. Measurement of the basal secretion is helpful in the diagnosis of these tumors. If a basal hypersecretion is found and this is not reduced by more than 25 percent as a result of the administration of propantheline bromide (Pro-banthine), one may conclude that a Zollinger-Ellison tumor is probably present. If the hypersecretion is of nervous origin, probantheline bromide will usually reduce it from 50 to 75 percent.

The beneficial effect of vagotomy in those ulcer patients in whom a hypersecretion of gastric juice of nervous origin has been found is readily accounted for. Why do a vagotomy in those gastric ulcer patients in whom the basal secretion is already subnormal, indicating that a hypotonus of the vagus secretory mechanism is probably present? It has been found both in man and animals that after vagotomy the response of the gastric glands to histamine, gastrin, and probably other similar stimulants is profoundly reduced.[14] Vagus impulses stimulate gastric secretion by causing a release of gastrin from the antrum in addition to the direct stimulating effect on the gastric glands. At the present time it is not known how significant this vagal release of gastrin is. Some workers believe that it represents a very considerable share of the total amount of gastric juice secreted. This vagal release of gastrin would, of course, be eliminated by vagotomy, and this factor may contribute to the beneficial effect of the operation. Recent experience with vagotomy and gastroenterostomy in the treatment of gastric ulcer indicates that this procedure is more effective than gastroenterostomy alone.

TRANSABDOMINAL VAGOTOMY

While division of the vagus nerves by a left transthoracic approach was the operation first performed by me, it has now been practically abandoned except for those patients who have had repeated gastric resections with subsequent jejunal ulcer formation. General anesthesia with ether or cyclopropane and curare is commonly employed. It is important to secure good relaxation. A long midline or left paramedian incision is made, extending from the xyphoid cartilage to 2 or 3 cm below the umbilicus. The stomach, duodenum, and other abdominal organs are then inspected and palpated. The left lobe of the liver is secured by the surgeon and pulled downward into the operative field (Fig. 1). This maneuver exposes the coronary ligament to the left lobe of the liver, and this can then be most easily divided with scissors by the assistant surgeon. After division of the ligament, the left lobe of the liver is retracted to the right by a gallbladder retractor. The upper part of the stomach and the lower end of the esophagus then come into view. A small transverse incision is made in the diaphragm about 1 cm above the esophageal hiatus (Fig. 2). This opening is enlarged by blunt dissection with the scissors and fingers. If a Levin tube has previously been introduced into the stomach, palpation of the esophagus is facilitated. The surgeon's index finger is then introduced over

the esophagus into the mediastinum. By gentle finger dissection the lower portion of the esophagus is separated from the surrounding loose areolar tissue. Care must be taken at this point not to penetrate the pleura. As the surgeon's fingers surround the esophagus, the vagus nerves can be felt posteriorly as they extend downward to the lesser curvature of the stomach. The esophagus is pulled downward into the abdomen for a distance of 6 to 8 cm (Fig. 3). When this is done, the left or anterior vagus nerve usually comes into view, extending along the front of the esophagus toward the lesser curvature of the stomach. The right, or posterior vagus nerve is felt as a firm cord posterior to the esophagus and usually close to its right border. It is usually convenient to separate the right vagus nerve from the esophageal wall by finger dissection and to pull this trunk around to the left or splenic side of the esophagus, where it can be ligated and divided. In most instances, the right vagus nerve is exposed for a distance of 6 to 8 cm above its entrance into the wall of the stomach along the posterior portion of the lesser curvature. A clamp is placed on this nerve as far superiorly as possible, and the nerve is then divided between silk or linen ligatures (Fig. 4). At this stage, a segment of 4 to 6 cm of the nerve may be resected if desired. The left vagus nerve is similarly freed from the anterior wall of the lower esophagus by finger dissection and cut between ligatures. This nerve also is divided 6 to 8 cm above its entrance into the stomach along the lesser curvature. Following division of the nerves, it will usually be possible to pull the esophagus still farther into the abdomen. This permits a careful review of the anterior and posterior wall to make certain that all vagus fibers have been divided. In about 50 percent of cases, only two large trunks are seen; in the remaining 50 percent, the anterior vagus nerve may be represented by two or more main branches, and in a smaller number, the right or posterior vagus may be found as two or more trunks. The esophagus and proximal end of the cut and tied vagus nerves are then allowed to retract upward into the mediastinum. The opening in the diaphragm is closed with several interrupted catgut sutures. The left lobe of the liver is then placed in its previous position,

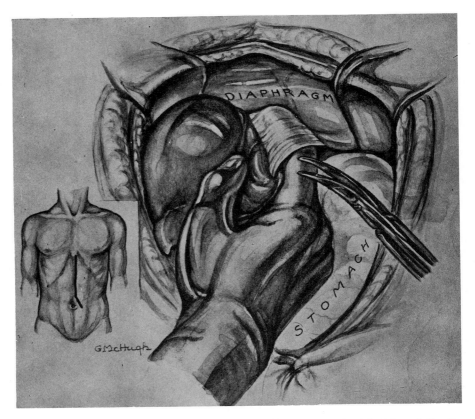

FIG. 1. Subdiaphragmatic vagotomy. The coronary ligament to the left lobe of the liver is divided.

but it is usually unnecessary to suture the coronary ligament. A posterior gastroenterostomy is now performed, making the anastomosis within 6 cm of the pylorus. The stoma should not be larger than 1.5 cm in diameter, to prevent the dumping syndrome. A pyloroplasty of the type described by Weinberg [15] may be substituted in place of the gastroenterostomy. Some surgeons prefer a pyloroplasty of the Finney type, believing that it provides better drainage of the vagotomized stomach. Postoperative decompression of the stomach is secured by means of a Foley bag inserted into the fundus of the stomach along the greater curvature by two infolding purse-string sutures. The catheter is wrapped with omentum and led through a stab wound to the left of the incision. Complete decompression of the stomach is secured by continuous suction applied to this tube for 5 days after the operation. During this time, the patient is given 3,000 cc of physiological salt solution intravenously each 24 hours. The 12-hour night secretion is collected in the usual way and the acid output determined. In the usual case, the output of acid will be found to be less than 10 mEq in a 12-hour period. If values higher than 20 mEq are repeatedly found, it is likely that all vagus fibers have not been divided or that the patient has a hypersecretion owing to a tumor of the type described by Ellison and Zollinger. On the sixth day, the patient is permitted small amounts of liquids, and this feeding is gradually increased by the addition of semisolid food. Satisfactory emptying is determined by aspiration on the gastrostomy tube in the evening. Some surgeons have stated that postoperative decompression of the stomach after vagotomy is not necessary and should be avoided. I am persuaded that this is a mistake. It is true that many patients get along well without decompression, but the occasional patient

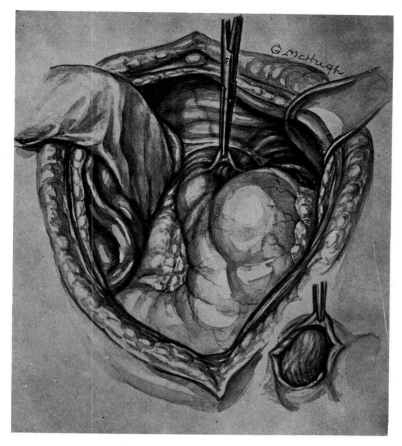

FIG. 2. Subdiaphragmatic vagotomy. The exposure of the esophagus. (From Dragstedt et al. *Ann. Surg.* 126:691, 1947.)

who develops a dilated stomach causes great anxiety and trouble and may continue to have unpleasant symptoms. Adequate decompression until the stomach has regained its tone and normal peristaltic activity has in our experience been the most important factor in postoperative management. A final determination of the night secretion is made on the eleventh postoperative day and the tube removed. The patient is brought back for subsequent measurements of the nocturnal gastric secretion at intervals of 6 months, 1 year, and 2 years. If the fasting nocturnal gastric secretion still yields values below 20 mEq of acid, and if x-ray examination shows no stasis of food in the antrum, the patient will probably remain free of recurrent ulceration.

SELECTIVE GASTRIC VAGOTOMY

Griffith, Harkins, Burge, Holle, Franksson, and others have demonstrated that it is possible and practical to divide the vagus nerves to the stomach alone and spare vagus fibers to the gallbladder, duodenum, pancreas, small intestines, and colon. This is of course theoretically desirable because, so far as we know, the beneficial effect of vagotomy is limited to its effect on the secretory and motor function of the stomach. Present techniques for selective vagotomy are more difficult and time-consuming than truncal vagotomy, as previously described. There is also

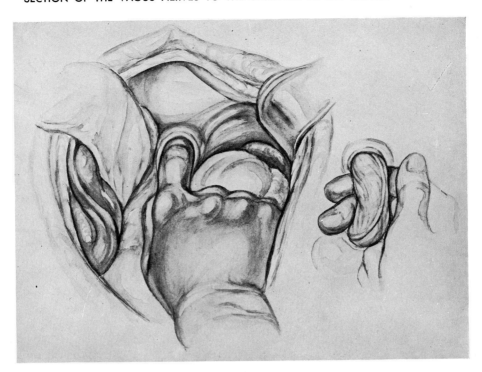

FIG. 3. Subdiaphragmatic vagotomy. Mobilization of the esophagus. (From Dragstedt et al. *Ann. Surg.* 126:691, 1947.)

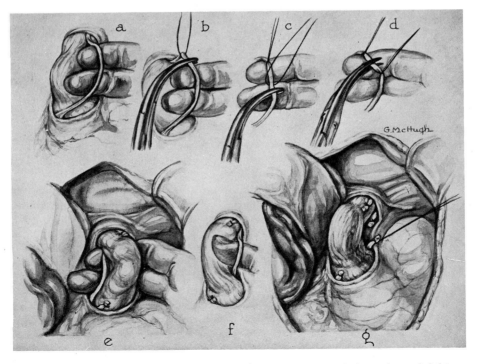

FIG. 4. Subdiaphragmatic vagotomy. The isolation and division of the right and left vagus nerves. (From Dragstedt et al. *Ann. Surg.* 126:691, 1947.)

the hazard of hemorrhage from the left gastric artery. These considerations must be balanced against the advantages that have been claimed for selective vagotomy. It was originally claimed that steatorrhoea and diarrhea were common complications of truncal vagotomy and were caused by impaired pancreatic function as a result of division of the vagus nerves. There was little direct evidence in support of this view. Subsequently it has been found that there is no significant difference in the quantity of fat in the stools of patients undergoing vagotomy of either type. I suspected that this would prove to be the case in view of the large factor of safety in pancreatic digestion. It is possible to remove up to two-thirds of the pancreas in animals without producing a defect in pancreatic digestion—provided the remnant of pancreas is supplied by a pancreatic duct. It also appears doubtful that division of the vagus nerves to the gallbladder causes any serious impairment of gallbladder function. The chief stimulant for gallbladder contraction is the hormone cholecystokinin, which is released from the duodenal mucosa on contact with fat or other substances in the diet. Fear that patients who have had a truncal vagotomy might display an increased incidence of gallstones in subsequent years has not been borne out by our experience. Nevertheless, it would appear wise at the present time for the surgeon who does a great deal of work in this area to familiarize himself with the detailed anatomy of the vagus supply to the stomach. He would then be in a position to employ selective vagotomy in those patients in whom, in his judgment, the procedure appears safe and easy to accomplish. When, however, adequate exposure is difficult to secure because the patient is fat, a truncal vagotomy should certainly be done, as the presumed advantages of selective vagotomy are meager and debatable.

POSTOPERATIVE COMPLICATIONS

In addition to the complications incident to laparotomy with manipulation of the upper viscera, a varying proportion of patients complain of symptoms that appear to be directly referable to the division of the vagus nerve supply to the gastrointestinal tract. These are usually trifling and inconsequential, and several writers have magnified them unduly. The most common complaints include sensations of distension in the upper abdomen, frequent belching (often of malodorous gas), and episodes of diarrhea. It is quite probable that the marked reduction in the acidity of the gastric content following vagotomy materially reduces the resistance of these patients to diarrheas of bacterial origin. They are also undoubtedly more susceptible than they were before to the ingestion of spoiled or contaminated foods, and this is especially true if abnormal stasis in the stomach occurs. Under these conditions, fermentation and bacterial putrefaction of food may occur with the resultant production of irritant chemical substances that cause diarrhea when they are discharged into the intestines. The vagus nerves are known to exert a tonic, augmenter effect on the motility of the stomach, and after their division the inhibitory effect of the sympathetic nerves prevails. If the stomach is permitted to become overdistended with gas or accumulated secretion in the immediate postoperative period, this overdistension further decreases gastric tonus and motility and is probably of greater significance than the inhibitory action of the sympathetic nerves. If overdistension is carefully prevented by gastric decompression for 4 or 5 days after the operation, the motility of the stomach gradually returns toward the normal level. In my experience, this prolonged decompression and gradual resumption of feeding with small amounts of food at first has practically eliminated diarrhea, distension, and belching as complications of truncal vagotomy.

A few patients have complained of dysphagia during the first 2 to 6 weeks after the operation. In most instances, this has been a result of trauma to the lower esophagus produced by separation and division of the vagus branches.

Esophagoscopic examination has revealed unilateral edema of the mucous membrane in several cases, and the esophagoscope has passed readily into the stomach with subsequent complete relief of symptoms. In many patients with duodenal ulcer, peptic esophagitis of varying degree is an associated lesion. We have encountered several patients with duodenal ulcers and simultaneous ulcers in the lower esophagus that healed after vagotomy with subsequent organic obstruction in the region of the cardia. A true cardiospasm has not so far been encountered in our series of vagotomy patients. Indeed, in my experience, one of the fringe benefits of vagotomy has been the relief of symptoms referable to a hiatal hernia. While division of the vagus nerves has permitted the stomach to be drawn downward into the abdomen, nevertheless I believe that the benefit has been obtained from reduction in the corrosive properties of the gastric content, brought about by the vagotomy. The relief of peptic esophagitis produced by the vagotomy has probably been more important in these patients than has prevention of reflux of gastric content into the esophagus.

I have never encountered serious symptoms associated with the separation, clamping, and division of the vagus nerves in the region of the cardia, and I believe that whatever reflex effects may be produced by the operation are inconsequential. It has not been my practice to infiltrate the vagus nerves with cocaine before division. Cases of sudden death during the course of a vagotomy operation have, however, been reported and have been attributed to vago-vagal reflexes. In view of the rare occurrence of this catastrophe, the possibility must be considered that these deaths were caused by the anesthetic rather than by the vagal trauma.

Concern has been expressed by some writers that vagotomy may lead to anesthesia of the stomach or duodenum together with the overlying peritoneum so that a painless progression or perforation of the ulcer might occur following the operation. This fear is probably groundless. The prompt disappearance of ulcer pain following vagotomy owes to the marked reduction in the concentration of free acid in the stomach and to a decrease in gastric tonus and motility and not to anesthesia of the gastric wall. Typical ulcer pain can be reproduced immediately after complete vagotomy for active duodenal ulcers if acid is instilled into the stomach. Crushing the vagus trunks at the level of the lower esophagus in conscious patients does not produce pain. The evidence is now fairly complete that sensory fibers conveying a sense of pain from the stomach, duodenum, and neighboring peritoneum pass to the sympathetic trunks and not to the vagus nerves.

GASTRIC VAGOTOMY FOR GASTRIC ULCERS

In 1943, when I first began performing supradiaphragmatic vagotomy for the treatment of peptic ulcers, I did not appreciate the necessity for combining the operation with an adequate drainage procedure. One hundred fifty-eight ulcer patients were treated by vagotomy alone, usually by a transthoracic approach. Many of these patients developed the unpleasant symptoms of gastric distension, belching, and diarrhea, and seven of them who were operated upon for duodenal ulcers subsequently developed typical gastric ulcers. When the transabdominal approach was adopted, and gastroenterostomy, pyloroplasty, or antrum resection was added to the vagotomy, I was impressed with the fact that gastric ulcers failed to develop as a complication in these patients. Indeed, some eight patients with gastric ulcers were treated by vagotomy and gastroenterostomy in this early period. I was gratified to see even large gastric ulcers on the lesser curvature heal promptly after this procedure. The operation was criticized, however, on the basis that it was unwise not to remove a gastric ulcer as it might be malignant or subsequently become malignant. At that time, several surgeons reported that from 15 to 20 percent of stomachs that were resected with a diagnosis of benign gastric ulcer actually turned out to be carcinomas when examined by the pathologists. In the intervening years since then, the situation has changed in two respects. The incidence of carcinoma of the stomach in the United States has declined. In a recent survey of 3,000 gastric resections performed for gastric ulcers in the Veterans Administration Hospitals, only 4 percent of the specimens revealed the presence of carcinoma. A second factor influencing surgical treatment has been the demonstration by Dorton,[16] Faris, as well as ourselves, that biopsy of gastric ulcer through a gastrotomy incision is a fairly dependable method for determining whether the ulcer is malignant. It is important in this connection that the hospital pathologist become expert in the diagnosis of gastric carcinoma from study of frozen sections.

I have accordingly advocated prompt operation in patients with gastric ulcers, at the same time assuring the internist that his patient will not be subjected to radical surgery unless microscopic proof can be obtained that the suspected ulcer is actually a carcinoma. If a carcinoma is found, a radical cancer operation is performed. If, however, it is not possible to secure microscopic evidence of malignancy, the gastrotomy wound is closed and a vagotomy combined with a gastroenterostomy is done. As the stomach with a gastric ulcer is often dilated and atonic, pyloroplasty is not recommended as a drainage procedure. Antrum resection or gastroenterostomy in the most dependent portion of the stomach is the better procedure.

The effectiveness of gastroenterostomy in healing most gastric ulcers was documented in the early surgical literature. The operation was abandoned, probably because gastroenterostomy proved to be inadequate treatment for duodenal ulcer, and the difference in pathogenesis between duodenal and gastric ulcers was not appreciated. It was probably also felt that partial gastrectomy might prove of some value should subsequent examination of the resected specimen prove it to be a carcinoma. The value of vagotomy and a drainage procedure in the treatment of duodenal ulcer has now been adequately demonstrated. This is not yet true of vagotomy and gastroenterostomy in the treatment of gastric ulcer. Balfour reported that 95 percent of gastric ulcer patients treated by simple gastroenterostomy were free of ulcer 5 years later. Vagotomy should contribute significantly to the beneficial effect of gastroenterostomy in the treatment of gastric ulcer in that it lessens the secretion of gastric juice. As mentioned earlier, this is accomplished by abolition of the vagal release of gastrin and reduction in the responsiveness of the gastric glands to humoral stimulation.

RECURRENCE OF ULCER AFTER VAGOTOMY

Gastrojejunal ulcer was early recognized as a frequent complication of gastroenterostomy for duodenal ulcer, and it was also noted that this lesion was rarely seen after gastroenterostomy for gastric ulcer.

These findings should have directed attention to the corrosive properties of the gastric content in gastric ulcer versus duodenal ulcer and lessened interest in decreased local resistance to the digestive action of gastric juice as the cause of ulcer. The finding of a high incidence of gastrojejunal ulceration after gastroenterostomy for duodenal ulcer is in harmony with the view that these lesions are produced by a hypersecretion of vagus origin. This hypersecretion would be unaffected by gastroenterostomy and the hyperacid gastric content might be expected to produce a new ulcer in the jejunum. The rare occurrence of gastrojejunal ulcer after gastroenterostomy for gastric ulcer is in accord with the concept that gastric ulcer is usually caused by a hypersecretion of gastric juice of hormonal origin brought about by stasis of food in the stomach. The gastroenterostomy might be expected to relieve the stasis and so correct the hypersecretion. It is probable that the few gastrojejunal ulcers that were found after gastroenterostomy for gastric ulcer occurred in patients in whom the basal gastric secretion was abnormally high either as a result of an Ellison-Zollinger tumor or excessive vagus impulses operating on an atonic stomach.

In my experience, 6 percent of patients with duodenal ulcers operated upon by vagotomy and gastroenterostomy or pyloroplasty developed recurrent duodenal ulcers or gastrojejunal ulcers at varying intervals after the operation. In my early experience, the most common cause of recurrent ulceration was incomplete vagotomy. After the first 2 or 3 years, however, the most common cause was an inadequate drainage operation with stasis of food in the antrum, sometimes distal to the gastroenterostomy that had been too highly placed in the stomach. Incomplete vagotomy is usually indicated by a 12-hour nocturnal gastric secretion of greater than 20 mEq of free hydrochloric acid and by a positive response to insulin hypoglycemia. In a few patients, persistent or recurrent ulceration associated with fasting hypersecretion of gastric juice is a result of gastrin released by a special type of tumor of the pancreas and duodenum described by Ellison and Zollinger. I have not yet seen a duodenal ulcer that has persisted or has recurred when the reaction to the insulin test was entirely negative on repeated testing, when the night secretion of gastric juice was at the normal level, and where stasis of food in the stomach was not present. In some cases, a gastrojejunal ulcer may form after complete vagotomy if an enteroenterostomy has been added to the drainage procedure. This diverts the alkaline duodenal secretions away from the gastroenterostomy stoma and thus produces a situation resembling that which obtains in the Mann-Williamson procedure for the production of experimental ulcers in animals. It is now quite evident that even a complete vagotomy cannot be relied upon to heal or prevent this type of ulcer in either man or experimental animals. The Roux-en-Y type of gastroenterostomy was rightly abandoned when Exalto [17] demonstrated the high incidence of gastrojejunal ulcer that regularly follows this procedure. It is thus clear that whenever operation for peptic ulcer is performed whereby a new outlet at the stomach is produced, the surgeon must be careful not to deflect the alkaline juices of the duodenum away from the region of the anastomosis.

REFERENCES

1. Dragstedt, L. R., and Vaughn, A. M., Arch. Surg. 8:791, 1924.
2. Matthews, W. B., and Dragstedt, L. R., Surg. Gynecol. Obstet. 55:265, 1932.
3. Dragstedt, L. R., Am. J. Roentgenol. 75:219, 1956.
4. Henning, N., and Norpoth, L., Dtsch. Arch. Klin. Med. 172:558, 1932.
5. Hay, L. J., Varco, R. L., Code, C. F., and Wangensteen, O. H., Surg. Gynecol. Obstet. 75:170, 1942.
6. Dragstedt, L. R., Ann. Surg. 102:563, 1935.
7. Dragstedt, L. R., and Owens, F. M., Jr., Proc. Soc. Exp. Biol. Med. 53:152, 1943.
8. Ohsawa, Arch. Jap. Chir. 10:605, 1933.
9. Dragstedt, L. R., Oberhelman, H. A., Jr., and Smith, C. A., Ann. Surg. 134:332, 1951.
10. Gregory, R. A., and Tracy, H. J. The preparation and properties of gastrin. J. Physiol. 149:70-71, 1959.
11. Dragstedt, L. R., Doyle, R. E., and Woodward, E. R. Gastric ulcers following vagotomy in some. Ann. Surg. 170:75, 1969.
12. Hurst, A. F. New views on the pathology, diagnosis, and treatment of gastric and duodenal ulcer. Brit. Med. J. 1:559, 1920.
13. Dragstedt, L. R. II, Lulu, D. J., Riley, W. J., and Lawson, L. J. Cephalic hypersecreting primary gastric ulcer patients. Arch. Surg. 102:462, 1971.
14. Oberhelman, H. A., and Dragstedt, L. R. Effect of vagotomy on gastric secretory response to histamine. Proc. Soc. Exper. Biol. Med. 67:336, 1943.
15. Weinberg, J. A. Modified Heineke-Mikulicz pyloroplasty with vagotomy in treating duodenal ulcers. In Maingot, Abdominal Operations, 6th ed. New York, Appleton-Century-Crofts, 1973.
16. Dorton, H. E. Vagotomy, pyloroplasty, and suture for bleeding gastric ulcer. Surg. Gynec. Obstet. 122:1015, 1966.
17. Exalto, J. Ulcers jejuni nach gastroenterostomie mitt Grenggeted d. Med. u. Chir. 23:13, 1911.

15

TYPES OF VAGOTOMY: PREFERENCE FOR THE SELECTIVE PROCEDURE

CHARLES A. GRIFFITH

As used herein, selective gastric vagotomy means transection of all the gastric vagi with preservation of both and all the hepatic and celiac vagi; total abdominal vagotomy means transection of all abdominal vagi. Two modifications are also recognized: (1) anterior selective-posterior total vagotomy (preservation of only the hepatic vagi) and (2) anterior total-posterior selective vagotomy (preservation of only the celiac vagi).

THE CONTROVERSY

The claim that selective vagotomy is a worthwhile refinement of total vagotomy continues to raise the three controversial issues that concern all the criteria for evaluating all operations for peptic ulcer: (1) completeness of vagotomy and recurrent ulcer; (2) technical difficulty and mortality; and (3) the functions of the hepatic and celiac vagi and gastrointestinal dysfunction. Critical evaluation of the controversy, therefore, entails consideration of all three issues and criteria.

COMPLETENESS OF SELECTIVE VAGOTOMY

We have investigated the completeness of the vagotomy by means of insulin tests and motility studies in dogs. Selective vagotomy was found to provide consistently negative insulin tests.[1, 2] Also, selective vagotomy completely eliminated the motile response of the stomach to electric stimulation of the vagal trunks.[3] From these results in dogs we concluded that neither the hepatic nor celiac vagi carry efferent secretory or motor fibers to the stomach and, therefore, the selective technique results in as complete a vagotomy of the stomach as the total or truncal technique.

The same results have been found in man. Burge[4] has shown that selective vagotomy completely eliminates the gastric motile response to electric stimulation of the vagal trunks. In addition, we, and several others, have found negative insulin tests after selective vagotomy. Furthermore, we have found by the insulin test that the selective technique provides a significantly lower rate of incomplete vagotomy than Dragstedt's total technique.[5] In the following section, the anatomical basis for a lower rate of incomplete vagotomy with the selective technique is described.

The Anatomical Levels of Vagotomy

The essential difference between Dragstedt's technique and the selective technique is the different anatomical level at which the vagotomy is performed. As evolved through Dragstedt's experience, total vagotomy is performed at or just above the level of the esophageal hiatus. In contrast, the selective technique is performed at the gastric cardia. Quite pertinent to the discussion is the fact that at the gastric cardia either total or selective vagotomy may be performed (Fig. 1).

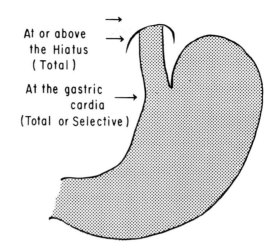

FIG. 1. The anatomical levels of vagotomy: *at or just above the hiatus* (total vagotomy by Dragstedt), and *at the gastric cardia* (total or selective vagotomy).

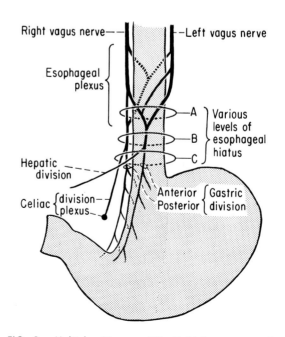

FIG. 2. Multiple Nerves. (A) Multiple nerves of esophageal plexus. (B) Two trunks (anterior and posterior). (C) Multiple nerves of truncal divisions.

Anatomical Variations at the Hiatus

From the left and right vagus nerves below the pulmonary plexus to the abdominal viscera, the vagal system consists of three constant components: (1) the esophageal plexus; (2) the two trunks; and (3) the four truncal divisions (the hepatic, the celiac, and the anterior and posterior gastric divisions). This system has no embryological or anatomical relationship with the diaphragm. Consequently, the vagal system may descend through the esophageal hiatus in the form of any one of its three constant components. Failure to emphasize this fundamental anatomical fact has led to the anatomically meaningless concept of "multiple nerves" (Fig. 2).

The vagi at the hiatus are also notorious for their extreme variations in position. These variations owe to the effects of embryologic rotation of the stomach (Fig. 3).

Anatomical Constants at the Gastric Cardia

Below the hiatus and within the abdomen, the hepatic and celiac vagi pursue constant anatomical courses. The hepatic division always runs within the lesser omentum to the porta hepatis. The celiac division always runs within the pancreatic-gastric fold to the celiac autonomical plexus. Lastly, the anterior and posterior gastric vagi always reach the stomach at the gastric cardia (Fig. 4).

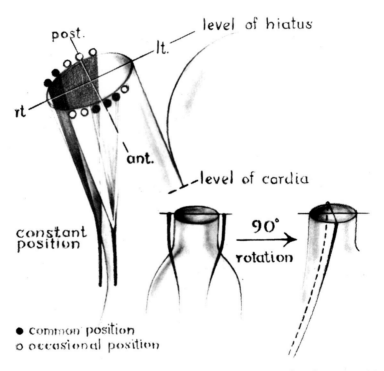

FIG. 3.   The effect of embryological rotation of the stomach upon the ultimate positions of the gastri vagi at the cardia and at the hiatus: Prior to rotation, one vagal trunk lies to the left of the esophagus and its gastric division goes to the left half of the stomach at the cardia and proximal lesser curve; the other trunk and its gastric division are in identical positions on the right. After rotation of 90 degrees, the left and right gastric divisions assume constant anterior and posterior positions, respectively, at the cardia and down the lesser curve. At the higher level of the hiatus, however, the vagal trunks are quite removed from the effect of rotation and therefore may rotate through a variety of degrees to assume a variety of positions.

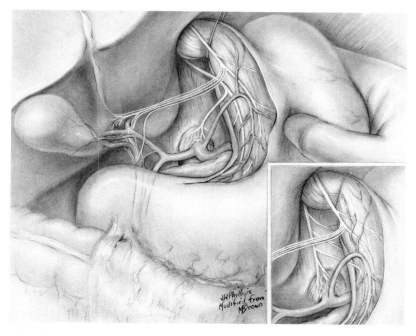

FIG. 4. The abdominal vagi. Note the variable position of the celiac vagal division—adjacent to the left gastric artery in the main illustration, and adjacent to the right diaphragmatic crus in the inset.

Cause of Incomplete Vagotomy

The surgical accomplishment of complete vagotomy requires that (1) all gastric vagi must be included in the tissue that is encircled with the esophagus and (2) all gastric vagi must be transected in the encircled tissue. Although these two requirements may seem all too simple, attention is drawn to the fact that past emphasis on the second requirement has detracted from the importance of the first. In other words, rather than stressing a technique by which all gastric vagi may be encircled with positive anatomical assurance, emphasis has been placed upon encircling the esophagus and then conducting a meticulous dissection in search for nerves that may be lurking within the esophageal facia propria and muscularis. As a result, failure to meet the first requirement, i.e., failure to encircle all gastric vagi, is the primary cause of incomplete vagotomy today.

If the vagal system is dissected within the confines of the hiatus and is not identified as the esophageal plexus or the two trunks or the four truncal divisions, the vagotomy must be conducted with the aim of finding unknown and variable numbers of nerves (Fig. 2) in unknown and variable positions (Fig. 3). With regard to the variable positions of the nerves at the hiatus diagramed in Figure 3, all nerves are shown lying closely applied to the esophagus. In this respect the illustration is in error, for in actual fact in some patients one or more nerves may be quite removed from the esophagus and lie more closely applied to the hiatal margins and aorta. Consequently, incomplete vagotomy occurs when the encircling finger excludes one or more of these nerves (Figs. 5 and 6).

Surgical Technique

CERTAIN ENCIRCLEMENT OF
ALL GASTRIC VAGI AT
GASTRIC CARDIA

The cardia is the one and only area where all gastric vagi gather to innervate the stomach. The key to the dissection is the ap-

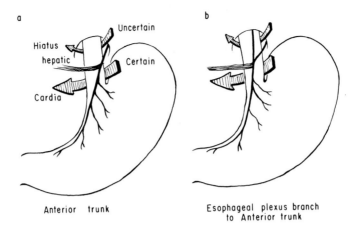

FIG. 5.   Encirclement of the anterior vagi. At the hiatus the anterior trunk (A) or a branch of the esophageal plexus contributing to the anterior trunk (B), may lie well to the (patient's) left of the esophagus. Failure to encircle the trunk (A) should lead to continued search for it. The encirclement of a branch of the esophageal plexus, however, may discourage further search, and the remaining branch is overlooked (B). In contrast to this uncertain encirclement at the hiatus, the encirclement of all gastric vagi at the cardia is certain.

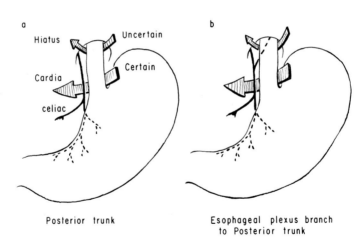

FIG. 6.   Encirclement of the posterior vagi. At the hiatus, the posterior trunk (A), or a branch of the esophageal plexus contributing to the posterior trunk (B), may lie well posterior to the esophagus in an extremely dorsal position adjacent to the right diaphragmatic crus, and continues in this extremely dorsal position as the celiac division to the celiac autonomic plexus (cf. inset, Fig. 4). In this circumstance, the posterior trunk (A) or a contributing branch of the esophageal plexus (B) may be excluded from the encirclement at the hiatus, but at the gastric cardia may always be included by virtue of the fact that at the lower level of the cardia the celiac vagal division may always be positively identified by palpating its course to the celiac plexus.

plication of the hepatic and celiac vagi as constant anatomical landmarks for the certain encirclement of all gastric vagi.

Step 1. For the encirclement of all gastric vagi on the patient's right, the landmark is the hepatic vagal division. The stretched-out lesser omentum is incised in its avascular area below the hepatic vagal division, well to the right of the gastric cardia. No gastric vagi lie to the patient's right of this incision in the lesser omentum.

Step 2. For the encirclement of all gastric vagi on the patient's left, the landmark is the cardioesophageal angle of His. The peritoneum is incised over this angle, and a finger is insinuated into the crotch between the esophagus and the gastric fundus. No gastric vagi reach the fundus to the patient's left of the angle of His.

Step 3. For the encirclement of all gastric vagi posteriorly, the landmark is the posterior trunk and its continuation as the celiac division. Finger dissection at the angle of His is therefore started not with the aim of encircling the esophagus but with the aim of palpating the posterior trunk-celiac division posterior to the esophagus. Once the posterior trunk-celiac division is positively identified by palpating its course to the celiac plexus (Figs. 4 and 6), the finger is dissected through the areolar tissue in the pancreatic-gastric fold posterior to the posterior trunk-celiac division. By encircling the posterior trunk-celiac division, all gastric vagi are encircled posteriorly. No gastric vagi lie posterior to the posterior-trunk celiac division.

Step 4. After the finger is dissected posterior to the posterior trunk-celiac division, the fingertip encounters the peritoneum covering the patient's right surface of the pancreatic-gastric fold in the lesser peritoneal space. At this point, the fingertip may be seen, or at least palpated with a finger of the other hand,

through the incision in the lesser omentum initially made below the hepatic vagal division. The fingertip is then worked into the lesser peritoneal space through the peritoneum covering the pancreatic-gastric fold, and emerges through the incision in the lesser omentum below the hepatic vagal division. The encirclement of all gastric vagi with the most distal esophagus is thereby accomplished.

At this stage, when one is certain that all gastric vagi are encircled, a soft rubber urethral catheter or Penrose drain may replace the encircling finger to maintain the encirclement and exposure. The operation next proceeds according to the decision of selective or total vagotomy.

THE SELECTIVE TECHNIQUE

Selective gastric vagotomy essentially entails ligation and transection of all of the aforementioned encircled tissue except the esophagus and the hepatic and celiac vagi. In addition, the descending branch of the left gastric artery must also be ligated and transected in order to interrupt those posterior gastric vagi that may arise quite distally from the posterior trunk-celiac division and go to the stomach with the left gastric artery. Neither the hiatus nor the vagal trunks are dissected or exposed. Furthermore, the gastric vagi are not purposely exposed or identified. Instead, all tissue known to contain the gastric vagi is clamped, ligated, and transected.

Step 1. By finger dissection, separate the posterior trunk-celiac division from the distal esophagus so that the posterior trunk-celiac division may be gently displaced to the patient's right and the most distal esophagus to the patient's left.

Step 2. Through the aforementioned aperture in the lesser omentum below the hepatic vagi, separate the tissue containing the descending branch of the left gastric artery from the lesser curve. This tissue also contains the greater anterior and posterior gastric nerves of Latarjet. Clamp, transect, and ligate this tissue. The muscle of the lesser curve is then bared at the point of this dissection.

Step 3. By finger dissection, encircle all remaining tissue between the posterior trunk-celiac division and the proximal lesser curve—from the initial point of separation between the posterior trunk-celiac division and the distal esophagus superiorly (Step 1) to the point of transection of the descending branch of the left gastric artery and the nerves of Latarjet inferiorly (Step 2). This tissue contains the ascending esophageal branch(es) of the left gastric artery, and also may contain remaining fibers of the posterior gastric vagi. Clamp, transect, and ligate this tissue.

Step 4. With the finger dissect from the distal esophagus all tissue remaining anterior to the esophagus. The line of dissection is below the hepatic vagi. This tissue contains the residual anterior gastric vagi. Clamp, transect, and ligate this tissue, taking care to avoid injury to the hepatic vagi.

Step 5. At this point of the operation, the hepatic and celiac vagi and their parent trunks are completely separated from the distal esophagus and proximal gastric cardia. The only intact gastric vagi that can possibly remain are those that may arise from the esophageal plexus or the trunks above the level of the dissection (Fig. 2). Consequently, the most distal esophagus must be inspected and palpated for residual gastric vagal fibers. These fibers usually lie within the esophageal fascia propria, and are transected by a final dissection that lays bare the longitudinal muscle of the esophagus in its entire circumference. It is our belief, and there is no evidence to the contrary, that no vagi reach the stomach via a course deep to or within the esophageal muscle. Complete vagotomy of the stomach may be accomplished without circumcising or transecting the esophagus in both dogs and man.

The Total Technique at the Cardia

Total vagotomy essentially entails ligation and transection of all tissue encircled at the gastric cardia except the esophagus. The descending branch of the left gastric artery need not be ligated, and the dissection may be conducted without regard for the hepatic vagi. Again, the vagal trunks and gastric vagi are not purposely exposed or dissected. Instead, all of the encircled tissue containing the vagi is clamped, ligated, and transected so that only the bared distal esophagus remains.

Comments

With the selective or total techniques of vagotomy at the gastric cardia as described, inadequate incomplete vagotomy with recurrent ulcer caused by an overlooked branch of the esophageal plexus or a trunk is impossible because the vagotomy is performed at the lower level of the truncal divisions. The only type of incomplete vagotomy that may occur is a small twig to the proximal fundus described in Step 5.

In regard to the incomplete vagotomy due to an intact twig to the gastric fundus, Pritchard et al.[6] showed that only a small area of gastric mucosa remained vagally innervated. Legros and Griffith [7] next demonstrated that this small area of residually innervated mucosa was capable of providing only a small and delayed response to insulin. This type of response indicates an incomplete but adequate vagotomy. Lastly, Jones and Griffith [8] showed that the small area of residually innervated mucosa remains small and does not increase in size by vagal reinnervation. Thus, the adequate vagotomy remains adequate, and does not become inadequate by vagal reinnervation.

THE ISSUE OF TECHNICAL DIFFICULTY

Total vagotomy at the gastric cardia is considered no more difficult, time-consuming, or hazardous than total vagotomy at the hiatus. Selective vagotomy, however, is unquestionably more difficult and time-consuming than total vagotomy, and therefore is more hazardous in some patients.

Obesity increases the technical difficulty of any abdominal operation, and selective vagotomy is no exception. In our initial experience, we therefore limited the selective technique to thin patients undergoing elective operation. As experience increased, we gradually extended the operation to include more obese patients. Total vagotomy, however, still remains a wiser choice in some obese and poor-risk patients undergoing urgent operation.

The presence of a large left hepatic artery arising from the left gastric artery (10 to 15 percent) also increases technical difficulty. Although the presence of this aberrant artery is not considered a definite contraindication to selective vagotomy, great care must be taken to preserve it in order to avoid necrosis of the left hepatic lobe.

Anterior selective vagotomy is usually technically easy. In some patients, however, the fibers of the hepatic division arise quite low —at or just above the cardia—and anterior selective vagotomy must be performed with meticulous technique across the anterior surface of the gastric cardia. In these patients, total anterior vagotomy is easier because the tissue anterior to the esophagus may be transected without regard for low-lying fibers; the result is often a complete anterior gastric and incomplete hepatic vagotomy.

For surgeons experienced in gastric resection, posterior selective vagotomy is usually not particularly difficult or hazardous. Nevertheless, clearing the proximal lesser curvature of all omental attachments, with ligation and transection of the descending branch of the left gastric artery, is clearly a more extensive dissection than that required for posterior total vagotomy.

The use of selective vagotomy has not increased our rate of operative morbidity and mortality. We emphasize, however, that we have applied the selective technique only when the specific operative circumstances have indicated its safe performance. Under adverse operative circumstances as, for example, in obese patients undergoing operation for massive hemorrhage, we have performed total vagotomy at the cardia.

FUNCTIONS OF THE HEPATIC AND CELIAC VAGI

Some critics antagonistic to selective vagotomy claim that the hepatic and celiac vagi have no significant functions and may be transected by total vagotomy with impunity in all patients. Other critics recognize the functions of the hepatic and celiac vagi, but do not believe the functions are significant enough to warrant the tedium of the more difficult selective technique. Our rebuttal to these views is as follows. Although there is no evidence that selective vagotomy is superior to total vagotomy on the basis of digestion, absorption, and overall nutrition, three known effects of transecting the hepatic and celiac vagi seem significant.

First, and in the only study of its kind reported in the American literature to date— namely, routine cholecystograms upon a sizable number of patients taken in the long term after total vagotomy—Clave and Gaspar [9] found that approximately one out of four of their patients had developed gallstones 2 to 4 years after operation. This lithogenic effect of total vagotomy was formerly believed to be due solely to biliary stasis consequent to either or both decreased flow of bile and dilatation of the gallbladder (Fig. 7). More recent studies by Fletcher and Clark [10] have shown that total vagotomy also lowers the concentration of cholates in the bile, which predisposes to the precipitation of cholesterol. This latter effect may well explain the findings of Barnett and Hilbun [11] as diagramed in Figure 8. Our long-term results indicate that the sequelae of biliary tract disease consequent to total vagotomy may be

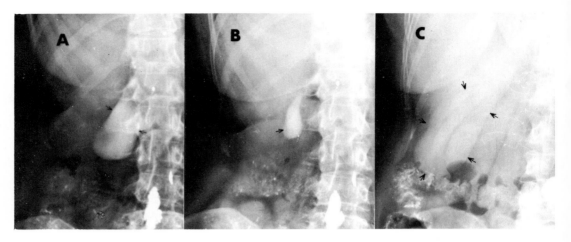

FIG. 7. The effects of complete hepatic vagotomy. The patient underwent transabdominal repair of a hiatal hernia, during which all hepatic vagi were transected in order to gain adequate exposure of the diaphragmatic crura. The gastric and celiac vagi were preserved. Cholecystograms before operation demonstrate normal functions of concentration (A) and contraction in response to a fatty meal (B). Four years after operation, the patient suffered an attack of typical biliary colic that subsided spontaneously. Subsequent cholecystograms failed to reveal the gallbladder on two successive days, but on the third day a faint concentration of dye was demonstrated in a dilated gallbladder (outlined by *arrows;* C). No contraction occurred after a fatty meal. During the following year, the patient had repeated attacks of biliary colic, which necessitated cholecystectomy. At operation the gallbladder was unusually large and contained inspissated biliary sludge ("mud"). (The patient had previously undergone myelography several years prior.)

eliminated by selective vagotomy.[12]

Second, case reports of prolonged and se-

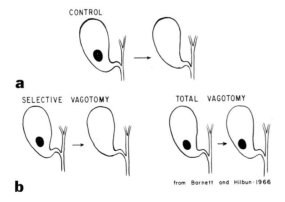

FIG. 8. (A) Human gallstones dissolve in normal canine gallbladders. (B) Human gallstones also dissolve in the gallbladders of dogs with selective vagotomy. (C) Human gallstones do not dissolve in the gallbladders of dogs with total vagotomy.

vere postvagotomy ileus have appeared sporadically in the literature ever since Dragstedt introduced vagotomy. This ileus is due to hypotonicity of the midgut consequent to its vagal denervation by hepatic and celiac vagotomy, and may be avoided by selective vagotomy (Fig. 9). Long-term and perhaps permanent motile dysfunction of the small intestine has also been observed, but its clinical significance or insignificance remains unknown. It is known, however, that this dysfunction with intestinal stasis is a common denominator in many syndromes (e.g., sprue) manifested by diarrhea. At any rate, this intestinal dysfunction does not occur after selective vagotomy.[12]

Third, in Heidenhain pouch dogs with and without various drainage procedures, pouch secretion is at least 2 times greater after total vagotomy than after selective vagotomy.[13, 14, 18] The cause of this effect remains unknown, but it is postulated that the hepatic and celiac vagi inhibit gastric secretion (perhaps by a chalone from the viscera of the midgut that is under vagal control). If appli-

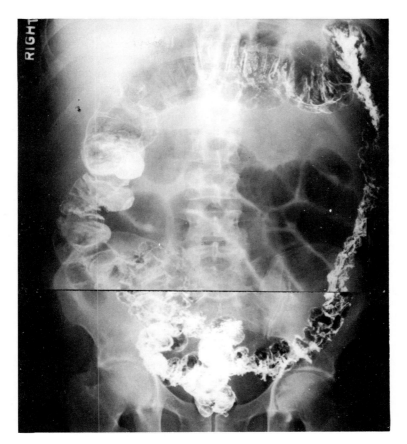

FIG. 9. Barium enema in patient with severe postoperative ileus 8 days after anterior selective-posterior total vagotomy (hepatic vagi preserved, celiac vagi transected). The entire midgut (small intestine and colon to the splenic flexure), denervated by celiac vagotomy, is dilated. The hindgut (splenic flexure to colon), innervated by the sacral parasympathetics, is collapsed. Spontaneous expulsion of flatus did not occur until the twelfth postoperative day, at which time gastric suction was no longer necessary and the patient could first retain oral feedings.

cable to man, selective vagotomy may well lower gastric secretion more effectively than total vagotomy which, in turn, may be a definite factor for our low rate of recurrent ulcer observed to date.[15]

DUMPING AND DIARRHEA

From our experience with the Billroth I and II resections, and with total and selective vagotomy plus simple drainage or antrectomy, we have come to recognize four general groups of patients; Group I, no dumping and no diarrhea; Group II, mild to moderate dumping and no diarrhea; Group III, severe dumping with diarrhea; Group IV, no dumping but with diarrhea. Groups I and II are the most common. Group III usually occurs after extensive gastric resection; the fact that in this group the diarrhea is apparently a consequence of dumping is basic to evaluating the great debate about postvagotomy diarrhea. Group IV (no dumping but with diarrhea) consists of patients with total vagotomy but not patients with selective vagotomy. The cause(s) of this type of diarrhea after total vagotomy and its elimination by selective vagotomy remain unknown (see Chap. 27).

Dumping is the only undesirable side-effect

observed after selective vagotomy plus pyloroplasty or antrectomy. Although the exact cause of dumping remains unknown, there is general agreement that pyloric dysfunction and consequent alteration in gastric emptying are prime factors. We therefore investigated the effects of selective vagotomy plus Maki's [16] pylorus preserving resection (or suprapyloric antrectomy) in Heidenhain pouch dogs. When all the proximal antrum was removed, and the distal 1.5 cm of antrum and pylorus were preserved, the results were marked decrease in pouch secretion and preservation of normal rhythmic gastric emptying without dumping or stasis.[17, 18]

With these experimental results, plus the fact that removal of 90 to 95 percent of the antrum should provide additional protection against recurrent ulcer, selective vagotomy plus suprapyloric antrectomy have been evaluated in man. Preliminary results have shown a marked reduction in gastric secretion, no stasis, and no dumping in response to provocative meals.[19] These early results have encouraged continuation of the evaluation of selective vagotomy plus suprapyloric antrectomy, but I cannot recommend the operation to others until more patients have been followed for longer periods of time.

SUMMARY

We recognize three general techniques of vagotomy: (1) selective at the gastric cardia, (2) total at the gastric cardia, and (3) total at or just above the hiatus. By the criteria of recurrent ulcer, mortality, and gastrointestinal dysfunction, the advantages and disadvantages of these three techniques are summarized below.

In comparing total vagotomy at the cardia with total vagotomy at the hiatus, the technical difficulty and side-effects are equal. By virtue of the certain encirclement of all gastric vagi at the cardia, however, in contrast to the uncertain encirclement at the hiatus, the rate of incomplete vagotomy at the cardia is less than it is at the hiatus. We have therefore abandoned vagotomy at the hiatus in favor of vagotomy at the cardia.

In comparing selective with total vagotomy

at the cardia, the rates of incomplete vagotomy are the same. The decision to perform selective vagotomy, therefore, becomes a compromise between the advantages of preserving the hepatic and celiac vagi and the disadvantages of a more difficult dissection. The latter disadvantages preclude the safe performance of selective vagotomy in all patients (e.g., obese and poor-risk patients undergoing urgent operation). In those patients upon whom selective vagotomy may be safely performed, we preserve the hepatic and celiac vagi in order to (1) eliminate the sequelae of stasis in the gallbladder and bowel, (2) prevent the lithogenic biochemical effect in the biliary tract consequent to total (hepatic) abdominal vagotomy, and (3) preserve the apparent inhibition of gastric secretion by the hepatic and celiac vagi.

REFERENCES

1. Griffith, C. A., and Harkins, H. N., Gastroenterology 32:96, 1957.
2. Pritchard, G. R., Griffith, C. A., and Harkins, H. N., J. Surg. Res. 8:68, 1968.
3. Stavney, L. S., Kato, T., Griffith, C. A., Nyhus, L. M., and Harkins, H. N., J. Surg. Res. 3:390, 1963.
4. Burge, H., Vagotomy, Baltimore, Williams & Wilkins, 1964.
5. Griffith, C. A., J. Dig. Dis. 12:333, 1967.
6. Pritchard, G. R., Griffith, C. A., and Harkins, H. N., Surg. Gynecol. Obstet. 126:791, 1968.
7. Legros, G., and Griffith, C. A., Ann. Surg. 168:1030, 1968.
8. Jones, W. M., and Griffith, C. A., Ann. Surg. 171:365, 1970.
9. Clave, R. A., and Gaspar, M. R., Am. J. Surg. 118:169, 1969.
10. Fletcher, D. M., and Clark, C. G., Br. J. Surg. 56:103, 1969.
11. Barnett, W. O., and Hilbun, G. R., Surgery 60:840, 1966.
12. Griffith, C. A., Am. J. Surg. 118:251, 1969.
13. Shiina, E., and Griffith, C. A., Ann. Surg. 169:326, 1969.
14. Everett, M. T., and Griffith, C. A., Ann. Surg. 171:31, 1970.
15. Griffith. C. A., Leyse, R. M., Davis, D. R., and Magoon, C. C., Am. Surg. 1972.
16. Maki, T., Shiratori, T., Hatafuku, T., and Sugawara, K., Surgery 61:835, 1967.
17. Everett, M. T., and Griffith, C. A., Ann. Surg. 171:36, 1970.
18. Kilby, J. O., and Griffith, C. A., Surgery 69:702, 1971.
19. Griffith, C. A., Northwest Med. 68:927, 1969.

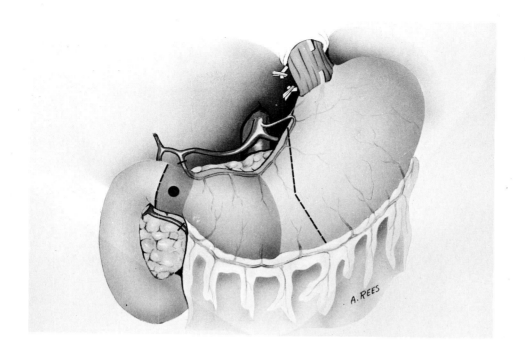

16

VAGOTOMY AND ANTRECTOMY

J. LYNWOOD HERRINGTON, JR.

HISTORICAL NOTES

The combination of bilateral truncal vagotomy and a conservative resection of the distal stomach has been shown over the past two and one-half decades to be an effective means of controlling the complications of duodenal ulcer. Each component of the combined operation has truly a fascinating history, and it would seem worthwhile to review briefly the historical development of distal gastric resection and to cite the early observations regarding the role of the vagus nerves in promoting gastric secretory activity. As a result of contributions by innumerable investigators on the physiology of the gastric antrum and the influence of the vagus nerves on the stomach in both control subjects and ulcer preparations, the operation of *vagotomy and antrectomy* evolved.

Distal gastric resection. According to Temkin,[1] the first proposal to remove the distal portion of the stomach was made by Michaelis in 1780, then professor of surgery and anatomy at the University of Marburg. In 1810 Daniel Merrem,[2] a youthful and brilliant student of Michaelis, published a dissertation on several surgical subjects which included a report of three experimental animals subjected to pylorectomy after which the proximal stomach pouch was invaginated into the duodenum. Only one of the three animals survived. In 1811, Conrad Langenbeck[3] of Gottingen stated: "I consider the operation of pylorectomy a means of expediting from this world more quickly, but in an excruciating manner, a man who is past saving." These words, uttered by one of the greatest professors of his time, created such an impasse that no significant progress was made in experimental gastric surgery for the following six decades, and the dreams of Michaelis and Merrem were either ridiculed or ignored.

In 1874, Gussenbauer and von Winiwarter,[4, 5] both assistants to Theodore Billroth of Vienna, undertook an experimental study of pylorectomy and published their results in 1876. They also carried out distal gastric resection on cadavers. Both investigators exercised praiseworthy caution in the clinical application of their work, for up to that time no one had dared to attempt such a procedure in a human being. They did state, however, that the procedure was possibly applicable to certain cases of pyloric carcinoma, and even more justifiable for benign stenosing lesions of the distal pylorus and duodenum.

The first attempt at resection of the distal stomach in a human being was made by the famous French surgeon, Jules Péan[6] in 1879, but unfortunately the patient did not survive. It is of extreme interest to note that Péan had not taken the problem to the experimental laboratory before embarking upon an endeavor of this magnitude. In 1880, Ludwig Rydygier[7] likewise performed an unsuccessful pylorectomy. The first successful, and the third attempt, at pylorectomy is credited to Theodore Billroth[8] in 1881. After removing the pylorus, Billroth anastomosed the duodenum to the lesser curve of the gastric pouch, but in subsequent operations he employed the greater curve for the reconstruction. During the ensuing two decades, pylorectomy was carried out by many European surgeons, largely for carcinoma of the pylorus. At the turn of the century, the operation began to be employed with increasing frequency for benign ulceration of the distal stomach and duodenum. Such outstanding surgeons as Rydygier, Jedlicka, von Haberer, Clairmont, and Finsterer made valuable contributions and pioneered distal gastric resection for the surgical treatment of duodenal ulcer.

The outstanding experiments by Edkins[9] in 1905, in which he isolated a crude extract (gastrin) from the mucosa of the gastric antrum of the cat, which proved to be a potent gastric secretagogue, represent some of the greatest contributions to the subsequent development of the current surgical therapy for ulcer disease. In 1915, Schur and Plaschkes,[10] in an elaborate discussion of the physiology of the gastric antrum, stressed the importance of antrectomy in reducing gastric acidity in the patient with duodenal ulcer and its effect upon ulcer-healing and prevention of recurrence. The subsequent sophisticated studies of Boller and Pilgerstorfer,[11] Komarov,[12] and Uvnäs[13] with isolated gastrin and its stimulating effect on the parietal cell mass truly defined the role of the gastric antrum. These studies were of major importance to surgeons who later developed the concept of the combined operation.

Vagotomy. In 1814 Benjamin Brodie[14] made the astute experimental observation that dogs exterminated by an intravenous injection of arsenic, at sacrifice, demonstrated copious amounts of fluids in the gastric contents. In addition, if the vagus nerves were divided prior to the drug administration, at autopsy the dog's stomach was found empty of secretions. Claude Bernard,[15] in 1858, noted an arrest of gastric contractions and lack of gastric secretion following vagal denervation. Pavlov,[16] in 1894, described the absence of hydrochloric acid in the fasting gastric secretions following vagotomy, but was able to produce an acid response with subsequent feedings. He later showed that the vagus nerves supply secretory fibers to the gastric glands and constitute the pathway for stimuli that excite the cephalic phase of gastric secretion. Schiff[17] likewise recorded a fall in gastric secretory response following vagotomy.

In 1914, Exner and Schwarzmann[18] were the first to perform vogotomy in a human being via the abdominal route. The operation was done mainly for tabetic crisis and functional gastrointestinal disorders. Gastric atony was clearly recognized as a significant postoperative complication, and a tube was passed through the pylorus via a gastrostomy route to control the complication. Later these investigators added gastroenterostomy. Latarjet,[19] in 1922, advocated vagotomy for benign gastric outlet obstruction and was the first to combine vagotomy with a limited pylorec-

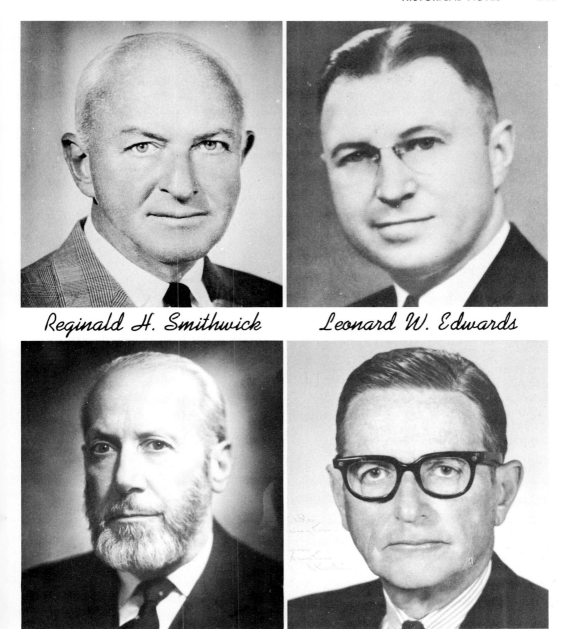

Reginald H. Smithwick   *Leonard W. Edwards*

H. Daintree Johnson   *Henry N. Harkins*

FIG. 1. The illustrious surgeons who developed and pioneered the operation of vagotomy and a conservative distal gastrectomy.

tomy. Schiassi,[20] in 1925, added a drainage procedure to vagotomy in cases with obstruction. Aside from the physiological studies of A. J. Carlson [21] in the 1920s demonstrating the continuous secretion of gastric juice throughout the fasting state, and later experiments showing that hypersecretion of gastric juice in the duodenal ulcer patient was of cephalic origin, few experimental and clinical articles appeared in the literature regarding the effects of the vagus nerves on the stomach.

Thus, the initial clinical trials with vagotomy were short-lived and follow-up data went largely unpublished. The operation received severe criticism, for in many instances it was performed for various functional disorders with poor results. In addition, during the 1920s the rise in popularity of simple gastroenterostomy championed by Berkeley Moynihan of Leeds and William J. Mayo of Rochester, and during the 1930s the pleas for adequate gastric resection by Strauss, Berg, and Lewisohn, did much to bury vagotomy for the time being. About the only significant clinical reports that appeared during these times were those by Klein,[22] in 1929, who performed left vagus section with adequate gastrectomy, and Winkelstein,[23] in 1938, who likewise utilized a generous distal resection with anterior vagotomy. Follow-up reports were lacking.

In 1943, Dragstedt [24] produced a real awakening and challenge to members of the surgical world when he and Owens published an account of two patients with duodenal ulcer treated by transthoracic vagotomy which resulted in prompt ulcer-healing and a marked diminution in gastric acid secretion with a rise in intragastric pH. Similar findings were observed by subsequent investigators. It was soon recognized, however, that gastric atony and stasis were prominent postoperative complications requiring a drainage procedure in about two-thirds of the cases. In ensuing years, vagotomy received harsh criticism from various sources, but these were later overcome mainly as a result of the persistent efforts by many experimental and clinical investigators and particularly through the noteworthy factual contributions of Lester Dragstedt.

The combined operation. With full appreciation of the physiological effects of vagotomy and the further reduction of gastric acidity afforded by antrectomy, Farmer and Smithwick [25] of Boston treated 18 patients with duodenal ulcer by vagotomy and removal of an estimated 50 percent of the distal stomach. This combined procedure resulted in a marked reduction of both the quantity of free acid and hydrogen ion concentration. The reduction exceeded that obtained with other conventional operations. In addition, they observed that distal resection in excess of more than an estimated 50 percent did not result in further lowering of free acid output or pH change. Their preliminary results were presented before the American Surgical Association in 1951. It is of historical interest that Smithwick performed the first such procedure in October of 1946 and termed the distal resection a *hemigastrectomy*. This particular patient had developed a stomal ulcer following simple gastroenterostomy. Smithwick dismantled the gastroenterostomy, performed a bilateral truncal vagotomy with an estimated 50 percent resection, and reestablished alimentary continuity with a posterior Hofmeister reconstruction.

In January of 1947, Leonard Edwards [26] of Nashville, unaware of Smithwick's combined operation performed 3 months previously, along the same line of reasoning carried out truncal vagotomy with an estimated 40 percent resection for a complication of duodenal ulcer. He termed the resection an *antrectomy* and constructed a retrocolic Billroth II type anastomosis. In 1952, before the Southern Surgical Association, he reported encouraging results among a group of 34 patients.

Credit should also be extended the outstanding British surgeon, H. Dantree Johnson [27] of London, who in 1947, unaware of the operation performed by both Smithwick and Edwards, carried out vagotomy-antrectomy using a Hofmeister-type reconstruction. The operation was later mentioned at a meeting of the Royal Society of Medicine. The late Henry Harkins [28] introduced a significant and worthwhile modification to the combined procedure when he advocated alimentary reconstruction with terminoterminal gastroduodenostomy in preference to gastrojejunostomy (Fig. 1).

To complete the historical story of the combined operation, attention should be directed to the work of Colp,[29] in 1948, who reported satisfactory results with truncal vagotomy and gastrectomy, but the resection entailed removal of approximately 75 percent of the distal stomach. Follow-up data were subsequently reported by Druckerman et al.[30] in 1952. The procedure devised by Colp did indeed combine resection with vagotomy but the concept was not to employ a conservative resection but to add vagotomy in order to prevent recurrent ulceration, which in his experience had been prevalent following high gastric resection alone. Palumbo [31] expressed the same philosophy when he reported 25 cases in 1951 with no ulcer recurrence and complete gastric achlorhydria.

Thus, Smithwick, Edwards, and Johnson must each be extended full credit for independently developing the combined operation of conservative distal resection and bilateral truncal vagotomy. In the minds of each observer, the operation eliminated both the neurogenic and hormonal phases of gastric secretion, but left the patient with a sizable gastric reservoir which they hoped would protect against long-term ill effects. The combined operation also possessed the advantages of being applicable not only to patients undergoing definitive operation for the complication of ulcer intractability, but also to the emergency massive bleeder, to patients with gastric outlet obstruction, and even to selected cases of acute ulcer perforation.

IMPORTANCE OF THE GASTRIC ANTRUM IN ULCEROGENESIS

Although the role of vagal activity in the genesis of duodenal ulcer has been dealt with extensively elsewhere in this text, its importance cannot be overemphasized. It has become increasingly apparent in recent years, through extensive experimental work, that the vagus nerves exert an even more profound influence on gastric secretion than was originally believed. In addition to their role of mediating the interdigestive and nocturnal secretions of gastric juice, the vagus nerves are capable of producing the release of gastrin when the antrum is at an alkaline pH. Also, the principal stimuli for pepsinogen secretion are mediated by the vagi. Following vagal denervation, there is a diminution in the release of antral gastrin and likewise a decreased secretory response of the parietal cell mass to histamine and parasympathomimetic drugs. The intact vagus potentiates the response of parietal cells to all stimuli. It has been shown that vagotomy of the main stomach has no significant effect on the augmented gastric phase of secretion produced by antral exclusion. Vagotomy reduces the acid response to gastrin to a greater degree than to histamine.

Pavlov first noted the stimulating effect of food and water in the stomach on the secretion of hydrochloric acid. As mentioned, Edkins, in 1906, isolated a substance from the pyloric mucosa of both cats and dogs which, when injected intravenously, caused a marked increase in the secretion of gastric juice. He called this substance gastrin and elaborated his hypothesis of the hormonal or gastric phase of secretion.

Komarov, in the early 1940s, isolated gastrin from the pyloric mucosa of the experimental animal and found it to be a protein-like substance free of histamine. It has been shown that the release of gastrin from the antrum, with subsequent stimulation of gastric secretion, takes place in the presence of an alkaline or slightly acid medium. This stimulation continues until the acidity of the gastric pH approximates a pH of 2.5 or 3.0. Then further liberation of gastrin ceases and the humoral phase of secretion becomes quiescent.

When 24-hour quantitative collections of gastric secretions from Pavlov or Heidenhain pouch animals were made, complete removal of the gastric antrum with reconstruction of continuity by anastomosing the body of the stomach to the side of the duodenum produced a profound reduction in the gastric juice secreted by the isolated pouch. Following complete vagotomy in Pavlov pouch dogs, subsequent removal of the antrum almost completely terminated the secretion of gastric juice from the isolated stomach pouch.[32] Thus, it is felt that the vagus nerves and the gastric antrum contain the key to the secretory activity of the gastric glands. The secretory importance of the antrum has been further exemplified by transplantation experiments in which the antrum was transplanted into the side of the duodenum or into the transverse colon as a diverticulum, with resultant augmentation of gastric secretion from a Pavlov pouch.[33] Following antral extirpation, these secretions were reduced. Schmitz [34] concluded that gastric drainage procedures that permitted increased antral stimulation and an alkali-acid rebound caused an increase in Heidenhain pouch hydrochloric acid secretions. The high incidence of recurrent ulceration following antral exclusion operations further attests to the importance of the gastric antrum as a potent source of acid stimulation.[35, 36]

Perhaps one of the most convincing experiments depicting the role of the antrum as an important factor in the possible genesis of ulcer disease is the ingenious three-phase total parietal cell pouch devised by Sauvage,[37, 38] who has demonstrated that this procedure is a potent ulcerogenic mechanism. Vagotomy alone did not decrease the incidence of ulceration in the pouch dogs in this experimental procedure, but antral extirpation did. Antrectomy combined with vagotomy offered a marked degree of protection against the development of stomal ulceration.

Storer[39] showed that vagotomy and antral resection afforded protection against the development of stomal ulceration in the Mann-Williamson preparation. Vagotomy alone afforded protection against ulceration in 55 percent of the animals; antral resection alone gave protection to two-thirds of the animals; but a combination of the two procedures offered complete protection to 83 percent of the animals.

Kay[40] of Glasgow found that antrectomy reduced gastric secretion by 70 percent, and that vagotomy alone likewise reduced the total acid output by some 60 to 70 percent. A combination of the two procedures resulted in a 95 percent reduction in acid output. Although the parietal cell population is virtually unaltered after antrectomy and vagotomy, the acid-secretory cells no doubt become definitely less responsive to histamine stimulation. Following complete vagotomy and antral resection in patients with duodenal ulcer, achlorhydria is usually found during the fasting state and also after test meal stimulation. The majority of the patients have no hydrochloric acid response to histamine, and when a response is elicited, it usually ranges from 5 to 10 clinical units or less than 2 mEq of total acid output. The quantitative hourly fasting secretory volumes of gastric juice obtained after the combined procedure usually range from 0 to 20 ml, and the hourly basal output of hydrochloric acid is usually less than 0.5 mEq. Under these

circumstances, the patient should, theoretically at least, be protected against the development of recurrent ulceration.

Gregory and Tracy,[41] in 1961, using extraction methods, were able to isolate gastrin I and gastrin II, each peptide having identical amino-acid compositions but differing in electrophoretic and chromatographic properties. Each gastrin was many times more potent than histamine in stimulating acid secretion from a Heidenhain pouch. Both gastrins, under experimental conditions, not only stimulated acid secretion, but also stimulated pepsin secretion, pancreatic flow, pancreatic enzyme secretion. and gastrointestinal motility. One unusual finding was that acid secretion produced by the subcutaneous injection of either one of the gastrins could be inhibited by the rapid intravenous injection of the other gastrin.

Woodward and co-investigators[32] have demonstrated that antrectomy was followed by 74 percent decrease in the volume of gastric output, a 51 percent drop in acid concentration, and an 86 percent reduction in total mEq of hydrochloric acid by Heidenhain and Pavlov pouches.

In recent years, the antrum of the stomach has assumed added importance as an endocrine organ, and gastrin has been associated with or implicated in several pathological states. Of particular interest along this line has been the isolation of a powerful gastrin-like substance from pancreatic islet adenomas in patients with the Zollinger-Ellison syndrome.[42, 43]

Various mechanisms have been shown to be responsible for the release of gastrin from the pyloric antrum. The presence of food in the antrum, mechanical and chemical stimulation, vagal impulses, and pH content of the antrum are each important factors in exciting antral secretory activity. Dragstedt demonstrated that the antrum may undergo constant 24-hour stimulation with neutral liver extract without showing signs of decreased secretion from a Heidenhain pouch.[44] Recent evidence has shown that gastrin is also present in the alimentary tract distal to the pylorus, and this extra-antral gastrin may possibly be under vagal control.[45]

It is only recently that the exact source of gastrin within the antrum has been identified. Formerly it was shown by indirect methods that the source of gastrin was either in the antral mucosa or submucosa because resection of antral mucosa or submucosa would abolish the gastrin mechanism. Likewise, mechanical or chemical antroneurolysis would interfere with its production. Woodward [46, 47] suggested that gastrin elaboration and release might possibly be closely associated with the submucosal plexus of Meissner. Reynolds [48] believed that the submucosal interstitial substance was the site of origin of antral gastrin. Pearce and Friesen [49] recently made a noteworthy contribution when they identified the endocrine polypeptide cells by optical microscopic, cytochemical, and electron microscopic techniques. These investigators recognized four cellular types in the stomach and three in the small intestine. The gastrin (G) cells were observed as large oval-shaped cells among the mucous epithelial cells located at the junction of the middle and deep mucosa of the gastric antrum. These cells were seen to contain granules of varying size and densities. The cells appeared to be fully granulated in patients with active duodenal ulcer and empty of granules in patients with achlorhydria. Broome [50] showed that following antrectomy there is a marked reduction in peak gastric acid response to histamine. There was even a greater reduction with the addition of vagotomy.

Some investigators [51, 52] have proposed the existence of an inhibitory antral hormone that acts in the presence of an antral pH of 2.5 or less and inhibits parietal cell secretion. Others [53] feel that no such inhibitory hormone exists, but that gastrin elaboration merely stops in the presence of a low antral pH, presumably through local neural reflexes. Harrison [54, 55] demonstrated evidence for the existence of a true inhibitory hormone with divided antral preparations. His data were interpreted as evidence that the antrum in situ, bathed in acid, elaborated a hormone which inhibited gastric secretion. Upon excision of this segment, acid output increased as the Heidenhain pouch was freed from the inhibitory action of this chalone. Jordan,[56, 57] using acid profusion of antral cutaneous fistulas, felt that an inhibitory hormone existed. Duval [58] using cross-circulation or cross-transfusion experiments, suggested the existence of such a hormone.

Byrnes [79, 80] investigated 41 normal patients, 27 patients with duodenal ulcer, 5 patients with recurrent ulcer, 12 patients with benign gastric ulcer, and 8 postgastrectomy patients with a negative insulin test. Gastrin was assayed using antiserum raised against pentagastrin. Normal patients were found to have a serum gastrin level of 0.4 $\mu\mu$g per milliliter. Duodenal ulcer patients had an elevated level of 1.3 $\mu\mu$g per milliliter, and patients with recurrent ulcer following operation were found to have a gastrin level of 1.0 $\mu\mu$g per milliliter. Patients with gastric ulcer were found to have normal serum gastrin levels. Patients with complete vagotomy had serum gastrin levels lower than normal individuals. Following a protein meal, both normal controls and duodenal ulcer patients demonstrated a significant rise in serum gastrin levels, with the duodenal ulcer group demonstrating a greater rise. Gastric ulcer patients showed fasting and postfeeding serum gastrin levels not significantly different from normal individuals. Hyperglycemia suppressed serum gastrin levels in all groups. Byrnes further showed that 8 postvagotomy patients with complete denervation had a mean gastrin level of only 0.15 $\mu\mu$g per milliliter as compared to a level of 0.4 $\mu\mu$g per milliliter in normal controls. Three patients with incomplete vagotomy demonstrated a fasting hypergastrinemia. Atropine was successful in producing a transit reduction in serum gastrin levels in patients with intact vagi. Byrnes concluded that hypergastrinemia could be abolished by either medical or surgical vagotomy. He also suggested that serum gastrin levels may in the future be of benefit in assessing the completeness of vagotomy. There have been no studies yet in the human to show the effect of vagotomy on the gastrin content of antral tissue, but it has been shown experimentally that extrinsic antral denervation decreases the gastrin response following antral profusion with acetylcholine.

An exciting discovery was made by McGuigan [59, 60] in 1968, when he developed the radioiodine immuno-assay of gastrin. Jaffe and McGuigan,[61] using insulin-induced hypoglycemia in the dog, were able to show that vagal stimulation resulted in an increase in serum gastrin in portal vein blood. This was the first documentary evidence showing the measurement of the hormone by a direct method. Heretofore other methods of measurement were indirect, using gastric secretory studies and experimental pouches. Charters and Thompson [62] have measured serum gastrin levels in venous blood from isolated canines' antra during acid secretion. A radio-immuno-assay was used that is based on competitive inhibition of a reaction between isotope-labeled gastrin and antigastrin antibodies or unlabeled gastrin.

Trudeau and McGuigan [63, 64, 65, 66] state that gastrin is the most important humoral agent in the regulation and stimulation of acid secretion. In their experience the mean fasting serum gastrin concentration in patients with duodenal ulcer averaged 78 $\mu\mu$g per milliliter, and similar levels were found in normal control patients. On the other hand, mean serum gastrin concentrations in patients with gastric ulcer were significantly greater, averaging 159 $\mu\mu$g per milliliter. An inverse relationship existed between the fasting serum gastrin levels and the rates and concentration of hydrochloric acid secretion. The patient with an active duodenal ulcer who demonstrated an increase in gastric acid secretion was found to have a low serum gastrin level; whereas the patient with benign gastric ulcer who demonstrated normal or hypoacid secretion had a high level of serum gastrin. In patients without gastrointestinal tract disease, elevated serum gastrin levels were observed with increasing age. McGuigan and Trudeau [67, 68, 69] observed that fasting gastrin concentrations are reduced in patients following vagotomy-antrectomy by 77 percent. In contrast, there was no reduction, but actually a rise in fasting gastrin concentrations following vagotomy-pyloroplasty. The latter findings were similar to duodenal ulcer patients who had not been subjected to operation. In addition, vagotomy-antrectomy reduced mean basal and maximum stimulated acid output over 90 percent. There was less acid reduction following vagotomy-pyloroplasty (Figs. 2 and 3).

Yalow and Berson [70] found high values of plasma gastrin among five patients with the Zollinger-Ellison syndrome, and the values were likewise elevated in 17 patients with pernicious anemia. The administration of oral hydrochloric acid to pernicious anemia

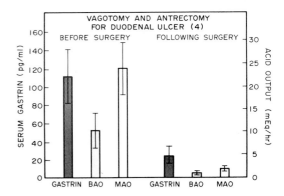

FIG. 2. Following vagotomy-antrectomy there occurs a marked reduction in serum gastrin levels, as well as a profound reduction in both basal acid output and maximal acid output. (From Trudeau and McGuigan, New Engl. J. Med. 286:184, 1972.)

patients produced an acute fall in plasma gastrin concentration. These findings are in keeping with the concept that in the acidified antrum, gastrin release is inhibited.

In studies to the contrary, Reeder, Thompson and co-workers [71, 72, 73] demonstrated in an experiment with a small group of control patients and patients with duodenal ulcer that the ulcer patients demonstrated a higher level of serum gastrin, both fasting and postprandial, than did control patients.

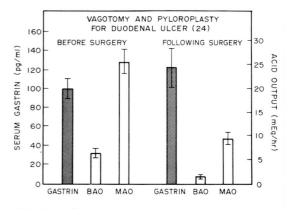

FIG. 3. Following vagotomy-pyloroplasty there actually occurs a rise in serum gastrin levels, but an appreciable fall in both basal and maximal acid output, as depicted. (From Trudeau and McGuigan, New Engl. J. Med. 286:184, 1972.)

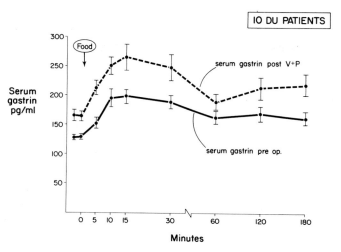

FIG. 4. The rise in serum gastrin levels following vagotomy-pyloroplasty. (Unpublished data; courtesy of Dr. J. C. Thompson and co-workers.)

Further unpublished experiment suggests that the difference may not be statistically significant but that gastrin levels in duodenal ulcer patients tend to be higher. This would indicate that the normal closed-loop relationship in which high levels of acid secretion suppress gastrin release is lost in patients with duodenal ulcer. These co-workers have also recently studied the serum gastrin response to a test meal in ulcer patients before and after operation; ten patients underwent vagotomy-pyloroplasty and seven patients underwent vagotomy-antrectomy. The fasting preoperative serum gastrin levels were again higher among ulcer patients than among the control subjects. The serum gastrin values rose after vagotomy-pyloroplasty, and after vagotomy-antrectomy the serum gastrin levels

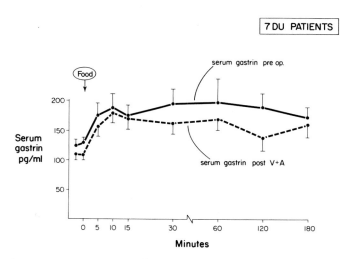

FIG. 5. Following vagotomy-antrectomy there occurs only a slight fall in serum gastrin levels. (Unpublished data; courtesy of Dr. J. C. Thompson and co-workers.)

reduced only slightly, this indicating the importance of extra-antral sources of gastrin (Figs. 4 and 5).

Reeder and Thompson [74] also found consistent increases in serum gastrin concentration and gastric acid secretion during the infusion of calcium in both normal individuals and in patients with duodenal ulcer. The calcium-induced secretory response was abolished by atropine. The serum gastrin levels, however, did not diminish even 3 hours after the initial atropine injection. They concluded that in man the stimulation of gastric secretion during calcium infusion is caused by the elevation of the serum concentration of gastrin, and that calcium potentiates the action of gastrin on the parietal cell.

It has been shown that the maximal acid response to calcium infusion is about one-third the maximal response to betazole (Histalog). In patients with the Zollinger-Ellison syndrome, calcium infusion has proved to be a potent stimulus for both acid secretion and gastrin release, producing a response of 75 percent or more of the maximal response to betazole. Hypercalcemia produced by calcium infusion has also been shown to be associated with an increase in serum gastrin concentration of over 200 percent in normal individuals and a lesser increase noted in patients with duodenal ulcer.[75, 76, 77, 78]

Among patients with duodenal ulcer the G-cells of the antrum have been shown using electron microscopic techniques to be filled with cytoplasmic granules, while the G-cells in patients with gastric ulcer or pernicious anemia demonstrated cytoplasm void of granules.[49]

It is indeed difficult to explain the diverse gastrin levels observed by different investigators in patients with benign gastric ulcer and duodenal ulceration. The methods and agents employed in the various immunoassays have differed and the conflicting results may perhaps not be statistically significant. No doubt, in the future a universally employed standardized assay would shed more light on this perplexing and intriguing problem.

One cannot question that the clinical importance of the gastric antrum is exemplified by the fact that patients who develop recurrent ulceration following complete vagotomy and juxtapyloric gastroenterostomy can be cured by simply removing the gastric antrum. Also, recurrent ulcers that develop after complete vagotomy and patulous pyloroplasty are corrected by removing the antral segment. Both the experimental and clinical importance of the gastric antrum in ulcerogenesis and its removal in combination with vagotomy for treatment of duodenal ulcer have been beautifully documented by the studies of Thompson and Peskin.[52]

EXPERIENCES WITH VAGOTOMY-ANTRECTOMY

From January 1947 through December 1971 a total of 3,584 patients have undergone vagotomy-antrectomy for complications of duodenal ulcer on our services. The youngest patient was 8 years of age and the oldest was 94 years. The ratio of men to women was 7 to 1. The average patient age was 47 years, and the length of ulcer history prior to surgical intervention among the entire series averaged 12 years.

Among the 3,584 patients, pain refractory to prolonged medical management was the indication for operation in 51 percent. In 32 percent of the patients, a single massive hemorrhage along with a past ulcer history or repeated minor bleeding was the reason for operation. Fifteen percent of the patients

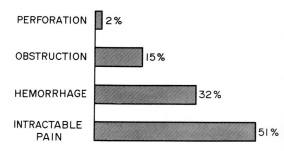

FIG. 6. Indications for operation among 3,584 patients undergoing vagotomy-antrectomy.

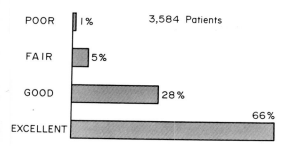

FIG. 7. Overall clinical results among the entire series of patients followed from January 1947 through December 1971.

presented with gastric outlet obstruction and a small group of selected patients (2 percent) with an acute perforation were considered suitable candidates for definitive surgical therapy. There were no postoperative deaths in this latter group of patients (Fig. 6).

The follow-up among the entire series has been practically total and has consisted of frequent office visits, hospital outpatient studies, and hospital readmissions when deemed advisable. Some patients, of course, have subsequently died of unrelated causes since operation, but each was followed to the time of death, and have remained in the clinical study. Clinical results have been graded in four separate categories: (1) excellent, (2) good, (3) fair, and (4) poor. An excellent result is recorded only if the patient

55 (1.6%) deaths in 3,584 patients

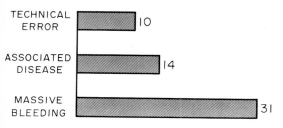

FIG. 8. The highest mortality has occurred in the elderly, poor-risk patient operated upon for massive hemorrhage.

3,584 Patients
January, 1947 - December, 1971

MORTALITY IN EMERGENCY
OPERATION FOR HEMORRHAGE
all ages - 3.4 %
over 60 years - 6.5 %

NON-FATAL COMPLICATIONS - 18.0 %

COMPLICATIONS DIRECTLY
RELATED TO STOMACH - 5.5 %

FIG. 9. Truncal vagotomy-antrectomy. The mortality for emergency operation and the percentages of nonfatal complications are depicted for 3,584 patients followed from January 1947 through December 1971.

is free of all digestive complaints and possesses a digestive apparatus comparable to that of a normal individual. A good result is listed if the patient experiences mild dumping symptoms, occasional epigastric distress, or mild and transient diarrhea. A fair result is given the patient who continues to complain of abdominal distress, not like ulcer disease, and moderate dumping symptoms. Many of this group in spite of their new set of symptoms state that they benefited from the operation. A result is recorded as poor if the patient has received no improvement from the operation, if he has a distressing new set of symptoms, or if a recurrent ulcer develops.

According to the above criteria, the clinical results have been excellent in 66 percent, good in 28 percent, fair in 5 percent, and poor in 1 percent (Fig. 7).

Among the group of 3,584 patients there were 55 postoperative deaths either in the hospital or within 30 days after dismissal from the hospital (mortality rate, 1.6 percent). The majority of deaths [31] occurred in elderly patients in the seventh and eighth decades of life who were operated upon as an emergency procedure for control of massive hemorrhage. Frequently many of these pa-

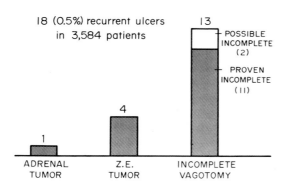

18 (0.5%) recurrent ulcers in 3,584 patients

FIG. 10.   The rate of recurrent ulceration among the entire series has been less than 1 percent and a proved incomplete vagotomy has been the leading cause of recurrence.

tients were transferred to the surgical service late, usually 48 to 96 hours after having received 8 to 12 units of blood. It is felt that had the operation been advised earlier after the onset of bleeding some members of this group would have survived. Disabling-associated disease in the elderly patient with massive bleeding or obstruction was the reason for operative death in fourteen cases. In

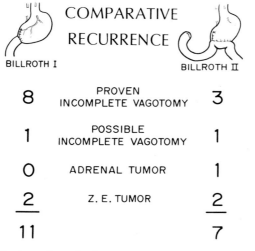

FIG. 11.   The Billroth I reconstruction with vagotomy has proved as effective as a Billroth II resection with vagotomy in controlling recurrent ulceration.

ten cases, a simple technical or judgment error on the part of the surgeon in carrying out the combined operation was alone responsible for death. In each case, this could have been avoided had the operator paid closer attention to minor technical details (Fig. 8). The incidence of nonfatal significant hospital complications among the 3,584 patients has been 18 percent. The mortality rate for emergency operation for control of hemorrhage including all ages has been 3.4 percent and the mortality rate for massive hemorrhage in patients over age 60 has been 6.5 percent. For nonfatal complications related directly to the stomach, such as an anastomotic leak or stomal obstruction, the rate has been 5.5 percent (Fig. 9). Over the follow-up study, symptoms of the dumping syndrome have occurred in 30 percent of patients but have proved severe in only 1 percent. Weight losses below ideal level have occurred in 10 percent.

The recurrent ulcer rate during the follow-up period after vagotomy-antrectomy has been astoundingly low. There have been 18 proved recurrent ulcers and no additional case of a suspected recurrence among the 3,584 patients (incidence of recurrence, 0.5 percent). Approximately 1,500 patients have now been followed for 10 years and almost 500 patients have been observed from 15 to 25 years. Each of the 18 recurrences was manifested by recurrent pain, bleeding, or perforation which occurred within 24 months of operation. This has also been the experience of Smithwick and Farmer, and we have not seen recurrences develop during the long-range follow-up. This latter finding is a great endorsement for the operation and further attests to the effectiveness of the combined procedure in the prevention of recurrences.

Among the eighteen recurrent ulcers observed to date, four resulted from a Zollinger-Ellison tumor proved either at subsequent operation or at autopsy. Eleven patients had an incomplete vagotomy at the original operation, confirmed later by the Hollander test and at subsequent operation for correction of the recurrence. A functioning adrenal tumor was responsible for a recurrent ulcer in one patient. One patient is of interest in that she developed massive hematemesis several days after vagotomy-antrectomy performed for a penetrating duodenal ulcer. She had respiratory insufficiency and was quite ill. At emergency reoperation, multiple mucosal and submucosal ulcerations were found which literally filled the remaining gastric pouch. Unfortunately the patient did not survive total gastrectomy, and autopsy was not permitted. Either this patient had additional parasympathetic innervation or presented some bizarre endocrine abnormality such as a Zollinger-Ellison tumor, or else some type of stress phenomenon occurred. We have included this case in our recurrent ulcer data, but no recurrence of a duodenal ulcer was noted. One additional patient rebled massively several months after vagotomy-antrectomy and required emergency reoperation. Because of the desperate situation in each case, a high resection of the stomach was done, and the periesophageal area was not explored. The patient has not re-bled during a long-range follow-up. However, the small gastric pouch which remains with its small parietal cell mass is incapable of responding to insulin hypoglycemia. Thus the status of vagal nerve activity cannot be correctly determined. It is quite possible that incomplete vagotomy was carried out at the initial operation (Fig. 10).

Of the 18 recurrences, 11 followed vagotomy-antrectomy and a Billroth I reconstruction, and 7 followed a Billroth II type anastomosis. It should be stressed that the Billroth I anastomosis in our hands has been used most frequently and is considered our procedure of choice since its introduction with vagotomy in 1951 by Harkins (Fig. 11).

ACCUMULATED CLINICAL DATA

Several years ago Thoroughman published a complete and comprehensive retrospective study analyzing the 504 patients who had undergone truncal vagotomy and hemigastrectomy. The overall hospital mortality rate, including both elective and emergency cases, was 1.6 percent. For patients undergoing elective operation, the mortality rate was 0.54 percent and for emergency bleeding patients it was 5 percent. Ninety-one percent of the entire series experienced

satisfactory long-term results over a 2- to 14-year follow-up. Only two recurrent ulcers developed among the 504 patients (incidence of 0.4 percent), and each recurrence was due to an unrecognized Zollinger-Ellison tumor. During the long-term postoperative evaluation, over 90 percent of patients were achlorhydric to histamine stimulation. Postoperative weight losses occurred in only 26.5 percent of patients, and in most instances the loss was due to a chronic debilitating illness and was not the direct result of vagotomy-hemigastrectomy. Diarrhea occurred in 4.1 percent of patients, but was severe in only one patient. Symptoms of the dumping syndrome occurred in 10.5 percent of cases. At the present time Thoroughman is even more enthusiastic with the combined procedure, and the overall mortality rate continues to be under 2 percent, the recurrent ulcer rate 0.05 percent, and overall patient satisfaction over 90 percent.[81, 82]

Another outstanding retrospective study of vagotomy and distal gastrectomy is that of Palumbo. His series is perhaps the most carefully studied and documented analysis of the problem to appear in the American literature. From 1952 to June 1972 Palumbo has carried out vagotomy and distal gastrectomy on 611 patients: 558 patients were operated upon on an elective basis and 53 patients were operated upon as an emergency. The overall mortality rate has been 2.3 percent (14 deaths). The combined emergency and elective mortality rate among 417 patients under age 60 was 1.4 percent, and the mortality rate in patients over age 60 was 4.1 percent. Among 51 patients undergoing emergency operation for massive hemorrhage, there were 3 deaths (mortality rate, 5.9 percent). The 3 deaths were due to postoperative pulmonary complications. Among 558 patients undergoing the combined procedure on an elective basis there were 11 deaths, or a mortality rate of 1.9 percent. Among the elective group, the mortality rate in those patients below 60 years of age was 1.2 percent, and in those over 60 years it was 3.8 percent. During the follow-up period, 62.4 percent of patients maintained their preoperative weight, 21 percent gained weight following operation, and 16.6 percent lost weight after surgery. Weight loss due solely

Table 1.   ACCUMULATED DATA

Studies	Number of Cases	Mortality (percent)	Satisfactory Results (percent)	Recurrence (percent)	Follow-Up (years)
Thoroughman, J. C. (elective and emergency cases)	504	1.6	91	0.4	2 to 14
Palumbo, L. T. (elective and emergency cases)	611	2.3	90	0.6	1 to 20
Farmer, D. A. (elective and emergency cases)	622	1.9	92	1.4	1 to 26
Jordan, P. H. (elective cases)	90	0	89	1.1	1 to 8
Wolf, J. S. (elective and emergency cases)	547	1.1	90	0.6	1 to 10

to the operative procedure, however, was only 3.1 percent; the remainder of the weight losses were related to chronic constitutional illnesses. The ulcer recurrence rate in Palumbo's series, over a follow-up of 1 to 20 years, has been 0.6 percent. Of 476 patients undergoing postoperative gastric secretory studies, 94.8 percent showed no free hydrochloric acid in the gastric contents.[83, 84]

Farmer has continued to follow the cases reported by himself and Smithwick in the early 1950s, and of 752 patients, 622 have been followed from 1 to 26 years. The overall operative mortality rate among the group of 622 patients was 1.9 percent and the current recurrent ulcer rate is 1.4 percent. Among the 15 patients comprising the series of 622 who have developed a recurrent ulcer, 14 recurrences were due to a proved incomplete vagotomy, and one was the result of a Zollinger-Ellison tumor. Farmer has observed that each recurrence occurred during the early follow-up period and he has not observed a recurrent ulcer over the long-range study of his patients.[85, 86]

Jordan [87, 88] recently published a perspective, randomized study of vagotomy-antrectomy that comprised a series of 90 patients undergoing elective operation. There was no death in the entire group and 89 percent of the patients have experienced a satisfactory result. Only one recurrent ulcer has developed over an 1- to 8-year follow-up. Jordan concluded that vagotomy-antrectomy was superior to lesser operations as the treatment of choice for the elective management of duodenal ulcer in the majority of patients because of its low recurrent ulcer rate with-

out the association of increased morbidity or mortality. He felt the operation contraindicated when highly technical problems were encountered at operation.

Wolf,[89] in a recent retrospective study, performed vagotomy-antrectomy among 547 patients including both elective and emergency cases, with an overall mortality rate of 1.1 percent. During a follow-up study from 1 to 10 years, the recurrent ulcer rate has been 0.6 percent, and 90 percent of patients expressed satisfaction with the procedure. It is of interest that during the past 5 years the operative mortality rate among elective cases in Wolf's group has dropped from 0.8 percent to 0.3 percent (Table 1).

TECHNIQUE

The type of abdominal incision is strictly a matter of personal preference. We prefer a long midline incision extending from the ensiform process to below the umbilicus (Fig. 12). In extremely obese individuals, a high bucket handle type incision affords excellent exposure. We feel that either a right or a left subcostal incision leaves much to be desired. After a thorough abdominal exploration is made, the duodenal ulcer is evaluated as to its penetrating effect into the pancreas, and its relationship to surrounding structures, particularly the common bile duct. Added attention is given to examination of the pancreas, especially if a Zollinger-Ellison tumor is suspected from the preoperative work-up.

In the combined operation, vagotomy is

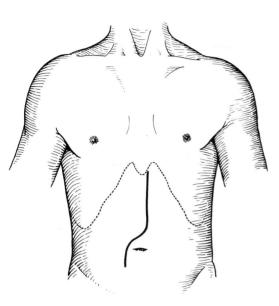

FIG. 12.   The abdominal incision must be generous, for adequate exposure is mandatory.

carried out first. Although some surgeons, notably Crile and Weinberg, prefer to elevate the left lobe of the liver superiorly to gain access to the distal esophagus, our preference is to divide the avascular triangular ligament and to retract the left hepatic lobe to the right. Care must be exercised, however, and the ligament should not be divided as far back as its origin or troublesome bleeding will ensue from the phrenic veins. It is our feeling, however, that division of the avascular ligament and retraction of the left lobe to the right inflicts less trauma to the liver than does forcefully elevating the left lobe superiorly, leaving the avascular ligament intact. In the latter circumstance, we have seen subcapsular hematomas result. Division of the ligament also gives added exposure to the distal periesophageal area. In our opinion, it is important to have two assistants to retract the costal arches in addition to a first assistant whose sole duty it is to assist the operator. This facilitates greatly the execution of the operation and diminishes the likelihood of injury to the spleen, liver, and other structures. Of course, excellent anesthesia is mandatory, as proper relaxation of the patient is an all-important factor in the performance of the procedure.

The spleen is covered by a moist lap-

arotomy pack, and gentle downward traction is applied on the cardia and lesser curve of the stomach. One should avoid downward traction on the greater curve to prevent splenic injury. A small transverse incision is made in the peritoneum overlying the esophagus approximately 2 cm below the inferior edge of the diaphragm. The operator's right index finger is then introduced into this incision and with careful and gentle blunt dissection, the esophagus is completely encircled. The right vagal nerve, which usually lies posterior and to the right of the esophagus, is identified by palpation and freed up. An assistant then places three long clamps on the nerve over a distance of approximately 2 inches and the nerve is divided between the superior and the most distally placed clamp, thus removing a section of the nerve with the middle clamp. As small veins usually accompany the nerve, the cut ends of the divided nerve are ligated with silk sutures or else secured with a metal clip.

The left vagus nerve, the smaller of the two, is more constant in location, being imbedded in the anterior musculature of the esophageal wall. This nerve is sectioned, a segment removed, and the nerve ends are ligated or clipped. A careful search is then made by each member of the operating team for any additional nerve fibers which, if found, are divided. Frequently the left nerve will divide above the esophageal hiatus and two long filaments will have to be dealt with. In performing vagotomy, we do not divide the esophageal branches of either the right or left nerve which enter the esophageal wall at the level of the hiatus. Division of these twigs is unnecessary and usually results in esophageal motility disturbances. Some surgeons prefer not to free the esophagus from its bed in performing vagotomy but rely on a nerve hook to free up both the right and left vagi without disturbing the posterior fibrous attachments about the esophagus and the posterior layer of the phrenicoesophageal ligament. By gently encircling the esophagus as described, we have not encountered the complication of posterior gastroesophageal reflux or the subsequent development of a sliding esophageal hiatal hernia. Lastly, if there is any attenuation of the right crural sling, this structure is approximated posterior to the esophagus with several interrupted sutures of No. 2–0 silk (Fig. 13). If a sliding

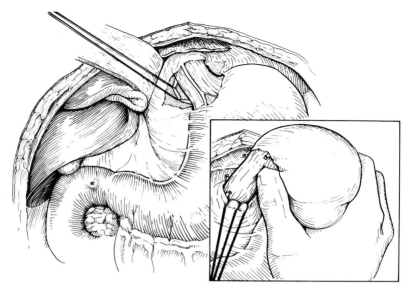

FIG. 13. A long segment is removed from both the right and left vagal nerve trunks. Esophageal fibers, if present, are preserved. The right crural sling, if attenuated, is approximated with interrupted No. 2–0 silk sutures. If a sliding esophageal hiatal hernia exists, either a Hill gastropexy or a Nissen fundoplication is carried out.

esophageal hiatal hernia is present, in addition to repairing the crural sling, we also perform a posterior gastropexy after the method of Lucius Hill.

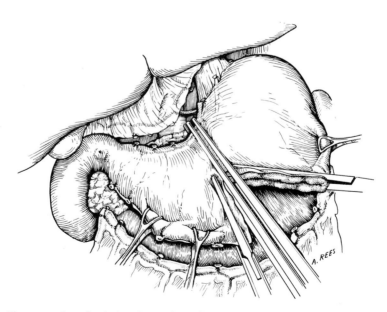

FIG. 14. The stomach is divided midway along the greater curve, and the greater curve is used later for anastomosis to the duodenum. Clamps are placed obliquely and higher on the lesser curve according to the principle of Schoemaker.

The peritoneum overlying the esophagus is not reapproximated, and after being certain that hemostasis is complete, the left hepatic lobe is allowed to assume its normal anatomical position without suture. This technique employing vagotomy has worked well in our experience, and we have not employed transabdominal supradiaphragmatic vagotomy as advocated by Dragstedt.

Attention is now directed to the stomach, and the greater curve of the organ is gently grasped with several Babcock clamps and fanned out, with moderate traction. The vessels along the greater curve are isolated, divided, and tied with silk. The dissection along the greater curve extends to the junction of the right and left gastroepiploic vessels, which is about midway the distance of the greater curve. Distally on the greater curve, the dissection is next taken to the pylorus, where the right gastroepiploic artery vessels are divided and secured with silk. At this stage, the distal half of the stomach along the greater curve is entirely free and can be fanned out further and elevated with Babcock forceps so that the underlying pancreas can again be thoroughly examined for the possibility of an adenoma or other abnormality. With the lesser sac opened, the fibrous anatomical adhesions between the posterior wall of the stomach and the pseudocapsule of the pancreas are now severed, thus allowing the lesser curve of the stomach to be entirely free.

Attention is now directed to the lesser gastric curve, and a point approximately 3 cm proximal to the angularis is selected for ligation of the vascular bundle along the curve. This ligation includes division of the descending branches of the left gastric artery and vein. Fanning out the greater curve with moderate tension, using Babcock forceps held by an assistant, greatly facilitates the dissection of the vessels along the lesser curve. After this dissection, the distal half of the stomach is now ready for division and extirpation.

On the greater curve of the stomach, the point of the transection is approximately 2 cm distal to that on the lesser curve. The stomach is divided between two straight Allen or Glassman clamps placed at right angles to the long axis of the stomach at the point selected midway on the greater curve. These clamps define the size of the gastroduodenal or gastroenteric stoma. After division of the stomach between these two clamps, another pair of similar but longer clamps is placed

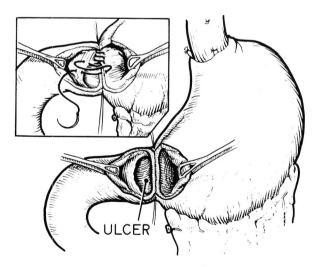

FIG. 15.   With deep, penetrating posterior wall ulcers, a Billroth I reconstruction may still be carried out in many instances. In such situations, the ulcer is left attached to the pancreas and the gastric wall is anastomosed to the duodenal wall below the site of the ulcer, thus excluding the ulcer from the alimentary stream.

from this point of division in similar fashion across the gastric wall up to the point previously selected on the lesser curve. The stomach is next divided between these two clamps, which completes the entire division of the stomach. This is the operative technique originally described by Schoemaker of the Hague. The extent of the distal resection encompasses the antral segment and amounts to about a 40 percent resection in terms of total gastric mucosal surface area (Fig. 14).

The stomach pouch along the lesser curve, still held with the Allen clamp, is closed beneath the clamp with one hemostatic layer of continuous chromic catgut. The clamp is then removed, the crushed tissue excised, and a second layer of interrupted 2–0 silk sutures is placed beneath the previous catgut suture. Next, the original catgut suture is returned along the length of the lesser curve as a continuous Lembert suture. One seromuscular suture of silk is placed at the junction of the lesser curve closure and the tip of the Allen clamp applied to the greater curve for future reference. The antral segment is now reflected to the right and serves as a handle for the operator in facilitating the dissection of the distal

pylorus and duodenal bulb. The right gastric artery is ligated and divided as well as the several small veins encountered on the posterior wall of the distal pylorus and proximal duodenum. The ulcer is removed if it is easily accessible, but if it is deeply embedded in the pancreas or located low in the duodenum, removal is contraindicated, for carrying the dissection too far down onto the duodenum is conducive to significant complications. Routine removal of the ulcer, as advocated by some gastric surgeons, is, in our opinion, to be condemned. If there is a recent history of hemorrhage or if the patient is bleeding at the time of surgery, a more aggressive attempt is made to remove the ulcer or at least to obliterate the ulcer crater with interrupted sutures of heavy silk. On many occasions we have removed the proximal one-half or more of a deep penetrating ulcer and have left the distal portion of the ulcer attached to the pancreas. In such instances, providing the patient has a normal or near-normal anterior duodenal wall, we do not hesitate to proceed with end-to-end gastroduodenostomy. When encountering large and deep posterior penetrating ulcers that have completely destroyed the posterior

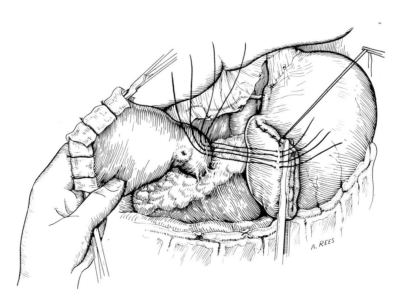

FIG. 16. The lesser gastric curve has been closed. A posterior row of interrupted seromuscular sutures is placed between the greater curve of the gastric pouch and duodenal wall distal to the ulcer.

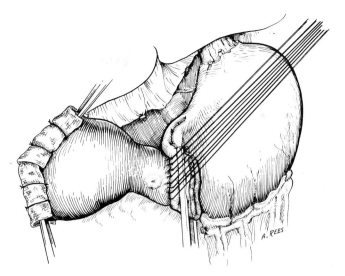

FIG. 17.   The silk sutures have been tied individually, thus approximating the gastric pouch to the second portion of the duodenum.

wall of the duodenal bulb, we still in many cases perform end-to-end gastroduodenostomy by gently freeing the posterior duodenal wall distal to the ulcer and bringing the posterior wall of the gastric pouch over the ulcer crater and suturing the gastric pouch to the duodenum below the ulcer site. Thus, the anastomosis overlies the ulcer crater and

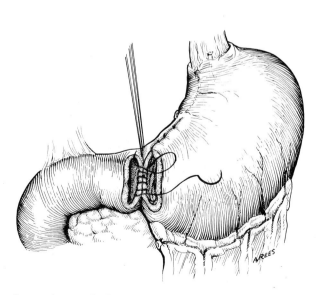

FIG. 18.   The specimen, along with the clamp on the greater curve of the gastric pouch, has been removed, and any crushed tissue excised. The posterior gastric and duodenal walls are being approximated with a continuous suture of fine chromic catgut, the suture encompassing the full thickness of both the gastric and duodenal walls.

leaves the crater excluded on the head of the pancreas (Fig. 15).

In the usual case after we have freed the duodenum the satisfactory distance, gastroduodenal continuity is next reestablished. The first step is begun by setting a row of interrupted seromuscular sutures of fine silk between the posterior wall of the greater curve of the gastric pouch, still occluded by the Allen clamp, and the posterior aspect of the duodenum (Fig. 16). After placement of the final suture, the gastric pouch and duodenum are brought into apposition by the first assistant and the sutures are individually tied (Fig. 17). The clamp is next removed from the greater gastric curve and the crushed tissue excised. The duodenum is then transected and the antral segment and bulb are removed. A continuous layer of fine chromic catgut suture is next placed, further uniting the gastric and duodenal walls. This suture commences posteriorly at the greater curvature aspect of the anastomosis and incorporates all layers of the opposing gastric and duodenal walls. As the running catgut stitch advances, the previously placed silk sutures are cut close to the knots (Fig. 18). The catgut suture when completed posteriorly is then advanced anteriorly as an inverting suture to approximate the anterior gastric and duodenal walls. It is imperative that bits of tissue be taken near the cut ends of the opposing gastric and duodenal walls so that a minimal cuff is inverted (Fig. 19). A final row of fine interrupted silk sutures placed anteriorly completes the anastomosis. Care is taken to place a special *angle stitch* at the lesser curve of the gastroduodenal anastomosis. This silk suture includes both anterior and posterior gastric walls and the lesser curve of the duodenum, to ensure against postoperative leakage. The reference suture, previously referred to, is of great importance in defining the exact position to place this triangular stitch (Fig. 20). As a final step, the greater omentum is brought up and interposed between the gastroduodenal suture line and the inferior aspect of the liver (Fig. 21). This maneuver will ensure against the anastomosis adhering to the right hepatic lobe, producing angulation and kinking with resultant obstruction. Before this step was utilized, we encountered several cases of postoperative stomal obstruction on this basis. Particularly did this complication occur in several instances where concomitant

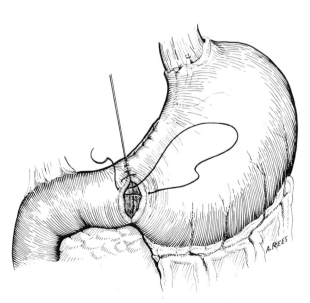

FIG. 19. The chromic catgut suture is being advanced anteriorly as a continental stitch, thus inverting the gastric and duodenal walls. Note that very small bits of tissue are being taken to allow for an adequate lumen.

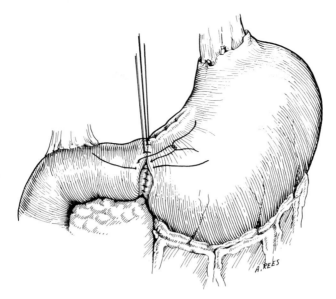

FIG. 20. An anterior seromuscular layer of interrupted silk sutures completes the anastomosis. A triangular stitch at the lesser curve of the anastomosis ensures against leakage at this critical angle.

cholecystectomy was performed. At reoperation the gastroduodenal anastomosis was found adherent to the gallbladder fossa. Since interpolating the omentum between these structures this complication has not occurred, however.

As a rule, we do not insert Penrose drains to the right upper quadrant following the alimentary reconstruction. In a small percentage of cases, however, where the anastomosis is technically difficult. or where there is extreme edema about the pancreas and

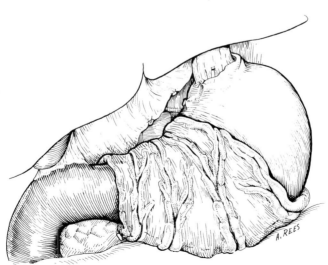

FIG. 21. The greater omentum is shown brought up and interpolated between the gastroduodenal suture line and the undersurface of the right hepatic lobe. Prior to utilizing this step, we have had the gastroduodenal suture line adhere to the liver and produce gastric outlet obstruction.

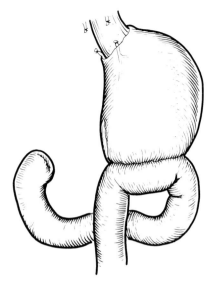

FIG. 22. Bilateral truncal vagotomy with a left-to-right, short-loop gastrojejunostomy. This reconstruction is used in selected circumstances.

related structures, drainage is instituted for several days. In several technically difficult cases in which drainage was instituted, we have observed a minimum of bile leakage about the drains, and in such situations, drainage has proved to be of great value.

Should the pathological condition encountered about the duodenum not lend itself to reconstruction by end-to-end gastroduodenostomy, we close the duodenal stump using a standard three-layer technique and restore continuity with a short-loop retrocolic gastrojejunostomy (Fig. 22). Currently we are employing end-to-end gastroduodenostomy as the preferred method of reconstruction and are using the Hofmeister anastomosis in only 2 percent of cases. This latter reconstruction is employed with deep penetrating posterior wall ulcers in which the anterior duodenal wall is also involved in extensive scar tissue and in cases of extreme obesity where exposure is difficult. Also, if there is stenosis in the second and third duodenum, obviously a Billroth I reconstruction is contraindicated.

The laparotomy wound is closed in layers with interrupted silk sutures. Retention sutures are used almost routinely except in young, slender individuals.

DISCUSSION

Within recent years, experimental work has shown a definite interrelationship between the cephalic and the hormonal phases of gastric secretion. Stimulation of the vagus nerves causes the release of gastrin from the antrum, and the release of gastrin potentiates the response of the parietal cell mass to vagal stimulation. Removal of the cephalic phase of secretion by complete vagotomy reduces to some extent the response of the hormonal phase by diminishing the release of gastrin and likewise renders the parietal cells less responsive to all stimuli. Removal of the hormonal phase of secretion materially reduces the effectiveness of the cephalic phase.[90]

The suggestion that the gastric antrum is a perpetuating factor in the development of duodenal ulcer has gained widespread general support, for there appears to be convincing clinical and experimental evidence that the antrum plays an important role in duodenal ulcer as well as in stomal ulceration.[91, 92, 93] Much discussion has arisen as to the anatomical extent of the distal resection necessary to ensure complete antral extirpation. The limits of the antrum are variable, and antral mucosa is known to extend higher on the lesser curvature than on the greater curve. Indeed, on the lesser curve, antral tissue has been found to extend to the esophagus. In recent years several sophisticated methods of defining the antral limits at the time of operation have been described. These methods, for the most part, employ staining with Congo red and also pH determinations have been used.[94, 95, 96, 97]

Our landmarks used in removing the antrum have been the points of oblique division of the stomach at the lesser curvature several centimeters above the angle, and about midway along the greater curve. This actually entails approximately a 40 percent distal resection and encompasses somewhat more than the antral segment, for as a rule the antrum is usually restricted to the distal 25 to 30 percent of the stomach. We have not felt it important to use Congo red staining at the time of operation, for in our opinion precise delineation of the antrum is unnecessary. If a Billroth II type reconstruction is employed after vagotomy-antrectomy, it is imperative of course, to remove the distal extent of the antrum, as the antrum in exclusion constitutes a potent ulcerogenic situation. If a cuff of proximal antral tissue is left attached to the gastric pouch following a Billroth II type anastomosis, it is of far less clinical importance. Provided there is no obstruction at the gastroenterostomy site, and provided the gastric pouch empties readily after a Billroth II type reconstruction, the leaving behind of a small segment of proximal antral tissue is of no consequence. This feeling is also shared by Palumbo. Should obstruction subsequently develop at the stoma, however, stasis will occur and the small retained proximal antrum will become ulcerogenic. We stress that we prefer to remove the entire antrum, but if one leaves behind a small segment of antral tissue, either proximally or distally after vagotomy-antrectomy, and a classic Billroth I reconstruction,

no particular hazard is created provided the gastroduodenostomy empties readily and no stasis occurs. In a normally emptying gastroduodenostomy with a small amount of antral tissue retained proximally or distally, the small residual secretions of acid from the gastric fundus and particularly the inhibitory action of the duodenal hormones constituting the duodenal break on gastric secretion, although altered somewhat by vagotomy, renders innocuous any small residual antral tissue.

Currently, vagotomy-antrectomy appears to be the most effective procedure yet devised to control the duodenal ulcer diathesis.[81, 83, 85, 87, 89, 98, 99, 100, 101] In our current series totaling 3,584 patients, an operative mortality rate of 1.6 percent is not at variance with reports of other series from similar university and teaching centers. An analysis of etiological factors influencing our mortality rate revealed that the greatest risk

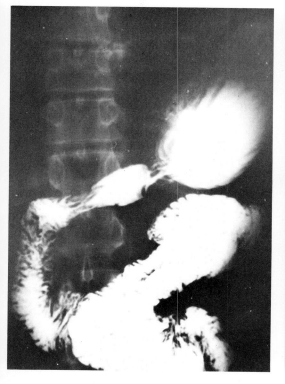

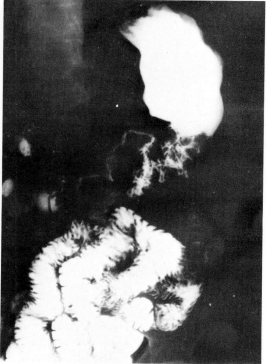

FIG. 23. Postoperative barium study showing a normal gastric pouch and normal gastroduodenal outflow tract following bilateral truncal vagotomy-antrectomy and a Billroth I reconstruction.

FIG. 24. Postoperative normal barium study following bilateral truncal vagotomy-antrectomy with a short-loop retrocolic Hofmeister type reconstruction.

of the procedure has been in its application to the elderly poor-risk individuals who experience near-exsanguinating hemorrhage, elderly patients with severe constitutional disease, and those who present severe ulcer processes that render duodenal dissection hazardous. Earlier operation in the elderly patient with massive hemorrhage may lower the mortality. We feel strongly that proper timing and early operation are more important than the choice of operation when one is confronted with the elderly poor-risk bleeder. As a result, we have been employing vagotomy and pyloroplasty less in such circumstances. Our results with vagotomy-pyloroplasty have in general been disappointing, but we believe it still has a limited application in highly selected instances.[102, 103]

It is indeed gratifying to note that 94 percent of the patients undergoing vagotomy-antrectomy have experienced a satisfactory clinical result. It should be emphasized that many of the patients who had an unsatisfactory result were benefited by the operative procedure, and except for the 18 patients who developed recurrent ulcerations, each has been relieved of ulcer distress.

During the past 15 years on our service, an increasing number of patients have been subjected to a Billroth I reconstruction following vagotomy-antrectomy. In our early experience, the Billroth II reconstruction was employed exclusively. At present the Billroth I reconstruction has been used in approximately 2,800 cases. The latter type of reconstruction is our current method of choice; and as experience with end-to-end gastroduodenostomy has increased, we have found it safe to adapt the principle to the vast majority of the large posterior penetrating ulcers. As stated elsewhere, it is our firm belief that the Billroth I reconstruction can be safely carried out in most instances and now only a very small percentage of our patients undergo the Billroth II type anastomosis (Figs. 23 and 24). If there is any discrepancy in the size of the duodenal opening to be anastomosed to the gastric pouch, the Horsley maneuver of longitudinally incising the antimesenteric duodenal border for a centimeter or two may be readily performed. Also, in the majority of our patients being operated upon for gastric outlet obstruction, we perform end-to-end

gastroduodenostomy and routinely carry out a long Horsley incision on the antimesenteric border of the descending duodenum (Fig. 25). It is rare that we Kocherize the descending duodenum during our dissection, and we particularly feel that it is contraindicated in most instances when performing end-to-end gastroduodenostomy. If the duodenum is Kocherized, in our opinion it disturbs duodenal peristalsis, presents problems in duodenal emptying, and actually causes reflux of duodenal contents into the gastric pouch, with resultant bilious vomiting in some instances. Routine Kocherization of the duodenum has also been condemned by Weinberg.

Interest in the Billroth I reconstruction has been experienced by many gastric surgeons during the past decade, and it is being used throughout the country with increasing frequency. As with any other type operation, one becomes more proficient in its use as experience accumulates. It is extremely important, however, that one be able to recognize the extensive inflammatory duodenal ulcer process which should not be treated by Billroth I reconstruction. We have had no experience with the Finney-von Haberer modification of the Billroth I and I feel it is seldom indicated. The instances of postoperative stomal obstruction following gastroduodenostomy have been limited almost entirely to our early experience, and at present this complication is rarely encountered.[104, 105] We have experienced a few anastomotic leaks after a Billroth I reconstruction in difficult cases, but in no instance has a fatality resulted. In each case the possibility of postoperative leakage was appreciated at the time of operation, and in these cases generous right upper quadrant drainage was instituted. Leakage following a Billroth I anastomosis has been associated with less morbidity than leakage from a duodenal stump closure, for in the former reconstruction the leaks are apparently small and the majority of the duodenal contents drain back into the gastric pouch and are removed through the indwelling nasogastric tube. It would appear to be indeed rare for a gastroduodenostomy completely to disrupt as is frequently the case when a duodenal stump closure breaks down.

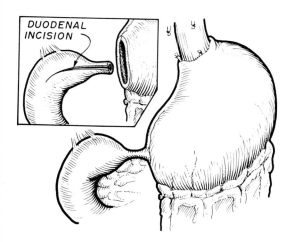

DUODENAL INCISION

FIG. 25. The Horsley maneuver is depicted, in which the lumen of the duodenum is increased by dividing it along the antimesenteric border. This maneuver is particularly applicable when operating upon the patient with gastric outlet obstruction where there is marked stenosis of the duodenal bulb.

Symptoms suggesting the dumping syndrome have occurred in 30 percent of patients who underwent a Billroth I reconstruction on our service and also in approximately 30 percent of those with a Billroth II reconstruction. The clinical results following the Billroth I and Billroth II reconstruction in our experience are also about equal. The Billroth I is more expedient, and is a more physiological and anatomical reconstruction, since it preserves the duodenal outflow tract, preserving to some extent the humoral factor of duodenal inhibition. Of course, duodenal hormonal inhibition is somewhat diminished by bilateral truncal vagotomy. The Billroth I reconstruction also allows for more thorough mixing of the gastric contents with bile and pancreatic juices. Postoperative weight status has been equal among the Billroth I and Billroth II groups; but the Billroth I reconstruction is particularly preferred when operating upon the slender and malnourished individual and also in women with complications of ulcer. In approximately 10 percent of patients, those with the Billroth I and Billroth II reconstruction have lost weight to a figure below the ideal level.

Vagotomy-antrectomy appears to have stood the test of time. Many of its former critics now heartily endorse the operation. The combined procedure is currently the most effective operation at the surgeon's disposal to control the complications of duodenal ulcer. The combined procedure, when properly and skillfully executed, can be performed with a low morbidity and low mortality rate. The significant long-term adverse side-effects are small, indeed. In our opinion, the operative mortality rate following surgery for duodenal ulcer in large series, even in the hands of the most skilled, will never approximate zero percent. The mortality rate can, however, be kept at a respectably low figure if surgical consultation from our medical colleagues is requested earlier in chronic duodenal ulcer cases of long-standing, with good surgical indications. When severe constitutional disease and old age overcome the patient, the mortality rate rises when ulcer complications develop. Irrespective of the type of operation carried out in such circumstances, the mortality rate will be high.

Considering all factors involved, vagotomy-antrectomy is now recognized over the surgical world as the most effective therapeutic procedure for control of the complications of duodenal ulcer.

REFERENCES

1. Temkin, O., Merrem's youthful dream: The early history of experimental pylorectomy. Bull. Hist. Med. 31:29, 1957.
2. Merrem, D. C. T., Animadversiones quaedeum chirurgicae experimentils in animalibus factis illustratae, Giessae, Taché et Mueller, 1810.
3. Langenbeck, C. J. M., Bibliothek fur die chirurgie, Gottingen, 1811, cited by Temkin, 1957.
4. Gussenbauer, C., Ueber die erste durch Th. Billroth am Menschen ausgefuehrte Kehlkopf Exstirpation und die Aneuendung eines Kunstlichen Kehlkopfes, Arch. Klin. Chir. 17:343, 1874.
5. Gussenbauer, C., and Von Winiwarter, A., Die partielle mangenresection. Arch. Klin. Chir. 19:347, 1876.
6. Péan, J. E., De l'ablation des teemeurs de l'estomas par la gastrectomie, Gaz. d. hop. 52:473, 1879.
7. Rydygier, L., Extirpation des carcinomatosen pylorus, Tod nach Zwolf Stunden, Dtsch. Z. Chir. 14:252 1880.
8. Billroth, T., Clinical Surgery. Translated by C. T. Dent. London, New Sydenham Soc., 1881.
9. Edkins, J. S., J. Physiol. (Lond.) 34:133, 1906.

10. Schur, H., and Plaschkes, S., Mitt. Grenzgeb. Med. Chir. 28:795, 1915.
11. Boller, R., and Pilgerstorfer, W., Klin. Wochenschr. 15:1608, 1936.
12. Komarov, S. A., Rev. Can. Biol. 1:191, 1942.
13. Uvnäs, B., Acta. Physiol. Scand. 6:97, 1943.
14. Brodie, B. C., Philos. Trans. R. Soc. Lond. [Biol. Sci.] 104:102, 1814.
15. Bernard, C., Lecons sur la Physiologie et la Pathologie du Systeme Nerveux, Paris, Balliere, 1858.
16. Pavlov, I. P., The Work of the Digestive Glands, 2d ed. Translated by W. H. Thompson, London, Griffin, 1910.
17. Schiff, M., Neue Untersuchungen uber den Einfluss des Nerves Vagus auf die Magentatigkeit. Monatschrift fur Proktische Medizin. Jg. V. M. 11 and 12, 1867, pp. 321–366.
18. Exner, A., and Schwarzmann, E., Mitt. Grenzgeb. Med. Chir. 28:15, 1914.
19. Latarjet, A., Bull. Acad. Natl. Med. (Paris) 87:681, 1922.
20. Schiassi, B. M., Ann. Surg. 81:939, 1925.
21. Carlson, A. J., Physiol. Rev. 3:1, 1923.
22. Klein, E., Ann. Surg. 90:65, 1929.
23. Winkelstein, A., and Berg, A. A., Am. J. Dig. Dis. 5:497, 1938.
24. Dragstedt, L. R., and Owens, F. M., Jr., Proc. Soc. Exp. Biol. Med. 53:152, 1943.
25. Farmer, D. A., Howe, C. W., Porell, W. J., and Smithwick, R. H., Ann. Surg. 134:319, 1951.
26. Edwards, L. W., Herrington, J. L., Jr., Ann. Surg. 137:873, 1953.
27. Johnson, H. D., Proc. R. Soc. Med. 41:649, 1948.
28. Harkins, H. N., Schmitz, E. J., Harper, H. P., Sauvage, L. R., Moore, H. C., Storer, E. H., and Kanar E. A., West. J. Surg. 61:316, 1953.
29. Colp, R. P., Klingenstein, L. J., Druckerman, V. A., and Weinstein, A., Ann. Surg. 128:470, 1948.
30. Druckerman, L. J., Weinstein, V., Klingenstein, P., and Colp, R., Ann. Surg. 136:211, 1952.
31. Palumbo, L. T., Marquis, F. M., and Smith, A. N., Arch. Surg. 62:171, 1951.
32. Woodward, E. R., Bigelow, R. B., and Dragstedt, L. R., Am. J. Physiol. 162:99, 1950.
33. Dragstedt, L. R., Woodward, E. R., and Smith, C. A., Am. J. Physiol. 165:386, 1951.
34. Schmitz, E. J., Kanar, E. A., Storer, E. H., Sauvage, L. R., and Harkins, H. N., Surg. Forum 3:17, 1952.
35. Bales, H. W., Schilling, J. A., Ann. Surg. 143:531, 1956.
36. Schilling, J. A., and Pearse, H. E., Surg. Gynecol. Obstet. 87:225, 1948.
37. Sauvage, L. R., Schmitz, E. J., Storer, E. H., Kanar, E. A., Smith, F. R., and Harkins, H. N., S.G.O. 96:127, 1953.
38. Sauvage, L. R., Schmitz, E. J., Storer, E. H., Smith, F. R., Kanar, E. A., and Harkins, H. N., Proc. Soc. Exp. Biol. Med. 79:436, 1952.
39. Storer, E. H., Woodward, E. R., and Dragstedt, L. R., Surgery 27:526, 1950.
40. Kay, A. W., J. Roy. Coll. Surg. (Edinburgh) 7:275, 1962.
41. Gregory, R. A., and Tracy, H. J., J. Physiol. (Lond.) 156:523, 1961.
42. Lowicki, E. M., Surgery 57:602, 1965.
43. Gregory, R. A., Ir. J. Med. Sci. 6:443, 1964.
44. Dragstedt, L. R., Quintana, R. B., de la Rosa, C., and Linares, C. A., Arch. Surg. 89:1043, 1964.
45. Jordan, G. L., Jr., Quast, D., and Johnson, R., Am. J. Gastroenterol. 35:546, 1961.
46. Woodward, E. R., Park, C. L., Jr., Schapiro, H., and Dragstedt, L. R., Arch. Surg. 87:512, 1963.
47. Woodward, E. R., and Eisenberg, M. M., Surg. Clinic. North Am. 45:327, 1965.
48. Reynolds, B. L., Am. Surg. 33:352, 1967.
49. Pearce, A. G. E., Coulling, I., Weaver, B., and Friesen, S., Gut 11:649, 1970.
50. Broome, A., and Olbe, L., Scand. J. Gastroenterol. 4:281, 1969.
51. Thompson, J. C., Davidson, W. D., and Miller, H. H., Surg. Forum 15:317, 1964.
52. Thompson, J. C., and Peskin, G. W., S.G.O. 112:205, 1961.
53. Longhi, E. H., Greenlee, H. B., Bravo, J. L., Guerrero, J. D., and Dragstedt, L. R., Am. J. Physiol. 191:164, 1957.
54. Harrison, R. C., Lakey, W. H., and Hyde, H. A., Ann. Surg. 144:44, 1956.
55. Harrison, R. C., Williams, H. T. G., Pisesky, W., Husian, S., Silbermann, O. H., Francis, G. J., and Irvine, J. W., Surgery 50:151, 1961.
56. Jordan, P. H., Jr., and de La Rosa, C., Ann. Surg. 160:978, 1964.
57. Jordan, P. H., Jr., and Sand, B., Surgery 42:40, 1957.
58. Duval, M. K., Jr., and Price, W. W., Ann. Surg. 152:410, 1960.
59. McGuigan, J. E., Gastroenterology 54:1005, 1968.
60. McGuigan, J. E., Gastroenterology 55:315, 1968.
61. Jaffe, B. M., McGuigan, J. E., and Newton, W. T., Surgery 68:196, 1970.
62. Charters, A. C., Odell, W. D., Davidson, W. D., and Thompson, J. C., Surgery 66:104, 1969.
63. McGuigan, J. E., and Trudeau, W. L., Gastroenterology 58:139, 1970.
64. Trudeau, W. L., and McGuigan, J. E., Clin. Res. 17:312, 1969.
65. Trudeau, W. L., and McGuigan, J. E., New Engl. J. Med. 284:408, 1971.
66. McGuigan, J. E., and Trudeau, W. L., New Engl. J. Med. 282:358, 1970.
67. McGuigan, J. E., and Trudeau, W. L., New Engl. J. Med. 286:184, 1972.
68. Trudeau, W. L., and McGuigan, J. E., Gastroenterology 59:6, 1970.
69. McGuigan, J. E., Personal communication, 1972.
70. Yalow, R. S., and Berson, S. A., Gastroenterology 58:1, 1970.
71. Reeder, D. D., Jackson, B. M., Ban, J. L., Davidson, W. D., and Thompson, J. C., Surg. Forum 21:290, 1970.
72. Thompson, J. C., Ann. Rev. Med. 20:291, 1969.
73. Thompson, J. C., Personal communication, 1972.
74. Reeder, D. D., Jackson, B. M., Ban, J. L., Clendinnen, B. G., Davidson, W. D., and Thompson, J. C., Ann. Surg. 172:540, 1970.
75. Turbey, W. J., and Passaro, E., Arch. Surg. 105:62, 1972.
76. Passaro, E., Basso, N., and Sanchez, R. E., Am. J. Surg. 120:138, 1970.

77. Basso, N., and Passaro, E., Arch. Surg. 101:399, 1970.
78. Trudeau, W. L., and McGuigan, J. E., New Engl. J. Med. 281:862, 1969.
79. Byrnes, D. J., Lazarus, L., and Young, J. D., Aust. Ann. Med. 19:240, 1970.
80. Byrnes, D. J., Young, J. D., Chisholm, D. J., and Lazarus, L., Br. Med. J. 2:626, 1970.
81. Thoroughman, J. C., Walker, L. G., and Raft, D., S.G. & O. 119:257, 1964.
82. Thoroughman, J. C., Personal communication, 1972.
83. Palumbo, L. T., Sharpe, W. S., Lulu, D. J., Bloom, M. H., and Dragstedt, L. R., II, Arch. Surg. 100:182, 1970.
84. Palumbo, L. T., Personal communication, 1972.
85. Farmer, D. A., Harrower, H. W., and Smithwick, R. H., Am. J. Surg. 120:295, 1970.
86. Farmer, D. A., Personal communication, 1972.
87. Jordan, P. H., and Condon, R. E., Ann. Surg. 171:547, 1970.
88. Jordan, P. H., Personal communication, 1972.
89. Wolf, J. S., Bell, C. C., and Zimberg, Y. H., Am. Surg. 38:187, 1972.
90. Dragstedt, L. R., Oberhelman, H. A., Jr., Woodward, E. R., and Smith, C. A., Am. J. Physiol. 171:7, 1952.
91. Dragstedt, L. R., Arch. Surg. 75:552, 1957.
92. Dragstedt, L. R., Oberhelman, H. A., Jr., and Woodward, E. R., J.A.M.A. 147:1615, 1951.
93. Woodward, E. R., Lyon, E. S., Landor, J., and Dragstedt, L. R., Gastroenterology 27:766, 1954.
94. Bergstrom, H., and Broome, A., Acta. Chir. Scand. 128:526, 1964.
95. Capper, W. M., Butler, T. J., Buckler, K. G., and Hallet, C. P., Ann. Surg. 163:281, 1966.
96. Moe, R. E., Nyhus, L. M., and Harkens, H. N., Bull. Soc. Int. Chir. 22:424, 1964.
97. Osborne, M. P., and Frederick, P. L., Surg. Gynecol. Obstet. 121:592, 1965.
98. Edwards, L. W., Scott, H. W., Jr., Edwards, W. H., Sawyers, J. L., Gobbell, W. G., and Herrington, J. L., Jr., Am. J. Surg. 105:352, 1963.
99. Farmer, D. A., Hanover, H. W., and Smithwick, R. H., Am. J. Dig. Dis. 7:195, 1962.
100. Scott, H. W., Jr., Sawyers, J. L., Gobbell, W. G., Herrington, J. L., Jr., Definitive surgical treatment in Duodenal Ulcer Disease: Current Problems in Surgery. Chicago, Year Book, 1968.
101. Herrington, J. L., Jr., Surgery of the Stomach and Duodenum by Harkins, H. N., and Nyhus, L. M., Vagotomy and antrectomy. Boston, Little, Brown, 1969.
102. Herrington, J. L., Jr., Surgery 68:587, 1970.
103. Herrington, J. L., Jr., Am. J. Surg. 121:215, 1971.
104. Herrington, J. L., Jr., Classen, K. L., and Edwards, L. W., Ann. Surg. 153:575, 1961.
105. Herrington, J. L., Jr. Ann. Surg. 157:83, 1963.

17

MODIFIED HEINEKE-MIKULICZ PYLOROPLASTY WITH VAGOTOMY IN TREATING DUODENAL ULCER

JOSEPH A. WEINBERG

Modified Heineke-Mikulicz pyloroplasty combined with vagotomy constitutes a radical departure in the surgical treatment of duodenal ulcer. The procedure, based on physiological principles, has proved to be an effective means of healing the ulcer and its complications with a reasonable degree of predictability, and more importantly, it accomplishes this with minimal surgical mortality and morbidity, and with minimal disturbance of the vital functions of digestion and metabolism.

With the introduction of the Dragstedt operation of vagotomy in 1943, it became possible to reduce excessive gastric acidity, the responsible factor in chronic duodenal ulceration, to nonulcerative levels and in this way control the disease. It was soon realized, however, that vagotomy has the additional effect of reducing the gastric muscular contractility and tonicity and of altering the pyloric sphincteric mechanism to a degree that markedly interferes with gastric emptying; and because of this, some type of emptying procedure must accompany vagotomy to make it satisfactory for practical use. A simple pyloroplasty fashioned on the Heineke-Mikulicz principle has proved to be an effective means of dealing with the problem. By making a longitudinal incision across the pyloric ring and closing it in a transverse direction, a large enough lumen to restore adequate gastric emptying is obtained. Thus the Heineke-Mikulicz pyloroplasty, one of the first procedures to be used for the surgical treatment of duodenal ulcer (1886) and long abandoned because of its ineffectiveness as a cure for ulcer when used by itself, now returns for use as an adjunctive emptying procedure with vagotomy.

NEW ROLE OF HEINEKE-MIKULICZ OPERATION

For the Heineke-Mikulicz type of pyloroplasty to be effective in the new role, a simple but important modification is necessary. In the original operation described by Heineke [7] in 1886, and by Mikulicz [10] in 1888, the multiple rows of sutures used in closing the pyloroplasty incision cause an infolding of tissue which impairs the lumen and tends to make the pyloroplasty ineffective. The handicap imposed by the infolding of tissue is not as pronounced if the nerve supply of the stomach and the pyloric ring is intact; but with the reduced muscular activity of the stomach induced by the vagotomy, the infolding becomes a definite barrier to adequate emptying. The fault is readily corrected by the simple device of closing the pyloroplasty incision with a single row of sutures instead of the conventional multiple rows. As a further means of assuring patency, the practice of turning in the "dog-ear" projections at each end of the converted pyloroplasty incision is omitted.

Single-row closure of incisional wounds of the gastrointestinal tract is a safe procedure. Halsted,[6] in 1887, conducted animal experiments in which single- and multiple-row suturing in intestinal anastomoses were compared. He found that leakage, obstruction, and excessive adhesions are more prone to occur with multiple-row than with single-row closure. Concerning the effect of multiple-row closure on healing, he states ". . . perhaps the greatest danger of turning in too much is that the circulation at the site of the suture may be so much interfered with that union will not take place." The evidence which

Halsted presents in favor of single-row closure is so convincing that even the most avowed skeptic must be convinced of its superiority. Gambee,[4] reporting on single-layer intestinal anastomosis, states: "The method has proven most satisfactory in our hands and those associated with us over a period of years and under a great variety of circumstances. We use it in repairing the small as well as the large intestine, and anastomose the gallbladder to the open end of the jejunum and the esophagus to the jejunum in this way. It lends itself to precision and can be done under the most difficult circumstances."

ADVANTAGES OF PYLOROPLASTY

There are important practical reasons for using pyloroplasty as an emptying procedure with vagotomy. Most important of all from the physiological standpoint, the normal continuity of the gastrointestinal tract is retained. It is probably for this reason that the incidence of dumping and other disturbing postoperative sequelae is low compared with that in procedures involving resection or gastrojejunostomy. The evidence based on long-term appraisal indicates that late malnutrition and anemia, which are not uncommon following gastrectomy, are unlikely occurrences with pyloroplasty.

The operation is simple in comparison with other procedures and the surgical mortality and morbidity are accordingly low. Too little attention has been given to this aspect of ulcer surgery, which should be the first consideration in a disease of the benign nature of duodenal ulcer.

Pyloroplasty provides an opportunity to inspect the pyloroduodenal mucosal lining for assessment of the extent of disease. This advantage finds especial usefulness in cases in which the diagnosis is not definitely established before operation. If no evidence of ulcerative disease is found, the patient is spared an unnecessary vagotomy.

In operations for bleeding ulcer, the eroded vessel may be exposed early in the operation through the pyloroplasty incision and ligated with a transfixion suture directly in the ulcer bed. It is in this role that the procedure of pyloroplasty with vagotomy finds one of its most important applications.

If, for any reason, a second operation is necessary, revision is easily accomplished, unlike the difficulties of revision after gastrectomy or gastrojejunostomy.

Indications. The indications for pyloroplasty with vagotomy are much the same as the indications for other procedures used in the treatment of duodenal ulcer. *The operation finds its best use in ulcers complicated by bleeding, obstruction, perforation,* or *deep penetration.* The results are less satisfactory in patients in whom the manifestations are largely "psychosomatic" with little supporting objective evidence of ulceration. The results are apt to be poor when the indications are vague.

Special mention should be made of duodenal ulcer complicated by obstruction. Whether or not pyloroplasty with vagotomy is used will depend on the degree of distortion and constriction present. If it appears that a suitable pyloroplasty cannot be made, gastrojejunostomy or resection is used instead.

Contraindications. *Pyloroplasty is generally contraindicated if there is excessive scarring, thickening, and narrowing of the pyloroduodenal channel.* An exception is ulcer complicated by massive hemorrhage, in which case it is better to risk the possibility of a poorly functioning pyloroplasty than to prolong the operation with a more complex procedure. If the pyloroplasty should fail to function properly, revision can be made at an appropriate later time.

Obstruction beyond the first 2 cm of the duodenum is an absolute contraindication. Distal constriction is not always recognizable in the preoperative examination; for this reason, the pyloroduodenal canal should always be tested for patency at the operating table by probing with the index finger well into the second portion of the duodenum after making the pyloroplasty incision. If distal obstruction is present, gastrojejunostomy or other indicated procedure is added.

Ulceration associated with the Zollinger-Ellison syndrome is not amenable to vagotomy and pyloroplasty. The neoplasm which characterizes the disease should be looked for in patients with extremely high gastric acidity (see Chapter 13).

TECHNIQUE

Preparation. The patient is given a clear, bland liquid diet beginning the morning of the day before the operation. A nasogastric suction tube is inserted the evening before the operation, to be left in place until the operation has been completed. The tube serves to keep the stomach empty during the preoperative and operative periods, and acts as a guide for manipulation of the esophagus during the performance of the vagotomy.

Anesthesia, abdominal incision, and general abdominal exploration. The anesthesia should be one that will provide thorough relaxation for work in the subdiaphragmatic area. A high transverse abdominal incision with moderate curvature upward will give good exposure for both the vagotomy and the pyloroplasty. However, the type of incisional approach—transverse or longitudinal—will be determined largely by the surgeon's individual preference.

The general examination of the abdominal viscera is done in a systematic manner with little handling of structures, as excessive handling may cause disturbing postoperative intestinal stasis and distension. This precaution, always good practice in abdominal surgery, is especially important in operations involving vagotomy, because of the tendency to temporary inactivity and distension of the stomach and small bowel following vagal denervation.[8]

The vagotomy. The vagotomy usually precedes the pyloroplasty. This order of procedure originated as an intended safeguard against infection of the mediastinum which might occur as the result of contamination by escaped gastroduodenal content if the pyloroplasty were to be performed first. Experience has shown that the possibility of mediastinitis with the reverse order is so remote, however, even in cases of perforated ulcer, that it should not be a consideration if there is special reason to reverse the order. The pyloroplasty should always be performed before the vagotomy in cases of actively bleeding ulcer in order to accomplish arrest of hemorrhage by transfixion ligation early in the operation. In cases of perforation, early arrest of leakage is accomplished by making the closure a part of the pyloroplasty which precedes the vagotomy. A third reason for reversing the usual order is uncertainty regarding the diagnosis. In this situation, by performing the pyloroplasty first, one may inspect the inner surface of the pyloroduodenal segment through the open pyloroplasty incision for the presence or absence of ulcer disease.

The technique of vagotomy is described in Chapters 14 and 15.

The pyloroplasty. The modified Heineke-Mikulicz pyloroplasty is used solely as a gastric emptying procedure in combination with vagotomy and is not, by itself, a curative procedure for chronic duodenal ulcer.

The pyloroduodenal area is first examined to make sure that there is no contraindication to pyloroplasty. Constriction and adhesions are not necessarily contraindications. A lumen reduced to no more than a centimeter in diameter may be enlarged to adequate size if there is no great distortion of the involved segment.

The Kocher maneuver of mobilizing the duodenum is not used in the operation. It offers no advantage, and may actually cause harm by laying the groundwork for obstructing adhesions, because of the raw unperitonealized surfaces which it creates. The Kocher maneuver also introduces the hazard of injury to the common biliary duct and to major blood vessels in the area, especially if the field is obscured by inflammatory congestion and fibrous thickening.

To begin the pyloroplasty (Fig. 1), two guide sutures are placed a centimeter apart at the level of the pyloric ring anteriorly, midway between the upper and lower borders of the pyloroduodenal canal. The guide sutures, which are to serve as tractors, are inserted deeply to prevent their pulling out when traction is applied.

A longitudinal incision is now made across the pyloric ring through all layers, extending approximately 3.5 cm on the gastric side and 2.5 cm on the duodenal side. The greater length on the gastric side is to allow for the greater thickness of the gastric wall, in making the alignment for closure of the pyloroplasty incision in the transverse direction.

If there is difficulty in recognizing the pyloric ring as a landmark because of obscuration by inflammatory changes, a short incision (not more than 2 cm) is made over its probable location so that identification can be made by palpation from within the canal. The incision can then be extended to the proper length on the gastric and duodenal sides of the ring. In this way, the error of making too long an incision, owing to miscalculation, is avoided. An incision which is too long will result in an inadequate pyloroplasty lumen, just as too short an incision will. The total length of the incision is ordinarily not less than 5.5 cm and not more than 7 cm. The incision is sometimes made longer, up to 8 cm, in cases of actively bleeding ulcer, to allow working space for ligation of the eroded vessel. Here the risk of too long an incision is justified by the urgency of the situation, even though a corrective procedure may be necessary at a later time.

If the ulcer lesion is in the line of the pyloroplasty incision, it is transected and not excised. This will avoid irregular alignment in the pyloroplasty closure. There has been secure healing without exception in cases in which the transected ulcer has been included in the suture line.

Immediately after the pyloroplasty incision is made, the stomach is emptied of its content by aspiration through the open incision to prevent flooding of the operative field. The lining of the pyloroduodenal segment is inspected to determine the extent of ulcerative disease, and the canal is probed with the index finger well into the second portion of the duodenum to determine whether distal impairment is present which would defeat the purpose of the pyloroplasty.

The longitudinal pyloroduodenal incision is now converted to a transverse direction in preparation for the closure of the pyloroplasty incision. Traction is applied on the guide sutures previously placed at the level of the pyloric ring. The guide suture tractors are supplemented by Allis forceps tractors placed on each side of the divided pyloric ring.

Interrupted surgical cotton sutures, No. 0000, are used for the closure. Gut suture material is contraindicated because of its susceptibility to the lytic action of the digestive juices. The closure is started at the upper (subhepatic) end of the converted wound. With this order, and with continu-

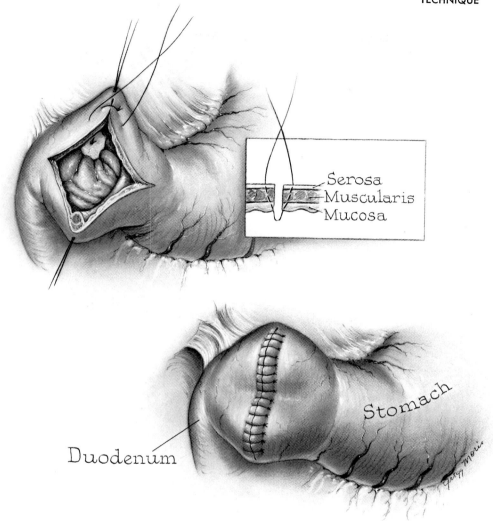

Serosa
Muscularis
Mucosa

Stomach

Duodenum

FIG. 1. Pyloroplasty with one-row closure of the pyloroplasty incision. Longitudinal pyloro-duodenal incision has been converted to transverse direction for closure. (From Weinberg, *Am. J. Surg.* 102:158, 1961.)

ous suction during the closure, contamination of the field by escaped gastric content is reduced to a minimum without the use of surrounding gauze packs. The interrupted sutures are placed approximately 3 mm apart, with each suture inserted in the following manner: The needle enters the serosa on one side about 3 mm from the cut edge and is directed obliquely through all layers to emerge at the cut edge of the junction of submucosa and mucosa. The needle then enters the opposite side of the incision, at the junction of mucosa and submucosa, to emerge on the serosal surface 3 mm from the cut edge (insert, Fig. 1). With the placement of the sutures in this manner, the corresponding layers are accurately approximated when the sutures are tied, thus reducing the possibility of emergence of mucosal tissue onto the serosal surface. The latter point is especially important as a guard against postoperative adhesions, which sometimes form between the line of closure and the undersurface of the liver. While such occurrences are uncommon, they are to be avoided because of the impairment of the

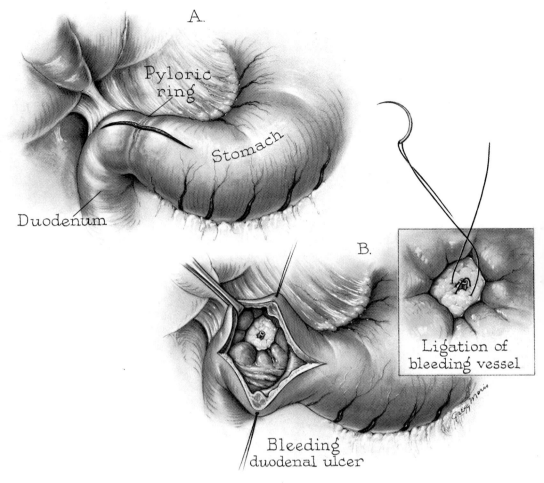

FIG. 2.   Ligation of bleeding vessel through open pyloroplasty incision. (From Weinberg, *Am. J. Surg.* 102:158, 1961.)

pyloroduodenal channel they may cause. An additional advantage of including all layers in each stitch is that dead space between layers is obliterated, leaving no opportunity for the accumulation of serum and blood clot between the layers, an advantage which is not realized with separate closure of the submucosal-mucosal and musculo-serosal layers. The close placement of the sutures, 3 mm apart, provides adequate hemostasis for the most part, and few divided vessels will require ligation. Continuous suturing is never used with single-row intestinal closure, if for no other reason than that the entire suture line would be no more secure than its weakest point.

After the closure has been completed, areas of protruding raw tissue which may be present along the suture line are peritonealized with fine superficial stitches. The projections at each end of the closed wound are not turned in, as to do so would narrow the lumen. (It should be mentioned that these projections may give a false impression of ulcer in postoperative radiographic studies unless the radiologist is aware of the technique used in the pyloroplasty operation.)

Before the abdomen is closed, a gastrostomy is established for drainage during the early postoperative period. This is accomplished by insertion of a Foley balloon catheter through a stab wound in the anterior wall of the stomach midway between the greater and lesser curvatures. The stab incision is closed around the tube with an absorbable purse-string suture and the balloon is distended with water to assure its retention within the stomach. The free end of the tube is then brought to the outside through a small stab incision in the anterior abdominal wall. The stomach is anchored to the peritoneal surface of the abdominal wall around the emerged tube with several fine absorbable sutures to prevent the interposition of intestinal coils around the tube. The tube is withdrawn on the sixth postoperative day. The small opening on the abdominal wall left after withdrawal of the tube closes spontaneously within several days.

CONTROL OF ULCER HEMORRHAGE BY LIGATION, PYLOROPLASTY, AND VAGOTOMY

Transfixion ligation added to pyloroplasty with vagotomy has proved to be an effective means of dealing with uncontrolled hemorrhage complicating duodenal ulceration.[11, 12] This complication, occurring as it often does in elderly individuals with associated debilitating disease, accounts for most of the surgical mortality and morbidity of duodenal ulcer disease. The operation avoids a hazardous dissection in the immediate area of penetrating ulceration and hemorrhage, with the result that surgical trauma and operative time are greatly reduced in an emergency in which these factors have an important bearing on recovery.

The preparation for the operation is the same as with other surgical procedures for the arrest of ulcer hemorrhage.

The ligation is performed as the first step in the operation, in order to hold blood loss to a minimum. The technique of abdominal approach, pyloroplasty (Fig. 1), and vagotomy are the same as for elective duodenal ulcer operations except that the pyloroplasty precedes the vagotomy, and the pyloroplasty incision is made a centimeter or two longer to provide working space for ligation of the bleeding vessel.

As soon as the pyloroplasty incision is made,

blood clots are evacuated by compression on the stomach and by suction. The ulcer is exposed, and a finger is placed over the bleeding site while adequate exposure is being obtained by encirclement of the pyloroplasty incision with several Allis forceps for retraction. Further exposure may be obtained by placing Allis forceps around the thickened margin of the ulcer for traction.

A specific type of needle is necessary for the transfixion ligation (Fig. 2). It must be small enough and curved enough for easy manipulation in the small working space, and stout enough to resist breakage in the indurated ulcer floor. A half-circle Mayo needle No. 4 or 5 will meet the requirements in most cases. Nonabsorbable suture material is used for the transfixion ligation, preferably stout (No. 30) surgical cotton, which will not break in making a firm tie over the bleeding site. Surgical gut suture in any form should never be used, because of its susceptibility to the lytic action of the digestive secretions. Horsley,[13] in his book on operative surgery (1921), cautions against absorbable suture for ligation in this area and cites a fatality resulting from its use: "Death occurred on the ninth day as a result of hemorrhage. . . . The post mortem examination . . . showed where the catgut was digested and absorbed . . . probably silk sutures in this area would be preferable to catgut." We had a similar experience in our own clinic before we were fully aware of the hazard of using absorbable suture material for ligation in this area.

A figure-of-eight transfixion suture is used to ligate the bleeding vessel (Fig. 2). If the erosion is large, two or even three additional sutures may be needed to control the bleeding. Failure to arrest the bleeding with one figure-of-eight suture, however, is usually an indication that the suture has not been placed completely around the bleeding vessel.

Regarding the possibility of injury to the pancreas with the passage of the transfixing ligature around the bleeding vessel, there has been no clinical evidence of traumatic pancreatitis in the more than 100 ligations we have performed by this method. Also, there have been no injuries to the common biliary duct. While injury to the duct must always be regarded as a possibility, however remote, if the relationships are obscured by the congestion and edema of inflammation, the risk is an acceptable one considering the gravity of the emergency.

Failure to obtain permanent arrest of bleeding by direct transfixion ligation in combination with vagotomy and pyloroplasty is almost invariably due to one of three causes: (1) the wrong kind of needle, (2) the wrong kind of suture material, (3) failure to insert the suture completely around the bleeding vessel.

After it is certain that bleeding has been arrested, the pyloroplasty is completed and the vagotomy performed. The vagotomy should be performed at the same session, as postponement may result in rebleeding before healing of the ulcer takes place.

POSTOPERATIVE DIETARY MANAGEMENT

The postoperative dietary program plays an important role in lessening the incidence of the digestive disturbances of dumping and diarrhea which tend to follow operations involving the stomach and duodenum.

Nothing is given by mouth during the first 5 days after the operation. Appropriate intravenous fluids are given to maintain fluid balance and to provide vitamin and electrolyte needs. Oral feeding is started on the sixth postoperative day, at which time the gastrostomy tube is removed. The oral intake begins with 2 or 3 ounces of bland sugar-free fluids at intervals of several hours during the day. If this is well tolerated, the diet is increased during the next 6 weeks with the gradual addition of semiliquid and soft foods including eggs, gelatin, gruels, pureed vegetables, and tea. Sugar and simple starches are rigidly excluded because of their tendency to cause dumping in the early stage of dietary adjustment. The main reliance is on protein foods, with fats and complex starches permitted in moderation. After the sixth week, gradual change is made to a normal diet, adding items as they are tested by the patient for tolerance. This general dietary program can be adjusted to meet special needs in problem situations. For example, in one patient a problem of severe and persistent dumping was solved by limiting the breakfast to a small broiled steak, followed by less restrictive noon and evening meals. Each patient is interviewed by the hospital dietitian before leaving the hospital, preferably with a member of the family present, and the reasons for the restrictions are explained. He is given a printed postoperative diet list and is advised to communicate with his doctor without delay in the event of dietary disturbance. Judging from our own experience gained through trial and error and through the helpful advice of Dragstedt (personal communication) and Lieber,[9] the planned dietary program described here will reduce the disturbing sequelae of dumping and diarrhea to unusual and relatively minor occurrences.

GENERAL APPRAISAL

More than 1,300 operations of the modified Heineke-Mikulicz pyloroplasty combined with vagotomy have been performed at the Long Beach Veterans Administration Hospital since the inception of the operation in 1947. The overall recurrence incidence is estimated at 5 percent. Most of the recurrences have been controlled by medical therapy. The overall surgical mortality rate is less than 0.5 percent. Postoperative sequelae of dumping and diarrhea are infrequent occurrences, as compared with their incidence in other procedures. Goligher et al.,[5] in a 1972 article entitled *Five to Eight-year Results of Truncal Vagotomy and Pyloroplasty for Duodenal Ulcer,* found the incidence of proved or *suspected* recurrent ulcer to be, respectively, 6.7 and 7.3 percent. It is possible, however, that a number of patients suffering from recurrent ulcer were subjected to what may be termed "inadvertent incomplete vagotomies" as, at a second operation, no technical defects could be attributed to the pyloroplasties per se.

In emergency cases of hemorrhage complicating the duodenal ulcer, there have been 4 deaths in 111 operations of pyloroplasty and vagotomy with added ligation of the bleeding vessel. Similar results are reported by others using the operation.[1-3]

A trend toward the use of pyloroplasty with vagotomy as a preferred procedure in the surgical treatment of duodenal ulcer is seen in the statewide study being conducted by the Ohio Chapter of the American College of Surgeons under the chairmanship of Stanley Hoerr, in which selected private, public, and university hospitals representative of surgical practice in the state report at 5-year intervals on the frequency of use of the several established surgical procedures for duodenal ulcer. In the first survey, covering the period 1956–60, the combination of vagotomy with pyloroplasty was used in 1 percent of 2,561 operations. In the second survey, 1961–66, the procedure was used in 26 percent of 6,259 operations performed. The summarizing paragraph of the recent report in the Bulletin of the American College of Surgeons, September–October 1967, states "It is clear that Ohio surgeons are performing drainage procedures with vagotomy more frequently than before, and gastrectomy with or without vagotomy less frequently; pyloroplasty has become a popular drainage procedure. . . ."

REFERENCES

1. Brizzolara, Am. J. Surg. 102:258, 1961.
2. Farris and Smith, Am. J. Surg. 105:388, 1963.
3. Foster, Hickock, and Dunphy, Surg. Gynecol. Obstet. 117:257, 1963.
4. Gambee, West J. Surg. Obstet. Gynecol. 59:1, 1951.
5. Goligher et al., Br. Med. J. 1:7, 1972.
6. Halsted, Surg. Papers John Hopkins Press, 1924.
7. Heineke, Fron Müller Mang Dissert Furth, 1886.
8. Isaac et al., Am. J. Roentgenol. 63:66, 1950.
9. Lieber, J.A.M.A. 176:208, 1961.
10. Mikulicz, Arch. Klin. Chir. 37:79, 1888.
11. Weinberg, Am. J. Surg. 102:158, 1961.
12. Weinberg, Monthly Clin. Managr. Chicago, Year Book, 1964.
13. Horsley, J. S., Operative Surgery. St. Louis, C. V. Mosby, 1921, p. 561.

18

THE PYLOROPLASTIES AND GASTRODUODENOSTOMIES

RODNEY MAINGOT

PYLOROPLASTY

In the surgical treatment on duodenal ulcer, the advent of vagotomy was largely responsible for the survival of pyloroplasty. One of the effects of vagotomy is a reduction in the tone of the gastric musculature and alteration of the pyloric sphincteric action, with the result that emptying of the stomach is interefered with. Because of this, some type of drainage procedure, such as pyloroplasty, gastroduodenostomy, or gastrojejunostomy, must be carried out to prevent stasis.

Heineke-Mikulicz Pyloroplasty

The Heineke-Mikulicz pyloroplasty, as modified and practised by Weinberg, is by far the most popular of the procedures that *enlarge the gastric outlet* and provide good drainage of the stomach (see Chap. 17).

One other pyloroplasty will be described in this chapter, namely, that of Judd, and two gastroduodenostomies, namely, Finney's and Jaboulay's.

HISTORICAL NOTE

Heineke in 1886 was the first surgeon to perform pyloroplasty for pyloric stenosis caused by duodenal ulceration.

Mikulicz,[12] a keen observer and one who was constantly alert to the possibilities of a new operation, performed a number of pyloroplasties after the Heineke plan with immediate gratifying results. His article dealing with this pyloroplasty, which was published in 1888, did much to popularise the operation.

In the original Heineke-Mikulicz operation a longitudinal incision, about 2 in. (5 cm.) long, was made through all the coats of the pyloroduodenal segment, and the wound was then sutured transversely with multiple rows of interrupted stitches of silk. Unfortunately the over-zealous introduction of a large number of interrupted sutures often caused infolding of the suture line, valve formation, and partial obstruction from the resulting oedema of the stoma. Leakage, pyloric stenosis, recurrent ulceration, or activation of the original ulcer were common post-operative sequelae, and the operative death-rate was not inconsiderable.

Weinberg [13] first introduced his modification of the Heineke-Mikulicz about 26 years ago.

When this procedure is combined with truncal or, preferably, with *selective* vagotomy in the treatment of duodenal ulcer, the immediate and late results have been excellent and the mortality rate less than 0.5 percent.

Statistics prove that it is a highly efficient "drainage" procedure.

Judd's Pyloroplasty

Judd [8] first performed this operation in 1920, and it soon became popular in America owing to the forceful personality of its originator, to the simplicity of the technical steps, and to the encouraging immediate results that were obtained. Judd was a superb teacher and one of the leading surgeons of his day.

It is significant that at the Mayo Clinic in 1934, for no fewer than 30 percent of the chronic duodenal ulcers submitted to operation, Judd's pyloroplasty was the selected procedure, while in 1936 the figure dropped to 10 percent, and in 1942 to 1.3 percent. There is no mention of Judd's operation in the *Report of Surgery of the Stomach and Duodenum for 1944* submitted by Counseller, Waugh, and Clagett in 1946.[1]

Judd's pyloroplasty is occasionally performed today following selective vagotomy for duodenal ulcer. The immediate results of this pyloroplasty *alone* were promising; but the late results were disappointing owing to recurrent ulceration and scar stenosis.

It served to prove what I have said before, namely, that every operation upon the stomach or duodenum for peptic ulceration is a success until it is found out.

Technique. The operation consists of vagotomy followed by mobilisation of the duodenum by Kocher's method, and wide removal of the anterior two-thirds or more of the pyloric sphincter, an adjacent portion of the antrum, and also the anterior wall of the bulb including an ulcer when present at this site. When this excision is completed, the openings at the distal end of the stomach and at the upper end of the duodenum appear like the openings of a gastrojejunostomy after the posterior layer of sutures has been introduced (Fig. 1 [2]). The gaping oval or circular aperture that results from this excision is closed in the transverse axis with two layers of sutures, using a continuous suture of 0 or 00 chromic catgut for an accurate approximation of the apposing margins of the antrum and duodenum and a final row of interrupted reinforcing serosal stitches of 000 Dexon or 4–0 Deknatel or Mersilk (Fig. 1 [3]).

GASTRODUODENOSTOMY

There are many ways of performing this operation, but only two well-known methods—that of Finney and that of Jaboulay—need concern us.

Finney's Operation

Finney [2] first performed the gastro-duodenostomy, which now bears his name, over 70 years ago, and his original description of the operation is rewarding and worthy of renewed study. Few abdominal operations have been better described or more accurately illustrated.

It would repay the surgeon to study once more the superb drawings of this operation, which were executed in 1907 by Max Brödel, the greatest medical artist of all time.

Finney's operation [3] has never at any time been widely practised in European countries. I have rarely seen the operation performed by other surgeons; this is probably owing to the fact that most British surgeons prefer gastrojejunostomy to any form of gastro-duodenostomy when a short-circuiting operation is indicated, and that most of those who favour gastroduodenostomy usually choose the method of Jaboulay on account of its greater simplicity.

Finney [4] writes as follows:

If the pylorus and first portion of the duodenum are so bound down with scar tissue of a chronic ulcer, or too densely attached to undersurface of liver and common duct to be properly freed, or if the seat of an ulcer, perforating into and inti-

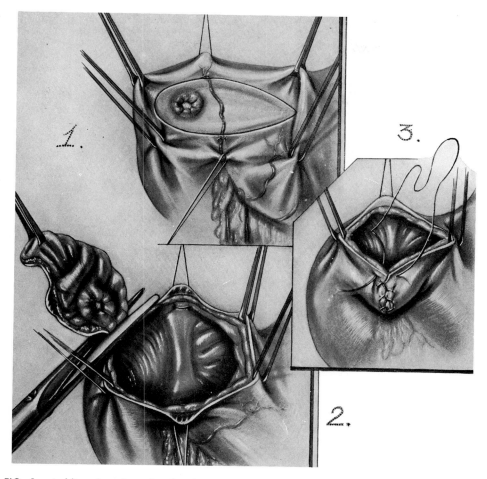

FIG. 1. Judd's pyloroplasty for chronic anterior-wall duodenal ulcer. This operation is combined with selective vagotomy.

mately involving the head of the pancreas behind, interferes with proper mobilisation for the performing of a pyloroplasty or prohibits a resection, then quite frequently one can still mobilise the second and third portions to allow of a subpyloric Jaboulay type of gastroduodenostomy, which has all the advantages referred to above. Incidentally, this is an operation which in our opinion is far too seldom used, which is simple to perform, and which accomplishes everything that a gastrojejunostomy does without many of the latter's objectionable features.

It is interesting to note that this gastroduodenostomy was popularised and cogently advocated some 17 years ago by Lischer and Burford.[10] These surgeons have been employing Finney's operation in the treatment

of peptic oesophagitis that is caused by transcardial reflux of gastric acid pepsin, into the distal portion of the oesophagus.

Nissen's operation, as described by John Borrie in Chapter 74, often affords considerable relief of this distressing condition.

Lischer and Burford [11] write:

We have subjected 16 patients with hiatal hernia of the short type associated with esophagitis to Finney pyloroplasty. All of these patients had a longstanding history of "heart burn", regurgitation and inability to sleep in a recumbent position. Dietary and medical management had failed to produce lasting remissions. All patients were proved by esophagoscopy to have esophagitis. In none had the disease progressed to frank stenosis, but three had ulceration of the esophago-gastric junction. The Finney type of pyloroplasty was the only treatment employed. . . . None of the patients had postoperative dietary restrictions or were placed on medical management.

The results have been strikingly good. The follow-up study has extended from four to 18 months. Fifteen of the 16 patients have had encouraging results—10 excellent and five good.

The one failure in the entire group occurred in a patient who, on subsequent eaxmination, was found to have a paraesophageal type of hernia, the repair of which resulted in relief of symptoms.

The rationale for pyloroplasty in the treatment of peptic esophagitis is to decrease the resistance at the pylorus and in so doing enhance the chances for continuous gastric outflow. The Finney type of pyloroplasty is a means of gaining

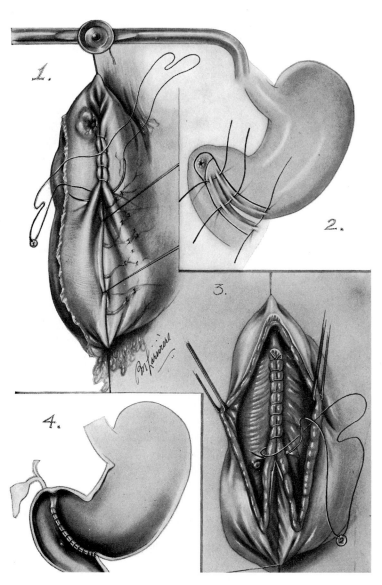

FIG. 2.   Finney's operation for chronic duodenal ulcer. (1) First continuous posterior suture is being introduced. (2) Position of three stay sutures and horseshoe-shaped incision. (3) Second posterior through-and-through all-coats suture is being introduced. Note position of papilla of Vater. (4) Section through stoma shows large size of stoma and position of papilla of Vater. This operation is preceded by selective vagotomy.

a wide gastroduodenal opening and thus assuring the most efficacious method of increasing gastric outflow. Our results to date seem to justify this procedure and to verify the reasons for its success. It is a simple operation with little risk, and, in our subjects, has produced gratifying results. (See Nissen's method, and Chap. 74).

Technique of Finney's operation.
There are two essential steps of the opera-

tion: (1) thorough mobilisation of the pylorus and the first three portions of the duodenum and (2) the making of an ample stoma. The stoma must be large and must extend well below the level at which the common bile duct enters the duodenum through the papilla of Vater, to allow a free and ready interchange of gastric and duodenal contents, thus counteracting any free hydro-

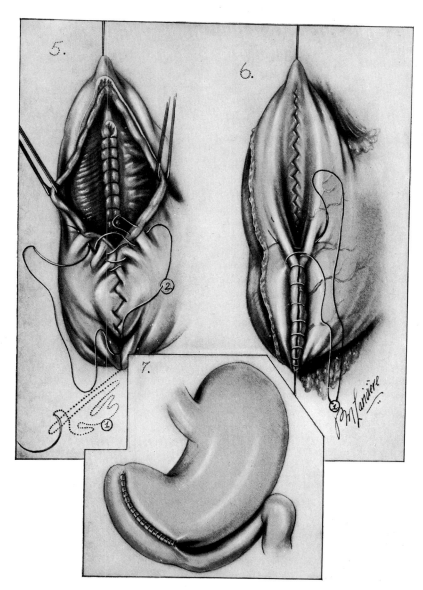

FIG. 3.   Finney's operation. (5) First anterior suture is being introduced as loop-on-the-mucosa stitch. (6) Second anterior suture is being introduced as Lembert suture. (7) Appearance of parts after operation.

chloric acid that may be present in the stomach. Above all, it must be supple and free from any tension, and able to move facilely with the contraction of its component parts.

The operation is started by mobilising the first and second parts and *the commencement of the third part of the duodenum* and of the pylorus itself by Kocher's method. This is accomplished by dividing the peritoneum and fascia propria on the outer aspect of the duodenum, by freeing any adhesions that exist, and by gently coaxing the bowel medialward with gauze or finger dissection. Unless a free and complete mobilisation can be achieved, the operation should be abandoned, as recommended by Finney himself, who attached the utmost importance to this preliminary step.

When therefore the pylorus and duodenum have been freed and the abdominal field packed off with Lahey's cellophane pads [9] or thin plastic sheets, three sutures of 00 silk are passed to act as guides and as tractors. The first is introduced close to the greater curvature of the stomach at a point about 3½ inches (8.9 cm) proximal to the pylorus, and then picks up a corresponding point on the inner border of the duodenum just above where the second part merges into the horizontal third part. This suture is tied and clipped with a haemostat. The second suture is inserted immediately below the pylorus, while the third (the middle one) is placed midway between the other two, about the level of the ampulla of Vater. These sutures, too, are knotted and clipped. Two additional temporary sutures are next inserted, one at the uppermost border of the pylorus and the other about 1 inch (2.5 cm) below the first guide suture. Intestinal clamps are not used (Fig. 2 [*1* and *2*]).

Traction is now made on the guide sutures while the first (posterior) continuous Lembert suture is introduced, commencing at the pylorus and ending just below the first guide suture. When this point is reached, the suture is laid aside for the moment, to be used again as the anterior invaginating stitch (Fig. 3 [*1*]). An inverted U- or horseshoe-shaped incision is made parallel with the posterior line of sutures through all the coats of the stomach, the pylorus, and the duodenum. If an ulcer is found on the anterior wall of the duodenum, it can be excised easily with scissors, as much scar tissue as possible being removed with it. An ulcer on the posterior wall of the duodenum should be inspected, carefully palpated, and left undisturbed, unless it is actively bleeding. When this is the case, the ulcer crater should be obliterated by introducing three or four well-placed deep sutures of 1 mersilk mounted on atraumatic Mayo No. 1 needles and by tying these firmly —but not too tightly.

The posterior through-and-through (all coats) suture is then applied, starting at the divided pylorus and proceeding downward to the lower angle of the incision. From this point, it is carried upward without interruption as a Connell or loop-on-the-mucosa stitch, uniting the anterior edges of the stomach and duodenum and the divided pylorus, beyond which point it is tied (Fig. 3 [*5*]).

The first posterior seromuscular suture is then taken up again and continued anteriorly to reinforce and invaginate the first row of sutures (Fig. 3 [*6*]). A few interrupted stitches of fine silk are placed here and there where the suture line requires strengthening, and adjacent tags of omentum are drawn across and anchored to the anterior suture line to prevent the gut from adhering to the parietal peritoneum, the liver, or the gallbladder.

When the operation has been completed, it will be seen that the duodenum assumes its original position, dragging the stomach with it. The raw space on the outer surface of the duodenum occasioned by the preliminary mobilisation can with advantage be likewise covered with a portion of the greater omentum.

I have often felt uneasy about obtaining a secure and "waterproof" closure of the top end of the anastomosis. Nevertheless, there have been no significant postoperative complications or any fatality to report in my small series of 35 cases. This operation, when performed for duodenal ulcer, should always be combined with selective vagotomy; in fact, vagotomy has been instrumental in keeping Finney's drainage procedure "alive"! Hendry [5] has given a good account of this operation and his satisfactory late results.

Jaboulay's Subpyloric Gastroduodenostomy

This operation was first described by Jaboulay[6] in 1892 and slightly modified by him and his associates 2 years later.[7] It is indicated in those cases of duodenal ulcer in which gastrojejunostomy (with vagotomy) is the operation of choice but is impracticable owing to the presence of massive adhesions involving the upper jejunal coils. It may also occasionally be carried out where Finney's operation is contraindicated on account of

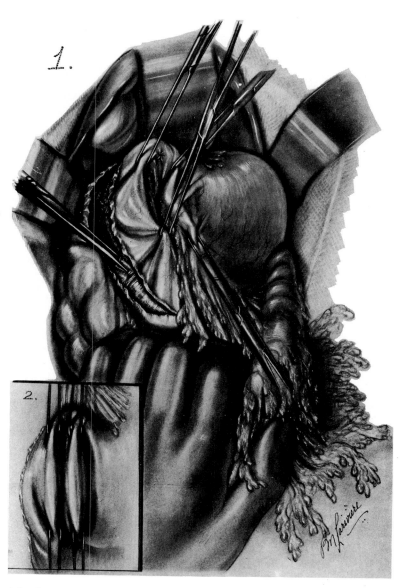

FIG. 4. Jaboulay's operation for chronic duodenal ulcer. (1) Duodenum is being mobilized by Kocher's method. (2) Adjacent portions of stomach and duodenum are held in Allis forceps and are ready to be anatomosed. Selective vagotomy precedes this operation.

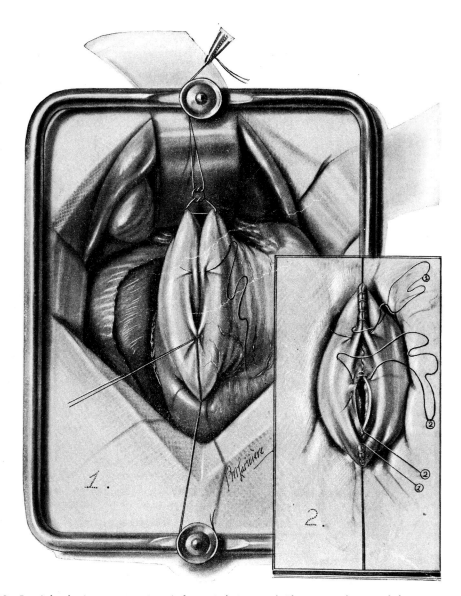

FIG. 5. Jaboulay's operation. Lang's frame is being used. The principal steps of the anastomosis are depicted. Selective vagotomy is carried out before the performance of this operation. (From Madden, 1964. *Atlas of Technics in Surgery*, 2d ed. Courtesy of Appleton-Century-Crofts, New York.)

fixation of the duodenum by a large oedematous penetrating ulcer.

This operation had at one time the distinguished patronage of Moynihan and Wilkie. Wilkie [15] found, on reviewing 180 of his cases, that the results were excellent in 64 percent, 25 percent of the patients were relieved but not cured, and in 11 percent symptoms of dyspepsia persisted. *This was before the days of vagotomy!*

Technique of Jaboulay's gastroduodenostomy. The first step, as in Finney's operation, consists of mobilising the duodenum by Kocher's method (Fig. 4 [1]). Two tractor sutures are then inserted. The first is passed close to the greater curvature of the antrum just short of the pyloric ring, and picks up a point on the anterior wall of the duodenum immediately below the scarred area of the bulb. The second stitch is introduced near the greater curvature about 3½ inches (8.9 cm) away from the pylorus, and then picks up a point on the medial margin of the lowest portion of the second part of the duodenum. When these sutures have been tied and slung to the Lang's frame, the whole of the second portion of the duodenum and some 3 inches (7.6 cm) or so of the anterior wall of the vestibule of the stomach are snugly drawn together side by side and are ready for the process of anastomosis.

The use of clamps is unnecessary; in fact they often prove cumbersome. Two continuous sutures are used for making the anastomosis; the first is a seromuscular stitch that unites the adjacent portions of the stomach and duodenum, while the second is a through-and-through suture of 00 or 0 chromic catgut, which is inserted after the stomach and duodenum have been incised (Fig. 5). This latter stitch is now carried anteriorly as a Connell suture which approximates the anterior margins of the stomach and duodenum, while the first stitch further invaginates the anterior suture line. At the end of the operation, the scarred area of the bulb is invaginated with a few interrupted sutures of 00 silk and covered with omentum. This simple, safe, and efficient drainage operation (combined with selective vagotomy) appears to be gaining in favor at the present time.

REFERENCES

1. Counseller, Waugh, and Clagett, Proc. Mayo Clin. 21:17, 1946.
2. Finney, Johns Hopkins Hosp. Bull. 13:155, 1902.
3. Finney, Surg. Gynecol. Obstet. 43:508, 1926.
4. Finney, Am. J. Surg. 40:121, 1938.
5. Hendry, Surg. Gynecol. Obstet. 116:657, 1963.
6. Jaboulay, Arch. Prov. Chir. 1:1, 1892.
7. Jaboulay, Gaz. Hebd. méd. 31:89, 1894.
8. Judd, 42:381, 1922.
9. Lahey, J.A.M.A. 104:1990, 1935.
10. Lischer and Burford, Ann. Surg. 144:647, 1956.
11. Lischer and Burford, Modern Surgical Management, Chicago, Year Book, 1957.
12. Mikulicz, Arch. Klin. Chir. 37:79, 1888.
13. Weinberg, Am. J. Surg. 92:202, 1956.
14. Weinberg, Am. J. Surg. 105:401, 1963.
15. Wilkie, Br. Med. J. 1:535, 1929.

19

VAGOTOMY AND GASTROJEJUNOSTOMY FOR DUODENAL ULCER

RODNEY MAINGOT

HISTORICAL NOTE

Since its introduction by Wölfler (*Zbl Chir 8*:705, 1881) at Nicoladoni's suggestion in 1881, gastrojejunostomy has passed through many variations in the method of its performance until it has become more or less standardised and is practiced in much the same manner in almost every clinic throughout the world. Wölfler's first operation was an *anterior* long-loop antiperistaltic gastrojejunostomy, and this in 1883 gave place to Courvoisier's posterior gastrojejunostomy (*Zbl Chir 10*:794, 1883). Von Hacker (*Arch Klin Chir 32*:616, 1885) recommended a posterior antiperistaltic gastrojejunostomy with the use of a long proximal jejunal loop and the construction of a large stoma placed right across the posterior wall of the stomach. As obstructive symptoms were common after Wölfler's method, Braun in 1892 (*Zbl Chir 19*:102, 1892), and later Jaboulay, introduced the addition of a lateral entero-anastomosis between the proximal and distal jejunal limbs to overcome regurgitant vomiting, which was a common sequel to the long-loop method. According to Watson (*Int Abstr Surg 98*:521, 1954), the use of a mechanical device for gastrointestinal anastomosis was an important advance in spite of the failure of decalcified bone plates, which had been introduced by Senn (*Ann Surg 7*:171, 1888), and rapidly followed by the introduction of various plates, bobbins, and buttons, the most successful of which were the Murphy button (*Med Record 42*:665, 1892) and the Mayo-Robson bone bobbin (*Brit Med J 1*:688, 1893).

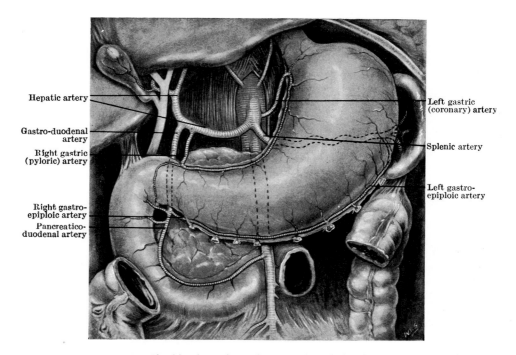

Hepatic artery

Gastro-duodenal artery

Right gastric (pyloric) artery

Right gastro-epiploic artery

Pancreatico-duodenal artery

Left gastric (coronary) artery

Splenic artery

Left gastro-epiploic artery

FIG. 1.   The blood supply to the stomach and the duodenum.

Roux's anastomosis en-Y (*Rev Gynéc Chir Abd 67*:122, 1897) was first performed in 1897, and it was hoped that this operation would solve the problem of vicious-circle vomiting. But it was followed by such a high percentage of stomal ulcers that it was abandoned. Brenner (*Wien Klin Wschr 5*:375, 1892) was the first surgeon to perform a retrocolic anterior long-loop isoperistaltic gastrojejunostomy, the long proximal jejunal loop being brought through an opening in the mesocolon and gastrocolic ligament and the jejunum anastomosed to the anterior wall of the pyloric segment of the stomach.

Stiles and Sherren, and at a later date Wilkie, improved upon Brenner's method by performing the operation without a loop and making a junction either to the anterior wall of the stomach or to its posterior surface parallel with and close to the greater curvature. Petersen (*Beitr Klin Chir 29*:597, 1900; and *Arch Klin Chir 62*:94, 1900) laid the foundation of the modern operation of posterior no-loop gastrojejunostomy. W. J. Mayo (*Ann Surg 43*:537, 1906) and Moynihan (*Ann Surg 47*:481, 1908) were among the first to observe the enormous advantages of Petersen's method, which overcame in a most successful manner the great bugabear of the long-loop operation—vicious-circle vomiting—and they, by their masterly skill and judgment, evolved a technique which was widely adopted for over a quarter of a century (Figs. 1 and 2).

INDICATIONS

In the surgical treatment of duodenal ulcer, *vagotomy should be performed before any emptying or drainage procedures*, which include gastrojejunostomy, pyloroplasty, gastroduodenostomy, and antrectomy (Figs. 3 and 4). *When the drainage operation is gastrojejunostomy, the stoma should always be constructed in the antrum itself.* The stoma, when completed, can be vertical, oblique, or longitudinal. My preference is for a longitudinal stoma made in the posterior wall of the antrum and close to the pyloric outlet (Fig. 5). Some surgeons prefer a longitudinal stoma fashioned at the greater curvature of the antrum or at the anterior or posterior wall of the antrum. (Tanner)

The indications for gastrojejunostomy may be outlined as follows:

Chronic duodenal ulcer. (1) In selected cases in infancy and childhood. (2) in characteristically thin, underweight, and introspective patients; (3) in debilitated pa-

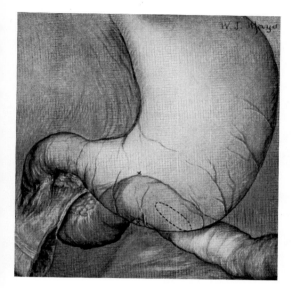

FIG. 2. No-loop gastrojejunostomy after the posterior method (W. J. Mayo). By preserving the normal direction of the uppermost portion of the jejunum, a kink has been avoided; x and x mark the commencement of the jejunum. (Courtesy of the Mayo Clinic.)

tients with callous lesions who in addition have some complicating constitutional dis-

order; (4) in those cases in which, owing to the position and physical characteristics of the ulcer, the risks associated with partial gastrectomy appear to be prohibitive; for instance, the ulcer may be unusually large, deeply eroding the pancreatic head, or it may be involving the vital structures in the right border of the hepatoduodenal ligament in a dense mass of inflammatory tissue (Fig. 6); (5) in certain cases of *advanced pyloric stenosis in aged patients* and in postbulbar duodenal ulcer, more particularly where the crater lies in the substance of the pancreas.

Cancer of the stomach. The best palliation is afforded by subtotal gastrectomy. When this operation is not feasible, anterior gastrojejunostomy may provide some temporary respite.

Cancer of the head of the pancreas or lower end of the common bile duct. Where eradication of the malignant mass is not possible or is deemed inadvisable, anterior gastrojejunostomy combined with hepaticojejunostomy, should be performed to relieve jaundice and to forestall duodenal obstruction.

Pressure on stomach or duodenum from without. In certain cases in which the

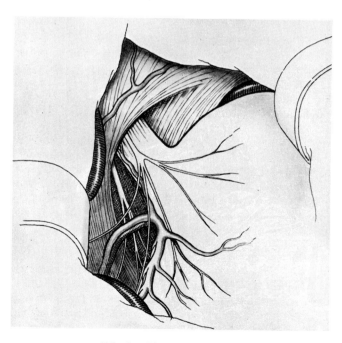

FIG. 3. The vagus nerves.

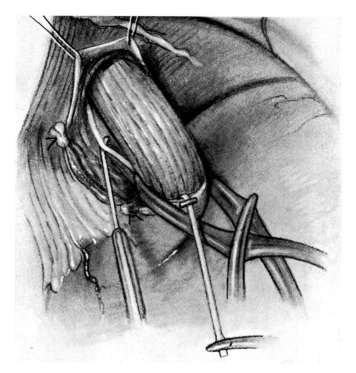

FIG. 4. Truncal vagotomy. This is performed before carrying out the gastrojejunostomy.

duodenum or distal half of the stomach is partially or wholly occluded by pressure from without, such as may be occasioned by *severe* inflammatory adhesions or compression by a tumor that defies removal.

Trauma to pylorus or duodenum. Following certain traumatic lesions of the pyloric region of the stomach or duodenum —e.g., some types of retroperitoneal rupture of the duodenum. I believe that *short-loop anterior or posterior gastrojejunostomy,* with the stoma placed in the antrum, affords excellent drainage of the stomach (see Fig. 5). A satisfactory stoma should admit the tips of two fingers.

Factors relating to the aetiology, pathogenesis, and choice of vagotomy—truncal or selective—and of operation in cases of peptic ulcer and to the immediate and late results of elective procedures are considered comprehensively by C. V. Mann in Chapter 11 and by other contributors in this Section.

TECHNIQUE OF POSTERIOR GASTROJEJUNOSTOMY

The operation of posterior gastrojejunstomy is performed as follows: The abdomen is opened through a median or paramedian incision of ample length to permit easy exploration of the abdominal viscera and the performance of vagotomy (See Figs. 3 and 4; and also Chaps. 14, 15 and 16). After the scarred first portion of the duodenum has been inspected, the entire stomach, the remainder of the duodenum, and the duodenojejunal flexure are methodically scrutinised for evidence of any other pathological lesion. The stomach, transverse colon, and greater omentum are then drawn through the wound and held upward by an assistant to

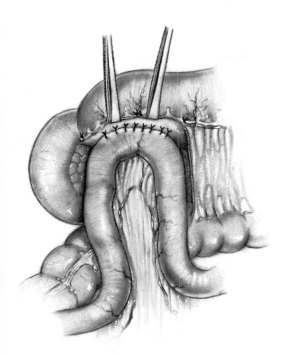

FIG. 5. Anterior short-loop retrogastric gastrojejunostomy with stoma fashioned in the posterior wall of the antrum, close to the pyloric outlet.

allow inspection of the undersurface of the mesocolon and the position of the middle colic artery and its arching branches. The surgeon then passes his right hand along the posterior surface of the mesocolon toward the left of the spine to pick up and identify the ligament of Treitz, after which he withdraws some 6 to 8 inches (15 to 20 cm) of proximal jejunum through the wound, wraps it in a small towel soaked in warm saline solution, and lays it aside on the abdominal wall for use at a later stage in the operation.

Any slight adhesions found attaching the jejunum to the undersurface of the mesocolon are divided. When, however, these adhesions are *very* extensive—the aftermath of peritonitis, if there are many congenital bands and membranes, or if the jejunum is fixed to the mesocolon for several inches—it is better to leave the parts undisturbed and to abandon the posterior operation.

The blood vessels in the mesocolon are carefully observed; if these are numerous, aberrant, or irregular in their arrangement or are obscured in fat, if an adequate bloodless space cannot be found in which to make

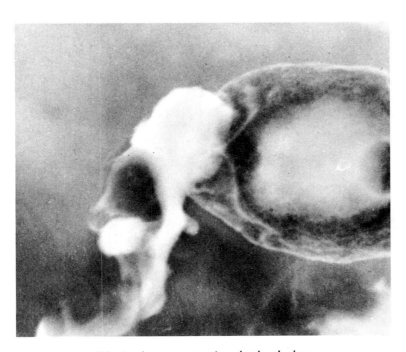

FIG. 6. Large penetrating duodenal ulcer.

the opening into the lesser peritoneal sac, or if the mesocolon is short or fused to the peritoneum of the stomach bed, thus obliterating the omental bursa, the posterior operation should not be attempted. In such circumstances it might be preferable to perform Jaboulay's gastroduodenostomy (see Chap. 18).

When the vertical stoma is selected—and this is the method I shall now describe—two pairs of forceps are fixed to the curvatures, one on the lesser curvature of the antrum, about 1 inch (2.54 mm) proximal to the pylorus and the other exactly opposite on the greater curvature. When these Allis forceps are in position, the surgeon draws the stomach, the transverse colon, and the greater omentum through the wound and holds the

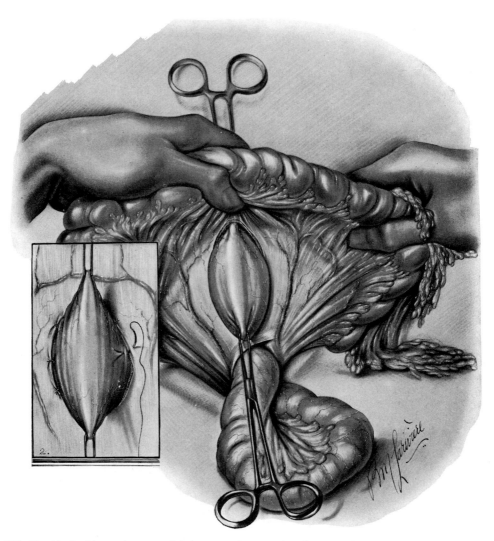

FIG. 7. Vertical posterior gastrojejunostomy. Opening has been made in mesocolon through a wide arch of the middle colic artery. Duodenojejunal flexure and first loop of jejunum have been withdrawn from abdomen. Vertical pouch of posterior wall of antrum has been drawn through opening of mesocolon. Allis forceps are acting as guides. Inset shows edge of mesocolon being sutured to posterior wall of the antrum.

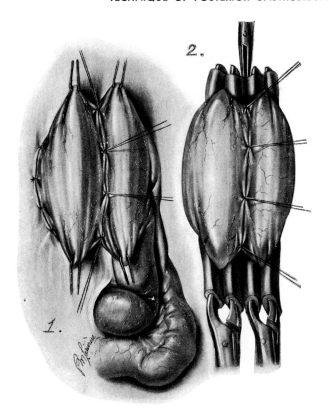

FIG. 8. Vertical posterior gastrojejunostomy. (1), Operation *without* aid of clamps (2); *with* clamps.

transverse colon upward to display the full face of the mesocolon. An opening is then made through the mesocolon into the lesser sac in a bloodless space that exists to the left or right of the middle colic artery and beneath an anastomotic arch. This is done by drawing the mesocolon away from the stomach and clipping it with a haemostat at a bloodless spot. A snip is then made with scissors by the side of the clip into the lesser sac, after which the opening is further enlarged vertically to admit three or four fingers. This opening must not be too niggardly, never less than 3 inches (7.6 cm) long, and should permit a complete exploration of the posterior aspect of the stomach and its bed. If any adhesions exist between the antrum and the pancreas, these should be freed and the organ adequately mobilised before proceeding with the anastomosis.

The portion of the antral wall needed for the anastomosis is then drawn through the opening in the mesocolon. The Allis forceps on the greater curvature will now be seen at the upper end of the opening (near the colon), while the pair of Allis forceps on the lesser curvature guide and bulge a fold of stomach through at the lower end of the opening. The fold of stomach to be utilised in the anastomosis is again freely mobilised by division of any filmy adhesions and is drawn further through the opening in the mesocolon. The Allis forceps at the selected points on the greater and lesser curvatures at the extremities of the fold of stomach to be used in the anastomosis are elevated, while the edges of the opening in the mesocolon are stitched all around the stomach with a series of interrupted sutures (Fig. 7 [*inset*]). It is better to anchor the edges of the opening in the mesocolon to the stomach at this stage, as the suturing can be done more easily and more accurately than when the jejunal loop is in the way, as it will be

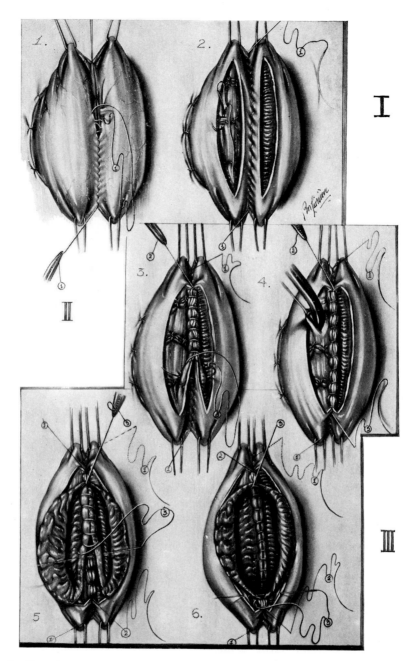

FIG. 9. Posterior gastrojejunostomy: method of introducing three posterior rows of sutures.

at the end of the operation.

It should be noted especially that the mesocolon is stitched to the stomach wall itself, well beyond the area to which the jejunum will be attached and not to the finished suture line of the gastroenteric stoma. It was formerly sutured in the latter position to act as a reinforcement, but this practice has now been abandoned. By the former method the anastomosis is placed well into the greater peritoneal cavity, this method of suturing rendering constriction of the stomach impossible.

If enterostomy clamps are used, the gastric fold is raised and clamped, the tips of the blades pointing to the patient's chin and the handles towards the pubes. The selected coil of jejunum is picked up and the portion chosen for the anastomosis, about 2 inches (5 cm) from the duodenojejunal flexure, is likewise clamped, after which the two clamps are brought together, side by side, and the parts are ready to be anastomosed (Fig. 8).

When clamps are not employed, the antimesenteric border of the portion of jejunum chosen for the anastomosis is picked up with Allis forceps which are placed 3 inches (7.6 cm) apart (Fig. 8 [1]). The proximal point of the jejunal loop engaged in the anastomosis is applied to the lesser curvature of the stomach, while the distal point is applied to the greater curvature. The transverse colon, the omentum, and any intestines which have prolapsed through the wound are now replaced in the abdominal cavity and are prevented from protruding into the field of operation by means of suitably placed abdominal packs. The only portions of the viscera which are allowed to remain outside the abdomen are those about to be anastomosed.

The operative field is isolated with large,

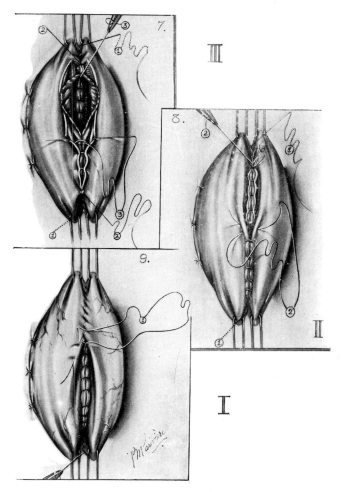

FIG. 10.   Posterior gastrojejunostomy: method of introducing three anterior rows of continuous sutures.

moist abdominal packs. The folds of stomach and jejunum are now kept taut and in close apposition and are steadied by an assistant who holds the upper and lower sets of Allis forceps in his fingers. Four interrupted sutures of 000 silk are introduced to approximate the adjacent walls of stomach and jejunum, to prevent rotation of the jejunum, and to act as suitable tractors. The first posterior suture, 000 chromic catgut, is now introduced as a Cushing right-angled stitch which unites the contiguous seromuscular coats of the stomach and jejunum from the lesser to the greater curvature. When it reaches the greater curvature, it is locked and laid aside to be used again at a later stage in the operation (Fig. 9 [1] .

Two longitudinal incisions are now made with a knife through the seromuscular coats of the stomach and jejunum down to the mucosae, parallel with and 1/4 inch (6.3 mm) from the posterior suture line. The mucous membrane of the stomach and jejunum will pout through these incisions as the seromuscular coats retract and as they are freed by gentle dissection. A few large blood vessels, which can be seen coursing over the exposed surfaces of the gastric and jejunal mucous membranes, are underrun and ligated with fine plain catgut on each side of the line of the proposed incision through the mucosae (Fig. 9 [2]).

The second posterior stitch starts at the greater curvature end and is introduced as a continuous through-and-through all-coats suture. When it reaches the lesser curvature, it is locked and put on one side. A small incision is made through the gastric mucous membrane, large enough to admit a suction tube, which is used to aspirate the contents of the stomach (Fig. 9 [4]). The mucous membrane of the stomach is picked up with forceps and divided with scissors for almost the full length of the seromuscular incision. The jejunal mucous membrane is similarly picked up and incised and the gut thoroughly sponged. Redundant gastric and jejunal mucous membrane is not excised.

The third continuous suture of 000 chromic catgut approximates the margins of the mucous membranes of the stomach and jejunum posteriorly, and when the suturing has been completed along the posterior margin of the incision, it turns the corner at the lesser curvature and returns along the anterior margin as the first *anterior* stitch, without interruption, locking, or knotting, until the end that was left long is reached. A double knot is tied and the ends are cut short (Fig. 9 [5]).

The second posterior suture is then taken up and returned as the second anterior suture, being passed as a closely applied continuous Lembert suture which invaginates the anterior suture line. When it reaches the greater curvature, it is knotted and cut short.

The third posterior suture is now picked up once more and introduced anteriorly as a Cushing right-angled stitch, and when it reaches the lesser curvature is tied to the point where it was started (Fig. 10 [9]).

Curved or straight (eyeless) intestinal needles are used and are threaded with 000 chromic catgut or Dexon.

Four interrupted sutures of fine silk are introduced to reinforce further the anterior suture line. *The surgeon and his assistants then change their gloves, and fresh instru-*

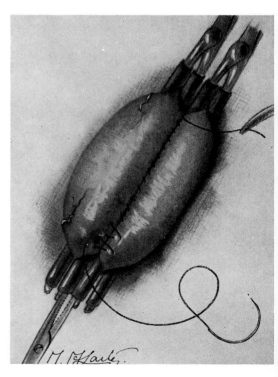

FIG. 11. Posterior gastrojejunostomy with two rows of continuous sutures. First posterior continuous suture is being introduced.

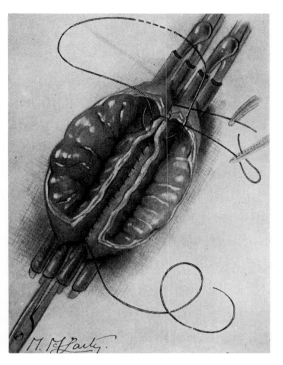

FIG. 12. Posterior gastrojejunostomy with two rows of continuous sutures. Second posterior all-coats continuous suture is commenced.

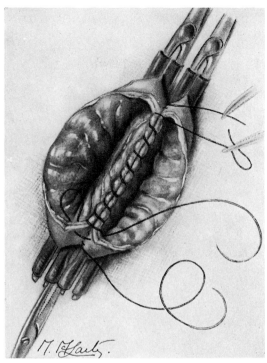

FIG. 13. Posterior gastrojejunostomy with two rows of continuous sutures. Second posterior suture is turning corner.

ments are used for closing the abdominal incision.

The operation is completed by replacing the colon and omentum in their normal positions and by testing with the fingers the size of the stoma. A good stoma will admit two fingers.

This method of performing posterior gastrojejunostomy with *three rows of anterior and posterior continuous sutures* has been criticised on the grounds that it is unnecessarily complicated and protracted. It has, however, its advantages, since bleeding from the suture line and leakage do not occur when this method is correctly executed. My operative mortality rate is less than 0.5 percent. Again, there is much to be said in favour of *precision* in the technique of abdominal operations.

The method of performing gastrojejunostomy with clamps and by two rows of continuous sutures of 0 or 00 chromic catgut, which was popularised by Moynihan and W. J. Mayo and which is favoured by most surgeons, is illustrated in Figures 11 to 15.

ANTERIOR GASTROJEJUNOSTOMY

In recent years, when performing vagotomy and a short-circuiting procedure for duodenal ulcer, I have almost invariably selected anterior gastrojejunostomy in preference to the posterior methods of anastomosis. Anterior gastrojejunostomy is simple, safe, and efficient, has an operative death rate of less than 0.5 percent, and can be performed in a short time. Furthermore, should an anastomotic ulcer appear at some later date, the taking down of the anastomosis and the subsequent gastroduodenal resection will present few, if any, technical difficulties. On the other hand, the combination of anastomotic ulcer and a short-loop posterior gastrojejunostomy may be, and often is, a formidable condition to rectify.

The essential points of the anterior operation are the use of a *short* isoperistaltic

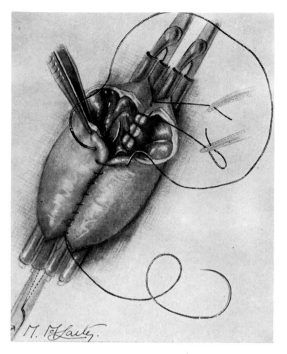

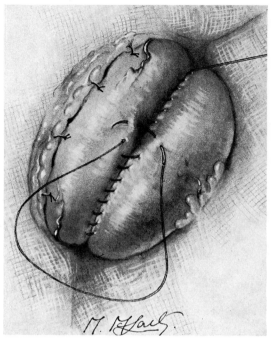

FIG. 14. Gastrojejunostomy with clamps and two rows of continuous sutures. First anterior suture is introduced as Connell loop-on-the-mucosa suture.

FIG. 15. Posterior gastrojejunostomy with two rows of continuous sutures. Second anterior seromuscular culture is nearing completion.

jejunal loop and the fashioning of the antral stoma at or just anterior or posterior to the greater curvature. Except when performing the anterior procedure the greater omentum should be detached from the distal one-third of the greater curvature of the stomach (see Fig. 16).

In performing anterior gastrojejunostomy for duodenal ulceration, the proximal jejunal loop is picked up and drawn taut to the proximal portion of the antrum and a point on the jejunum some 2 inches (5 cm) *beyond* this is chosen for the anastomosis. The portion of small bowel selected for anastomosis is usually some 4 inches (10 cm) from the ligament of Treitz. The jejunal loop is brought from the patient's left side to the right so that an isoperistaltic junction is constructed. The jejunal loop should be unrestrained and mobile and should not compress

the underlying transverse colon. It should take a graceful curve from the ligament of Treitz to its point of attachment to the stomach.

The stoma should be at least 2 inches (5 cm) long and should be placed longitudinally in the distal portion of the antrum.

The suturing is conducted as in the posterior operation except that, in order to avoid obstructive kinking of the jejunum, the first continuous seromuscular suture of 000 chromic catgut unites the stomach and jejunum over a much wider area than is required for the vertical posterior opening.

The important technical steps of *retrogastric anterior gastrojejunostomy* will be appreciated by referring to Figure 16. The operation here described is, in many ways, similar to the one practised by Colcock and Braasch.[4]

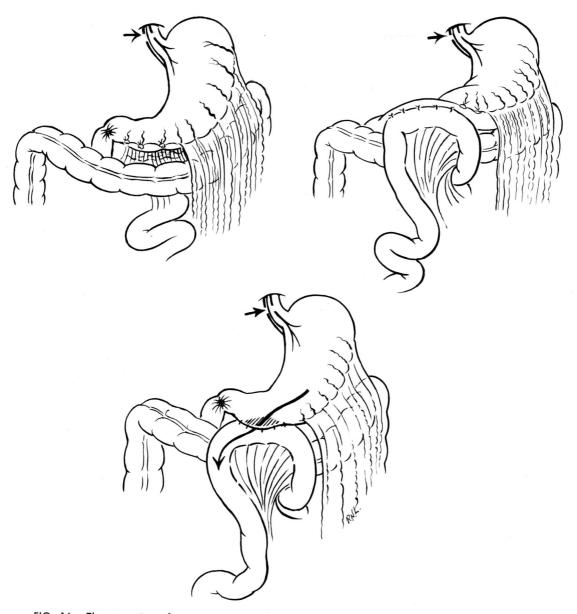

FIG. 16. The operation of anterior retrogastric gastrojejunostomy with stoma fashioned in the posterior wall of the antrum, close to pyloric outlet. Note truncal vagotomy.

THE RESULTS OF VAGOTOMY AND GASTROJEJUNOSTOMY FOR DUODENAL ULCER

Goligher et al.,[6] wrote:

From our data we believe that if the surgeon wishes to continue practising truncal vagotomy with a gastric drainage procedure, vagotomy and gastroenterostomy is in general preferable to vagotomy and pyloroplasty, for disturbances of alimentary function are only marginally more frequent after it, and it seems to afford somewhat better protection against the tendency to recurrent ulceration if the vagotomy should be incomplete. In addition, gastroenterostomy is nearly always applicable in practice, while a pyloroplasty may sometimes be technically difficult and possibly less safe.

Acting on the advice of Lester Dragstedt, I have performed truncal vagotomy, in preference to selective vagotomy, for the majority of my cases. Selective vagotomy may be a difficult and, in a few instances, a hazardous procedure in very obese and broad-chested muscular patients.

In most series of duodenal ulcer patients treated by vagotomy and gastrojejunostomy the mortality rate is reported to be 0.5 percent or even lower, the recurrent ulcer rate 2.5 to 5 percent, and the results following a 5-year follow-up are stated to be good or highly satisfactory in approximately 80 percent. My results show a mortality of 0.5 percent and a *proved* recurrent ulcer rate of 3 percent.

INADVERTENT GASTROILEOSTOMY

Inadverent gastroileostomy is a preventable error in gastric surgery.

Since the first description of gastroileostomy in 1915 by Martin and Carroll,[11] over 80 additional cases have been reported in the literature. Deaver[5] reported 35 instances in the literature to that time. It seems certain that it must have occurred many more times but, understandably, many instances have not come to light (Jesseph, 1962). Marshall and O'Donnell,[10] in a well-documented article, state that its incidence is far greater than the reported cases would indicate be-

cause of the reluctance of surgeons to report these surgical errors. Moretz[13] believes that the original operation is always performed by some surgeon other than the one reporting the case and that unreported cases in which both operations are carried out by the same surgeon may be quite unknown. Marshall and O'Donnell[10] write on this matter as follows:

The main interest of this syndrome lies not in the numbers involved but in its preventability and remediability. Many cases were reported during the heyday of gastroenterostomy but the complication was not a serious one with the short circuit procedure as some of the gastric contents continued to go through the pylorus. The mistake continues to be made at gastric operations, however, and it is a much more serious matter when a subtotal gastrectomy is performed and the gastric remnant is anastomosed to a lower ileal loop.

We have seen seven cases of this syndrome in the Lahey Clinic during the past 28 years. In all seven cases the initial operation had been done elsewhere and the patients were referred to the clinic for treatment. Four of the patients had had subtotal gastrectomy and in the three remaining patients gastroileostomy had occurred during the attempted performance of a gastroenterostomy.

Excellent accounts of gastroileostomy, gastroileal ulcer, and gastrocolostomy are given by the following authors, from whose writings I have obtained valuable information for this article: McKenzie and Robertson,[12] Barritt,[1] Boice,[2] Gross and Waugh,[7] Konarow,[8] and Parys.[14]

Signs and symptoms. An analysis of the cases shows that the most common complaints are gaseous distention, foul eructations, borborygmi, and bloating of the abdomen. According to Castleton and Bailey,[3] in addition to the above symptoms the classical features are those of *diarrhoea and weight loss*. Steatorrhoea as a rule begins immediately after the first operation, and the stools are frothy, pale, bulky, and malodorous. Weight loss is most noticeable in those patients who have had a partial or a subtotal gastrectomy for benign ulcer and in whom the gastric remnant has been anastomosed to the lower ileum. Weight loss again is marked and progressive, and steatorrhoea severe in all the patients who develop a gastroileal ulcer. Macrocytic anaemia, a sprue-like state, manifestations of the deprivation of Vitamin B complex, oedema of the lower extremities due to hypoproteinaemia, and alkalosis are observed in many of these unfortunate patients.

Boice [2] gives an interesting account of one of his patients who was admitted to hospital with abdominal colic, nausea, vomiting, and carpopedal spasm, and who presented the picture of small-gut obstruction, alkalaemia, and tetany.

Pain is a common feature. It may manifest itself as a sullen paraumbilical ache, as intestinal colic, or as a severe burning pain such as is not uncommonly observed in certain cases of extensive peptic ulceration of the stomach. Again, the pain may be constant and excruciating and stab through to the back or to the left side of the chest when an anastomotic ulcer of some proportions develops following subtotal gastrectomy and union of the lower ileum to the gastric remnant.

Diagnosis. The majority of such patients are gravely ill, anaemic, dehydrated, wasted, and lethargic. The tongue is often bright red or crimson, denoting a lack of Vitamin B. The abdomen is protuberant; loud rumblings of the intestines and belching of evil-smelling gas are troublesome features; weight loss is apparent and the legs are frequently swollen consequent upon hypoproteinaemia.

A history of a previous gastric operation, repeated blood investigations, and barium-meal X-ray examinations is routinely obtained. The diagnosis is clinched by carrying out barium-meal studies followed by a barium enema. It seems apparent from a study of a large series of cases that no case was misdiagnosed when both of these radiological studies were performed, but more often than not barium-enema X-ray examination alone will yield a correct diagnosis.

Treatment. As many of these patients are poor surgical risks, an attempt should be made to correct dehydration, electrolyte loss, nitrogen balance, avitaminosis, and anaemia, which is so often of the secondary, macrocytic type. Food by mouth has obvious limits, but some patients tend to gain weight when a high-calorie diet rich in proteins is administered at frequent intervals. Barritt considers that the nutrition of the patient is often improved by a preliminary jejunostomy and milk-drip feedings through the indwelling intestinal tube, McKenzie and Rocke Robertson have suggested that the prescription of cortisone is of value in preparing these patients for major sugery.

As I have stated, inadvertent ileostomy is a tragic and preventable complication of gastric surgery. It seems incredible to me that any surgeon should perpetrate such a misdemeanour as to anastomose the ileum (or even the colon) to the stomach during the performance of any gastric operation which is conducted for the cure of chronic peptic ulceration. Prophylaxis is the key word!

Before performing gastrojejunostomy or partial gastrectomy, the surgeon should display and demonstrate to an assistant the ligament of Treitz and the fixed portion of the duodenojejunal flexure. The Babcock forceps are clipped to the first loop of the jejunum some 6 or 8 inches (15 to 20 cm) away from the ligament of Treitz and then placed under the outer layer of large swabs on the abdominal wall. This serves as an invaluable marker. It should be stressed that the ligament of Treitz is the one and only dependable landmark in choosing the correct jejunal loop.

The operation of choice for gastroileostomy (with or without stomal ulceration) depends upon the condition of the patient and the presence or absence of pathological lesions in the stomach or duodenum. For instance, when there is no evidence of gastric or duodenal ulcer, the correct procedure would be simple lysis of the gastroileostomy and the restoration of gastrointestinal continuity. When, on the other hand, a gastric or duodenal ulcer is found to be present, the operation recommended would consist of taking down the gastroileostomy, followed by the Billroth II plan.

For those patients who were subjected to gastric resection with gastroileostomy (with or without stomal ulceration), the best procedure would entail lysis of the gastroileostomy, adequate gastric resection, followed by the ante-colic Schoemaker-Billroth II method of repair.

Gastrocolostomy. Peptic ulceration of the colon is, of course, invariable, and in addition to diarrhoea and loss of weight, there may be occult or massive bleeding. Recognition of this grave error in technique can be demonstrated by barium-meal X-ray studies—that is, barium meal of the stomach and duodenum followed by barium enema. Treatment is the same as for gastroileostomy —namely, prompt reestablishment of normal continuity followed by appropriate surgical measures for any concomitant lesion in the stomach or duodenum when present.

REFERENCES

1. Barritt, Lancet 2:564, 1952.
2. Boice, Am. J. Roentgenol. 66:601, 1951.
3. Castleton and Bailey, Am. J. Surg. 79:736, 1950.
4. Colcock and Braasch, Surg. Clin. North Am. 45:585, 1965.
5. Deaver, Surg. Gynecol. Obstet. 100:621, 1955.
6. Goligher et al., Br. Med. J. 1:7, 1972.
7. Gross and Waugh, Arch. Intern. Med. 102:722, 1958.
8. Konarow, Chirugija 40:53, 1964.
9. Landry, Surgery 30:528, 1951.
10. Marshall and O'Donnell, Surg. Clin. North Am. June, 665, 1951.
11. Martin and Carroll, Am. Surg. 61:551, 1915.
12. McKenzie and Rocke Robertson, Ann. Surg. 138:911, 1953.
13. Moretz, Ann. Surg. 130:124, 1949.
14. Parys, Wiadomósci Lekarskie 24:777, 1971.

20
THE BILLROTH I OPERATIONS

RODNEY MAINGOT

HISTORICAL NOTE

This historical note on gastric resection based on the Billroth I principle is founded on information culled from the papers of the following authorities: Narath (*Deutsche Ztschr Chir 136*:62, 1919); Spivack (*The Surgical Technic of Abdominal Operations*, 1955); Moore and Harkins (*The Billroth I Gastric Resection*, 1954); Waugh and Hood (*Quart Rev Surg Gynaec Obstet 10*:201, 1953, and *11*:1, 1954); and Harkins and Nyhus (*Surgery of the Stomach and Duodenum, Churchill*, 2d ed., 1969).

Merrem (*Med Doct Gissae*, 1810, cited by Rydygier in 1881) is accredited with being the first surgeon to perform pylorectomy and end-to-end gastroduodenostomy in dogs. He suggested that this operation might be applied to humans suffering from cancer of the pyloric segment of the stomach. Gussenbauer and von Winniwarter (*Arch Klin Chir 19*:347, 1876), following a meticulous study of the morbid anatomy of gastric cancer and the performance of seven pylorectomies in dogs, came to the conclusion that in some instances of malignant pyloric obstruction resection of the tumour and axial union between the antrum and duodenum was a feasible procedure and was worthy of a trial in human beings. Péan (*Gaz des hôp 52*:473, 1879) at the Hospital of Saint Louis performed the first recorded pyloric resection for carcinoma on a human. His patient died on the fourth postoperative day. Rydygier (*Arch Klin Chir 26*:731, 1881), on Nov. 16, 1880, performed the second pyloric resection on a human for carcinoma of the pylorus. He reestablished continuity by gastroduodenal anastomosis with a series of interrupted silk sutures. This patient collapsed and died some 12 hr. following the operation.

The first successful resection for cancer of the stomach was accomplished by Billroth in 1881 (*Wien Med Wschr 31*:161, 1881). Rydygier (1881) stated that Billroth performed the third pylorectomy with gastroduodenostomy for an obstructing carcinoma of the pylorus in the human. Billroth had no knowledge of Rydygier's case when he successfully carried out this operation on Jan. 29, 1881. The patient was a woman, aged 43, and the pyloric tumour was mobile and lent itself readily to resection. She unfortunately died four months after the operation, from liver metastases.

In this operation, after resecting the pyloric segment of the stomach and a small portion of the first part of the duodenum, Billroth closed the greater curvature side of the stomach and then anastomosed the open end of the duodenum to the lesser curvature side of the stomach. Silk sutures were used in fashioning the anastomosis.

In Billroth's second operation, the patient succumbed from obstruction of the stoma. In consequence of this he performed his third, fourth, and fifth resections of the pylorus for carcinoma by anastomosing the open end of the duodenum to the greater curvature side of the gastric stump after closing the redundant lesser curvature. All these patients died in the early postoperative stages.

Bardenheuer (1881) performed the sixth pylorectomy on the human, and based the steps of his operation on the lines previously suggested by Billroth. His patient did not survive the shock of the resection for more than 2 days.

Rydygier, on Nov. 21, 1881, performed pylorectomy with gastroduodenostomy for a *benign chronic pyloric ulcer* which was producing obstructive symptoms. The patient lived to be discharged from the hospital in a highly satisfactory condition. According to Moore and Harkins (1954), Rydygier reported this case under the title of *The First Resection for Stomach Ulcer,* and when this article was abstracted in another journal two months later, the editor wrote a footnote as follows: "And I hope the last!"

Kocher (1893) implanted the end of the duodenum into the posterior wall of the stomach (after the open mouth of the stomach had been closed) in order to avoid the "angle of sorrow"—*Jammerecke;* but this operation was rarely practised by his contemporaries. Von Haberer (*Zbl Chir 49*:1321, 1922) and Finney (*Tr South S A 36*:576, 1924) sutured the entire open end of the stomach to the side of the second portion of the duodenum after the duodenal stump had been securely closed and inverted. Finney was performing this operation in 1922 at a time when he had no knowledge that von Haberer was carrying out the same procedure for benign and malignant lesions of the stomach.

Schoemaker (*Arch Chir 94*:541, 1911) was among the first surgeons to extend gastric resection both for malignant and benign lesions of the stomach (as well as for duodenal ulcer) and to excise practically the whole of the lesser curvature prior to the performance of end-to-end gastroduodenostomy. He himself had no trouble from leakage at the *Jammerecke,* and his immediate and late results were most gratifying.

Von Haberer (*Munchen Med Wschr 80*:915, 1933) performed his *reefing and narrowing* of the mouth of the gastric stump after partial gastrectomy long before the publication of his paper in 1933. He ligated or transfixed and tied all the blood vessels lying on the submucosa of the stomach, with the prime object of controlling bleeding from the severed end of the gastric remnant, and to his satisfaction he found that this manoeuvre reduced the gastric stoma to such proportions that it made end-to-end gastroduodenal anastomosis a relatively simple operation.

Horsley (*JAMA 86*:664, 1926) described splitting the anterior duodenal wall to allow of the fashioning of a larger gastroduodenal stoma. He anastomosed the open end of the duodenum to the lesser curvature portion of the gastric stump after the greater curvature portion had been closed and inverted.

INDICATIONS FOR THE BILLROTH I OPERATION

The indications for the performance of the Billroth I operation may be summarised as follows (Fig. 1):

1. In the majority of cases of *chronic gastric ulcer* where the duodenum is

normal. When a duodenal ulcer is present in addition to a gastric ulcer—i.e., combined ulcers, the Schoemaker-Billroth II procedure is to be preferred. Likewise, in those cases in which the first and second parts of the duodenum appear to be unduly shortened and narrowed or show evidence of fibrotic distortion from past or present ulceration.

Orr,[13] a leading British surgeon who is an authority on the aetiology, pathogenesis, and treatment of peptic ulceration, writes:

So far as gastric ulcer is concerned (unless it is combined with duodenal ulcer) surgical opinion is unanimously in favour of the Schoemaker modification of the Billroth I procedure.
This is probably the most entirely satisfactory gastric operation at our disposal.
The operative death-rate is less than 0.5 percent, the recurrence rate is under 1 percent, the physiological disturbance is minimal and it removes the ulcer and the ulcer-bearing area.
Acid secretion is cut down but not eliminated by virtue of the antrectomy, and the acid chyme passes into the duodenum invoking the inhibitory mechanism and causing the release of hormones which stimulate biliary and pancreatic secretion, and mixing of the gastric contents with the duodenal secretions takes place at the site and at the time nature intended. There is no loop to become kinked and no risk of stasis.

In a general way, it may be stated that in approximately 80 percent of cases of gastric ulcer the Billroth I operation would be the one of choice. Furthermore with "high cardial" ulcers, Pauchet's operation, which is in fact a modification of the Schoemaker procedure, should in many instances be completed by an end-to-end gastroduodenal anastomosis rather than by a terminolateral gastrojejunosotomy.

The Kelling-Madlener operation for *high gastric "cardial" ulcers* is discussed in Chapter 21. The operation of choice for *combined ulcers* is the Schoemaker-Billroth II procedure (see Chap. 21).

Personal experience has proved that in 96 percent of cases of gastric ulcer it is possible by adequate mobilisation of the stomach and for the first two portions of the duodenum to perform a partial gastrectomy and an end-to-

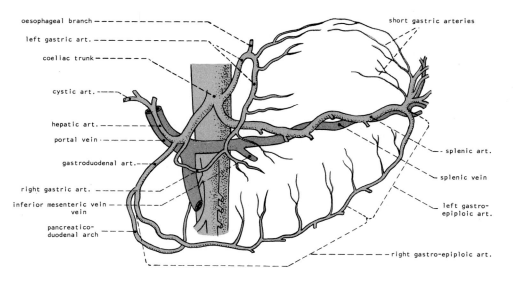

FIG. 1. The arterial supply to the stomach and duodenum. (After *Gray's Anatomy.*)

end anastomosis without any tension; but the *Billroth I operation should never be forced,* and where there is any likelihood of tension or strain on the suture line, the surgeon should not hesitate to carry out the Billroth II operation, which yields results that are in many respects comparable with those which follow the Billroth I procedure.

2. *Duodenal ulcer.* The most popular operations today for *chronic duodenal ulcer* are truncal or selective vagotomy and antrectomy (or hemigastrectomy) (Chap. 16), partial gastrectomy (excision of 65 to 75 percent of the distal portion of the stomach plus two-thirds of the lesser curve) by the Schoemaker-Billroth II procedure (Chap. 21), and vagotomy combined with such *drainage operations* as pyloroplasty (Chap. 17), gastrojejunostomy (Chap. 19), or gastroduodenostomy (Finney and Jaboulay techniques) (Chap. 18) and proximal selective vagotomy.

Most of the so-called antrectomies are, in fact, hemigastrectomies, as at least 70 percent of the vertical part of the lesser curvature of the stomach has to be excised when the antrum is being removed for duodenal ulcer. Antrectomy, per se, entails resection of about 40 to 45 percent of distal stomach.

Partial gastrectomy, in which 65 to 75 percent of the stomach is removed must be distinguished from *subtotal gastrectomy,* in which about 80 percent or more of the distal stomach is resected (Fig. 2). *Subtotal gastrectomy* followed by the Billroth I methods of anastomosis should not be carried out for duodenal ulceration, as serious

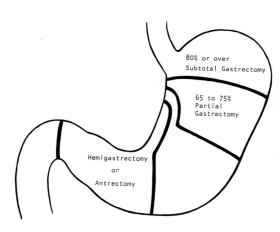

FIG. 2. The amount of stomach removed in antrectomy or hemigastrectomy; 65 to 75 percent partial gastrectomy; and subtotal gastrectomy. Note that most of the lesser curvature of the stomach is excised in all these resections.

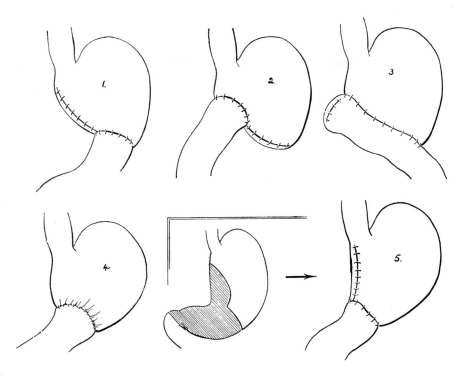

FIG. 3. Billroth I operations: (1) Billroth I; (2) Horsley; (3) von Haberer-Finney; (4) von Haberer; (5) Schoemaker.

postoperative complications, including the dumping syndrome, loss of weight, metabolic disturbances, etc., are commonly observed (see Chap. 27).

It should be noted here that the Billroth I and II operations for duodenal ulcer are followed by a recurrent ulcer rate of 0.8 to 4 percent, whereas when these operations are carried out for gastric ulcer, the recurrent ulcer rate is less than 0.5 percent. Statistical figures relating to recurrent ulcer rates are discussed by Grassi,[6] Goligher et al.;[5] by C. V. Mann (Chap. 11); and by the writer in Chapter 24.

It is necessary to repeat and also to emphasise that the surgeon would be well advised to abandon gastric resection, with its concomitant hazards, and to select vagotomy combined with a gastric drainage operation when the patient is aged, emaciated, or suffering from a concomitant medical disease, such as diabetes or nephritis; when the first portion of the duodenum is grossly deformed and contracted; when there is a marked degree of inflammatory oedema or periduodenal infection; or where the bulb is the seat of a large, deeply penetrating, and adherent crater capable of compromising the duct of Santorini or the lower portion of the choledochus.

The *choice of operation* and the *results of elective operations for peptic ulcer* are fully discussed in Chapter 11; and detailed descriptions of the techniques of vagotomy are submitted in Chapters 15, 16, 17, and by Lester Dragstedt in Chapter 14.

3. *Cancer of the distal portion of the stomach.* In elderly or debilitated patients suffering from cancer of the antrum, the Billroth I operation may be entertained, when the time-saving element is an important consideration.

The operation entails removal of the first portion of the duodenum, *subtotal gastrectomy* after the Schoemaker plan, and excision of the greater omentum, the gastrohepatic omentum, and all adjacent visible and palpable lymph nodes. In certain instances, splenectomy may facilitate the mobilisation of the upper end of the stomach and at the same time render it possible to perform a more radical operation which, nevertheless, is confined to the supracolic department.

The objection to the Billroth I procedure in cases of gastric carcinoma is the possible *tendency* to limit the scope of the operation. This objection is, of course, valid only if the operation is used indiscriminately or injudiciously.

The following types of repair will be described later in this chapter: (1) Schoemaker-Billroth I operation; (2) Pauchet's modification of the Schoemaker operation; (3) modification of Billroth I operation as practised by Finsterer; (4) von Haberer-Finney operation; (5) von Haberer's "reefing" of the mouth of the gastric pouch followed by end-to-end gastroduodenostomy; (6) Horsley's modification of the Billroth I procedure; and (7) Finochietto's method. Some of these are illustrated in Figure 3.

GENERAL CONSIDERATIONS OF THE BILLROTH I OPERATION

Protection of Vital Structures

In the surgical treatment of gastric and duodenal ulcer the importance of meticulous identification of the adjacent structures to be preserved cannot be sufficiently stressed. The vital structures include the lower reaches of the common bile duct, the pancreatic ducts, the pancreas itself, the common hepatic artery, the middle colic artery, and the spleen.

Undue traction on the greater curvature of the stomach, the gastrocolic ligament, or gastrosplenic omentum is sufficient at times to cause tearing of the splenic capsule or of the pulp of the spleen itself, with consequent troublesome oozing of blood. When bleeding is brisk or impossible to control, as will often be the case, immediate splenectomy should be performed.

This mishap does not increase the hazards of partial gastrectomy, but it is nevertheless a surgical blemish.

The middle colic artery may become adherent to a gastric ulcer or may be tethered to the posterior wall of the antrum in cases of penetrating duodenal ulcer. A good view of the interior of the omental bursa and of the entire course of the middle colic artery should always be obtained before freeing the mesocolon from its attachments; otherwise this important vessel may be mistaken for the right gastroepiploic artery and be severed during the liberation of the stomach. Ligation of this vital artery may lead to gangrene of the transverse colon, although this is not by any means always the case.

In cases in which the lesser peritoneal sac is obliterated by adhesions, a segment of the right colic vessels or the middle colic artery may be picked up, clipped, and ligated during the devascularisation of the greater curvature which precedes gastric resection. If the middle colic artery is inadvertently crushed or ligated during the performance of partial gastrectomy, no immediate decision should be made concerning the viability of the transverse colon. The surgeon should proceed with the liberation of the stomach and duodenum, and after deciding upon the type of anastomosis, he should then examine critically the suspected segment of bowel for any telltale signs of vascular interference. When the inaugural signs of gangrene are present or when a portion of colon is thought to be "doubtful," the peccant segment of bowel should be resected forthwith and continuity restored by the open end-to-end method. Under no condition should an ulcer, whether it be gastric or duodenal, which has penetrated the substance of the pancreas be excised or cauterised. However, in some cases, a four-quadrant "biopsy" may be taken to clinch the diagnosis of simple ulcer or ulcerating carcinoma. The common bile duct, the pancreatic ducts, and the hepatic artery are likely to be subjected to injury—contusion, division, ligation, or partial excision—when a surgeon obstinately attempts to liberate the first part of the duodenum in the face of insurmountable obstacles associated with a large, deeply excavating ulcer and a mass of inflammatory tissues which extends almost to the porta hepatis.

General Abdominal Exploration and Assessment of Pathology

Exploratory laparotomy has already been discussed in Chapter 10, but it is necessary to repeat that when operation is advised in chronic gastric or duodenal ulcer, the surgeon should conduct a thorough routine examination, not only of the stomach and duodenum but also of the remaining abdominal viscera.

The local and total pathology must be carefully assessed.

The organs are best investigated in the following order: cardia and lower end of the oesophagus; oesophageal hiatus, spleen, liver, gallbladder, and bile passages; stomach and duodenum; omental bursa; pancreas; duodenojejunal flexure (the ligament of Treitz) and small intestine; the ileocaecal region, terminal ileum, appendix, caecum and adjacent mesentery; the colon; the pelvic organs and kidneys.

A search should always be made for a diaphragmatic hernia, and the oesophageal hiatus should be tested with the fingers of the right hand. Should the oesophageal hiatus readily admit three or more fingers, the diagnosis of hiatal hernia can be made with assurance.

The size, consistency, and mobility of the spleen should always be ascertained, because when the spleen is mobile the approach to the left gastroepiploic artery, the short gastric vessels, and the fundus of the stomach is a simple undertaking. On the other hand, if the spleen is anchored by adhesions in its hidden retreat, it is liable to injury when the greater omentum or the greater curvature of the stomach is pulled upon, and also when a moderate degree of traction is applied to the vasa brevia before they are secured by ligatures. Laceration of the splenic pulp during the course of partial gastrectomy demands immediate splenectomy.

Adhesions, which frequently exist between the gallbladder and the first part of the duodenum and the hepatic flexure of the colon, should be divided with scissors to ensure a good view of the common bile duct, the pyloric zone, and the duodenal bulb.

The whole of the stomach and duodenum must be methodically examined; the anterior surface of the stomach, the greater and lesser curvatures, the omenta with their lymph nodes, and the cardiac and pyloric regions are palpated and carefully visualised, after which the posterior surface of the stomach and the gastric bed are explored, either through an incision made in the lesser omentum or, preferably, through a wide opening in the gastrocolic omentum.

It is advisable to mobilise the duodenum by Kocher's method [12] in order to facilitate a thorough examination of the entire duodenum, as well as to elevate the bulb so that it can be readily tested for any scarring, distortion, pouching, narrowing, ulceration, or thickening of the bowel (Fig. 3). The presence of an active ulcer or the ravages of past ulceration either in the first or second portion of the duodenum can be detected by external inspection and palpation. At times a posterior-wall duodenal ulcer or a gastric ulcer may be identified by feeling the crater through the wall of the duodenum or stomach.

If a preoperative diagnosis of chronic duodenal ulcer cannot be upheld on abdominal exploration—and the combined clinical and radiological evidence is wrong in about 3 percent of cases—the surgeon would be well advised to perform duodenotomy with division of the pyloric sphincter in order to inspect the posterior wall of the first part of the duodenum. When no lesion can be detected, the Heineke-Mikulicz pyloroplasty

with transverse closure of the pyloroduodenotomy incision should complete the enquiry (see Chap. 17).

The first loop of jejunum should be picked up and drawn through the wound to allow of inspection of the ligament of Treitz, to ascertain whether any congenital or inflammatory bands bind it to the mesocolon, and to find out whether the superior mesenteric vessels unduly compress the third portion of the duodenum and have produced duodenal ileus.

The entire colon is next examined for any evidence of diverticulitis or malignant disease.

The liver is easily explored by slipping a hand over its exposed surface and palpating it to test its consistency.

I should like to emphasise again that small haemangiomas and subserous cysts of the liver are commonly observed at laparotomy—an estimate would be about 10 percent. Superficial cysts of the liver can be readily dispersed by compression with the index finger.

The gallbladder and bile ducts should be examined, and a search should be made for the presence of gallstones. Cholecystectomy for calculous cholecystitis does not increase the risks of partial gastrectomy for benign ulcer. In recent years, following the practice of Zollinger, I have routinely examined the pancreas to exclude the presence of ulcerogenic tumours. When the acid values are unusually elevated, a small biopsy of the tail of the gland is carried out.

TYPES OF REPAIR

The Schoemaker-Billroth I Operation

If, after conducting a methodical examination of the abdominal viscera on the lines indicated above, the surgeon decides that a gastric resection is indicated—for instance, *for a chronic gastric ulcer in the region of the incisura*—the operative steps usually follow these lines:

A large gauze pack is introduced behind the spleen to thrust it forward in order to facilitate the isolation and ligation of the vessels along the greater curvature of the stomach. The greater omentum and transverse colon are then drawn through the wound, placed on the abdominal wall, and covered with large abdominal packs. An avascular area in the gastrocolic omentum is picked up with haemostats and incised in order to gain access to the lesser sac. This opening is enlarged to the right and left by underrunning, ligating, and dividing portions of the omentum below the curving gastro-

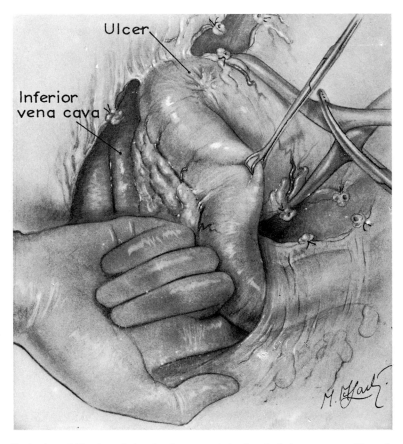

FIG. 4. Kocher's mobilisation of the duodenum and the head of the pancreas. Note that in some cases the proximal portion of the third part of the duodenum is mobilised.

epiploic arch (Figs. 4 to 6).

A Deaver retractor is now inserted into the omental bursa, and the stomach is retracted upward whilst the transverse colon, mesocolon, and body of the pancreas are drawn downward. A good view is thus obtained of the lesser sac, which facilitates the division of adhesions, of the *suspensory ligaments of the left gastroepiploic vessels,* and of the bands which tether the gastric ulcer to the pancreas or to the mesocolon itself. It also brings to view the scarred surface of a small lesser-curve ulcer, inflammatory bands which accompany perforation into the pancreas, and the angry oedema which may surround and obscure the vulnerable middle colic artery.

At this stage, following sharp dissection with scissors, the semiadherent leaf of the mesocolon can be stripped downward, thus exposing the posterior aspect of the antrum, the pylorus, and the first inch (2.4 cm) or so of the posterior wall of the duodenum and the gastroduodenal artery where it lies in its shallow groove of pancreatic tissue.

A penetrating gastric ulcer can be surrounded by the index finger and pinched off (Figs. 7 and 8).

The hole in the stomach is then closed with strong sutures and the crater mopped dry with gauze swabs. The crater with its rim of fibrotic or granulation tissue which remains in the pancreatic substance should not be excised, excavated, curetted, or cauterised, as any such interference would predispose to the formation of a pancreatic fistula.

If an unduly large gastric ulcer is encountered and it defies the "pinching off" method, the stomach wall around the ulcer

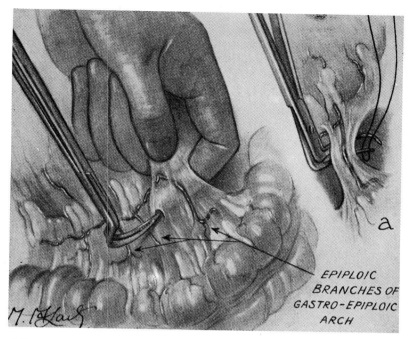

FIG. 5.   Schoemaker-Billroth I operation. Method of making an opening in the gastrocolic omentum to gain access to the lesser peritoneal sac. (From Maingot, 1950. *Techniques in British Surgery.* Courtesy of W. B. Saunders Company, Philadelphia.)

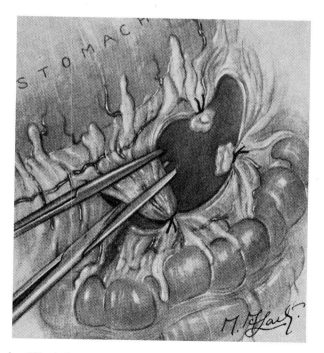

FIG. 6.   Schoemaker-Billroth I operation. An opening is made in gastrocolic ligament to gain access to the lesser peritoneal sac. (From Maingot, 1950. *Techniques in British Surgery.* Courtesy of W. B. Saunders Company, Philadelphia.)

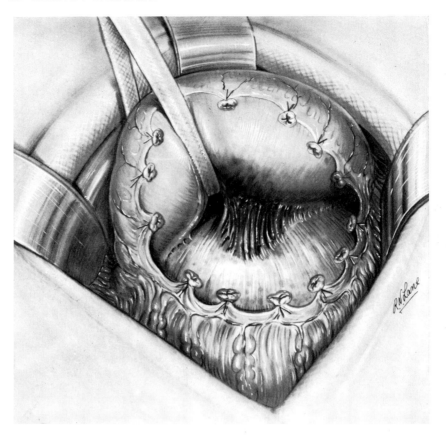

FIG. 7.   Exposure of the bed of the stomach. A gastric ulcer is present and firmly attached to the body of the pancreas.

should be cautiously cut through circumferentially with a scalpel. The gastric contents should be completely removed by aspiration, after which the stomach cavity should be lightly packed with a roll of gauze to prevent subsequent oozing and also to aid in a small measure in the mobilisation of the viscus.

The dissection now proceeds along the greater curvature towards the inferior surface of the first portion of the duodenum. After isolation of the right gastroepiploic vessels at the lower border of the pylorus, they are ligated in continuity and divided. The greater curvature (i.e., inferior border) of the first part of the duodenum is partially liberated after underrunning, ligating, and dividing the thickened ridge of omentum which is constantly found close to the inferior border of the pyloric outlet. The second and third por-

tions of the duodenum are further mobilise by Kocher's method, after which the righ gastric artery is isolated with dissectin forceps, underrun with aneurysm needle threaded with silk or catgut, doubly ligatec and divided. The shorter anterior duodena vessels should be displayed *close to the duc denal wall* before being secured by slende pointed haemostats and divided on the duc denal wall itself. (See Fig. 4.)

The flimsy gastrohepatic omentum is ir cised and a gauze sling is slipped around th stomach to aid in the mobilisation of th duodenum. It is always advisable to mobilis the lesser curvature of the duodenum thor oughly, particularly when the surgeon antici pates performing a Billroth I operation, a such mobilisation renders easier the intro duction of a purse-string suture at the *Jam merecke*.

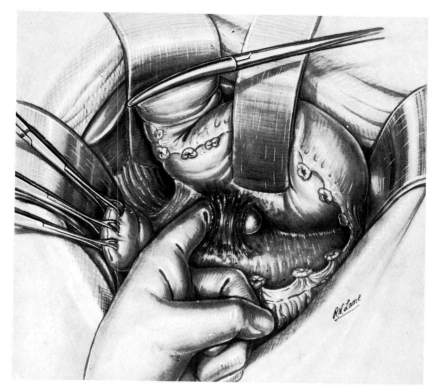

FIG. 8.   Schoemaker-Billroth I operation. Liberation of stomach and method of surrounding penetrating gastric ulcer with index finger. Ulcer will subsequently be pinched off from the pancreas thereby gaining further mobility of the stomach.

After the first part of the duodenum has been adequately mobilised, two straight clamps are applied side by side close to the pyloric outlet, and the bowel is transected with a knife. When the first part of the duodenum is short, it is advisable to conserve as much healthy tissue as possible.

A large swab soaked in warm saline solution is then placed over the duodenum while the stomach is lifted up and drawn over to the right in preparation for the isolation and ligation of the left gastroepiploic artery and the lower two or three vasa brevia. High ligation of the vasa brevia imparts a wide range of mobility to the stomach and is an essential step in the operation. The upper portion of the stomach becomes more tubular and elongated after these short gastric vessels have been tied and divided.

The identification and ligation of the left gastric artery are difficult in many cases of gastric ulcer, owing to the deposition of fat high up on the lesser curvature, the surrounding oedema, and the enlargement of the related lymph nodes; but in cases of duodenal ulcer, the securing of this large vessel is comparatively easy.

The stomach is drawn vertically through the wound and then folded over the left costal margin to display the upper third of the posterior wall of the stomach. The position of the first posterior transverse branch of the left gastric artery is noted; the groove between the edge of the lesser curvature and the main vascular bundle is felt between the index finger and the thumb of the left hand; dissecting forceps are insinuated between the lesser curvature and the main descending branch of the left gastric artery to provide sufficient room for the passage of two ligatures of strong silk or catgut, which are slipped upward and tied firmly; a large

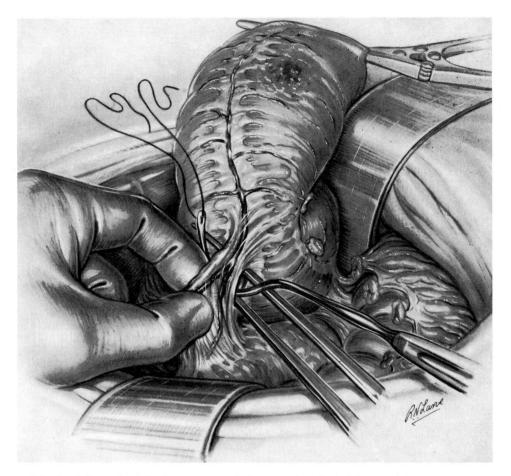

FIG. 9. Schoemaker-Billroth I operation. Isolation and method of ligating left gastric artery.

haemostat is clamped to the pedicle below the ligatures, and the left gastric vessels are divided; the haemostat is drawn downward for 1 to 2 inches (2.5 to 5 cm) towards the incisura to expose the bared lesser curvature, which is immediately reperitonealised; and, after it is certain that haemostasis is complete, the mobile stomach is ready for resection (Figs. 9 and 10).

Before ligating the left gastric artery, the surgeon should remember that an *accessory hepatic artery or the main hepatic artery* may arise from the left gastric artery or coeliac axis and is then in danger of being clamped and ligated during division of the left gastric artery (Fig. 9). This anomaly is found in about 5 percent of subjects, and when it is present, care should be taken to preserve this important nutrient vessel to the liver. During the performance of partial gastrectomy for gastric ulcer, I have on three occasions observed the common hepatic artery arising from the main trunk of the left gastric artery or from the short stem of the coeliac artery.

In gastric ulcer cases, the ideal amount of stomach to excise is approximately 60 to 70 percent; as a rule, about 75 percent of the vertical portion of the lesser curvature is resected, as this area may contain a "tongue-like" projection of antral mucosa.

The main principle of partial gastric resection for gastric ulcer is to conserve a good portion of the stomach—i.e., towards the greater curvature area, while removing the antrum and most of the lesser curvature, together with the ulcer.

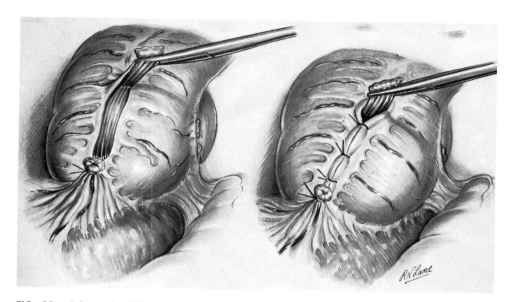

FIG. 10. Schoemaker-Billroth I operation. After securely ligating and dividing left gastric artery, raw surface high up on the lesser curvature of stomach is reperitonealised.

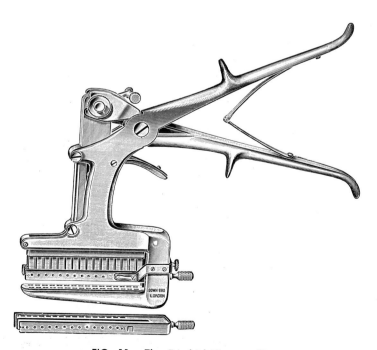

FIG. 11. The Friedrich-Petz machine.

There are various methods of performing the *Schoemaker-Billroth I operation,* but the one that I have employed most frequently and with great success is the one I shall now describe.

A pair of Babcock forceps is affixed to a point on the greater curvature to mark the distal line of transection and also to steady the stomach while a small Payr clamp is applied perpendicularly to the greater curvature, extending to the width of the body of the stomach for a distance of 2½ to 3 inches (6.3 to 7.6 cm). Large Kocher forceps are placed just distal and parallel to the first Payr clamp. The whole thickness of the stomach between these clamps is incised with a knife to a point of ½ inch (1.27 cm) beyond the tips of the proximal Payr clamp. The two clamps are now widely separated, and another Payr clamp is crushed home obliquely across the anterior and posterior walls of the stomach from the tips of the Payr clamp applied to the greater curvature portion of the stomach to a point on the lesser curva-ture which is 2 inches (5 cm) below the oesophagogastric junction, after which the portion of the stomach distal to this clamp is cut adrift and removed (Fig. 13).

The gastric resection may be performed with the aid of a *Petz sewing clamp* or, prefer-ably, the *Friedrich-Petz machine* (Figs. 11 and 12).

The technique is as follows:

When the site of transection has been selected, a Babcock clamp is clipped to the greater curvature just distal to the chosen site. A small Payr clamp is then applied perpendicularly to the greater curvature at the selected level and extending across the width of the body of the stomach for a dis-tance of about 2½ to 3 inches (6.3 to 7.6 cm). Large Kocher forceps are placed just distal to the Payr clamp and parallel with it. The stomach between these two clamps is incised with a knife, and after separating the clamps a Petz machine is applied obliquely across the anterior and posterior walls of the stomach from the tip of the small Payr clamp

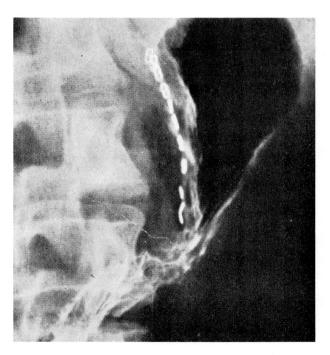

FIG. 12. Gastrografin view of stomach and duodenum taken some 5 years after Schoemaker-Billroth I resection for gastric ulcer. Note that Petz clips are still in position on reconstructed lesser curvature.

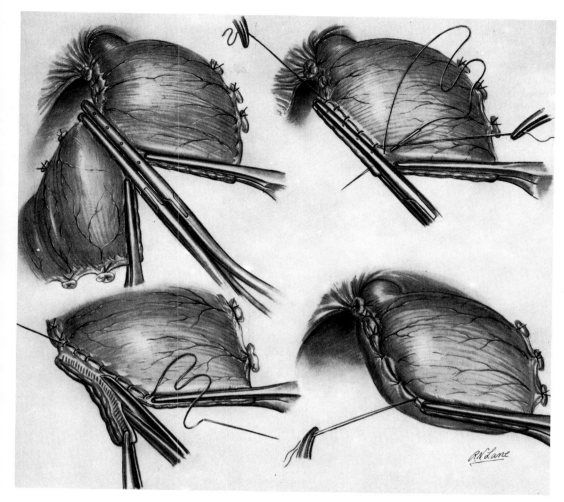

FIG. 13. Schoemaker-Billroth I operation. Method of preparing gastric pouch and extent of resection prior to anastomosing gastric remnant to duodenum. Note also that author's gastric clamp has been applied to lesser curvature and that a sewing-machine stitch has been inserted below this clamp. The final steps in closing the "new" lesser curvature are shown.

to a point on the lesser curvature that is approximately 2 inches (5 cm) below the cardiac orifice. The Petz machine is crushed home and a double row of fine metallic staples is passed along the line of application of the clamp. The Petz machine is removed. The stomach is then transected by cutting through the middle of the crushed groove between the double row of Petz clips.

By this plan, most of the lesser curvature of the stomach is removed with the specimen. The new "lesser curvature" with its contained Petz clips is oversewn with a running Cushing stitch and then inturned by intro-

ducing a series of interrupted Lembert sutures of 00 Mersilk or Dexon on 30- to 37-mm half-curved atraumatic (eyeless) intestinal needles. The end of the stomach embraced by the Payr clamp is drawn across and applied to the clamp on the duodenal stump to test the feasibility of performing an axial union. If there is no tension and a gastroduodenal anastomosis can be performed, this should be carried out (Fig. 12).

In most cases I do not use a Petz instrument for removing the lesser curvature, but employ the Payr clamp method. The Payr clamp, which is affixed to and extends across the stomach to a point below the cardiac orifice, is oversewn with a continuous catgut suture or closed with a sewing-machine stitch beneath the clamp, after which the Payr clamp is removed and the suturing is continued (Fig. 13).

After inserting the continuous suture of 0 chromic catgut and closing the new lesser curvature, the curvature is securely inturned with a series of closely applied interrupted sutures of fine silk or with a series of mattress sutures of the same material. These sutures extend almost to the tips of the Payr clamp, which has been affixed to the end of the gastric remnant.

At this stage of the operation, the Payr

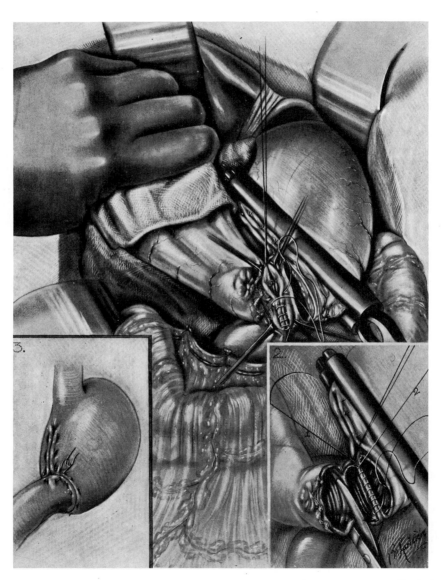

FIG. 14. A simplified method of conducting the gastroduodenal anastomosis. A Billroth I type of repair for duodenal ulcer. (1) First continuous posterior seromuscular suture is being introduced. (2) Duodenum is being cut adrift just as second posterior all-coats through-and-through suture is about to be completed. (3) Arrangement of parts at completion of operation.

clamp at the end of the gastric remnant is rotated to expose the posterior surface of the stomach, and a transverse incision is made parallel with and ⅓ inch (8.4 mm) proximal to the Payr clamp through the seromuscular coats down to the exposed submucosa. Each blood vessel that is seen lying on the submucosa is individually transfixed and ligated with 000 plain catgut to ensure absolute haemostasis. The Payr clamp is once again rotated to display the anterior wall of the gastric pouch, and another transverse incision is made through the seromuscular layer of the stomach as close to the clamp as is possible.

All the exposed blood vessels lying on this area of the mucosa are likewise transfixed and ligated seriatim. When this step in the operation has been completed, the ends of the stomach and duodenum are once again approximated to test the mobility of the parts about to be engaged in the anastomosis. If everything is satisfactory for an end-to-end union, the first posterior layer of interrupted suture of 000 silk is inserted and the two stay sutures at each end are clipped with haemostats and retained as tractors.

The small rim of stomach embraced by the Payr clamp and mucosa distal to the haemostatic sutures is cut away with a knife, after which the gastric pouch is aspirated with a Shepherd suction instrument. After the clamp on the duodenal stump has been removed and the rim of crushed tissues trimmed away, the second posterior layer of an all-coats, through-and-through continuous suture of 0 or 00 chromic catgut is inserted. The anterior sutures are now inserted as a continuous Connell suture to ensure a neat and watertight turn-in, not only at the superior and inferior corners of the anastomosis but also in its central portion.

The second anterior suture line consists of a series of interrupted Lembert seromuscular sutures of fine silk which invert the first row of sutures. A special type of purse-string suture is now introduced at the "angle of sorrow" in the manner shown in Fig. 14 (*3*).

After it is certain that there is no tension at the site of anastomosis, and after the patency of the gastroduodenal stoma has been tested with the thumb and index finger, a portion of the greater omentum is drawn over the anastomosis to act as a cloak and a guard against the possibility of the subsequent development of adhesions between the gastric pouch and the line of anastomosis itself, on the one hand, and the incision in the abdominal wall, on the other.

Following the Schoemaker-Billroth I operation, drainage of the operative field is as a rule undesirable. The abdominal incision is finally closed in the manner previously described (see Chap. 1).

Pauchet's Operation

On occasion the ulcer is situated too high on the lesser curvature or too high on the posterior wall of the stomach to permit the use of two Payr clamps or the Schoemaker clamp to remove the lesser curvature of the stomach. In such instances, a modification of the Schoemaker operation, as first devised by Pauchet, is advisable. (See also Chap. 21.) The dissection proceeds as described above, up to the point where the two small Payr clamps are applied across the stomach, and the greater curvature half of the stomach is divided between them with a knife. The stomach is surrounded by packs and then held upward with the Payr clamps. The lesser curvature is rotated medially and is excised with scissors, the cutting being adjusted to remove more or less of the anterior or posterior wall according to the position of the lesion.

The excision can be made high enough to excise an ulcer an inch or two (2.5 to 5 cm) from the oesophageal margin. On occasion, where the ulcer is very large and is penetrating the pancreatic substance, the stomach wall should be cut adrift from the ulcer crater after the left gastric artery has been secured near its origin.

The surgeon should next insert a finger into the stomach and pass it into the oesophagus to verify the position of the cardiac orifice.

There is little bleeding and soiling by this method if the stomach contents are continuously aspirated and the snipping with scissors is done little by little, each short segment of the anterior and posterior wall of the stomach being sutured with a through-and-through running stitch of 0 chromic catgut before division (Fig. 15). *If by chance the*

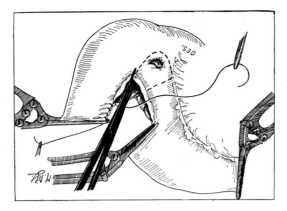

FIG. 15. Pauchet's operation for high gastric ulcer. With distal half of stomach firmly lifted up with Payr clamp, a tonguelike piece of lesser curve containing ulcer is removed. Short segment is then cut and immediately sutured with continuous stitch. (From Maingot, 1950. *Techniques in British Surgery.* Courtesy of W. B. Saunders Company, Philadelphia, and Mr. Norman Tanner.)

cardiac orifice is involved, the suturing should be performed with a large stomach tube placed in the stomach by the anaesthetist.

When the lesser curvature incision has been closed, it is next inverted by a series of Lembert or mattress fine silk sutures and the operation is completed as a Billroth I or Billroth II repair. In those rare instances in which the right margin of the oesophagus needs "repairing" it is advisable to bring up the afferent jejunal loop and suture it over the lower end of the oesophagus and the newly fashioned "lesser curvature" (Billroth II operation). This tubular form of gastric remnant has excellent function and proves satisfactory even with excisions as high as the cardia. Transient dysphagia may be experienced by some patients, but this does not last any length of time. When, however, there has been some evidence of stenosis, recourse should be made to intermittent dilatation of the cardiac orifice with graduated oesophageal bougies.

A Modification of the Billroth I Operation by Employing the Two Large Payr Clamp Method as Practised by Finsterer

Most operations performed today on the stomach and duodenum are in fact modifications of those practised by our intellectual surgical forebears. The same applies to the Billroth I operation in which the open mouth of the duodenum is anastomosed to the greater curvature portion of the gastric stump and the lesser curve portion is closed and inverted.

In this operation, the numerous small vessels on the upper (gastric) side of the epiploic arch, as well as a few of the lower vasa brevia, are individually seized, ligated, and divided in order to liberate the greater curvature, after which the right and left gastric arteries are isolated, doubly ligated, and then cut so that the lesser curvature can be mobilised. Two large Payr clamps are next applied horizontally across the body of the stomach, on a line indicated in the inset of Figure 16.

Another large Payr clamp is placed parallel to this but on the distal or pyloric side, and the stomach is transected between them. The distal portion of the stomach with its attached clamp is covered with a waterproof square and drawn across to the right, thus exposing the pancreas and the posterior surface of the pylorus as well as the commencement of the first part of the duodenum.

The distal portion of the stomach is then laid aside on the abdominal wall while the upper half of the margins of the gastric pouch embraced by the large Payr clamp is undersewn with a continuous suture of 0 chromic catgut or, preferably, with a sewing-machine stitch, after which the clamp is removed and a small Payr clamp is affixed to the greater curvature portion of the stomach.

The suture line along the new lesser curvature is now inverted with interrupted mattress sutures of fine silk, while the snout of stomach which results at the greater curvature and which is steadied with the Payr clamp is amputated in order to facilitate the anastomosis of this region of the stomach with the first part of the duodenum. (See Fig. 16 inset.)

In cases of gastric ulcer, the dissection and the liberation of the first portion of the duodenum present little if any difficulty, but in duodenal ulcer cases the anterior duodenal arteries which run into the upper border of the bulb should be secured, divided, and ligated. Where there is much scarring and shortening of the duodenum, as may occur

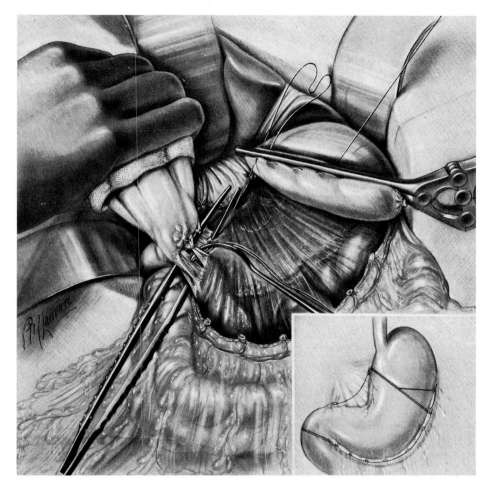

FIG. 16. The Billroth I type of operation in which two large Payr clamps are employed for the gastric transection. The stomach has been clamped with two Payr enterotomes and then transected. The first portion of the duodenum is being mobilised by the division of numerous bands which anchor this part of the duodenum to the pancreas. *Inset* shows the amount of stomach and duodenum excised. The vascular epiploic arch, in this instance, is preserved. (After Finsterer.)

in some examples of duodenal ulcer, there is some danger in clamping near the common hepatic artery or the choledochus.

For safety, fine artery forceps are used, and one pair at a time is placed on the tissues *flush against the duodenal wall*. With a sharp scalpel the vascular tissue is divided between the duodenum and the artery forceps. Often it will be found that there is no great bleeding from the duodenum, the tissue being mainly fibrous, but occasionally a vessel may have to be caught on the duodenal wall. Keeping thus snugly against the duodenum is, I believe, the main secret in the safe dissection of duodenal ulcer, for even if the bile duct or common hepatic artery is aherent to the duodenum, such close dissection will still be safe. The dissection is continued until a short length of normal duodenum beyond the ulcer is mobilised.[16]

When the duodenum has been rendered sufficiently mobile, it is approximated to the lower cut end of the stomach and the anastomosis is performed with two posterior and two anterior rows of continuous sutures of 0 or 00 chromic catgut.

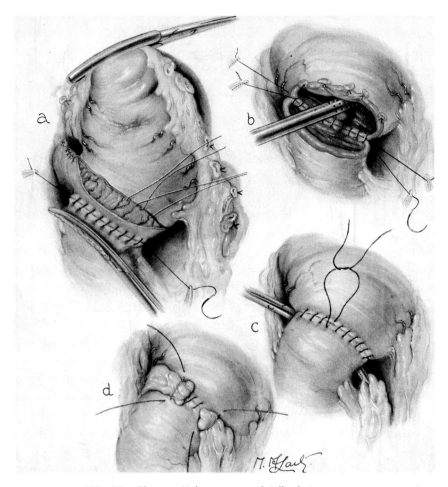

FIG. 17. The von Haberer type of Billroth I operation.

A final row of interrupted Lembert sutures of fine Mersilk is introduced to support and invert the suture lines.

If there is any tension on the line of anastomosis, it may be reduced by further mobilisation of the greater curvature of the stomach and of the duodenum itself.

At the completion of this operation, a purse-string suture is passed just above the anastomosis through the anterior and posterior walls of the stomach and the duodenum at the spot where the suture lines converge. Before closing the abdominal incision, the greater omentum is drawn through the wound and is then folded over the duodenum, and a portion is packed so as to cover the raw surface left behind by the

Kocher mobilisation of the duodenum. Von Haberer's modification of the Billroth I operation is illustrated in Figure 17.

Tanner's technique of the Billroth I operation will be appreciated by referring to Figure 18.

Von Haberer-Finney Operation

This procedure extends the scope of the Billroth I operation. The operation is particularly applicable after the gastric remnant has been "tubed" on the lines described under the Schoemaker-Billroth I operation and the duodenum and the head of the pancreas have been fully mobilised. When, how-

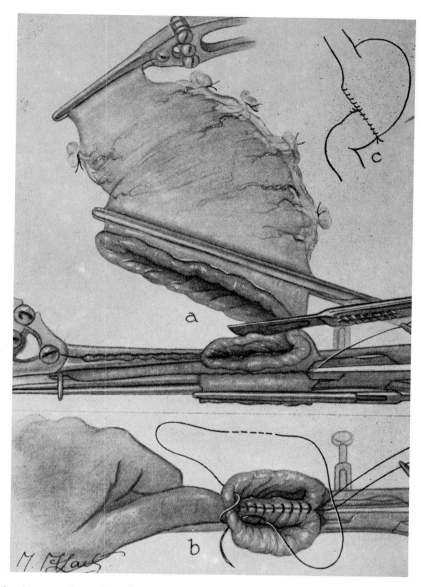

FIG. 18. Norman Tanner's technique of performing the Billroth I operation with the aid of Lane's intestinal clamps. (From Maingot, 1950. *Techniques in British Surgery.* Courtesy of W. B. Saunders Company, Philadelphia.)

ever, the whole of the open end of the stomach is used for this type of terminolateral union, its calibre should be reduced circumferentially by *von Haberer's method of "reefing"* and narrowing of the cut end of the stomach (Fig. 17).

In the von Haberer-Finney operation, the end of the duodenum is closed as, in the circumstances, it is considered unsuitable for anastomosis to the mouth of the gastric pouch.

An end-to-side anastomosis is carried out between the mouth of the gastric remnant and the second portion of the duodenum, employing two rows of interrupted sutures for the posterior union and two rows for the anterior suture line. When this terminolateral junction is affected, the stoma should

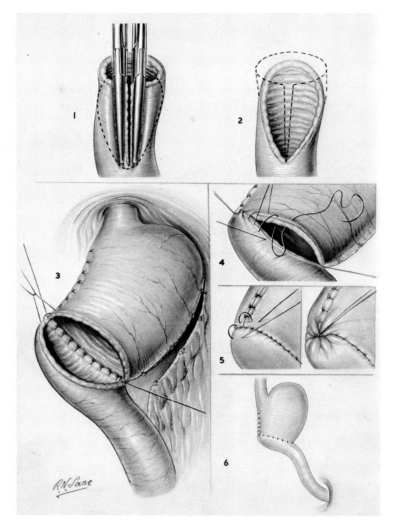

FIG. 19.   The author's modification of the von Haberer-Finney operation.

be capacious enough to admit two fingers (see Fig. 3).

If, following gastroduodenal resection, the calibre of the remaining portion of the bulb and the second portion of the duodenum itself are narrow, this operation is rendered possible and is, in fact, simplified by adopting the writer's plan.

This entails making a longitudinal incision 2½ inches (6.3 cm) long in the antero-superior wall of the duodenum, extending from the open end of the first part of the duodenum to a point below the papilla of Vater; excising a triangular area from both the lateral and the medial margins of the duodenal wall; and performing an end-to-end anastomosis without the encumbrances and disadvantages associated with a blind end.

Figure 19 (1–6), which was drawn from sketches made during an operation for duodenal ulcer performed by the writer, gives the artist's impression of the technique employed at the time.

In a personal series of 38 operations performed by this modified von Haberer-Finney procedure during the last 7 years, the results have all been satisfactory (Fig. 20).

Support of the views expressed by the

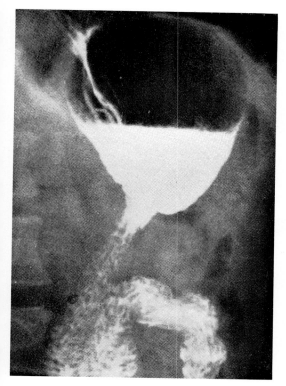

FIG. 20. The author's modification of the von Haberer-Finney operation for chronic duodenal ulcer. Appearance (on barium-meal x-ray) about 7 years after the operation.

writer will be found in the following contributions. Feggeter and Pringle;[2] Tanner;[16] Savage et al.;[14] Tanner;[17] Dragstedt;[1] Goligher et al.;[3-5] and Herrington[7] (see also Chap. 16).

Horsley's Operation

Horsley[9, 10, 11] recommended his modification of the original Billroth I resection in which the end of the duodenum is anastomosed to the lesser curvature side of the stomach in order to preserve all peristaltic activity. He believed that it would be easier and safer to close the "critical angle" with such an anastomosis, as when the greater curvature part of the stomach was employed in an axial union with the duodenum this critical angle was, in the past, an occasional source of peritonitis from leakage.

Horsley also advocated an incision in the anterior duodenal wall in order to produce a larger duodenal stoma, thereby minimising the chances of obstruction.

The essential steps of Horsley's operation will readily be appreciated by referring to Figures 21 to 24.

At the completion of the Horsley-Billroth I procedure, a Levin tube is guided through the gastroduodenal stoma into the second portion of the duodenum, and a serosa-lined Stamm gastrostomy is performed to ensure complete decompression of the small gastric segment during the first few postoperative days.

Gastrostomy following operations for peptic ulcer may be indicated: (1) where the patient cannot or will not tolerate the presence of an indwelling nasogastric tube; (2) in aged and decrepit subjects; (3) where following the anastomosis the stoma is judged to be too tight or strained; and (4) after vagotomy and a drainage procedure such as gastrojejunostomy have been conducted for advanced pyloric stenosis caused by a long-standing cicatrising duodenal ulcer and associated with gross distension and atony of the stomach.

In response to the controversy of whether or not *postoperative gastric suction* should be used, the words of Sprong[15] come to mind: "Some patients are going to need decompression and should have it. Many others will do fine without it and should not be subjected to it. Thus avoid routinely using it and avoid routinely not using it." Some surgeons believe that gastrostomy, as a method of decompression of the stomach (and for feeding purposes) following gastric operations is being carried out much too frequently in clinics throughout the world. In most instances, it is an unnecessary refinement, and it is often followed by fixation of the stomach to the anterior abdominal wall, which subsequently might give rise to constant or intermittent epigastric pain and to other symptoms. On occasion, after removal of the gastrostomy tube, severe infection of the stab wound and leakage of gastric contents leading to chemical peritonitis have been reported. A few fatalities, too, have been recorded. I also maintain, with Herrington and his colleagues[7, 8] that the time has come when the *routine* use of gastric decompression by means of a nasogastric tube following opera-

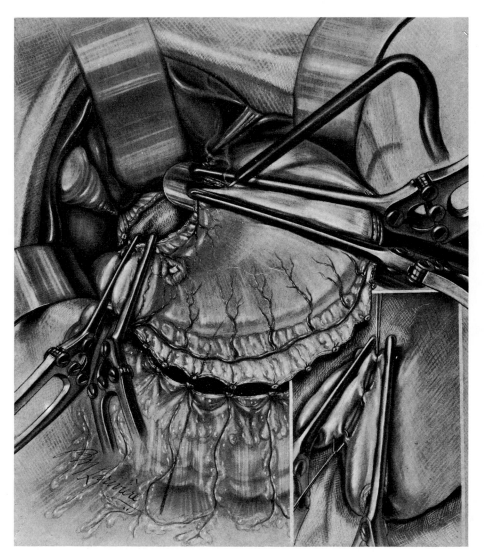

FIG. 21. Horsley's technique of Billroth I type of repair for gastric ulcer.

tion for gastroduodenal ulcer should be strictly limited or even eliminated.

At present, my line of management may be outlined as follows:

1. One to two days before operation: give liquid diet only.
2. Six hours before operation: insert nasogastric tube. Make sure that stomach is empty before, during, and for a short period after operation.
3. In recovery room: continue blood transfusion and/or parenteral infusions. Aspirate gastric contents hourly. Remove nasogastric tube 10 hours postoperatively.
4. For 72 hours: give nothing by mouth, and continue intravenous therapy.

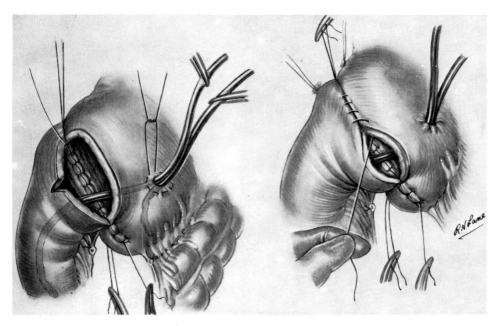

FIG. 22. Horsley's technique of the Billroth I operation. Note catheter-duodenostomy and catheter-gastrostomy.

5. Third day: give water only.
6. Fourth day: give clear fluids.
7. Fifth day: give frequent soft feeds.
8. Ninth day: discharge from hospital!

In the rare event of abdominal distention, ileus, or repeated vomiting, the reinsertion of a nasogastric Levin tube will, of course, be necessary. *So "avoid routinely not using it," as advised by wise Dr. Sprong.*

Finochietto's Method

Enrique Finochietto was an outstanding Argentinian who practised surgery with great skill and distinction for many years in Buenos Aires. He invented many ingenious surgical instruments, operating tables, and orthopaedic apparatus. He wrote several books on operative surgery; his technique was precise, safe, and superb; and he was well known and admired for his skill and character by all eminent surgeons of his day. He made a practice of spending several months each year during his busy profes-

sional life attending surgical clinics in various parts of the world, and most especially in North America and Great Britain. It was during one of these visits to me at the Southend General Hospital that, with the master by my side to guide and encourage me, I learned the steps of his technique of the Billroth I operation (Figs. 25–27). The following is an extract of what he wrote for me:

In the Péan-Billroth I operation I attach the greatest importance to a most liberal mobilisation of the duodenum. Instead of dissecting the peritoneum on the outer border of the duodenum I commence by severing the filamentous bands and adhesions over the very middle of the gut by means of a blunt instrument and by enlarging the opening thus made, both upward and downward. Along the outer border of the duodenum the mobilisation proceeds until the colon is displaced downward. I divide the right colophrenic ligament which slings the hepatic flexure of the colon upward to obtain the best possible view of the duodenum. The duodenum is mobilised by what I have termed the "extended" Kocher procedure. The duodenum and the head of the pancreas when freed can be turned over and carried towards the middle line. Behind it can

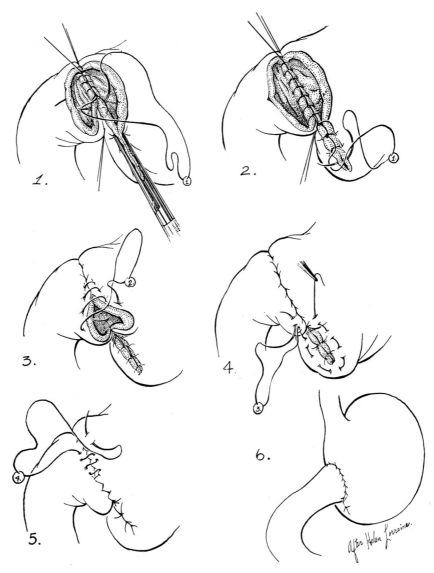

FIG. 23.   Horsley's technique of Billroth I type of repair. Method of anastomosing the upper cut end of the stomach to the cut end of the duodenum.

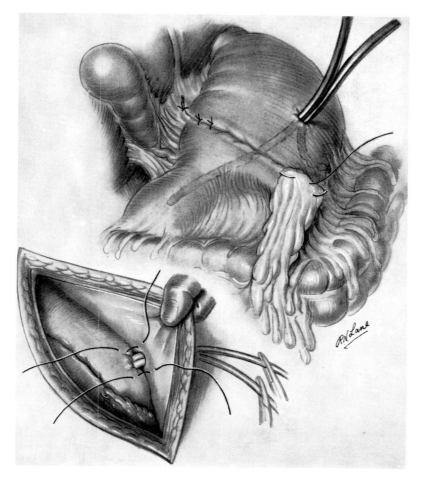

FIG. 24.   Horsley's technique of the Billroth I operation.

be seen the inferior vena cava in all its width and about 7 to 8 cm of its length. The adhesions and bands are firmer and more vascular at the upper part, where most of them require two ligatures. The freed duodenum permits of a more thorough eaxmination of any duodenal ulcers which may be present, of the head of the pancreas, and of the structures contained in the right border of the gastrohepatic omentum. It is very dangerous to remove any portion of the pancreas whilst resecting a peptic ulcer; if, therefore, an ulcer has penetrated the pancreas, it is best to sacrifice a portion of gut and to leave the ulcer attached to the pancreas, rather than to attempt local excision of a portion of the gland.

In actual practice, if I cannot free the duodenum well away from the gland, I often desist from this type of operation.

Before proceeding further with the operation

and after ensuring a complete haemostasis, I place a gauze swab to cover the raw surface which has resulted from the mobilisation of the duodenum, and this swab I leave in position, not removing it until the operation is nearly complete.

Next comes the division of the right part of both omenta. Ligatures are placed on each vessel before it is cut. The vessels are tied in continuity. The vessels attached to that portion of the stomach or duodenum about to be resected are ligatured and tied with two knots, and a little further away two ligatures are placed on the same vessel, each tied with three knots. I invariably try to preserve the vascular epiploic arch, thereby ensuring a good blood supply to the great omentum.

Figure 28 shows the stage in the operation

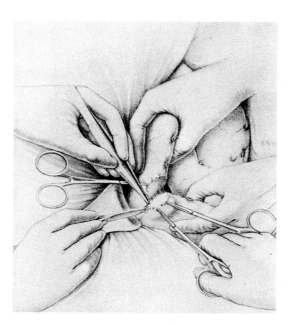

FIG. 25. Finochietto's technique of the Billroth I operation. Mobilisation of the first portion of the duodenum.

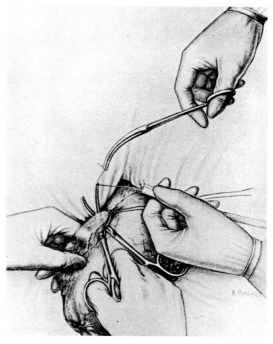

FIG. 27. Finochietto's technique of the Billroth I operation. Ligation of the left gastric artery.

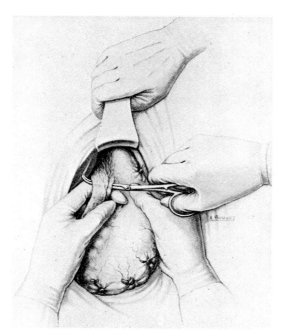

FIG. 26. Finochietto's technique of Billroth I operation. Ligation of the left gastric artery.

when, following high ligation of the right and left gastric arteries, and some of the vasa brevia, the stomach and duodenum have been completely mobilised, and Finochietto's special duodenal clamp is being applied to the duodenum distal to the ulcer. In the inset, the duodenum is shown in the process of being cut across.

The further steps of Finochietto's method of end-to-end gastroduodenostomy are so clearly depicted, step by step, by such superb artists as Mr. A. Bouvet and Miss P. Larivière that a detailed description here would be superfluous (Figs. 29, 30); but the reader should observe how particular Finochietto is to free the seromuscular layers from the underlying mucosa on the gastric side prior to inserting the long continuous master suture, and how this suture is applied.

Finochietto performed this operation in more than 400 cases with only five fatalities, and he assured me that the late results were excellent in 80 percent of his cases. The danger of axial rotation, flattening of the second portion of the duodenum against the

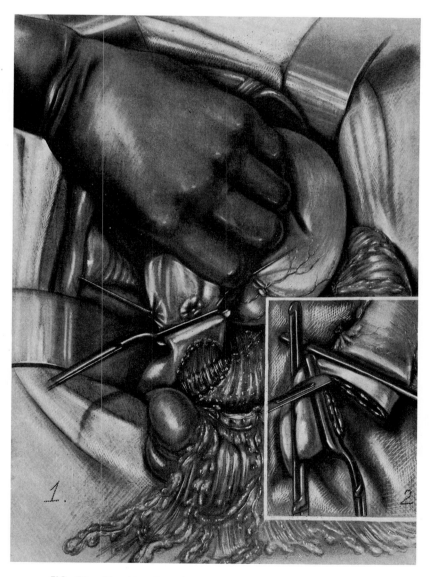

FIG. 28. Finochietto's technique of the Billroth I operation.

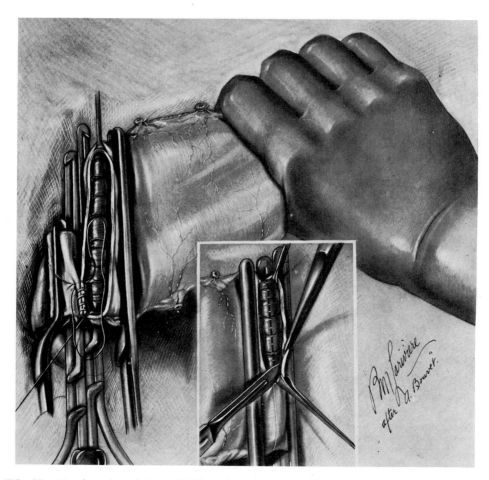

FIG. 29.   Finochietto's technique of Billroth I operation. First through-and-through posterior continuous suture is being introduced. Note gastric mucous membrane is not included in suture. Inset
shows seromuscular coat of stomach being divided anteriorly down to mucous membrane. Dotted
line indicates line along which mucosa will subsequently be divided.

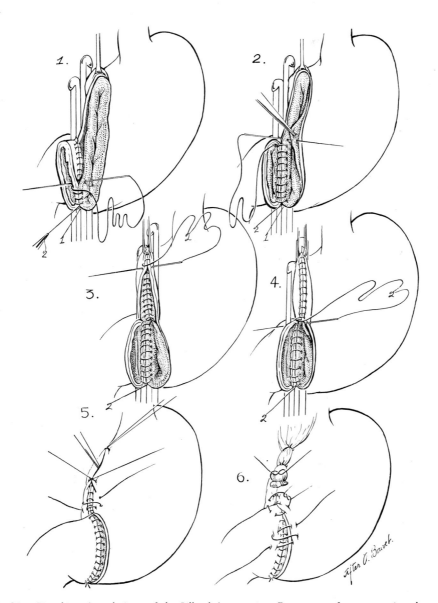

FIG. 30.   Finochietto's technique of the Billroth I operation. Every step of anastomosing the gastric pouch to the mouth of the duodenum is well depicted. (1) The second continuous through-and-through suture is being introduced. (2) When the second continuous suture has reached the upper end of the duodenum, it picks up both margins of gastric mucous membrane. (3) Continuous suture on returning approximates seromuscular edges of the stomach. (4) Continuous suture has been completed down to the upper margin of duodenum. (5) Lesser curvature is being reconstituted and invaginated by series of interrupted cross-sutures. (6) Anterior edge of seromuscular coat of stomach is being sutured to anterior wall of duodenum by series of interrupted cross-sutures. Purse-string suture is inserted to close so-called dangerous angle.

spinal column, or kinking of the commencement of the third portion of the duodenum can be circumvented by a thorough mobilisation of the duodenum.

REFERENCES

1. Dragstedt, Arch. Surg. 91:1005, 1965.
2. Feggeter and Pringle, Surg. Gynecol. Obstet. 116:175, 1963.
3. Goligher et al., Br. Med. J. 1:455, 1966.
4. Goligher et al., Br. Med. J. 2:787, 1968.
5. Goligher et al., Br. Med. J. 1:7, 1972.
6. Grassi, Br. J. Surg. 58:187, 1971.
7. Herrington et al., Ann. Surg. 159:807, 1964.
8. Herrington et al., Surg. Gynecol. Obstet. 121:351, 1965.
9. Horsley, J.A.M.A. 86:664, 1926.
10. Horsley, Surgery of the Stomach and Small Intestine, 1926.
11. Horsley, Surg. Gynecol. Obstet. 44:215, 1927.
12. Kocher, Zbl. Chir. 30:33, 1903.
13. Orr, Ann. R. Coll. Surg. Engl. 34:314, 1964.
14. Savage et al., Am. J. Surg. 107:283, 1964.
15. Sprong, Am. J. Surg. 94:257, 1957.
16. Tanner, Br. J. Surg. 51:5, 1964.
17. Tanner, Ann. R. Coll. Surg. Engl. 37:150, 1965.

21

THE BILLROTH II OPERATIONS

RODNEY MAINGOT

HISTORICAL NOTE

Billroth, on Jan. 15, 1885, performed the first gastric resection with closure of the cut end of the stomach and anterior gastrojejunostomy. He reported the clinical and operative details of the case before a meeting of the Royal Medical Society at Vienna on Feb. 20, 1885. As his patient was emaciated and a poor surgical risk owing to the presence of a pyloric cancer, Billroth originally planned to perform a two-stage operation. He envisaged that the first stage would be an anterior gastrojejunostomy and that after a short interval the second stage could be an antrectomy with closure of the open ends of the stomach and duodenum. As the patient withstood the short-circuiting procedure satisfactorily, he proceeded with the gastric resection and with the closure of the ends of the stomach and duodenum.

Von Hacker (1885), who reported Billroth's case, suggested that it would simplify the operation if the end of the stomach were anastomosed to the side of the proximal jejunum—i.e., by a terminolateral anterior gastrojejunostomy.

This advice was accepted by Krönlein, who, on May 24, 1888, carried out this one-stage partial gastrectomy with an antecolic anastomosis. Antecolic anastomoses predominated in the early Billroth II variations, but were later replaced by the retrocolic type of anastomosis.

During the last 20 years or so, however, there has been a definite return to the antecolic procedures.

According to Narath (*Deutsch Z Chir 136*:62, 1916) von Eiselsberg (1889) was the first to close the upper end of the gastric pouch to reduce the size of the orifice and then to perform an anterior anastomosis between the greater curvature portion of the stomach with a loop of proximal jejunum. Braun and Jaboulay (1892) performed the same procedure as von Eiselsberg, but the operation was completed by the performance of an entero-anastomosis between the afferent and efferent limbs of the jejunum.

The retrocolic anastomoses were first sponsored by Hofmeister (*Beitr Klin Chir 15*:351, 1896). After gastric resection he sutured the upper end of the gastric opening and then anastomosed the first loop of proximal jejunum to the greater curvature portion of the stomach. The opening in the mesocolon was sutured around the anastomotic line to add further support to the junction.

The same procedure was carried out by Finsterer in 1914 (*Deutsch Z Chir 128*:514, 1914).

Reichel (1908) and Polya (1911) performed partial gastrectomy with retrocolic gastro-enterostomy in which the entire open end of the stomach was anastomosed to the side of the proximal loop of jejunum. Here the afferent limb was affixed to the lesser curvature (Fig. 1).

Polya (*Zbl Chir 38*:89, 1911) was one of the first to write about the technical details of partial gastrectomy with retrocolic end-to-side gastrojejunostomy. Reichel (1908) was performing the identical operation in 1907, and published his method three years before the description of Polya's memorable article appeared in the literature.

It would seem to me that we name certain operations after certain well-known surgeons merely because it is customary and more convenient, but it is often the best-known sponsor rather than the originator of a particular operation who receives all the praise and credit.

Hofmeister (1908), and six years later Finsterer (*Deutsch Z Chir 128*:514, 1914), slightly modified the original Hofmeister procedure. They performed a retrocolic anastomosis, uniting the proximal jejunum to the lower half of the open end of the stomach after closing the top half of the stomach. *The short afferent limb of jejunum was buttressed to the closed upper half of the stomach, thus producing a valve effect.* This operation is often referred to in the literature as the Hofmeister-Polya operation.

Balfour (*Surg Gynec Obstet 25*:473, 1917) reported his modification of the Krönlein operation, in which a long proximal jejunal loop was brought over the colon (antecolic from right to left and anastomosed to the whole of the cut end of the stomach. This operation was completed by the performance of a side-to-side entero-anastomosis to overcome the possibility of any vicious-circle vomiting. This procedure was widely used for some years following *subtotal gastrectomy for cancer* of the distal half of the stomach.

Moynihan (1923) reversed the position of the jejunal loop: in other words, he brought the loop from the left to the right with the afferent limb to the greater curvature. In Moynihan's original account the anastomosis was antecolic, the proximal jejunal loop was short, certainly not more than 5 in. (12.7 cm.) from the ligament of Treitz to the greater curvature, and the whole width of the divided end of the stomach was anastomosed to the jejunum.

A few years after the publication of Moynihan's operation it became customary to reduce the size of the gastric stoma by closing the upper third or upper half of the mouth of the gastric remnant towards the lesser curvature, the lower portion of the open end of the stomach towards the greater curvature being used for the gastrojejunal anastomosis (Fig. 1).

While paying tribute to the great pioneer gastric surgeons who have been listed above, we should also bear in mind many of those who followed them, who by their courage, skill, and judgment, have modified and in certain instances improved the technical details of the operations for the destructive lesions of the stomach and duodenum. To mention but a few names: Sherren, Moynihan, W. J. Mayo, C. H. Mayo, Lewisohn,, Berg, Strauss, Lake, Schmieden Friedemann, Dragstedt, Wangensteen, Harkins, Judd Lahey, Visick, Marangos, Tanner, Goligher, and Herrington, Jr.

INDICATIONS

Gastric ulcer. Although it is my practise to select the Billroth I operation in preference to the Billroth II methods of repair in cases of *gastric ulcer,* in analysing my series I find that in some 20 percent of cases of gastric ulcer the Billroth II operation is carried out.

I have said that the Billroth I operation should never be "forced." I also believe that in cases of *combined ulcers* and in those instances in which the duodenum appears to be unduly narrowed or scarred, it is unwise to perform the Billroth I operation, as the Billroth II methods will yield better results in such circumstances.

Duodenal ulcer. The term *partial gastrectomy* implies the excision of 65 to 75 percent of the distal portion of the stomach including a sizeable portion of the first part of the duodenum. In *subtotal gastrectomy,* 80 percent or more of the distal stomach is resected. This latter procedure followed by a Billroth II method of anastomosis is the best operation for malignant lesions of the pylorus, the antrum, and the body of the stomach (see Chap. 28). In all cases of chronic duodenal ulcer where it is possible to mobilise the first portion of the duodenum *with safety and security,* I would most cogently advise the surgeon to perform the antecolic Schoemaker-Billroth II operation, employing a short loop of jejunum for the anastomosis. After many years, this operation has come, once again, into its own. The mortality rate is 0.8 to 2.5 percent and the recurrent ulcer rate varies from 0.9 to 4.5 percent. In my experience, the proved recurrent ulcer rate has been 2 percent and the mortality 1 percent.

Gastric cancer. Most of the subtotal gastrectomies performed for cancer of the stomach are completed after the Billroth II types of repair. This subject is discussed in Chapter 28.

Where, at operation, tumours of the stomach of doubtful pathology are found, or again in cases of sarcomatous lesions, subtotal gastrectomy followed by a Billroth II procedure is advocated. The Schoemaker-Billroth II operation, with or without selective vagotomy, is the procedure of choice for recurrent ulcer (stomal ulcer) and is discussed in Chapter 24.

CHOICE OF OPERATIONS

Some varieties of Billroth II operations are as follows:

1. Partial gastrectomy with *retrocolic anastomosis:* Polya; Hofmeister-Finsterer; and Schoemaker-Billroth II.

2. Partial gastrectomy with *antecolic anastomosis:* Moynihan; Krönlein; Balfour; and Schoemaker-Billroth II.
3. Operations for "difficult" duodenal ulcers: Bancroft-Plenk; Nissen's procedure; Lahey's method; partial gastrectomy with external duodenal catheter drainage—duodenostomy, and Kelling-Madlener operation.

Lester Dragstedt and Woodward [6] write: "When operating for *chronic gastric ulcer* the surgeon must make sure that the lesion is not a carcinoma. After this is done his choice of a definitive operation to cure the disease perhaps lies between (a) partial gastrectomy, (b) vagotomy and dependent gastroenterostomy or, (c) resection of the antrum (*the Kelling-Madlener operation*) if the ulcer is high on the lesser curvature and biopsies have proved it to be benign."

The subject of highly selective, parietal cell vagotomy, or proximal selective vagotomy is discussed in a number of chapters in this Section. The reader is also referred to the article by J. Lynwood Herrington, Jr. on "Current operations for duodenal ulcer" in *Current Problems in Surgery,* Year Book Medical Publishers, Inc., July, 1972, Wirthlin and Malt (*Surg. Gynec. Obstet. 135:913, 1972*), and to Annotation in *Brit. Med. J. 1:256, 1973.*

TECHNIQUES

Partial Gastrectomy with Retrocolic Anastomoses

POLYA OPERATION

In the original Billroth II operation, 1885, the distal portion of the stomach was resected, the duodenal stump was closed, and the cut end of the stomach was sutured and inturned; an antecolic gastrojejunostomy was then carried out with the afferent limb at the greater curvature.

In the Polya operation, the whole of the open end of the stomach pouch is anastomosed to the first loop of the jejunum behind the colon (posterior end-to-side gastrojejunostomy), the afferent limb of jejunum being short and attached to the lesser curvature (Fig. 1).

The posterior Polya operation is especially indicated when the patient is young, as in infancy and childhood, and in cases in which the body of the stomach is narrow or somewhat contracted, as has been observed in subjects who are very thin and emaciated. The size of the stoma may appear to be large, but it is governed by the calibre of the jejunum engaged in the anastomosis. Strangely enough there is little or no regurgitation of gastric contents into the duodenum. Figure 2 confirms this statement.

It should be noted once again that when the upper end of the cut stomach is closed, the anastomosis is made at the lower cut end of the gastric pouch, and the short afferent jejunal loop is brought up behind the transverse colon and attached to the whole of the reconstructed "lesser curvature," the procedure is correctly termed the *Hofmeister-Finsterer method.* (See Fig. 17.)

In the retrocolic Polya operation, the vascular gastroepiploic arch may be preserved, as shown in Figures 3 and 4, or the gastrocolic ligament may be divided below the arch and the right and left gastroepiploic vessels ligated.

The liberation of the greater curvature is more exacting and tedious when the main gastroepiploic vessels are preserved. Today it is not customary to keep this vascular arc intact, as it has been shown that necrosis of the greater omentum very rarely follows judicious ligation of the blood vessels in the gastrocolic ligament (Fig. 4). When this step has been completed, the pylorus and the first portion of the duodenum are mobilised by underrunning of the numerous vascular bands and adhesions on the superior, inferior, and posterior aspects of the bowel. The adhesions or bands that exist posteriorly are isolated with a grooved director or with long nontoothed dissecting forceps prior to ligaturing and dividing them seriatim (Fig. 4 [2]).

When a *posterior-wall duodenal ulcer* is attached to the pancreas, the dissection must be cautious, else the pancreas may be inadvertently injured or a brisk troublesome haemorrhage be produced by the laceration of a large vessel. There are manifold unnamed arteries in this region which are hidden in dense, stumpy, fibrous bands, each of which must be individually isolated and ligatured.

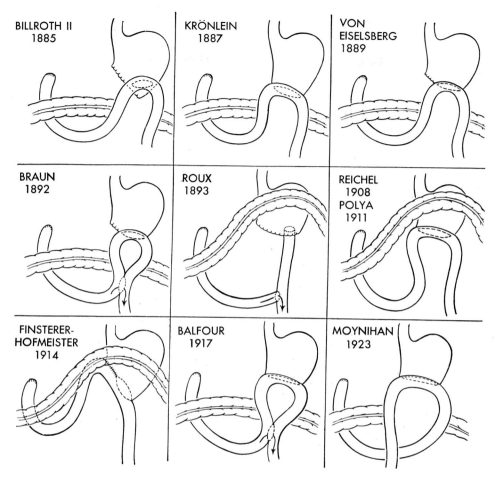

FIG. 1. Billroth II operation and some modifications.

After visualisation of the course of the common bile duct, the right gastric vascular pedicle is isolated and divided. Figure 5 illustrates how this may be done. The proximal end of the artery is doubly ligated with strong silk or catgut, as any slipping of the ligature here would have serious consequences (Fig. 5). If a posterior-wall ulcer has penetrated deeply into the pancreas, the duodenum should be dissected free, leaving the ulcer crater in the substances of the pancreas. *Under no circumstances should this ulcer crater be excised or cauterised, owing to the risk of subsequent pancreatitis or pancreatic fistula* (see Fig. 10).

It is necessary to free the duodenum for at least ½ inch (1.27 cm) beyond the scarred or ulcerated area in order to leave sufficient healthy tissue for an easy and safe inversion of the cut end.

There are many ways of closing the duodenal stump.

In the average case, two straight clamps are placed on the duodenum, side by side, distal to the ulcer, or clamped to its fibrotic base, and the bowel is divided between them, pains being taken to pack off the operative field, as is shown in Figure 6.

A warm pad is spread out underneath the duodenum and pyloric segment of the stomach, and on top of this is placed a Sargent retractor to act as a guard while the bowel is being transsected. The clamp on the gastric side of the duodenum is covered with a small waterproof square or a plastic bag which is tied in position, after which the

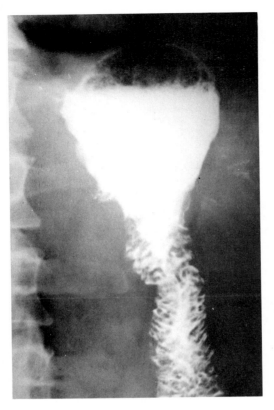

FIG. 2. Barium-meal x-ray examination appearances 2 years following the performance of a posterior Polya operation as described in the text.

stomach is drawn over to the left and away from the field of operation, while the other clamp is rotated to expose the undersurface of the duodenal stump, which is then sutured over with a right-angled continuous stitch, this being drawn tight as the clamp is released. This Cushing or Mikulicz stitch produces a neat inversion of the margins of the duodenum and is carried back to its starting point and tied firmly. When this suturing has been completed, the end of the duodenum is further inturned with a purse-string suture or with a series of closely applied interrupted sutures of fine silk, and pads of adjacent omenta are drawn across the suture line and tied in position to afford the maximum degree of protection against leakage (Fig. 7).

The Allis forceps method, which is some-times used to aid the closure of the end of the duodenum, has many supporters, includ-ing the surgeons at the Lahey Clinic. Here again the end of the duodenum supported by a series of Allis forceps is elevated and a continuous suture is inserted, starting from the greater-curvature end of the duodenum and to the lesser-curvature end. As the sutur-ing proceeds from one end to the other, the forceps are removed seriatim. When the first suture line has been completed, it is rein-forced with a series of closely applied Lem-bert sutures or, better still, with mattress sutures of fine silk. The various techniques employed in secure closure of the duodenal stump are shown in detail in Figures 7, 8, and 9.

The application of a clamp to the liber-ated first portion of the duodenum and at a point distal to the ulcer may be impossible to accomplish owing to the foreshortening of the gut. In such circumstances it is often wise merely to transect the duodenum distal to the ulcer or its scarred face and to effect the closure by means of an economical Con-nell loop-on-the-mucosa stitch of 0 chromic catgut, after which a series of interrupted mattress sutures of fine silk is introduced to strengthen and protect the inverted suture line.

This simple method of closing the duo-denal stump is shown in Figure 8 (top three figs.).

The left gastric artery must now be se-curely tied. In cases of duodenal ulcer, this presents no difficulty, but in gastric ulcer, ow-ing to inflammatory thickening and oedema of the lesser omentum, to the presence of large inflammatory nodes, and to the fixa-tion of the stomach to the pancreas by an eroding ulcer and to surrounding adhesions, it is often an anxious and arduous dissection.

With *penetrating gastric ulcers* it is better to pinch off the ulcer or to cut the stomach. adrift from its attachment to the pancreas (Fig. 10). This liberation of the stomach will, of course, facilitate the isolation and ligation of the left gastric pedicle. By far the best method of securing and ligating the left gastric vascular stump is by what may be called the three-clamp method, shown in Figure 11 (*3*). By this method, the partially mobilised stomach is drawn upward and over

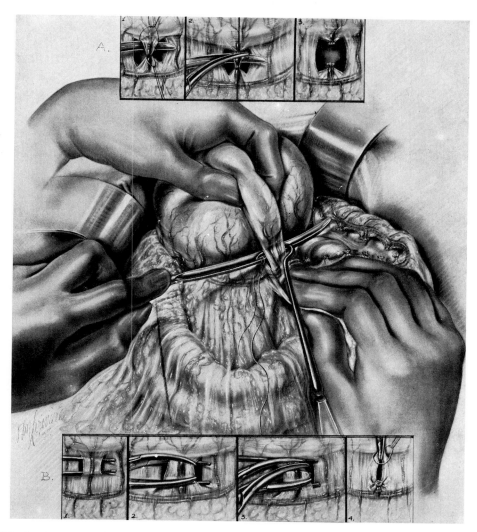

FIG. 3. Posterior Polya partial gastrectomy for chronic duodenal ulcer. The vascular epiploic arch is being detached for the greater curvature. It is not essential to preserve this arch of blood vessels intact. Most sugeons gain access to the lesser sac (to free adhesions in the gastric bed) by dividing and ligating the gastrocolic omentum *below* the gastroepiploic arch.

the left costal margin so that the left gastric vascular pedicle comes into view. Anomalies of the left gastric artery are searched for, and particularly any accessory hepatic artery that may run in the lesser omentum to the liver substance. When such an accessory artery is sizeable, it should be carefully preserved; if, on the other hand, it is minute, it may be sacrificed.

The left gastric vascular pedicle is best ligated where the artery divides into the small ascending and the large descending branches. The fatty tissues of the gastro-hepatic ligament with the left gastric artery and its descending branch are separated from the lesser curvature with long dissecting forceps which are passed between the gastric wall and the artery.

During this dissection, care should be taken not to push the forceps into the muscular coats of the stomach or even into the cavity of the stomach.

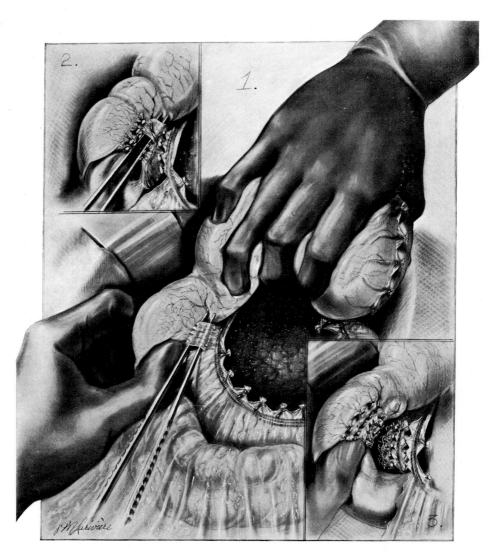

FIG. 4.   Posterior Polya partial gastrectomy for duodenal ulcer. Mobilisation of posterior aspect of the first part of the duodenum.

The point selected for ligation of the left gastric artery is usually 2 inches (5 cm) below the cardio-oesophageal junction, and should be above the level of the majority of resectable gastric ulcers.

With the dissecting forceps in position, an aneurysm needle threaded with strong catgut or silk is passed and the gastric pedicle is ligated high up at the point previously indicated. A second ligature is then applied close to the first one, after which the pedicle is seized with a haemostat and divided with scissors (Fig. 12).

By the three-clamp method, two haemostats are applied to the artery at the selected point, and another one a little lower down, and the artery is divided between the distal and middle haemostats. The topmost artery forceps are removed, leaving the middle ones in position, and two ligatures are slipped into the groove and tied securely. The middle haemostat is then surrounded with a liga-

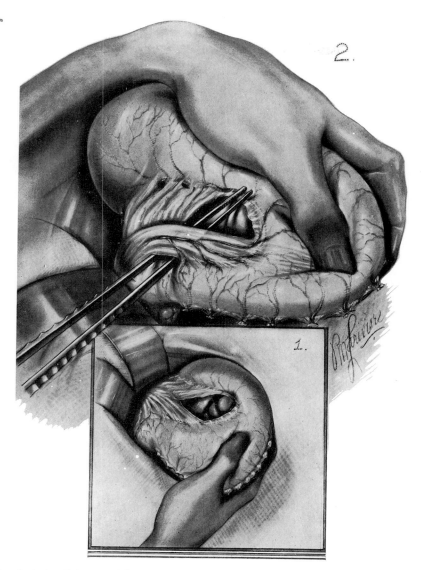

FIG. 5. Posterior Polya partial gastrictomy for chronic duodenal ulcer. Isolation and ligation of right gastric vessels.

ture which is firmly tied and the ends cut (Fig. 11).

The forceps that are grasping the lower end of the vascular pedicle are now drawn downward toward the incisura for a distance of about 2 inches (5.08 cm) or more to permit the lymph nodes and fatty tissues in this region to be dissected downward for a short distance. A raw surface will result on the lesser curvature from the stripping of the peritoneum from this region. This area should be oversewn and reperitonealised with a continuous suture of fine chromic catgut or with silk carried on small curved atraumatic (eyeless) needles. If this is done at this stage, it will greatly facilitate the introduction of sutures in this region after the stomach has been cut adrift. For added security, the suture line should be reinforced with a series of closely applied noncapillary sutures of 00 silk.

In order to effect a wide range of mobility

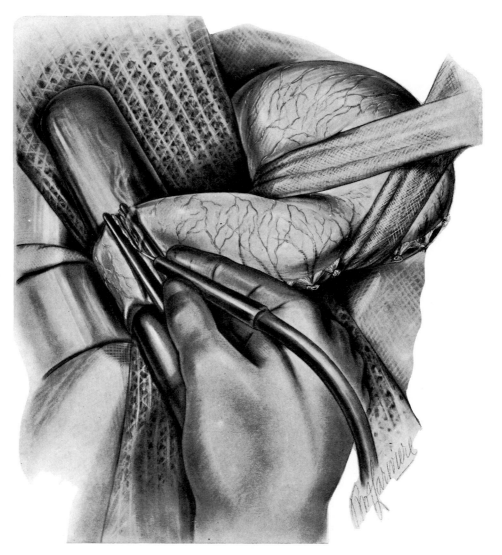

FIG. 6. Posterior Polya partial gastrectomy for chronic duodenal ulcer. The duodenum is being divided with a diathermy needle. Note how the operative field is carefully packed off; also note the position of the Sargent retractor.

of the stomach, it is often necessary to isolate, underrun, ligate, and divide at least two or three of the lower short gastric blood vessels which lie in the flimsy gastrosplenic omentum. These vessels are best secured after the left gastric pedicle has been dealt with (Fig. 12).

During the mobilisation of the fibrofatty tissue high up on the lesser curvature, one or two posterior transverse branches of the left gastric artery will need transfixion sutures to prevent the formation of haematomas in this area.

It will now be seen that the stomach is freely mobile and ready for anastomosis with the jejunum.

In the posterior Polya or the Hofmeister-Finsterer operation, an opening is next made in the mesocolon through one of the wide avascular areas which exist to the left or

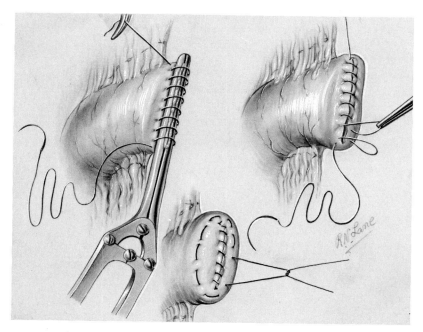

FIG. 7. A reliable method of closing the duodenal stump.

right of the main branch of the middle colic artery, in the manner shown in Figure 13, and the proximal jejunal loop is drawn into the supracolic compartment after the ligament of Treitz has been identified.

At this stage, it is well to suture the left margin of the mesocolon to the posterior surface of the stomach about 1 inch (2.5 cm) proximal to the proposed line of transection; when the anastomosis has been completed, the right margin of the mesocolon is fixed to the anterior surface of the gastric remnant ½ inch (1.27 cm) above the anterior row of sutures, thus placing the stoma in the infracolic compartment of the abdominal cavity (Figs. 14, 15, and 16).

I prefer to perform the anastomosis without any appreciable loop, as it is easier to approximate the short proximal limb of jejunum to the lesser curvature with the distal end at the greater curvature; in other words, the loop of proximal jejunum is drawn from right to left across the portion of stomach to which it will be united.

In making the anastomosis without the aid of intestinal or other clamps, two, three,

or *even* four rows of sutures can be used. In the operation here illustrated, and which was drawn during the performance of a posterior Polya procedure, four rows of sutures were employed for the anastomosis, the first posterior row of interrupted sutures of fine silk being inserted with great care to prevent axial rotation of the intestine and to simplify the introduction of the posterior continuous sutures.

Three continuous sutures of 0000 chromic catgut on atraumatic (eyeless) ½-circle taper 30-mm intestinal needles are used, *but there can be no objection to the employment of only two rows of sutures provided the stitching is carried out very accurately.*

The first posterior continuous suture, which starts at the greater curvature, is a right-angled stitch of the Cushing type, and approximates the adjacent margins of the jejunum and stomach. When it reaches the lesser curvature, care is taken to place one or two closely applied locking sutures (Fig. 15 [2]).

An incision extending from the lesser to the greater curvature is now made through

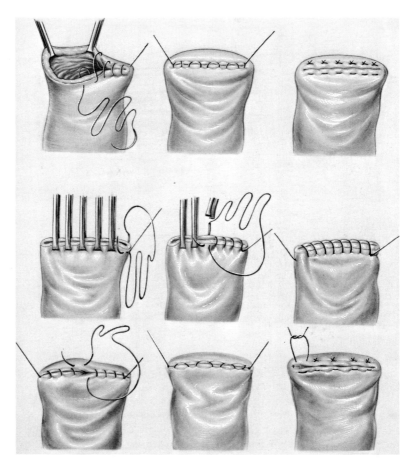

FIG. 8.   Closure of the duodenal stump: two methods.

the seromuscular coats of the stomach, down to the mucosa, about ¼ inch (6.3 mm) distal to the suture line, and the numerous blood vessels which are displayed lying on the mucosa are individually underrun and tied as they emerge from under the seromuscular flap that lies closest to the line of sutures (Fig. 15 [4]). This is the surest method of controlling bleeding from the stomach and keeping the field of operation neat and tidy.

The seromuscular coats of the jejunum are likewise incised for a length corresponding to the incision in the stomach, and any brisk bleeding points are controlled with a ligature.

The second posterior suture, which is a through-and-through all-coats stitch, starts at the greater curvature and finishes at the lesser curvature, where it is locked (Fig. 15 [5]). The mucous membrane of the jejunum is incised for the full length of the incision and the interior of the intestine is aspirated and then cleansed with small swabs that have been soaked in warm normal saline solution. The mucosa of the stomach is punctured and a suction tube inserted through the hole to withdraw any remaining gastric secretion, after which the mucosa is divided for the full length of the incision.

The third posterior suture approximates the cut edges of the mucous membrane of the stomach and jejunum, and when it reaches

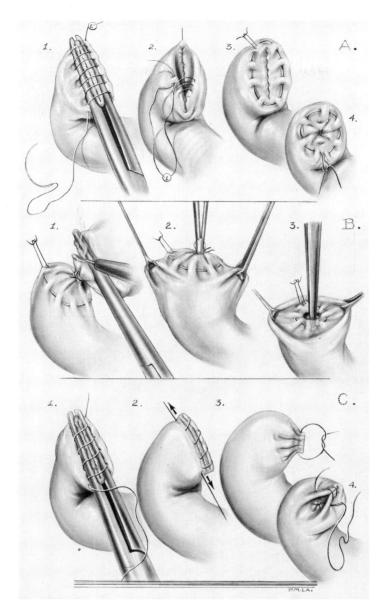

FIG. 9. Closure of the duodenal stump: three methods of closure and inversion of the stump are depicted.

the lesser curvature it is locked, like the former two sutures (Fig. 15 [8]). A large square pack is placed over the gaping mouths of the stomach and jejunum, and the stomach is turned over to the right, as if it were on a hinge, to expose its anterior surface, where a transverse incision is made with a knife down to the submucosa to permit easy ligaturing of the numerous vessels that are found here. At the lesser and greater curvatures, this incision joins the now-sutured posterior margins.

The stomach is put on the stretch and cut adrift by snipping through the mucosa with scissors. The third posterior stitch is continued as the first anterior stitch, and unites the cut edges of the mucosae of the stomach and jejunum; when it reaches the greater

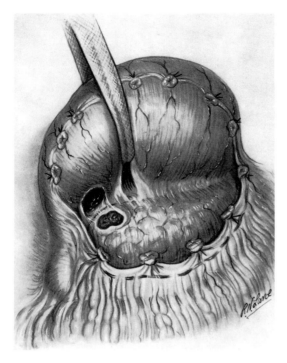

FIG. 10. Pyloric ulcer attached to the pancreas has been pinched off or cut free.

curvature, it is knotted to the point where it started (Fig. 16 [9]. Likewise, the second posterior stitch, on turning the corner at the lesser curvature, picks up all the coats of the anterior margin of the stomach and jejunum, and proceeds to the greater curvature, where it is tied.

The third anterior suture finishes as it started—i.e., as an inverting seromuscular Cushing stitch (Fig. 16 [11].

When the anastomosis has been completed, a few interrupted sutures of fine silk are placed here and there on the anterior suture line, and especially in the region of the lesser curvature, to afford additional security. The retrocolic Polya operation has been criticized on the following grounds:

1. It is time-consuming.
2. Four layers of sutures for fashioning the anastomosis is unnecessary, as two layers are sufficient.
3. The stoma is unusually large.
4. There is a tendency of food to re-

gurgitate into the afferent limb of the jejunum and into the duodenum.
5. The production of a *valve* may interfere with the emptying of the gastric pouch.

Most of these criticisms are unwarranted as, in my series of some 200 cases, there were no instances of bleeding or leakage from the suture lines, no regurgitation into the duodenal loop, and barium-meal x-ray investigations did not show any evidence of valve formation. (See Fig. 2.) The mortality rate was 1 percent for gastric ulcers and 2 percent for duodenal ulcers; the proved recurrent ulcer rate was 2 percent for duodenal ulcer and 0 for gastric ulcer; and the late results were good or satisfactory in approximately 90 percent.

HOFMEISTER-FINSTERER OPERATION

This popular operation is ascribed to Hofmeister (1908), but it was developed independently by Finsterer (1914). It is frequently termed the *Hofmeister-Finsterer operation* and sometimes the *Hofmeister-Polya operation.*

The Hofmeister-Finsterer procedure is a retrocolic end-to-side gastrojejunostomy in which the upper end of the cut stomach is closed and the anastomosis carried out between the lower cut end of the stomach and jejunum. As in all these posterior reconstructions, the afferent loop is short and is attached to the lesser curvature of the stomach. The important steps in the posterior Hofmeister-Finsterer operation are depicted in Figure 17.

At the completion of the Hofmeister operation, there is only partial buttressing of the inturned upper end of the stomach, whereas in the Finsterer method the whole of the closed top end of the stomach is buttressed with afferent jejunum. Finsterer produced this valve-like effect with the object of deflecting the gastric contents directly into the efferent jejunal limb. He hoped by this valve formation to prevent any of the gastric contents from passing into and filling up and distending the duodenum (Fig. 18 (*1*)).

In this operation, the liberation of the

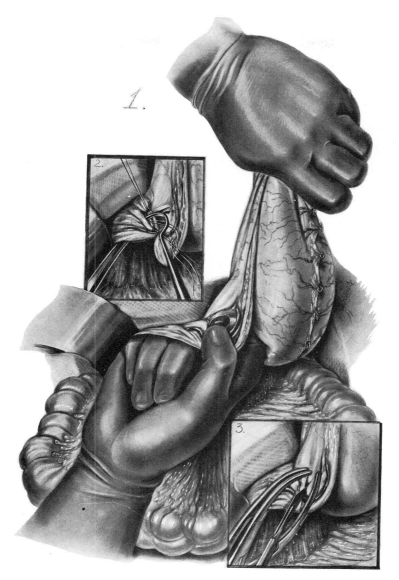

FIG. 11. Posterior Polya partial gastrectomy for chronic duodenal ulcer. Ligature of the left gastric artery. (1) The index finger of the right hand has been insinuated between the main branch of the left gastric artery and the lesser curvature of the stomach high up. (2) The artery is being tied off with the aid of a curved director and the aneurysm needle. (3) Three-clamp method of securing left gastric artery.

stomach proceeds as in the one just described, and the stomach is transected obliquely between two large Payr clamps at the selected site, gauging (and it is often a guess!) that approximately 70 to 75 percent of the stomach will be removed.

If the duodenum has not been divided between clamps, after cutting across the stom-

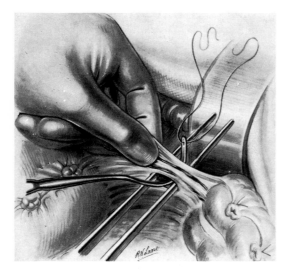

FIG. 12.   Isolation, ligation, and division of the left gastrocolic vessels.

ach between the large Payr clamps the distal clamp should be surrounded with a swab or a plastic purse and the stomach should be lifted up to facilitate the ligation of the right gastric artery.

At this stage, with the distal portion of stomach fully elevated, the adhesions that bind the posterior wall of the duodenum to the pancreas should be individually secured and ligated, and when the first portion of the duodenum has been adequately mobilised it can, at this stage, be transected between two large haemostats. The cut end of the duodenum is then closed by one of the methods previously described.

The large Payr clamp, which has been crushed home to the proximal segment of stomach, is next removed and the agglutinated margins of stomach are caught and elevated by a row of Allis forceps, which will reduce leakage and prevent any bleeding. The upper half of the cut end is now turned in. The first row of sutures is introduced as a continuous all-coats suture of 0 chromic catgut which ensures haemostasis and an even approximation of the posterior and anterior walls of the stomach.

The second row of sutures consists of a series of closely applied Lembert or mattress sutures of fine silk. The Allis forceps remain

on the lower half of the cut end of the stomach while the left margin of the incised mesocolon is sutured to the posterior wall of the stomach and while the short loop of proximal jejunum is being anchored to the lower half or more of the posterior aspect of the stomach about ¾ inch (19 mm) from the site of the proposed new stoma (see Fig. 17).

The Allis forceps are now removed, the crushed area in the stomach wall is cut away with scissors, and an opening is made in the anterior wall of the jejunum which will be of the same length as the gastric stoma; after gastric and jejunal contents have been sucked out, the anastomosis is carried out with a continuous posterior lockstitch of 00 or 0 chromic catgut which is carried anteriorly as a Connell suture. When this has been introduced, the posterior and anterior suture lines are strengthened by the insertion of a series of closely applied interrupted sutures of fine silk or 000 Deknatel.

The edge of the right half of the opening in the mesocolon is then sutured with interrupted stitches to the anterior aspect of the stomach, fully 1 inch (2.5 cm) away from the newly constructed suture line. In some instances it may be advisable, as Finsterer urged, to reinforce the entire closed upper end of the gastric pouch by suturing the afferent jejunum over this area. The mouth of the new gastroenteric stoma should be at least 2 inches (5 cm) in length, or should admit two fingers.

POSTERIOR SCHOEMAKER-BILLROTH II OPERATION

After the stomach has been prepared as in the Billroth I operation, and the duodenal stump closed and invaginated by one of the methods previously described, the small Payr clamp attached to the end of the *tubed stomach* is drawn through an opening in the mesocolon made to the left of the arching middle colic artery. The left margin of the opening in the mesocolon is sutured to the posterior aspect of the stomach about 1 inch (2.5 cm) or so from the proposed site for the stoma, after which the operation will proceed, on the lines already described.

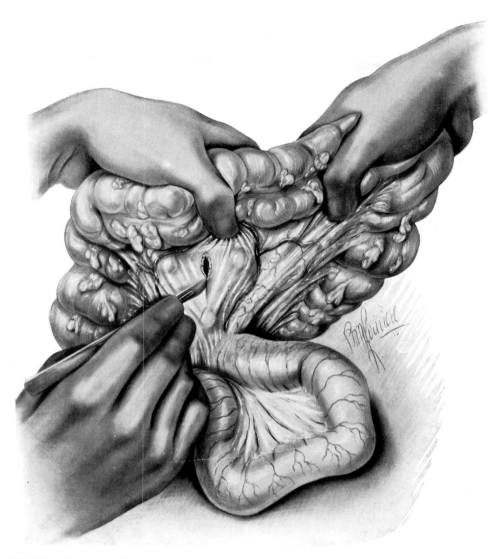

FIG. 13.   Posterior Polya partial gastrectomy for chronic duodenal ulcer. In posterior operation opening is made in mesocolon through one of the wide avascular areas which exist to right or left of middle colic artery. It is usually advisable to make opening in mesocolon to left of main trunk of middle colic artery.

Partial Gastrectomy with Antecolic Anastomosis

MOYNIHAN'S OPERATION

In Moynihan's operation the selected jejunal loop is anastomosed to the whole of the cut end of the stomach. The jejunal loop is short, rarely exceeding 4 to 5 inches (10 to 12.7 cm), and is brought from the fixed point on the duodenojejunal flexure across the colon as close to the splenic flexure as possible and applied to the whole cut end of the stomach from left to right, two rows of continuous sutures being employed in restoring the continuity of the alimentary canal. *Moynihan (1917) did not in fact close the upper end of the gastric pouch, but many surgeons now prefer to do this in order to reduce the size of the stoma.*

This operation is particularly applicable where the stomach is small and where any *reduction in its calibre would appear to be unnecessary.*

A modification of this operation may be performed with the *Petz sewing machine,* in which case, following the transection of the stomach between the row of metal staples, the upper half or so of the remaining gastric

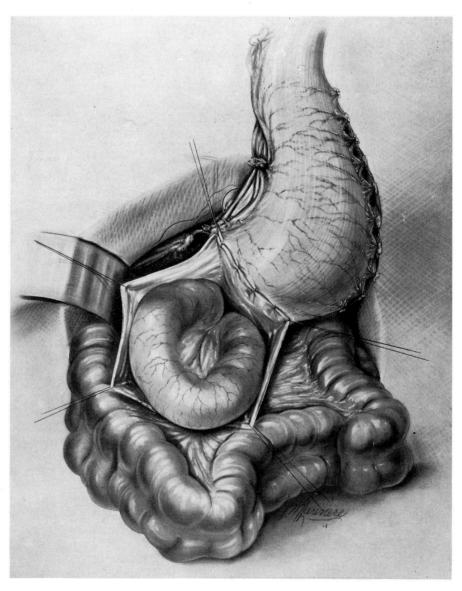

FIG. 14.   Posterior Polya partial gastrectomy for chronic duodenal ulcer. In the retrocolic operation the left cut margin of the mesocolon is stitched to the posterior surface of the stomach about 1 inch (2.5 cm) proximal to the proposed line of transection.

pouch is closed and the staples are buried with a continuous inverting right-angled stitch of catgut and reinforced with a number of mattress sutures of the same material or of fine silk.

After the clips are cut away from the lower portion of the gastric pouch and haemorrhage is controlled, the anastomosis is constructed with two rows of anterior and posterior sutures. The first posterior row should consist of interrupted sutures of fine silk or catgut; the second posterior is introduced as a continuous all-coats lockstitch which is carried anteriorly as a Connell suture, and when this has been inserted the anterior suture line is strengthened and

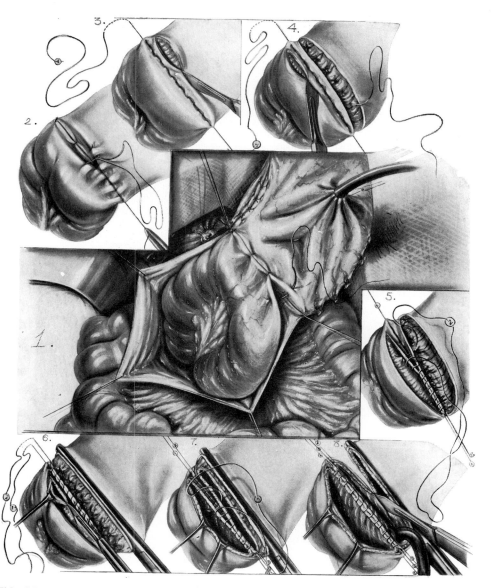

FIG. 15.   Posterior Polya partial gastrectomy for chronic duodenal ulcer. A retrocolic operation is being conducted *without* the aid of intestinal clamps. Details of suturing of individual layers of stomach and jejunum while making anastomosis are shown step by step.

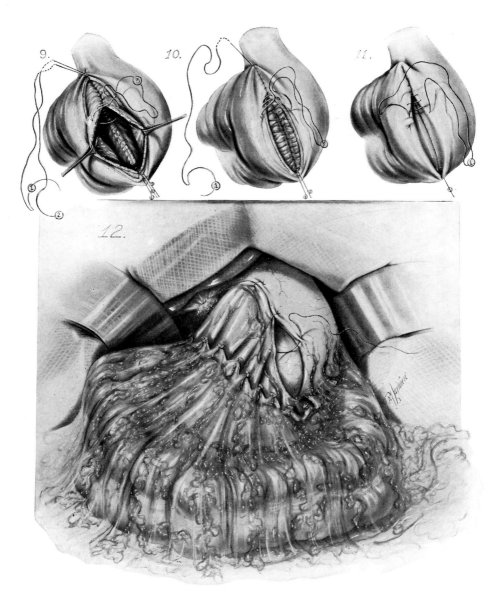

FIG. 16. Posterior Polya partial gastrectomy for chronic duodenal ulcer. Three anterior continuous sutures are shown in 9, 10, and 11. In 12, right margin of the opening in the mesocolon is being sutured to the anterior wall of stomach just above anastomotic line. The greater omentum, with its blood supply intact, is shown spread out over the transverse colon.

inverted with a series of mattress sutures of fine silk.

The points to note in this operation are partial buttressing of the closed upper end of the stomach; the relatively short loop, not exceeding 5 inches (12.7 cm)—i.e., from the ligament of Treitz to the greater curvature;

and a stoma that will admit two fingers.

BALFOUR OPERATION

In this operation, about 75 percent of the stomach is excised and the proximal jejunum is brought over the transverse colon

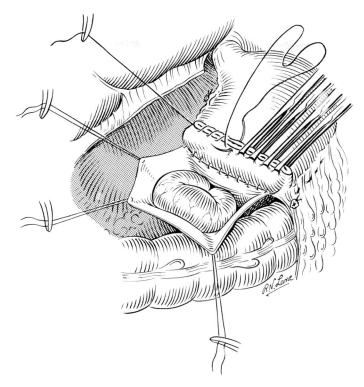

FIG. 17.   The posterior Hofmeister-Finsterer operation.

and anastomosed to the *whole of the cut end of the stomach*, the jejunal loop being taken from right to left. In other words, the afferent limb is attached to the lesser curvature (Fig. 18, *Inset 3;* see also Fig. 1).

In the *Krönlein operation* (1888), the loop is short, rarely exceeding 5 inches (12.7 cm), whereas in the Balfour procedure the afferent limb is moderately long, being about 8 inches (20 cm) in length. Balfour (1923), again, performed an *enteroanastomosis* between the afferent and efferent limbs of the jejunum, especially following resection for gastric ulcer and malignant lesions of the stomach.

When either of these operations is performed, it is important to anchor the afferent limb of jejunum to the remnants of the gastrohepatic omentum, or perhaps to the capsule of the pancreas, in order to prevent undue rotation of the jejunal loop or even volvulus formation.

With these anterior operations, one would have thought that the incidence of small-gut obstruction would be fairly common; in practice, however, it is exceptional for a loop of small bowel to force its way behind the jejunal loop and become entrapped in this area (see Chapter 27).

Von Eiselsberg's Operation: Hofmeister's Operation

Von Eiselsberg (1889) was the first to suggest an antecolic anastomosis in which the upper half of the cut end of the stomach was closed and the lower half toward the greater curvature was employed for fashioning the stoma. This operation now bears Hofmeister's name, and in many clinics it is termed the anterior Hofmeister-Polya method. In many teaching centres in London, it is often referred to as the anterior Polya operation. (See Fig. 1.)

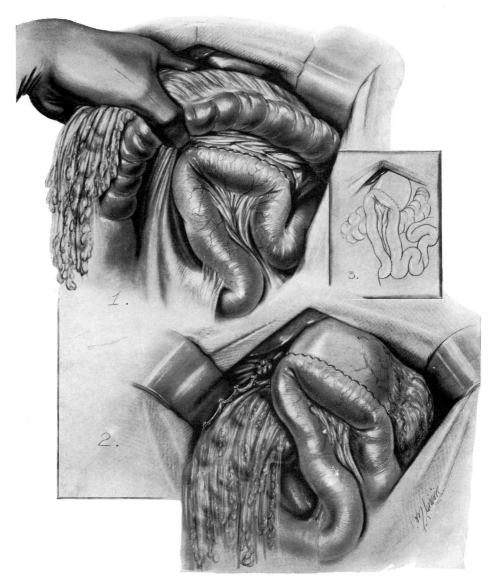

FIG. 18. Anterior and posterior Polya types of partial gastrectomy for chronic duodenal ulcer. Balfour's operation is shown in *inset* 3.

In this procedure, following gastric resection the upper half of the stomach is closed and inverted, and the greater-curvature portion of the stomach is anastomosed to a short loop of proximal jejunum, which is drawn over the transverse colon from right to left with the efferent limb at the greater curvature itself. Most surgeons buttress the upper closed end of the stomach with afferent jejunum, not only to reinforce what may be a weak area but also to produce a valve which some believe is instrumental in directing the gastric contents directly into the efferent jejunal limb.

Schoemaker-Billroth II Operation

Here again, when performing a variation of the Billroth II operation, I frequently employ this procedure.

The stomach is "prepared" as in the Schoemaker-Billroth I operation, and the open end of the tubed stomach is anastomosed to the proximal jejunal loop which is drawn from left to right with the *short afferent limb,* not exceeding 10 cm, attached to the greater curvature. The important steps in this operation are illustrated in Figures 19 to 22 inclusive.

It is important at the completion of this operation to insert a purse-string suture at the so-called critical angle. This purse string picks up the anterior and posterior walls of the stomach and takes a generous bite of the anterior wall of the jejunum just about where the three suture lines converge.

Emphasis is laid on the following points: excision of most of the lesser curvature, a short loop, a small stoma, and insertion of the purse-string suture at the critical angle.

Operations for Difficult or Irremovable Gastric and Duodenal Ulcers

Difficult Gastric Ulcers

Gastric resection will prove difficult and exacting where the ulcer is very large, where it has penetrated deeply into the pancreas, liver, or abdominal wall, or where again it is located high up near the cardia, either on the lesser curvature itself close to the oesophagogastric junction or on the posterior wall of the stomach close to the fundus, or at least in the proximal one-fifth of the stomach.

Operations for gastric ulcer are, as a rule, straightforward, as the majority of such ulcers are situated in a readily accessible portion of the viscus—namely, in the region of the incisura angularis or in the lower third of the vertical portion of the lesser curvature. Some of these ulcers appear at operation as small puckered scars in the region

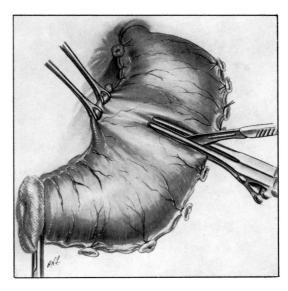

FIG. 19.   Schoemaker-Billroth II operation.

of the lesser curvature; some are attached by filamentous bands or adhesions to the pancreas or even to the mesocolon. Some again, have a narrow or wide isthmus where the ulcer has penetrated into the pancreatic substance.

There are some gastric ulcers which may be described as "giant" sized and which may occupy as much as one third of the posterior wall of the stomach. Most penetrating gastric ulcers can be readily "pinched off" from their base; if, however, they are large, the crater should be left in situ in the pancreatic substance after cutting around its base with a knife or diathermy needle. Under no condition, as I have said, should the crater which remains in some adjacent viscus such as the pancreas or liver be *excised* or *cauterised,* as such interference may give rise to haemorrhage or to a subsequent attack of acute pancreatitis, or even to a troublesome or possibly fatal pancreatic fistula. In some instances, however, a four-quadrant "biopsy" may be indicated.

The most difficult of all gastric ulcers are those which are situated high up near the cardia, the so-called *cardial ulcers,* for which Pauchet's operation is the best and safest.

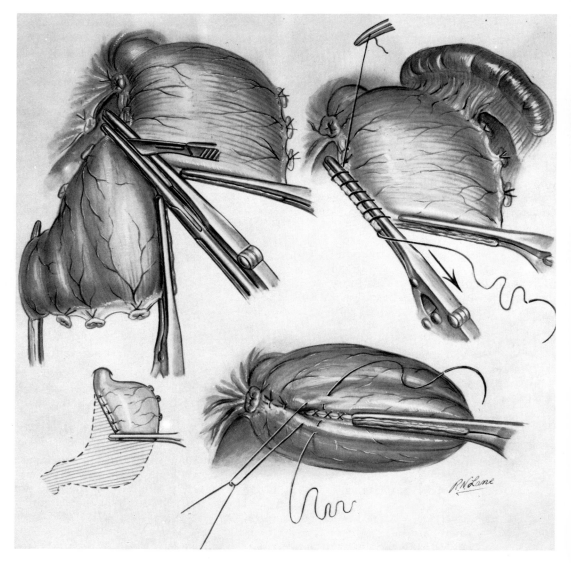

FIG. 20.   Schoemaker-Billroth II operation. Note extent of resection.

PAUCHET'S OPERATION

This operation is in fact a modification of Schoemaker's method, and it entails the mobilisation of the greater curvature, the pyloric region of the stomach, and the first part of the duodenum.

After the duodenum has been transected between clamps, the stomach is drawn firmly upward to the right and two small Payr clamps are applied to the greater curvature and body of the stomach at a point opposite to but well above the angulus. These Payr clamps are placed side by side horizontally across the stomach at the site indicated and with their tips about 1 inch (2.5 cm) or so distant from the lesser curvature. The stomach is divided between the Payr clamps, and a good rim of lesser curve is cut away a few centimetres short of the ulcer. It may be possible to include the cardial ulcer in the

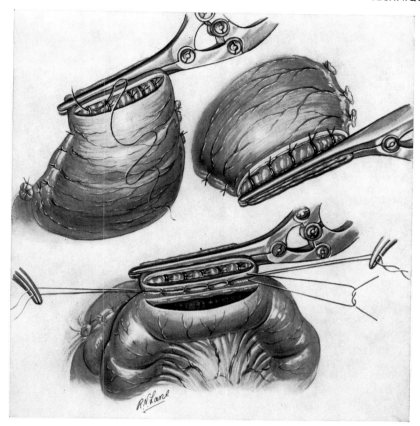

FIG. 21. Schoemaker-Billroth II operation: antecolic method.

segment which is excised. If this is impossible, owing to deep penetration of the ulcer, the lesser curvature should be trimmed away from the crater. A new "lesser curve" is reconstructed by snipping through the anterior and posterior walls of the lesser curve of the stomach toward the cardia and introducing a continuous through-and-through all-coats suture of 0 chromic catgut, the suture being continued step by step with the snipping process.

With the truly high cardial ulcers, the anaesthetist should be instructed to pass a large stomach tube, which acts as a useful guide and facilitates the suturing at the dangerous cardiooesophageal junction.

When this continuous suture has been inserted, the suture line should be oversewn and be inverted with great caution and meticulous care so as not to produce any constriction in the region of the cardia. It is

best to use interrupted mattress sutures of fine silk placed close to one another and tied with a moderate degree of tension.

When this newly fashioned lesser curvature is considered to be watertight, the surgeon has a choice of completing the operation by the Billroth II or Billroth I method of anastomosis (Fig. 23).

TOTAL GASTRECTOMY

This procedure for a *benign* cardial ulcer is, in my opinion, an unjustifiable operation; except, perhaps in exceptional circumstances. (See Chap. 13 by Zollinger.)

KELLING-MADLENER OPERATION

With certain high cardial ulcers, some surgeons prefer to resect about 65 percent of the stomach distal to the ulcer, and to anas-

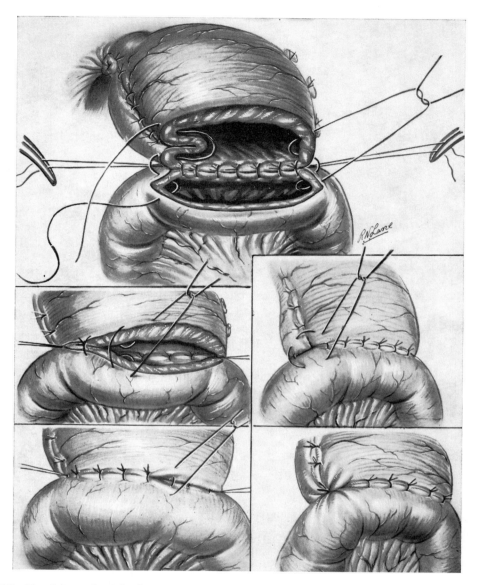

FIG. 22.   Schoemaker-Billroth II operation: antecolic method. Some important steps in fashioning gastrojejunal stoma.

tomose the cut end of the gastric pouch to the first loop of proximal jejunum. Today, vagotomy sometimes precedes the resection.

This is termed the *Kelling-Madlener procedure*.

Kelling[11] described this operation about 6 years before Madlener[14] published his paper (Fig. 24).

I have rarely adopted this technique, because in spite of early relief of symptoms, the persistence of gastric ulceration is high. Again, in some instances, failure is heralded by the sinister onset of cancer of the cardia. This emphasises the point made by Zollinger et al.[27] that a preliminary transgastric *four-quadrant frozen-tissue examination of the* ulcer must be undertaken before deciding upon the correct procedure to adopt in cases of ulcerative lesions close to the cardiac orifice (Fig. 25).

A

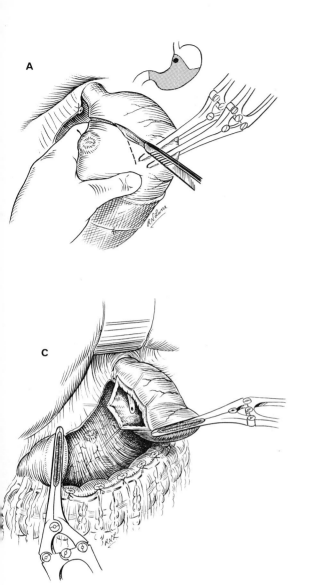

B

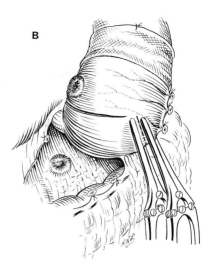

C

FIG. 23.   Pauchet's operation.

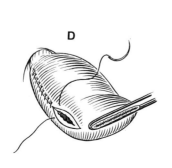

D

E

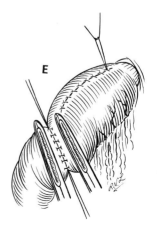

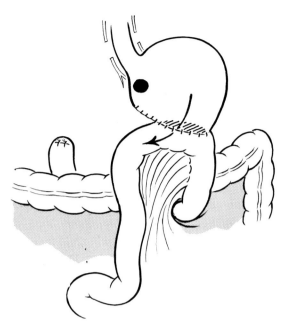

FIG. 24. The Kelling-Madlener procedure for high cardiac ulcer. In *most instances* selective vagotomy may be indicated.

Zollinger adds vagotomy to antral resection when there is histological proof that the ulcer is benign.

In some clinics, however, vagotomy and pyloroplasty or gastroenterostomy is preferred to distal gastric resection (Dorton,[5] Gammie,[9] Dragstedt and Wordward,[6] and Lewis and Qvist [13]). (See Fig. 25).

Further matters concerning "cardial" peptic ulcers may be found in Chapters 11, 14, 15, and 19.

DIFFICULT OR "IRREMOVABLE" DUODENAL ULCERS

The number of difficult or "irremovable" duodenal ulcers diminishes in direct proportion to the surgeon's skill and experience.

The technical management of the duodenal stump is not difficult when partial gastrectomy has been performed for gastric ulcer or cancer; but, with partial gastrectomy for duodenal ulcer, success or failure often depends on the way in which the surgeon deals with mobilisation of the first portion of the duodenum and of the duodenal stump itself.

Although on many occasions the liberation and safe closure of the first portion of a fibrotic, scarred, or ulcerated duodenum present technical difficulties, it is nevertheless true to state that less than 5 percent of duodenal ulcers are "irremovable."

In certain instances, in which a duodenal ulcer is situated in the distal part of the bulb, it is possible to perform a *proximal closure*— i.e., to transect the duodenum just beyond the pyloric ring and to mobilise the segment of gut proximal to the ulcer and invert and close it securely. The ulcer, bathed in alkaline juices, invariably heals, although, on occasion, postoperative haemorrhage from the ulcer bed may be a troublesome complication (Fig. 26).

The surgeon should remember that inflammation and ulceration may shorten the duodenum so that the ampulla may be 2 inches (5 cm) or even less distal to the pylorus rather than 3 or 4 inches (7.6 to 10 cm).

The majority of duodenal ulcers exposed to view at operation give the impression of being easier to remove than they actually prove to be when dissection is started. If the surgeon is confident that such dissection can be readily carried out past the duodenal ulcer, it is best to excise the ulcer and close the duodenum distal to it.

If resection "looks difficult," if the crater of the ulcer is unduly large, if the duodenum is markedly shortened, if periduodenal inflammation extends to and implicates such vital structures as the hepatic artery or the lower portion of the choledochus, the surgeon would be well advised to perform gastrojejunostomy combined with vagotomy rather than hazard gastroduodenal resection, which involves risking such grave complications as rupture of the duodenal stump, duodenal fistula, subhepatic abscess, spreading peritonitis, or injury to the common bile duct or even to the duct of Wirsung.

As an alternative procedure to gastrojejunostomy combined with vagotomy, the surgeon may elect to perform the *Bancroft-Plenk operation*.[2, 22] If a decision is made to employ this operation, the blood supply to the pyloric zone of the stomach should not

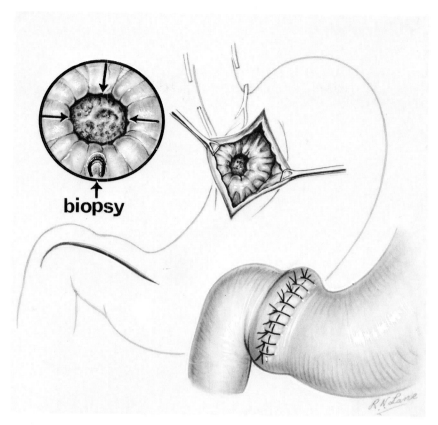

biopsy

FIG. 25. Transgastric technique for four-quadrant biopsy of high gastric ulcer situated close to the cardia. In a few instances, if the ulcer proves to be benign, the operation can be completed by performing vagotomy and pyloroplasty, but in some instances Pauchet's procedure is preferable. Note truncal vagotomy.

be interfered with. In other words, this operation would not be safe if the pyloric region and a segment of the first portion of the duodenum were devascularised.

In those instances in which the surgeon stubbornly persists with the dissection and liberation of the duodenum in the face of the great difficulties enumerated, he may have to have recourse to *Lahey's procedure* [12] of intubation of the common bile duct with a Cattell T tube in order to help in the palpation and visualisation of its course or to *Nissen's method* [19, 20] if the duodenum has been literally torn away from a huge fibrotic crater. Again, *catheter duodenostomy* may be the only procedure open to the surgeon where he finds it otherwise impossible to effect a satisfactory closure of the duodenal stump (see Chap. 9).

I have on many occasions been able to free the posterior wall of the duodenum from a large crater by inserting the index finger into the lumen of the bowel, and by sharp-knife dissection, separating the wall of the gut from its dense posterior attachments (Fig. 27).

The secret of successful liberation of the first portion of the duodenum lies in *dissection close to the duodenal wall*, clamping the blood vessels just distal to the wall of the gut, and avoiding ligation of any bleeding points on the surface of the gut.

In all cases in which it has been possible to liberate only a small segment of duodenum, the closure should be effected with an economical Connell suture followed by a row of reinforcing mattress sutures of fine silk (Fig. 28).

THE BANCROFT-PLENK OPERATION

This operation was first practised by Wilmanns in 1923, and was modified by Bancroft [2] and by Plenk. [22] Valuable contributions on the subject of this operation will be found in articles by Allen and Welch, [1] Wangensteen, [24] Makkas and Marangos, [15] Welch, [26] and Tanner. [23]

This operation has one great advantage in that in cases of difficult or irremovable duodenal ulcer, the implicated zone of the duodenum is not disturbed, the gastrin-producing pyloric mucous membrane is excised, and partial gastrectomy can be conducted with a low death rate. For instance, Makkas and Marangos reported a series of 415 cases with 9 deaths—2.1 percent—and satisfactory late results in 90 percent of the cases. In a personal series of 120 cases there were 2 deaths from peritonitis due to leakage of the duodenal stump, and the late results were on the whole gratifying. The recurrent-ulcer rate was approximately 4 percent.

There are, however, certain *disadvantages:* Leakage and peritonitis may be distressing sequelae and perhaps occur more frequently than has been indicated in the literature.

During the pyloric dissection, some of the antral mucous membrane may be left behind, and this at a later date may favour the production of a stomal ulcer. Again, instances have been recorded in which the excluded duodenal ulcer has perforated or bled postoperatively.

It must be emphasised once again that in

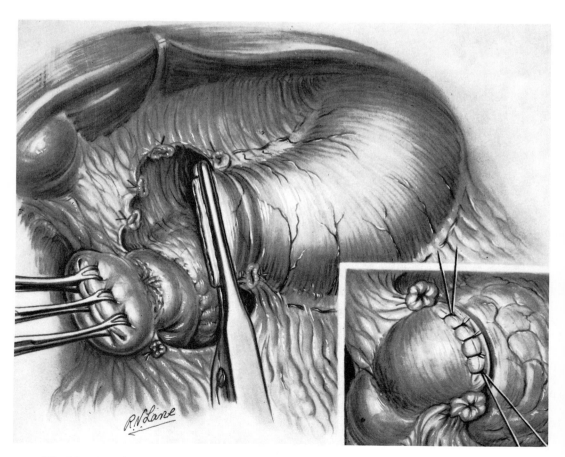

FIG. 26. Partial gastrectomy for duodenal ulcer in the distal portion of the bulb or in the second portion of the duodenum. Method of proximal closure of the duodenal stump.

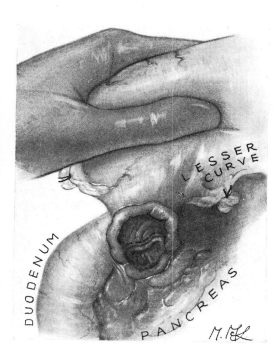

FIG. 27. Large penetrating duodenal ulcer.

seeking to ensure an adequate blood supply to the stump, the right gastroepiploic and right gastric vessels must not under any condition be separated from the pyloric zone.

The Bancroft-Plenk operation is conducted as follows: After partial mobilisation of the greater and lesser curvatures, a circular incision is made through the seromuscular coats of the antrum about 3 inches (7.62 cm) proximal to the pyloric sphincter. The seromuscular layer is picked up with Babcock or Allis forceps and, by gauze and scissors dissection, the mucosa is stripped off the muscular coat as far as the pyloric ring itself (Fig. 29).

The dissection is carried to the point where the mucosa disappears through the narrow pyloric canal. The cuff of pyloric muscle is folded over the pyloric sphincter, and a purse-string suture of 000 chromic catgut mounted on a small, curved, eyeless intestinal needle is inserted just proximal to the point at which the mucosal cuff enters the tunnel (Fig. 30). In surrounding the tube of liberated mucosa, the purse-string suture should be introduced in such a way that the

needle picks up *only* small bites of *submucosa*. Under no condition should this cuff of mucosa be transfixed and ligated or be underrun with continuous sutures.

After the mucosal tube has been cut away proximal to the purse-string suture, the margins are gathered together and invaginated into the pyloric canal as the purse-string suture is being tied. This is a safe, watertight closure and ensures that no damage is done to this delicate and friable structure. To tie off the mucosal cuff is to court disaster, as a ligature thus applied becomes a necrosing one which will cut through in 4 to 5 days (Figs. 31 and 32).

After the introduction of the purse-string suture, as described above, the major portion of the seromuscular cuff is excised and then closed with clips introduced by a small Petz clamp or by means of a sewing machine stitch of 00 chromic catgut, after which the suture line is protected with omentum. The seromuscular tube plays no part in the safe closure of the pyloric canal; in fact, it may necrose and slough away, particularly when it is inturned with a series of strangling purse-string sutures (Figs. 33 and 34).

The operation is completed by performing the antecolic Schoemaker-Billroth II procedure (see Figs. 19–22 and 34).

Ample drainage should always be provided following this procedure, owing to the possible danger of subsequent leakage.

Nissen's Method

When trouble is experienced in dissecting the posterior duodenal wall from the pancreas, Nissen's method of suturing the cut duodenal-wall edges opposite the crater to the undissected distal crater edge, followed by the burying of the suture line in the ulcer crater, can be employed (*Duodenal and Jejunal Peptic Ulcers*, 1945, p. 50, Heinemann).

This method is particularly applicable to large callous posterior-wall ulcers in which the posterior wall of the duodenum, the distal edge of the ulcer, and the pancreas are all welded together. The writer's modification of Nissen's method is illustrated in Figure 35.

Following this operation, the operative field and the right subhepatic space should be drained, as leakage has been known to

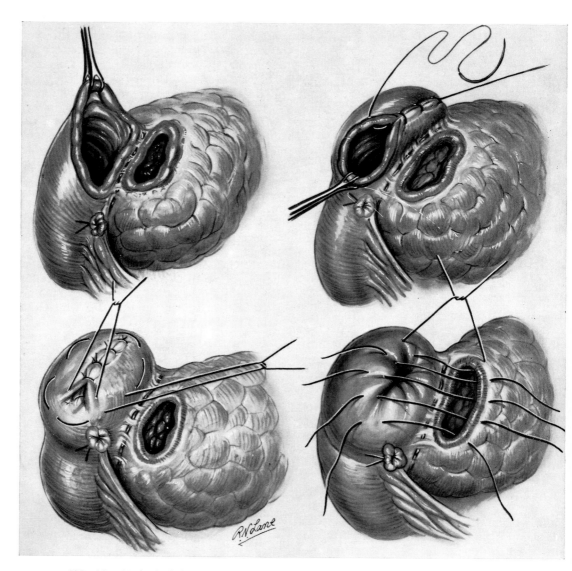

FIG. 28.   Method of closing the duodenal stump in some cases of difficult duodenal ulcer.

occur following the adoption of this method of closure.

LAHEY'S METHOD

Lahey [12] advocated his method in those cases in which the dissection of the duodenal stump proved difficult and in which the common bile duct may be injured either by partial section or by the application of a ligature or transfixion suture to a portion of the wall of the duct. Such damage to the choledochus may of course have fatal consequences unless recognised early and corrected within a few days of operation (Fig. 36).

To avoid these complications Lahey advised that choledochostomy with T tube drainage should be carried out in all difficult cases. By his plan the common bile duct is displayed, opened, and probed, after which one limb of a long T tube is passed into the duodenum, and the upper limb of the T tube is cut short in order to enable it to lie in the common hepatic duct. The opening in the

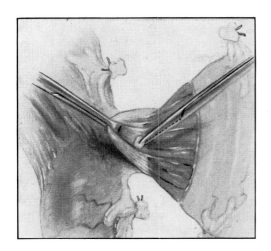

FIG. 29. Bancroft-Plenk operation.

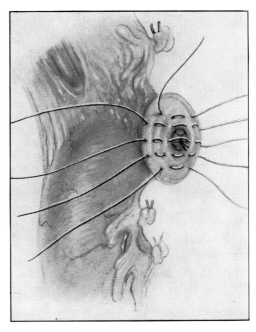

FIG. 31. Bancroft-Plenk operation.

duct is then closed around the issuing limb of the tube, which is led to the exterior for drainage purposes. With the T tube in place, it is possible to visualise and to avoid "vital" structures and to proceed with the duodenal dissection and closure with greater safety. The T tube is removed on the eighth postoperative day (Figs. 36 and 37).

CATHETER DUODENOSTOMY COMBINED WITH PARTIAL GASTRECTOMY

Catheter duodenostomy combined with partial gastrectomy may be indicated

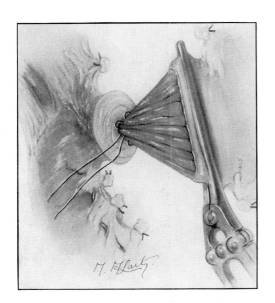

FIG. 30. Bancroft-Plenk operation. Note the introduction of the purse-string suture.

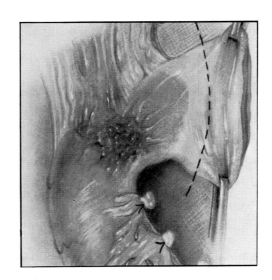

FIG. 32. Bancroft-Plenk operation.

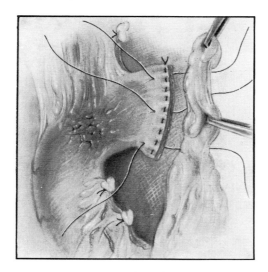

FIG. 33. Bancroft-Plenk operation.

when, following gastroduodenal resection for a large and inflamed duodenal ulcer, the secure closure of the stump seems to be well-nigh impossible. A full account of the operation is given in Chapter 9 by James Priestley of the Mayo Clinic.

Miscellaneous Gastric Operations

CONNELL'S OPERATION

This operation was devised by Connell[3] and consists in excising a huge V-shaped wedge from the body of the stomach. At the apex of the V excision the lesser curvature is left intact. Two-thirds of the greater curvature and a large triangular portion of the anterior and posterior walls of

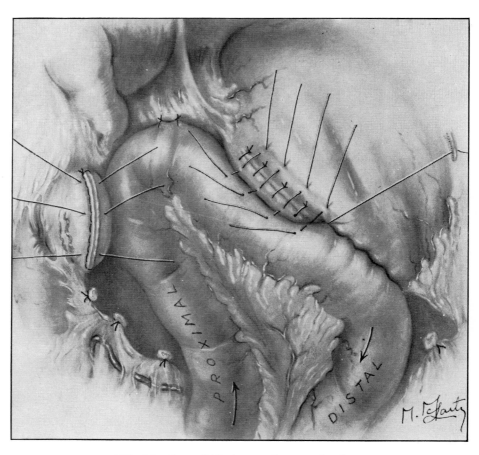

FIG. 34. Bancroft-Plenk operation completed.

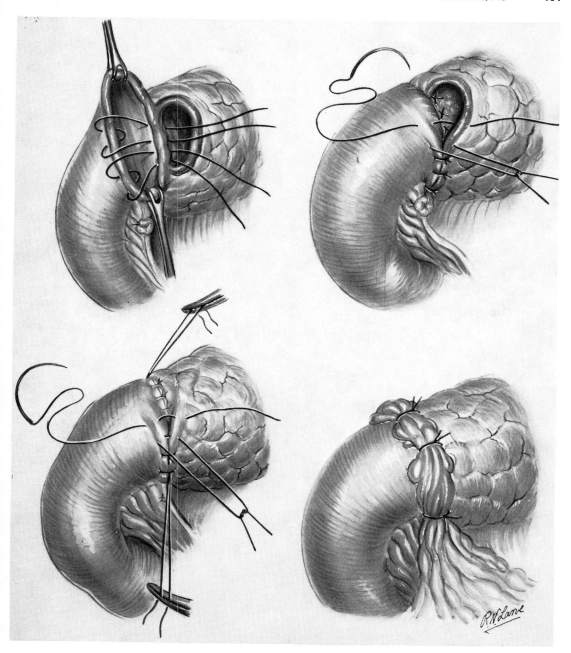

FIG. 35.   Nissen's method.

the stomach are removed in one piece, after which the defect in the gastric wall is repaired at right angles to its longitudinal axis so that no narrowing results.

The excision of an extensive portion of gastric wall, including a large area of principal glands, combined with vagotomy and pyloroplasty, aims at reducing gastric acidity and at the same time overcoming obstruction at the gastric outlet. The operation, so far as I am aware, had few supporters. I have had no experience of this procedure.

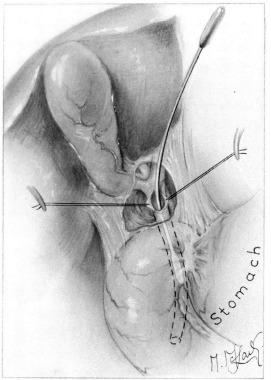

FIG. 36. Lahey's method of dealing with a difficult duodenal ulcer. The common bile duct is exposed, opened, and Bakes' dilators are passed into the duodenum to dilate the ampullary region. The dilator serves as a useful guide.

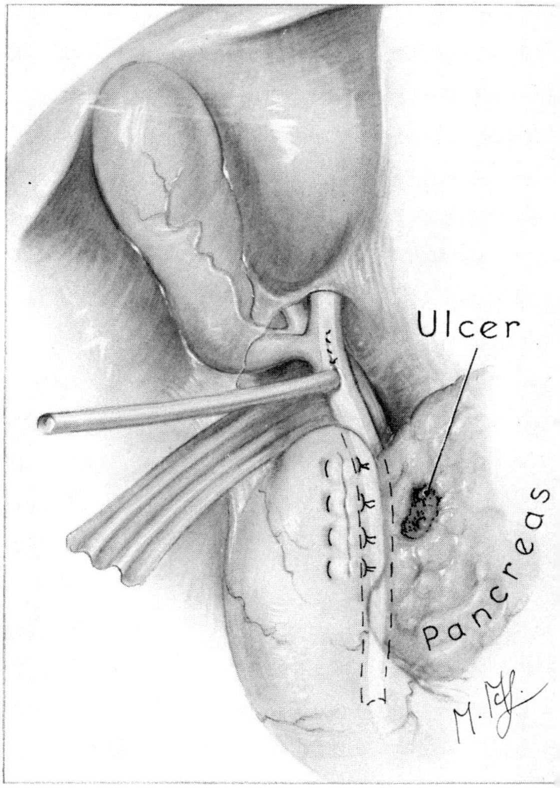

FIG. 37. Lahey's method of dealing with a difficult duodenal ulcer. The operation of gastroduodenal resection, followed by an antecolic Polya anastomosis, is completed. Note the closure of the duodenal stump, the anatomical relations of the long T tube, and the corrugated rubber drain. The ulcer, which remains in the head of the pancreas, should not be cored out or fulgurated. It should be left undisturbed.

WANGENSTEEN'S PROCEDURES

Wangensteen, in 1940, performed a similar but more radical operation than Connell's for acid reduction, in which he excised the major portion of the greater curvature of the stomach, most of the fundus, and more than half of the anterior and posterior walls of the stomach. The defect from this excision, when sutured, produced a tubular effect.

Wangensteen at a later stage sutured the gaping defect in the stomach transversely, thereby facilitating the suturing of the huge gap in the gastric wall. He completed his operation by performing pyloroplasty to aid in the emptying of the reduced gastric pouch.

In 1952 Wangensteen[24] performed a segmental gastric resection in which the body of the stomach was excised between clamps, the remaining proximal segment of stomach being anastomosed end-to-end to the cut end of the antrum, after which a Heineke-Mikulicz pyloroplasty was carried out.

These operations of Wangensteen for reduction of the acid-pepsin ratio in the treatment of peptic ulceration have received scant support from surgeons in Britain, although he himself has been well pleased with the results of this segmental resection combined with pyloroplasty.

DELOYERS' OPERATION

Deloyers [4] recommended a "reverse" gastrectomy—resection of the whole body of the stomach, followed by oesophagoantral anastomosis. This operation is in some respects akin to some of the procedures that are performed for growths involving the upper fifth or so of the stomach, including the juxtacardial area.

Despite the good results and the low mortality rate reported by Deloyers, the operation has without any doubt worse functional results than any other form of gastrectomy for duodenal ulcer, and it also carries a higher mortality rate. Tanner believes that its wide use for an innocent condition such as duodenal ulceration would be disastrous.

"ASEPTIC" GASTRIC RESECTION

Gastric resection followed by anastomosis of the stomach to the jejunum by the closed or aseptic method has been advocated and was at one time recommended by Wangensteen (1940), Culligan (1944), and Pannett (1945). It is claimed that the closed or aseptic method of gastrojejunal union reduces the incidence of postoperative peritonitis (!) and infection of the wound, as well as shock and the length of time expended on the operation. As, however, the procedure is not truly aseptic and the measures taken to prevent postoperative haemorrhage are not satisfactory, and as the sutures cannot be introduced with the same accuracy and precision as by the open technique, this closed method has been abandoned.

REPLACEMENT OPERATIONS

Primary partial gastrectomy with jejunal replacement, as described by Henley,[10] and partial gastrectomy with colonic replacement of the stomach, as sponsored by Moroney,[18] in the treatment of peptic ulceration,

are no longer practised, owing to the high incidence of early and extensive anastomotic ulceration and to the frequent advent of widespread inflammatory or chemical fibrotic contraction of the replaced loop of bowel.

In the past I had occasionally performed partial gastrectomy with colonic replacement for gastric and duodenal ulcer, but *invariably with subsequent regret*. In nearly every instance in which I employed this procedure, a difficult and hazardous secondary operation for excision of the blighted replaced segment of intestine proved necessary. I have had no personal experience with jejunal interposition apart from reoperation for stomal ulceration on patients who were referred to me from elsewhere.

REFERENCES

1. Allen and Welch, Ann. Surg, 115:530, 1942.
2. Bancroft, Am. J. Surg. 16:223, 1932.
3. Connell, Surg. Gynecol. Obstet. 49:696, 1929.
4. Deloyers, Ann. R. Coll. Surg. 18:277, 1956.
5. Dorton, Am. Surg. 30:561, 1964.
6. Dragstedt and Woodward, Scand. J. Gastroenterol. Suppl. 6, 243, 1970.
7. Edkins, J. Physiol, 34:133, 1906.
8. Finsterer, Zentralbl. Chir. 45:438, 1918.
9. Gammie, Proc. R. Soc. Med. 56:500, 1963.
10. Henley, Br. J. Surg. 40:118, 1952.
11. Kelling, Arch. Klin. Chir. 134:755, 1918.
12. Lahey, Surg. Gynecol. Obstet. 76:641, 1943.
13. Lewis, A., and Qvist, G., Br. J. Clin. Prac. 25:9, 1971.
14. Madlener, Zentralbl. Chir. 50:1313, 1923.
15. Makkas and Marangos. Br. J. Surg. 37:206, 1949.
16. Marshall and Reinstine, Surg. Clin. North Am. 35:711, 1955.
17. McKittrick, Moore, and Warren, Ann. Surg. 120:531, 1944.
18. Moroney, Lancet 1:933, 1955.
19. Nissen, Zentralbl. Chir. 60:483, 1933.
20. Nissen, Duodenal and Jejunal Peptic Ulcers. London, Heinemann, 1945, p. 50.
21. Ogilvie, Lancet 2:295, 1938.
22. Plenk, Zentralbl. Chir. 63:3019, 1936.
23. Tanner, Br. J. Surg. 51:5, 1964.
24. Wangensteen, Surgery 12:731, 1942.
25. Wangensteen, J.A.M.A. 149:18, 1952.
26. Welch, Surgery of the Stomach and Duodenum, Chicago, Year Book, 1966.
27. Zollinger et al., Gastroenterology 35:521, 1958.

22

ACUTE PERFORATED PEPTIC ULCERS

ANDREW M. DESMOND

Perforation constitutes one of the major complications of gastric, duodenal, or gastro-jejunal ulcers. Prompt recognition of the condition is of paramount importance, as only by early diagnosis and treatment is it possible to reduce the still relatively high mortality. For some reason not fully understood, the base of the ulcer suddenly ruptures with the result that the contents of the stomach, duodenum, or jejunum escape into the peritoneal cavity, initiating a train of events which, if not properly managed, may lead to general bacterial peritonitis and the death of the patient. Sometimes, especially if the stomach is relatively empty, the perforation may become sealed off and the peritoneum may be able to deal with the contamination so that spontaneous recovery occurs. On occasion, the perforation may be shut off from the peritoneal cavity and a localised abscess develops in the lesser sac, Morison's pouch, the subphrenic spaces, or the right paracolic region.

Acute perforation of a peptic ulcer is a relatively common complication. About 100 years ago it was rare and Brinton, in 1857, was able to collect only 234 cases from the literature. Up to the mid-1950s there was a progressive increase in its frequency, but there is ample evidence that since about 1955 there has been a steady decline in its incidence. Illingworth et al. (1944) have shown that there was more than a fivefold increase in Glasgow between 1924 and 1944, and that a similar rise was observed in other large cities in Great Britain during the same period. Weir (1960), in a survey of 1,390 cases in northeast Scotland, and MacKay, reviewing 5,343 in western Scotland, found that a peak incidence was reached in about 1953 and that since then there has been a steady decline. The writer, in a personal study of 750 patients treated between 1946 and 1966, found a similar fall. The cause may be either that peptic ulceration is becoming less com-

mon or that a higher proportion of patients is presenting earlier for medical or surgical treatment, for there is no doubt that the neglected and untreated ulcer is more liable to complications, especially perforation and haemorrhage.

Perforated peptic ulcer is more common in men than in women and perforated duodenal ulcers more common than perforated gastric ulcers, but it is important to realise that there is considerable variation in statistics throughout the world. MacKay found that the ratio of males to females had fallen from 19:1 in 1953 to 6:1 in 1963. In the writer's series it was 12:1 in 1953 and 6:1 in 1966. Thus, it would seem that in London and Scotland, while there is an overall decline in incidence, there is, nevertheless, an increasing percentage of women who perforate their ulcers. In the Scottish series, the ratio of duodenal to gastric ulcers was 18:1; in contrast, in London it was nearer 7:1.

Illingworth, in analysing a series of 7,156 patients with perforated peptic ulcers treated in hospitals in the West of Scotland, found that the mortality rate had fallen from 25.7 percent in 1924 to 14.1 percent in 1943 and to 5 percent in 1953. Avery Jones et al. (1953) state that in the 5 years from 1947 to 1951 the total fatality in 340 cases, including those undiagnosed until after death, was 7.9 percent. The operative mortality in 335 cases was 3.1 percent. In 1970 the mortality from the same source had fallen to less than 2 percent in the patients operated upon. Nevertheless, all are agreed that the mortality in patients over 60 years of age remains high and that an increasing number of elderly patients in an aging population perforate peptic ulcers. Furthermore, a disconcertingly high number of patients arrive at hospital moribund because of perforation. Kozoll and Meyer, in their series of 1,904 cases, state that 78 were discovered at autopsy and that 188 patients were so ill on arrival at hospital that only conservative treatment was possible, with 123 deaths. Thus, if only those fit for surgery are considered, the mortality rate is low, but it remains high when the aged and moribund are included in the statistics. This emphasizes the importance of early diagnosis.

The liability of a peptic ulcer to perforate is difficult to assess. In a series of 33,439 cases of gastroduodenal ulcers collected from the literature by DeBakey (1940), there were 4,410 perforations, an incidence of 13.3 percent. Bager (1929) found that perforation occurred in 18.1 percent of 9,475 cases of peptic ulcer. Most statistics are, however, based on the proportion of peptic ulcers which perforate in patients attending or admitted to hospital for treatment. If one takes into account the large numbers who are treated outside hospitals, it is probable that the likelihood of a peptic ulcer to perforate is considerably lower than this. Nevertheless, perforation is still a common cause of death and this must be seriously considered when advising a patient whether or not to have elective surgical treatment for his ulcer.

AETIOLOGICAL FACTORS

Sex incidence. When a large series of cases is studied, the striking fact emerges that there is a preponderance of men over women. Up to the mid-1950s most published series reported 85 to 95 percent males, but recent literature has shown an increasing proportion of females. The cause of this is difficult to determine, but in the last 25 years women have more and more undertaken the tasks and responsibilities or even manual occupations of men, and a higher proportion of them are heavy smokers.

Although perforated duodenal ulcer is more common in both sexes, undoubtedly a higher proportion of perforations in females are gastric ulcers. Perforated gastric ulcer is more common in older patients. In the author's series of 511 perforations, treated between 1953 and 1966, 11 percent of the 421 males and 28 percent of the 90 females had perforated gastric ulcers. Furthermore, of these, 72 percent of the males and 92 percent of the females were over 50 years of age (Fig. 1).

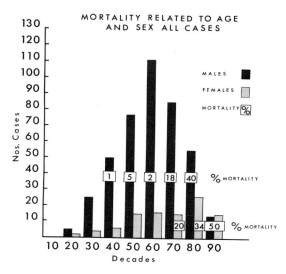

FIG. 1. Mortality related to age and sex, all cases.

Age incidence. Up to the last war, about 75 percent occurred in the third to fifth decades, inclusive, and about 5 percent in the first and second decades, but in the last 25 years, probably owing to the fact that we are all living longer, an increasing percentage of perforations occurs in the sixth, seventh, and eighth decades, so that there has been a shift in age incidence towards the

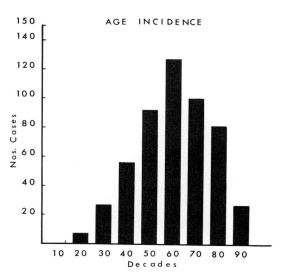

FIG. 2. Age incidence.

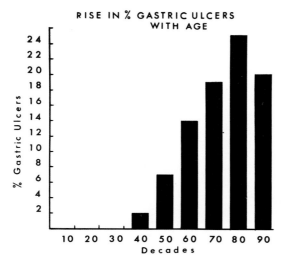

FIG. 3.   Rise, in percent, of gastric ulcers with age.

older age groups. Gastric ulcers are much more common in older people and this, partly at least, accounts for the higher incidence of perforated gastric ulcers today as compared with the mid-1950s (Figs. 2 to 4). Perforations may occur in the *neonatal period* or in extreme old age. Bird et al. (1941), in a comprehensive review of the literature, found reports of 18 neonates, 15 aged 15 days to 1 year, and 44 between 1 and 15 years. Only 37 were operated on, with 8 deaths. All the others died and only 1 in 5 neonates

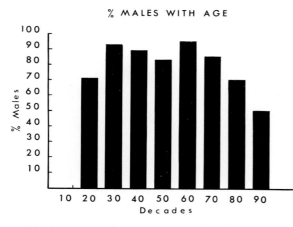

FIG. 4.   Gastric ulcers, in percent, of males with age.

survived. Reams et al. (1963) report a mortality of 57 percent in 39 neonatal perforations. Kennedy (1954), Moncrief (1954), and Millar Bell (1953) have also given comprehensive accounts of acute perforated ulcers in infancy.

Occupational incidence. It is commonly stated that perforation is more likely to occur in those engaged in heavy manual work, and that the lifting of weights or strenuous exercise, by causing a rise of intra-abdominal pressure, predisposes a patient to perforation who is suffering from a peptic ulcer. Weir (1960), in reviewing 1,390 cases in northeast Scotland, found the highest incidence in fishermen, farm labourers, and heavy manual workers; less than half the numbers were in professional or sedentary occupations. Kozoll and Meyer (1960), in reporting 1904 perforations, put the occupational incidence as follows: dependents, 12.9 percent; nonskilled, 27.9 percent; semiskilled, 14.5 percent; skilled, 11 percent; and "white collar" workers, 3.8 percent. *Only 16 of the total were professionals.* Tilton (1936) found that over 50 percent of his patients were of the sedentary class. It would appear that when a series is reported from a general hospital which has a high intake of manual workers the incidence in the professional and sedentary groups is low, whereas in a "private" practice the reverse is the case.

Weir's figures, covering a large geographical area with a mixed population, are more likely to be correct. Strang and Spencer (1950), in a collected series of 1,349 cases, found that 29 percent of the patients were heavy smokers and 10 percent were alcoholics.

Trauma. Occasionally a patient with a perforation may give a convincing history of abdominal trauma. In my series I have been unable to obtain such a history in 750 cases. Most patients try to relate their acute pain to some possible causal incident, and the occurrence of a traumatic incident to the abdomen can sometimes be foremost in their minds, especially if they are heavy manual workers. Fallis (1938) gives the incidence as 2 percent in 100 cases.

Iatrogenic perforations. *Certain drugs* are known to be causative in the production of peptic ulcer, notably phenylbutazone (Butazolidin), steroids, and aspirin. A patient with a duodenal or gastric ulcer who regularly takes these substances is more likely to have a perforation or a haemorrhage than one who does not. It is important to exclude the presence of a peptic ulcer before prescribing such drugs; and, in addition, if a patient with a perforated ulcer is taking cortisone, adequate preoperative and postoperative steroid cover must be undertaken. Spiro and Milles (1960) reported that peptic ulcer occurs in about 5 percent of patients with rheumatoid arthritis, but where such patients are being treated with cortisone, the incidence rises to 12 percent and a significant number of these ulcers perforate. This complication they find far more common in women (see Chap. 11).

Seasonal incidence. Many writers have sought to show that there is an increase in ulcer symptoms and in ulcer perforations in the winter. Jamieson (1947) stated that the incidence was uniform throughout the spring and summer but dropped in the autumn, only to rise again to *a peak in winter.* Moore (1950) believes that twice as many ulcers perforate in the winter months as in the summer. My own experience in London is that the more severe the winter the higher the number of perforations. Perforation occurs most commonly in the early evening (MacKay, 1966; Maingot, 1973).

Geographical incidence. There are great variations in the incidence of perforations in various parts of the world, but it is particularly common among Westernised civilisations and practically unknown among more primitive populations, such as the Bantu in South Africa. When primitive peoples move to and work in areas of Western civilisation and adopt Western dietary and social habits they become more likely to develop peptic ulceration and perforation.

TYPES OF PERFORATION

Acute. The ulcer perforates and the general peritoneal cavity becomes flooded with gastric and duodenal contents. This is by far the most common presentation.

Subacute. In subacute perforations, only a circumscribed area of the peritoneal cavity becomes contaminated by the leakage —the so-called leaking peptic ulcer. Such localisation may be dependent upon a number of factors, such as the limited size of the perforation, the emptiness of stomach, adhesions around the ulcer, or the plugging or sealing-off of the opening shortly after perforation either by omentum or a neighbouring viscus.

Chronic. When an ulcer perforates but the area is walled off by adhesions or by such viscera as the liver, colon, or omentum (or when a gastric ulcer perforates into the omental sac with a sealed omental foramen), a chronic abscess may form and give rise to considerable confusion in diagnosis. These patients usually present with an abdominal mass and/or signs of a subphrenic abscess.

PATHOLOGY

Acute perforation may occur in acute or chronic duodenal ulcers. It is my opinion that acute gastric ulcers never perforate and that all gastric ulcers that do so are of the chronic type. The reports of the incidence of acute perforated duodenal ulcer vary in the literature. In the writer's series, 30 percent of 609 perforated duodenal ulcers were *acute*—that is, there was no antecedent history of peptic ulcer and, at operation, the first part of the duodenum was mobile (with absence of fibrosis) and only a small perforation was found on its anterior wall.

Sometimes it is difficult to determine, at operation, whether the ulcer is actually acute or chronic, as even in the absence of an antecedent history, there may be oedema and swelling around the ulcer which has the appearance of chronicity. I believe these should be classified as chronic ulcers and, in fact, if they are treated by simple suture, a high proportion of the patients will subsequently develop symptoms of chronic ulceration. If a true acute ulcer, as described above, is treated by simple suture, only a small proportion will recur.

Peptic ulcers that perforate into the general peritoneal cavity are situated on the anterior or anterosuperior walls of the duodenum or on the lesser curvature of the stomach (see Chaps. 11 and 12).

The site of the ulcer is obvious in the majority of cases. It is either gastric or duodenal. In some cases, the anatomy of the pylorus and of the duodenal bulb may be greatly distorted.

It may be impossible to identify the veins of Mayo which mark the dividing line between stomach and duodenum, and the region may be so obscured by oedema and adhesions that it may be difficult to be sure whether the ulcer is duodenal, pyloric, or prepyloric. Perforated pyloric and prepyloric ulcers are rare. If they can be confidently identified as such, they should be treated as gastric ulcers. When the site cannot be identified by sight and touch, it is probably wiser to classify and treat ulcers as duodenal. If they are treated by simple suture, subsequent investigations or operation usually shows that such is indeed the case.

At operation or at autopsy in cases of perforated duodenal ulcer, the site of the perforation was found by Kozoll and Meyer (1960) to be on the anterior wall in 92 percent, on the posterior wall in 2 percent, and on or about the pyloroduodenal junction (classified as duodenal ulcers) in 6 percent.

An encircling ulcer, penetrating into the pancreas in its posterior part, may perforate in its anterior part.

Two duodenal ulcers, an anterior one which has perforated and a posterior penetrating one, are commonly found at operation. When haemorrhage coexists with perforation, it is usually the posterior one that bleeds. Rarely, a posteriorly situated ulcer may perforate extraperitoneally and the extravasated fluids may collect in the region around the kidney, giving rise to signs of perinephric abscess. If the fluid tracks downward still further, a mass may appear in the right iliac fossa, simulating an appendix abscess. The drainage of such abscesses may result in a duodenal fistula.

The *size of the perforation* in a duodenal ulcer varies from 3 mm to over 1 cm in diameter and may be even greater in a perforated gastric ulcer.

The majority of perforated ulcers of the stomach are found on the anterior or anterosuperior surface of the lesser curvature. Only exceptionally do ulcers of the upper portion of the stomach and cardia perforate. When

they do, the operation of simple suture or resection may be very difficult.

Kozoll and Meyer (1960) emphasise the fact that the higher the perforation the greater the mortality and that perforations involving the upper portion of the stomach may be associated with a mortality as high as 80 percent.

The indurated ulcer situated on the greater curve is probably malignant and calls for radical measures, whenever possible.

Doll (1950) found that of 86 acute perforations in men, diagnosed as simple gastric ulcer at operation, 7 (8.1 percent) proved to be malignant within a period of three years. Aird (1935) found in the literature 71 cases of perforated carcinoma of the stomach simulating perforated gastric ulcer, to which he added 7 cases from the records of the Edinburgh Royal Infirmary and 1 patient of his own.

McNealy and Hearn (1935) reported 133 cases, and Boyce (1946) 36 similar cases. Kennedy (1951) stated that in his series of 111 cases of acute perforations there were 6 cases of perforated malignant gastric ulcer. The writer, in a retrospective study of 240 perforations treated between 1946 and 1953, found that there were 52 patients with gastric ulcer and of those who survived 5 died of carcinoma of the stomach within 18 months. In a prospective study of 511 perforations treated from 1953 to 1966, during which time 72 perforated gastric ulcers were treated by gastric resection, 9 were cases of carcinoma in situ. This represents an incidence of 11 percent. Seven of the 9 patients had further operations, within 2 months, in order to convert a partial gastrectomy into a subtotal one (with lymphatic gland clearance). All these patients have survived, free of malignant disease, for 1 to 8 years.

Large ulcers of the stomach usually perforate anteriorly and associated bleeding may occur from the posterior penetrating part. However, perforation may occur into the lesser sac or even between the layers of the gastrohepatic omentum. *Multiple perforations are described but must be extremely rare.* There have been no cases in the writer's series. A gastric ulcer associated with a perforated duodenal ulcer or vice versa is, however, not an uncommon finding, and such an association must be sought for at operation.

The larger the perforation and the older the patient, the higher the morbidity and mortality. Gastric perforations are usually larger than duodenal perforations and as these are more common in elderly patients the prognosis is always more grave and the mortality considerably higher than is the case with perforated duodenal ulcer.

Perforation is a rapid process, even in chronic ulcers, and is due to the sudden sloughing of an unsupported portion of the floor of the ulcer, probably due to impairment of blood supply by infective endarteritis.

Immediately after the perforation has occurred, chemical peritonitis develops as a result of the irritant action of the contents of the stomach or duodenum. It is difficult to determine how long it takes for the chemical peritonitis to develop into a frank bacterial one. Theoretically, it should depend on such factors as the size of the perforation, the magnitude of the spillage, the reaction and composition of the gastric contents, the general condition of the patient, and his resistance to infection. Hamilton and Harbrecht (1967) and Kincannon et al. (1963) have demonstrated that the spillage is nearly sterile and furthermore that cultures taken at operations performed even after 24 hours were more often negative and less often grew pathogens than at earlier operations. They also conclude that the magnitude of the spillage does not influence the development of peritonitis. The preoperative use of antibiotics may play a considerable part in this finding. It appears that bacterial peritonitis will supervene only in the grossly neglected case or in the debilitated patient with poor resistance to infection.

Paralytic ileus and intestinal obstruction will supervene if bacterial peritonitis becomes established and then the clinical picture will be similar to that in peritonitis from other causes (see Chaps. 61 and 64).

When large accumulations of fluid are found, however, it would be reasonable to suppose that defensive adhesions are unable or sluggish to form, and the contamination will be more widespread. It has been the writer's experience that the more massive the spillage the longer it takes to resuscitate the patient before operation, and the higher

the incidence of residual subphrenic and pelvic abscesses.

CLINICAL PICTURE

Acute Perforation

A history of peptic ulceration is not necessarily of importance in the diagnosis of acute perforation. Only about 50 percent of patients with perforated ulcer give a history of symptoms suggestive of chronic peptic ulcer when they are questioned during the acute episode. Careful questioning after recovery, however, increases this number to about 70 percent; 15 percent of patients give a short history with symptoms for a week or two prior to perforation; the remaining 15 percent give no history of ulcer at all—even when questioned closely after recovery. In those patients with a history of previous ulceration, usually there has been an acute exacerbation of symptoms immediately preceding the perforation.

In any large series it is common to find that few of those who perforate have had a well-supervised, systematic course of medical treatment. Perforation is rare when the patient is undergoing strict medical treatment in hospital, but when it does occur it is the most lethal form (Vale and Cameron, 1936).

Finsterer's aphorism that *"bleeding ulcers rarely perforate and perforated ulcers rarely bleed"* is, alas, untrue! A history of gastrointestinal haemorrhage can be obtained in a significant number of cases, and patients without such a history who are anaemic at the time of perforation can usually be assumed to have had occult bleeding. In all, about 25 percent of patients with acute perforations have bled preoperatively, but, fortunately, the compound catastrophe of perforation and massive haemorrhage is rare, occurring in less than 2 percent of cases.

Although partaking of a large meal, having a barium-meal x-ray examination, straining, coughing, strenuous exercise, or trauma to the epigastrium may play a part in precipitating perforation, it is just as likely to occur while the patient is resting or even asleep.

From the moment of perforation, the clinical course can be divided into three stages, each of variable duration: (1) *the primary stage, or stage of peritoneal irritation,* (2) *the secondary stage, or stage of peritoneal reaction, and* (3) *the tertiary stage or stage of bacterial peritonitis.* If the condition remains untreated, there is usually a gradual transition through these stages, but the pathological processes and clinical pictures tend to overlap.

The clinical picture of a perforation is generally unmistakable. The patient can usually recall the actual *moment of perforation* very vividly. At that moment he is suddenly seized with an acute agonising upper abdominal pain, which usually becomes rapidly generalised. He is plunged into a state of prostration and may be rendered immobile and helpless. The pain may be of a more intense, lancinating character in the epigastrium. In some cases, where the perforation is small and leaking minimally, the pain may be more localised, tending to be felt on the right side of the epigastrium when the ulcer is duodenal and on the left when gastric. Occasionally, the initial pain is felt only in the chest.

Primary stage. This follows immediately upon perforation. The symptoms, which arise with dramatic suddenness, are due to the intense irritation of the peritoneum by the escape of gastric and duodenal contents. This sudden and violent irritation of the peritoneum produces an immediate reflex on the circulatory and nervous systems, commonly referred to as primary or "neurogenic shock." Occasionally, the patient may die at this stage, particularly an elderly patient with a perforated gastric ulcer, or one in whom perforation is associated with massive haemorrhage. Usually, however, this state of so-called shock is transient and most patients when first seen in hospital have a relatively normal pulse and blood pressure, although they are obviously in considerable distress. In the early stages, nausea and vomiting are uncommon, although retching may be troublesome. In addition to the abdominal pain, there may be referred pain, felt over one or both shoulders, as a result of diaphragmatic irritation. If present on the right side, it suggests a perforated duodenal ulcer; if bilateral, a perforated anterior or lesser-curve gastric ulcer. Such referred pain may

also be present in other conditions, such as diaphragmatic pleurisy, coronary thrombosis, ruptured ectopic gestation, acute cholecystitis, and acute pancreatitis. It is rare, however, in acute appendicitis.

On examination it will be seen that the patient lies almost rigid, with his legs drawn up and his hands held tensely to his side. He is afraid to move, for the slightest movement aggravates the pain. In a few instances the patient may be extremely restless, or again, he may lie curled up in bed in a position of flexion with his hands grasping his epigastrium. The face is pale and sweating, and the expression is one of anxiety or fear. The extremities are pale, cold, and moist with sweat.

The temperature during the primary stage may be subnormal, as low as 95° to 96° F, or normal; occasionally, it is slightly raised. The pulse rate, as mentioned before, is normal or only slightly increased. The respiratory rate is always increased, and the respiratory excursions are shallow and thoracic in nature, owing to the immobility of the diaphragm.

On inspection, the abdomen will be seen to be immobile, there being no movement on respiration. In a thin patient it is retracted—the scaphoid abdomen—with the rectus muscles thrown into prominence, but in a fat patient these appearances are less obvious.

On palpation, the muscles are tensely rigid and board-like. This rigidity is universal and extends into the flanks. On the most prolonged and searching examination, relaxation will not occur, even for a fleeting moment. There is marked tenderness, and usually also "release tenderness," which likewise extends to all parts of the abdominal wall. It is essential, therefore, that palpation be done slowly and carefully. In the early stage, the muscle overlying the perforation itself is particularly metal-like, and the tenderness is more exquisite in this region. In multiparous women and old people, the rigidity may be less board-like because of poor musculature, but the tenderness is no less marked. Auscultation usually reveals a total absence of bowel sounds. The rigidly of the abdominal muscles arises immediately after perforation and persists throughout the primary and secondary stages into the tertiary stage, only lessening in the more advanced state of septic peritonitis. The administration of morphine has the effect of numbing the pain and rendering the patient more comfortable and less apprehensive, but it has little or no direct influence upon the stubborn rigidity of the abdominal muscles.

Sometimes the fluid escaping from a perforated duodenal ulcer may trickle down the right paracolic gutter, producing signs suggestive of acute appendicitis, with tenderness and rigidity limited to the right side of the abdomen. Many such patients would no doubt develop generalised abdominal signs before long, if left untreated.

When a gastric ulcer perforates into the lesser sac, the patient may complain of a pain in the back and a feeling of suffocation. While the irritant gastric contents are contained within the sac, there may be very little guarding of the abdominal muscles; however, when the fluid escapes into the general peritoneal cavity—and this usually happens soon—the symptoms and signs become indistinguishable from those of a perforated ulcer at any other site.

From the moment of perforation, the transition through the primary stage to the secondary stage takes 2 to 6 hours, depending on the size and site of the perforation, and the magnitude of the peritoneal soiling. It is during this stage that spontaneous sealing-off of the perforation may occur. If there is gross leakage of gastric contents, however, the patient may pass rapidly to the stage of septic peritonitis.

The length of the *stage of reaction,* although variable, rarely exceeds 6 hours. The pain, which is most intense at the moment of perforation and during the stage of peritoneal irritation, tends to ease off somewhat during this stage. *For this reason the stage of reaction has sometimes been called the stage of delusion.* There is, to all appearances, a general improvement in the patient's condition. He will state that he feels better, and that he thinks the crisis has passed. The sharp edge of pain has been dulled. He feels warmer, and his colour and general mien have improved. He may still be sweating but the extremities are no longer chilled. The temperature is normal or only slightly raised, the pulse shows little if any change in rate, but the respirations remain hurried. He is thirsty and often asks for a drink—

which of course must be refused.

This improvement in his well-being may cause the patient to delay calling for medical assistance, and it is in this stage also that most of the errors in diagnosis occur. On careful examination, however, it will be seen that the *alae nasi* are working vigorously, that the respirations are still shallow, laboured, and costal in type, and that the patient lies completely motionless with the knees drawn slightly upward. He is still afraid to move for fear of aggravating the pain.

The abdominal physical signs usually leave no room for doubt. The tenderness and rigidity are still present to a marked degree. The pelvic peritoneum is exquisitely tender on rectal examination, and there may be some diminution of liver dullness to percussion, especially with perforated gastric ulcers. On auscultation the abdomen is silent.

One of the most reliable diagnostic procedures in acute perforated peptic ulcer is *the x-ray demonstration of a penumoperitoneum.* Scout x-ray films of the patient in

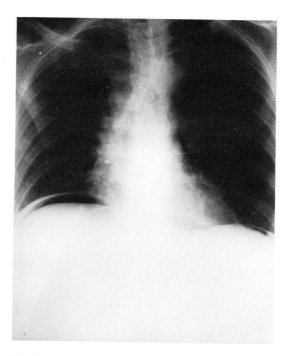

FIG. 5. Perforated gastric ulcer showing gas under the right cupola of the diaphragm (straight x-ray picture).

the erect or sitting position will show gas under one or both diaphragms in some 80 percent of cases of perforation. *A small amount of gas between the liver and the right side of the diaphragm is usually associated with a perforated duodenal ulcer* (Figs. 5 and 6). A lateral x-ray film with the patient on one side may show that the gas bubble has shifted, but it still assumes the highest level. Edwards and Foster (1962) found this sign positive in 66 percent of cases. Kozoll and Meyer (1962) found subphrenic gas in 85 percent; they also found that when pneumoperitoneum was absent, the mortality was less. *It must be emphasised, however, that negative x-ray findings do not exclude a diagnosis of perforation.*

Some clinics have used x-ray pictures of the abdomen following the injection of 60 ml of 50 percent Gastrografin down a nasogastric tube. Jacobson et al. (1961) report a high rate of success. The dye escapes through the perforation, thus making it possible to identify its exact site. This test is invaluable where *conservative treatment* of perforated peptic ulcer is carried out on a large scale,

as failure to demonstrate escape of dye suggests sealing-off of the perforation, and perforated gastric ulcers, which always require surgical treatment, can be identified. The author has no experience of this investigation but, without condemning it, would suggest that it throws an unnecessary burden upon the patient, unless conservative treatment is being considered.

The tertiary stage—the stage of bacterial peritonitis—does not usually supervene until 12 or more hours after perforation; indeed, it seems that it is not always an inevitable sequel to the secondary stage, as was once thought, since many patients coming to operation long after such a time lapse have been found to have a relatively sterile peritoneal exudate. Today, patients are seen and treated during the first and second stages, so that this final stage rarely should be seen. The mortality of patients who are not admitted to hospital until they are in the tertiary stage is inevitably high, for many are already beyond the help of medical or surgical treatment.

The clinical picture of the tertiary stage of a perforated peptic ulcer is essentially the

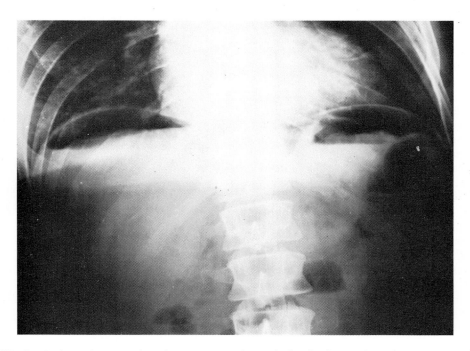

FIG. 6.   Perforated peptic ulcer showing gas underneath the diaphragm (straight x-ray picture). Gas under both diaphragms usually indicates a perforated gastric ulcer.

same as that of a generalised bacterial peritonitis from any other cause. Pain, although still present, is less severe; vomiting is now frequent, while hiccoughs may further distress the patient. As a result of sweating, vomiting, and the outpouring of fluid into both the peritoneal cavity and the distended paralysed intestine, dehydration and electrolyte depletion become more evident. The patient complains of an insatiable thirst. Fever is present, the temperature is usually above 100° F, and the body is dry and flushed, while the lips and tongue are dry and coated. Urinary output almost ceases. The pulse steadily rises and becomes small and thready, and respiration is shallow and rapid. With the rising pulse, the blood pressure starts to fall, indicating that a hypovolaemic shock with circulatory failure has supervened.

Examination of the abdomen will show certain important differences between this and the preceding stage. With the accumulation of gas and fluid in the paralysed intestine, the abdomen begins to distend. The abdominal muscles are still "guarded" but no longer board-like; they are nevertheless tense enough to limit the distention to some degree. Tenderness is still generalised but the palpating hand is no longer resented. On auscultation, an occasional "obstructive tinkle" is heard. The characteristic picture of intestinal obstruction due to paralytic ileus, with effortless regurgitation of dark faecal-smelling fluid and meteorism, takes 36 to 48 hours to develop.

The terminal phase is a complex clinical state in which toxaemia, dehydration, paralytic ileus, oligaemia, and hypovolaemic shock with circulatory failure, all contribute. The patient is overwhelmed and a fatal outcome is inevitable. He may either drift into delirium followed by coma or may remain acutely conscious to the end. Death usually takes place some 4 to 5 days after perforation (see Chaps. 61 and 64).

Subacute perforation. An ulcer may perforate and the perforation may seal rapidly before there is spillage of gastric and duodenal contents into the general peritoneal cavity. There is a sudden onset of acute upper abdominal pain, often more severe in the right upper quadrant. It may radiate through to the back, to the pericardium or to the left scapular region. Respirations will be shallow and deep inspiration may be associated with an abrupt "catch" in the breath.

On examination, there is local tenderness and rigidity but the rest of the abdomen will be "soft" to palpation and nontender. On occasion, an x-ray film will reveal a small amount of gas under the diaphragm. The condition closely simulates acute cholecystitis. but there is no pyrexia and a history of chronic peptic ulceration may be obtained. After an hour or two, with bed rest, the pain will usually subside. Rarely, the tenderness and rigidity may extend and the signs of an acute perforation develop.

Chronic perforation. When an ulcer perforates into an area that is walled off by adhesions or by adjacent viscera such as the colon or greater omentum, or, again, where a gastric ulcer perforates into the omental sac with a sealed-off omental foramen, a *chronic abscess will form* and will give rise to considerable confusion in diagnosis. As these patients do not present with the signs and symptoms of general peritonitis, they are seldom diagnosed as having perforated peptic ulcer.

A subphrenic abscess may form. Occasionally x-ray films of the abdomen may reveal a cavity containing gas, or the radiological signs of subphrenic abscess may be demonstrated with a raised fixed diaphragm on x-ray screening (see Chap. 67). The common sites for an abscess to form are Morison's pouch, the right infrahepatic subphrenic space, the omental bursa, and the left infrahepatic subphrenic space. Usually the true diagnosis is made only on exploratory laparotomy, performed to drain the abscess.

Perforation associated with haemorrhage. The association of a perforation with massive haemorrhage is a grave but fortunately rare complication. It may present in one of three ways (Gordon-Taylor, 1937): (1) haemorrhage and perforation occurring concomitantly; (2) haemorrhage following a recently sutured perforation; and (3) perforation occurring during the medical treatment of haemorrhage.

The *first* way is associated with an extremely high mortality; it accounts for a considerable number of patients brought to hospital moribund, and may be the cause of sudden death in an elderly patient. In the *second* and *third* ways, the prognosis is much better, as these patients are already under medical observation and can be resuscitated and treated surgically before shock becomes irreversible. Nevertheless, the mortality is high. In the author's series it was over 30 percent. In most of these cases, the ulcer is large and deeply penetrates the pancreas, the liver, or the left gastric pedicle. The ulcer ruptures where it is relatively unsupported but the bleeding arises from erosion of a large vessel, such as the gastroduodenal, the splenic, or the left gastric artery, or, in the case of a perforated stomal ulcer, the middle colic artery or one of its large branches.

The clinical picture is that of acute perforated peptic ulcer associated with signs of haemorrhage. The patient is usually pale, and severely "shocked" with a rapid pulse and a low blood pressure. Energetic resuscitative measures are required and, in most cases, urgent surgery is mandatory, usually a partial gastrectomy.

Perforation of an intrathoracic gastric ulcer. Fortunately this is rare. The ulcer is in a hiatal hernia which is fixed in the mediastinum and, unless the existence of the hernia is known, it is extremely difficult to make a correct preoperative diagnosis, as the symptoms and signs point to some grave intrathoracic lesion, such as a coronary thrombosis, acute pericarditis, pulmonary embolism.

The outstanding clinical features are dysphagia, cyanosis, dyspnoea, shock, and immobility of the chest, diaphragm, and upper abdominal muscles.

An x-ray picture may reveal a quantity of gas in the mediastinum and, if there has been previous vigorous vomiting, spontaneous perforation of the oesophagus may have to be considered. Diagnosis is frequently delayed as the patients are commonly admitted to hospital as *acute medical emergencies*. Exploratory laparotomy will reveal the site of the lesion, and a thoracoabdominal incision may be required to gain access to it.

Pseudoperforation. Most surgeons at some time have operated on patients, having made a confident diagnosis of perforation, and at laparotomy found the abdominal cavity to be normal. With modern diagnostic techniques, such as radiology, this should seldom occur. Rarely is the cause of the pain discovered but occasionally an intrathoracic lesion is discovered postoperatively, such as spontaneous pneumothorax or a small coronary occlusion. In those geographical areas where neurosyphilis is still relatively common, the gastric crisis of tabes dorsalis should be considered.

DIAGNOSIS

In 95 percent of cases, the diagnosis presents little difficulty. The existence of concomitant disease may cause confusion. It is not rare for a perforation to occur in a patient under treatment in a medical ward who is suffering from cardiac or pulmonary disease, or advanced neurological disorders. The physician must be alert to this possibility and regard with suspicion acute abdominal pain occurring during the course of another illness.

Where it is impossible to make an accurate diagnosis, it is important to recognise that an acute abdominal catastrophe has occurred which requires immediate surgical treatment.

If the patient gives a history of previous gastric trouble, the advent of a sudden agonising abdominal pain followed by collapse, abdominal rigidity, and tenderness should leave no doubt in the mind of the clinician that the case is one of acute perforation. The value of x-ray examinations has already been stressed.

Differential diagnosis falls into two main categories.

1. *Acute medical conditions.* These include acute thoracic diseases (acute diaphragmatic pleurisy, lobar pneumonia, acute pericarditis, coronary thrombosis); food poisoning; gastric crises of tabes; acute alcoholism; meningitis; the preeruptive stage of herpes zoster; acute phlegmonous gastritis; and acute porphyria.

2. *Acute surgical conditions.* These include acute appendicitis; acute pancreatitis; acute intestinal obstruction; acute cholecystitis; mesenteric thrombosis; ruptured ectopic gestation; acute peritonitis from any other cause; spontaneous rupture of the oesophagus; and ruptured or dissecting aortic aneurysm.

Peritonitis from acute appendicitis. This condition may be confusing as there is usually a longer history, onset is less dramatic, fever and foetor of the breath are present and pain referred to the shoulder is unusual. Nevertheless, most surgeons have either explored the right iliac fossa, only to find that the patient has a perforated ulcer, or made an upper abdominal incision only to find that the cause of the peritonitis was in the appendix. Free air in the peritoneal cavity should *never* be present in appendicitis and an x-ray examination in the erect position will help in the diagnosis.

Acute pancreatitis. This condition simulates perforation very closely. The treatment is conservative in the first instance and most surgeons believe that immediate operation increases the mortality. Serum amylase estimations will differentiate the two in most instances. Rogers (1961) reports the results of serum amylase estimations in 1,000 perforations and in only 16 percent was it over 200 Somogyi units, and never more than 250. In the majority of cases of acute pancreatitis, figures of 600 or more are recorded, so that this investigation should be carried out as a routine procedure in all cases of suspected perforated peptic ulcer (see Chap. 36).

Intestinal obstruction. Apart from clinical differences, the abdominal x-ray scout films will often show dilated loops of intestine with fluid levels and no intraperitoneal free gas. In *acute cholecystitis,* it is rare for there to be generalised abdominal rigidity unless the gallbladder has ruptured, in which case preoperative diagnosis is purely an academic exercise. *Mesenteric thrombosis or embolism* may well be confused with perforation. *A cardiovascular lesion* and the occurrence of melaena will suggest the diagnosis. In addition, these patients are often profoundly "shocked" at the outset.

Spontaneous rupture of the oesophagus. This condition is always preceded by vigorous retching and vomiting—unusual in perforations. Gas in the mediastinum can often be demonstrated by radiology.

Ruptured aortic aneurysm. This is usually palpable. Tenderness is often maximal in the flanks or groins, and although the abdomen is guarded it is seldom, if ever, rigid. An outstanding symptom is intense back pain and the patient is usually profoundly "shocked." An anteroposterior x-ray film may reveal calcification in the aneurysm and a lateral x-ray film may show a "soft shadow" on the posterior abdominal wall with gas-containing gut in front of it (see Chap. 56).

Dissecting aneurysm. This condition may present with abdominal rigidity before the dissection has burst. Backache is intense and there may be reduction or inequality of the femoral pulses. X-ray pictures may reveal the widening of both the abdominal and the thoracic aortas and, of course, there will be no free intraperitoneal gas.

PROGNOSIS

Prognosis will depend on:

1. *The amount and nature of the fluid in the stomach at the moment of perforation.* The fuller the stomach and the greater the amount of free fluid and gas in the peritoneal cavity, the worse the prognosis.

2. *The size of the perforation.* The larger the perforation, the poorer the prognosis.

3. *The chronicity of the ulcer.* It is exceptional for a patient with a perforated *acute ulcer* not to recover. The great majority of the deaths occur when chronic ulcers perforate (Gilmour, 1953, and Desmond, 1962).

4. *The position of the ulcer.* As has been stated, the higher the ulcer is situated on the lesser curvature, the greater the postoperative mortality (Kozoll and Meyer, 1960).

5. *The age of the patient.* Under the age of 60 years the mortality is negligible but with each increasing year of age the prognosis worsens (see Fig. 1).

6. *Associated diseases.* A high proportion of older patients will have serious disease such as hypertension or cardiovascular and pulmonary conditions and will thus be less able to withstand the rigours of perforation and its associated operation. Many will die of pulmonary or cardiac complications, although recovery from the perforation is "pathologically" complete.

7. *Sex.* The postoperative mortality is higher in men although the incidence of gastric ulceration is higher in women.

8. *The time factor.* The time that has elapsed between perforation and treatment is one of the most important factors in prognosis. The longer the interval between the rupture and the operation, the higher the mortality. After 12 hours the death rate rises steeply. The "golden time" for

treatment is between 6 and 12 hours after perforation.

9. *Associated haemorrhage.* As has been stated, this considerably prejudices the patient's chance of recovery. The incidence is about 2 percent (Slater, 1951, and Avery Jones et al., 1953). A more radical surgical approach and the substitution of partial gastrectomy for simple suture has reduced the mortality considerably but this association is probably the greatest factor in prognosis.

10. *The preoperative and postoperative management.* The marked reduction in overall mortality is due to the following:

a. Improved methods of preoperative treatment, especially gastric suction, intravenous fluid and electrolyte replacement, antibiotic therapy, and blood transfusion (see Chaps. 106 and 107).

b. Improved methods of anaesthesia, especially muscle relaxants and positive-pressure pulmonary ventilation.

c. Better postoperative management, particularly greater control over infection by means of chemotherapy and antibiotics (see Chap. 107).

d. Improved operative technique and the adoption of a more radical approach to the treatment of perforated ulcer.

TREATMENT

The treatment of acute perforated ulcer in most large general hospitals is operative. Some surgeons use conservative treatment in selected cases, but, as a rule, it is adopted only for those patients who are not considered fit enough to withstand an abdominal operation.

Preoperative Management

It is mandatory that a short time be spent on resuscitation of the patient prior to operation. Precipitate surgery often leads to increased mortality, whereas preliminary attention to restoration of fluid, electrolyte, and blood loss will make surgery much safer and prevent many of the possible postoperative complications. Wound healing especially will be more certain and infection less likely.

This regime may occupy 2 or 3 hours, but if the patient is bleeding vigorously, it is essential to operate earlier.

The regimen suggested is as follows:

1. It is better to treat the patient in the supine position with only one or two pillows. If he is *in a state of shock,* the foot of the bed must be raised.

2. As soon as the diagnosis is made, pain and anxiety are relieved by an injection of Pethidine (meperidine) or Omnopon.

3. The stomach is emptied by syringe aspiration through a nasogastric tube. Mechanical suction is unreliable and the full attention of an experienced nurse is required to ensure that the stomach is completely emptied. If solid food is present, it may be necessary to pass a large stomach tube to aspirate as much as possible. Lavage should not be performed as it may open a sealed perforation or further increase the amount of peritoneal soiling. A tube should be left in the stomach during the operation and postoperatively.

4. No fluids are given by mouth, although thirst should be treated by saline mouth washes. An intravenous infusion of 0.18 percent saline in 4.3 percent glucose solution should be commenced and, provided renal function is normal, a litre may be safely given in the first hour. A specimen of blood is taken for blood count, blood grouping, electrolyte estimations, and serum amylase estimations. If the patient is anaemic or there is associated haemorrhage, a slow blood transfusion is commenced. Deficiency in chloride should be rectified by infusions of normal saline. Where shock is severe, plasma or plasma expanders such as dextran are given until blood is available.

5. If the patient is unable to pass urine and the bladder is distended, a catheter should be inserted. The urine must be tested, especially for sugar.

6. The blood pressure and pulse rate should be taken and recorded at half-hourly intervals.

7. It is probably inadvisable to administer an antibiotic—e.g., penicillin and/or streptomycin, at this stage, as a routine procedure.

8. Preparation of the abdomen is better postponed until the patient is anaesthetised. Not until the clinician has satisfied himself that the patient is in as good a condition as possible should he be taken to the operating room.

Surgery

For many years the treatment of perforated peptic ulcer consisted (almost exclusively) of suturing the perforation with or without drainage of the peritoneal cavity. Occasionally, in the presence of pyloric stenosis a gastroenterostomy was performed and rarely a tube gastrostomy or duodenostomy was carried out.

Simple suture remains the standard treatment today but many clinics have found that, in selected cases, more radical treatment by emergency gastric resection or by vagotomy associated with a gastric drainage procedure is not associated with increased mortality, and some authors report a decline in both mortality and morbidity. Keetley (1902) was the first to perform gastric resection in perforated ulcer, but it was von Haberer who popularised the operation in 1919.

Simple suture.   Until the turn of the century perforation of peptic ulcer was usually a fatal event. Isolated cases of recovery after operation were recorded and, no doubt, a number of patients recovered spontaneously. The first operations consisted of simple suture of the rupture with two rows of Lembert sutures, washing out the peritoneal cavity with warm water or antiseptic solutions, and inserting rubber or glass drainage tubes down to the site of the ulcer, to the pelvis and sometimes to the loins. We now realise that peritoneal lavage is unnecessary and often harmful and that drainage is required only in the presence of established bacterial peritonitis.

Bennett (1896) first suggested that in some cases in which the perforation was very large and the opening difficult to suture owing to the friability of the parts, omentum could be used to plug the defect. Today, it is found more satisfactory to introduce three interrupted sutures, one at the top, one in the middle, and one at the bottom of the perforation and, after bringing up a portion of the greater omentum and laying it over the defect, to tie them, in order to hold it in position (Fig. 8). Cellan-Jones (1929) and Roscoe (1937) emphasised the simplicity and effectiveness of this procedure and maintained that it never produced duodenal stenosis.

The operation of simple suture is straightforward and quick to perform; it seldom takes more than a few minutes after the abdomen has been opened and does not require any special experience or skill in abdominal surgery, nor does it subject the patient to prolonged anaesthesia or shock. It aims solely at warding off the immediate danger in a patient who is seriously ill and whose life is threatened, while subjecting him to the minimum amount of operative trauma.

The object is not to cure the ulcer; this can be deferred to a later date. *Nevertheless cure can be achieved in 85 percent by this simple technique if the ulcer is acute, and in 25 percent if it is of the chronic type.*

Many large series of cases of perforated ulcers treated by simple suture have been reported and the results show great variation. Gilmour and Saint (1932) reported a mortality of 4.7 percent, while Houston (1946) gives the Newcastle figures for 1943 as 184 cases with 8.2 percent mortality and for 1944 as 190 cases with 6.3 percent mortality. Avery Jones (1957) reported a 4.9 percent mortality in 365 cases. The writer's figures (Desmond, 1957) show a mortality of 5.8 percent in duodenal ulcers and 21 percent in gastric ulcers when treated by simple suture. Kingsbury and Pennoyer (1962) report a mortality of 12 percent in 506 operations.

These figures can hardly be considered entirely satisfactory and have led many surgeons to try other methods, some more conservative and some more radical. Attention has also been drawn to the late results in perforated *chronic* duodenal ulcers. Approximately 3 percent reperforate and 75 percent of the patients will continue to have symptoms; about 50 percent will require further surgery. The high incidence of perforated gastric ulcers that are found to be malignant has also caused much concern.

Finally, when patients in whom perforation is associated with haemorrhage are treated by simple suture, the incidence of postoperative haemorrhage is high, sometimes necessitating a second operation in a few days.

With these considerations in mind, many surgeons are now performing simple suture only in selected cases and are employing a more radical procedure, such as partial gastrectomy or vagotomy plus a drainage operation, in others. They have been gratified to find that the mortality is no higher and is in many instances even lower than with simple suture.

Technique of simple closure.   The choice of anaesthetic must be left to the expert anaesthetist. Muscle relaxants have added greatly to the ease of performance of the operation and the peritoneal toilet and wound closure simplified. As these patients are unprepared and many are heavy smokers with chronic respiratory disease, tracheobronchial toilet is essential during and after the operation.

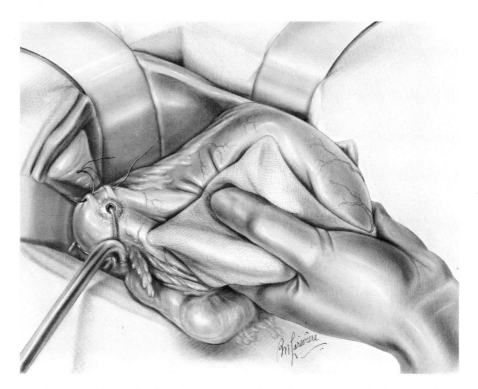

FIG. 7.   Acute perforated duodenal ulcer. Note method of exposure. Aspiration of fluid in right subhepatic space.

There is a *choice of two epigastric incisions:* midline or paramedian. I prefer the midline, as it is the most rapid method of "entry"; it is easy to close; and, in a potentially infected area, it does not lay open the rectus sheath. On opening the peritoneal cavity there is often an escape of gas and the wound may be quickly flooded with fluid. The edges of the wound should be gently retracted and the right lobe of the liver drawn upward with a suitable retractor, so as to bring the lesser curvature of the stomach, the pylorus, and the first part of the duodenum into view.

In most cases the perforation is readily seen (Fig. 7). It may be oval or circular and punched out, and of variable diameter. Through this opening the stomach contents will be seen to pour intermittently or continuously. In duodenal perforations, the escaping fluid is usually bile-stained and somewhat frothy. The gut around the perforation is injected and oedematous in many cases.

In the *acute ulcer,* the duodenum is mobile and there are no adhesions. In *large chronic ulcers* the first part of the duodenum seems to be but part of a chronic inflammatory mass consisting of greater omentum, the pancreatic head, the lower portion of the stomach, and sometimes the liver and the hepatic flexure of the colon. All variations between these two extremes may be encountered. In many the perforation will be sealed at the time of laparotomy and may not be obvious without a careful search. Occasionally omentum, some viscus, or the anterior abdominal wall seals the hole and only separation of one or other of these structures will reveal the perforation. If the perforation is so obscured, gentle dissection with the finger will produce some welling-up of fluid and thus reveal it.

A perforated gastric ulcer may be immediately revealed on gently drawing down the stomach. It is commonly situated on the anterior part of the lesser curvature. If the site of the perforation is not immediately obvious,

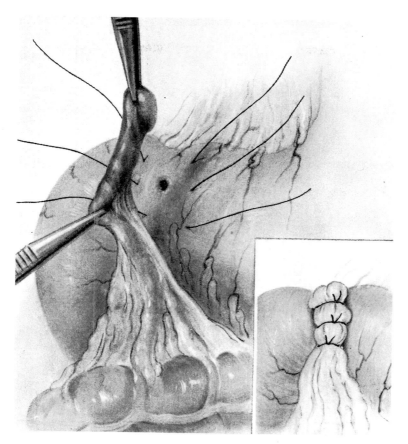

FIG. 8. Perforated duodenal ulcer. Simple suture by Roscoe Graham technique. Three sutures of silk or cotton are introduced through the duodenal wall one above, one below, and one through the perforation. A portion of omentum is drawn across the perforation and the sutures are tied in the manner depicted in the *inset*.

a careful search may reveal a posterior gastric ulcer that has ruptured into the lesser sac. It is possible for such an ulcer to rupture, for the contents of the stomach to distend the omental bursa, and for the fluid to drain through the omental foramen and contaminate the general peritoneal cavity. The exact site of the perforation is difficult to find in these cases and simple closure may be a hazardous undertaking.

On occasion, perforation of an ulcer of the second part of the duodenum may be unmasked by mobilising of the duodenum by Kocher's method.

There are many ways of closing a perforation. Perhaps the simplest is to introduce three interrupted sutures of 0 chromic cat-

gut or silk mounted on atraumatic (eyeless) needles, the first above, the second below, and the third through the opening. A convenient portion of the greater omentum is laid over the perforation and the sutures tied gently to maintain it in place. Too much tension on the sutures may cause them to cut out, especially if the gut wall is oedematous and fixed (see Fig. 8). This method is applicable to all acute or chronic perforations. Where the ulcer is acute and the gut mobile, the hole can be more meticulously sutured, but usually this is unnecessary.

A purse-string suture is not recommended, except perhaps where there is a very small hole due to an acute ulcer. Certainly it should never be employed in perforation of large chronic gastric or duodenal ulcers, as the suture will cut out through the friable tissues.

It is very rare that suture by such a technique produces more than a temporary pyloric obstruction. Although postoperative gastric retention may occur for a while, the oedema around the ulcer soon subsides and normal gastroduodenal flow is restored. Thus it is unwise to add gastrojejunostomy at this stage. It is better to suture the perforation and await events. In rare cases in which obstruction persists, a definitive and curative operation can be carried out a week or so later.

Peritoneal toilet should then be carried out. It is remarkable how the patient's general condition will improve when excess fluid has been sucked out of the peritoneal cavity. It should be done meticulously, to a fixed routine, and with an efficient suction apparatus, thus:

1. The subphrenic spaces should be gently revealed by drawing down the liver.
2. Rutherford Morison's pouch and the right paracolic gutter are exposed by retracting the intestines medially.
3. A hand should draw up the intestines while the fluid is removed from the pelvis.
4. The spleen should be retracted medially and the left subphrenic area and the paracolic gutter sucked out.
5. No attempt should be made to remove fluid from amongst the coils of small intestine, but solid pieces of food or debris should be removed if found during these manipulations.
6. Swabbing with gauze should be minimal, as it is traumatic to the inflamed visceral peritoneum and may encourage the formation of adhesions.
7. A specimen of the fluid should be taken for bacteriological examination.

Drainage is necessary only when frank pus is present in the peritoneal cavity, in which case a latex drainage tube should be placed in the pelvis through a suprapubic stab wound and, if the infection is gross, another inserted in Morison's pouch through a right subcostal stab wound.

In addition, it is wise to drain the superficial layers of the abdominal incision in obese patients with frank peritonitis.

After meticulous haemostasis, the abdominal incision is closed by one or other of the methods described in Chapter 1.

PERFORATED GASTROJEJUNAL ULCERS

Perforated stomal ulcers pose a more complicated problem, as, owing to adhesions from previous partial gastrectomy or gastrojejunostomy, it may be difficult to find the perforation; such is especially the case if a posterior (retrocolic) anastomosis has been fashioned. The transverse colon and greater omentum overlie the anastomosis, and careful mobilisation may be required to reveal it. Suture closure of the perforation must be performed with great care; otherwise there is danger of narrowing or distorting the anastomosis and of causing postoperative efferent or afferent loop obstruction (see Chap. 24).

Simple suture in the presence of stenosis. When a perforated duodenal ulcer is associated with a severe degree of pyloric stenosis, simple closure of the perforation may aggravate the obstruction. In such cases, it is probably better to perform either a partial gastrectomy or a vagotomy with a drainage procedure, such as pyloroplasty or gastrojejunostomy.

In desperate cases of gastric ulcer perforations, it may be wiser to perform *catheter gastrostomy* using a No. 16 Foley catheter, and, if a subsequent operation becomes necessary, the patient will be in good shape to withstand partial gastrectomy.

Simple suture in perforations associated with haemorrhage. When haemorrhage is combined with acute perforation, it is better that a radical operation be performed as an emergency procedure. As a posterior duodenal ulcer is usually the site of the bleeding when an anterior one perforates, or part of a peptic ulcer perforates and another part bleeds, simple suture is likely to be followed by postoperative bleeding in a high proportion of cases. When suture is performed as a matter of expediency, it should be realised that this may be a *temporary measure* and, if the patient's general condition improves sufficiently, early reoperation may be necessary to carry out the radical procedure.

Emergency Radical Treatment

Partial gastrectomy. According to Sir Zachary Cope (1965), Keetley in 1902 had to operate upon a large perforated ulcer situated near the pylorus for which he thought fit to perform a pyloroduodenectomy. The patient made an excellent recovery and in consequence Keetley warmly advocated this procedure. However, few surgeons practised partial gastrectomy for ruptured peptic ulcer until recent years. From 1919 onwards, von Haberer and other Continental surgeons were urging the adoption of gastric resection for both perforated gastric and duodenal ulcer.

It is not surprising that partial gastrectomy should be tried in certain cases of perforated ulcer. While at first it was performed only in patients who came to operation soon after perforation, it was discovered that successful results might be obtained even in later cases. Bisgard (1945), for example, stated that gastric resection can be performed in good-risk patients (even in the presence of diffuse peritoneal soiling) within 12 hours after perforation, with a lower mortality than simple suture, and that this particularly applied to cases of gastric perforations.

Sirgrist (1957) reported that 195 of 302 patients with an acute perforation had a primary gastric resection with a 5 percent mortality and 90 percent excellent postoperative results. Nuboer (1951) reported 131 patients so treated, with 5 deaths, and Lowden (1952) reported 57 cases with no fatality. Jordan and DeBakey (1963) carried out 317 partial gastrectomies and 22 antrectomies combined with vagotomy, and state that their mortality was no higher than in elective cases. In the author's series, there have been 305 gastric resections for acute perforations: 202 patients were under 60 years of age, with only 1 death; 268 were under 70 years of age, with 11 deaths (4 percent mortality), and, when the 37 patients over 70 years of age are included in the series, the mortality for the 305 resections was 6.2 percent.

It is therefore clear that gastric resection for acute perforated peptic ulcer is a safe operation, but certain provisos must be laid down:

1. First and foremost, the facilities must be ideal.
2. The surgeon must be experienced in gastric surgery.
3. The patient should be in reasonably fit condition to withstand the operation.

With these in mind I would advocate the method:

1. In all cases of perforated gastric ulcer, because 10 percent are malignant. Furthermore, in many cases, the ulcer is a large one eroding into the pancreas, and simple suture is unlikely to be successful.
2. Where haemorrhage and perforation occur concomitantly.
3. In cases of perforated duodenal ulcer associated with stenosis.
4. Where the patient has had a previous perforation which was treated by simple suture.
5. In all cases of *chronic* duodenal ulcer, as evidenced by the length of history and/or the appearance of the ulcer at operation.
6. In the presence of combined gastric and duodenal ulcer, one of which has perforated.

I would add two contraindications to gastric resection. (1) In patients below the age of 30 years, the approach should be less radical. These young patients should be given a chance to cure their ulcer by medical means. Unless the ulcer is gastric, or a duodenal ulcer has been present for many years, they should be treated by simple suture. (2) In young patients suffering from an acute duodenal ulcer perforation, who give a short history of dyspepsia, and who at operation have a mobile duodenum and minimal induration and oedema, simple suture is unquestionably preferred to radical measures.

In my opinion the operation of choice for perforated duodenal ulcer is an antecolic Polya-Hofmeister type of operation with the shortest possible afferent jejunal loop, and for gastric ulcer a Billroth I operation with an end-to-end gastroduodenal anastomosis. However, it matters little what type of gastrectomy is used provided it is one known to have a low incidence of postgastrectomy syndromes.

Vagotomy and drainage procedures. In recent years, vagotomy combined with pyloroplasty, gastroenterostomy, or antrectomy has in large measure replaced gastric resection in the treatment of duodenal ulcer.

The technique, apart from meticulous peritoneal toilet, differs in no way from elective procedures, and fears that mediastinitis may be caused following vagotomy have not been fulfilled. A pyloroplasty is usually added to the vagotomy where this is technically feasible but, when there is gross induration and oedema of the duodenum, it is better to suture the perforation, and perform a gastrojejunostomy combined with vagotomy. When haemorrhage is associated with the perforation, vagotomy plus antrectomy with a gastroduodenal or a gastrojejunal anastomosis is advocated.

Hamilton and Harlbrecht (1967) report 36 such patients, with no deaths, and of these 28 percent were operated upon between 13 and 24 hours after the perforation: 27 had vagotomy and pyloroplasty, 3 had partial gastrectomy, and 6 antrectomy with complementary vagotomies, the reason for the associated resections being concomitant haemorrhage.

Pierandozzi et al. (1960) performed vagotomy plus a drainage procedure on 75 good-risk patients, all with acute perforations of under 12 hours, with 1 death. Kincannon et al. (1963) report 34 selected cases, all with perforations under 12 hours and no deaths; 15 percent of their patients were over 60.

The writer has had experience of 20 cases, all of which were unselected and in all age groups. The patients have all done well with minimal postoperative complications and a reasonably good follow-up.

I would not, however, recommend vagotomy plus pyloroplasty for perforated gastric ulcers, particularly in view of the high association of carcinoma with these lesions.

Selective vagotomy and drainage. Recently there has been a swing away from truncal or total vagotomy in the treatment of duodenal ulcers, to the technique of selective vagotomy, in which the nerves to the stomach are severed and the hepatic and coeliac branches preserved (see Chap. 15).

Although this is technically a more difficult and tedious procedure, the efficacy of which is still under review, it could be that in due course this method may replace truncal vagotomy, in which case one can see no reason why it should not be performed as an emergency procedure.

In summary, it may be said that whilst simple suture still remains the most commonly employed method, radical treatment of perforated gastric ulcers by partial gastrectomy and perforated duodenal ulcers by antrectomy plus vagotomy is justified in the hands of experienced surgeons. There is no doubt that vagotomy plus a draine procedure carries a lower mortality rate than partial gastrectomy alone, and it is a matter of personal choice as to which radical operation is used. When a massive indurated duodenal ulcer has perforated, partial gastrectomy may be, and often is, a hazardous procedure and vagotomy plus gastroenterostomy (with the stoma fashioned in the antrum) is the treatment of choice. (Chap. 19.)

Similarly, when the perforated ulcer is gastrojejunal, gastric resection may be difficult and complicated. Vagotomy, again, would be the treatment of choice, but care must be taken not to obstruct the stoma when suturing the perforation.

POSTOPERATIVE COMPLICATIONS

Peritonitis. This accounts for the majority of the fatalities, but it must be remembered that a large number of elderly patients with cardiovascular and respiratory diseases perforate peptic ulcers. The cooperation of an experienced physician in the postoperative period may prevent many deaths from *cardiac failure* or overwhelming *chest infections.*

Subphrenic and pelvic abscesses. These are not uncommon; but all surgeons who have had experience of gastric resection for acute perforations have noted the dramatic fall in the number of residual abscesses when compared to those encountered with simple suture. *Postoperative haemorrhage* is always a risk after simple suture and may require further urgent surgery. After a gastric resection, this may occur from the suture line and is seldom severe (see Chap. 26).

Gastric and duodenal fistulas. These

may occur after simple suture but with modern techniques should not occur after gastric resection or vagotomy plus a drainage operation. The *wound infection* rate is high, whatever the method of treatment used, especially where bacterial peritonitis is established, but wound disruption, postoperative phlebothrombosis, and pulmonary embolism follow the same patterns as in elective surgery (see Chaps. 9, 26, and 57).

Postoperative care after simple suture. The patient returns to bed with nasogastric tube still in situ and the intravenous infusion still running. He is nursed flat in the supine position until consciousness is fully regained, after which he should be gradually raised into the sitting-up posture. Subject to the degree of shock and restoration of normal blood pressure, an half-hourly pulse chart is kept. Gastric aspirations are continued until the returning fluid becomes clear, and auscultation of the abdomen reveals the return of peristalsis. An accurate fluid-balance chart and daily electrolyte estimations will regulate the quantity and quality of the intravenous fluid. Vitamins B and C should be given intramuscularly. Anaemia should be rectified by blood transfusions. Antibiotics should not be given routinely. The specific indications for such therapy are where bacterial peritonitis is present or where a chest infection coexists. The result of the cultures taken at operation will dictate the use of a specific antibiotic agent (see Chap. 107).

Regular physiotherapy to promote chest expansion and good bronchial drainage should be started as soon as possible. Early ambulation will reduce the liability to postoperative thromboembolic complications. Adequate analgesia is essential to facilitate this regime.

As soon as the gastric aspirations are satisfactory and there are signs of returning intestinal activity, 2-hourly milk feeds are commenced with alkalis, anticholinergic, and sedative drugs.

The late presentation. Occasionally a patient with a perforated ulcer is admitted to hospital in a late stage of the disease, with established peritonitis and circulatory failure. The mortality rate is very high in such cases and treatment presents a formidable problem. As previously stated, Kozoll and Meyer (1960) found 188 such patients in their series of 1904 perforations; with conservative management 123 of these died.

The first consideration in the management of such patients is vigorous *resuscitation*. They are usually in a state of severe shock and require intravenous infusions of plasma or blood, followed by normal saline, to restore their blood volume and peripheral circulation. Large doses of antibiotics should be administered. *Oxygen therapy has proved beneficial.* Such resuscitative measures must necessarily be modified according to the age and general condition of the patient, since too rapid a transfusion may precipitate left ventricular failure in the elderly or in those with poor cardiac function. The use of a central venous pressure manometer is of the utmost value in regulating the rate of infusion.

In some cases these measures will improve the patient's condition sufficiently to allow operative treatment to be carried out. In many patients, however, although there may be some improvement, a degree of circulatory failure will persist. In such instances a choice has to be made between early surgery and stubborn armed expectancy.

The accepted routine is to perform a laparotomy under local anaesthesia and remove as much purulent fluid as possible with minimal operative manipulation, suture the perforation, and insert drainage tubes into the pelvis, into Morison's pouch, and elsewhere, if required. My experience with this method has not been associated with much success and, in 1953, I decided to adopt a more radical approach to the problem, as illustrated by the following case report.

CASE REPORT

A man, aged 64, was admitted pulseless, with no recordable blood pressure, and with clinical peripheral circulatory failure. He had a rheumatic mitral valvular lesion, chronic bronchitis, and emphysema. A perforation had occurred 24 hours before and the abdomen was distended and silent. Resuscitation restored the blood pressure to 60 mm Hg systolic, but the diastolic pressure remained unrecordable. Under local anaesthesia, a laparotomy revealed a large perforation of a massive duodenal ulcer measuring 7 by 4 cm, encircling the duodenum, and penetrating the pancreas, liver, and gallbladder. A thorough peritoneal toilet was carried out, after which it was observed that the patient's general condition improved dramatically. A *Polya-Hofmeister partial gastrectomy was performed and the peritoneal cavity drained.* At the end of the operation the blood pressure had risen to 110 mm Hg systolic, the peripheral circulation was normal, and the pulse was of good volume, but rapid. He made an uninterrupted recovery.

Since 1953 I have treated several patients in a similar fashion with a satisfactory fall in mortality.

Medical or Conservative Management

If operative interference is withheld and medical treatment is undertaken, one of three results may be expected:

1. The abdominal tenderness and rigidity may gradually disappear and the perforation close.
2. A localised abscess—perigastric or subphrenic—may form.
3. The patient may die of septic peritonitis.

Studied conservatism may be justifiable in certain circumstances: in the early acute case in which the diagnosis is in doubt, when the patient is a poor operative risk, in aged and infirm patients, and in some cases, in subacute peptic ulcer perforations. Nonsurgical methods of treatment may be carried out in such cases provided that all facilities are at hand for immediate operation, should this prove to be necessary.

Again, if the patient is seen for the first time some days after perforation has occurred and there is sufficient evidence that the infective process is definitely limited and well confined, more is to be gained by waiting than by performing an injudicious exploration for a condition that is likely to resolve itself. When operation is undertaken at a later date in such cases, operative measures for the cure of the condition are rendered easier and more satisfactory by the reduction in the size of the ulcer. On the other hand, if a perigastric or subphrenic abscess does not resolve, expectant treatment will ensure its being securely shut off.

I must emphasize that if the diagnosis remains uncertain for 6 hours or so, if the patient has x-ray evidence of a gastric ulcer or gives a history of a previous operation, or again, if he shows no improvement after a trial of aspiration treatment, abdominal exploration should be carried out without delay.

Conservative (expectant, nonsurgical, or aspiration) treatment consists of continuous effective gastric aspiration, combined with antibiotic agents, adequate intravenous fluid administration, and sedation. It requires constant and skilful watchful care, enthusiasm, and at least two straight x-ray film checks (with the patient in the sitting-up position) to determine the amount of air (if any) beneath the right cupola of the diaphragm, and the correct positioning of the nasogastric tube in the pyloric antrum. No fluids are permitted by mouth for the first 48 hours. Laparotomy is performed if there is no obvious clinical improvement.

The chief *objections* to the nonoperative treatment are:

1. *Uncertainty or error in diagnosis.* Bertram (1957) rightly states that if the diagnosis is not clear and if the possibilities of atypical coronary thrombosis and other nonsurgical diseases and acute pancreatitis have been carefully excluded, exploratory operation is imperative. In actual experience the errors in diagnosis are nearly always in the direction of conditions requiring urgent surgical intervention rather than conditions that are usually treated conservatively.
2. *The site of the perforation is unknown.* It is agreed that acute perforated gastric ulcers result in a higher death rate than do perforations of duodenal ulcers when medical management is employed for these cases. The same is in all probability true of treatment by suction.
3. *The possibility of treating a perforated gastric carcinoma.*

The medical management of acute perforated peptic ulcer has been discussed in a most comprehensive manner by Chamberlain (1951), Heslop et al. (1952), and Taylor (1957). Taylor reported a mortality of 9.6 percent, which should be contrasted with the mortality following simple suture and immediate partial gastrectomy. Seely and Campbell (1956) reported a collected series of 139 such cases, with a mortality rate of 5 percent.

The adoption of this method of treatment has proved successful in *some hospitals* but *most* surgeons agree that early operative treatment is preferable.

REFERENCES

Aird, I., Br. J. Surg. 22:545, 1935.

Armitage, G. H., Br. Med. J. 1:615, 1953.

Avery Jones, F., and Doll, R., Br. Med. J. 1:122, 1953.

Avery Jones, F., Br. Med. J. 1:786, 1957.

Bager, B., Acta Chir. Scand. 64:5, 1929.

Bird, C. E., Lumper, M. A., and Mayer, J. M., Ann. Surg. 114:526, 1941.

Bisgard, J. D., Surgery 17:498, 1945.

Boyce, F. F., Surg. Gynec. Obstet. 83:718, 1946.

Cellan-Jones, C. J., Br. Med. J. 1:1076, 1929.

Chamberlain, D., Proc. R. Soc. Med. 44:273, 1951.

Cope, Z. V., Proc. R. Soc. Med. 31:465, 1938.

Davison, M., Aries, L. J., and Pilot, I., Surg. Gynecol. Obstet. 68:1017, 1939.

DeBakey, M. E., Surgery 8:852, 1940.

Desmond, A. M., and Seargeant, P. W., Br. J. Surg. 45:283, 1957.

Desmond, A. M., Calif. Med. 96:315, 1962.

Doll, R., Br. Med. J. 1:215, 1950.

Edwards, R. H., and Foster, J. H., Am. J. Surg. 105:551, 1962.

Estes, W. L., and Bennett, W. A., Ann. Surg. 119:321, 1944.

Fallis, L. S., Ann. Surg. 41:427, 1938.

Gilmour, J., and Saint, J. H., Br. J. Surg. 20:78, 1932.

Gilmour, J., Lancet 1:870, 1953.

Gordon-Taylor, G., Br. J. Surg. 25:403, 1937.

Hamilton, J. E., and Harbrecht, P. J., Surg. Gynecol. Obstet. 124:61, 1967.

Heslop, T. S., Bullough, A. S., and Brun, C., Br. J. Surg. 40:52, 1952.

Houston, W., Br. J. Surg. 2:221, 1946.

Illingworth, G. P. W., Scott, L. D. W., and Jamieson, R. A., Br. Med. J. 2:617, 1944.

Jacobson, G., Berne, G. J., Meyers, H. I., and Rossoff, L., Am. J. Roentgenol. 86:37, 1961.

Jamieson, R. A., Br. Med. J. 2:289, 1947.

Jordan, G. L., and DeBakey, M. E., Calif. Med. 98:7, 1963.

Keetley, C. B., Lancet 1:885, 1902.

Kennedy, R. L. J., J. Pediat. 2:641, 1933.

Kennedy, T., Br. Med. J. 2:1849, 1951.

Kincannon, W. N., McLenathin, C. W., and Weinberg, J. A., Ann. Surg. 29:692, 1963.

Kingsbury, H. A., and Pennoyer, D. C., Postgrad. Med. 31:364, 1962.

Kozoll, D. D., and Meyer, K. A., Surg. Gynecol. Obstet. 111:607, 1960.

Kozoll, D. D., and Meyer, K. A., Arch. Surg. 84:646, 1962.

Lowden, A. G. R., Lancet 1:1267, 1952.

MacKay, C., Br. Med. J. 1:689, 1966.

McNealy, R. W., and Hearn, R. F., Surg. Gynecol. Obstet. 67:818, 1938.

Maingot, R., Personal communication, 1973.

Millar Bell, D., Lancet 2:810, 1953.

Moncrief, W. H., Ann. Surg. 139:99, 1954.

Moore, S. W., Surg. Clin. N. Amer. 429:30, 1950.

Nuboer, J. F., Lancet 2:952, 1951.

Picrandozzi, J. S., Himshaw, D. B., and Stafford, C. E., Am. J. Surg. 100:245, 1960.

Reams, G. B., Dinnaway, J. B., and Watts, W. L., Pediatrics 31:97, 1963.

Rogers, F. A., Ann. Surg. 153:228, 1961.

Roscoe, G. R., Surg. Gynecol. Obstet. 64:235, 1937.

Seeley, S. F., and Campbell, D. C., Surg. Gynecol. Obstet. 102:435, 1956.

Sirgrist, J., Am. J. Surg. 94:911, 1957.

Slater, N. S., Br. Med. J. 2:1257, 1951.

Spiro, H. M., and Milles, S. S., N. Engl. J. Med. 263:286, 1960.

Strang, C., and Spencer, I. O. B., Br. Med. J. 1:873, 1950.

Taylor, H., Gastroenterology 33:353, 1957.

Tilton, B. T., Am. J. Surg. 32:238, 1936.

Vale, C. F., and Cameron, D. A., Ann. Surg. 103:353, 1936.

von Haberer, H., Wien Klin. Wochenschr. 32:413, 1919.

Weir, R. D., Scot. Med. J. 5:257, 1960.

23

ACUTE HAEMATEMESIS AND MELAENA FROM PEPTIC ULCERATION
Aetiology, Diagnosis, Medical and Surgical Management

SIR FRANCIS AVERY JONES and **JOHN W. P. GUMMER**

The management of acute haematemesis and melaena necessitates close cooperation between the physician and the surgeon. The physician has much to offer in diagnosis and the emergency management of the bleeding, but the surgeon must be kept appropriately in the picture, as the timing of surgical intervention is very important if the best results are to be achieved. The clear objective of every hospital must be that a maximum possible number of medical and surgical patients leave the hospital. Haematemesis with melaena is a complication that carries a significant mortality rate, particularly in older age groups—a mortality rate that can be reduced not only by technical skill, but also by good organization. An effective way of providing good organization is for all the patients admitted to one hospital to be admitted under one medical unit, and to have the patients remain in this department if surgery is needed. This has been the practice at Central Middlesex Hospital for over 30 years, and during this time over 4,500 patients have been so treated. The medical team have the urgent responsibility of resuscitation and of going as far as possible in diagnosis. In seriously ill patients, emphasis must be kept on restoring the blood volume, and, in the case of catastrophic bleeding, the arrest of haemorrhage surgically. Diagnostic measures may not even be possible, as they could delay urgent treatment. The advantage of centralizing the management of these patients is that the team becomes very experienced in their management, surgical cooperation is streamlined, and excellent opportunities are provided for clinical research studies. Clinical vigilance can pay big diagnostic dividends,

as all members of the team are on the lookout for the occasional unexpected diagnosis. Although the majority of these patients are admitted for peptic ulceration, there are a number of occasional causes when accurate diagnosis is essential in order to achieve the best results.

In approaching the problem, it is of some value to have a mental picture of the relative incidence of different diagnoses, and the experience at Central Middlesex Hospital has been as shown in Table 1.

Table 1. ADMITTED FOR HAEMATEMESIS MELAENA, 1941-70, INCLUSIVE

Lesion	Number	Percent
Chronic gastric ulcer	741	16.3
Duodenal ulcer	1,593	35.1
Postoperative	271	6.0
Acute gastric lesions	1,111	24.5
Hiatal hernia	120	2.6
Unclassified	134	3.0
Total	3,970	
Malignant gastric neoplasms	120	2.6
Portal hypertension	233	2.9
Other causes	316	7.0
	4,639	100.0

An alternative mental approach is to have a picture of the mechanisms of alimentary bleeding clearly in the mind. The mechanisms may be classified as follows:

Erosion and/or rupture of blood vessels, associated with:

Peptic or pancreatic digestion
Pressure necrosis, e.g., aneurysm

Hypertension—systemic or portal

Angiectasis

Abiotrophy, e.g., pseudoxanthoma elasticum

Infiltrations, e.g., amyloid

Atherosclerosis

Bacterial inflammation

Trauma, e.g., Mallory-Weiss

Gastrostaxis or enterostaxis:

Idiopathic

Secondary

It is important to emphasize that bleeding can occur not only from a single bleeding point but from a diffuse mucosal haemorrhagic reaction, gastrostaxis or enterostaxis. Doig and Shafar [4] presented an admirable study of the disturbed haemodynamics associated with superficial mucosal haemorrhages following intracranial vascular accidents. They pointed out that venules forming the source of the haemorrhages were often much dilated, and there were perivascular haemorrhages that tended to coalesce to form typical wedge-shaped superficial mucosal haemorrhages, and some of these could develop into small acute ulcers. There is still insufficient knowledge of these diffuse haemorrhagic reactions. Some may be due to a pinpoint vascular accident in the hypothalamus, and some may be due to an acute disruption of the normal defence mechanism of the mucosa—a defence which depends on the integrity of the mucus coating. The defence mechanism can be impaired by vitamin deficiencies, and also by anti-inflammatory drugs that may increase the permeability of the mucus protective layer to hydrogen ions, which may then reflux back through the mucosa and so damage the gastric epithelial cells.

There are four clinical groups of special interest to surgeons:

1. Patients with sudden, unheralded, life-threatening bleeding.
2. Patients with steady, slow, continued bleeding.
3. Patients with recurring, separate crises of bleeding.
4. Patients with known peptic ulcer.

CLINICAL GROUPS

Patients with Sudden, Unheralded, Life-Threatening Bleeding

These are patients in whom the severity of the haemorrhage may necessitate an early decision to operate, and, in spite of rapid transfusion, CVP (central venous pressure) measurements may indicate failure to restore or to maintain blood volume. The majority of these patients will have acute or chronic painless peptic ulcers. Fibre-optic endoscopy is invaluable in demonstrating these ulcers, which are commonly found high up on the posterior wall, associated with varying degrees of gastric mucosal atrophy. They will be impalpable from the outside of the stomach, but the bleeding vessel may be felt, like a lead shot, when the mucosa is palpated. Posterior wall duodenal ulcers may also be impalpable, and their presence may not be appreciated until the duodenum is opened through a pyloroplasty incision. Sometimes a large, chronic ulcer will be found in spite of the absence of any dyspeptic history. This can occur particularly in those patients who are relatively pain-insensitive to normal stimuli—a point which can be demonstrated clinically.

Mallory-Weiss syndrome. The important clue to the diagnosis in these patients is the fact that they have vomited food first and then, perhaps several hours later, have had a haematemesis. The physical strain of vomiting has caused a laceration at the junction of the oesophagus and the cardia—a situation more liable to happen if there is some degree of atrophic gastritis, and if there is a sliding hiatal hernia as well, which means that the pressure in the lower oesophagus can build up more quickly and reach a point where the mucosa splits. The lesion can also occur in patients who have had severe coughing bouts or status epilepticus. Endoscopy can demonstrate the lesions quite clearly, but it is necessary to get the stomach well blown up with air as the instrument is withdrawn. Bleeding is not controlled by tamponage, and the tear may need surgical underrunning. As it is a lesion easily overlooked at operation, it is one which must always be kept in mind when operating in these circumstances.

Portal hypertension. The diagnosis of portal hypertension can fortunately be made clinically in the majority of patients, as hepatosplenomegaly may be found, together with cutaneous manifestations of parenchymatous liver disease. In this group of patients it is well worthwhile making every attempt to control bleeding with vasopressin (Pitressin) or balloon pressure on the cardia, and, if the bleeding stops, to investigate in more detail the possibility of pathological lesions of the liver. Although the majority of patients are postsinusoidal, intrahepatic, and there is also an association with cirrhosis, thus carrying a poor prognosis, it must be remembered that the presinusoidal causes, including splenic or portal block, primary portal hypertension, congenital hepatic fibrosis, and schistosomiasis carry a better prognosis, and elective surgery may prove very successful.

Leiomyoma. This condition can cause a sudden, entirely unheralded, severe haematemesis, but the diagnosis does not normally present difficulties, as the smooth tumour can be easily visualized gastroscopically or radiologically, or easily felt at laparotomy. Some difficulties may occur, however, when a leiomyoma is present in the jejunum, as it may give rise to postprandial pain. A diagnosis of duodenal ulcer may be readily accepted, as the tumour may be very difficult to palpate, particularly in the region of the duodenojejunal flexure.

A solitary, abnormally large, submucosal artery. This condition again can cause sudden, entirely unheralded, massive bleeding, and it is due to rupture of a single abnormally large artery in the submucosa, usually in the stomach, but it has been reported in the upper intestine as well. Such arteries appear to be otherwise normal and do not show any arteriosclerotic changes. One such patient has been seen in this series, and Goldman [6] reviewed twenty-four patients described in the literature. The mucosal defect may be very small—only 2 to 5 mm in diameter—and merely exposing the large artery, which a surgeon may be able to feel after opening the stomach. Similar bleeding

from ruptured normal-sized blood vessels may occur in patients with pseudoxanthoma elasticum (Grönblad-Strandberg syndrome) and in the Ehlers-Danlos syndrome. In pseudoxanthoma elasticum, there is alteration of the elastic tissue of the body, and the characteristic skin changes greatly facilitate this diagnosis: the skin is coarse and thicker than normal, looking rather like a crepe bandage, with the elevations being slightly yellow; there is loss of skin elasticity, and it tends to form folds easily. These changes are found particularly in the neck, axillae, antecubital areas, inguinal folds, and the periumbilical region. Angioid streaking of the optic fundus may be seen. In the Ehlers-Danlos syndrome, there is a generalized defect in the organization of the connective tissue, resulting in hypermotility of the joints, hyperextensibility of the skin, and wide, thin scars which frequently overlie the bony prominences. These haemorrhages from abiotrophy of the gastrointestinal blood vessels underline the need for routine careful inspection of the skin.

Aneurysm. An arteriosclerotic aneurysm of the aorta may cause pressure necrosis, and the third part of the duodenum is at particular risk and is the most common site. The diagnosis is an important one to keep in mind, as successful excision of a bleeding aneurysm has been reported by Law et al.[12] It must be remembered that such aneurysms do not always pulsate, as they may contain laminated clots, and there may be a history of episodes of quite intense pain, usually associated with phases of enlargement.

Biliary diseases (Haemobilia). Massive, unheralded bleeding can occur into the biliary tree as a result of gallstone cholecystitis, aneurysm of the hepatic artery, and biliary tract tumours. A case of a patient surviving rupture of an aneurysm of the hepatic artery has been reported by MacKay and Gordon Page.[13] Haemobilia is characteristically associated with upper abdominal pain and some degree of jaundice, both of which arise from blood clots in the common bile duct. Bleeding into the alimentary tract can also occur from the erosion of a large gallstone through the gallbladder into the duodenum, and bleeding can occur as well from within the pancreas and come down the pancreatic duct. This is particularly apt to happen when there is pancreatic lithiasis associated with pancreatitis. Chronic pancreatitis may indirectly give rise to alimentary bleeding by causing splenic vein compression or thrombosis, and massive bleeding may follow cysto-gastrostomy for pancreatic cyst. A direct expansion of carcinoma of the head of the pancreas, or bile duct carcinoma relating to the duodeum, may also cause massive bleeding.

Carcinoma of the stomach. Brisk bleeding may be the very first symptom of carcinoma of the stomach and may present without any previous digestive symptoms. The reason for this is the peptic digestion of a small malignant plaque in the stomach with exposure of submucosal blood vessel. Such patients are very apt to be mistakenly diagnosed as suffering from simple gastric ulceration. Brisk bleeding can also occur in patients with an advanced carcinoma, but the clinical picture then does not offer any particular difficulties in diagnosis.

Patients with Steady, Slow, Continued Bleeding

These patients present difficult diagnostic and management problems and are found to have a spongy, haemorrhagic mucosa affecting part or all of the stomach or in the region of a stoma. Such patients will bleed at the rate of about 500 ml a day, and this may persist for days; daily blood transfusion may be needed for 1 or even 2 weeks. These patients may be found to have achlorhydria and severe chronic atrophic gastritis, and there has presumably been a failure of the normal defence mechanism of the stomach. The best policy is to persevere with medical management and not to operate.

Patients with Recurring Separate Episodes of Haematemesis and Melaena

These patients have recurring episodes of acute bleeding, usually at intervals of months or several years, and routine investigations have not provided a satisfying explanation for their bleeding. The causes that should be kept particularly in mind are:

Postbulbar duodenal ulcer. Ulcers in this situation can escape radiological diagnosis, unless particular attention is focused on the postbulbar area. Otherwise, the very normal and indeed sometimes large duodenal bulb may dominate the radiological picture and conceal the ulcer just distal to it. Unless the duodenum is opened at operation, again such ulcers may not be seen or felt. It is to be hoped, however, that with endoscopic duodenoscopy, such ulcers will no longer escape detection before operation.

Meckel's diverticulum. This remains a significant cause of recurrent episodes of melaena. Such patients are liable to have a tender point in the right lower abdomen. It is exceptional for x-ray visualization to be achieved, but recently a scanning technique has been introduced that may facilitate the identification of acid-secreting Meckel's diverticula.[9]

Hiatal hernia. There is a small group of patients with hiatal hernia, who present with recurring episodes of haematemesis and melaena. The milder forms of bleeding tend to be associated with particularly sensitive oesophageal mucosa, with an erosion oesophagitis causing bleeding and melaena. The more severe examples with haematemesis and melaena tend to be those patients with a fixed hiatal hernia and a gastric ulcer in relation to the ring constriction at the level of the diaphragm.

Leiomyoma. Leiomyoma must be kept in mind. Although the diagnosis is relatively easy in most patients, nevertheless occasionally a leiomyoma in the upper small intestine may escape detection. Indeed, one such patient was seen, in whom the diagnosis was only made at urgent laparotomy, when the tumour had become distended with blood.

Angioma. Angioma constitutes the most difficult diagnostic group. Characteristically, the capillary telangiectasia will be associated with recurring epistaxis and with cutaneous manifestations. The cavernous group, however, may present no clues, but angiography at the time of bleeding may provide the necessary evidence for locating bleeding. Even so, at operation they may be very difficult to detect. Plain x-ray of the abdomen may demonstrate calcification in relation to the haemangioma. Some of these patients are particularly sensitive to aspirin, which may in some way precipitate bleeding.

Aneurysm. Aneurysm of the aorta,

or aneurysm within the biliary tree, may sometimes leak blood intermittently, but sooner or later catastrophic haemorrhage may occur. The diagnostic pitfall is the lack of pulsation which will result from laminated clots forming within them.

There is a very definite group of patients who have had previous gastric surgery, who present with recurring episodes of bleeding. Some of these patients may be shown to have unabsorbed catgut at the stoma. Sometimes endoscopy may demonstrate spongy bleeding mucosa, again relating to the stoma and without frank ulceration. A stomal ulcer, or a persistent duodenal ulcer may be the explanation.

Blood diseases are an important medical group, particularly von Willebrand's disease, a condition in which there is deficiency of antihaemophilic globulin (AHG, or Factor VIII). Alimentary bleeding is usually mild, and the clinical picture is very variable, with a tendency to ready bruising, epistaxis, and prolonged bleeding, but the only bleeding manifestation may sometimes present as episodes of alimentary haemorrhage. Thrombocytopenic purpura and qualitative platelet disorders due to abnormal clotting function of platelets (thrombocytopathy) or defective platelet clumping (thrombasthenia) are very rare causes of recurrent episodes of melaena.

Medical disorders, such as primary amyloidosis, chronic renal failure, reticulosis, regional enteritis, and renal carcinoma eroding the duodenum, are all occasional causes.

Patients with Known Peptic Ulcer

The most common cause of bleeding, as can be seen in Table 1, is peptic ulceration. This can cover a wide spectrum, from a small, acute ulcer to a large, deep, penetrating crater. X-ray negative gastric ulcers that can be diagnosed gastroscopically make up at least one-third of the acute lesion group which includes also gastrostaxis and the Mallory-Weiss syndrome. The sex ratio of patients with these acute gastric ulcers is roughly equal. The history of dyspepsia is often indefinite and may go back some years, but in the majority it is usually very short, or entirely absent. These ulcers are found particularly on the upper part of the lesser

curve and the adjacent posterior wall of the stomach. Men often return for further treatment a few years after treatment for the primary condition; they now tend to have typical chronic gastric ulcers. Women show no such tendency, but they may have further acute episodes of bleeding. These gastric ulcers often develop against a background of chronic gastritis.[11] Langman's study showed that the patients seemed to fall into two groups: (1) about two-thirds were found to be abnormal on gastric biopsies and showed low acid secretion, with the possibility of an acute gastric ulcer and (2) about one-third were found to be normal on biopsy and showed a high acid secretion, with the possibility of an undetected duodenal ulcer. Rather unexpectedly, these patients with a normal mucosa seemed at greater risk from aspirin than those who had severe gastritis, and it has been suggested that they may protect themselves against adverse factors by their very rapid cellular turnover.[17] Bleeding from these erosions can be extremely severe and life-threatening, necessitating surgical intervention. Sixty patients out of a series of 1,030 were operated on at the Central Middlesex Hospital. In 33, a single small acute ulcer was found; in eight, there were two ulcers; 13 had three to five acute ulcers; in five, there was diffuse, haemorrhagic, erosive gastritis; and in one, no abnormality was found. In a high proportion of these acute ulcers, there was an exposed and often vigorously spurting artery in the base of a small ulcer. The mortality rate for these acute ulcer patients, under age 60 was very low (0.75 percent), but in the over-60 age group it rose to 6.3 percent.

Chronic ulcers of the stomach and duodenum will normally show up radiologically, but it must be remembered that there is a proportion of both gastric and duodenal ulcers that fail to be seen radiologically; they may, however, be found by endoscopic examination. The diagnostic problem may be accentuated because sometimes chronic gastric or duodenal ulcers can be painless, particularly in patients whose pain threshold is high. In dealing with bleeding from peptic ulcer, it is important to decide whether the patient comes in a high-risk group, as these are the ones who particularly may need surgical intervention.

PHYSIOLOGICAL EFFECTS AND COMPLICATIONS

The effects of haemorrhage on the circulatory system depend on the volume and rate of bleeding and the condition of the circulatory system prior to the haemorrhage. If the patient is otherwise healthy, the fall in blood volume resulting from the haemorrhage causes a diminished cardiac output with lowered pressure in the right atrium, and this is largely compensated for by peripheral and splanchnic vasoconstriction. With very severe bleeding, there may be loss of this peripheral resistance, leading to a marked fall in blood pressure and loss of consciousness. With lesser degrees of bleeding, transient syncope with vasovagal reaction, initially associated with a slowing of the pulse, can occur. Bleeding tends to be associated with rapid, shallow, sighing breathing, and the onset of such breathing may be an early indication of further bleeding. With the restoration of blood volume by taking up fluid from tissue spaces, a hyperkinetic state may develop as the result of compensatory mechanisms attempting to overcome the diminished oxygen-carrying capacity. In this state, the pulse is full and bounding. Both blood pressure and jugular pressure are raised, and transfusion at this stage may precipitate cardiac failure, as a result of an increase in jugular pressure. This, however, can be prevented by the administration of diuretics before and during the transfusion.

Clinically, both the pulse and systolic blood pressure may give a misleading impression of blood loss, as both can be well maintained in the normal range, in spite of quite appreciable bleeding, in view of the efficiency of the compensatory mechanisms. A useful clinical guide at the bedside is the diastolic pressure, and a fall to 65 mm indicates moderate to severe bleeding, except in hypertensive patients who maintain their diastolic pressure better than normal. The colour of the hands is particularly useful in diagnosis; a waxed appearance, with ivory-like nails, and dark constricted veins may indicate a severe loss of blood, and this is a particularly ominous sign. The fact that the patient has vomited blood will indicate that at least a litre has been lost already. On the other hand, a melaena stool can be caused by as little as 50 ml of blood.

MEDICAL MANAGEMENT

The management of patients with a serious degree of blood loss has been enormously improved by the use of a CVP line which enables the CVP to be recorded and rapid transfusions given, sufficient to bring the CVP back to normal levels. It also enables a fairly accurate titration of blood loss to be undertaken. Furthermore, the CVP is an excellent indication of recurrent bleeding. This may enable emergency surgery to be undertaken without any further delay, if it has been decided on as a policy. Many hospitals are now introducing CVP techniques in the management of the more severe cases of gastroduodenal haemorrhage, and the technique has not yet been standardized. The supraclavicular subclavian vein technique is on that can be readily acquired by resident staff, using preferably the large size intracath, and aiming to have the tip in the superior vena cava. It is essential that the patient be tipped head down to prevent any risk of air embolus during the introduction of the catheter, and it is very advisable for blood warmers to be used, so that large volumes of cool blood are not quickly introduced, as this may cause cardiac embarrassment. The patient needs quick restoration of blood volume, and this in fact is more important initially than the restoration of the oxygen-carrying capacity. For this reason, a plasma expander should be given while the blood is cross-matched. Saline in practice is perfectly efficient in this respect, and, unlike dextrans, does not cause any subsequent complications with blood cross-matching, but there may be occasions when plasma is preferred. Under certain clinical circumstances, it may be decided to use unmatched universal donor blood, and normally it is sufficient to use half-hourly matched blood for the initial units. If haemodilution has already taken place and the CVP has returned to normal, it is necessary to give intravenous Frusamide (Lasix) 80 to 120 mg to ensure adequate diuresis, and higher amounts may sometimes be indicated. In practice, the increased potassium content of stored blood does not seem to constitute a problem, possibly because the blood is coming initially into contact with the endocardium and not initially affecting the coronary artery circulation. In practice, also, calcium injections are not necessary, although perhaps this might be kept in mind when really massive repeated transfusions have been required, for example, in patients with portal hypertension.

The serious complications of anoxaemia remain a constant spur for prompt adequate replacement of blood loss, so that, if a patient should bleed again, he is in a position to withstand further loss. Anoxaemia may impose serious added strains on the myocardium, particularly when there is preexisting myocardial insufficiency, and it may precipitate myocardial infarction. Cerebral vascular accidents may also complicate acute alimentary bleeding. Amaurosis, sometimes permanent blinding, is a particularly serious consequence of the vasoconstriction associated with recurrent bleeding in an already anaemic individual. The accurate replacement of blood following acute haemorrhage also has the great advantage of avoiding the hyperkinetic phase which would otherwise occur during haemodilution. This phase, with its increased CVP, increases the problems of blood transfusion and can lead to acute failure of the left side of the heart. There is no doubt that the use of the central venous line into the subclavian vein with monitoring of the CVP has been a very considerable advance in the management of the more - severe cases of haematemesis and melaena, and it makes a very real contribution towards the success of surgery, when it is needed.

The restoration of the blood volume and the institution of such steps as are necessary for the cessation of bleeding are the first priorities in management, and these have precedence over all special investigations needed for accurate diagnosis, other than a simple clinical history and physical examination. Nevertheless, there is a basic responsibility for trying to determine the cause of bleeding as quickly as possible, and in practice this may mean urgent fibre-optic oesophagogastroduodenoscopy, or emergency barium meal. Each patient must be reviewed on individual merits. There is no doubt that

urgent endoscopy can be a great help in identifying acute ulcers, which particularly in older age groups may indicate surgery, if further rebleeding occurs. It is a great help for the diagnosis of portal hypertension, although the majority in fact can be diagnosed by the bedside. Endoscopy also may provide the answer for bleeding from chronic ulceration or neoplasm, both simple and malignant, and may confirm a diagnosis of Mallory-Weiss syndrome. With the modern fibre-optic endoscopy technique, and the use of intravenous Diazepam, there is no doubt that the patient can tolerate the examination very well, but every examination, however carefully done, can carry some slight risk of mishap, and any such investigation should be done only when there will be therapeutic advantage to the patient commensurate with any discomfort or risk. An urgent barium meal is the simplest, safest investigation, and it can be given even when bleeding is continuing, but there are important pitfalls in diagnosis, and acute gastric ulcers can very easily be overlooked as can postbulbar ulcers. In order that emergency investigations bring maximum benefit to the patient, the effective organization of team care is necessary. The following points summarize the basic management:

1. Take a basic medical history and physical examination, and interview any friends or relatives who may accompany the patient.
2. Reassure the patient. Explain to him that an ulcer has caught a small blood vessel, and that treatment is highly successful in the majority of patients, but blood transfusions may be needed, and occasionally, but not often, an operation. Tranquilizers may be given, if thought necessary, either soluble phenobarbital or Diazepam by injection.
3. Order complete bed rest and ask for bed blocks to be available.
4. Request an hourly initial blood pressure chart and pulse chart. If the clinical impression is one of serious blood loss, set up a central venous line, recording pressures half-hourly to one-hourly, and start with saline infusion, pending a supply of blood.
5. Arrange for haemoglobin and blood

urea determinations and cross-matching, and proceed, if appropriate, with half-hourly blood cross-matching unit.

6. Request soft diet, two-hourly feeds with milk or other fluids on the locker, restricting intake only if the patient is nauseated.

7. Review the need for further diagnostic measures, including Hess test for capillary fragility, screening of blood for coagulation or bleeding defects, sulfobromophthalein (Bromsulphalein) test for liver dysfunction, emergency endoscopy, and emergency barium meal.

8. If all investigations have proved negative, ensure that a follow-up appointment is arranged, as a proportion of such individuals will come back with gastric or intestinal neoplasm, or definite peptic ulcer which has not shown on the initial studies.

The following points are particularly important to keep in mind in relation to prognosis. Age is a particularly important factor, rather than duration of history. In patients over age 60, the risk increases sharply. The prognosis is much better in acute than chronic ulcer under the age of 60, but this difference becomes much less marked in the older age groups, where acute ulcers without previous history can cause very serious bleeding necessitating surgical intervention. The prognosis of gastric ulcer is twice as poor as with duodenal ulcer, and the finding of a definite gastric ulcer with recurrent bleeding after admission is an absolute indication for surgery.

If the initial bleeding is severe, causing shock, and needing six or more units of blood to restore CVP, emergency surgery should be undertaken forthwith.[14] The association of other disease processes is to be noted and taken into consideration, and there may be circumstances in which they entirely exclude surgical intervention. Recurrence of bleeding after admission is the most important single prognostic factor, and being 60 years of age or more at once brings the patient into the 20 percent or higher mortality risk.

SURGICAL MANAGEMENT

Surgical treatment is mainly reserved for patients with recurrent haemorrhage, particularly those over the age of 60 and who are known to have a chronic ulcer. Medical management in such cases is not satisfactory and the mortality rate in this group is high, although many of these patients will recover. The mortality rate from emergency surgery in these circumstances is also high and for a number of reasons. Shock from repeated haemorrhage, arteriosclerosis, coronary artery disease, and prostatic enlargement all make a contribution to the mortality. Many of the ulcers are large and have penetrated to involve adjacent organs, so that mobilization and closure of the duodenal stump may be difficult. In order to overcome this difficulty, many surgeons now advocate transduodenal suture of the bleeding point combined with vagotomy and pyloroplasty and claim better results for this procedure than for partial gastrectomy. The highest mortality rates for emergency partial gastrectomy for haemorrhage occur in cases of chronic duodenal ulcer, and the mortality rates are lowest in those cases when an acute gastric ulcer is responsible for the bleeding.

The adoption of a policy of selective surgery for the treatment of recurrent haemorrhages has not resulted in an overall reduction in the mortality of ulcer haemorrhage when compared with the results obtained by purely medical management. Despite this, there has been a general move away from an entirely medical management to one of selective surgery, and for several reasons.

Medical management alone for the treatment of recurrent haemorrhage may necessitate giving very large transfusions of blood, and with the increasing demands that are being made on blood banks it may be impossible for the bank to supply the required volume of blood. The adoption of a selective surgical policy will reduce the demands on the blood bank; from time to time it is necessary to advise an operation to control bleeding because the patient is of an unusual blood group and it is impossible to obtain a sufficient quantity of blood of this group. It is, of course, essential not to run out of blood and then to attempt an emergency operation.

Tanner [16] has expressed the view that any patient with severe bleeding, a known history of chronic ulcer, and over the age of 45 should be operated on as soon as he is resuscitated, and every patient must be reviewed as an individual problem.

The pattern of disease is constantly changing and this is certainly true of ulcers. Peptic ulcer is not as common as it was and there has recently been a falling-off in the number of admissions to hospital for the treatment of chronic duodenal ulcer. In most instances, the comparison between a policy of medical management and selective surgical management covers many years, and whilst the adoption of a policy of selective surgery has not resulted in any appreciable reduction in the overall mortality, it is possible that owing to a change in the pattern of the disease, without this policy there would have been an increase in the mortality rate.

There is an even more important consideration. The successful medical management of ulcer haemorrhage does not cure the patient of his ulcer, and whilst it enables the patient to leave hospital and probably return to his work, there is a very real risk that the patient will suffer further complications from his ulcer and may well have another haemorrhage, which could be fatal. Against this, those who have had a successful emergency gastrectomy are usually cured of their ulcer and do not suffer any further complications. If this can be achieved without adding to the mortality rate, and possibly reducing the amount of blood required, the policy of selective surgery obviously has advantages.

Harvey and Langman [7] have studied the late results of medical and surgical treatment for bleeding duodenal ulcer and they concluded that the relapse rate was markedly greater in medically than in surgically treated patients. It is of interest that the risk of relapse appears to be less in women than in men.

Timing of Operation

If it is decided that the haemorrhage requires surgical treatment, this should be carried out as soon after the patient has been adequately resuscitated as is possible. Delay at this stage only increases the risk of another haemorrhage with subsequent deterioration in the general condition of the patient. A report by Cocks, Desmond, Swynnerton, and Tanner,[3] from St. James's Hospital, Balham, has confirmed this view and has shown that the operative mortality rates more than double if emergency operations are performed later than a few days after the admission of the patients.

Choice of Operation

It has already been stressed that there is a difference in the mortality rates of emergency operations for chronic duodenal ulcer and for gastric ulcer. This difference is very largely due to the difficulty of mobilising and closing the duodenal stump when a large duodenal ulcer is present, penetrating deeply into the pancreas and often eroding the gastroduodenal artery. With the increasing adoption of vagotomy and pyloroplasty for the treatment of uncomplicated duodenal ulcer, many surgeons have had little experience in the management of a difficult duodenal stump. In an attempt to overcome this difficulty when dealing with a case of ulcer haemorrhage, many surgeons advocate transduodenal suture of the bleeding point and then vagotomy and pylorplasty [2] (Fig. 1). This technique, however, is not always successful in controlling the haemorrhage: Akin and Sullivan [1] have reported a series of 20 patients so treated in which three had further massive bleeding and two of these had to undergo emergency partial gastrectomy. Silen and Moore [15] have made a plea for caution in the adoption of this technique, for they too fear the risk of further bleeding. They point out that side-wall injuries in arteries do not stop bleeding as readily as transections and that it is not surprising that suture through inflammatory ulcerating tissue is not always successful.

Just as the mobilisation and closure of the duodenal stump may be a very difficult procedure, so too may be the performance of an adequate pyloroplasty when a large penetrating ulcer is present, particularly if the ulcer is on the superior border of the duodenum.[8] The authors have a strong personal prefer-

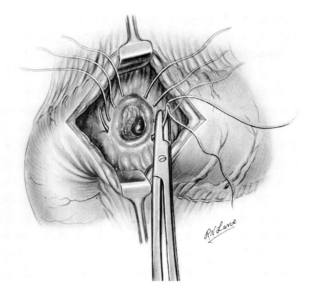

FIG. 1. Bleeding from the base of a large chronic duodenal ulcer on the posterior wall. The anterior wall of the first part of the duodenum has been incised and retracted. Sutures of strong silk are inserted deeply through the edges and base of the ulcer before they are tied one by one. The bleeding artery (itself) was not visualised.

ence for carrying out partial gastrectomy in these cases and in the report from St. James's Hospital already quoted, it is of interest that all 566 patients were treated by emergency partial gastrectomy.

It is obviously impossible to set out hard and fast rules as to whether a bleeding duodenal ulcer should be treated by suture, vagotomy and pyloroplasty, or by partial gastrectomy. The skill and experience of the operator in dealing with a difficult duodenal stump, and the extent of the ulcer, must be weighed against the possible risk of further bleeding and its effects.

More recently transgastric suture, combined with vagotomy and pyloroplasty, has been advocated as the emergency treatment for bleeding from a gastric ulcer.[5] The advantage of this procedure over the more usual Billroth I type partial gastrectomy, which gives good results, is not evident. Even for high gastric ulcers, a reconstruction using the Schoemaker technique usually leaves an adequate gastric remnant. There may be a place for such a procedure in the management of bleeding from an acute gastric erosion.

Technical Considerations

PREOPERATIVE MANAGEMENT AND ANAESTHESIA

Once the decision to operate has been made, every effort should be made to bring the patient to the theatre in the best possible condition. Bleeding from a peptic ulcer is usually intermittent rather than continuous and it is often possible, and indeed advisable, to spend a few hours following a haemorrhage in improving the general condition with adequate transfusions before submitting such a patient to an operation. It is only occasionally that bleeding is so profuse and continuous as to make this impossible. Also, an adequate supply of blood must be available.

Every effort should be made to empty the stomach through a nasoduodenal suction tube or a Senoran's evacuator, but this is not always effective, for the stomach may be full of clot. Because of this, it is important to have .the services of a skilled anaesthetist who is able to pass a cuffed endotracheal tube quickly and before there is a risk of the patient's vomiting and inhaling some of the clot.

Chronic duodenal ulcer. For a bleeding chronic duodenal ulcer, the treatment of choice is partial gastrectomy with reconstruction by the Polya method, the exact technique being that to which the surgeon is most accustomed. When mobilising the duodenum, it is most important in these difficult cases to go on until there is an adequate length of duodenum available for closure and oversewing. If this is not persevered with, there is a great risk that leakage will take place from the duodenal stump. Even with extensive posterior ulcers that have penetrated into the pancreas, it is usually possible to obtain a good plane of separation from the pancreas beyond the ulcer. At the end of the operation, a drain should be put down to the duodenal stump through a stab incision separate from the main wound and this should be left in position for at least 5 days. The alternative is underrunning the bleeding point, pyloroplasty, and vagotomy; the indications for this procedure as opposed to partial gastrectomy have already been discussed.

Haemorrhage from a postbulbar duodenal ulcer is a particularly difficult problem, for partial gastrectomy with removal of the ulcer may incur a real risk of damage to the common bile duct, though if this can be avoided, partial gastrectomy is the treatment of choice. Division of the duodenum proximal to a postbulbar ulcer is often possible and may be successful in preventing further haemorrhage, but failing this, suture, pyloroplasty, and vagotomy may be advisable.

Chronic gastric ulcer. If surgery is necessary for the control of bleeding from a chronic gastric ulcer, partial gastrectomy should be performed. The reconstruction should be by the Billroth I end-to-end gastroduodenal method or by the Schoemaker modification of this if the ulcer is situated high in the stomach.

Acute gastric ulcer. Surgery is not often needed for the control of bleeding from an acute gastric ulcer, but when it is necessary, it is probably wise to carry out a Billroth I partial gastrectomy in exactly the same way as for a chronic gastric ulcer. It has been

suggested that local excision or simple underrunning of the bleeding point is all that is required. Certainly such a procedure will be effective in controlling the immediate bleeding, but at least in men there is a considerable risk that further chronic ulceration will occur at some future date and possibly be complicated by another haemorrhage.

Stomal ulcer. Severe and recurrent bleeding from a stomal ulcer usually means that the anastomosis must be unpicked, the ulcer excised and some form of reconstruction carried out. If the ulcer has developed after gastroenterostomy, this should be converted into a partial gastrectomy. If the previous operation was a partial gastrectomy, it may have been unsatisfactory in some way. It is well recognised that stomal ulcers may develop when a Billroth I gastrectomy has been performed for a duodenal ulcer. If this is the case, the anastomosis should be unpicked and the ulcer excised, and after the duodenal stump has been closed, a Polya reconstruction should be performed. If the previous operation was a Polya-type partial gastrectomy for duodenal ulcer, the stomal ulcer may have developed because a small segment of pyloric antrum has been left with the duodenal stump. Under these circumstances not only should a further resection be performed but the antral segment must also be removed. Whenever a stomal ulcer is being dealt with, it is most important to examine the pancreas in case an adenoma is present which may be causing the Zollinger-Ellison syndrome.

Impalpable ulcer. When performing laparotomy for ulcer haemorrhage, it is sometimes impossible to palpate an ulcer. It is always important to carry out a full intra-abdominal examination in case there should be some ohter cause for the bleeding, and this is particularly so in these circumstances. If no lesion can be found, a so-called blind gastrectomy should not be performed. Often in these cases the stomach is grossly distended with clot. Under these circumstances, there should be no hesitation in opening the stomach and evacuating the clot. After this has been done, it is often possible to palpate a shallow ulcer that had previously been missed. If it is still impossible to palpate an ulcer, the gastrotomy opening should be ex-

Table 2.   MORTALITY RATE FROM HAEMATEMESIS AND MELAENA, CENTRAL MIDDLESEX HOSPITAL, LONDON, 1960 TO 1970

Lesion	Age	Number	Deaths	Mortality Rate (percent)	Age	Number	Deaths	Mortality Rate (percent)	Total Number	Total Deaths	Mortality Rate (percent)
Chronic gastric ulcer	−60	88	5	5.7	60+	164	22	13.4	252	27	10.7
Duodenal ulcer	−60	380	8	2.1	60+	244	21	8.6	624	29	4.7
Acute gastric	−60	145	1	0.75	60+	142	9	6.3	287	10	3.5
Post operative	−60	42	2	4.8	60+	42	3	7.1	84	5	6.0

Table 3.   HAEMATEMESIS AND MELAENA OVERALL INFLUENCE OF AGE ON MORTALITY RATE, CENTRAL MIDDLESEX HOSPITAL, LONDON, 1960 TO 1970

Age	Number	Mortality Rate (percent)	Age	Number	Mortality Rate (percent)	Age	Number	Mortality Rate (percent)
−60	665	2.4	+60	592	9.3	All	1,247	5.7

tended to permit careful examination of the inside of the stomach. In the majority of cases, the source of the bleeding will be seen: it may be a small acute lesion with a hardened vessel in its centre which is often more easily detected by palpation from within than visually. It may be a shallow and quite extensive ulcer with soft edges that was impossible to feel from the outside. If such a lesion is discovered, it is a simple matter to carry out a gastrectomy in such a way as to include the lesion. Many of these lesions are situated high in the stomach and may be multiple; they could easily be left behind in the gastric remnant if a blind gastrectomy is performed.

If no lesion is seen inside the stomach, the duodenum should be mobilised, opened, and examined from within in exactly the same way; a shallow duodenal ulcer may be exposed and can then be dealt with. If such an examination still fails to reveal the cause of the bleeding, the oesophagogastric junction should be inspected for varices or for bleeding lacerations of the Mallory-Weiss syndrome.

RESULTS

The results of a policy of selective surgical management can be seen from a study of Tables 2 and 3, which show the results of such a policy as carried out at the Central Middlesex Hospital, London, from 1960 to 1970. Because of the influence that age has on these results, two groups of patients are reported, those under 60 years of age, and those aged 60 and over. The total mortality rate for the younger age group was 2.4 percent, whereas in the over-60 group it was 9.3 percent.

These figures do not show the purely operative mortality rate, which in gastric ulcer is comparatively low—whereas in chronic duodenal ulcer emergencies, it is high. Thus it can be concluded that recourse to surgery should be early if the bleeding is known to be from a chronic gastric ulcer, but that in a chronic duodenal ulcer, a rather more conservative policy might be adopted.

REFERENCES

1. Akin, J. M., and Sullivan, M. B., Surgery 54:587, 1963.
2. Clark, C. G., Postgrad. Med. J. 44:590, 1968.
3. Cocks, J. R., Desmond, A. M., Swynnerton, B. F., and Tanner, N. C., Gut 13:331, 1972.
4. Doig, A., and Shafar, J., Q. J. Med., N.S. 25:1.
5. Dorton, H. E., Surg. Gynecol. Obstet. 122:1015, 1966.
6. Goldman, R. L., Gastroenterology 46:589, 1964.
7. Harvey, R. F., and Langman, M. J. S., Q. J. Med., N.S. 30:539, 1970.
8. Jensen, H. E., and Amdrup, E., Scand. J. Gastroenterol. 4:667, 1969.
9. Jewett, T. C., Duszynski, D. O., and Allen, J. E., Surgery 68:567, 1970.
10. Avery Jones, F. Fifth Symposium on Advanced Medicine (Royal College of Physicians), 48–71, 1969.
11. Langman, M. J. S., Hansky, J. H., Drury, R. A. B., and Avery Jones, F., Gut 5:550, 1964.
12. Law, S. W., Garrett, H. E., and De Bakey, M. E., Gastroenterology 43:680, 1961.
13. Mackay, A. G., and Gordon Page, H., N. Engl. J. Med. 260:468, 1959.
14. Northfield, T. D., and Smith, T., Lancet 2:584, 1970.
15. Silen, W., and Moore, F. D., Ann. Surg. 160:778, 1964.
16. Tanner, N. C., Br. J. Surg. 51:754, 1964.
17. Valman, H. B., Parry, D. J., and Coghill, N. F., Br. Med. J. 4:661, 1968.

24

ANASTOMOTIC (STOMAL) ULCERATION

RODNEY MAINGOT

Anastomotic ulcer (syn: postoperative ulcer, jejunal ulcer, marginal ulcer, stomal ulcer, gastrojejunal ulcer, recurrent ulcer, or secondary peptic ulcer) can follow any operation in which gastric and jejunal mucosa become continuous, e.g., gastrojejunostomy and Billroth II methods. Again, such ulcers may arise following pyloroplasty, gastroduodenostomy, or the Billroth I types of repair.

Anastomotic ulcer is the most common of the remote complications of gastric surgery for benign peptic ulceration of the duodenum. Lowdon [14] points out that it is a man-made disease and represents a serious failure of surgical treatment, and, in addition, is often a more troublesome and dangerous condition than the original disorder.

AETIOLOGY AND PATHOGENESIS

The aetiology and pathogenesis of peptic ulcer, the choice of operation, results of elective procedures, and incidence and treatment of anastomotic ulcerations are also discussed in Chapters 11 and 13.

Causes of anastomotic ulceration are as follows:

1. Inadequate surgical procedure
   Incomplete vagotomy
   Inadequate gastric resection
   Long afferent loop (Fig. 1)
2. Hypersecretion of gastric juice
   Retained gastric antrum
   Zollinger-Ellison syndrome
3. Ulcerogenic medication

Incidence of Anastomotic Ulcer

It is universally agreed that gastrojejunostomy alone for duodenal ulcer is the operation most frequently followed by anastomotic ulcer. Next in order of frequency are vagotomy anl pyloroplasty for duodenal ulcer. Most recurrent ulcers observed following truncal, selective or superselective vagotomy are a result of *incomplete vagotomy*. This complication, arising after partial gastrectomy for gastric ulcer, is extremely rare. For instance, Balint et al.[2] report a series

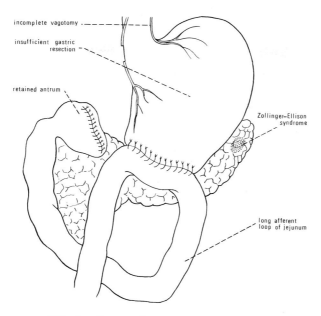

incomplete vagotomy

insufficient gastric resection

retained antrum

Zollinger–Ellison syndrome

long afferent loop of jejunum

FIG. 1.   Causes of anastomotic ulceration.

of 160 cases of anastomotic ulcer following surgery for duodenal ulcer and found that only two had followed partial gastrectomy for gastric ulcer. They state that in view of the very great rarity of anastomotic ulcer after partial gastrectomy for gastric ulcer, it is reasonable to suggest that an undetected or unrecorded duodenal ulcer may have been present as well, in these two patients.

Tanner [25] informed me that in a series of his, in over 1,000 operations for gastric ulcer there were only two patients who subsequently developed stomal ulceration. Both recurrent ulcers followed the Billroth I type of operation.

He writes: [24]

Occasionally a recurrent ulcer is gastric. Because a gastric ulcer is very rarely seen in association with a Polya type of gastrectomy, the almost certain cure is to carry out a gastrectomy completed with a gastrojejunal anastomosis.

In a personal series of 433 gastric excisions for gastric ulcer, there has, so far, been no case of anastomotic ulcer.

Age.   Anastomotic ulcer can occur at any age. It has been reported in patients from 2 to 81 years of age. The youngest patient in my series was a youth of 17 who had had a gastrojejunostomy performed for duodenal ulcer 3 years previously, and the oldest was a man of 78 upon whom I had performed vagotomy and anterior gastrojejunostomy under local anaesthesia for pyloric stenosis. The latter developed a huge jejunal ulcer 9 months later, for which an antecolic Schoemaker-Billroth II procedure was carried out, and when he was examined 10 years later, he appeared to be in excellent health.

Most of the cases of anastomotic ulcer are observed between the ages of 42 and 55, the average age being 48. Thus, in Marshall's series [18] of 200 cases the average age was 48.2 years. Balint et al.[2] recorded the average age in their series of 156 cases to be 46. It is interesting to note that in all the reported series there is a larger proportion of patients over the age of 60 in the postgastrojejunostomy group than there is in the partial gastrectomy group.

Sex.   Anastomotic ulcer occurs most frequently in men, in the proportion of approximately 4 to 1. This ratio correlates well with the predominance of duodenal ulcers in men.

Anastomotic ulcer may, for all practical purposes, be considered never to occur after operations for *cancer of the stomach*. Judd reported 1 case, and other instances may be found in the literature; but Garnett Wright [7] was unable to find a single case out of 436 which was traced, and offers the following possible explanation for the absence of this complication:

1. That carcinoma patients are immune from secondary ulceration.
2. That the majority of these patients do not live long enough for secondary ulcers to develop; but this is only true in part, since secondary ulcers may appear very soon after operation.
3. That symptoms of secondary ulcer are likely to be masked by those of carcinoma.

Family history. The tendency for duodenal ulcer to occur in families has already been mentioned, but a family history is still more commonly obtained in cases of anastomotic ulceration. Arthur Allen reported a family in which the father and five sons all had an ulcer history with numerous gastric operations.

Type of Ulcer and Type of Operation

Anastomotic ulcer may develop after anastomosis of the stomach to any part of the intestinal tract; but, as has been stated in the introductory remarks to this chapter, it occurs most commonly after simple gastro-jejunostomy for duodenal ulcer (Table 1). Tanner [23] reported that after a 10-year period anastomotic ulceration developed in over 50 percent of his cases in which posterior gastro-jejunostomy was performed for duodenal ulcer. Lewisohn [13] was one of the first to draw attention to the frequency of recurrent ulceration following simple gastrojejunostomy for duodenal ulcer and assessed the incidence at 34 percent.

In many cases, anastomotic ulcer has developed after *inadequate resection of the*

Table 1.   INCIDENCE OF ANASTOMOTIC ULCER FOLLOWING OPERATIONS FOR DUODENAL ULCER

Authors	Type of Operation	Recurrent Ulcer (in percent)
Lewisohn, 1925	Simple gastrojejunostomy	34
Tanner, 1954	Simple gastrojejunostomy	50
Harkins et al., 1960	Vagotomy and antrectomy	0.5
Herrington Jr., 1969	Vagotomy and antrectomy	0.5
Herrington Jr., 1972	Vagotomy and antrectomy	0.3
Burge, 1959	Vagotomy and gastrojejunostomy	3.8
Goligher, 1972	Vagotomy and gastrojejunostomy	2.5 to 5.9
Burge, 1959	Vagotomy and pyloroplasty	3.1
Weinberg, 1969	Vagotomy and pyloroplasty	4.5 to 5.0
Dragstedt, 1969 and 1972	Vagotomy and drainage operation	5 to 8
Goligher, 1972	Vagotomy and pyloroplasty	6.7 to 7.3
Harkins and Nyhus, 1969	Partial gastrectomy, Billroth I	3.5
Marshall and Reinstine, 1955	Partial gastrectomy, Billroth II	2.3
Orr, 1964	Partial gastrectomy, Billroth II	3.5
Goligher, 1972	Partial gastrectomy, Billroth I and II	0.9 to 3.7
Maingot, 1961 and 1972	Partial gastrectomy, Billroth II	2
Allen and Welch, 1942	Antral exclusion (von Eiselsberg, and Devine)	80
Ogilvie, 1938	Antral exclusion (Devine)	80

Partial gastrectomy = Excision of 65 to 75 percent of the distal portion of the stomach plus a variable amount of the first part of the duodenum.
Subtotal gastrectomy = Removal of more than 75 percent of the stomach.
Many surgeons describe a three-quarter excision of the stomach as a subtotal gastrectomy.

stomach, such as hemigastrectomy, and frequently after partial gastrectomy in which *a portion of the pyloric antrum had not been excised.*

The recurrence rate following Billroth I operations is higher than after the Billroth II methods. This statement is confirmed by Cooper and Welbourn,[29] who reported proved anastomotic ulcers in 8.2 percent of their cases after Billroth I operations for duodenal ulcer, and in only 1.8 percent after Billroth II procedures.

During the last 5 years, statistical data indicate a high ulcer recurrence rate of 5 to 10 percent for vagotomy and pyloroplasty. This is probably accounted for by the "inadvertent" or *incomplete section of the important vagal branches* that supply the stomach. The best results for duodenal ulcer are recorded after antrectomy and vagotomy or partial gastrectomy by the Schoemaker-

Table 2. INTERVAL FROM INITIAL OPERATION TO ONSET OF ANASTOMOTIC ULCERATION

Operation	Interval (years)
Gastroenterostomy	7.4
Gastric resection	1.9
Gastroenterostomy and vagotomy	1.7
Gastric resection and vagotomy	1.1

Note: Six years is the average time lapse between surgery and the onset of symptoms with a gastrojejuno-colic fistula.[3]
Source: Wychulis, Priestly, and Foulk. Surg. Gynecol. Obstet. 122:89, 1966.

Billroth II procedure. The nutritional and metabolic consequences associated with the "dumping syndrome" can be mitigated by ensuring that not more than three quarters

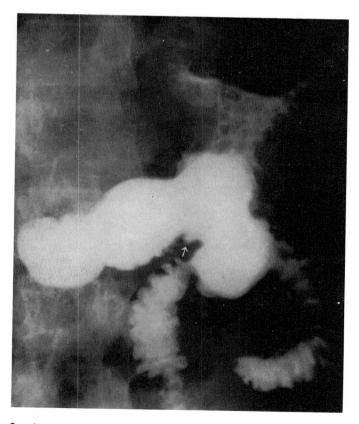

FIG. 2. Anastomotic ulcer following gastrojejunostomy for duodenal ulcer.

of the stomach is resected when carrying out the Billroth II procedure. Table 2 shows the interval from initial operation to the onset of anastomotic ulceration. It is based on an article written by Wychulis, Priestly, and Foulk.[30]

ULCEROGENIC TUMOURS OF THE PANCREAS

The reader is referred to Chapter 13 by Zollinger et al.

DIAGNOSIS

Symptoms and signs. *Pain* is the most prominent symptom and is more severe and persistent than in cases of primary peptic ulcer. In most cases of anastomotic ulcer following gastric resection, the pain is situated in the upper portion of the epigastrium and more particularly below the left costal margin. In some patients, the pain is experienced to the right of the xiphoid process, while in others it is referred to the lower part of the left side of the chest or even as high up as the shoulder region. In the gastrojejunostomy group, the pain is felt over a wide area of the epigastrium, but it is rarely referred to the left side of the chest, to or below the umbilicus, or to the back.

But pain may occur atypically anywhere in the abdomen, including the left upper quadrant. The pain and dyspepsia may be nocturnal and they are usually relieved by antacids.

Penetration of the ulcer may be indicated by *backache,* or by pain over the lower ribs on the left side.

Vomiting, which varies in intensity and frequency, takes place in 50 percent of the cases. It is often self-induced and is the most speedy method of obtaining relief from pain. Vomiting is usually preceded by nausea and anorexia. Constipation is common, but when a gastrojejunocolic fistula develops, there is usually a very persistent diarrhoea and steatorrhoea.

Haemorrhage is the most common symptom of anastomotic ulceration, and this occurs in about 60 percent of patients. Bleeding (haematemesis and/or melaena) that ensues some time after an operation for duodenal ulcer may be taken as good evidence of anastomotic ulceration. Bleeding is more likely to be chronic than massive, and therefore the patient often presents with *anemia.* Less than 10 percent of anastomotic ulcers perforate.

Radiological findings. Positive proof of an anastomotic ulcer is obtained when x-ray studies show the presence of a crater at or near the stoma. It must be emphasised here that x-ray diagnosis of recurrent ulceration is difficult, and negative findings do not exclude the presence of an ulcer, as has al-

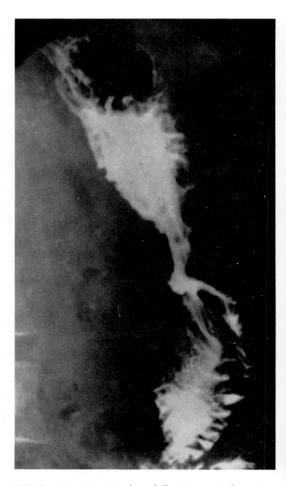

FIG. 3. Anastomotic ulcer following partial gastrectomy of Billroth II type for chronic duodenal ulcer.

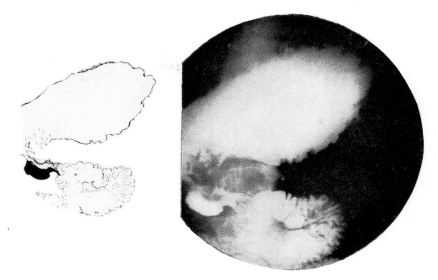

FIG. 4. Anastomotic ulcer following gastrojejunostomy for duodenal ulcer. Note large crater and scarring associated with some obstruction of stoma.

ready been stated. Walter et al.[28] found that only 40 percent of anastomotic ulcers following partial gastrectomy were detected by means of barium-meal studies. In Marshall's series [18] (1960), positive radiological evidence of an anastomotic ulcer was elicited in 70 percent of the cases. Dr. W. Young (1971/ 1972) of the Royal Free Hospital, Diagnostic Radiological Department, informs me that the figure now approximates 80 percent.

A diagnosis is made by one or a combination of two of the following findings: (1) persistent tenderness over the site of the stoma; (2) gross deformity of the stoma; (3) stenosis of the stoma; (4) residue in the region of the stoma; (5) marked delay in emptying of the stomach; (6) deformity of the efferent limb of jejunum close to the stoma; and (7) the presence of a crater (Figs. 1 through 5).

Gastroscopy and gastrophotography. A marginal ulcer can often be detected by means of fibre-optic endoscopy and gastrophotography (see Chap. 4).

COMPLICATIONS

The following complications can occur: (1) perforation; (2) haemorrhage; (3) stenosis or obstruction; (4) the onset of carcinoma of the stomach or of the gastroenteric stoma; (5) gastrojejunocolic fistula.

Perforation in an anastomotic ulcer. This occurs in about 10 percent of cases after vagotomy and a drainage operation, and in approximately 2 percent of cases after partial gastrectomy (Fig. 5).

Some surgeons recommend simple closure as *treatment of perforated anastomotic ulcer;* and if there is considerable contamination of the peritoneal cavity, drainage also will be required.

Following the operation, the patient should be put on a special diet and treated with the medicines that are employed in the management of peptic ulcer cases. But if no improvement results, which is likely, hemigastrectomy combined with vagotomy will prove necessary.

Condon and Tanner [5] operated upon 198 patients with anastomotic ulcer with a mortality rate of 4.5 percent. Thoroughman et al.[26] found 8,779 anastomotic ulcers reported in the literature, of which 472 were characterised by perforation into the peritoneal cavity. When simple closure was performed, the mortality rate was 20 percent and the ulcer recurred in 89 percent. On the other

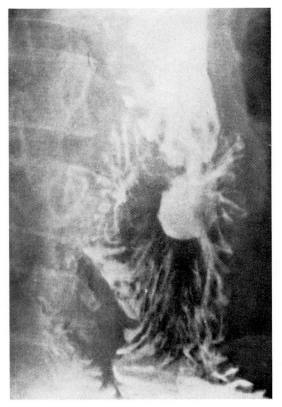

FIG. 5. Anastomotic ulcer following partial distal gastrectomy for duodenal ulcer.

hand, gastric resection was followed by an 8 percent mortality rate.

Haemorrhage. As stated above, haemorrhage *may be so severe* as to demand immediate surgical intervention (see Chap. 23).

Obstruction of the stoma. This occurs in 4 to 8 percent of cases and generally denotes the presence of marginal ulceration. Other causes of obstruction at or about the stoma include faulty operative technique, adhesions and bands, jejunogastric intussusception, volvulus of the jejunal loop, or herniation of the afferent and/or efferent limbs of the jejunum through defects in the mesocolon.

A nonfunctioning stoma, as revealed by x-ray pictures, usually implies chronic anastomotic ulceration with cicatrisation or other mechanical causes. (see Chap. 27).

Ulcerogenic drugs. The *corticosteroids* are known to increase the secretion of acid-pepsin and, therefore, to increase ulceration (see Chap. 107).

Aspirin and *phenylbutazone,* by their local effects on the gastric mucosa, and *caffeine, histamine, phenylbutazone,* and *rauwolfia,* by their stimulation of increased gastric secretion, also cause an increase in peptic ulcer.[12]

The management in these cases consists of discontinuance of the ulcerogenic drug and efficient medical treatment of the ulcer (Frederick, 1964).

If complications occur, such as recalcitrant haemorrhage, surgery should be carried out.

Gastrojejunocolic fistula. Cases of *gastrocolic fistula* and one case of *gastrojejunocolic* fistula due to benign gastric ulcer with no previous surgery have been reported by Sterns and Bird,[22] Ger et al.,[8] and Friedman et al.[6] Sterns and Bird state that only 37 cases of *gastrocolic fistula* (with no previous surgery) arising from benign gastric ulcers have been reported since the original recognition of this fistula as a clinical syndrome in 1775. In a review of the literature from 1920 to 1968 they found only 13 cases. Further cases have been reported by Blumen and Weber [4] in 1970 by Ger et al.[8] in 1971.

Friedman et al.[6] reported the first case of *gastrojejunocolic fistula,* in a woman heroin addict aged 44, who had a benign gastric ulcer and *who had not had previous gastric surgery.*

At operation, he performed partial gastrectomy (Billroth II) accompanied by limited segmental resections of the jejunum and colon which were involved in the ulcerated and inflammatory mass. His patient made a good and uneventful recovery.

Gastrojejunocolic fistula is the most serious late complication of peptic ulcer surgery. This grave complication may follow vagotomy and a drainage operation or partial gastrectomy when performed for chronic duodenal ulcer. The condition is rarer after the Billroth II operation. Gray and Sharpe [9] and Aird [1] have each described a case of *duodenocolic fistula* following the Billroth II type of anastomosis.

Gastrojejunocolic fistula is seldom encountered after any type of operation for gastric ulcer and is unknown following palliative or radical procedures for gastric cancer.

Table 3.   INCIDENCE OF GASTRO-
JEJUNOCOLIC FISTULA CAUSED BY
ANASTOMOTIC ULCER

Author	Incidence (in percent)
Verbrugge, 1925	11.3
Judd and Hoerner, 1935	8.7
Wright, 1935	8.7
Lahey, 1936	11.0
Walters and Clagett, 1939	13.6
Allen, 1937	14.0
Marshall, 1957	15.1
Lowdon, 1948	22.4
Lowdon, 1962	10.0
Hardy and Oates, 1966	10.0
Harkins and Nyhus, 1969	9.0
Tanner, 1972	8.0

As I have reported,[17] it may occur as late as 37 years after the performance of gastrojejunostomy for hypertrophic infantile pyloric stenosis.

A fistula between the stomach, transverse colon, and jejunum occasionally results from carcinoma of the stomach or of the colon and has, on rare occasions, been reported in cases of ulcerative colitis. It is most frequently observed following simple gastroenterostomy for duodenal ulcer (Fig. 4).

Incidence. The risk of gastrojejunocolic fistula following anastomotic ulceration appears from the published figures to be about 10 percent (Table 3).

According to Lowdon,[16] estimates vary from 7.5 percent to 22.4 percent, but all refer to the incidence of fistula in patients returning to hospital for treatment of anastomotic ulcer and *presumably* exaggerate the true incidence of the complication.

Czerny, Simon and Arnsperger (*Beitr Klin Chir. 37:765,* 1903) were the first surgeons to report a case of gastrojejunocolic fistula following gastrojejunostomy. Hamann (*Trans Amer Surg Ass 33:358,* 1915) described the first case in America and Barling (*Brit J Surg 5:343,* 1917) the first case in Great Britain. By 1940, Thomas (*Mil Surgeon 87:232,* 1940) had collected 207 cases of gastrojejunocolic fistula. Bornstein and Weinshel (*Surg Gynec Obstet 72:459,* 1941) reviewed 332 collected cases.

This serious condition can occur at any age. It has been reported in children and in extremely old patients. The peak incidence is between 50 and 70 years of age.

Lowdon,[16] who has operated in 50 such cases, writes:

A fistula may develop at any age and at almost any time after the gastrojejunostomy is made. One of my patients developed the fistula three weeks after operation and another developed symptoms of fistula 30 years after gastroenterostomy.

Some 97 percent of the patients are males. Lowdon[15] reported 41 patients with gastrojejunocolic fistula; only one of these was a woman.

In 1962, he wrote: "A striking feature is the rarity with which the condition affects women. In over 500 reported cases there have been only 8 female patients!"

Pathological Conditions. As stated above, in the majority of cases the fistula followed simple *posterior gastrojejunostomy,* which was, for many years, the most common type of anastomosis. The proximity of the stoma to the colon is an important factor; for instance, fistula formation is a comparatively rare complication of anastomotic ulcer following the Billroth I types of gastroduodenal anastomoses.

On occasion, an active ulcer becomes attached to, and then perforates in, the adjacent colon, but in the majority of cases a gradually enlarging abscess forms and bursts into the colon, and a fistula of some length through scar tissue results. In either case, the walls of the fistulous tract are soon lined by epithelium so that spontaneous closure is impossible.

The size of the fistula varies from a few millimetres up to 5 cm in diameter. The size of the fistula bears no relation to the severity of the symptoms.

In about 80 percent of the cases, the communication is between the jejunum (just distal to the stoma) and the colon; in 15 percent of the cases, it is at the anastomosis itself; and in 5 percent it is gastrocolic.

Severe gastritis and jejunitis are usually present. The jejunitis is an important feature of the pathologic condition.

The presence of *two fistulas* occurring simultaneously was reported by Haufmann and Gosset in 1925.

Diagnosis. The common symptoms are abdominal pain, diarrhoea, loss of weight, faecal breath and vomiting, rumbling bowel sounds, flatulence, melaena, and anaemia.

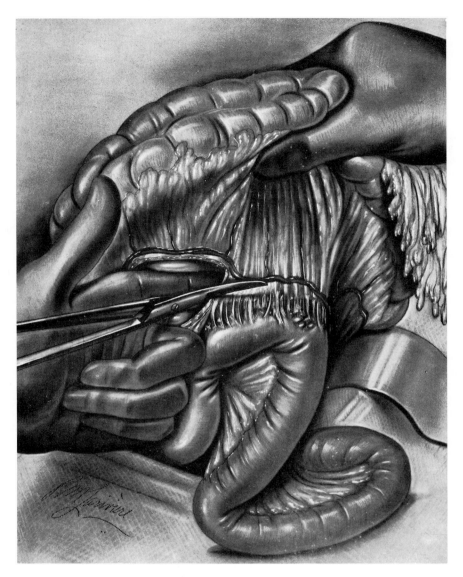

FIG. 6. Operation for anastomotic ulcer. Disconnecting posterior gastrojejunostomy. Shows stage in operation when mesocolon is being detached from region of gastroenteric stoma.

As soon as the fistula has become established, there is frequent belching of foul-smelling gas and intractable diarrhoea.

Vomiting of "faeculent" or yellowish "pea-soup" material occurs in over 60 percent of the cases and may be truly faecal in character.

Nausea, anorexia, loss of weight, extreme emaciation, a sullen ache in the epigastrium or left upper quadrant, backache, and the manifestations that accompany the deprivation of vitamins B and C, latent tetany, hypoproteinaemia, oedema of the lower extremities, and mental depression associated with a feeling of hopelessness are some of the leading clinical features. On the other hand, some patients with gastrojejunocolic fistula have had relatively mild and short or

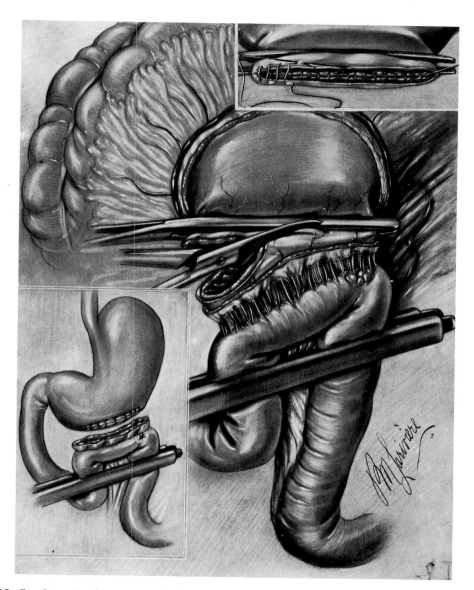

FIG. 7. Operation for anastomotic ulcer. Gastrojejunal anastomosis is being disconnected. There was no evidence of duodenal ulceration and the pylorus was patent. Opening in stomach was closed, and after trimming away the gastric remnant, which was attached to the jejunum the opening in the jejunum was likewise sutured and the parts restored to normal conditions.

intermittent symptoms and their general health is not seriously affected.

An x-ray examination after the administration of a barium meal or preferably of a *barium enema* confirms the presence of a fistula between the colon and stomach. *Of all investigations, a barium enema offers the most accurate means of diagnosis.* A barium-meal follow-through x-ray examination will fail to show the fistula in more than 30 per cent of cases.

Whenever this symptom complex develops, a faulty anastomosis, such as gastroileal or gastrocolic, must also be considered (see Chap. 19).

Preoperative investigations will include

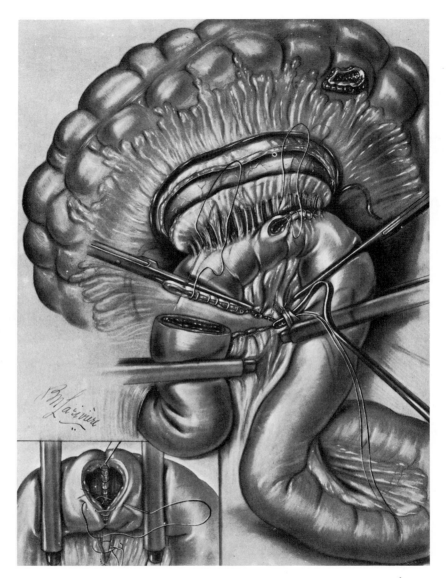

FIG. 8.   Operation for anastomotic ulcer. Portion of the jejunum engaged in anastomosis is hopelessly contracted, oedematous, and inflamed. This portion of jejunum is therefore excised and jejunal continuity is restored by end-to-end anastomosis. Note that the base of the anastomotic ulcer is attached to a portion of the transverse colon which was freed from the anastomotic junction. Note also that the mesocolon has been mobilised below the arching middle colic artery.

complete examination of the blood, faeces, and urine; blood urea estimations; liver function tests; determination of calcium loss, etc. The value of fibre-optic endoscopy has already been stressed (Chap. 4).

The *treatment of gastrojejunocolic fistula* is discussed later in this chapter. It may, how-ever, be stated here that the treatment is surgical and in *most* cases will consist of dismantling of the gastrojejunostomy, resection of the fistulous tract and implicated jejunum, axial anastomosis of the jejunum, closure of the defect in the colon, and partial gastrectomy followed by the antecolic method of anastomosis (Schoemaker-Billroth II).

In those patients who are gravely ill, wasted, and suffering from devastating diarrhoea, a three-stage operation is the right treatment. A preliminary defunctioning colostomy constructed just proximal to the hepatic flexure of the colon has the immediate effect of relieving diarrhoea and other symptoms, and in rendering the patient fit for major surgery in a few weeks' time, as suggested and practiced by Pfeiffer.

OPERATIONS FOR ANASTOMOTIC ULCER

Prophylactic Measures

When gastrojejunostomy is being carried out for a feeble, aged, poor-risk patient suffering from an intractable or penetrating duodenal ulcer, it should be combined, when conditions permit, with the relatively quick operation of vagotomy, since anastomotic ulceration does not necessarily spare the patient·because he happens to be in the winter of his life. Davey wisely remarks that confusion often comes from consideration of the decrease of acidity with advancing age, forgetting that mucosal resistance also declines and the end-result is still peptic ulceration.

Anastomotic ulcer occurs after partial gastrectomy for duodenal ulcer, but its incidence can be markedly reduced by removing *at least* 75 percent of the stomach and by performing a Schoemaker-Billroth II operation. When, at reconstruction, antrectomy or hemigastrectomy is. undertaken, vagotomy is a mandatory procedure, but the surgeon must also assure himself that vagotomy is *complete*.

Every possible source of infection in the mouth and pharynx must be removed before the operation, and at exploration any associated disease of the appendix, gallbladder, and the like, must be dealt with as seems best in the circumstances.

Preoperative Treatment

Medical treatment is the best preoperative treatment!

Gastrojejunocolic fistula is a fatal disease unless it is treated by timely surgical intervention. Preoperative treatment includes the

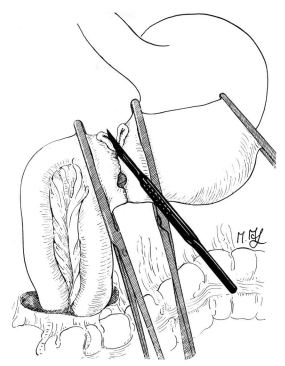

FIG. 9. Anastomotic ulcer following *low gastric resection plus* posterior gastrojejunostomy for duodenal ulcer. Note the following points: anastomosis freed from mesocolon and drawn into supracolic department; precise and bloodless incision through old suture line; too little stomach removed at previous operation. Correct procedure is closure of opening in jejunum, vagotomy, and three-quarter gastric resection followed by antecolic gastrojejunostomy based on Schoemaker-Billroth II plan.

correction of malnutrition, dehydration, anaemia, and vitamin and electrolyte deficiencies. Chemotherapy to reduce the infectivity of the large bowel content should be used and may itself help to produce some temporary improvement.

The patient should be admitted to hospital at least 1 week prior to operation to ensure that he is rendered as fit as possible to withstand a major abdominal procedure.

Operative Treatment of Anastomotic (Recurrent) Ulcer

In the treatment of gastrojejunal ulceration, the surgeon must adapt the second operation to the individual case, taking into

Table 4.   OPERATIONS FOR
ANASTOMOTIC ULCERATION

First Operation	Procedures Advised at Second Operation
Pyloroplasty or gastrojejunostomy with vagotomy	Hemigastrectomy—but check on thoroughness of vagotomy
Gastric resection with vagotomy	If vagotomy not complete, further transection of remaining nerves may be sufficient If no nerve fibres remain, do three-quarter partial gastrectomy by the antecolic Schoemaker-Billroth II procedure
Gastric resection alone	When previous gastric resection is considered inadequate, do three-quarter partial gastrectomy If amount of stomach resected and the anastomosis appears to be entirely satisfactory, and functioning well, do vagotomy alone
Partial or subtotal gastrectomy with or without vagotomy in the presence of Zollinger-Ellison syndrome	Do *total* gastrectomy plus removal of ulcerogenic pancreatic tumour or tumours, or abnormal nonbeta islet-cell pancreatic tissue

account (1) the operation previously performed, (2) the pathological findings at the second operation, and (3) the suspected cause of the recurrence.

If the anastomotic ulcer occurred after gastrojejunostomy or pyloroplasty with vagotomy, the 65 percent hemigastrectomy or 75 percent partial gastrectomy is indicated with vagotomy, if not accomplished at the first operation.

If vagotomy was carried out at the first operation, most often gastric resection is the operation of choice. But the surgeon must also assure himself that vagotomy is complete.

When gastrojejunal ulcer follows gastric resection, vagotomy or re-resection may be used, or both.[3] (See Table 4.)

Today, the operative mortality rate following the procedures varies from 0.5 to 4.5 percent.

POSTOPERATIVE MORTALITY RATE AND LATE RESULTS

In Marshall's Lahey Clinic series [18] of 200 cases there were 2 deaths following re-resection of the stomach in 57 patients, 3 deaths following gastric resection for anastomotic ulcer after gastrojejunostomy in 118 patients, and 1 death in 25 cases of vagotomy plus excision of the ulcer. There were, therefore, 6 deaths in 200 cases, a hospital mortality rate of 3 percent. A follow-up study of 168 of these cases revealed recurrent ulceration in 12 instances.

At the present time, the mortality rate varies from 0.5 to 4.5 percent, and depends on the type or extent of operation carried out at the *second operation*, for instance the mortality rate following vagotomy alone is not higher than 0.5 percent whereas partial gastrectomy or re-resection is associated with a hospital mortality rate of 2 to 4 percent.

OPERATIONS FOR GASTROJEJUNOCOLIC FISTULA

In the management of these difficult cases, the writer has gained much inspiration and help from the valuable papers of Pfeiffer and Kent,[19] Skoog-Smith et al.[21] and Nyhus in Harkins and Nyhus.[10]

Preoperative Treatment

The patient should be prepared for operation as soon as the diagnosis is established by opaque meal and enema. The preoperative management usually takes about 1 week. The patient should be confined to bed for most of the time; he is given deep-breathing exercises by a physiotherapist; the stomach is irrigated twice daily with warm saline solution; the diet is of high calorific value and large doses of vitamins A, B, C, and K are given; several blood transfusions are

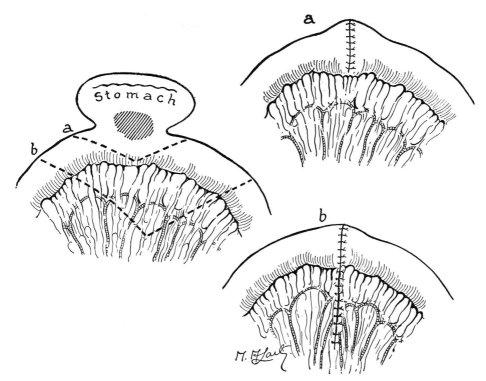

FIG. 10. Anastomotic ulcer. (A) Wedge excision with transverse suiture; (B) excision and axial anastomosis. (After Lahey.)

necessary, as anaemia and hypoproteinaemia are usually marked features; intravenous preparations of protein, glucose-saline solutions, and Hartmann's fluids are given according to the protein, salt, and water requirements; the stomach and bowel are rendered as sterile as possible by the oral administration of neomycin, kanamycin, with or without sulphathalidine; and sleep is ensured with the aid of one of the long-acting barbiturates.

Choice of Operation

The *choice of operation* will depend upon the following: (1) *the age and general condition of the patient;* (2) the extent of the inflammatory matting together of the implicated viscera; and (3) the nature of the primary operation.

If the patient's general condition is satisfactory and:

1. *If the previous operation has been a gastrojejunostomy,* the abdomen should be opened through a long left paramedian or vertical rectus muscle-splitting incision to afford the maximum exposure. The operation should be completed in *one stage* if the scarring is not too extensive and the implicated viscera are not so inextricably welded together as to obscure the usual landmarks. The colon should be separated from the jejunum and stomach. This will leave a gaping hole in the stomach and the attached jejunum, through which the gastric and intestinal contents are removed by suction. The margins of the aperture in the colon are trimmed, after which the hole is closed in such a manner that no narrowing or stricture is produced. If the hole in the colon is extensive, if it is close to or involves the mesenteric attachment of the bowel, or if it is impossible to suture the defect with safety and in a watertight fashion or it is apparent

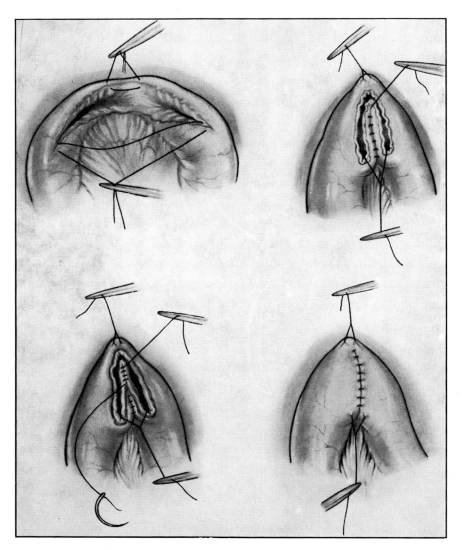

FIG. 11.   Method of closing a defect in the proximal jejunum by modification of the Finney method. (After Devine.)

that approximation of the margins of the opening will result in stricture of the bowel, the fistulous segment of the bowel should be resected and axial anastomosis should be performed.

The next step consists of freeing the jejunal loop from the stomach, after identification of the middle colic artery. The gastrojejunostomy is undone and the defects in the stomach and jejunum are closed. The opening in the jejunum may be closed by the Lahey or Finney methods, but if it is extensive it is safer to resect the segment of jejunum and to perform an end-to-end union. Gastroduodenal resection, in which at least 75 percent of the stomach is resected, is then carried out, after which any gap in the mesocolon is closed and an antecolic Schoe-

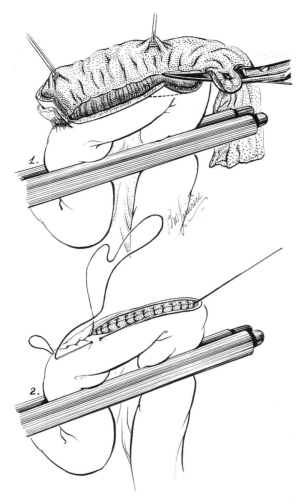

FIG. 12.   Closure of the jejunum.

maker-Billroth II type of anastomosis is constructed. Vagotomy completes the operation, if it is estimated that the gastric resection is less than 65 percent.

2. *If the previous operation has been a Billroth II partial gastrectomy,* after dismantling the colon from the stomach pouch and the jejunum and *after dealing with the involved colon on the lines already described,* the afferent and efferent limbs of the jejunum are divided between clamps close to the gastroenteric stoma, and end-to-end anasto-

mosis is performed, thus restoring jejunal continuity. After reducing the gastric pouch to the desired size (i.e. leaving at least 25 percent in situ), an antecolic Schoemaker-Billroth II anastomosis should be fashioned.

If the patients's general condition is poor, weight loss is marked, diarrhoea intractable, his response to preoperative treatment tardy, and the surgeon regards a one-stage operation with misgivings, it is advisable to employ a three-stage operation.

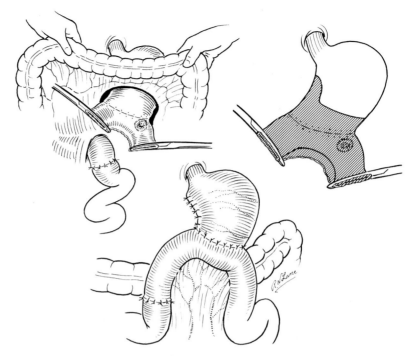

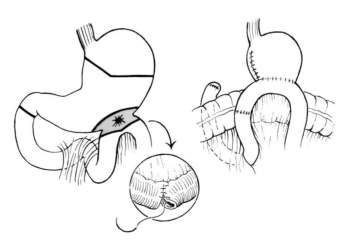

FIG. 13.   Operation for anastomotic ulcer. The previous operation was a posterior Billroth II.

FIG. 14.   Operation for anastomotic ulcer. The previous operation was a gastrojejunostomy.

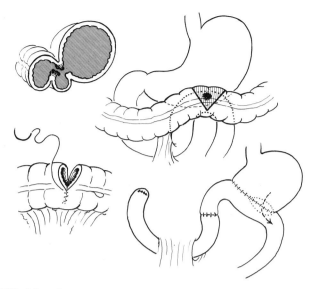

FIG. 15.   One-stage operation for a gastrojejunocolic fistula.

Staged Resection— Pfeiffer's Operation

The *first-stage operation* is used to divert the faecal stream away from the fistula, thus preventing the regurgitation of colonic contents into the stomach and jejunum and relieving the deleterious effects of prolonged acute gastroenteritis.

Proximal colostomy—sited just proximal to the hepatic flexure of the colon—is per-

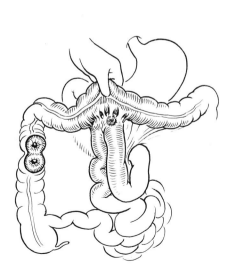

FIG. 16.   Gastrojejunocolic fistula. Pfeiffer's operation. First-stage procedure—defunctioning colostomy.

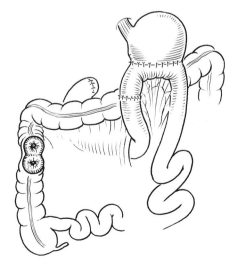

FIG. 17.   Gastrojejunocolic fistula. Pfeiffer's operation. Second-stage procedure—partial gastrectomy and antecolic Billroth II procedure.

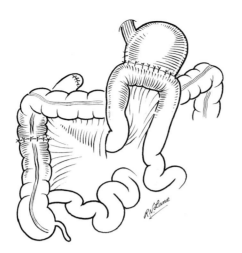

FIG. 18. Gastrojejunocolic fistula. Pfeiffer's operation. Third-stage procedure, completion—closure of the colostomy.

formed. The second and major portion of the operation is carried out—2 to 3 weeks following the fashioning of the diverting colostomy, and includes segmental colectomy and jejunectomy (followed by end-to-end unions of the colon and of the jejunum) and subtotal gastrectomy. The operation is completed by the Schoemaker-Billroth II procedure. About 2 to 3 weeks following these resections and reconstructions, the loop colostomy is closed (see Figs. 16, 17, and 18).

I recommend the operation of primary resection (Schoemaker-Billroth II) whenever the patient can be adequately prepared and is fit to withstand a long and difficult major surgical procedure.

Today, the operative mortality for Pfeiffer's staged operations is about 3 to 6 percent.

REFERENCES

1. Aird, Companion of Surgical Studies, 2d ed. London, Churchill Livingstone, 1957.
2. Balint et al., Lancet 2:551, 1957.
3. Behars, Surg. Clin. North Am. 51:879, 1971.
4. Blumen and Weber, J.A.M.A. 214:2335, 1970.
5. Condon and Tanner, Gut 9:438, 1968.
5a. Frederick. Surg. Gynecol. Obstet. 118:1093, 1964.
6. Friedman et al., N. Y. State J. Med. 15:854, 1951.
7. Garnett Wright, Br. J. Surg. 22:433, 1935.
8. Ger et al., Am. J. Surg. 122:115, 1971.
9. Gray and Sharpe, Arch. Surg. 43:850, 1941.
10. Harkins and Nyhus, Surgery of the Stomach and Duodenum, 2d ed., Boston, Little, Brown, 1969.
11. Johnston and Ferris, Surg. Clin. N. Am. 51:871, 1971.
12. Leurat and Lambert, Am. J. Dig. Dis. 5:623, 1960.
13. Lewisohn, Surg. Gynecol. Obstet. 40:70, 1925.
14. Lowdon, Edinb. Med. J. 55:533, 1948.
15. Lowdon, Br. J. Surg. 41:113, 1953.
16. Lowdon, Proc. R. Soc. Med. 55:196, 1962.
17. Maingot, Lancet 2:910, 1952.
18. Marshall, Surg. Clin. North Am. 40:673, 1960.
19. Pfeiffer and Kent, Am. J. Surg. 46:94, 1939.
20. Scobie, Lancet 1:370, 1969.
21. Skoog-Smith et al., Surg. Gynecol. Obstet 91:447, 1950.
22. Sterns and Bird, Can. J. Surg. 11:199, 1968.
23. Tanner, Postgrad. Med. 30:124, 1954.
24. Tanner, Proc. R. Soc. Med. 59:20, 1965.
25. Tanner, Personal communication, 1970.
26. Thoroughman et al., Ann. Surg. 169:790, 1969.
27. Van Heerden, Bernatz, and Rovdstad, Mayo Clin. Proc. 46:25, 1971.
28. Walters, et al., Surg. Gynecol. Obstet. 100:1, 1955.
29. Welbourn and Cooper, Lancet 2:193, 1954.
30. Wychulis, Priestly, and Foulk, Surg. Gynecol. Obstet. 122:89, 1966.

25

CHRONIC DUODENAL ILEUS: VOLVULUS OF THE STOMACH

RODNEY MAINGOT

CHRONIC DUODENAL ILEUS

Types

Chronic duodenal ileus is a condition in which there is a constant or intermittent delay in the passage of duodenal contents, resulting in dilatation of the duodenum.

Cases of chronic duodenal dilatation associated with stasis but occurring without any evidence of mechanical obstruction may be due to a congenital absence of ganglion cells in Auerbach's plexus.

Any obstructing agent is capable of producing duodenal stasis, and this may (and often does) lead to dilatation or megaduodenum.

Duodenal ileus may be *congenital* or *acquired*.

Classification of Chronic Duodenal Ileus
I. *Congenital*
    (a) *Megaduodenum congenitum*, in which it is thought that some form of neuromuscular incoordination exists.
    (b) Malrotation.
    (c) Folds and bands.
    (d) Duodenal diverticula.
    (e) Arteriomesenteric occlusion.
    (f) Duodenal stenosis.
    (g) Annular pancreas.
II. *Acquired*
    (a) Extrinsic lesions
        (1) Aneurysm.
        (2) Cysts and tumours of the pancreas.
        (3) Enlarged lymph nodes and neoplasms.
    (b) Intrinsic lesions
        (1) Ulcer.
        (2) New growths.
        (3) Inflammation, e.g., regional enteritis.
        (4) Foreign bodies.

This section deals mainly with two types of duodenal ileus: (1) megaduodenum congenitum and (2) arteriomesenteric occlusion (Wilkie's disease).

CONGENITAL TYPE

In this type—*megaduodenum congenitum*—the condition is primarily a vago-sympathetic incoordination comparable with oesophageal achalasia or with megacolon (Hirschsprung's disease). In these cases, there is a congenital absence of ganglion cells in the myenteric plexus, which accounts for the marked stretching of the thickened atonic coats of the gut and the gross dilatation that ensues.

In some cases, there is a history of indigestion and vomiting dating back to childhood. Dubose [6] recorded a case in an infant. Downes [5] described the condition in a child of 4½ years of age, and Balfour and Gray [1] reported the case of a patient aged 41 in whom the presence of *megaduodenum congenitum* was confirmed by x-ray examination and by operation. In none of these reported cases was there any demonstrable mechanical obstruction.

Barnett and Wall [2] described a case of megaduodenum resulting from the absence of the parasympathetic ganglion cells in Auerbach's plexus. Up to 1955 these authors could collect only 35 cases, but suggest that the disease is more frequent and has been misdiagnosed often as other forms of duodenal ileus. Harkins and Nyhus [8] confirm this view.

I have encountered only two cases in my surgical career. Both patients were females, aged 9 and 22 respectively, and, following the construction of jejunoduodenostomy (with an unduly large stoma) in both patients, the immediate and late results were unsatisfactory. Microscopical investigation of biopsies taken from the duodenal walls failed to display the presence of ganglion cells.

ACQUIRED TYPES

The obstructing agent may be a result of:

Intrinsic lesions. (1) innocent or malignant growths—e.g., cancer of the distal duodenum; (2) peptic ulcer; (3) foreign bodies, such as gallstones, hairballs, or *Taenia saginata;* or (4) congenital defects.[9]

Extrinsic lesions. (1) pressure of the superior mesenteric artery (arteriomesenteric ileus). (2) congenital or acquired periduodenal bands or adhesions causing angulation of the duodenum, the duodenojejunal flexure, or the first loop of the jejunum; (3) malrotation of the intestines and colon [7]—an incompletely rotated caecum may lie across the third part of the duodenum and obstruct it by bands or extrinsic pressure; (4) cancer of the tail or body of the pancreas, cancer of the stomach, malignant lymph nodes in the root of the mesentery, tuberculous or lymphadenomatous nodes lying along the superior mesenteric blood vessels as they cross the duodenum; (5) cicatrisation following stomal ulceration after gastrojejunostomy; (6) lordosis; and (7) visceroptosis.

HISTORICAL NOTE

Rokitansky in 1849 was the first to suggest that compression of the duodenum by the superior mesenteric vessels might be responsible for dilatation of and stasis within the duodenum.
But Wilkie was the first to give a detailed and accurate account of the pathophysiology of *arteriomesenteric ileus.* Chronic duodenal ileus was ably described by Petit (*Paris Thesis 67:* 1900), Dwight (*J Anat Physiol 31*:516, 1897), and Glenard (*Presse Méd Belge 41*:57, 1889), but we are indebted chiefly to the following surgeons for a correct understanding of the causes and of the

methods of treatment: Finney (*Bull Johns Hopkins Hosp 17*:37, 1906); Stavely (*Bull Johns Hopkins Hosp 19*:252, 1908); Wilkie (*Brit J Surg 9*:204, 1921); Robertson (*Surg Gynec Obstet 40*: 206, 1925); and Barnett and Wall (*Ann Surg 141*:527, 1955).

In the type due to *mechanical obstruction,* as a result of the continued intermittent blockage, the duodenal wall becomes thickened and the pylorus stretched. Wilkie, a great surgeon and teacher whose brow wore many laurels, regarded chronic duodenal ileus as a predisposing cause of duodenal and gastric ulceration, and this view is supported by modern gastroenterologists. *Wilkie found evidence of chronic peptic ulceration in 35 out of 135 patients with chronic duodenal ileus operated upon by him.* He also considered regurgitant vomiting following gastrojejunostomy to be in some cases due to a preexisting duodenal ileus, although it is important to remember that the obstruction may be of a temporary nature. In Friedenwald and Feldman's series of 80 cases of chronic duodenal ileus, duodenal ulcer was noted in 35 instances and gastric ulcer in 8.

Diagnosis of Arteriomesenteric Ileus. Diagnosis is made on the history of the case, the physical examination of the patient, the radiological examination of the stomach and duodenum, and if necessary, by exploratory operation. Although, as I have shown, there are many causes of chronic duodenal ileus and many clinical pictures may be presented, the following account may be taken to be more or less characteristic of that large group of cases in which the compression of the distal duodenum is by the superior mesenteric artery; these comprise 75 percent of all cases, and are sooner or later referred to the surgeon for advice.

The patient is usually, although by no means always, a thin woman of 20 to 40 years of age in whom visceroptosis is present. The symptoms often date back to infancy, and the patient regards herself as having a "weak stomach" which is easily upset by certain items of diet. The early symptoms include gastric flatulence, nausea, epigastric discomfort, and mild attacks of bilious vomiting; but when adult life is reached the symptoms become more severe and persistent and do not respond readily to treatment. Epigastric pain and distention arise during or shortly after the intake of food and are aggravated by standing or by exercise. The patient will often complain that she is unable to finish her meals as there is a sense of insufferable oppression in the abdomen which feels tight to bursting point. On such occasions, she will often resort to self-induced vomiting, and large quantities of gas will be belched up together with thin, bitter-tasting, bile-stained fluid. Every few weeks there will be an exacerbation of symptoms—bilious attacks in which the patient will feel ill and be prostrated by severe bouts of colicky pain and vomiting. Constipation is a troublesome feature, as are also the loud splashing and gurgling noises which may be heard in the abdomen.

The patient will derive little or no benefit from many and varied courses of medical treatment, from the wearing of special abdominal belts, from massage, or from special diets, but will, however, obtain some relief from postural treatment—i.e., by lying face downward or by assuming the genupectoral position when the pain is at its height.

Physical examination rarely reveals any positive sign, but epigastric distention may be observed in extreme cases.

Radiological examination of the stomach and duodenum following the administration of a barium meal is of all methods of investigation the most valuable and reliable. Duodenography, as described by Kreel in Chapter 4, is a helpful aid to diagnosis. In a well-established case, marked dilatation of the duodenum with statis, often with a "mo-

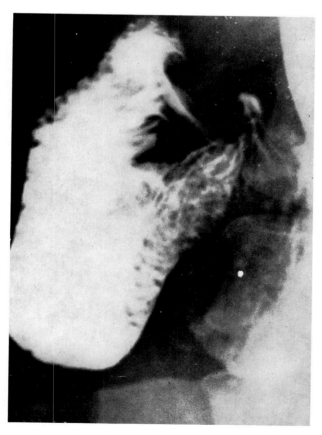

FIG. 1. Arteriomesenteric ileus. Third portion of duodenum was obstructed by superior mesenteric blood vessels. (Author's case.)

saic" pattern of the mucosa, will be observed, and reverse peristalsis may be noted (Fig. 1). In addition, the presence of visceroptosis may give an indication of the causal factor.

In the differential diagnosis, the following conditions will have to be considered: chronic peptic ulcer, duodenal diverticulum, chronic cholecystitis, malrotation of the colon, congenital bands and adhesions, visceroptosis, and neurosis.

The Technique of Duodenojejunostomy

Medical treatment should be given a trial and will consist of the following: rest in bed with the foot of the bed elevated, abdominal massage, a high-caloric nonresidue diet, administration of atropine and phenobarbital, duodenal aspiration followed by lavage, abdominal exercises, and special abdominal binders and supports.

Such remedies may yield relief in some of the *milder* cases, but it is very doubtful whether they will have any effect upon the *severe cases associated with obstruction*. For the latter, the operation of duodenojejunostomy, as first suggested by Finney in 1906 and as first performed by Stavely in 1908, should be carried out.

This operation is a simple undertaking, and when the indications are indisputable the immediate and late results are good. It should, however, be remembered that in cases of *megaduodenum congenitum* the late results of this emptying procedure are usually disappointing. In certain instances a definite band or adhesion may be the causative factor, and when such is found, simple division of the obstructing agent will, in the majority of cases, suffice to effect a cure. When, however, the obstruction is due, as it often is, to compression of the third portion of the duodenum by the superior mesenteric blood vessels, duodenojejunostomy should be performed. The transverse colon is drawn through the wound and elevated, thus exposing the prominent, bulging, third part of the duodenum; the peritoneum over it is incised and the gut freely mobilised. The first loop of the jejunum some 3 to 4 inches (7.6 to 10 cm) from the ligament of Treitz is then brought over to the right and anastomosed to the mobile duodenum as in the performance of a gastrojejunostomy.

At the completion of the operation, the anterior and posterior margins of the mesocolon are stitched to the duodenum to obliterate any dangerous gaps in the mesentery. The stoma should be at least 2 inches (5 cm) wide, and the suturing should be performed with 00 chromic catgut mounted on atraumatic (eyeless) needles (Fig. 2).

Gastrojejunostomy has no place in the treatment of chronic duodenal ileus.

The results that follow gastrojejunostomy are disappointing because this short-circuiting procedure does not relieve the reverse peristalsis in the duodenum or the sullen ache in the epigastric region. The patients feel full shortly after commencing a meal, and most of them lose weight. When there is a marked degree of mobility of the caecum or ascending colon, some surgeons recommend that colopexy be carried out, but I have not found this added procedure advantageous.

The *after-treatment* is conducted on the same lines as for gastrojejunostomy. Immediate relief is usually experienced and in clear-cut cases this proves to be of a permanent nature (Fig. 3).

Wilkie performed duodenojejunostomy in 127 cases with a mortality of 6.5 percent. He considered that operative treatment gave, on the whole, a "gratifying impression." The writer, up to the present time, has performed this operation in 41 selected cases with no hospital mortality rate. The late results have been satisfactory in 29 instances, but in the remaining 12 cases dyspepsia, periodical bouts of vomiting, and weight loss have been constant features. The 2 cases of *megaduodenum congenitum* which I have described are not included in the above series. Tyson and Keegan,[12] in an instructive and comprehensive paper, have reported cases that were treated successfully by means of duodenojejunostomy; and so have Harkins and Nyhus,[8] Farquharson (1966), Qvist (1970), and Gracey (1972).

In infants suffering from duodenal obstruction due to congenital bands or to an incompletely rotated caecum lying across the third part of the duodenum and obstructing it by extrinsic pressure, the results of opera-

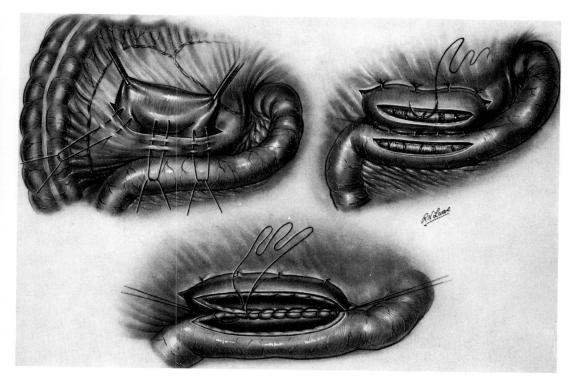

FIG. 2.   Duodenojejunostomy for chronic duodenal ileus.

tive intervention, as pointed out by Nixon, in Chapter 76, are good to excellent.

In nervous young adults suffering from chronic ill health and recurrent attacks of dyspepsia and in whom x-ray studies reveal a *mild or moderate degree of duodenal stasis* associated with visceroptosis, the results of this short-circuiting operation are very disappointing.

The best results follow duodenojejunostomy when the obstructed duodenum is grossly distended and vomiting is a prominent feature.

VOLVULUS OF THE STOMACH

Historical Note

The first case of *acute* gastric volvulus was described by Berti *(Gass Med Ital Prov Venet 9:*139,

1866), who found the condition at postmortem examination. Berg *(Nord Med Ark 19:*1, 1897) was the first to operate for this rare accident. Payr *(Mitt Grenzgeb Med Chir 20:*686, 1909) reported 22 cases, whilst Deaver and Ashurst *(Surgery of the Upper Abdomen,* 1921) were able to trace 35 cases, in 22 of which operations were performed, with a mortality of 60 percent. Laewen *(Deutsche Zt Chir 206:*319, 1927) in reviewing the literature reported 40 cases and included those of Thorek *(JAMA 81:*636, 1923) and Nockolds *(Brit J Surg 11:*774, 1924). Laewen estimated the death rate of gastric volvulus at 40 percent. Readers interested in this subject are referred to a series of instructive and interesting papers by Schatzki and Simone *(Amer J Dig Dis 7:*213, 1940), Hamilton *(Amer J Roentgenol 54:*30, 1945), Palumbo *et al. (Gastroenterology 45:*505, 1963), Lewinson *et al. (Henry Ford Hosp Med Bull 11:*357, 1963), and Maurer *(Tex J Med 60:*589, 1964).

Gosin and Ballinger *(Amer J Surg 109:*642, 1965) state that since the publication of Berg's paper in 1897 some 200 cases have been described in the literature. The number of case reports increase yearly; 13 reports can be found in the literature for 1963 and over 40 for 1970–71. Many patients with chronic recurrent volvulus, the common variety, have only minimal symptoms and require no treatment.

Acute gastric volvulus, leading to *gangrene*, is a rarity, and most surgeons will deal only with two or three such patients in a professional lifetime. Volvulus of the stomach is an abnormal anterior or posterior rotation of a portion of or the whole of the stomach about either the coronal or the sagittal axis of the body. Buchanan [3] in a classic article, pointed out that *total* gastric volvulus is not strictly a *complete* volvulus from the anatomical point of view, as the gastrohepatic ligament is sufficiently strong to anchor firmly the uppermost part of the fundus even in extreme torsion.

The stomach is limited in its excursions between its two fixed points—the gastrophrenic ligaments above and the peritoneal coverings of the pylorus and duodenum below—by the length of the gastrohepatic omentum and the lesser curvature of the stomach itself, and may be displaced within these limits by intrinsic or extrinsic pressure.

Pressure displacement of the stomach is of common occurrence and is frequently observed on radiological investigation of the viscus, but *torsion of almost the whole of the stomach* is rare; in fact, so rare that only about 300 authentic cases have so far been recorded.

Classification

Singleton (1940) and Wastell and Ellis [13] offer the following classification:

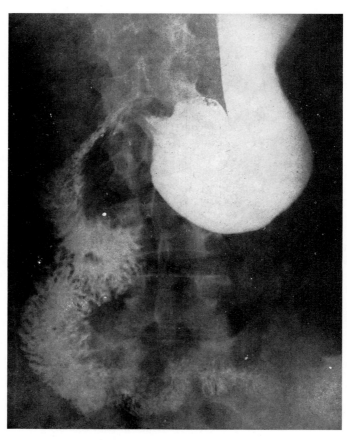

FIG. 3. Arteriomesenteric ileus. Same case as in Figure 1. Barium-meal x-ray appearances 3 months after duodenojejunostomy. Note that the emptying procedure has proved successful. (Author's case.)

1. Type:
   a. *Organo-axial.* Rotation of the stomach upward around the longitudinal axis—i.e., around the coronal plane and cardiopyloric line. Here the stomach becomes a closed loop, distending rapidly, producing acute symptoms, and requiring immediate decompression.
   b. *Mesenterio-axial.* Rotation of the stomach from right to left or very rarely from left to right around the sagittal plane. This type is often chronic or intermittent and is more common than (a).
2. *Extent:*
   a. *Total*—cases in which the whole stomach except the part attached to the diaphragm rotates forward and upward so that the greater curvature lies superiorly between the liver and diaphragm, and the posterior wall of the stomach faces anteriorly.
   b. *Partial*—where the rotation is limited to one segment of the stomach, this being nearly always the pyloric portion.
3. Direction:
   a. *Anterior*—cases in which the rotation passes forward.
   b. *Posterior.*
4. Severity:
   a. *Acute*—with signs and symptoms of an acute upper abdominal catastrophe.
   b. *Chronic*—associated with persistent or recurrent symptoms suggestive of a gastric ulcer or hiatal hernia.

In Wastell and Ellis' review of 8 patients (7 female and 1 male), they found 59 percent to be of the organoaxial type and 29 percent mesenteroaxial; the remainder were either mixed or unclassified.

Dalgaard [4] collected 150 cases of volvulus of the stomach, including about 100 cases of acute volvulus.

Tuffier, in 1907, is credited with the first report of a case of *chronic gastric volvulus* in which at operation the distal segment was found to be sharply twisted on an axis at right angles to a line joining the cardia to the pylorus. Rosselet (1921) was the first to diagnose chronic gastric volvulus by means of fluoroscopy, and he, with Gilbert in 1922, described the details of another case that was demonstrated radiologically. Since these reports, a number of cases have been shown on x-ray investigation, and radiographs have been well reproduced in Shanks and Kerly's *A Textbook of X-ray Diagnosis, Vol. 5, The Abdomen.*

Aetiology

Gastric volvulus may occur at any age, but the majority of recorded cases were found in patients between the ages of 50 and 60. The sex incidence is about equal.

For volvulus to occur, there must be some ligamentous laxity, for the stomach is held at its oesophageal end by the ligaments around the hiatus and at its distal end by the descending portion of the duodenum becoming retroperitoneal. There is usually an obvious predisposing cause. The *causes* of volvulus of the stomach may be enumerated as follows: (1) para-oesophageal hiatal hernia, (2) other diaphragmatic hernias resulting from trauma or congenital defects, (3) eventration of the left diaphragm—the most common cause, (4) pyloric and duodenal obstruction, which produces chronic dilatation of the stomach, and, (5) a heavy meal—which may predispose to the condition of approximating the pylorus and cardia.

Aerocoly, or distention of the large bowel with gas, was at one time considered to be an important aetiological factor. While distention of the transverse colon will undoubtedly cause displacement of the stomach, it is impossible for volvulus to occur if the ligamentary supports of the stomach are normal and staunch. The degree of twisting appears to be variable, the average being about 180 degrees. Thorek, Pendle, and Kocher mentioned 270 degrees and Niosi 360 degrees, but it seems that figures estimated by surgeons operating rapidly should be accepted with reservations.

Clinical Picture

In *chronic* cases, the symptoms are frequently those of a mild continuous or intermittent dyspepsia resembling in many respects the so-called peptic ulcer syndrome. Some patients with chronic mesenterioaxial volvulus will complain of distress or bloating during meals or shortly after the intake of food, whilst others again suffer from short or prolonged attacks of recurrent cramp-like epigastric pains accompanied by vomiting or retching. In such cases a correct preoperative diagnosis is often rendered possible by repeated barium-meal x-ray examinations.

In *acute* cases, the clinical features are so characteristic and the symptoms occur in such a definite sequence that, provided surgeons bear this accident in mind, it should in most instances be readily recognised and appropriate treatment be instituted without undue delay.

The three typical findings are:

1.   Early vomiting followed by intractable retching and inability to vomit.
2.   Severe epigastric pain associated with rapidly increasing distention of the epigastrium, but the iliac fossae remain flat.
3.   Inability to secure the passage of a stomach tube.

The sequence of events is:

1.   Pyloric occlusion (incessant vomiting of high obstruction).
2.   Obstruction of the cardia (inability to vomit or to obtain the passage of a stomach tube).
3.   Distention of the stomach with gas and fluids (the closed-loop type of obstruction).

Attempts to investigate the patient by barium or other contrast media show complete obstruction at the lower end of the oesophagus.

Urgent exploration is required, otherwise gangrene of the stomach is likely to necessitate gastric resection. The operative mortality rate has been assessed at 30 to 40 percent.

Operative Treatment

When symptoms of chronic recurrent volvulus—the commonest variety—are dis-abling, operative measures should be directed towards removing the cause. Para-oesophageal or other hiatal hernias are dealt with by reduction and repair. (See Chap. 74.) Relief of pyloric or duodenal obstruction is needed, if present. For those patients with *eventration of the diaphragm,* various methods of treatment such as gastropexy, partial gastrectomy, and gastrojejunostomy have all been tried with different degrees of success. According to Norman Tanner, the most logical and most successful operation is the so-called colonic displacement of the stomach. In this operation, the greater curvature of the stomach is completely freed from the colon so that the transverse colon can roll up under the left cupola of the diaphragm without dragging the stomach after it. A gastropexy is added after this procedure. At a long-term follow-up, 12 out of 14 patients operated upon by Tanner showed a successful result after this procedure.

This gastropexy yields results that are superior to those that follow the various types of gastropexy advocated in many textbooks, in which the stomach wall itself is sutured to the parietes or to the diaphragm.

When chronic gastric volvulus is complicated by the presence of intrinsic benign or malignant lesions of the stomach or of the first portion of the duodenum, the operative procedure of choice would be partial or subtotal gastrectomy by the Billroth I or II methods.

REFERENCES

1.   Balfour and Gray, Surg. Clin. North Am. 12:862, 1932.
2.   Barnett and Wall, Ann. Surg. 141:527, 1955.
3.   Buchanan, Br. J. Surg. 18:99, 1930.
4.   Dalgaard, Acta Chir. Scand. 103:131, 1952.
5.   Downes, Ann. Surg. 66:436, 1917.
6.   Dubose, Surg. Gynecol. Obstet. 29:278, 1919.
7.   Gross, The Surgery of Infancy and Childhood, Philadelphia, W. B. Saunders, 1953.
8.   Harkins and Nyhus, Surgery of the Stomach and Duodenum, London, Churchill, 1969.
9.   Ladd, J.A.M.A. 101:1453, 1933.
10.   Leading article, Br. Med. J. 2:446, 1971.
11.   Tanner, Am. J. Surg. 115:505, 1968.
12.   Tyson and Keegan, J.A.M.A. 165:1665, 1957.
13.   Wastell and Ellis, Br. J. Surg. 58:557, 1971.

26

A. COMPLICATIONS AND SEQUELAE OF GASTRIC OPERATIONS

RODNEY MAINGOT

Every operation for ulcer appears to be a success until it is found out.—SIR HENEAGE OGILVIE

The complications that can occur after gastric operations may be classified as immediate and remote.

Immediate Complications

1. Chest complications, such as bronchitis, lobar pneumonia, lobar atelectasis, and lobular atelectasis; cardiovascular accidents; and pulmonary embolism.
2. Haemorrhage; shock.
3. Complications attributable to the administration of the anaesthetic or to specific anaesthetic agents.
4. Fluid, electrolyte, and nutritional problems; acidaemia and alkalaemia; uraemia.
5. Acute retention of urine; anuria; cystitis; pyelonephritis.
6. Venous thrombosis—phlebothrombosis and thrombophlebitis.
7. Wound infection and disruption of the abdominal wound.
8. Dumping syndrome; stomal obstruction due to oedema or technical defects; acute obstruction and intestinal strangulation. Volvulus of the stomach or of the jejunal limbs engaged in the anastomosis.
9. Acute dilatation of the stomach.
10. Acute peritonitis and subphrenic abscess. Perforation of a suture line, particularly the duodenal stump or of an oesophageal anastomosis. Necrosis of the gastric remnant.
11. External fistula from (a) blown-out duodenal stump following the Billroth II operation; (b) anastomotic junction; (c) pancreatic and biliary fistulas.
12. Acute postoperative pancreatitis.
13. Jaundice.
14. Acute perforation of a new or old peptic ulcer.
15. Diarrhoea; steatorrhoea.
16. Acute pseudomembranous enterocolitis.

Remote Complications

1. Anastomotic ulcer, including gastrojejunocolic fistula. Acute perforation or massive haemorrhage from an anastomotic ulcer.
2. Acute intestinal obstruction.
3. Jejunogastric intussusception.
4. The onset of gastric cancer or gastric ulcer following gastrojejunostomy with or without vagotomy. Cancer in the gastric stump following partial gastrectomy.
5. Gastroileostomy, gastroileac ulcer, and gastrocolostomy.
6. Incisional hernia.
7. Haemorrhage from: (a) erosions in acute hypertrophic gastritis; jejunitis or duodenitis; (b) carcinoma or benign ulcer of the stomach; (c) anastomotic ulcer; (d) oesophageal peptic ulcer; (e) the erosion of a large artery —e.g., gastroduodenal, which has been incorporated and buttressed to the duodenal stump during partial gastrectomy for duodenal ulcer.
8. Cholangitis; gallstones; choledocholithiasis; bile peritonitis.
9. Functional gastrointestinal complaints.
10. The "dumping" syndrome—mechanical and metabolic aspects.
11. Anaemia and deficiency states.

465

A large number of these complications may follow *any* abdominal operation but are here included to make the classification as comprehensive as possible. These complications can be reduced to a minimum by good anaesthesia, careful preoperative and postoperative management, proper selection of patients for operation, the appropriate operation, meticulous technique, complete haemostasis, the judicious use of chemotherapeutic agents, and the maintenance of fluids and electrolytes before, during, and after intricate and protracted operations upon the stomach, duodenum, and proximal jejunum.

Priestley[29] points out that many other factors exist that may contribute to the likelihood of complications following gastric operations, but these vary in significance from patient to patient. The important consideration is to bear in mind the possibility of these factors and to make every effort to correct them before operation is undertaken. At the present time our main endeavour should be directed toward the *prevention* of these complications. Recognition and treatment then become necessary in a decreasing number of patients and only when prophylactic measures fail.

Certain complications that occur after gastric operations will now be discussed.

HAEMORRHAGE AFTER GASTRIC OPERATIONS

Haemorrhage following gastric operations for benign or malignant lesions is a rare complication and may be intraperitoneal or intraintestinal. It may occur as haematemesis and/or melaena in the early or the late postoperative phase.[35]

Immediate causes. In the postoperative period, bleeding is usually due to faulty haemostasis in the gastroduodenal or gastrojejunal suture line.

Oesophageal varices, either unsuspected or coincidental may bleed.[33]

There may be oesophageal peptic ulcer in association with hiatal hernia, or multiple acute erosions of the gastric mucosa.[21]

Unsuspected blood dyscrasias may cause postoperative haemorrhage, as described by McLaughlin and Coe.[26]

Anastomotic ulceration may have an early onset. This complication in the immediate postoperative phase is most frequently witnessed following the first-stage operation of the two-stage partial gastrectomy procedure described by McKittrick, Moore, and Warren.[25]

There was a case at the Southend General Hospital in which a large stomal ulcer developed within two weeks of the performance of the first-stage operation of McKittrick's two-stage partial gastrectomy, and in which a massive haematemesis was the first evidence of the lesion. The stomal ulcer rapidly healed following excision of the antrum and the first portion of the first part of the duodenum with its contained ulcer.

Littler,[23] in a well-documented article, states that there are many recorded cases in which *severe* haemorrhage occurred 10 to 20 days after partial gastrectomy for peptic ulcer. He believes that bleeding in these cases was due to secondary haemorrhage. He says that a possible explanation of its cause lies in the development of sepsis in and around the gastrojejunostomy suture line, with the production of submucous abscesses and consequent erosion of thrombus and of blood vessel walls in the vicinity of proteolytic ferments. He describes an interesting case in which a perigastric abscess developed after subtotal gastrectomy, and played a major part in the causation of repeated severe attacks of haematemesis.

Late causes. May include bleeding (1) from the original ulcer bed; (2) due to anastomotic ulcer or gastrojejunocolic fistula; (3) due to cancer of the stomach; (4) from erosive gastritis or multiple acute erosions of the efferent limb of the jejunum; (5) due to retrograde jejunogastric intussusception; or (6) from the duodenal stump following gastric resection caused by erosion of the gastroduodenal artery and in all probability produced by transfixion sutures that picked up the vessel and buttressed it against the closed end of the duodenum.

Following most gastric operations, and particularly those in which some form of anastomosis has been undertaken, the first few ounces of fluid aspirated are usually blood-stained, and this is due in most instances to a slight oozing of blood from the suture line in the stomach. Sometimes, however, haemorrhage may be caused by rough or repeated handling of a fixed duodenal ulcer which has, on exploration, proved to be irremovable. Should the patient continue to vomit bright blood or become blanched, a serious view of the case must be taken. Postoperative haematemesis or melaena is nowadays a rare occurrence, as special precautions are taken in suturing to prevent the likelihood of haemorrhage at the anastomotic line.

Immediate measures. If the patient continues to bleed, proceed as follows:

1. Morphine should be given liberally to allay anxiety.
2. Blood transfusions are given and often prove successful either in helping to "arrest" the haemorrhage or in rendering the patient fit to withstand a second operation, should it prove necessary. Large quantities of compatible blood must always be available for the treatment of these patients.
3. A nasogastric tube is passed and the gastric contents are aspirated hourly. The appearance of fresh blood in the aspirating syringe will often be the first warning of another brisk haemorrhage, and resuscitative measures should be put in train at once in such instances.
4. One to two ounces of water is given orally each hour.
5. Antibiotic agents are injected in full dosage.
6. Ample doses of vitamins B, C, and K are introduced into the intravenous drip daily.
7. Barium- or Gastrografin-meal x-ray investigation may prove of diagnostic help in certain selected cases, but is by no means a routine procedure.

Operative treatment. If, in spite of the above emergency measures, shock is present, the pulse rate continues to rise steadily, the patient continues to vomit bright blood, and the systolic blood pressure progressively deteriorates, the abdomen should be opened. The abdominal wall is painted with cetrimide and Hibitane. The skin sutures are removed, the wound edges retracted, and tetracloths affixed to the margins. The sutures in the abdominal wall are then snipped with scissors and removed, and the abdominal cavity is opened.

If the previous operation has been a *posterior gastrojejunostomy*, the transverse colon and greater omentum are drawn through and lifted upward over the edges of the wound and the stitches in the mesocolon are snipped. The anterior row of sutures in the anastomosis is cut through with scissors and is extracted. The outer margins of the wounds in the stomach and jejunum are held apart with Babcock forceps and the area is thoroughly cleansed. A through-and-through all-coats suture of 0 chromic catgut is inserted, starting at one end of the posterior suture line and proceeding to the opposite end. It then continues anteriorly, uniting the anterior margins of the stomach and jejunum firmly and evenly in such a way that the risk of further haemorrhage is eliminated. This anterior suture line is further reinforced and invaginated by a continuous Lembert or Cushing suture of 00 Dexon or chromic catgut and then reinforced with a few well-placed interrupted sutures of fine silk, after which the margins of the opening in the mesocolon are again stitched to the stomach on each side.

If the previous operation has been an *anterior gastrojejunostomy,* the anterior row of sutures should be removed to permit inspection of the posterior suture line. A new through-and-through haemostatic suture should be introduced, embracing all the coats of the stomach and jejunum, after which the anterior row of sutures is further reinforced and invaginated by a continuous Lembert suture.

If the previous operation has been a *gastroduodenostomy,* the anterior row of sutures is unpicked, any bleeding point is underrun, and the posterior layer is reinforced with interrupted sutures of 00 chromic catgut. From this point onward the steps of the operation are precisely similar to those of an ordinary gastroduodenostomy.

Massive haematemesis and/or melaena immediately following *partial or subtotal gastrectomy* is rare, but when it occurs it is usually safer to control the bleeding point by a direct surgical attack than to rely upon blood transfusions and medical management.

Where severe haemorrhage occurs, necessitating emergency operation, I employ a left-sided subcostal incision (Kocher) to display the small gastric pouch and the anastomosis, as the stomach is usually tucked away under the left cupola of the diaphragm. Gentle traction is exerted on the efferent limb of the jejunum and the gastric remnant to coax them toward the abdominal incision. Here again all the anterior rows of sutures are cut and removed, and the interior of the stomach and the posterior anastomotic line are carefully inspected to detect the bleeding point or points. A few interrupted sutures of 0 chromic catgut or Dexon are inserted to control any area from which the bleeding appears to be arising, after which a continuous posterior lockstitch suture of 00 chromic catgut is introduced and then continued anteriorly as a through-and-through all-coats suture, the loops being placed close to one another before being drawn firmly into place. The operation is completed by inversion and strengthening of the anterior suture line with a series of closely-applied Lembert sutures of fine Mersilk.

Gilchrist and DePeyster [13] state that during the previous 9 years eight of their patients developed massive postoperative haemorrhage from the stomach *following operation upon other organs*. None treated solely by medical measures survived, whereas three patients who had subtotal gastric resection for this complication were cured.

Dumping and other syndromes associated with mechanical factors, and the nutritional and metabolic consequences of surgery for peptic ulcer are discussed in Chapter 27.

Necrosis of the gastric remnant. This is reviewed by Harkins,[17] Jackson,[20] Hardy,[15] and by Harkins and Nyhus (1969), in *Surgery of the Stomach and Duodenum*.

Necrosis of the gastric stump is a rare complication of subtotal gastrectomy. It is prone to occur after high resections for carcinoma of the stomach and in aged patients suffering from arteriosclerosis.

Casebolt (1959) reported 2 cases. He showed that the gastric remnant obtains its blood supply from the ascending branch of the left gastric artery, the inferior phrenic,

and the vasa brevia arteries, and suggested that at least one of these arteries and preferably a branch of another be kept intact. Harkins stated that in a series of 500 subtotal gastrectomies he has seen 2 cases of what he terms the *blue stomach syndrome* after division of the left gastric artery and all the vasa brevia. He also pointed out that it was important to avoid any tension on the suture line of the anastomosis, as this may obstruct a somewhat compromised circulation.

Few patients have survived this catastrophe. It is a wise precaution to insert a drainage tube close to the newly constructed stoma following the performance of subtotal gastrectomy carried out on the Billroth II plan. Should the patient subsequently develop a gangrenous patch in the gastric remnant and this sloughs away and gives rise to an external gastric fistula, the surgeon would be well advised to act promptly and courageously: he should explore the abdomen through a left subcostal incision and perform *total* gastrectomy. It is only by these means that a few of these unfortunate patients can be saved.

Spencer [34] successfully performed total gastrectomy for pouch necrosis 40 hours after an initial subtotal gastrectomy with a gastrojejunostomy—Billroth II type of repair.

Late causes of obstruction following gastric operations. Obstruction occurring months or even years after gastric operations is always a very grave symptom and may be due to one of the following causes:

1. The formation of a new peptic ulcer in the stomach or duodenum.
2. Stomal ulceration: gastrojejunocolic fistula.
3. The onset of malignant disease of the stomach.
4. Intestinal obstruction due to bands and adhesions.
5. Contraction of the aperture in the mesocolon following posterior gastrojejunostomy.[6]
6. Erosive "spongy" jejunitis (Fig. 1) and gastrojejunitis.
7. Retrograde jejunogastric intussusception.

Retrograde jejunogastric intussuscep-

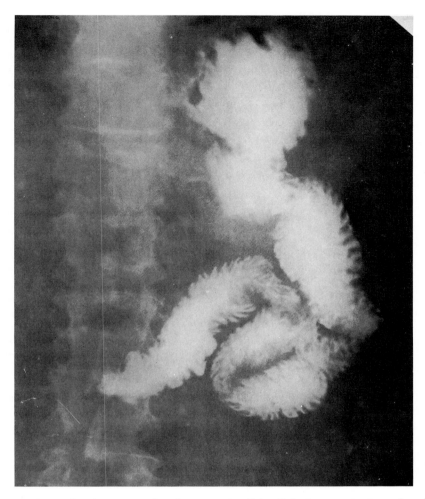

FIG. 1. Radiograph taken 3 months after posterior Polya-Hofmeister gastrectomy for chronic duodenal ulcer in a man aged 42. Note the presence of jejunitis of the efferent limb of the jejunum. The main postoperative symptoms were anorexia, nausea, epigastric distention, and attacks of bleeding. Symptoms were relieved by performance of vagotomy.

tion. This is well recognised as a rare complication after gastrojejunostomy and the Billroth II operations.

Reyelt and Anderson (*Surg Gynec Obstet 119*:1305, 1964) state that although Wölfler performed the first gastrojejunostomy in 1881, it was not until 33 years later that Bozzi reported this complication following this operation. According to Shackman (*Brit J Surg 27*:475, 1940) there were no further reports in the literature dealing with this subject until von Steber (*München Med Wschr 20*:648, 1917) in Germany recorded his experience with a case. Richard Warren (*Lancet 2*:615, 1919) was the first British surgeon to oper-

ate on a case of jejunogastric intussusception in which a large segment of the efferent limb of the jejunum had prolapsed into the gastric cavity. Hamilton Drummond (*Brit J Surg 11*:79, 1923), who was an accomplished surgeon, reviewed 13 cases to date, and added one of his own. Von Brunn published the first radiological diagnosis of the condition in 1924.

Lundberg (*Acta Chir Scand 54*:423, 1922) was the first to describe this condition complicating partial gastrectomy. His patient was a woman aged 41 who, 10 years after the performance of a Billroth II procedure for pyloric carcinoma, developed a retrograde jejunogastric intussusception. Smith (*Brit J Surg 42*:654, 1955) reviewed 16 cases occurring after partial gastrectomy and described a further case of his own. According to Early *(Postgrad Med 33*:193, 1957) it would appear that this complication, although showing a steady increase in recorded incidences during recent years, is still rare. Recently, Restogi, et al. *(Cleveland Clin Quart, 35*:33, 1968) stated that in the American literature only 45 cases have been reported.

The most common type of retrograde intussusception, according to Irons and Lipkin,[19] who collected reports of 100 cases, is the one in which the *efferent loop* of jejunum prolapses into the stomach. This occurrence accounts for 75 percent of all cases.

Intussusception of the *afferent loop* into the stomach is the next most common, while in the third and final type, which is distinctly rare, both loops undergo intussusception. This type, the least common form (10 percent of all cases), occurs early during the postoperative period. All three types have followed gastrojejunostomy, but only type 2 (intussusception of the *afferent* loop into the stomach) has been reported after a partial gastrectomy.

Ryelt and Anderson [31] have pointed out that although early reports indicate a predominance of intussusception following gastrojejunostomy, the trend in the surgical treatment of peptic ulcer has changed, so that within the past 6 years 8 of the 13 cases reported in the American literature alone followed gastric resection with the Billroth II type of anastomosis. Recently, Christeas and Sfinas [5] reported a case of jejunojejunal intussusception, which developed acute obstruction 6 years after a *total gastrectomy*. Following resection of the gangrenous intussuscepted bowel, the patient made a good recovery. They claim that their case was the first to be recorded in medical literature. Up to 1964, 145 cases of jejunogastric intussusception had been reported in the world literature. This figure has increased to about 170 cases by the end of 1971.

Jejunogastric intussusception may be acute or chronic; the sex incidence is equal; the peak age incidence is about 50; the condition may arise from 5 days to 30 years after operation; and a correct preoperative diagnosis is rarely made, the usual one being that of acute high gut obstruction or severe bleeding from secondary peptic ulceration.

Adams[1] recognized two *clinical types:*

1. That in which the patient is suddenly seized with an acute attack of epigastric pain followed by a sensation of severe constriction in the upper abdomen, and by vomiting. On examination of the abdomen, there is visible peristalsis, and a tumour can often be palpated in the epigastrium. Since these cases are diagnosed as an acute intestinal obstruction, operation is usually performed without any delay, thus rendering the prognosis favourable. The mortality rate, however, is almost 100 percent if surgical exploration is not attempted (Fig. 2). In contrast, early operation has proved life-saving in 90 percent of the patients treated surgically.

2. In the other type, which closely resembles a bleeding anastomotic ulcer, the dumping syndrome, proximal loop obstruction, or obstruction due to adhesions, vomiting is frequent and becomes first blood-stained and then definitely haemorrhagic. A provisional diagnosis of bleeding recurrent ulcer is usually made and the patient receives treatment by medical measures accordingly, thereby leading to delay in operation with a consequently high mortality.

As spontaneous reduction never occurs, unless operation is performed in all such cases, the patients will die within a few days. If, however, early operation is carried out, the prognosis is good. Shackman (1940) stated that of fifteen patients operated upon within 48 hours of onset, all recovered, whereas in ten patients operated upon after 48 hours there was a mortality rate of 50 percent. Vink [36] recorded a mortality rate of 10 percent for those patients who were operated upon within 48 hours and of 50 percent after that time.

From the literature, Adams [1] reported thirty patients who were subjected to operation; nine of these died and twenty-one recovered. He also reported one successful case of his own. Debenham [7] recorded an interesting case of retrograde intussusception of the jejunum following gastrojejunostomy, and offers many useful suggestions with regard to

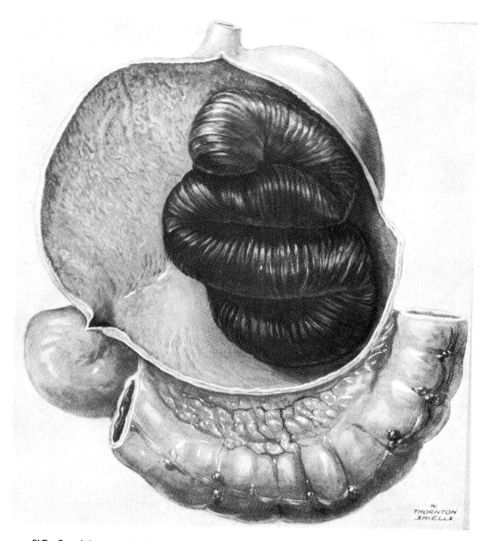

FIG. 2. Jejunogastric intussusception. (Museum, St. Bartholomew's Hospital, London.)

operative treatment. Instructive articles by the following surgeons should also be consulted: Douglas,[9] Prokasha et al.,[30] and Gerber and Pinsky.[12]

The *chronic variety* is characterised by epigastric distress, nausea, colicky pains, and intermittent and sometimes severe vomiting occurring at a remote date after gastrojejunostomy. *A barium-meal x-ray examination is useful in confirming the diagnosis, as the intussusception displaces the barium and so produces a marked filling defect.* A rounded shadow produced by the ectopic coils of jeju-

num in the stomach tends to change its position on palpation, and is marked with striations due to the folds of jejunal mucosa. In a few cases, *gastroscopy* has been instrumental in clinching the diagnosis.

The following points should be emphasised in connection with this rare complication following gastrojejunostomy:

1. Jejunogastric intussusception is a well-established late complication of gastrojejunostomy or the Billroth II operations for peptic ulcer. It occurs in

acute or chronic forms, the former being fatal apart from operation.

2. Diagnosis is possible, dependent upon the rule: "Where haematemesis or obstructive symptoms appear after a gastrojejunostomy, think of intussusception." [1]

3. If, in a patient with acute intestinal obstruction, the following triad is present, acute retrograde intussusception should be diagnosed: (a) epigastric scar; (b) visible peristalsis, the waves passing from left to right; (c) a palpable mobile swelling about the mid-abdomen.

4. The chronic or intermittent form is to be remembered as one of the causes of recurrent vomiting after gastrojejunostomy or partial gastrectomy. Early radiography is demanded in such cases, and will reveal the intussusception, if present, and pave the way for a curative operation.

Treatment. The following operative procedures have been practised:

1. Reduction of the intussusception.
2. Revision of the anastomosis.
3. Suturing together the efferent and afferent limbs after reduction of the intussusception.
4. Entero-anastomosis, the afferent limb being anastomosed to the efferent limb.
5. Resection of the anastomosis followed by partial gastrectomy, gastrointestinal continuity being established by the Billroth I type of repair or by the Schoemaker-Billroth II method.

According to Early, no operative procedure has been shown to prevent recurrence, which, however, is rarely seen after simple reduction of the intussusception. *Where the intussusceptum is gangrenous, resection and revision of the anastomosis is the correct treatment.* Recurrence after operative reduction is exceptional and the only instances so far reported are those of Baumann,[2] Hublin,[18] and Douglas.[10]

Suturing the afferent and efferent limbs together after reduction of the intussusception or the construction of an entero-anastomosis does not prevent the possibility of recurrence, as Hublin [18] has shown. Even the

Billroth II methods are no guarantee against future intussusception, for this complication has occurred after the antecolic as well as the retrocolic types of operation. Intussusception has taken place even after subtotal gastrectomy, and instances of such complications following the radical types of subtotal gastrectomies have been recorded by MacNamara (1944), Grimes (1949), and Welbourn (1955). The performance of the Billroth I operation renders complete immunity.

GASTRIC CARCINOMA FOLLOWING OPERATIONS FOR PEPTIC ULCER

This subject is discussed by Gray and Lofgren,[14] Orringer,[27] Bennett and Rossmiller,[3] Franchini et al.,[11] Lacache and Van Kemmer,[22] and Burns and Taubman.[4] The last-mentioned authors state that carcinoma of the stomach developing after gastric surgery for *duodenal ulcer* is well recognised, and that the incidence has been found to be almost identical to the expected frequency for the intact stomach in the general population. If the previous operation has been carried out for *gastric ulcer,* however, the risk of subsequent gastric cancer is increased. Coexisting duodenal ulcer and gastric carcinoma in the absence of previous gastric surgery is much less common. Burns and Taubman [4] have been able to find only 78 definite cases in the literature. They describe two cases of their own in which gastric carcinoma was associated with duodenal ulceration.

Gastric ulcer and gastric cancer are uncommon complications in patients who have undergone gastrojejunostomy. Gray and Lofgren [14] found 26 cases of gastric ulcer and 17 cases of carcinoma in 825 instances in which exploration of a previously performed gastrojejunostomy was undertaken. It is important to exclude the possibility of gastric cancer before instituting medical therapy for a gastric ulcer developing after gastrojejunostomy.

The occurrence of carcinoma of the stomach after partial gastrectomy for gastric ulcer is rare. Debray et al.[8] observed 11 cases of gastric carcinoma occurring after gastric resection for gastric ulcer. They have also collected reports of 113 similar cases from the literature. There was an average of about 14 years between the time of resection and the development of the tumour, the periods ranging from 3 to 37 years.

The onset of carcinoma is heralded by epigastric pain, anorexia, vomiting, dysphagia, loss of weight, haematemesis, and anaemia. In 49 cases, the cancer was situated remote from the anastomosis, while in 31 cases the growth was found at the line of anastomosis.

The diagnosis is often suspected on clinical grounds and clinched by x-ray studies and fibregastroscopy. The prognosis here, following radical subtotal gastrectomy or total gastrectomy, is grave.

Pack and Banner [28] report 25 cases of gastric cancer that subsequently developed in stomachs surgically treated by gastrojejunostomy or partial gastrectomy for chronic duodenal ulcer. The time elapsing between the original operation and the onset of the carcinoma varied from 8 to 25 years. These authors believe that the oft-repeated statement that duodenal ulcer and gastric cancer seldom occur in the same subject should be modified to state that a previous duodenal ulcer confers no immunity against the subsequent development of gastric cancer.

JAUNDICE FOLLOWING PARTIAL GASTRECTOMY

Jaundice occurring in the early postoperative stage is always an occasion for alarm. It may be caused by:

1. Injury to the common bile duct (see Chap. 48).
2. Occlusion of the papilla of Vater by inturned duodenal wall, following Billroth II procedures for duodenal ulcer.
3. Blood transfusion.
4. Viral hepatitis or homologous serum hepatitis.
5. Calculous cholecystitis or cholangitis.
6. Acute pancreatitis (see Chap. 36).
7. Obstruction of the afferent limb of the jejunum following gastrojejunostomy or the Billroth II methods of partial gastrectomy (see Chap. 27).
8. Obstruction of the choledochus caused

by the reactivation of a large penetrating posterior wall duodenal ulcer following inadequate gastric surgery.

The reader is referred to an excellent article by Sales,[32] which deals with all the important aspects of jaundice and duodenal ulceration.

When jaundice ensues *early*, that is, a few days after the performance of gastroduodenal resection for a penetrating duodenal ulcer, the usual diagnosis made is injury to the choledochus or acute viral hepatitis. If a blood transfusion has not been given and if "toxic" hepatitis can be excluded with a high degree of certainty, the surgeon should assume that acute obstruction of the proximal loop of the jejunum is present or that the common bile duct has been traumatised. During operation for a large posterior-wall duodenal ulcer, the lower end of the choledochus may be: crushed, divided, incised, excised, or occluded by a ligature or suture, or the papillary region may be compressed by inverted duodenal wall following a Billroth II operation for duodenal ulcer or for cancer of the pyloric portion of the stomach.

Volvulus of the jejunal loop engaged in the anastomosis, if not corrected by immediate detortion, may give rise to portal thrombosis which, in turn, may account for severe icterus.

A lethal cause of jaundice arising in the early days after a Billroth II partial gastrectomy is *obstruction of the gastroenteric stoma or of the afferent or efferent limb of the jejunum* (see Chap. 27). It is an example of the closed-loop type of obstruction. Bile and pancreatic and duodenal juices are poured into the occluded segment of intestine, and a stage is reached when the pressure inside the tightly distended loop—which is, in a sense, a continuation of the choledochus—is greater than the biliary pressure. The pent-up juices in the engorged and bloated coil of intestine are forced into the duct of Wirsung and the biliary passages and test the integrity of the duodenal closure. Jaundice ensues if the duodenal stump does not blow out. The condition is, of course, not compatible with life and, if the obstruction is not rectified by an immediate operation, death from acute liver failure will ensure in a few days.

I have previously drawn attention to the mechanics of this grave complication of gastroduodenal resection, in my work, *The Management of Abdominal Operations*.[24] The surgeon should be on the alert to recognise and appreciate the true significance of this complication. Therefore, in those cases in which jaundice is detected after gastric surgery, the surgeon should order plain x-ray films of the abdomen in order to clinch or refute a diagnosis of high, small-gut, closed-loop acute obstruction. It may be argued that such a method of investigation is superfluous in a seriously ill patient who, in any case, will have to be subjected to laparotomy for suspected trauma to the bile ducts. However, radiological investigation may be the means of supplying an important clue to the true state of affairs. To be forewarned in such instances will prove helpful to the surgeon at exploration and curtail intra-abdominal manipulations.

If, on the other hand, the continued pressure of the imprisoned fluid in the closed loop is sufficient to cause disruption of the suture line of the inturned duodenal stump, the patient will develop general peritonitis, a subhepatic abscess, or an external duodenal fistula. The jaundice, as a rule, slowly wanes when the bowel contents are free to pour through the hole in the disrupted suture line of the duodenum.

The *treatment*, then, of jaundice caused by obstruction of the stoma or the loops of jejunum engaged in the anastomosis following a Billroth II partial gastrectomy or gastrojejunostomy, is immediate exploration at which the cause of the block is determined and corrected by the simplest procedure compatible with safety. The treatment of *external duodenal fistula* is described in Chapter 9.

The subject of jaundice occurring after gastric operations receives the expert attention of Hardy and State.[16]

REFERENCES

1. Adams, Br. Med. J. 1:388, 1935.
2. Baumann, Arch. Klin. Chir. 111:504, 1919.
3. Bennett and Rossmiller, Cleve. Clin. Q. 9:116, 1952.
4. Burns and Taubman, Br. J. Surg. 54:174, 1967.
5. Christeas and Sfinas, Br. J. Clin. Pract. 22:439, 1968.
6. Cleator et al., Br. Med. J. 1:530, 1968.
7. Debenham, Br. Med. J. 1:388, 1935.
8. Debray et al., Schweiz. Med. Wochenschr. 88:631, 1958.
9. Douglas, Postgrad. Med. 30:200, 1954.
10. Douglas, Postgrad. Med. 30:204, 1954.
11. Franchini et al., Arch. Ital. Patol. Clin. Tumori. 5:495, 1962.
12. Gerber and Pinsky, Calif. Med. 98:221, 1963.
13. Gilchrist and DePeyster, Ann. Surg. 147:728, 1958.
14. Gray and Lofgren, Surg. Gynecol. Obstet. 89:285, 1949.
15. Hardy, Am. J. Surg. 108:699, 1964.
16. Hardy and State, Surg. Clin. North. Am. 44: 371, 1964.
17. Harkins, Ann. Surg. 150:1074, 1959.
18. Hublin, Acta. Chir. Scand. 101:3, 1951.
19. Irons and Lipkin, Ann. Surg. 141:541, 1955.
20. Jackson, Ann. Surg. 150:1071, 1959.
21. Jankelson and Milner, J.A.M.A. 145:17, 1951.
22. Lacache and Van Kemmel, Arch. Chir. 26:618, 1966.
23. Littler, Br. J. Surg. 45:277, 1959.
24. Maingot, The Management of Abdominal Operations, 2d ed., London, Lewis, 1957.
25. McKittrick, Moore, and Warren, Ann. Surg. 120:531, 1944.
26. McLaughlin and Coe, Arch. Surg. 60:378, 1954.
27. Orringer, Surgery 28:680, 1950.
28. Pack and Banner, World Congr. Gastroenterol, 2:1016, 1958.
29. Priestley, Surg. Gynecol. Obstet. 107:375, 1958.
30. Prokasha et al., Arch. Surg. 68:491, 1954.
31. Ryelt and Anderson, Surg. Gynecol. Obstet. 119: 1305, 1964.
32. Sales, Br. J. Clin. Pract. 26:103, 1972.
33. Sedgwick and Vernon, Surg. Clin. North Am. 48: 523, 1968.
34. Spencer, Arch. Surg. 73:844, 1956.
35. State, Surg. Clin. North Am. 44:371, 1964.
36. Vink, Acta Chir. Neerl. 2:377, 1950.

B. POSTOPERATIVE ENTEROCOLITIS

SIR FRANCIS AVERY JONES

Enterocolitis is a broad term which covers a number of different pathological conditions: some have an ischaemic origin due to atherosclerotic mesenteric disease with or without occlusion (see Chap. 82). This is an unlikely but perhaps occasional complication of abdominal surgery. Among the infective causes, staphylococcal enterocolitis is the most important in relation to abdominal surgery. Pseudomembranous or necrotising enterocolitis of unknown but possibly vascular aetiology is another possibility.

STAPHYLOCOCCAL ENTEROCOLITIS

Patients receiving broad-spectrum antibiotics by mouth are at risk of developing staphylococcal enterocolitis. The danger arises when the patient becomes cross-infected in hospital with a resistant staphylococcus that can then multiply rapidly while other organisms are being killed off by the oral antibiotic. The risk may be greater in patients who are given preoperative wide-spectrum antibiotics, a common procedure before colonic operations, although seldom before gastric operations. Tetracycline or Ampicillin excreted in the bile may reach a higher than usual concentration in the intestine if the patients are starved.

The *clinical picture* is dominated by the rapid onset of profound shock associated with a remarkable degree of mental alertness. It comes on usually between the second and fifth postoperative day. The diagnosis must be kept in mind whenever a postoperative patient becomes unexpectedly and unaccountably ill, and it is essential that a diagnosis be established as rapidly as possible. This may be achieved by immediately taking a rectal swab and using Gram's stain on it.

The illness is characterised by peripheral circulative failure but not always severe diarrhoea. Abdominal pain, distention, hypopyrexia, and anuria are common. If the diagno-sis is suspected, it is advisable to give Cloxo-cillin immediately by mouth (alternatively erythromycin) and also fluids intravenously. All treatment must be supervised hour by hour; carefully organised medical and nursing care may make all the difference between success and failure.

The *differential diagnosis* in these patients is between staphylococcal enterocolitis and nonspecific pseudomembranous colitis. The clinical pictures are in fact identical, but in pseudomembranous colitis no staphylococci are found on the Gram's smear or on subsequent culture. The immediate postoperative course is uneventful and then suddenly after the second postoperative day the patient becomes acutely ill with peripheral circulatory failure. Diarrhoea is less common than in staphylococcal enterocolitis, but can be very severe. It was a prominent symptom in only 4 of the 16 cases described in one series. Sometimes there is abdominal pain, distention, hyperpyrexia, and anuria, but the outstanding general feature is the rapid development of a state of profound shock associated with mental alertness. A plain x-ray of the abdomen may show dilatation of the small intestinal loops.

The *pathological changes* vary considerably in the extent and disribution of the lesion. In some patients, the entire intestinal tract is involved; in others, the lesions are limited to either the small or large bowel. Within the affected segments, the changes may be patchy and irregular. It is common to find considerable dilatation of the affected part of the bowel, particularly when the small intestine is involved. Externally the bowel shows a dusky purplish appearance owing to intense hyperaemia and stasis. There is often a small amount of serosanguineous fluid in the peritoneal sac. Within the small bowel, there is usually a large amount of faecalent fluid mixed with blood. On the other hand, the large bowel is frequently empty, apart from excessive secretion of mucus which may be bile-stained. When

475

mucosal necrosis is well established, the appearances are unmistakable: the necrotic mucosa presents a dull yellow appearance, sometimes stained green by bile or dark brown if there is much extravasation of blood. Exudation on the surface of the necrotic mucosa forms a pseudomembrane, which may be lightly or firmly attached. There is often an abrupt transition between normal mucosa and the damaged zones. With the progression of the condition, the mucosa undergoes coagulative necrosis and may then slough off, causing peritonitis. Histologically, the capillaries may be dilated but vasculitis is not usually found.

The relationship of this condition to *Clostridium welchii* remains uncertain. It is known that in various parts of the world a segmental necrotising enteritis occurs due to *C. welchii,* type C, which produces a beta toxin. Gas gangrene and food poisoning are due to type A, which produces an alpha toxin. It is likely that *C. welchii* may flourish in a milieu of necrosis, and it seems more likely that its presence, when noted, is a result and not a cause of the postoperative pseudomembranous enterocolitis.

Treatment. In a suspected case of enterocolitis, an immediate bacteriological study of the stool to exclude staphylococcal superinfection and to look for the presence of *C. welchii* is the initial step. Shock should be treated by intravenous therapy, including electrolyte normalisation and administration of blood, norepinephrine, and hydrocortisone as needed. Penicillinase-resistant antibiotics (Cloxicillin or Methicillin) may both be given, orally and parenterally, respectively. In the postoperative case, there is at present no evidence to show that *C. welchii,* type C plays any part, and tetanus antitoxin does not help. The possibility of its use must be reviewed in sporadic cases, however, particularly in regions where type C infection is known to occur. The use of antihistamine drugs has been suggested on the basis that acute necrotising enterocolitis is the result of an antigen-antibody response. In patients who have had a partial gastrectomy, there is a particularly difficult diagnostic dilemma, as high intestinal obstruction in the immediate postgastrectomy period may give a very similar clinical picture; in view of the extreme diagnostic difficulty, Kay and his colleagues advise laparotomy at once, in these circumstances.

REFERENCE

Kay et al., Br. J. Surg. 46:45, 1959.

C. ANAEMIA FOLLOWING OPERATIONS ON THE GASTROINTESTINAL TRACT

JOHN RICHMOND

Anaemia, a reduced haemoglobin level in the blood, arises either from a fall in the number of erythrocytes or a fall in their haemoglobin content, or a combination of the two. Of the various aetiological factors, only deficiency of iron, vitamin B_{12}, and folate are implicated in the types of anaemia that may follow operations on the gastrointestinal tract. Because of the different mechanisms involved, the relevant aspects of the metabolism of these haematinic substances are briefly reviewed.

PHYSIOLOGICAL CONSIDERATIONS

Iron. The iron content of the diet is very variable depending on personal and racial habits and economic status, but even from a good mixed Western diet only 2 to 4 mg per day can be absorbed.[1]

Although the body conserves iron very avidly, each individual requires about 1 mg per day to replace iron lost in desquamated cells, sweat, and hair.[2] Women of reproductory age require, on average, an additional 1 mg per day to meet menstrual loss of iron [3] and a further 1 mg per day to cope with iron requirements during pregnancy.[4] As 100 ml of blood contains 50 mg of iron, any abnormal bleeding seriously compromises iron balance; the same is true of frequent blood donation.

Iron is absorbed in the upper part of the small intestine, but diminishingly well below the level of duodenum and proximal jejunum. Iron compounds, with the exception of haem compounds, are dissociated and ionised in the stomach by gastric secretions. Haem is probably incorporated into the intestinal mucosal cell as such,[5] absorption being affected by substances that vary the degree of polymerisation. A substance has been identified in depepsinised gastric juice and in intrinsic-factor preparations that appears to enhance the absorption of haemoglobin iron.[6] For nonhaem iron,[7, 8] but not for haem iron,[9] gastric hydrochloric acid enhances absorption. A number of other intraluminal factors are known to be important; for example, ascorbic acid [10] and alcohol [11] improve iron absorption, while phytates [12] and phosphates [13] have a depressive effect. A heat-labile component of pancreatic juice, probably trypsin,[14] also has a depressive effect; in chronic pancreatitis, therefore, there is increased iron absorption, which is reduced by the administration of pancreatin.[15, 16]

Following gastrointestinal operations, iron deficiency might easily arise if nutritional intake of iron were reduced, if there were alteration in the normal effects of gastric juice on the digestion of iron-containing foods, or if there were any bypass of, or hurry past, the best absorptive areas for iron. The problem would be aggravated should there be any increase in iron loss from bleeding.

Vitamin B_{12}. The nutritional requirement of vitamin B_{12} in health is in the range 2 to 5 μg per day.[17] The greater part, about 70 percent, of that present in food is absorbed, and most mixed diets contain adequate supplies. Vitamin B_{12} is synthesised by microorganisms and is available almost exclusively in foods of animal origin; the tiny amounts in plant foods probably derive from contaminating soil, fungi, and bacteria.

One feature of vitamin B_{12} metabolism that is of clinical significance is the very slow turnover in the body. Vitamin B_{12} will be lost in the urine, faeces, and desquamated cells, as well as by breakdown, but studies both in pernicious anaemia patients [18] and in normal subjects [19] indicate a biological half-life of about a year.

Vitamin B_{12} appears to be unique in requiring an endogenous factor for its absorption. In man, Castle's intrinsic factor, a mucopolysaccharide not yet isolated in pure form, is secreted by cells of the body and fundus of the stomach, but not to any important extent in the antrum, and not by cells outside the stomach. Intrinsic factor binds vitamin B_{12} to form a firm complex; binding occurs mainly in the stomach, but also in the small intestinal lumen.[20, 21]

Vitamin B_{12} is also unique in that it is absorbed from a very small segment of the intestinal tract. Several experimental studies indicate that vitamin B_{12}-intrinsic factor complex is mainly, if not exclusively, absorbed from the ileum.[22, 23, 24] Booth and Mollin,[25] using radioactive labelled vitamin B_{12} in patients subjected to laparotomy, confirmed that in man, absorption was confined to the distal half of the small intestine and probably to the distal one-third.

Vitamin B_{12}-intrinsic factor complex is believed to be adsorbed to specific receptors on the brush border of ileal enterocytes,[26] and this process is dependent on the presence of calcium ions. It is still not certain whether the complex is absorbed as such or whether intrinsic factor is split off prior to the active transport of vitamin B_{12} into the mucosal cell. The process of assimilation of vitamin B_{12} does, however, seem to take several hours.[27]

Hence, after gastrointestinal surgery, it is unlikely that the small dietary requirement of vitamin B_{12} would be seriously affected, but vitamin B_{12} absorption could be impaired from loss of intrinsic factor, interference with intrinsic factor—vitamin B_{12} binding, or resection, or bypass of the ileum.

Some intraluminal factors that might affect vitamin B_{12} absorption have been identified. If divalent ions such as calcium are important, the availability of calcium in the gut could play a part, and it has been shown that the chelating compound EDTA[28] and hypocalcemia[29] both have an inhibitory effect. Vitamin B_{12} is better absorbed when taken with a meal,[30] possibly because of an enhanced secretion of intrinsic factor.[31] Many years ago[32] it was found that the effectiveness of vitamin B_{12}-intrinsic factor was reduced by acidification. This observation may explain why Veeger et al.[33] found that in chronic pancreatitis, when the duodenal contents are acid due to lack of bicarbonate, vitamin B_{12} absorption is reduced. The studies of Veeger et al.[33] suggested that one or more of the pancreatic enzymes might also be implicated in the absorption of vitamin B_{12}-intrinsic factor complex. Recently Henderson et al.[34] have confirmed malabsorption of vitamin B_{12} in a proportion of patients with chronic pancreatitis, the absorptive defect being corrected when vitamin B_{12} was given with food.

Folate. The daily nutritional requirement for folate to maintain folic acid balance is of the order of 150 μg. It goes up to 350 μg in the later stages of pregnancy.

The folate content of diets has been difficult to establish because of the many polyglutamate forms in food and the different assay techniques that have been used. Folate is present in a wide range of animal and plant foods and the free folate content of 24-hour food collections has been found in different studies to be in the range 100 to 300 μg per day;[35, 37] food treated with the enzyme conjugase indicates a total folate content in the range 450 to 650 μg per day. The amount of folate actually available to the individual, however, apart from socioeconomic considerations, depends very much on the freshness of food and the amount of cooking. For example, Hurdle[36] showed that 80 to 90 percent of the folate activity of many vegetables was lost after only a few minutes' boiling. In addition, although intestinal fluids have been shown to have conjugase activity,[38, 39] the polyglutamate forms of folate in the diet may be available for absorption only to a limited extent.[17, 40, 41]

The site of absorption of folate from the small intestine is uncertain, but in common with other water-soluble vitamins, it is probably mainly in the jejunum;[42] there is evidence, however, that folate is well absorbed throughout the small intestine.[43]

The biological half-life of folate seems to be measured in weeks. This is in accord with clinical experience, which indicates that folate deficiency develops much more readily than vitamin B_{12} deficiency. In one study, Herbert[44] found that in a healthy individual a folate-deficient diet led to early megaloblastic change in the bone marrow in about 4 months.

Folate deficiency develops easily when there is a poor diet and when there is an increased requirement, as in infection and chronic bleeding. On the other hand, folate differs from vitamin B_{12} in that it does not require intrinsic factor, or any equivalent and it is not absorbed from such a limited part of the gut.

It will be seen that there are several possible mechanisms by which an individual might become deficient of essential haematinic substances after gastrointestinal surgery. The main causes are nutritional insufficiency, maldigestion, and malabsorption; and in many patients there is a combination of factors.

INCIDENCE

Anaemia following gastrectomy was probably first described by Deganello,[45] but prior to World War II there were few reports of the association in the medical literature. In the last 20 years, gastric operations, particularly partial gastrectomy for peptic ulcer, have been commonplace; Johnson[46] estimated that 30,000 people per year in England and Wales were having some form of gastric surgery. It is now apparent that anaemia following gastric operations is a major clinical entity in developed countries. Indeed in adult males in these countries, postgastrectomy anaemia is probably the most common form of deficiency anaemia that is encountered. Other forms of gastrointestinal surgery are also important aetiologically in the genesis of anaemia, but are seen less frequently.

Partial gastrectomy. This operation has a number of obvious effects that could be relevant to the availability of essential haematinics. First, there is loss of reservoir function of the stomach which can not only interfere with the total intake of food, but also lead to the rapid passage of stomach contents into the small intestine before there has been time for adequate gastric digestion of food. Both effects are likely to be worse in the Polya than in the Billroth I type of operation. Second, there is loss of gastric secretory function from resection, the severity depending on the operation. A high proportion of the body and with it parietal cells and intrinsic-factor-secreting tissue is removed by partial gastrectomy. The antrum is also removed and the vagal control of gastric secretion variably interrupted. In the last 15 years, chronic duodenal ulceration has been treated mostly by vagotomy and some form of drainage of the stomach, posterior gastroenterostomy, pyloroplasty, or antrectomy. Although these operations aim to preserve the whole or the greater part of the stomach, they inevitably cause significant reduction in the secretion of hydrochloric acid. Third, in the Polya-type operation, the duodenum is bypassed. Not only is this the best absorptive area for iron, but exclusion of the duodenum leads to failure of proper mixing of food with pancreatic and biliary secretions and also to loss of the normal pancreatic secretory response to gastric emptying. Finally and again in the Polya-type operation, obstruction to emptying of the afferent loop may persist leading to stasis and the growth of bacterial flora. Capper and Welbourn [47] estimated that a blind or stagnant loop developed in some 5 percent of cases.

According to Chanarin,[17] the incidence of anaemia in published series of cases totalling over 7,000 patients who had had a partial gastrectomy was 28.8 percent. Morley and Roberts [48] first drew attention to what is now a widely held view, namely, that anaemia is much more common after the Polya-type partial gastrectomy than after the Billroth I operation; in the Morley and Roberts small group of patients, the relative incidence of anaemia was 3:1. Baird et al.[49] showed how anaemia was a function of time after surgery. In addition, females are much more rapidly and more frequently affected than males; the incidence in females is approximately 50 percent, whereas that in males is less than 20 percent.[50] Baird et al.[49] and Blake and Rechnitzer [51] indicate that the sex difference is due mainly to women

in the reproductive period and this is no doubt a reflection of the additional physiological requirements for iron in this group.

The majority of patients who have anaemia following partial gastrectomy have *iron deficiency anaemia*. The mechanisms of production of negative iron balance, poor nutritional intake, bleeding, and malabsorption are all relevant. Poor dietary intake is difficult to quantitate, but is likely to be found in those who have had chronic peptic ulceration and have followed an old-fashioned type of gastric diet obsessively over many years; such diets were low in iron content. Nutritional insufficiency might also be suspected in those with a small gastric remnant and small intake of food. Baird et al.[49] found a lower food intake of iron in their anaemic males compared with the nonaenemic group. Occult bleeding from erosive gastritis, recurrence of peptic ulceration, and carcinoma in the gastric remnant, has generally been regarded as an uncommon aetiological factor.[49, 52, 53] Whole-body counting techniques [54] suggest, however, that iron loss may be greater than has been appreciated.

Undoubtedly malabsorption of iron, singly or in combination with other factors, is now regarded as the most important mechanism in most patients. The fasting patient has no difficulty in absorbing inorganic iron,[55, 56] but inorganic iron taken with food and radioactive iron incorporated in food are less well absorbed in partially gastrectomised subjects than in controls; moreover, when iron deficiency develops, although the absorption of medicinal iron is enhanced, the usual increase in the absorption of iron taken with food does not occur.[57-63] This malabsorption is likely to arise from several effects of gastrectomy. After partial gastrectomy, there is loss of the effect of hydrochloric acid and the delay in the normal stomach for digestion. The gastric contents are hurried through the duodenum as in the Billroth I operation, or they bypass the duodenum and hurry down the upper jejunum as in the Polya operation, before the ingested iron can be made available for assimilation. Although both operations are associated with anaemia, Hallberg et al.[63] showed, as might be expected, that malabsorption of iron was more severe after the Polya operation than after the Billroth I operation.

Some of the earlier large series of post-gastrectomy anaemia [49, 51] found *megaloblastic anaemia* in only occasional patients; more recent studies put the incidence in the region 5 to 10 percent.[53, 64] Many reported investigations [17] on fasting patients have indicated malabsorption of vitamin B_{12} in well over one-third. The literature on megalobastic anaemia shows that this is a less straightforward problem than iron deficiency. First, the diagnosis may be obscured or confused by concomitant iron deficiency. Second, because of the very slow development of vitamin B_{12} deficiency, many patients have long since left the scrutiny of regular follow-up before megaloblastic anaemia develops. Third, it is only in the last decade that serum vitamin B_{12} assay, the ultimate criterion of vitamin B_{12} deficiency, has been freely available. The higher incidence of megaloblastic anaemia in recent years, compared with earlier series, may be a result of better diagnosis, but may also reflect the more extensive gastric resections of the postwar period. Nutritional deficiency of vitamin B_{12} is unlikely to play any part in the causation of megaloblastic anaemia. The most important factors are the extent of the removal of intrinsic factor secreting tissue [65] and the postoperative development of mucosal atrophy in the stomach remnant, perhaps from reflux of intestinal contents and from chronic iron deficiency. At all events, it is loss of intrinsic factor that leads to malabsorption of vitamin B_{12} in the majority of patients. The significance of removal of normal gastrin stimulation of intrinsic factor [66, 67] is not known. Vitamin B_{12} malabsorption due to a stagnant afferent loop syndrome following a Polya partial gastrectomy occurs, but is apparently not common.[17, 68]

The problem of megaloblastic anaemia following partial gastrectomy is further complicated by the finding in several series [69-71] that folic acid deficiency can occur and be the main cause of anaemia in as much as 20 percent. The reasons for this are obscure, since the intrinsic factor mechanism, vital to vitamin B_{12} absorption is not relevant to folic acid. One possibility is that nutritional insufficiency, which occurs very readily with folate, is significant in these patients. Alternatively, true gluten-sensitive enteropathy leading to small intestinal malabsorption of folate and other nutrients appears to develop after, or be unmasked by, gastric surgery in occasional patients.[72, 73]

Gastroenterostomy. Iron-deficiency anaemia is a common complication of this operation, an observation first made by Vaughan; [74] Weir and Gatenby [75] found this type of anaemia in more than one-third of their 60 patients. The same mechanisms that apply to the Polya-type partial gastrectomy apply also to gastroenterostomy. By contrast, megaloblastic anaemia due to vitamin B_{12} deficiency, apparently consequent on loss of intrinsic factor activity from gastric atrophy, has been reported rarely.[53, 76, 77] Presumably in patients with pyloric stenosis a blind afferent loop syndrome could develop, but this does not seem to have been described.

Total gastrectomy. Since in man, intrinsic factor is secreted exclusively by the stomach, vitamin B_{12} malabsorption is inevitable following total gastrectomy.[78, 79] Megaloblastic anaemia is also inevitable if the patient survives long enough. Chanarin [17] has shown from collected published data a peak incidence of megaloblastic anaemia at 5 years, but in some patients it has not developed for as long as 10 years. It is uncommon in less than 2 years and those patients who develop megaloblastic anaemia early may well have vitamin B_{12} deficiency at the time of operation. Shearman et al.[80] reported that in a series of thirty-five patients with gastric carcinoma, four had established "pernicious anaemia" at the time of surgery and two others had subnormal vitamin B_{12} levels. Nelson and Howe [81] found vitamin B_{12} malabsorption due to intrinsic-factor deficiency in 40 percent of 82 patients with gastric carcinoma; this appeared to be consequent on mucosal atrophy rather than tumour infiltration of the mucosa. Subacute combined degeneration of the spinal cord appears to occur just as frequently as in Addisonian pernicious anaemia.[17] Paulson and Harvey,[82] in regular follow-up of 27 patients with gastric neoplasm, reported the development of iron-deficiency anaemia in the very early months after operation, too early to be ascribed to nutritional insufficiency or malabsorption. These authors believed that blood loss from erosions in the oesophagus and jejunum were responsible. Conway and Conway,[69] and Izsak [83] and Adams,[84] report folic acid deficiency in occasional patients after total gastrectomy; Doig and Girdwood,[77] and Izsak,[83] have found normal absorption of folic acid in small numbers of patients, and the likelihood is that folate deficiency is mainly due to deficient nutritional intake and to the increased metabolic turnover of folic acid seen in malignant disease.

Miscellaneous. There are insufficient data available on the effects on the blood of vagotomy combined with the newer drainage operations. Usually there is insufficient resection of stomach to lead to critical loss of intrinsic factor activity. Bitsch et al.[85] and Adams et al,[86] however, have found some fall in the intrinsic factor output following histamine stimulation after such procedures. Feggeter and Pringle [87] suggest that iron deficiency may develop in as many as 10 percent of patients after 10 years, and Cox et al.[88] found reduction in serum iron values, particularly in women, in as much as 50 percent of cases.

The uncommon operation of bypass of the stomach with oesophagojejunostomy should, on theoretical grounds, not lead to anaemia because of preservation of intrinsic-factor secretion. Callender et al.,[89] however, found that although only one of twelve patients was anaemic at the time of study, all showed malabsorption of vitamin B_{12} and subnormal vitamin B_{12} levels. Moreover, the defect was not completely corrected by giving intrinsic factor.

Finally numerous clinical and experimental observations confirm that resection or bypass of the terminal ileum leads to malabsorption of vitamin B_{12}, but not of iron or folate. The critical amount of small-gut resection probably varies from individual to individual. It seems that vitamin B_{12} malabsorption is unlikely if less than 2 feet of ileum is removed, but inevitable if the resection exceeds 6 feet.[90, 91]

DIAGNOSIS OF ANAEMIA

Anaemia occurring after gastrointestinal surgery has some features that bear emphasis. First, the history of a previous operation is a vital diagnostic clue. A lot of time is saved by getting precise details of past surgical treatment. For example, resection of part of the ileum might lead to vitamin B_{12} deficiency, while resection of the jejunum should not. Total gastrectomy inevitably causes vitamin B_{12} deficiency, but subtotal gastrectomy does so only in a proportion of cases. Second, gastric operations frequently lead to a combined deficiency of iron and vitamin B_{12} and rarely of folate. This can give rise to a confusing haematological picture. Third, all the known causes of vitamin B_{12} deficiency can lead as in Addisonian pernicious anaemia, to vitamin B_{12} neuropathy, including subacute combined degeneration of the spinal cord.[92]

The diagnosis is suspected on clinical grounds from the usual nonspecific features of anaemia, namely, progressive tiredness and breathlessness. Anaemia following partial gastrectomy and ileal resection is often accompanied by diarrhoea and by clinical and biochemical steatorrhoea; after ileal resection, it may be very severe. An afferent loop syndrome following partial gastrectomy may be suggested by troublesome bilious regurgitation. Prolonged severe iron deficiency may be accompanied by brittle nails or flat nails, atrophy of the tongue and angular stomatitis. Both vitamin B_{12} and folate deficiency ultimately lead to glossitis; in patients with severe anaemia, there is usually slight hyperbilirubinaemia. As mentioned above, vitamin B_{12} deficiency can lead to symptoms and signs of neuropathy which, although rare, is potentially serious.

In patients with iron deficiency, blood examination will show a reduced mean corpuscular haemoglobin concentration (MCHC) below 30 percent and hypochromic cells in the blood film. In doubtful cases, the serum iron measurement may be helpful in that the serum iron level will be reduced below 60 μg per 100 ml and the total iron-binding capacity (TIBC) will be raised beyond 400 μg per 100 ml. Vitamin B_{12} and folate deficiency are suspected from a raised mean corpuscular volume (MCV) indicating the macrocystosis that should be seen in the blood film. If these deficiencies are at all likely, the diagnosis should be confirmed by microbiological assay of the serum levels of vitamin B_{12} and folate and by examination of the bone marrow. It may not be possible to repeat these investigations again for months or years once further tests and therapy have been initiated. Moreover, to begin therapy empirically is bad clinical practice because not only does it obscure the diagnosis, but also in the case of vitamin B_{12}, treatment usually has to be continued for life. The serum assays of vitamin B_{12} and folate are the most critical indicators of deficiency of these vitamins. The taking of other vitamins, antibiotics, and probably many drugs—e.g., chlorpromazine—may vitiate the result.

When iron and vitamin B_{12} or folate deficiency are combined, there is hypochromia of the erythrocytes and macrocytosis, a so-called dimorphic picture. It can be misleading and the bone marrow may not show classic megaloblastic erythropoiesis.

When there is iron deficiency, an essential investigation is stool examination for occult blood. This may be the guide to stomal ulceration, to carcinoma of the stomach remnant, or to diagnoses unrelated to past surgical treatment, e.g., carcinoma of the caecum. It may also explain failure to respond to apparently adequate therapy or early relapse after correction of anaemia. If the significance of blood loss is uncertain, the precise amount can be determined by labelling the patient's erythrocytes with ^{51}chromium and measuring the amount of radioactivity lost in the stools over a period of several days.

Patients with vitamin B_{12} deficiency usually require precise diagnosis of the absorptive defect. Provided the patient has normal renal function, the Schilling test will demonstrate malabsorption of vitamin B_{12}. The test can be repeated using intrinsic factor, and this should correct the malabsorption in most cases with vitamin B_{12} deficiency following gastric operations. In the rare case with a blind afferent loop following a Polya-type gastrectomy, intrinsic factor will have no effect, but malabsorption should be corrected after a course of antibiotic therapy, e.g., tetracycline or neomycin. In patients who have had ileal resection or bypass of the terminal ileum from an ileotransverse colostomy, neither intrinsic factor nor antibiotic therapy should have any effect. Since 1,000 μg of vitamin B_{12} is administered in the course of the Schilling test, serum assay of vitamin B_{12} and marrow examination must be done first.

In the few patients who develop folic acid deficiency after gastric surgery, if poor nutritional intake is not a satisfactory explanation, exclusion of a gluten-sensitive enteropathy becomes necessary.

Finally, if the haematological diagnosis has been made correctly, appropriate haematinic therapy will give confirmation in a reticulocyte response followed by a steady rise in haemoglobin level.

TREATMENT OF ANAEMIA

All patients who have had a total gastrectomy and resection or bypass of the terminal ileum are likely to develop vitamin B_{12} deficiency if they survive for long enough. They should therefore receive vitamin B_{12} therapy in the form of hydroxocobalamin, 1,000 μg I.M. every 2 months, prophylactically for life.

The high incidence of anaemia following gastric operations other than total gastrectomy is an indication that it should be anticipated. Annual review with full blood examination and preferably also with serum vitamin B_{12} estimation would go a long way to meeting the problem.

Profoundly anaemic patients may require blood transfusion, and this applies particularly to the elderly, for relief of cardiac failure. Patients with iron deficiency are usually cured by oral iron medication. Ferrous sulphate tablets are suitable for most people, but in the event of their having any adverse effects, there is a wide range of inexpensive alternatives, ferrous fumarate being the least troublesome. Contrary to what might be expected, the newer slow-release preparations, e.g., Slow-Fe appear to be absorbed satisfactorily also.[93] For the few patients who cannot take pills, the proprietary preparations, Sytron elixir or Plesmet syrup are palatable and well tolerated. Treatment should be continued until the haemoglobin level is normal and then for a further 3 months to replete the body stores. If the cause cannot be removed, anaemia is liable to recur and further iron therapy for one month in three, or three months per year, is a good plan.

Only rarely is iron deficiency difficult to correct using oral medication. If this occurs, occult bleeding should first be suspected and excluded. I recently had a patient who developed a carcinoma in the stomach remnant after a partial gastrectomy 30 years earlier. Several stool examinations for blood were negative and a barium meal also yielded negative results. The diagnosis was made only on gastroscopy. Failure to respond is otherwise likely to be because the patient is not taking his iron. There does, however, seem to be a small proportion of patients in whom the malabsorption of iron cannot be overcome with oral preparations. For this group, parenteral therapy either as a course of intramuscular injections using iron-sorbitol or as a whole-dose intravenous infusion of iron-dextran in saline or dextrose should be given. The amount of iron required varies with the severity of the anaemia, but is generally about 2 g.

In vitamin B_{12} deficiency hydroxocobalamin, 1,000 μg, should be given intramuscularly twice weekly until the haemoglobin level is corrected, and then, unless the cause can be removed by further surgical treatment, every 2 months for life. Folic acid deficiency, as has been emphasised, is rare. It will be corrected by giving folic acid tablets, 5 mg three times daily, but these should not be given alone unless it is absolutely certain that vitamin B_{12} deficiency does not coexist; there is a real danger of precipitating vitamin B_{12} neuropathy if it does.

Generally, when folic acid is required, iron and vitamin B_{12} supplements will be required as well. If, after investigation, a gluten-sensitive enteropathy becomes a likely possibility, trial of a gluten-free diet is also indicated.

A few patients ultimately require further surgical treatment for removal of the cause of anaemia. This applies, for example, when bleeding from stomal ulceration is identified. Conversion of a Polya-type gastrectomy to a Billroth I operation will remove a blind afferent loop if this is shown to be the cause of vitamin B_{12} deficiency. Sometimes careful investigation and examination of previous records have unexpected results. For example, Doig and Girdwood [77] reported the case of a girl who developed megaloblastic anaemia in pregnancy. This proved not to be due to the usual folate deficiency, but to vitamin B_{12} deficiency. Anaemia had been caused by an ileotransverse colostomy undertaken for "Crohn's disease" when the girl was 9 years old. Retrospectively, the diagnosis was more likely to have been the Schönlein-Henoch syndrome, however. Accordingly, the anastomosis was later undone with correction of the absorption defect.

REFERENCES

1. Finch, S., Haskins, D., and Finch, C. A., J. Clin. Invest. 29:1078, 1950.
2. Greer, R., Charlton, R., Seftel, H., Bothwell, T., Mayet, F., Adams, B., Finch, C., and Layrisse, M., Am. J. Med. 45:336, 1968.
3. Bothwell, T. H., and Finch, C. A., Iron Metabolism. Berlin, Springer Verlag, 1964.
4. De Leeuw, N. K. M., Lowenstein, L., Hsieh, Y-S., Medicine (Baltimore) 45:291, 1966.
5. Conrad, M. E., Benjamin, B. I., Williams, H. L., and Foy, A. L., Gastroenterology 53:5, 1967.
6. Waxman, S., Pratt, P., and Herbert, V., J. Clin. Invest. 47:1819, 1968.
7. Goldberg, A., Lochhead, A. C., and Dagg, J. H., Lancet 1:848, 1963.
8. Jacobs, P., Bothwell, T., and Charlton, R. W., J. Appl. Physiol. 19:187, 1964.
9. Biggs, J. C., Bannerman, R. M., and Callender, S. T., Proc. 8th Cong. Europ. Soc. Haematol., Basle, 1961.
10. Moore, C. V., Iron Metabolism. Berlin, Springer Verlag, 1964.
11. Charlton, R. W., Jacobs, P., Seftel, H., and Bothwell, T. H., Abstracts 8th Cong. Int. Soc. Haematol., Stockholm, 1964.
12. Sharpe, L. M., Peacock, W. C., Cooke, R., and Harris, R. S., J. Nutr. 41:433, 1950.
13. Hegsted, D. M., Finch, C. A., and Kinney, T. D., J. Expr. Med. 90:147, 1949.
14. Callender, S., Symposium: Disorders of the Blood. Royal College of Physicians, Edinburgh, 1965.
15. Davis, A., and Badenoch, J., Lancet 2:6, 1962.
16. Sephton-Smith, R., Br. Med. J. 1:608, 1964.
17. Chanarin, I., The Megaloblastic Anaemias. Oxford and Edinburgh, Blackwell, 1969.
18. Schloesser, L. L., Deshpande, P., and Schilling, R. F., Arch. Intern. Med. 101:306, 1958.
19. Glass, G. B. J., and Mersheimer, W. L., J. Lab. Clin. Med. 52:860, 1958.
20. Latner, A. L., Haematol. Lab. 2:209, 1959.
21. Highley, D. R., and Ellenbogen, L., Arch. Biochem. Biophys. 99:126, 1962.
22. Johnson, P. C., and Berger, E. S., Clin. Res. Proc. 4:234, 1956.
23. Citrin, Y., DeRosa, C., and Halsted, J. A., J. Lab. Clin. Med. 50:667, 1957.
24. Best, W. R., Frenster, J. H., and Zolot, M. M.,

J. Lab. Clin. Med. 50:793, 1957.

25. Booth, C. C., and Mollin, D. L., Lancet 1:18, 1959.

26. Donaldson, R. M., Mackenzie, I. L., and Trier, J., J. Clin. Invest. 46:1215, 1967.

27. Booth, C. C., and Mollin, D. L., Br. J. Haemat. 2:223, 1956.

28. Grasbeck, R., and Nyberg, W., Scand. J. Clin. Lab. Invest. 10:448, 1958.

29. Clarkson, B., Kowlessar, O. D., Horwith, M., and Sleisenger, M. H., Metabolism 9:1093, 1960.

30. Swendseid, M. E., Gasster, M., and Halsted, J. A., Proc. Soc. Exp. Biol. Med. 86:834, 1954.

31. Rune, S. J., Gut 7:344, 1966.

32. Castle, W. B., Heath, C. W., Strauss, M. B., and Heinle, R. W., Am. J. Med. Sci. 194:618, 1937.

33. Veeger, W., Abels, J., Hellemans, N., and Nieweg, H. O., N. Engl. J. Med. 41:1341, 1962.

34. Henderson, J. T., Simpson, J. D., Warwick, R. R. G., and Shearman, D. J. C., Lancet 2:241, 1972.

35. Butterworth, C. E., Santini, R., and Frommeyer, W. B., J. Clin. Invest. 42:1929, 1963.

36. Hurdle, A. D. F., The folate content of a hospital diet. MD Thesis University of London, 1967.

37. Chanarin, I., Rothman, D., Perry, J., and Stratfull, D., Br. Med. J. 2:394, 1968.

38. Santini, R., Berger, F. M., Sheehy, T. W., Aviles, J., and Davila, I., J. Am. Diet. Assoc. 14:562, 1962.

39. Klipstein, F. A., Am. J. Clin. Nutr. 20:1004, 1967.

40. Bethell, F. H., Meyers, M. C., Andrews, G. A, Swendseid, M E., Bird, O. D., and Brown, R. A., J. Lab. Clin. Med. 32:3, 1947.

41. Perry, J., and Chanarin, I., Br. Med. J. 4:546, 1968.

42. Hepner, G. W., Booth, C. C., Cowan, J., Hoffbrand, A. V., and Mollin, D. L., Lancet 2:302, 1968.

43. Burgen, A. S. V., and Goldberg, N. J., Br. J. Pharmacol. Chemother. 19:313, 1962.

44. Herbert, V., Trans. Assoc. Am. Physicians 75: 307, 1962.

45. Deganello, V., Arch. Ital. Biol. 33:118, 1900.

46. Johnson, H. D., Gut 3:106, 1962.

47. Capper, W. M., and Welbourn, R. B., Br. J. Surg. 43:24, 1955.

48. Morley, J., and Roberts, W. M., Br. J. Surg. 16:239, 1928.

49. Baird, I. M., Blackburn, E. K., and Wilson, G. M., Quart. J. Med. 28:21, 1959.

50. Hartfall, S. J., Guy's Hosp. Rep. 84:448, 1934.

51. Blake, J., and Rechnitzer, P. A., Quart. J. Med. 22:419, 1953.

52. Hobbs, J. R., Gut 2:141, 1961.

53. Weir, D. G., Temperley, I. J., and Gatenby, P. B. B., Ir. J. Med. Sci. Ser. 6 no 448:151, 1963.

54. Holt, J. M., quoted by Witts, L. J., Hypochromic Anaemia, London, Heinemann, 1969.

55. Smith, M. D., and Mallett, B., Clin. Sci. 16:23, 1957.

56. Baird, I. M., Podmore, D. A., and Wilson, G. M., Clin. Sci. 16:463, 1957.

57. Chodos, R. B., Ross, J. F., Apt, L., Pollycove,

58. Choudhury, M. R., and Williams, J., Clin. Sci. 18:527, 1959.

59. Baird, I. M., and Wilson, G. M., Quart. J. Med. 28:35, 1959.

60. Stevens, A. R., Pirzio-Biroli, G., Harkins, H. N., Nyhus, L. M., and Finch, C. A., Am. Surg. 149: 534, 1959.

61. Turnbull, A. L., Clin. Sci. 28:499, 1965.

62. Turnberg, L. A., Quart. J. Med. 35:107, 1966.

63. Hallberg, L., Sölvell, L., and Zederfeldt, B., Acta Med. Scand. 179 (Suppl. 445):269, 1966.

64. Deller, D. J., and Witts, L. J., Quart. J. Med. 31:71, 1962.

65. Posth, H. E., Pribilla, W., and Faillard, H., Med. Klin. 57:789, 1962.

66. Wangel, A. G., and Callender, S. T., Br. Med. J. 1:1409, 1965.

67. Irvine, W. J., Davies, S. H., Haynes, R. C., and Scarth, L., Lancet 2:397, 1965.

68. Hoffman, W. A., and Spiro, H. M., Gastroenterology 40:201, 1961.

69. Conway, N. S., and Conway, H., Br. Med. J. 1:158, 1951.

70. Deller, D. J., Richards, W. E. D., and Witts, L. J., Quart. J. Med. 31:89, 1962.

71. Mollin, D. L., and Hines, J. D., Proc. R. Soc. Med. 57:575, 1964.

72. Hedberg, C. A., Melnyck, C. S., and Johnson, C. F., Gastroenterology 50:796, 1966.

73. Mann, J. G., Brown, W. R., and Kern, F., Am. J. Med. 48:357, 1970.

74. Vaughan, J. M., Lancet 2:1264, 1932.

75. Weir, D. G., and Gatenby, P. B. B., Ir. J. Med. Sci., Ser. 6, no. 447:105, 1963.

76. Badenoch, J., Evans, J. R., Richards, W. E. D., and Witts, L. J., Br. J. Haematol. 1:339, 1955.

77. Doig, A., and Girdwood, R. H., Quart. J. Med. 29:333, 1960.

78. Swendseid, M. E., Halsted, J. A., and Libby, R. L., Proc. Soc. Exp. Biol. Med. 83:226, 1953.

79. Callender, S. T., Turnbull, A., and Wakisaka, G., Clin. Sci. 13:221, 1954.

80. Shearman, D. J. C., Finlayson, N. D. C., Wilson, R., and Samson, R. R., Lancet 2:403, 1966.

81. Nelson, R. S., and Howe, C. D., Cancer Res. 23:1756, 1963.

82. Paulson, M., and Harvey, J. C., J. Med. A. 220:310, 1954.

83. Izsak, F. C., Isr. Med. J. 22:21, 1963.

84. Adams, J. F., Scand. J. Gastroenterol. 3:145, 1968.

85. Bitsch, V., Christiansen, P. M., Faber, V., and Rodro, P., Lancet 1:1288, 1966.

86. Adams, J. F., Cox, A. G., Kennedy, E. H., and Thompson, J., Br. Med. J. 3:473, 1967.

87. Feggeter, G. Y., and Pringle, R., Surg. Gynecol. Obstet. 116:175, 1963.

88. Cox, A. G., Bond, M. R., Podmore, D. A., and Rose, D. P., Br. Med. J. 1:465, 1964.

89. Callender, S. T., Witts, L. J., Allison, P. R., and Gunning, A., Gut 2:150, 1961.

90. Kone, D. J., Cooke, W. T., Meynell, M. J., and Harris, E. L., Gut 2:218, 1961.

91. Booth, C. C., Absorption from the small intestine. Sci. Basis Med. An. Rev. 171, 1963.
92. Richmond, J., and Davidson, L. S. P., Quart. J.
Med. 27:517, 1958.
93. Parker, A. C., Simpson, J. D., and Richmond, J. Scot. Med. J. 17:314, 1972.

D. POSTOPERATIVE CHEST COMPLICATIONS

LORD BROCK

The importance of chest complications after abdominal operations is now widely appreciated, but only as a result of an increasing interest after a period of neglect. Surgeons themselves were largely to blame for this neglect because they had concentrated on the technical aspects of abdominal surgery, feeling that the chest was not their responsibility. It was often felt that the chief blame for complications rested with the anaesthetist rather than with the surgeon himself. As technical difficulties were overcome and the mortality and morbidity rates from purely abdominal causes fell, it became clear that chest complications were the chief remaining cause of morbidity and mortality and thus demanded the closest attention of the surgeon. It is essential that the anaesthetist too should understand the problem fully; the days when the interest of the anaesthetist began in the anaesthetic room and finished with the operation are past, and every good anaesthetist studies his patients before operation and watches their convalescence closely.

THE BASIC CAUSES

The old terminology of *postoperative chest, ether pneumonia,* and postoperative bronchitis reveals the earlier paucity of knowledge. In trying to understand the basic causes, it is necessary to consider certain facts and observations.

1. Chest complications are uncommon after operations on the head, neck, and extremities, with the exception of thyroidectomy, and are most likely to occur after operations on the abdomen, including those for hernia.
2. They occur just as commonly after local or spinal anaesthesia as after inhalation anaesthesia.
3. Men are affected more commonly than women.
4. Upper abdominal operations are more likely to be thus complicated than lower abdominal operations.
5. The incidence is increased when the operation involves section of the stomach or intestines, when sepsis is present, and in cases of malignant disease.
6. A preexisting respiratory infection, whether chronic, subacute, or acute, means a greatly increased risk.
7. Habitual or heavy smokers are much more prone to fall victims than nonsmokers, or light smokers, because of their chronic tracheopharyngobronchial irritation.
8. The time of year makes little difference except for a small increase at the time when catarrhal infections are more common.

A consideration of all these features has taught us that the main cause is sputum retention: that imperfect bronchial drainage leading to secondary atelectasis is the primary mechanism. This is the usual cause of the initial febrile disturbance in most cases, and although it may resolve spontaneously or respond to simple treatment, it may progress to grave or fatal pneumonia. Not all chest complications that follow abdominal operations are due to this cause; some, for instance, may be caused by grosser factors such as the inhalation of vomit, but bronchial retention is by far the most common and the most important.

It is essential to remember that there is rarely one single cause but usually many causes acting together. If it were possible to identify a single cause, it would be remedied with greater ease and more constant success. In almost every case, the several factors must be sought and considered. Again, it is important to recognise that certain types of patients are very prone to develop a chest complication under certain conditions; in fact, it may be impossible to prevent the development of a complication although its severity may be mitigated. Conversely, the risk in other types of patients may be negligible. Thus, if a healthy young woman with no respiratory infection, who is a nonsmoker, undergoes an operation on a leg it is very unlikely that her chest will suffer. In contrast, a middle-aged bronchitic man—especially if he has recently had an acute exacerbation of his respiratory infection and is a heavy smoker—who undergoes an upper abdominal operation such as gastrectomy for malignant disease or suture of a perforated duodenal ulcer, will be very lucky if he escapes without a chest complication.

PATHOLOGY

The fundamental pathological cause in most cases is a preexisting respiratory infection, acute, subacute, or chronic. The only practical alternative to this is infection of the air passages by material inhaled during anaesthesia. One of the most striking of the clinical features is the very early production of thick mucopurulent or purulent sputum at a time—e.g., 18 to 24 hours—when it would be very unlikely that a fresh infection could have caused it. Presumably the infection can be aggravated by inhaled anaesthetic agents which are irritants, but the problem is not quite so simple as this because other anaesthetic factors may not only cause increased production of secretion but also favour its early stagnation. Skill or want of skill in the administration is definitely important. Thus a badly administered anaesthetic, especially if accompanied by cyanosis, struggling, or obstructed respiration, is harmful, as is also prolonged deep narcosis. High spinal anaesthesia, deep basal narcosis from barbiturates or other drugs, or prolonged paralysis from curare are all unfavourable. Excessive administration of atropine, hyoscine, or scopolamine acts adversely by causing the bronchial secretions to become thicker and more tenacious and so more difficult to expel. In the same way a hot, dry atmosphere, profuse sweating, and excessive dehydration are harmful.

Next to the production of undesirable bronchial secretions is interference with their expectoration—that is, imperfect bronchial drainage. Prolonged deep narcosis enters into this, the other drug factor being unwise or excessive sedation, especially by morphine. Most of the other factors are, however, mechanical and, significantly, chiefly the responsibility of the surgeon himself. After every abdominal operation there is a certain amount of reflex immobility of the abdominal wall and of the diaphragm, especially on the side of the incision. This immobility is aggravated by conscious effort on the part of the patient if he feels undue pain or discomfort on breathing or coughing. Consequently, an ill-planned, roughly made incision, aggravated by excessive retraction and by rough handling of the viscera and the use of large intraperitoneal packs, is more harmful than a carefully planned and carefully made incision with gentle and considerate handling of the tissues. In this connection the transverse or oblique incisions are kinder than the vertical ones, with the possible exception of the midline supra-umbilical incision in which the recti are not directly interfered with. A drainage tube causes extra pain and so its use should be avoided whenever possible. The conservation of the function of the abdominal wall and diaphragm is of special importance in men, particularly middle-aged men of the labouring classes, because their thoracic respiration is usually deficient and sometimes entirely absent. The heavy worker learns to fix his chest to improve the power of his arm and shoulder muscles, and he breathes almost entirely with his diaphragm. If his abdominal respiration is interfered with as a result of an abdominal operation, the imperfect aeration of the lungs tends to promote atelectasis and makes coughing difficult and ineffective.

Difficulty with respiration and coughing is made worse by bandages or strapping being applied too tightly. The greatest care should be taken to see that these are not used in unnecessary amounts or applied too firmly. Postoperative distention aggravates constricting bandages further, and it should be a rule to loosen and readjust all bandages and strapping within 18 hours and then once daily.

During recovery from anaesthesia, posture is important. The usual position, flat on the back, has many disadvantages not the least of which is the large number of posteriorly directed bronchi which are favourably placed to receive and retain secretions or inhaled material. The ideal recovery position is prone with the foot of the bed slightly raised. This is, unfortunately, usually impracticable after a laparotomy, but a compromise may be made by arranging the patient in a semi-prone position with the operation side uppermost.

During the first days after operation, the factors already mentioned continue to act, especially excessive sedation and dehydration, but a very important one that now appears is undue immobility, and in the prevention of this, the nursing routine plays an important part. Some patients are active in bed from the start; some remain quite inert and semisomnolent from illness or from temperament; others are not moved enough, especially the fat, heavy patient; and others are even encouraged not to move, particularly if a diagnosis of pneumonia has been made. Indeed, the more ill the patient the more immobile he is allowed to remain, whereas it is often the case that the more ill he is the more essential it is that he should be made to move. This will be dealt with in more detail later, but the importance of postoperative immobility in the causation and aggravation of chest complications needs the greatest emphasis now.

Once the factors that cause the production of infected bronchial secretions and their retention have come into play, various secondary effects appear. The chief of these is atelectasis of the lung from absorption of air distal to the bronchial obstruction. The atelectasis causes a considerable rise in negative pressure within the pleura and bronchi which tends to suck secretions deeper in and makes the task of ciliary action much greater. In any case, ciliary action is rendered largely ineffective if it has to move a solid mass of thick mucus from a bronchus; it functions efficiently only in moving a surface layer of secretion. The absorption of air behind the obstruction removes the air necessary to provide the expulsive force for coughing. If retention of bronchial secretions continues, and especially if the patient's resistance is low or virulent organisms are present, a condition of simple atelectasis may proceed to simple bronchopneumonia, or abscess formation. Should inhaled vomit, infected blood clot, or actual shreds of tissue from the pharynx be present, the chances of septic pneumonia developing are great.

TYPES OF COMPLICATIONS

Simple Bronchitis

Simple bronchitis, of course, may occur without retention of sputum and consequent atelectasis.

Atelectasis

Atelectasis is usually described as massive, but the epithet is used far too loosely and without proper thought. Atelectasis may be: (1) lobular, (2) lobar, or (3) massive.

It is important to recognise that scattered or nonconfluent atelectasis is responsible for many of the milder forms of chest complication. Moreover, it may be present in the other lung when a lobar or massive atelectasis is present. Lobar atelectasis is uncommon but does occur. Massive atelectasis should be used to describe the condition when the greater part or the whole of a lung is affected.

Bronchopneumonia

Bronchopneumonia may be of a simple type developing from a bronchitis, especially in an enfeebled patient, but it more commonly follows bronchial retention and atelectasis. Some of the most severe chest complications are caused by septic bronchopneumonia.

Lung Abscess

Lung abscess may develop in an area of atelectasis following a simple bronchial retention of infected material as outlined above, especially if the organisms are of high virulence. More often, however, it follows the inhalation of particulate material or of infected blood clot or tissue fragments. If these come from the nose, mouth, or pharynx, the distribution is more likely to be confined to one bronchopulmonary segment. After abdominal operations, factors are present that tend to encourage the development of multisegmental basal involvement. The importance of avoiding operating in the presence of septic teeth, particularly when tartar masses and infected pockets are present, or in the presence of gross tonsillar and nasal sepsis, cannot be overemphasised.

Empyema

Empyema usually follows or accompanies one of the pneumonia processes, but it is as well to consider it separately, that we may be reminded to think of its presence, more particularly if the pneumonic process is prolonged. The overlooked empyema revealed in the postmortem room is an avoidable tragedy. Pleural infection may also follow an abdominal operation without a case of preceding penumonia, as a result of spread from a subphrenic inflammation or abscess.

CLINICAL FEATURES AND DIAGNOSIS

The diagnosis of simple bronchitis should occasion no difficulty, although the transition to atelectasis must be remembered.

By far the most important and dramatic picture is presented by atelectasis. In spite of clear descriptions of the condition at the end of the last century and at the beginning of this one, it is only too often misdiagnosed. This misdiagnosis is very likely to be made in children—children easily fall victims to atelectasis because of the smaller size of their bronchi and the consequent greater ease of bronchial retention.

The most characteristic feature of atelectasis is its early onset (Fig. 3). The temperature, pulse, and respiration rate begin to rise within 12 to 18 hours, and on the day following operation may be as high as 104° F. Tachycardia is often marked and may be disproportionately high. Atelectasis should always be considered in the differential diagnosis of a rising pulse rate. The patient presents a striking picture of respiratory distress; he is anxious and breathing in a rapid restrained fashion, and his face is often highly flushed or even slightly cyanosed. A feeling of illness and prostration is present, especially in children whose condition may appear alarming. A very characteristic feature is the presence of secretion in the trachea or larger bronchi. This is usually very obvious and it may be likened to the patient's gargling secretion in his trachea and large bronchi. He has a restrained and characteristic cough which can perhaps be best described by the slang term *fruity*. This sign or observation is so important that I hesitate to diagnose simple atelectasis unless I can detect it and thus satisfy myself that retained secretions are indeed present.

The patient may complain of considerable pain due probably to acute mediastinal displacement. He may be awakened from sleep by the pain, which is generally restrosternal. The physical signs in the chest are usually rich and abundant. The affected side of the chest moves poorly, unless of course the thorax is in any case fixed or rigid. The affected area is impaired or frankly dull to percussion; auscultation reveals absent or poor air entry, often with numerous added moist sounds and also often loud bronchial breathing. Bronchial breathing is, however, on the whole a good sign, as it indicates that the major bronchi are patent. A silent area may suddenly produce loud bronchial breathing after the patient has coughed up sputum.

The trachea and heart are characteristically displaced towards the affected side, but too much stress should not be laid on this as it may be difficult clinically to localise the apex beat accurately, and if both lungs are affected, even if one side is much worse than the other, the displacement is not likely to be great.

The diagnosis can usually be confirmed by radiography; there is never any objection to a radiograph being taken with a portable apparatus. Displacement of the mediastinum is noted and confirms the characteristic opacity of lobular, lobar, or massive atelectasis; the diaphragm is raised.

A very important diagnostic step is dem-

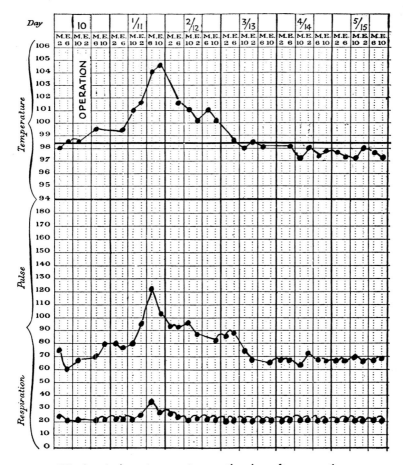

FIG. 3.   Atelectasis occurring on the day after operation.

onstration of the presence of retained viscid sputum and of the immediate, indeed often dramatic, change in the patient's general and local condition when it has been expectorated.

The patient should be made to lie down on the side, all pillows being removed except one under the head. The silent protestations of the nursing attendants should be ignored. If this change in position does not cause coughing and expectoration, the patient should be told to take a few deep breaths and then to cough. The wound should be supported by the hand. If coughing is still restrained, a CO_2 mixture (at least 30 percent) may be given to inhale, or in some cases the chest may be gently clapped or vibrated with the hand. The expectorated sputum

should be received into a dish; it can be demonstrated to be thick, glutinous, and purulent and will not move even if the dish is inverted.

Following this manoeuvre, the change in the patient's condition can be very dramatic. He loses his distressed, anxious expression, any tendency to cyanosis goes, his breathing is more free, and the "rattle" is no longer heard. Auscultation of the lung may show that an area previously almost silent may be full of showers of rales of all types or may exhibit loud bronchial breathing.

Finally, if adequate expectoration is maintained, the temperature and the pulse and respiration rates fall to normal within 24 to 48 hours.

Occasionally the onset of atelectasis may

be delayed for several days, but this is unusual.

A delay in rise of temperature, or slow rise over several days, or a late onset 10 to 20 days after operation, is much more suggestive of a true pneumonic process; the later pyrexia of the second or third week is suggestive of a lung abscess. The pyrexia of a true atelectasis may abate and then merge into the pyrexia of true subsequent bronchopneumonia. True pneumonia (usually confluent bronchopneumonia) should be suspected if the rise in temperature is slow or late *and if there is no definite evidence of retained secretion*. In the earlier stages of bronchopneumonia before suppuration has occurred, the expectoration of sputum is usually small in amount and not in thick viscid purulent masses as with atelectasis. The tracheal rattle of retained sputum is also not noticed early.

The diagnosis of lung abscess depends upon the later onset and also the expectoration of pus in sufficient quantity to suggest the emptying of a cavity. The sputum may or may not be foul. Radiography confirms the presence of an abscess in many cases but not in all.

The possibility of empyema should always be remembered, and although a swinging septic temperature and the characteristic signs of fluid may be present, the physical signs may be equivocal and the temperature may be normal or only slightly raised, particularly in elderly patients. It is quite wrong to philosophise from the foot of the bed as to the presence of an effusion or its nature. There is one way and one way only to be certain, and that is by diagnostic aspiration. Finally, it should be remembered that pulmonary tuberculosis may be the cause of a postoperative chest illness, especially in patients suffering from gastric or duodenal ulcer.

TREATMENT AND MANAGEMENT

The best treatment of a chest complication is preventive, and measures taken towards prevention should at any rate lessen the severity of the process even if they do not completely prevent it. It should be remembered that it may be impossible to prevent a chest infection from occurring in certain types of patients under certain conditions. Most of the principles of treatment follow naturally from what has already been said.

Preoperative Management

Except in operations of urgency, the teeth and nasal sinuses should be examined and treated. One so often sees grave or fatal suppurative pneumonia or lung abscess after operation for a perforated ulcer in the presence of dirty teeth that it would seem worthwhile, if facilities are available, to delay operation 15 to 20 minutes while simple scaling and cleaning of the teeth are done.

Again, unless the operation is urgent, it should not be carried out within 3 weeks of an acute respiratory infection or cold. It is not enough to wait a few days for the symptoms to settle; it is best to send the patient out of the hospital to return after a further wait. House surgeons in particular are liable to offend, owing to their eagerness to maintain adequate operating lists. If the patient has chronic bronchitis, preliminary treatment is indicated, including a course of a suitable antibiotic; the winter months should be avoided for an operation if possible.

Heavy smokers should limit their smoking or stop it completely; no more than three to five cigarettes a day should be allowed for 2 to 3 weeks before operation. Pipe-smoking is preferable to cigarettes.

Inspection of the chest movements and the type of respiration employed by the patient should be a routine, and a course of preoperative physical treatment and breathing exercises should be given. The physiotherapist should explain the need for postoperative deep breathing and coughing, and train the patient in the movements and manoeuvres necessary. The patient with chronic bronchitis should derive great benefit from this regime.

During Operation

The selection of the anaesthetic agent and of the anaesthetist is important, but there is little doubt that the skill of the anaesthetist is more important than the agent used. The good anaesthetist will not permit struggling and cyanosis and vomiting, nor will he cause his patient to be too deeply anaesthetised for a long time or be too deeply narcotised after the operation is over.

The surgeon should learn to choose his incision carefully and avoid undue trauma to the abdominal wall and careless powerful retraction and rough handling of the viscera. He should also see that the patient is not embarrassed by tight bandages and strapping when the dressings are applied. (Chaps. 1 and 2.)

Postoperative Management

After the patient is back in bed, everything must be directed toward the prevention of bronchial retention or to its relief if it supervenes. Excessive sweating should be avoided and dehydration controlled by the administration of rectal or intravenous fluids. A watch should be kept on bandages and strapping, and early and regular adjustments made to prevent restriction of breathing and of coughing. It is better to avoid encircling bandages entirely.

Sedation should be used intelligently. It is as wrong to underdose as to overdose. A patient whose cough reflex and respiration have been dulled by too much sedation is as badly off as the patient who is in too much pain and distress to breathe or cough with reasonable comfort. The ordering and administration of sedatives in the first 36 to 48 hours calls for great care and thought and not a little experience. Given in correct amounts, even morphine will help rather than hinder breathing and coughing. If it will allow a patient, with encouragement, to cough effectively without a sharp agonising stab of pain, then it can serve as a very useful expectorant.

It should be stressed that the patient must be *encouraged* to breathe deeply and to cough effectively. The need for this should have been explained to him before operation and he must be regularly reminded afterwards. While it is true that postoperative physical treatment comes into the realm of the physiotherapist, the part that the nurse plays is also important. The most fateful hours are the first 24 to 36 after the operation, and it is during these that the physiotherapist may not be present, and indeed if the patient is

ill or weak she may not be encouraged. The earlier and important management therefore falls into the sphere of nursing; this should be explained to the nurses and its recognition be *insisted upon*. When the patient is ill, and especially if he or she is fat and heavy, the tendency of the nurses to encourage immobility or their fear of disturbing the patient unduly should be corrected by definite and precise instructions from the surgeon. A great deal can be done by simple and intelligent means without adding any more strain to the patient.

The most important thing is to encourage and insist upon a simple routine of movement and postural drainage. At least twice a day every patient is washed, his bed made, and his back treated. These opportunities should be taken to perform a simple drill. All pillows should be taken away except one under *the head* (not under the shoulders); the patient should be laid flat and turned gently on the side. This position is excellent for treating the back, and if the movement does not start the act of coughing, the patient should be urged to cough while the nurse supports the wound or the patient supports it himself. A dose of sedative 10 to 20 minutes beforehand may enable the manoeuvre to be free from pain and much more effective. It will often be found that the dose of sedative is deliberately withheld until the patient has settled down. This is quite wrong and may be harmful if the sedation has not been preceded by coughing to empty the bronchi. Unless specifically instructed to put the patient flat and turn him on his side, the nurses may elect merely to raise an ill patient and treat his back from underneath while he is still upright. This may be the very patient in whom posturing is most important. If simple encouragement and instruction of the nursing staff fail to convince in any individual case, it is the duty of the surgeon or his deputy to stand by the patient and to lend the weight of his presence to the treatment. It may be necessary or even desirable to turn the patient on his side for no more than a minute or so; on the other hand, he may tolerate much longer, and if he can be arranged comfortably he may well lie in the position for 5 to 10 minutes. If there is definite expectoration, and more especially if there has been bronchial retention, he should certainly lie over for as long as possible, and during this time be encouraged to cough and breathe deeply at intervals. Gentle clapping or vibration may be useful, but the routine use of vigorous banging or pummeling is undesirable. It is usually unnecessary and may cause considerable pain and resentment.

If sputum retention and atelectasis have occurred, the surgeon, his deputy, or the anaesthetist should certainly supervise at least one therapeutic posturing of this sort to ensure that it is effective. A skilled physiotherapist can be very helpful, especially in continuing treatment.

It should be noted that the term *turning the patient* is preferred to *rolling*, which may well be misconstrued into literally rolling him backward and forward.

Atropine or belladonna is to be avoided, but stimulant expectorants can also be harmful by causing abundant frothy sputum. If any medicinal help is needed apart from proper sedatives, a simple inhalation is sufficient.

In addition to these postural manipulations, the patient should be encouraged to move about freely himself if possible and to enjoy the freedom of the bed. It has been noted that the poorer class of patient who is in an institution with a slender staff of nurses, who has to do more for himself in the way of stretching for things and giving himself food and drinks, often does better than the more fortunately placed patient with special nurses who attend to his every want and leave him with no movements to perform for himself.

The routine use of inhalations of CO_2 has been suggested as likely to be effective in diminishing the onset of atelectasis and of treating the condition if it has supervened. There is little evidence that it is in any way effective in lessening the incidence and indeed it has been shown definitely that the incidence after its use is, if anything, slightly greater than less. This may be because the hyperpnoea tends to cause secretions to be sucked in more deeply, or it may favour fatigue of the respiratory muscles. It is probable that it has some place in treatment of the established condition, for a few breaths may initiate the act of coughing in an otherwise reluctant patient.

A question of great importance is the use to be made of methods of direct suction of secretion, either by catheter or under direct vision by bronchoscopy. It can be said at once that after abdominal operations the need for these methods should scarcely ever arise. It is not justifiable to use them as a routine form of treatment in cases of atelectasis *when no attempt whatsoever has been made to prevent or treat the condition by simple posture*. The need for and the advantages which accrue from simple routine preventive postural manipulation are still too little known and used.

On the other hand, it is also desirable to recognise the occasional case in which bronchoscopic suction is indicated. It is quite often needed for the relief of bronchial retention after intrathoracic operations but rarely after abdominal operations as a therapeutic measure. It is chiefly needed after abdominal operations when there is doubt as to whether the condition is simple atelectasis, atelectasis complicated by progressive infection, or true suppurative bronchopneumonia from the start. If the patient is raising thick sputum that is moist and bubbly it does not follow that he is suffering from secretion retained in his larger bronchi with secondary peripheral effects. It is more likely that he has an infection of his smaller bronchi, possibly of his lung as well, which is producing the thick secretion that is embarrassing him. In other words, there is a source of secretion in the small bronchi beyond the reach of the suction tube, as opposed to accumulations in the larger bronchi. At bronchoscopy the large bronchi may be found to be almost or entirely empty.

As a general rule bronchoscopic suction under vision is to be preferred to blind suction with an intratracheal catheter. If performed by anyone with reasonable skill, it can be done with the patient sitting up in his own bed (the operator standing on a low platform at the head of the bed). The direct inspection of the bronchi is an advantage both for diagnosis and for more effective clearing of the bronchi than is possible with a simple catheter. The catheter is often only a means of provoking coughing.

DIFFERENTIAL DIAGNOSIS

In this section most stress has been laid on the part played by and the importance of bronchial retention and atelectasis in postoperative chest complications. There is no doubt that atelectasis in its various forms justifies this emphasis laid upon it. On the other hand it must always be remembered that nonatelectatic or purely pneumonic complications do occur, and it is just as undesirable to diagnose atelectasis when true pneumonia is present as to repeat the error, so often made in the past, of diagnosing pneumonia when simple atelectasis is present. At the same time the methods advocated for the prevention and management of simple atelectasis are not likely to harm a patient with a bronchopneumonia unless persisted in too actively, so as to cause exhaustion. Even with a true bronchopneumonic process, encouragement of free bronchial drainage is beneficial if used intelligently. In children, in particular, encouragement of expectoration is desirable. It has been said with justification that a diagnosis of bronchopneumonia in children is more of a prophecy than a present assessment.

The differential diagnosis and treatment of the various septic bronchopneumonic processes, including the earlier stages of lung abscess, are often difficult and complex, and fall more within the province of the physician or the surgeon specially trained in the diagnosis and management of thoracic diseases. In cases in which doubt or difficulties arise, it is a sound policy to cooperate early with a thoracic expert, rather than to leave the diagnosis in doubt and pursue an unsatisfactory line of treatment.

27

A. SOME SEQUELAE OF GASTRIC OPERATIONS, INCLUDING THE DUMPING SYNDROME AND METABOLIC DISORDERS

J. ALEXANDER-WILLIAMS

Surgeons have much to offer a patient with chronic or complicated peptic ulcer disease. *After gastric operations, most patients are cured and have no further dyspepsia.* Some die, however; and some have new or recurrent ulcers, some have new symptoms that are frankly iatrogenic, and others slip insidiously into a state of chronic malnutrition. These unwanted sequelae follow all types of gastric surgery from a three-quarter partial gastrectomy with gastrojejunostomy to a proximal gastric vatogomy (with preservation of antral vagal innervation) without pyloroplasty. This chapter is concerned with the cause, prevention, and correction of some of these complications.

Any classification of postoperative syndromes is arbitrary. If it were made comprehensive, it would have to range widely through such subjects as postoperative anastomotic leakage, thromboembolism, adhesion obstruction, and all types of postgastrectomy anaemia. Many of these subjects are covered in detail in other parts of this book. This chapter is not intended to be comprehensive but rather to select for detailed study subjects in which I have had particular experience or interest and in which there have been significant recent developments. Particular emphasis will be placed on complications susceptible to surgical correction.

SYMPTOMATIC DISORDERS AFTER GASTRIC OPERATIONS

In a comprehensive review of his experience in investigating patients referred for evaluation of symptoms after gastric surgery, Hirschowitz (1970) lists the symptoms as pain, vomiting, bleeding, dumping, diarrhoea, and weight loss; and he tabulates a cross-correlation between these (Table 1).

There will have been some selection of patients referred for investigation to Hirschowitz's specialised endoscopic unit with a reputation of elucidating complex referral problems. (See Chap. 4A.)

The relative incidence of the different symptoms in his patients does not reflect the "mix" found in other groups of patients followed after partial gastrectomy. Table 1 is reproduced merely to show the complexity of interrelationship of symptoms. Furthermore, it is clear from the data that most patients have a multiplicity of symptoms and so defy neat confinement to simple diagnostic categories. For example, of the 132 patients with *dumping*, 81 also had pain, 66 vomiting, 34 bleeding, 38 diarrhoea, and 55 weight loss. Despite the apparent impossibility of categorising polysymptomatic patients, most have one or two predominant symptoms, and so some working analysis will be attempted based on the presenting symptom.

Although most of the patients in Hirschowitz's series had a Billroth II operation or

vagotomy and antrectomy, he concludes, "No kind of operation was exempt from symptoms and no symptom was specific for any operation."

Pain

The patient who complains of continued or recurrent indigestion after an operation designed for the cure of this symptom needs careful investigation.

Once it is established that the pain or discomfort is associated with digestion and is not due to cardiac ischaemia or renal disease, it is then necessary to differentiate between recurrent peptic ulceration, oesophagitis, and biliary or pancreatic disease.

A carefully taken history and physical examination are essential, though these rarely establish the diagnosis with certainty. Special investigations are therefore required and should be comprehensive. For example, it is not safe to assume that the presence of oesophageal reflux on barium meal or the presence of gallstones on cholecystography necessarily means that the abnormality is the cause of the patient's symptoms. Other causes must be excluded.

After preliminary haematological and biochemical screening tests, all patients should have a plain abdominal x-ray examination. The erect and lateral films may show biliary or pancreatic calcification or distention of the gastric remnant or small bowel with air or fluid.

Biliary disease. A cholecystogram is advisable in all patients. I have seen patients who have had a vagotomy or even a revision gastrectomy in the mistaken belief that their persistent dyspepsia was due to recurrent ulceration or afferent-loop obstruction; in

Table 1.   PRESENTING SYMPTOMS IN 415 SYMPTOMATIC POSTGASTRECTOMY PATIENTS SHOWING THE NUMBERS OF EACH SYMPTOM ASSOCIATED WITH EACH OTHER. FIGURES REPRESENT NUMBER OF PATIENTS

Symptoms	Pain	Vomiting	Bleeding	Dumping	Diarrhoea	Weight Loss
Pain	249	130	76	81	30	82
Vomiting	130	189	60	66	33	76
Bleeding	76	60	139	34	16	42
Dumping	81	66	34	132	38	55
Diarrhoea	30	33	16	38	60	27
Weight loss	82	76	42	55	27	130

these patients, the symptoms were cured only after the detection and treatment of chronic biliary disease.

It has been suggested that gastrectomy and vagotomy both predispose to biliary disease (Manthorpe et al., 1966). Although the hypothesis lacks proof, the association is sufficiently common for the possibility of biliary disease always to be considered in a patient with dyspepsia after gastric operations.

Recurrent ulcer. For the proper diagnosis and evaluation of possible recurrent ulceration barium studies, fibre-optic endoscopy and acid secretion studies should always be performed. Barium studies are the simplest and least uncomfortable for the patient, and in my experience are successful in detecting more than 70 percent of patients ultimately proved to have recurrent ulceration. In recent years, the diagnostic accuracy of fibre-optic endoscopy has increased, and in our recent experience it has an even greater accuracy than barium meal. The value of acid secretion tests is to confirm that the patient has sufficient acid to produce a peptic ulcer and also to detect by the insulin test whether the vagotomy is complete. Although the problems of collection of secretions sometimes impair the accuracy of gastric secretion studies, most patients with recurrent ulcer after gastric surgery can be shown to be able to reduce the pH in their gastric remnant below pH 3.0. Most have a maximum acid output after pentagastrin of 15 or more mEq per hour, and the majority of patients with recurrence after vagotomy have a positive insulin test according to the criteria of Hollander (1948).

It is unwise to make a diagnosis of recurrent ulceration unless two of three methods of investigation are positive (barium-meal, endoscopy, or acid secretion studies). (See Chap. 24.)

Oesophagitis. In addition to the search for recurrent peptic ulceration, the barium meal also helps to provide evidence of hiatal hernia or oesophageal reflux. The definitive diagnosis of oesophagitis cannot be made on barium meal alone, although the complication of stenosis or oesophageal ulcer can occasionally be detected. A suspected diagnosis of oesophagitis should be confirmed by endoscopy. Mild oesophagitis, sufficient to

produce quite severe symptoms, may be associated with apparent normality on endoscopy. Biopsy should, therefore, always be performed, as this may show changes when the macroscopic appearances are normal.

If a patient is suspected of having pain of oesophageal origin, confirmation can be obtained by the acid provocation test. The lower oesophagus is slowly perfused through a nasogastric tube with a solution of N/10 HCl. If this produces the symptoms of which the patient is complaining, it is likely that these are due to oesophagitis. The test is also positive in patients with bile oesophagitis, so that although the site of the pain can be identified, the cause of the oesophagitis cannot. Overnight aspiration of lower oesophageal contents or overnight pH estimations help to elucidate the problem.

The subjects of management of recurrent ulceration and of acid oesophagitis are dealt with in Chapters 11, 24, and 74. The problems of bile oesophagitis will be further considered below (see Bile Vomiting).

Pancreatitis. Pancreatic pain may occur in some patients after gastric operations. Although acute traumatic pancreatitis occasionally complicates gastric operations, particularly those involving dissection of penetrating posterior ulcers, there is no evidence that gastric operations per se predispose to the development of pancreatitis. Some patients suffering from chronic pancreatitis, however, run the risk of being misdiagnosed as having chronic peptic ulceration, particularly if they also have duodenal scarring from an old healed duodenal ulcer. If such patients are treated by gastric surgery, then only naturally their symptoms will persist and present as postgastrectomy pain.

Recurrent or relapsing pancreatitis can usually be diagnosed with reasonable accuracy on clinical grounds, supplemented by the finding of abnormal serum amylase levels. (See Chap. 38.) Chronic pancreatitis is much more difficult to diagnose, especially if there is no calcification within the gland. Pancreatic function studies are not particularly reliable even in the presence of normal duodenal anatomy. In the patient with a gastrojejunal anastomosis, accurate pancreatic function studies are almost impossible because of the difficulties of intubation. Patients with persistent and undiagnosed post-gastrectomy pain are sometimes relegated to the diagnostic dustbin and their symptoms labelled chronic pancreatitis without the proof of positive findings.

Vomiting

Vomiting after gastric operations can be classified into four categories—easy regurgitation, bile vomiting, food vomiting, and nongastric nausea.

Easy Regurgitation

Competence of the gastrooesophageal mechanism that normally prevents regurgitation of gastric contents into the oesophagus may be damaged by gastric operations. Resections, particularly those with a Billroth I anastomosis, may open out and make obtuse the gastrooesophageal angle and so predispose to oesophageal regurgitation (Windsor, 1964). Truncal vagotomy may disturb the anatomical arrangements at the oesophageal hiatus and may also result in denervation of the lower oesophagus (Williams and Woodward, 1967). Removal of the antrum in gastric resection operations will also reduce the level of circulating gastrin, both in the resting state and after meals. This too may affect lower oesophageal sphincteric competence, as gastrin is known to increase muscular tone in the lower oesophagus.

Easy regurgitation may result in the patient's complaining of regurgitation of food or gastric contents into the mouth on stooping, bending, or lying down, or he may present with oesophageal pain, due to the irritant effects of gastric acid or alkaline duodenal contents on the lower oesophageal mucosa.

Bile Vomiting

Bile vomiting is a common and troublesome symptom after all forms of gastric surgery. In patients with this syndrome, the vomitus may be heavily bile-stained food or gastric mucus, but commonly and typically the syndrome consists of the vomiting of a clear yellow, or occasionally green, fluid. The patient may describe this fluid as "pure bile" or sometimes erroneously as "pure acid" be-cause of its bitter taste. The typical history of a patient with the bile vomiting syndrome is that shortly after a meal he begins to feel uncomfortably distended, he becomes nauseated, and then he vomits a large quantity of clear yellow bitter fluid. After vomiting, the symptoms are relieved. In some patients, the symptoms are present when they wake in the morning, the nausea continuing until they vomit spontaneously or induce vomiting. This syndrome was once labelled *the afferent loop syndrome,* as it was believed that the symptoms were due to the accumulation of bile within the afferent loop (Mimpriss and Birt, 1948). Because it was believed that the symptoms were due to the accumulation of bile within the afferent loop of patients with a gastrojejunal anastomosis, it was postulated that the distended loop emptied when the patient vomited (Wells and Welbourn, 1951; Wells and McPhee, 1952; Steinberg, 1954; Jordan, 1955; Stammers, 1961). The principal reason for questioning such a hypothesis is the finding of the bile vomiting syndrome in patients who had a Billroth I gastrectomy or after vagotomy and pyloroplasty. The relative incidences of bile vomiting after different operations for duodenal ulcer are shown in Table 2.

The hypothesis of the *afferent loop syndrome* was first questioned by Auguste and his colleagues (1963), who found that if patients with this syndrome were given a solid meal mixed with barium, on x-ray an accumulation of nonopaque layer was to be observed on top of the barium mixture.

We have confirmed this observation in

Table 2.   INCIDENCE OF BILE VOMITING AFTER DIFFERENT GASTRIC OPERATIONS (IN PERCENT)

Gastric Operation	Incidence of Bile Vomiting (Authors)	
	Nelson, 1968 (percent)	Goligher et al., 1972 (percent)
Billroth II gastrectomy	26.1	13.1
Vagotomy and antrectomy[a]	13.0	13.8
Vagotomy and gastrojejunostomy	6.1	14.5
Vagotomy and pyloroplasty	6.6	10.1

[a]*Usually with gastrojejunal anastomosis.*

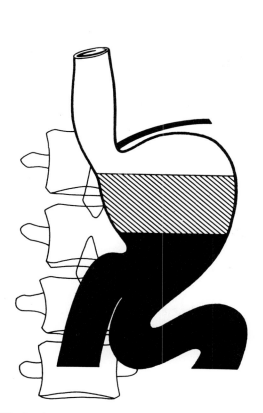

FIG. 1.   Barium/food meal findings in a patient with bile vomiting. The barium mixture is shown in black and the shaded area above depicts a layer of less opaque fluid which on aspiration was bile-stained.

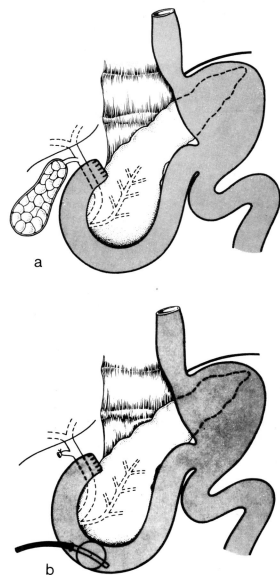

FIG. 2.   (A) Findings in a patient with the bile vomiting syndrome who also suffered from gallstones. (B) At the time of cholecystectomy a balloon catheter was placed in the duodenum and brought out through the abdominal wall.

several patients with bile vomiting syndrome after gastrectomy. We observed that when a layer of fluid accumulated on top of the barium, the patient experienced the symptoms of the syndrome (Fig. 1). If the layer of fluid is aspirated or was vomited, it was a clear yellow fluid. The observation was confirmed under experimental conditions; patients who experienced the symptoms after the meal had a nasogastric tube passed and the layer of clear yellow fluid aspirated. The symptoms then disappeared. If the aspirated fluid was replaced by an equal volume of normal saline, the patients experienced no symptoms. If, however, the saline was withdrawn and the original "bile" was reintroduced into the stomach, the symptoms returned.

Further observations that refute the con-cept of afferent loop distention were obtained by studying patients in our clinic with typical severe symptoms of bile vomiting after Billroth II partial gastrectomy. Three patients with the syndrome were also found to have cholelithiasis. The patients' permission was

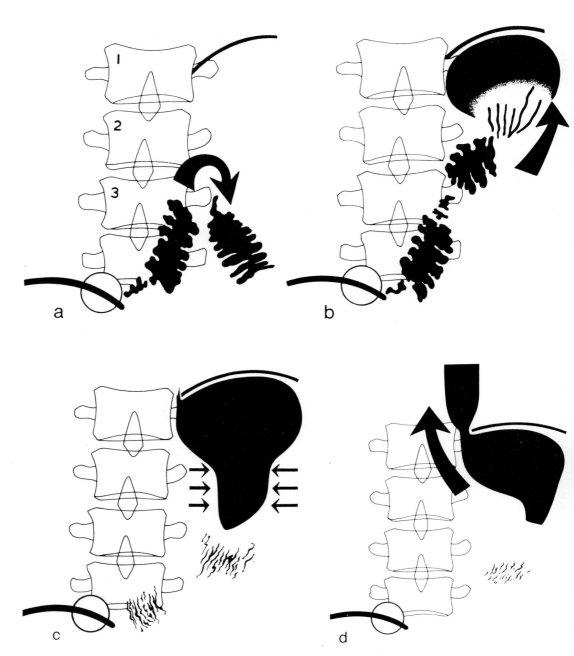

FIG. 3.   From a cineradiographic study of the patient shown in Fig. 2. (A) Instillation of saline/
gastrografin into the afferent loop led to immediate clearance via efferent loop. (B) Instillation
of bile/gastrografin led to accumulation in the gastric remnant. (C) 400 ml of opacified bile
all retained in gastric remnant. Patient experienced nausea and distal gastric remnant appeared to contract (Arrowed). (D) Fluid began to reflux into oesophagus. Patient experienced
severe symptoms of the bile vomiting syndrome and almost all the fluid instilled into duodenum
was vomited with relief of symptoms.

obtained to treat the problem surgically in two phases. First, removing the gallbladder and at the subsequent operation attempting to cure the bile vomiting (Fig. 2). At the cholecystectomy, a balloon catheter was placed in the duodenal loop and brought out through the abdominal wall. After recovery and return to a normal diet, the patients were further studied. With the catheter closed, the patients continued to suffer from the symptoms of bile vomiting, particularly after meals. If the duodenum was allowed to drain through the balloon catheter into a collecting bag, the patients did not experience the symptoms and observed that what was collected in the bag was identical to the substance they usually vomited. Two of these patients were then submitted to fluoroscopic examination during the installation, through the balloon catheter, of either normal saline or previously aspirated duodenal contents. Both fluids were opacified with one-quarter volume gastrografin to permit fluoroscopic examination. It was observed that when normal saline was introduced into the duodenum, the afferent loop could not be made to distend when even a volume as large as 200 ml was instilled rapidly. The saline merely emptied from the afferent loop and out through the efferent loop (Fig. 3A). If, however, the patients' own duodenal secretions were introduced rapidly into the duodenum, once again the afferent loop did not distend but the opacified fluid was ejected rapidly into the stomach; the stomach became larger and larger (Fig. 3B and C). The patients experienced the symptoms of the bile vomiting syndrome with nausea and distention and shortly afterwards vomited the fluid that

had been introduced into the duodenum (Fig. 3D). All three patients were subsequently cured of their bile vomiting syndrome by the jejunal interposition operation, described below.

Further important evidence in elucidating the cause of bile vomiting after gastrectomy was obtained from a study of two other patients with this syndrome who had originally been treated by conversion of their Billroth II anastomosis to a Billroth I anastomosis. This conversion operation did not relieve their symptoms; a second reconstructive operation was therefore performed and an isoperistaltic jejunal loop was interposed between the stomach and duodenum. As a result of this second reconstruction operation, both patients were completely cured of the symptoms of bile vomiting. In one of these patients, permission was obtained to drain the duodenum after operation through a balloon catheter. Once the patient had recovered from the jejunal interposition operation, she was studied cineradiographically to determine whether it was possible to induce fluid reflux back from the duodenum against "the peristaltic barrier" of the interposed loop. It was not possible to achieve more than a minimal reflux into the distal part of the jejunal loop even when the maximum tolerable volume of normal saline or bile was injected into the duodenum. This study confirmed the mechanical efficiency of the isoperistaltic loop. After 2 weeks, the balloon catheter was removed without complication.

As a result of these observations, we propose the following hypothesis: *The symptoms of bile vomiting reflux oesophagitis commonly found after partial gastrectomy are*

Table 3.   RECONSTRUCTION OPERATIONS FOR BILE VOMITING

Type of Reconstruction Operation	Number of Patients			Ages (in years)		Time Interval (in months)	
	All	Men	Women	Mean	Range	Initial Resection to Reconstruction Mean	Reconstruction to Assessment Mean
To Billroth I	15	10	5	53	41 to 67	79	103
Isoperistaltic loop of jejunum	18	10	8	51	39 to 62	94	75
Gastrojejunostomy to pyloroplasty	2	1	1	44 and 56		18	24
Conversion to Roux-en-Y anastomosis	2	2	—	50 and 59		70	110

not due to the accumulation of "bile" in the afferent loop but to the presence of "bile" in the stomach remnant. Bile in the stomach is an irritant, causes gastritis, and appears to interfere with normal gastric emptying (Williams, 1967). It follows therefore that to cure patients with the bile vomiting syndrome it is necessary to prevent bile refluxing into the gastric remnant.

Treatment.   Medical treatment of the symptoms of bile vomiting has been of very little value. If the patient sleeps well propped up in bed (as in the treatment of reflux oesophagitis), gastric emptying may be improved and some patients are helped. I have employed the oral administration of local anaesthetic agents, antispasmodics, and polysiloxane compounds, all with little effect. Patients usually revert to self-medication with antacids despite the fact that they are theoretically of no value. Metoclopramide (Maxolon) to promote gastric emptying has been claimed to be effective (Johnston, 1970).

Surgical treatment has been reserved for patients with severe disabling symptoms who were both fit and willing to undergo major gastric surgery. Details of the reconstructive operations in a series of my own are shown in Table 3.

The results of the two most common operations, *conversion* and *interposition* will be compared.

Conversion.   This group consisted of 10 men and 5 women with an age range of 41 to 67 years, and averaging 53 years of age. In addition to subtotal gastrectomy, four pa-

tients had already had further operations including enteroenterostomy, revision of the gastrojejunostomy, and relief of an acute afferent loop obstruction. Two patients had had a vagotomy. An average of 6.7 years elapsed between the initial gastric resection and the operation for bile vomiting.

Interposition.   This group was composed of 10 men and 8 women averaging 51 years of age (ranging from 39 to 62 years). Three patients initially had gastrectomies with gastroduodenostomies and had subsequent further resections with Billroth II anastomoses; 15 patients had Billroth II gastrectomies as the primary procedure. Two patients had had vagotomies. The mean interval between the initial gastric procedure and the operation for bile vomiting was 7.9 years. Complicating factors such as chronic pancreatitis, biliary disease, psychiatric illness, and previous operation for postgastrectomy symptoms are listed in Table 4.

Surgical technique.   *Conversion to Billroth I.*   The technique of conversion to a Billroth I anastomosis requires little ex-

Table 4.   COMPLICATING FACTORS BEFORE RECONSTRUCTION OPERATION

Factors	Conversion BII to BI	Jejunal Interposition
Number in group	15	18
Proven chronic pancreatitis	2	4
Past or present biliary disease	1	6
History of psychiatric illness	3	8
Previous constructive gastric operation	4	3

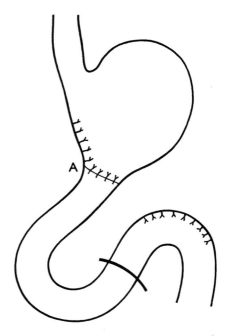

FIG. 4. The anastomosis after conversion of Billroth II to Billroth I anastomosis. The gastric remnant is anastomosed to the duodenum stump (A) and the jejunal stoma is closed.

planation. The Billroth II anastomosis was taken down and the defect in the jejunum closed transversely in two layers. The duodenal stump was identified (without difficulty in all but one patient), opened, and the gastric remnant anastomosed to the duodenum in two layers (Fig. 4). Vagotomy was performed in four patients; in three it had already been done.

Interposition. The ileal loop interposition operation will be described in greater detail (Fig. 5). In 14 of the 18 patients, a loop of jejunum 8 to 22 cm in length (average 18 cm) was mobilised with its blood supply from approximately 15 cm beyond the gastrojejunostomy. The jejunum was reconstituted with an end-to-end anastomosis. The gastrojejunal stoma was then taken down and the defect in the jejunum closed transversely with two layers of continuous suture. The duodenal sump was mobilised as before and the loop of jejunum brought up through a hole in the mesocolon and anastomosed between the duodenum and the gastric remnant. A stay suture was used to allow identification of the proximal end of the loop, which was anastomosed to the stomach so that peristalsis ran from the stomach to the duodenum (Fig. 5B).

In four patients, in the later part of the series, it was possible to simplify the technique by using the efferent loop still attached to the stoma and to swing this across to joint the duodenal stump anastomosing the afferent loop to the jejunum, so restoring bowel continuity (Fig. 5C). Two patients had a truncal vagotomy; in three it had already been performed. Three patients had a concurrent hiatal herniorrhaphy.

Other operations. The two patients with vagotomy and gastrojejunostomy had the gastrojejunostomy taken down. The hole in the stomach and the jejunum were closed with two layers of sutures and a one layer Heineke-Mikulicz pyloroplasty was performed. Both were relieved of their symptoms.

The Roux-en-Y anastomosis was performed by dividing the afferent loop at the level of the stoma and closing the gastric end. The proximal end was then anastomosed end to side to the jejunum 20 cm distal to the original stoma. Both patients had a truncal

vagotomy performed. The clinical result was good in both patients.

Results. Results of late follow-up evaluations on the patients in the conversion and interposition groups are listed in Table 5. Jejunal interposition was successful in 13 of 18 patients so treated (72 percent), whereas in only 8 of 15 patients (54 percent) in the conversion group was the treatment considered a success. Two patients following conversion to a Billroth I anastomosis continued to complain and were classified as failures. They were both later completely cured of their symptoms by jejunal interposition.

If either operation is to prove useful as a method of treating bile vomiting, any immediate improvement must be maintained over a long time. Therefore, the patients were asked whether they had immediate improvement following operation, and if they were improved, did this level of improvement maintain itself, improve still further, or regress. The results of this enquiry are listed in Table 6. Four fifths of all the patients who had initial improvement following surgery maintained this level or became progressively better; only three patients in the conversion group and two in the interposition group felt that they were improved shortly after surgery, but with the passage of time symptoms returned.

Twenty-nine of the 31 patients had lost considerable weight after their original ulcer operations. Only four of the 15 patients in the conversion group gained weight following the operation for bile vomiting; the mean weight gain was 1.1 kg. In contrast, two-thirds of the patients in the interposition group gained weight postoperatively; they gained an average of 7.1 kg.

Conclusions. The results of this study tend to support the hypothesis proposed earlier and demonstrate the beneficial results of operations designed to prevent bile regurgitation into the gastric remnant. The failures after conversion to Billroth I were associated with persistent influx of bile into the stomach and were later cured by the creation of an interposed loop. It appears that either jejunal interposition or a Roux-en-Y anastomosis is successful in relieving postgastrectomy bile vomiting, although my

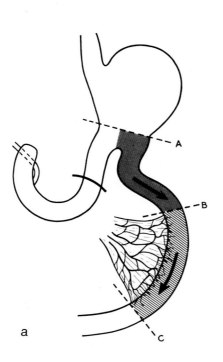

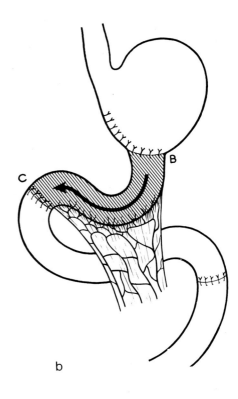

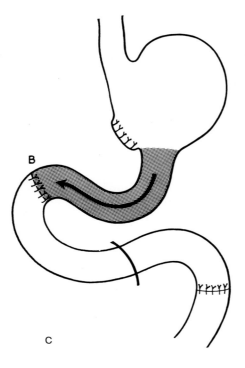

FIG. 5. Jejunal interposition conversion from Bill-roth II gastrectomy. (A) Either an isolated jejunal loop b-c or the immediate afferent loop a-b. A jejunal loop of 12 to 15 cm is prepared using either the immediate afferent loop (a-b) or a more distal loop with its blood supply (b-c). (B) An isolated loop with its mesentery is brought through a hole in the mesocolon and anastomosed between gastric remnant (b) and duodenal stump (c). The old jejunal stoma is closed. (C) Using the first 12 cm of the efferent loop to anastomose to the duodenal stump (b). The afferent loop is then anastomosed to the distal end of the divided efferent loop.

Table 5. FUNCTIONAL RESULTS OF OPERATIONS FOR AFFERENT-LOOP SYNDROME (AS ASSESSED BY PATIENTS AND "BLIND" BY AN INDEPENDENT PHYSICIAN)

Evaluations	Conversion Group	Interposition Group
Patient's		
Success	8	13
Improvement	2	1
Failure	5	4
Physician's		
Success	8	13
Improvement	5	1
Failure	2	4

experience of the latter operation is too small to permit a true evaluation. Vagotomy should always be added to any reconstruction operation; in four of the nineteen patients in this series who did not have a vagotomy, there was a recurrent ulcer in the juxtagastric jejunum and it necessitated a later vagotomy.

FOOD VOMITING

This problem is best considered in two phases, depending on the time of presentation after operation. The first, occurring immediately after the operation, is due to a delay in gastric emptying; and the second, occurring months or years later, is due to the development of obstruction at the stoma or distally in the bowel.

Delayed gastric emptying may occur as a complication of all gastric operations. Table 7 shows the incidence of this complication after five different operations in the series of Nelson (1968). Although many reports give an incidence of delayed gastric emptying after vagotomy and pyloroplasty as around

15 percent, in our experience the incidence is directly related to the experience in performing the operation. In our early experience, retention was relatively common. In 1962 we had a 17 percent incidence in our series of patients having vagotomy and pyloroplasty, but by 1965 the incidence had fallen to 3 percent (Barnes & Williams, 1967). Since 1965 the complication has rarely occurred.

Treatment of delayed gastric emptying depends to a certain extent on the type of operation used and on the nutrition and fortitude of the patient. The principal causes are stomal oedema and gastric atony, both of which will be expected to subside within the course of days rather than weeks after the operation.

In our patients who were able to tolerate nasogastric suction or who had gastrostomy drainage, we have used suction and intravenous therapy for periods up to 3 weeks, with eventual return to completely normal gastric emptying. In other patients submitted to reoperation after a week with apparently no gastric emptying, we have found the stoma to be completely patent, with no evidence of mechanical obstruction. Such a patient should probably have been treated conservatively for longer. In some patients, however, the stoma has been found to be hard, tight, and unyielding at reoperation. In such patients a reanastomosis or a proximal gastrojejunal drainage has been used.

Medical therapy may have something to offer in the management of delayed gastric emptying. Drugs aimed at reducing inflammatory oedema have been advocated, including steroids and phenylbutazone. I think that the theoretical disadvantages outweigh the advantages. Metoclopramide may be of value in accelerating gastric emptying and

Table 6. EFFECT OF PASSAGE OF TIME ON "GOOD RESULTS" AFTER RECONSTRUCTION OPERATIONS FOR BILE VOMITING — PATIENTS' ASSESSMENT

Assessment	Conversion Group	Interposition Group
No improvement at any time	1	2
After initial improvement		
Became even better	5 ⎫	8 ⎫
Maintained improvement	6 ⎬ 79 percent	6 ⎬ 87 percent
Regressed and became failures	3 ⎭	2 ⎭

Table 7.   DELAY IN GASTRIC
EMPTYING AFTER GASTRIC OPERATIONS

Operation	Incidence of Delay in Gastric Emptying (percent)
Billroth II gastrectomy	8
Vagotomy and antrectomy with gastrojejunal anastomosis	25
Vagotomy and antrectomy with gastroduodenal anastomosis	17
Vagotomy and gastrojejunostomy	16
Vagotomy and pyloroplasty	19

Source: After Nelson, Med. J. Aust. 2:522, 1968.

has been used in some patients in my series, apparently with the desired result. No comparative trials are available, however.

The diagnostic procedures that help in the assessment of the problem are: (1) The presence of bile in the nasogastric aspirate. In the absence of efferent loop obstruction, this indicates stomal patency and encourages continued conservative management. (2) A gastrografin contrast x-ray study. With the patient lying on the right side to facilitate gastric emptying, x-rays may show emptying to be present even in patients who continue to have large gastric aspirates. The radiological demonstration of emptying encourages conservative management. In the first few postoperative days, gastrografin may fail to leave the stomach and yet subsequent course shows normal emptying to be reestablished (Williams et al., 1968). (3) Gastroscopy may be helpful, particularly using the end-viewing fibre-optic instruments. This investigation will rarely be undertaken within the first postoperative week, but if a patient has failed to empty satisfactorily for 2 or more weeks after operation, the demonstration of a patent stoma would still encourage continued conservative management.

In summary, it can be said that delayed postoperative gastric emptying is usually the result of a technical error, and in the hands of an experienced surgeon this complication is rarely a problem.

Conservative management is associated with a high chance of success. Reoperation is rarely indicated and should not be undertaken before radiological and endoscopic studies have demonstrated a complete mechanical obstruction.

Late obstruction vomiting.   Patients who have had a normal postoperative course may later develop food vomiting from a mechanical cause. Mechanical obstruction due to band adhesions or volvulus obstruction are complications of all abdominal operations. The mechanical obstructions of specific interest after gastric operations are internal herniation and bolus obstruction.

Internal Herniation.   This was described exhaustively and comprehensively by Stammers in the fifth edition of this book and will not be discussed in detail here. Further reports, however, continue to appear in the literature and indicate that the complications of herniation still occur around the loops of a gastrojejunal anastomosis (Reding et al., 1967; Southam 1967; Frey and Coon 1968; Hedenstedt and Lindahl, 1968; and Cleator et al., 1968).

Although it is theoretically possible to prevent herniation by suturing the bowel or mesentery or omentum, the complication may occur even after careful closure, in my experience, particularly after a total gastrectomy with a Roux-en-Y anastomosis.

An interesting type of delayed mechanical obstruction after a Billroth I gastrectomy was described by Sim (1966), who suggested that gastroduodenal mucosal prolapse could occur as a late event after a Billroth I gastrectomy. He claimed that the syndrome was more common than had previously been recognised. The evidence he produces in his report, however, is equivocal and tenuous. In my experience the late development of mechanical stomal obstruction after a Billroth I gastrectomy is due usually to recurrent peptic ulcer at the stoma or rarely to the development of carcinoma. The late development of stenosis after vagotomy and pyloroplasty or gastrojejunostomy is almost always the result of recurrent ulceration and should be investigated and treated accordingly.

Bolus Obstruction.   After operations that remove the antrum, undigested large particles of food can pass into the small bowel and, if they collect into a semisolid bolus, can obstruct in the next narrow area of the bowel, usually at the ileocaecal valve. One of the most commonly reported types is an orange pulp bolus (Powley 1961; Knight and Scott, 1961; Nelson, 1968). The clinical presentation is of the subacute obstruction, similar to that seen in intestinal obstruction due to the passage of a large gallstone.

NONGASTRIC NAUSEA

Nausea and vomiting can occur in patients after gastric operations without any direct gastric cause. Vomiting may be associated with biliary or pancreatic disease. It is occasionally associated with severe states of malnutrition that can occasionally occur in patients, usually after an extensive gastrectomy. Vomiting may occur even in the absence of any organic disease. It can be associated with hysteria and sometimes even with malingering. One patient with persistent vomiting that occurred many years after a gastric operation was extensively investigated on my unit before it was discovered that the vomiting had its origin in labyrinthine disease.

DUMPING

The troublesome symptoms of the dumping syndrome occur 10 to 20 minutes after a meal. The syndrome is sometimes called *early dumping* to distinguish it from the somewhat similar symptoms of *late dumping,* which cocurs 60 to 90 minutes after a meal; the latter is due to hypoglycaemia. In this chapter we are concerned with the early postcibal symptoms, and I will use the term *dumping syndrome.*

Patients with the dumping syndrome experience two groups of symptoms—abdominal and systemic. The abdominal symptoms consist of abdominal fullness, sometimes accompanied by nausea, colic, and an attack of diarrhoea. The systemic symptoms include a feeling of weakness and even faintness, with sweating and palpitations in severe instances; the patient may have an irresistible desire to go to sleep. During the attack, the patient looks pale, and there is often a rise in the pulse rate, with hypotension and changes in the ECG (Sullivan, 1966).

INCIDENCE

The comparative incidence of the symptoms of dumping after different operations is shown in Table 8. The differences between the series are due to differences in definition or severity. It appears that dumping most commonly occurs after the Billroth II type of operation but it clearly occurs quite commonly after truncal vagotomy and simple drainage as well. It is claimed that proximal gastric vagotomy without pyloroplasty abolishes the complication of dumping (Humphrey et al., 1972).

AETIOLOGY

The abnormality involved in this syndrome is believed to be rapid "dumping" of food into the jejunum where isotonic equilibrium between intraluminal and extraluminal fluid can occur rapidly. Sugars and starches that are rapidly broken down into sugars exert a particularly strong osmotic effect so that there is net secretion of fluid into the lumen. This causes distention of the gut, which explains the abdominal symptoms of the dumping syndrome, the large

Table 8. INCIDENCE OF DUMPING AFTER DIFFERENT GASTRIC OPERATIONS (IN PERCENT)

Gastric Operation	Incidence of Dumping (Authors)		
	Nelson, 1968 (percent)	Cox et al., 1970 (percent)	Goligher et al., 1972 (percent)
Billroth II gastrectomy	47	15	21.5
Vagotomy and antrectomy (usually with Billroth II anastomosis)	36	26	8.5
Vagotomy and gastrojejunostomy	24	9	18.0
Vagotomy and pyloroplasty	29	11.5	12.0

volume of intraluminal fluid passing rapidly through the alimentary tract as does a saline cathartic.

The systemic symptoms experienced by patients with the dumping syndrome were originally also attributed to jejunal distention (Hertz, 1913). It is true that the symptoms can be reproduced by distending the gastric remnant or the jejunum with a balloon. This explanation is insufficient, however, to account for all the vasomotor symptoms. Le Quesne and his colleagues (1960) postulated that the symptoms are brought about by a decrease in plasma volume during the dumping syndrome, and they suggested that a rapid infusion of a plasma expander could control the postcibal symptoms. Later work by Butz, however (1961), showed that the dumping syndrome still occurred in susceptible patients even if the blood volume was maintained by infusion.

An alternative explanation of the vasomotor signs and symptoms was that a hormone or hormones, released from the wall of the distended gut, were responsible for the peripheral effects. 5-Hydroxytryptamine was first suggested by Bulbring (1958), and later by Johnson and Jesseph (1961). This hypothesis has recently received support from the work in Moscow by Sveshnikov and Stoilov (1968), who compared blood levels of 5-HT (serotonin) and urinary 5-hydroxyindoleacetic acid levels at rest and after a 75 g glucose load in normal patients, and in patients after gastrectomy with and without the dumping syndrome. They found that after glucose ingestion the 5-HT levels increased significantly in patients with moderately severe dumping but remained the same in the normal subjects and in gastrectomised patients without the dumping syndrome. Other workers have failed to show any correlation between blood 5-HT levels and the occurrence of the dumping syndrome (Silver and colleagues, 1965; Howe, 1964; and Zeitlin and Smith, 1966). Observations on patients in my own series tend to confirm the absence of a relationship between dumping and 5-HT levels.

The possibility that the humoral agent responsible for dumping is a plasma kinin was suggested by Zeitlin and Smith (1966) and confirmed recently by the work of Cuschieri and Onabanjo (1971).

PROVOCATION OF SYMPTOMS

A number of workers have found it possible to provoke typical dumping symptoms in unoperated subjects by instillation of a solution of hypertonic glucose through a tube directly into the small bowel. This individual susceptibility to dumping has led some investigators to use methods of assessing the "dumping threshold" before undertaking gastric surgery (Hinshaw et al., 1971). Fenger (1965) has advocated preoperative infusion into the duodenum of repeated doses of 50 g of glucose to identify patients with a low threshold. He suggested that if patients experienced severe dumping they might be rejected as candidates for gastric surgery or that they should have one of the less radical operations. Others have suggested that patients liable to develop dumping might be identified by psychological assessment or by evaluation of the sensitivity of the autonomic nervous system (Borgstrom and Bulow, 1967).

TREATMENT

Medical treatment. The most important virtue in the management of the dumping syndrome is patience; while many experience the symptoms of the dumping syndrome in the early weeks or months after operation, a decreasing number are troubled in the succeeding months and years. Many learn tricks of diet and posture to minimise the symptoms, but there also appears to be a natural tendency for the symptoms to decrease, suggesting that the body is adjusting to the abnormal physiological state.

Dietary advice can be of great help to patients with the dumping syndrome. While I generally advise patients to avoid sweet and starchy foods, I find that the most useful advice is to tell them to take their meals as dry as possible and to avoid drinking during the course of a meal. A relatively dry food mass empties very much less rapidly from the stomach than does a fluid meal.

Drugs may help in the management of the dumping syndrome, their rationale being based on the hypotheses of aetiology described above. Some drugs are thought to act by improving the rapidity of glucose absorp-

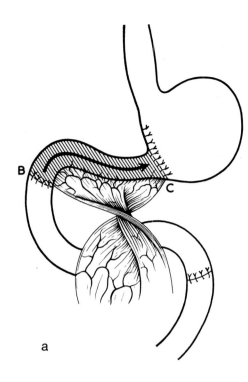

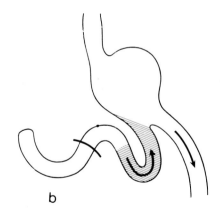

a

FIG. 6.   (A) The isolated jejunal loop is prepared as in Figure 5 but is reversed so that it lies in an anti-peristaltic direction.

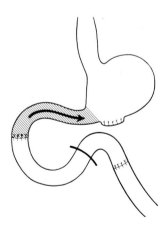

b

(B) It is sometimes possible, when there is a long afferent loop, to use part of the loop as an anti-peristaltic interposition.

tion through the jejunal mucosa and so giving it less time to exert an osmotic pressure within the lumen of the gut. Claims have been made that insulin or tolbutamide given before meals averts the symptoms (Le Quesne et al., 1960; Boss, 1966; Sullivan, 1966; and Magyar et al., 1966). The hypotensive agent reserpine has been advocated by Clemens (1966), while the antiserotonin drug cyproheptadine hydrochloride has been suggested by Sullivan (1966), but there is no evidence to support the latter view.

Table 9.   RECONSTRUCTION OPERATIONS FOR DUMPING

Type of Reconstruction Operation	Number of Patients			Ages (in years)		Time Interval (in months)	
						Initial Resection to Reconstruction	Reconstruction to Assessment
	All	Men	Women	Mean	Range	Mean	Mean
To Billroth I	9	6	3	50	41 to 58	60	99
Isoperistaltic loop of jejunum	12	8	6	51	41 to 62	80	71
Retroperistaltic loop of jejunum	6	5	1	44	27 to 59	71	12

Drugs have been used widely in the treatment of patients under my care and, of those mentioned, only insulin and tolbutamide have been effective in alleviating the dumping symptoms. When patients with severe dumping have been admitted to hospital and treated, it has almost always been possible to prevent the symptoms by diet and drugs. We have never been able to discharge the patient from hospital care, however, and continue successfully with hypoglycaemic therapy; eventually they have always considered the treatment worse than the complaint. Some of these patients have been sufficiently severely disabled to require reconstruction operations later.

Surgical treatment. As with bile vomiting, many surgeons have used reconstruction operation in an attempt to relieve severe dumping symptoms that have not responded to medical treatment and show no sign of spontaneous regression. My own experience is with three types of operation—conversion from Billroth II to Billroth I and interposition of a jejunal loop between the gastric remnant and duodenum, the loop being either isoperistaltic or retroperistaltic. Details of the patients to be reported here are given in Table 9 and the techniques of

the retroperistaltic operation are illustrated in Figure 6.

Results of reconstructive surgery. The patients were assessed clinically by an independent observer at varying intervals between 1 and 12 years after the reconstructive operation. As judged by the frequency and severity of their dumping symptoms, they were graded as being cured, improved, or showing no change. The results are shown in Table 10. Only one of the patients in the conversion group was cured of symptoms (11 percent), whereas five (46 percent) of the isoperistaltic interposition group and five (72 percent) of the retroperistaltic group were cured.

The number of patients in each group is small and the length of follow-up after retroperistaltic interposition is still short, so that no valid comparisons can be made. The results of the conversion operation are poor, however, when reviewed more than 5 years after the conversion. All nine patients in the conversion group claimed some improvement in the first 3 months after operation, but in the majority this improvement did not last more than 12 months. There is still time for the retroperistaltic conversion group patients to deteriorate symptomatically. The

Table 10.   RESULTS OF RECONSTRUCTION OPERATION FOR DUMPING

Physician's Evaluation	Conversion Group (9 patients)	Interposition	
		Isoperistaltic (12 patients)	Retroperistaltic (6 patients)
Success	1	5	5
Improved	3	5	1
Failure	5	2	0

isoperistaltic interposition patients have now been followed for more than 5 years, however, with only one patient out of twelve reverting to dumping after an initial improvement.

Discussion of results. The fact that the jejunal interposition operations gave better results than the simple conversion to Billroth I operation is consistent with the view that the aim of reconstructive surgery should be to slow down gastric emptying and thereby prevent excessively rapid entry of food into the small intestine. Although the series is small, the highest success rate was when the loop was reversed, which could be expected to have most effect on the rate of gastric emptying. Our isoperistaltic jejunal interposition results are similar to those reported from Russia by Kradinov and Volobuev (1966), who achieved good results in eighty patients and better than those experienced by Woodward and Hastings (1960), who cured only two of five patients with dumping by isoperistaltic jejunal interposition. Successful management of dumping by jejunal interposition has been achieved by several workers (Hedenstedt and Heijkenskjold, 1961; Kay and Cox, 1964; Gerwig et al., 1967). The reversed jejunal loop has been found to be effective in the control of dumping symptoms by Jordan and his colleagues (1963).

The relative lack of success of the conversion from a Billroth II operation to a Billroth I operation is in accordance with the experience of Borg and his colleagues (1968), who noted improvement in only six of sixteen patients. They concluded that surgeons should not employ this operation for the relief of dumping. The failure of this procedure for dumping symptoms has been reported previously by Andreassen (1961), who observed a recurrence of symptoms after initial improvement in 38 of 42 patients. Many workers have reported good results from this operation, however, as shown in Table 11. The different rates of success reported are probably due to several factors, including differing criteria for success, duration of follow-up, variations in operative technique, and difficulty in assessment of patients with multiple postgastrectomy problems.

Table 11.   RESULTS OF THE BILLROTH II TO I CONVERSION FOR DUMPING

Author	Patients (no.)	Cured or Improved	
		(no.)	(percent)
Perman (1947)	25	21	84
Bohmannson (1950)	24	24	100
Wallensten (1960)	18	18	100
Woodward and Hastings (1960)	11	8	73
Hinshaw et al. (1961)	13	12	92
Andreassen (1961)	42	38	90[a]
Borg et al. (1968)	16	6	38
Williams series	9	4	44

[a]*Andreassen noted a relapse after initial improvement in almost all these patients.*

Summary

From the evidence presented, it can be concluded that dumping symptoms are common after gastrectomy, occurring in about one-third of patients. They are particularly common after major Billroth II gastric resections. The frequency and severity of the symptoms are related to the rapidity of gastric emptying and determined, at least in part, by the individual susceptibility of the patient.

Most patients with dumping can be managed conservatively, and the symptoms improve with time in the majority. In severe and persistent cases, gastric reconstructive surgery can be effective in curing or improving the symptoms. In my hands, the conversion of a Billroth II to a Billroth I gastrectomy has a poor record in the management of dumping, but operations such as jejunal interposition, which delay gastric emptying, are effective.

DIARRHOEA

Although diarrhoea is often considered to be a problem peculiar to patients who have had vagotomy, it must be remembered that it occurs also after gastric operations without vagotomy. Table 12 shows the comparative incidence of diarrhoea after different gastric operations. It appears from these data that diarrhoea is 2 to 3 times as

Table 12.   INCIDENCE OF DIARRHOEA AFTER DIFFERENT GASTRIC OPERATIONS (IN PERCENT)

Gastric Operations	Incidence of Diarrhoea (Authors)	
	Nelson, 1968 (percent)	Goligher et al., 1972 (percent)
Billroth II gastrectomy	13 (0)	6.5 (0.9)
Vagotomy and antrectomy	30 (2.2)	23.2 (2.7)
Vagotomy and gastrojejunostomy	23 (2.1)	26.3 (5.1)
Vagotomy and pyloroplasty	33 (0)	21.0 (4.3)

Note: Incidence of severe diarrhoea is shown in brackets.

common after gastric operations associated with vagotomy as it is after operations relying on resection alone. Severe diarrhoea is rare after gastric resection but occurs in between 2 and 5 percent of patients after vagotomy.

While mild or moderate diarrhoea is usually tolerated by patients who consider that it is a small price to pay for the relief of their dyspeptic symptoms, severe diarrhoea seriously mars the beneficial effects of the operation. Therefore, surgeons have sought to minimise the ill effects of vagotomy by variations in the technique of vagotomy. The evidence available suggests that the incidence of diarrhoea is significantly reduced when selective vagotomy is used (Kennedy, 1973) and may be virtually abolished by proximal gastric vagotomy without pyloroplasty, preserving the vagal innervation to the antrum (Johnston, 1973).

Diarrhoea after gastric operations can be classified into two distinct types. *Continuous diarrhoea,* in which the patient has frequent loose stools every day, and *episodic diarrhoea,* in which there is a background of near-normal bowel habit with sudden unheralded attacks of urgent diarrhoea. Episodic diarrhoea is particularly characteristic in patients after vagotomy operations.

Aetiology

Despite exhaustive research, no simple answer has been found to explain diarrhoea after gastric operations. We have investigated many patients with continuous diarrhoea after gastric resection and have detected two patients with gluten-sensitive enteropathy (adult coeliac disease) and two patients with chronic pancreatitis and pancreatic exocrine insufficiency. In these patients, the defects were almost certainly present before operation and their effects merely accentuated by the gastric resection. We have also investigated other patients with diarrhoea after Billroth I gastrectomy and found gross colonisation of the upper gastrointestinal tract with colonic-type organisms. We have assumed that these patients have had a type of the intestinal blind-loop syndrome. Whether or not this theory is correct, long-term antibiotic therapy has failed to achieve anything more than temporary relief of the diarrhoea. In one patient, conversion from a Billroth II anastomosis to a Billroth I anastomosis was performed to abolish the "blind" duodenal loop. This procedure did not affect the flora of the upper gastrointestinal tract nor did it cure the diarrhoea.

A relatively rare but important cause of acute profuse diarrhoea is the development of a gastrocolic fistula due to stomal ulceration. I have treated three patients with a gastrocolic fistula: two after a Billroth II gastrectomy and one after a gastrojejunostomy. In all three, profuse debilitating diarrhoea was a major presenting symptom. It must also be remembered that diarrhoea may be a feature of the Zollinger-Ellison syndrome; an association between peptic ulcer and diarrhoea should lead to a consideration of this diagnosis. In some patients with continuous diarrhoea, no precipitating cause can be found.

The causes of episodic diarrhoea are less well understood. Three possibilities have been suggested: The first is that the stomach is unable to fulfill its bactericidal function, as a result of hypochlorhydria produced by the gastric surgery, so that the upper small bowel is susceptible to recurrent attacks of enteritis. Although this hypothesis seems logical, there has as yet been no conclusive evidence of any relationship between upper small intestine colonisation and the susceptibility to attacks of diarrhoea. Furthermore, the attacks of diarrhoea are so short-lived that the enteritis theory seems unlikely.

The other possibility is that diarrhoea may be related to the drainage operation, but the evidence on this point is confusing, some workers having claimed that too slow gastric emptying causes the diarrhoea and others that it is due to rapid gastric emptying (Cox, 1970).

A third and most logical possibility is that vagal denervation of the pancreas and biliary system and of the small intestine is the factor that is responsible for the diarrhoea. This hypothesis is supported by the finding that there is less diarrhoea after selective vagotomy or proximal gastric vagotomy than there is after truncal vagotomy. Although there is convincing evidence that the new variations of vagotomy are less disturbing to bowel habit than is truncal vagotomy, this still does not prove that diarrhoea is due to denervation of pancreas, biliary system, or small bowel.

TREATMENT

From our study of patients with episodic diarrhoea after truncal vagotomy, it appears that the symptoms become much less troublesome with the passage of time. Because of this continual improvement in the tendency towards attacks of episodic diarrhoea, the initial treatment should be symptomatic, the patients benefiting from dietary advice particularly directed towards the avoidance of milk products and wet, sweet foods. Symptomatic treatment with codeine and diphenoxylate (Lomotil) is of little value when attacks of diarrhoea are unheralded. Such simple treatment may tide the patients over the early difficult months, however, and should always be tried in preference to the more radical forms of reconstructive surgery that have been advocated. Some authors have recommended the interposition of reversed small-bowel loops in the attempt to control postvagotomy diarrhoea (Herrington, 1970). Although undoubtedly successful in some patients, radical surgical treatment should rarely be recommended.

METABOLIC DISORDERS

Malnutrition and deficiency states are well-recognised late complications of gastric surgery. Although observed initially after partial gastrectomy, it is now becoming evident that some deficiency diseases can also occur after the so called "conservative operations" such as vagotomy and pyloroplasty and vagotomy and gastrojejunostomy. The manifestations of malnutrition that occur after gastric operations are weight loss; anaemia with deficiencies of iron, vitamin B_{12}, folic acid; and metabolic bone disease. The problems of anaemia after gastric operations are considered elsewhere in this book so this chapter will therefore consider weight loss and bone disease. (See also Chap. 106.)

Weight Loss

Many patients lose weight or fail to gain weight after gastric operations. Those who are undernourished at the time of the operation seem to be at the greatest risk.

Weight loss is almost universal after total gastrectomy (Everson, 1952).

After Billroth I partial gastrectomy, it is reported in from 5 percent (Wallensten and Gothman, 1953) to 54 percent of patients (Harkins and Nyhus, 1956).

After Billroth II resection, it is reported by the same observers in 13 to 74 percent of patients. Weight loss also occurs after vagotomy and simple drainage procedures. In their comparison of the results of different operations, Goligher and his colleagues (1968) compared the actual weight of the patients in the series with the optimum weight and expressed the results as the actual and as a percentage of the optimum weight. When this index was used, Billroth II gastrectomy and vagotomy and antrectomy fared the same with the mean actual weight being 90 percent of the optimum weight. Patients who had had vagotomy and gastrojejunostomy fared better with a mean weight of 97 percent of their optimum weight. Various comparisons have been made between vagotomy and pyloroplasty and vagotomy and gastrojejunostomy (Cox, 1970). The results suggested that weight loss was less frequent or less substantial after vagotomy with pyloroplasty than when gastrojejunostomy was the drainage procedure.

AETIOLOGY

The cause of loss of weight after gastric operations is either (1) failure to eat enough food or (2) failure to absorb calories from the food.

Inadequate intake. Probably the most important cause is inadequate intake of food and this is due either to lack of appetite or fear of provoking postcibal symptoms.

Appetite is determined by a number of apparently unrelated factors including a low blood sugar, an empty stomach, and the feeling of mental and physical well being. A patient may have a poor appetite because he takes too much tobacco or alcohol and sometimes because he is deficient of minerals or vitamins. Iron deficiency is particularly likely to impair the appetite and so to a lesser extent is a deficiency of vitamin B_{12} or folic acid. In the correct evaluation of postoperative patients, all these factors must be assessed. Early satiation will depend on the size of the gastric remnant, its speed of emptying, and its ability to distend. The more radical the gastric resection, the greater the likelihood of weight loss. This generalisation, however, needs qualification, for some patients with an intact but denervated stomach feel full after a small quantity of food, while other patients with a total gastrectomy appear to have a normal appetite. The presence of gastritis often appears to be associated with anorexia. There is also some evidence to suggest that vagal sensory innervation may be important in normal relaxation of the stomach after a meal.

A fear of discomfort is often the major factor in limiting patients' food intake. Most of the severe cases of malnutrition that I have seen after gastric operations are in those patients with severe symptomatic disorders who sought relief from their distressing symptoms in the only way they found effective—by starvation.

Malabsorption. After partial gastrectomy, minor degrees of malabsorption are common; a faecal fat excretion of more than 6 g per day can be demonstrated in over 60 percent of patients. In the majority, the steatorrhoea is mild and perhaps only 1 percent have severe malabsorption; as a consequence, malabsorption is not thought to be a major cause of weight loss (Welbourn, 1967). Steatorrhoea after partial gastrectomy may have many causes, but in the majority of patients it appears to be related to interference with the normal mixing of the bile and pancreatic juices with food, the so called pancreatico-cibal asynchrony (Brain, 1953). In a detailed study of a group of patients with a weight loss of 6 kg or more after partial gastrectomy, Hilleman (1968) has shown that there was a delay of months or even years after operation before the weight loss became apparent. In every patient in his series, there was an increase in the faecal fat excretion, though fewer than half of the patients had diarrhoea. In addition, a careful dietary analysis showed that 25 percent of these patients had an adequate diet. Pancreatic insufficiency was considered a likely cause of the steatorrhoea in most and a therapeutic trial of pancreatic extract resulted in all patients gaining weight; in the majority there was a return towards normal of the faecal fat excretion. In a study of a similar group of patients, Clark (1963) found that in some patients weight loss was due to dietary deficiency but that in others on a good diet malabsorption was the only possible explanation for the weight loss.

Vagotomy and drainage operations are often followed by malabsorption, but it is usually of only a minor degree. Faecal fat output has been shown to be increased by vagotomy and gastrojejunostomy and to a lesser extent by vagotomy and pyloroplasty (Williams and Irvine, 1966). The incidence of steatorrhoea in 84 patients after vagotomy and jejunostomy studied by Cox and colleagues (1964) was 43 percent, although the actual levels of faecal fat excretion were not particularly high (mean of 7.5 g per day compared with an upper limit of normal of 7.0 g per day). Vagotomy alone or gastroenterostomy alone was not found to be associated with steatorrhoea in the group of patients studied by Butler and Eastham (1965). This finding suggests that it is a combination of vagotomy and the drainage which causes defective absorption.

Treatment of Weight Loss

Minor degrees of weight loss can be treated by advice on diet, correction of any associated mineral and vitamin deficiencies, taking snacks between meals, and possibly also a gastric stimulant such as sherry before meals. Johnston and his colleagues (1958) have shown that patients with weight loss after partial gastrectomy can regain lost weight if they are admitted to hospital and persuaded to eat sufficient food.

More severe degrees of weight loss where malabsorption is considered important should be investigated to exclude gluten-sensitive enteropathy. If pancreatic insufficiency is suspected, treatment with pancreatic extracts may be beneficial.

Patients with severe weight loss due to serious postcibal symptoms such as dumping or bile vomiting should be considered as candidates for gastric reconstructive surgery (see above).

Anaemia

A detailed account of anaemia after gastric operations is given in Chapter 26.

Bone Disease

Bone disease has only recently been recognised as an important complication of gastric surgery. After performing preoperative and postoperative calcium balance studies in patients undergoing partial gastrectomy, Nicolaysen and Ragard (1955) predicted that the negative balance induced by the operation must inevitably produce late metabolic deficiencies, Up to 1960, only 15 cases of bone disease following gastric surgery had been reported (Stammers and Williams, 1963), however. In the fifth edition of this book I reported on my series of 28 patients with postgastrectomy osteomalacia (see 5th ed., Chap. 28, pp. 516–517). Although there are now large numbers of well-documented cases of postgastrectomy osteomalacia, it must be emphasized that it is still a relatively uncommon complication of gastric surgery.

Types

Subclinical osteomalacia. Several authors have argued that if overt osteomalacia is rare, there must be a large group of patients with subclinical disease. Three independent surveys to determine the extent of the problem were undertaken in Aberdeen, Scotland; Adelaide, Australia; and Birmingham, England. Incidences of subclinical osteomalacia were reported in from 15 to 22 percent of patients many years after partial gastrectomy (Jones et al., 1962; Deller et al., 1963; Clark et al., 1964). Their assessments were based on evidence of diminished bone density on x-ray and on biochemical abnormalities such as a low serum calcium level and raised serum alkaline phosphatase level. Each of these groups of workers concluded that a raised serum alkaline phosphatase level was the first indication of metabolic bone disease after gastrectomy and suggested that in time a very large number of patients would develop osteomalacia.

This prediction was not substantiated by the observation of Morgan and his colleagues (1965), who found an incidence of raised serum alkaline phosphatase level in 18 percent of patients with gastrectomy over the age of 60 but concluded that this was not significant since a raised serum alkaline phosphatase level was also found in 20 percent of patients with vagotomy and drainage and in 9 percent of patients with a peptic ulcer but who had had no operation. Furthermore it was possible to find alternative explanations for most of the higher than normal enzyme levels and they concluded that a raised serum alkaline phosphatase level after gastrectomy was not a reliable indication of subclinical osteomalacia. They challenged the suggestion that subclinical disease existed. Since then other groups of workers at the Hammersmith Hospital, London, have shown that in the absence of Paget's disease of the bone or liver dysfunction a raised serum alkaline phosphatase level after gastrectomy is usually indicative of overt or subclinical osteomalacia (Thompson et al., 1966). The same group have also found that bone biopsy specimens from these patients, when examined by special histological techniques, give clear evidence of vitamin D deficiency (Bordier et al., 1968), and furthermore that these patients respond to a vitamin D challenge (Whittle et al., 1969). It is concluded, therefore, that although gross unequivocal osteomalacia is a relatively rare complication of partial gastrectomy, subclinical osteomalacia exists and is not uncommon. Our own observations of patients with raised serum alkaline phosphatase levels after partial gastrectomy have shown that they can remain asymptomatic and untreated for very many years without apparent deterioration. Some patients, however, have developed vague bone pains which have responded to vitamin D therapy.

Osteoporosis. One of the main difficulties in evaluating the problem of bone disease after gastric surgery is in distinguishing between the effects of the operation and the effects of aging. Alterations in calcium metabolism undoubtedly occur as the result of increasing age. Therefore, in any postoperative survey, the effects due to age have to be equated with those due to the operation. The changes that occur with age are usually considered to be osteoporosis; that is, loss of bone density without evidence of vitamin D deficiency. This can be detected on bone biopsy but is usually estimated radiologically by comparing the relative thickness of cortical bone to total bone width in a "standard bone," usually the second metacarpal or femur. Morgan and his colleagues 1965) found that the bone cortex after gastrectomy was thinner than normal in both sexes, but that this effect was apparent only after the age of 60 in men and 50 in women. They suggested that at those ages gastrectomy had the effect of accelerating the normal loss of bone. Nilsson and Wastlin (1971) found that the incidence of fractures in men 20 years after gastrectomy was almost double that in controls of the same age and that the type of fracture was similar to that seen in osteoporosis.

Bone disease after vagotomy. Metabolic bone disease might be expected to occur after any gastric operation. Duodenal bypass, however, appears to be one important associated factor, and many of the early case reports in the literature were in patients who had had gastroenterostomy alone.

As the result of a detailed study of 342 postgastrectomy and postvagotomy patients, Edie (1971) concluded that 30 percent of all patients after gastric operations developed some form of bone disease and that overt or subclinical osteomalacia is a significant component in approximately 25 percent of these. In his series, a raised serum alkaline phosphatase level usually indicated subclinical osteomalacia as shown by bone biopsy and response to vitamin D therapy. The incidence of a raised alkaline phosphatase level after Billroth II gastrectomy was 31 percent and after vagotomy and pyloroplasty it was 17 percent. The difference between the two operations was statistically significant (p < 0.005). Morgan and Pulvertaft (1969) found that the incidence of a raised alkaline phosphatase level was almost as high after vagotomy and gastrojejunostomy as it was after a Billroth II gastrectomy. On the contrary, Cox (1970) made a study of forty patients more than 8 years after vagotomy and gastrojejunostomy using measurements of serum calcium, phosphate and alkaline phosphatase, bone density, and phosphate excretion index and found no significant abnormality.

TREATMENT

There is no difficulty in formulating a policy for the treatment of the patient with gross osteomalacia after gastric operation. Oral doses of vitamin D 50,000 units once or twice daily may be given while the patient's response is carefully monitored to avoid vitamin D overdose. As there may possibly be associated calcium deficiency, it is advisable to give supplementary calcium therapy up to 1 g of calcium per day.

It is more difficult to know how to treat patients with minor degrees of osteomalacia; if the patient has a raised alkaline phosphatase level, minor histological abnormalities, and symptoms of bone pain, I advocate a trial of vitamin D therapy with careful monitoring of the serum calcium to avoid the dangers of overdose. If the patient's symptoms are relieved, a full dose of vitamin D is continued for 2 to 3 months, and the patient is then maintained on a dose of 500 units of vitamin D daily. In patients who have no conclusive evidence of vitamin D deficiency, there are dangers in giving large doses of vitamin D. It is extremely difficult to know whether it is advisable to treat post-gastrectomy patients prophylactically with vitamin D and calcium. I once believed that prophylactic therapy was essential, but after long experience with the problem of maintaining therapy I have come to realise that this counsel of perfection is impractical. Patients who are feeling well will not continue to take prophylactic medication. I now feel that it is more practical to advise regular screening tests of elderly patients after partial gastrectomy with estimations of the serum alkaline phosphatase level and occasional radiological measurement of bone density. A raised serum alkaline phosphatase level is the first and best index of bone disease, although if a raised phosphatase level is detected, Paget's disease or liver dysfunction must be excluded before it is assumed that this is due to metabolic bone disease.

REFERENCES

Andreassen, M., Acta Scand. (Suppl. 283):221, 1961.

Auguste, C., Ribet, M., Guerrin, F., and Lescut, J., Presse Med. 71:1021, 1963.

Barnes, A. D., and Williams, J. A., Am. J. Surg. 113:494, 1967.

Bohmannson, G., Acta Med. Scand. 138 (Suppl. 246):37, 1950.

Bordier, P. H., Matrajt, H., Hioco, D., Hepener, G. W., Thompson, G. R., and Booth, C. C., Lancet 1:437, 1968.

Borg, I., Borgstrom, S. G., and Haeger, K., Acta Chir. Scand. 134:655, 1968.

Borgstrom, S. G., and Bulow, K., Scand. J. Gastroenterol. 2:263, 1967.

Boss, M., Wiad. Lek. 19:1171, 1966.

Brain, R. F. H., Proc. R. Soc. Med. 46:438, 1953.

Bulbring, E., and Lynn, R. C., J. Physiol. 140:381, 1958.

Butler, T. J., and Eastham, R. D., Gut 6:69, 1965.

Butz, R., Ann. Surg. 154:225, 1961.

Clark, C. G., J. R. Coll. Surg. Edinb. 9:52, 1963.

Clark, C. G., Crookes, J., Dawson, A. A., and Mitchell, P. E. G., Lancet 1:743, 1964.

Clave, R. A., and Gaspar, M. R., Am. J. Surg. 118:169, 1969.

Cleator, I. G. M., Falconer, C. W. A., Small, W. P., and Smith, A. N., Br. Med. J. 2:530, 1968.

Clemens, M., Beitr. Klin. Chir. 213:26, 1966.

Cox, A. G., Prog. Surg. 8:45, 1970.

Cox, A. G., Bond, M. R., Podmore, D. A., and Rose, D. P., Br. Med. J. 1:465, 1964.

Cushieri, A., and Onabanjo, O. A., Br. Med. J. 2:565, 1971.

Deller, D. J., Edwards, R. G., and Addison, M., Aust. Ann. Med. 12:295, 1963.

Edie, R. L., Am. J. Med. 50:422, 1971.

Everson, T. C., Int. Abstr. Surg. 95:209, 1952.

Fenger, J. H., Acta Chir. Scand. 129:201, 1965.

Frey, C. F., and Coon, W. W., Am. J. Surg. 115:730, 1968.

Gerwig, H. W., Jr., Easley, G. W., and Mendoza, G. B., Arch. Surg. 95:631, 1967.

Goligher, J. C., Pulvertaft, C. N., de Dombal, F. T., Conyers, J. H., Duthie, H. L., Feather, D. B., Latchmore, A. J. C., Shoesmith, J. H., Smiddy, F. G., and Willson-Pepper, J., Br. Med. J. 2:781, 1968.

Goligher, J. C., Pulvertaft, C. N., Irvine, T. T., Johnston, D., Walker, B., Hall, R. A., Willson-Pepper, J., and Matheson, T. S., Br. Med. J. 1:7, 1972.

Harkins, H. N., and Nyhus, L. M., Bull. Soc. Int. Chir. 15:111, 1956.

Hedenstedt, S., and Heijkenskjold, F., Acta Chir. Scand. 121:262, 1961.

Hedenstedt, S., and Lindahl, C., Acta Chir. Scand. 134:581, 1968.

Herrington, J. L., Am. J. Surg. 119:342, 1970.

Hertz, A. F., Ann. Surg. 58:466, 1913.

Hilleman, H. S., Gut 9:576, 1968.

Hinshaw, D. B., Stafford, C. E., and Joergenson, E. J., Am. J. Surg. 94:242, 1952.

Hinshaw, D. B., Stafford, C. E., and Joergenson, E. J., Am. J. Surg. 94:242, 1952.

Hinshaw, D. B., Thompson, R. J., and Branson, B. W., Am. J. Surg. 122:269, 1971.

Hirschowitz, B. I., Prog. Gastroenterology 2:240, 1970.

Hollander, F., Gastroenterology 11:419, 1948.

Howe, C. T., Surg. Gynecol. Obstet. 119:92, 1964.

Humphrey, C. S., Johnston, D., Walker, B. E., Pulvertaft, C. N., and Goligher, J. C., Br. Med. J. 3:785, 1972.

Johnson, L. P., and Jesseph, J. E., Surg. Forum 12:316, 1961.

Johnston, D., In Vagotomy on Trial, A. G. Cox and J. A. Williams, eds., London, Heinemann, 1973.

Johnston, D., Humphrey, B. E., Walker, C. N. Pulvertaft, C. N., and Goligher, J. C. Br. Med. J. 2:788, 1972.

Johnston, I. D. A., Br. J. Surg. 57:787, 1970.

Johnston, I. D. A., Welbourn, R., and Acheson, K. Lancet 1:1242, 1958.

Jones, C. T., Williams, J. A., Cox, E. V., Meynell, M. J., Cooke, W. T., and Stammers, F. A. R., Lancet 2:425, 1962.

Jordan, G. L., Surgery 38:1027, 1955.

Jordan, G. L., Angel, R. T., McIlhaney, J. S., and Williams, R. K., Am. J. Surg. 106:451, 1963.

Kay, A. W., and Cox, A. G., Br. J. Surg. 51:673, 1964.

Kennedy, T., In Vagotomy on Trial, A. G. Cox and J. A. Williams, eds., London, Heinemann, 1973.

Knight, P. R., and Scott, P. J., Br. Med. J. 2:1150, 1961.

Kradinov, A. I., and Volobuev, N. N., Klin. Med. (Mosk.), 44:79, 1966.

Le Quesne, L. P., Hobsley, M., and Hand, B. H., Br. Med. J. 1:141, 1960.

Magyar, K., Rethely, J., and Kovacs, P. Z., Gesamte. Inn. Med. 21:629, 1966.

Manthorpe, R., Hagen, C., and Manthorpe, T., Ugeskr. Laeger 128:1563, 1966.

Mimpriss, T. W., and Birt, J. M. C., Br. Med. J. 2:1095, 1948.

Morgan, D. B., Patterson, C. R., Woods, C. G., Pulvertaft, D. N., and Fourman, T., Lancet 2:1085, 1965.

Morgan, D. B., and Pulvertaft, C. M., In After Vagotomy, J. A. Williams and A. G. Cox, eds., London, Butterworth, 1969.

Nelson, P. G., Med. J. Aust. 2:522, 1968.

Nicolaysen, R., and Ragard, R., Scand. J. Clin. Lab. Invest. 7:298, 1955.

Nilsson, B. E., and Wastlin, L. E., Acta Chir. Scand. 137:533, 1971.

Perman, E., Acta Med. Scand. 196 (Suppl.):361, 1947.

Powley, P. H., Br. Med. J. 2:1392, 1961.

Reding, R., Buschman, V., and Senst, W., Dtsch. Gesundheitsw. 22:553, 1967.

Silver, D., Andyan, W. C., Postlethwait, R. W., Morgan, C. V., and Mengel, C. E., Ann. Surg. 161:995, 1965.

Sim, G. P. G., Br. Med. J. 1:1517, 1966.

Southam, J. A., Ann. Surg. 165:323, 1967.

Stammers, F. A. R., Br. J. Surg. 49:28, 1961.

Stammers, F. A. R., and Williams, J. A., In Partial Gastrectomy. London, Butterworth, 1963.

Steinberg, M. E., Am. J. Gastroent. 22:273, 1954.

Sullivan, M. B., Surgery 59:645, 1966.

Sveshnikov, A. I., and Stoilov, L. D., Soviet Medicine 31:24, 1968.

Thompson, G. R., Neale, G., Watts, J. A. M., and Booth, C. C., Lancet 1:623, 1966.

Wallensten, S., Acta Chir. Scand. 118:278, 1960.

Wallensten, S., and Gothman, L., Surgery 33:1, 1953.

Welbourn, R. B., Review in Surgery 24:233, 1967.

Wells, C. A., and McPhee, J. W., Lancet 2:1189, 1952.

Wells, C. A., and Welbourn, R. B., Br. Med. J., 1:546, 1951.

Whittle, H., Layer, A., Neale, G., Thalassinos, N., McCloughlin, M., Marsh, M. N., Peters, T. G., Wedzicha, B., and Thompson, G. R., Lancet 1:747, 1969.

Williams, E. J., and Irvine, W. T., Lancet 1:1053, 1966.

Williams, J. A., Pacific Med. Surg. 75:105, 1967.

Williams, J. A., Barnes, A. D., and Toye, D. K. M., Am. J. Surg. 115:454, 1968.

Williams, J. A., and Woodward, D. A. K., Surg. Clin. N. Am. 47:1341, 1967.

Windsor, C. W. O., Br. Med. J. 2:1233, 1964.

Woodward, E. R., and Hastings, N., Surg. Gynecol. Obstet. 111:429, 1960.

Zeitlin, I. J., and Smith, A. N., Lancet 2:986, 1966.

B. METABOLIC SEQUELAE OF GASTRIC OPERATIONS

J. ALEXANDER-WILLIAMS

As we do not understand the primary cause of chronic peptic ulceration, there can be no direct attack on the cause. We therefore attempt to cure the disease surgically by artificially altering the patient's gastrointestinal physiology. The effect of the physiological alteration is to impair, if only to a minor degree, the normal digestion and absorption of calories, minerals, and vitamins. The human organism is able to compensate so that most of these impairments produce little or no demonstrable defect and any deficiencies that may develop usually take years to become manifest.

Some postgastrectomy deficiency states are difficult to detect in their early stages while in their later stages they are serious and irreversible.

It is therefore important for the surgeon to be aware of the dangers to which he submits those patients in whom he alters alimentary physiology.

The pathophysiology of peptic ulceration and the physiological effects of partial gastrectomy and vagotomy have been described elsewhere. In describing the metabolic sequelae of gastric operations, some repetition may be necessary. For this I make no apology, as the subject is sufficiently important to bear repeating.

The most important nutritional ill effects of gastric operations are weight loss, anaemia, bone disease, and nutritional neuropathy, while the complaints of "dumping" and diarrhoea have their basis in disturbed physiology. Postgastrectomy anaemia is discussed by John Richmond in Chapter 26C, and "dumping" and diarrhoea by me, in Part A of this chapter.

In this section, I propose to discuss the common problems of postoperative weight loss and some metabolic aspects of dumping and diarrhoea. Dumping and steatorrhoea in relation to the mechanical consequences of gastric resection have been discussed in the first half of this chapter. Both these complications are related to metabolic as well as to mechanical factors and will therefore be considered also below, where I will confine my remarks to the rationale of the dietetic and drug therapy. I will also describe the relatively uncommon but serious sequelae of gastrectomy: osteomalacia, osteoporosis, and nutritional neuropathy.

WEIGHT LOSS

Many patients lose weight or fail to gain weight after gastric operations. Weight loss is almost universal after total gastrectomy (Everson, 1952). After Billroth I partial gastrectomy, it is reported in from 5 (Wallenstein, 1954) to 42 percent of patients (Harkins and Nyhus, 1956). After Billroth II resection, it is reported by the same observers in 13 to 74 percent of patients. Weight loss occurs even after vagotomy and pyloroplasty. In my own series of 150 patients treated by vagotomy and pyloroplasty, 10 percent are below their preoperative weight or "ideal" weight. This can be compared with 59 percent of 772 postgastrectomy patients treated in the same centre who were underweight (Brookes et al., 1960). The cause of weight loss in patients after gastric operations is either their failure to absorb enough calories from the food they eat or their failure to eat enough food.

Digestion and Absorption of Food

ABSORPTION

Food is essentially a source of calories and amino acids. Its digestion and absorption need to be considered in relation to its three main components—carbohydrates, proteins, and fats—and each of these considered in the light of the postoperative physiology of the stomach, duodenum, and small bowel.

Stomach. The effect of all gastric operations is to reduce the acid-peptic secretion of the stomach, and all to some extent tend to decrease the length of time food remains in and is actively mixed in the stomach. These effects are least in vagotomy and pyloroplasty and greatest in extensive Billroth II or total gastric resections. Gastric digestion is therefore impaired by the same process that cures the ulcer.

Carbohydrates are the most easily digested and are not significantly affected by the new physiological state. Fats are not normally significantly affected by the altered gastric physiology, although there may be less effective liberation of fats from within animal or vegetable cells. Peptic breakdown of protein to polypeptides is the process most likely to be affected adversely by a short stay in less-active gastric milieu. Provided there is active tryptic digestion, however, even the total absence of peptic digestion is unimportant. There is a great deal of truth in the observation by Ivy (Lundh, 1958) that from a strictly digestive point of view the stomach is not an essential organ. It appears that the reservoir effect is the stomach function that is missed most after operations.

Duodenum. In the Billroth II type of operation, where the gastric remnant is anastomosed to the first few centimetres of the jejunum, food no longer passes into or through the duodenum. This manoeuvre has such profound physiological effects that it is surprising that the majority of patients so treated are so well nourished. The presence of food in the jejunum evokes the secretin-pancreozymin-cholecystokinin stimulation of biliary and pancreatic juice, but the stimuli are less effective than those evoked by food in the duodenum. There is, furthermore, a distance of several centimetres separating the digestive juices arriving in the duodenum and the food in the jejunum that stimulated their secretion. The food and the juice may then not mix adequately and so digestion is impaired; Brain and Stammers (1951) refer to this as *pancreatocibal asynchrony.*

As if this were not enough, further hazards lie in the path of the digestive juices. The afferent duodenal loop often contains organisms within its lumen. Operative aspiration and culture of the duodenal loop content in 12 of my patients with Billroth II anastomoses (reoperated on for reasons often unconnected with their original operation) has shown gross colonisation with large bowel organisms (*Escherichia coli, Klebsiella aerogenes, and Streptococcus faecalis*). In only one was the juice sterile. Similar findings with jejunal culture after gastrectomy were reported by Tabaqchali and Booth (1966).

These colonic organisms are not apparently directly harmful to the patient and only rarely give rise to the severe intestinal blind-loop syndrome with gross malabsorption, hypoproteinaemia, and failure to absorb vitamin B_{12}. They may, however, attack the bile salts and pancreatic enzymes. Experimental studies have shown that these organisms break down bile salts to free cholic acid and desoxycholic acid with reduction in the efficacy of the micellar formation and esterification of fatty acids (Donaldson, 1954). The pancreatic secretions do not fare much better at the hands of the afferent loop colonists. In the presence of these organisms, pancreatic lipase is readily inactivated and to a lesser extent trypsin and amylase are also inactivated (Lagerlöf, 1942; French and Crane, 1963).

The work of Butler (1961) has shown that fat absorption in man was significantly less after a Billroth II (with duodenal bypass) than after a Billroth I operation involving the same amount of gastric resection. He attributed this to a decrease in pancreatic digestion.

It is claimed by the advocates of the Billroth II type of operation in which the gastric remnant is anastomosed to the fourth part of the duodenum (Hermon Taylor, 1959) that the ill effects of duodenal bypass are avoided. The food from the gastric remnant is then directed into the duodenal loop and there mixed with the biliary and pancreatic secretions. The observed metabolic effects of this type of operation have been impressive (Higgins and Pridie, 1966), but so far there has been no controlled comparison with any other type of Billroth II anastomosis.

Small bowel. It is the reduction in intestinal transit time after gastric surgery that produces the most marked effect on jejunal absorption. Sugars in particular exert an osmotic effect and retain excessive fluid within the lumen of the gut. As absorption is not sufficiently rapid to keep pace with the equilibrium of tonicity, the large volume of fluid exerts a cathartic effect similar to that produced by magnesium sulphate. However, although passage through the jejunum is accelerated, the readily broken-down sugars are soon absorbed and passage through the ileum is normal or even slower than normal (Bruusgaard, 1946; Schlaeger,

1960). Rapid jejunal passage may adversely affect absorption of fats and proteins. As these appear to be absorbed during their passage through the ileum, however, there is usually no significant overall impairment of small bowel absorption.

Despite the many disturbances of physiology after gastric operations, the human digestive tract has so much reserve that there is usually little reduction in the proportion of calories absorbed from food. It is, even then, only fats that are grossly affected, and the daily absorption only reduced by a few grammes. The difference between fat absorption of 95 percent in normal subjects and 90 percent after gastrectomy represents a daily loss of less than 50 calories, a quantity easily made up by a slight increase in overall dietary intake. The main problem in postoperative weight loss is therefore not malabsorption but diminished dietary intake.

The causes of the diminished intake are: (1) lack of appetite, (2) early satisfaction after a small quantity of food, and (3) fear of provoking postcibal symptoms.

Lack of appetite. Appetite is determined by a number of apparently unrelated factors, including level of blood sugar, fullness or emptiness of stomach, and the feeling of mental and physical well-being. It is not the stomach alone that is the originator of the hunger or appetite signals. I have known patients with total gastrectomy who have a good appetite and experience hunger. The patient may have a poor appetite because he takes too much tobacco or alcohol or because he is deficient in minerals or vitamins. Iron deficiency is particularly likely to impair the appetite; so to a lesser extent do deficiencies of vitamin B_{12} and folic acid.

Early satiation will depend on the size of the gastric remnant, its speed of emptying, and its ability to distend. The more radical the gastric resection, the greater the likelihood of weight loss. This is a generalisation that needs qualification; it is unwise to suggest treating all patients with weight loss owing to a feeling of fullness after meals by reoperation to increase artificially the size of the gastric remnant.

The ability of the gastric remnant to dilate without symptoms may be related to the health of the gastric mucosa. There is a relationship between the presence on biopsy of atrophic or inflammatory gastritis and the symptoms of fullness after meals. It follows, therefore, that the general nutritional measures to improve appetite may also increase the capacity to take food. Nevertheless, the simplest way to overcome early satiation is to take small frequent meals.

Fear of discomfort. Some the most severe malnutrition I have seen in patients after gastrectomy has been those in whom alkaline oesophagitis and regurgitation were provoked by taking food; they then sought relief from these distressing symptoms in the only way they found effective—by starvation.

Treatment

Treatment is directed towards relief of the cause of the discomfort (e.g., dumping, bile vomiting, oesophagitis).

Severe malabsorption is relatively uncommon after gastrectomy and always suggests additional associated disease. This may be a pancreatic insufficiency, jejunocolic fistula, regional enteritis, gluten enteropathy, or the intestinal blind-loop syndrome.

DUMPING

The three essential features of the phenomenon of "dumping" are glucose intolerance, gut distension, and constitutional predisposition.

Features

GLUCOSE INTOLERANCE

The small bowel is unable to handle the glucose load of a meal "dumped" into it straight through the stomach. This results in the osmotic retention of large volumes of fluid in the gut with a consequent fall in blood volume, usually greater than 10 percent. The effect can be relieved or abolished by improving the rate of "handling" of glucose, by inducing hypoglycaemia with insulin or tolbutamide.

GUT DISTENSION

Another feature of the phenomenon is that symptoms are produced by distension of the small bowel and may occur even if the blood volume is maintained at normal levels by rapid transfusion. The humoral role of serotonin has been postulated but its aetiological significance is not proven. We have recently studied a patient with dumping in whom the free and platelet-bound 5-hydroxytryptamine (serotonin) did not significantly alter during a severe provoked dumping attack.

CONSTITUTIONAL PREDISPOSITION

Perhaps the most important feature of dumping is that the symptoms tend to occur in patients who can be shown preoperatively to have a predilection, by a provocative glucose meal. These same patients have a more-than-average incidence of allergic diseases such as hay fever or asthma. They are also said to have less-than-normal mental or emotional stability.

Certain additional observations about these patients cast further doubt on the prime importance of the purely mechanical changes brought about by operation.

1. Patients with dumping often develop these symptoms after several symptom-free years.
2. The symptoms are not always constant and patients may have weeks or even months of freedom.
3. Dumping is rarely seen in a patient who is otherwise fit and mentally stable.

These observations support Stammers' view that a purely mechanistic theory of aetiology cannot be the whole explanation. This may well be the reason why a purely mechanistic approach is unlikely to succeed.

I have seen a patient with severe fainting, palpitation, and sweating after meals, who was converted from a Billroth II to a Billroth I with a narrow stoma; he dramatically improved for 3 months and was then as bad as before. He was recognised as being emotionally unstable and in retrospect it was realised that he should not have had his second operation.

Special investigations in these patients are of little practical value in determining the type of treatment and should be employed only if their purpose is to advance knowledge. There is no practical value in determining whether during an attack a patient has hyperglycaemia or hypoglycaemia, or what type of glucose tolerance curve he has, or yet whether the barium meal empties rapidly from the stomach. Exactly comparable results to these tests would be obtained from many asymptomatic postgastrectomy patients.

Treatment

Treatment is empirical on a progressive scale (the first treatment for the least severe and earliest cases).

REASSURANCE

Most patients who, soon after operation, experience faintness after meals require nothing more than an explanation and reassurance. They may be reassured that their symptoms are likely to lessen and will probably disappear in the coming months.

CORRECTION OF DEFICIENCIES

It is essential in the management of any postgastrectomy problem to consider the possible role of mineral and vitamin deficiencies. Iron deficiency is the most common abnormality found after gastrectomy and may predispose to dumping symptoms. It is important to realise that iron deficiency may occur even without any obvious anaemia; a patient with a haemoglobin level of 13.0 g per 100 ml may be iron-deficient and with iron therapy may feel fitter and raise his haemoglobin level to 15.0 g per 100 ml. If the patient feels better, he is less likely to experience or be disturbed by dumping. Vitamin B_{12} and folic acid deficiencies should also be sought and corrected.

DIET

In addition to reassurance and iron therapy, simple dietary measures may be advised. These are sufficient to control most mild symptoms. Rather than eating, as many do, one protein-rich meal each day, the patient should be advised to take three such small meals, and, unless obesity is a problem, to take a small snack between each meal.

Large carbohydrate meals should be avoided and the caloric intake should be made up with fats and proteins. Restriction of fluid intake at mealtimes also helps to delay gastric remnant emptying and relieves symptoms.

The advice to lie down or rest after a meal may be useful in the immediate postoperative period, but it is impracticable once the patient returns to work.

DRUG THERAPY

The appreciation of the aetiological role of impaired intestinal handling of glucose, and the observation by LeQuesne and his colleagues (1960) that, in patients with dumping, insulin given before meals prevents symptoms, has led to a most significant new therapeutic approach with oral hypoglycaemic drugs. Tolbutamide 500 mg before each main meal, will often control symptoms and should be a first line of treatment in the patient with severe symptoms. Some success has been claimed with antiserotonin drugs, and Sullivan (1966) advocated 4 mg of Cyproheptadine before meals in addition to or instead of tolbutamide. My own experience with prescribing antiserotonin drugs for dumping has been limited to a few patients with rather atypical symptoms and one with a classic clinical picture, and in none was there any benefit.

OPERATIVE TREATMENT

The principles behind attempted surgical treatment of patients with dumping have already been described, earlier in this chapter. In the last edition of this book, I wrote that I thought that there was rarely, if ever, any need to operate on patients for dumping and that I had not seen a patient who could not be adequately controlled by nonoperative means. I now have to retract this view; although the vast majority of patients with dumping do not need reoperation, a few intractable sufferers have been treated successfully by jejunal interposition.

DIARRHOEA

In this section I will discuss only the rationale of the investigation and the treatment of diarrhoea that is found after gastrectomy and after vagotomy and "drainage" operations.

Features

It is interesting to note the observation that diarrhoea is more common after vagotomy and drainage than after gastrectomy. In the controlled clinical trial of Goligher, Pulvertaft, and Watkinson (1964), the incidence of diarrhoea after subtotal gastrectomy Billroth II was 10.7 percent, while after vagotomy and gastroenterostomy it was 27 percent, and after vagotomy and antrectomy with gastrojejunal anastomosis it was 20 percent.

The particular feature of postvagotomy diarrhoea is the susceptibility to episodes of diarrhoea at intervals of a week to a few months. The episodes last a few days and are characterized by the passage of frequent watery stools, often with a sense of urgency (Cox et al., 1964). Despite the fact that this problem of episodic diarrhoea is apparently not as common after gastrectomy as after vagotomy and gastrojejunostomy, Cox and his colleagues suggested that the gastrojejunal anastomosis was the major contributing factor. In our own series of patients with vagotomy and pyloroplasty, we found that 11 percent of patients complained of attacks of diarrhoea and 3 percent considered these attacks a drawback to the operation (Barnes and Williams, 1967). An earlier study of patients after partial gastrectomy (Jones et al., 1963) has shown that, more than 5 years after operation, only 6 percent of patients complained of diarrhoea and in none was this severe; none had the characteristic episodes of diarrhoea experienced after vagotomy. Our own experience, therefore, suggests that it is the vagotomy per se that is largely responsible for the diarrhoea, although the mechanism of its causation is not clear.

The foregoing remarks about management are formulated from experience with postgastrectomy patients but in practice they appear equally applicable to postvagotomy diarrhoea.

Some of the important causes of increased frequency and fluid consistency of stool after gastric operations are:

1. Increased small-bowel transit time, resulting from the loss of the gastric emptying regulation once the antrum and pylorus are removed.

2. The osmotic cathartic effect of large quantities of hypertonic foodstuffs arriving in the jejunum and attracting fluid into the lumen.

3. The production of large-bowel irritant within the gut. Probably an important factor in this mechanism is the breakdown of bile salts by bacteria. There may be some correlation between the number of organisms in a sample of jejunal aspirate and the degree of steatorrhoea (Tabaqchali and Booth, 1966). In addition to depriving the digestive tract of an effective emulsifying agent, the breakdown of bile salts liberates colonic irritants which cause diarrhoea. The impaired enzymatic digestion of foods provides more fuel for fermentation and bacterial breakdown in the gut.

As these three factors are present to some extent in all patients after gastrectomy, it is not surprising that mild upsets of bowel habit are common and the steatorrhoea is almost universal. *It is important to understand that there is no direct connection between steatorrhoea and diarrhoea; patients with gross steatorrhoea may have no diarrhoea.* Almost all patients after gastrectomy excrete a higher proportion of ingested fat in their faeces than do normal persons.

Treatment

When presented with the problem of a patient who complains of continued or episodic diarrhoea, the practical policy of management is first to treat all with simple empirical methods and to reserve sophisticated investigations for those with severe and unremitting symptoms. We have encountered 1 postgastrectomy patient with *gluten enteropathy* whose presenting symptom was diarrhoea, but this is not sufficient to advocate peroral jejunal biopsy in the evaluation of all patients with diarrhoea after gastrectomy.

The empirical regimen for the treatment of postgastrectomy diarrhoea is as follows.

Diet. The oldest gimmick known to gastroenterologists is to enquire if any particular food causes diarrhoea and advise its avoidance. Milk and milk products are the most common provoking agents. The avoidance of all milk products for a trial of 2 weeks and then observation of the provocative effect of a glass of raw milk should indicate those patients who are sensitive to milk.

Absorbents. The safest medicaments are the methylcellulose group of water-absorbing compounds. If they produce symtomatic control they can be used indefinitely.

Sedatives. Sedatives of the codeine or diphenoxalate type can be used and many patients are so controlled permanently. Because of the dangers of habituation they should be used with caution.

Antibiotics. A short course of broad-spectrum antibiotics will often control an attack of diarrhoea. The agents effective against the gram-negative organisms are the most useful, presumably because they abolish or alter the flora of the upper gastrointestinal tract, and in particular control those organisms that cause breakdown of bile salts.

Neomycin, not normally significantly absorbed from the alimentary tract, is the safest for prolonged administration, although even this drug may cause mucosal damage. Combinations of tetracycline and nystatin may also be used. Prolonged therapy rarely produces prolonged relief, but intermittent antibiotic therapy may help to control symptoms. (See Chap. 107.)

Pancreatic extracts. The results of treatment with pancreatin, bile salts, or both in patients with postoperative diarrhoea have been disappointing (Culver, 1962), although French and Crane (1963) reported the case of one patient in whom nutrition was improved. I have tried the effect of large doses of pancreatic and commercial pancreatic preparations in patients with severe diarrhoea after both gastrectomy and vagotomy. I have never succeeded in producing significant, lasting symptomatic improvement.

The investigation and treatment of severe or intractable diarrhoea are best accomplished in a specialised gastroenterological unit.

Some of the most important diagnoses to be considered are:

1. Gastrojejunocolic fistulas due to recurrent ulceration (see Chap. 24). This is investigated by barium enema and barium-meal examination as well as acid secretion studies to evaluate the cause of the ulceration.

2. Pancreatic insufficiency. This is investigated by pancreatic function studies with duodenal intubation and hormonal stimulation of the pancreas.

3. Gluten enteropathy as demonstrated by peroral jejunal biopsy.

4. Intestinal blind-loop syndrome studied by intestinal aspiration and culture and vitamin B_{12} absorption tests.

ABSORPTION OF CALCIUM AND VITAMIN D

A brief summary of the normal absorption of calcium and vitamin D will be given before consideration of the possible effects of gastric operations and the resultant changes in bone metabolism and structure.

Calcium

A normal adult diet in most parts of the Western world contains about 1,200 mg of calcium of which only about 200 mg are absorbed. An active transport mechanism for calcium exists in the small bowel. Absorption is greatest in the most proximal segments of the small intestine and decreases progressively in the more distal segments (Schachter, Dowdle, and Schenker, 1960). There appears to be facultative control of calcium absorption to meet individual needs, absorption increasing with growth and pregnancy as well as during periods of calcium depletion, while decreasing with age and a reduced calcium demand (Malm, Nicolaysen, and Skjelkvale, 1955). Schachter and Rosen (1959) suggested that the parathyroid hormone may play a part in regulating calcium absorption, but Fourman (1960) thought that there was little evidence of any endocrine control.

Vitamin D is essential for the normal absorption of calcium, but in healthy adults on an already normal diet, the daily administration of 2,000 I.U. of vitamin D does not increase the calcium absorption significantly (Jeans and Stearns, 1938; McCance and Widdowson, 1944).

The absorption of calcium may be en-

hanced by: acidity of the intestinal tract (Stewart and Percival, 1928; Kay, 1932; Schmidt and Greenberg, 1935; Bills, 1935); the presence of bile salts (Webling and Holdsworth, 1966); calcium depletion (Stearns and Moore, 1931); a high-protein diet (McCance, Widdowson, and Lehmann, 1942); or extra calcium needs, such as growth, pregnancy, and lactation (Liu and colleagues, 1941).

Although the evidence for this is not conclusive, the absorption of calcium is said to be *impaired* by the presence in the gut of substances which form insoluble calcium salts. These are:

1. *Dietary phytic acid.* Phytic acid occurs in the outer coats of the grains of many cereals, particularly wheat. It was for this reason that the wartime British 'National Loaf' had additional calcium added (McCance, 1946).
2. *Fatty acids* which form insoluble calcium soaps. However, a high-fat diet does not, in itself, interfere with calcium absorption (Aub, Tibbets, and McLean, 1937).
3. *Excess of dietary phosphorus.* This hypothesis, suggested by animal experiments, has not been supported by observations in man (Malm, 1958; Irving, 1957).

The effects of gastric operations on calcium absorption are:

1. Hypochlorhydria or achlorhydria achieved by the operation will reduce the degree of ionisation of calcium. Although absorption is favoured by gastric acidification, which renders dietary calcium more soluble, there is little evidence to show that, even in patients with an intact stomach, there is any correlation between calcium deficiency and the presence of achlorhydria or hypochlorhydria.
2. Duodenal bypass. The duodenum and upper jejunum appear to be the sites of optimal calcium absorption (Nicolaysen and Ragard, 1955; Schachter and Rosen, 1959). The Billroth II type of operation and gastroenterostomy both bypass this area and so might be expected to decrease calcium absorption. Hillemand and his colleagues (1960) believe that duodenal bypass is of prime importance as a cause of calcium deficiency and bone disease after gastrectomy, and claim to have cured a patient with osteomalacia by converting his Billroth II to a Billroth I anastomosis. Their case is not proven, however, as they started vitamin D therapy some weeks before conversion and continued it afterward. Recovery could have been due to a delayed response to vitamin D. I have previously reported the effect of conversion to Billroth I anastomosis in 2 patients with osteomalacia after gastrectomy (Williams, 1966). In one, conversion resulted in the calcium balance being altered from negative to positive, while in the other there was an apparent paradox as the symptoms and biochemical signs of osteomalacia did not develop until a year after the conversion.
3. The breakdown of bile salts to free cholic and desoxycholic acid by organisms found within the afferent loop and upper jejunum may impair the normal mechanism of calcium absorption.
4. Steatorrhoea. The impaired digestion and absorption of fats leads to an increased quantity of fatty acids in the small-bowel lumen. These may combine with calcium salts and form insoluble soaps. Most patients with osteomalacia after gastrectomy have steatorrhoea; however, most patients after gastrectomy have steatorrhoea and few of these develop osteomalacia. Furthermore, at least 7 of our patients with gross osteomalacia after gastrectomy had a normal faecal fat output.

Vitamin D

Little is known of the precise method of absorption of vitamin D. As a fat-soluble vitamin, its absorption might be expected to be similar either to that of triglycerides, which are absorbed in the jejunum after breakdown to fatty acids, or to cholesterol and related substances, which are probably absorbed predominantly in the ileum. Vitamin D malabsorption might be expected after partial gastrectomy, as a result of fat malabsorption, duodenal bypass, or both. It is of interest to note that of all the patients with postgastrectomy osteomalacia reported in the literature, 95 percent have had either a gastrectomy with gastrojejunal anastomosis or a gastroenterostomy. Thirty of our 32 postgastrectomy osteomalacia patients (see Table 16) had a duodenal bypass operation although during this same period in Birmingham about 20 percent of all gastrectomies were of the Billroth I (gastroduodenostomy type).

Vitamin D absorption tests have been performed in patients with osteomalacia after gastrectomy. Thompson, Lewis, and Booth (1966) have shown that the absorption of a single dose of 40,000 units is the same in these patients as in normal patients. Even if the absorption of free vitamin D is unaffected by operation, the absorption of vitamin D from food may well be impaired.

POSTGASTRECTOMY BONE DISEASE

Before 1962, bone disease complicating partial gastrectomy was considered to be a rare disease, sufficiently uncommon to warrant single case reports in the literature. There were at that time only 16 such cases reported in English, and all were then labelled "postgastrectomy osteomalacia." Table 13 shows the location of 14 of them in the literature.

A wider search of the literature, however, revealed that from Latin America and

Table 13. "POSTGASTRECTOMY OSTEOMALACIA" (AS REPORTED IN ENGLISH LANGUAGE)

Country	Author	Year	Cases
Great Britain	Nordin and Frazer	1956	1
Great Britain	Pyrah and Smith	1956	1
Great Britain	Baird and Oleesky	1957	5
Great Britain	Ellman and Irwin	1959	1
United States of America	Mellick and Benson	1959	2
Denmark	Harvald, Krogsgaard, and Lous	1962	3
Great Britain	Klipstein	1962	1

Table 14. FURTHER REPORTS OF BONE DISEASE COMPLICATING PARTIAL GASTRECTOMY

Country	Author	Year	Cases
Argentina	Udaondo and Castex	1947	41
France	Hillemand, Mialaret, and Boutelier	1960	39
France	Louyot, Mathieu, and Gaucher	1961	37
France	Lightwitz et al.	1961	42

France there were reports of large series (Table 14). In these reports the exact nature of the bone disease was not always defined; many of them appeared to be "malacic," but most were referred to as being of the "rarefying bone disease" type.

At about this time, three independent surveys of postgastrectomy patients were being conducted in Aberdeen, Scotland; Adelaide, Australia; and Birmingham, England (see Table 15). The results of these surveys were interpreted by the authors as indicating that 5 or more years after partial gastrectomy some abnormality of bone or of calcium metabolism could be detected in about 20 percent of cases.

In these three reports, the abnormality of bone was described as being a combination of osteomalacia and osteoporosis. It was further suggested by these authors that as time went by after operation, the abnormalities of bone became more severe. These reports created a certain amount of alarm, for it appeared likely that we were shortly to experience an "epidemic" of osteomalacia following 10 or more years in the wake of the postwar gastrectomy "bulge."

Although many of us interested in this problem are continuing to see new cases of gross bone disease following partial gastrectomy, there is still no sign of a rapid increase in numbers. Furthermore, in 1965 a report was made from York and Leeds, England, of the largest and most comprehensive long-term follow-up of partial gastrectomy patients so far conducted with the specific intention of detecting bone disease. This led the authors to conclude that postgastrectomy osteomalacia is a rare disease occurring in less than 1 percent of all patients, even many years after gastrectomy (Morgan et al., 1966).

Table 15.   RESULTS OF SURVEYS OF POSTGASTRECTOMY PATIENTS

Authors	City	Country	No. of Patients	Years Since Operation	Radiological Abnormality (percent)	Biochemical and Histological Abnormality (percent)
Clark, Crookes, Dawson, and Mitchell (1964)	Aberdeen	Scotland	53	7 to 16	14	28
Deller, Begley, Edwards, and Addison (1964)	Adelaide	Australia	76	6 to 15	53	25+
Jones, Williams, and Nicholson (1963)	Birmingham	England	52 / 32	5 to 6 / 10 to 12	Not studied	19.2 / 37.9

It would appear therefore that unequivocal osteomalacia is uncommon but that some bone abnormality is detectable in 20 to 30 percent of patients. What then is the nature of this bone abnormality?

Pathology

The first difficulty in understanding this problem is that our concept of the metabolic bone disease involves subdivision into two distinct pathological entities, osteomalacia and osteoporosis.

In normal bone, a little under half consists of mineral salts, chiefly calcium; about half the thickness of the shafts of long bone is made up of cortical bone and on biopsy the bony trabeculae of the medullary bone are substantial with only thin (less than 12μ) seams of uncalcified osteoid tissues.

In osteomalacia, the amount of bony tissue is not reduced, but the proportion of mineral salts is less. The cortices of the long bones are as thick as in the normal (although radiological definition of the trabeculae pattern may be reduced, giving a ground glass appearance on x-ray films). The trabeculae are not reduced in thickness but are lined with a thick layer of uncalcified osteoid tissue. Abnormalities of serum calcium, phosphorus, and alkaline levels are common, and there may be a low urinary excretion of calcium.

In osteoporosis, there is a reduction in the amount of bone with no change in the proportion of mineral salt to protein matrix. The cortices of the long bone are thin as are the bony trabeculae on bone biopsy. The

osteoid seams are absent or no greater than in the normal. There is usually no detectable abnormality of serum or urine biochemistry.

Osteomalacia

In Birmingham during the past years we have seen 28 cases of undoubted osteomalacia following gastrectomy (Table 16). From this experience, we can draw some conclusions about diagnosis.

Clinical features. Nine of the 28 patients were entirely asymptomatic; they had no abnormal physical or radiological signs. Seventeen complained of bone pain and 9 had bone tenderness. Five had pseudofractures, and pathological fractures occurred in 8.

It is of interest to note the common association between peripheral neuropathy and osteomalacia. Ten of our patients were investigated for neurological symptoms and found to have a neuropathy which did not respond at all or responded incompletely to vitamin B_{12}. In 6 patients idiopathic epilepsy occurred after the gastrectomy and in these no focal cause has yet been found.

Biochemical abnormalities. Serum calcium levels below 9.2 mg per 100 ml were found in 21 patients. Serum phosphorus levels below 3.5 mg per 100 ml were found in 22, and the calcium phosphorus product was below 25 in 120. A serum alkaline phosphatase level above 13 King-Armstrong units was present in 20 of 28 patients. The urine calcium was often below 60 mg per 24 hours; however, it was over 100 mg per 24 hours

Table 16.   FINDINGS IN

Factors	1	2	3	4	5	6	7	8	9	10	11	12	13
Sex	F	F	M	M	F	M	F	F	F	M	M	F	F
Age (yr.)	35	51	66	64	69	52	77	54	56	53	59	40	48
Ulcer	D	G	D	G	D	D	D	G	D	G	D	D	D
Operation	BII	BII	BII	BII	BII	BII	GE	BII	BII	BII	BII	BII	BII
Time interval (yr.)	5	10	12	11	12	11	30	7	18	5	9	2	8
Symptoms and signs													
Bone pains	+	−	−	+	−	+	−	+	−	+	+	+	+
Tenderness	−	−	−	+	−	+	+	+	−	+	−	+	+
Looser's zone	−	−	−	−	−	−	+	−	−	−	−	−	+
Fractures	−	−	−	+	+	+	−	−	−	+	−	+	+
Serum levels													
Calcium	9.7	10.1	10.1	8.7	8.3	8.6	8.4	9.1	8.8	8.0	7.8	8.8	7.8
Phosphorus	3.6	3.1	4.0	3.2	2.2	2.7	2.3	2.4	2.9	1.5	3.4	3.1	1.7
Ca X P	35	31	40	28	18	23	19	22	25.5	12	24	27	15
Alk. p'tse	2	20	17	11	9	37	22	31	22	25	17	13	20
Urinary													
Calcium	60	85	52	−	20	42	30	198	42	50	60	23	24
Steatorrhoea	+	−	−	−	+	+	+	+	NK	+	+	+	−
Osteoid seams (in μ)	40	25	30	NK	30	100	NK	30	NK	OM	OM (Gross)	OM	OM
Response to Vitamin D	NK	NK	Poor	Good	Good	Good	Good	Poor	Good	Poor	Poor	Good	Good
Associated deficiencies													
Iron	+	−	−	+	+	−	+	+	+	−	+	+	+
Vitamin B_{12}	−	−	−	+	−	+	+	+	+	−	+	+	+
Associated abnormalities													
Neuropathy	−	−	+	−	−	+	+	+	+	+	+	+	+
Epilepsy	−	−	−	−	−	−	−	+	+	−	−	−	+
Associated diseases	−	−	−	−	−	−	Panc.	−	−	−	Panc.	−	−
Diet	N	N	N	N	Poor	N	Poor	Poor	N	Poor	Good	Poor	Poor

NK indicates not known; plus sign, present; minus sign, absent; N, normal; Panc., ch. pancreatitis; and A.C.D., adult coeliac disease.

Source: Adapted from Postgraduate Gastroenterology, *Ballière, Tindall & Cassell, London, 1866, p. 292.*

28 CASES OF OSTEOMALACIA

14	15	16	17	18	19	20	21	22	23	24	25	26	27	28
F	F	F	M	M	F	F	F	F	M	F	M	M	M	M
43	38	55	48	61	42	55	59	62	49	60	69	55	64	47
None	D	D	D	D	D	None	G	D	G	D	D	D	D	D
BII	BII	BII	BII	BII	BII	BII	BI	BII	BI	BII	BII	BII	BII	BII
8	11	15	12	16	10	6	5	8	11	13	10	16	12	9
+	+	++	+	−	−	+	+	−	−	+	−	+	−	+
−	−	++	−	−	−	−	−	−	−	−	−	−	−	+
−	−	+	−	−	−	−	−	−	−	+	−	−	−	+
−	−	−	−	−	−	−	−	−	−	+	−	−	−	+
8.7	8.8	9.0	9.4	9.1	8.7	8.9	8.9	8.5	8.9	7.8	9.6	10.1	10.5	6.3
4.5	1.8	2.5	2.8	3.3	3.0	2.0	3.6	3.7	2.9	2.4	3.8	3.2	2.6	1.8
39	15.8	22.5	26.3	30	26.1	17.8	32	31	26	19	35	32	27	11.3
6	28	41	13	13	46	53	23	18	11	29	27	15	19	34
102	44	1	NK	NK	65	14	42	44	26	NK	111	44	109	45
+	+	+	NK	NK	+	+	−	NK	−	−	NK	NK	NK	+
25	50	100	45	30	50	60	50	40	25	40	25	25	35	55
Good	Good	Good	Poor	NK	Poor	Good	Poor	Good	NK	NK	Poor	Poor	NK	NK
+	+	+	+	+	+	+	+	+	−	−	+	−	−	−
+	−	+	−	−	+	−	−	−	−	−	−	−	−	−
−	−	−	−	−	−	−	+	−	−	−	−	−	−	−
+	−	−	−	−	−	−	−	−	−	−	+	+	−	−
−	−	−	−	−	−	ACD	−	−	−	−	−	−	−	Alcoholic
Poor	Poor	Poor	N	N	V.Poor	N	Poor	Poor	V.Poor	N	Poor	N	N	Poor

in 4 patients with definite osteomalacia.

The histological findings are usually considered to be the absolute criteria in the diagnosis of osteomalacia. In the recent report by Morgan and his colleagues (1965), the diagnosis of osteomalacia was not entertained unless there was histological evidence of increased thickness and increased lamination of uncalcified osteoid tissue lining the bony trabeculae. In 21 of our patients, the osteoid seams were 25μ or greater in thickness. In 4, the biopsy sections were no longer available for review but all had been reported as having gross osteomalacia with wide osteoid seams.

Vitamin D therapy. The rapid and satisfactory response to vitamin D therapy has been taken as the final means of diagnosing osteomalacia. In the York series, all 8 osteomalacia patients responded promptly to intramuscular injections of vitamin D (Morgan et al., 1965). The rapid response to injection therapy has also been reported by Thompson, Neale, Watts, and Booth (1966). Our experience with oral vitamin D has been that many months of intensive calcium and vitamin D therapy are often required before improvement can be detected. This delayed response is designated as "poor" on Table 16 and was observed in 8 patients.

In my opinion, there is no single test that will permit or refute the diagnosis of osteomalacia, but the finding of histological abnormalities of osteoid seams on bone biopsy is the only constant criterion.

OSTEOPOROSIS

As there is no serum or urinary biochemical abnormality detectable in osteoporosis, the diagnosis must be made radiologically or on bone biopsy. Since osteoporosis is common with increasing age and after the menopause, it is obvious that any estimation of the incidence after gastrectomy must be compared with that in an age- and sex-matched control group.

The incidence of radiological osteoporosis in the reports from Aberdeen and Adelaide had been estimated at about 20 percent, using as an index the metacarpal or the femoral score (see Table 15). The bone score is calculated from measurement of the midshaft of the bone and expressed as the percentage of the total thickness of the bone that is occupied by the dense cortical bone. The results of the radiological survey of metacarpal cortex in the York series of patients showed that the cortical thickness was significantly less in postgastrectomy patients over the age of 60 than in controls of the same age (Morgan, Pulvertaft, and Fourman, 1966).

In our clinic, we find that the femoral score is the most useful index of bone abnormality after gastrectomy. In our control series of femoral scores, we find no significant difference between males and females and very little decline with increasing age. In contrast the postgastrectomy patients have lower femoral scores, apparently decreasing with age or time since operation.

In conclusion, there appears to be a high incidence of bone rarefaction and abnormalities of serum calcium and alkaline phosphatase levels in patients many years after gastrectomy. Although frank osteomalacia is relatively uncommon, a "malacic" type of bone disease may be present in about 20 percent of cases. It seems likely that such a subclinical stage of the disease may continue for years without deterioration.

Other Gastric Operations

Metabolic bone disease might be expected to occur after any gastric operation, but as duodenal bypass seems to be one of the important associated factors, gastroenterostomy with or without pyloroplasty would seem to be a more likely cause than vagotomy and pyloroplasty. Morgan and his colleagues (1965) report that a raised alkaline phosphatase level is almost as common after vagotomy and gastroenterostomy (8.4 percent) as it is after partial gastrectomy (12.3 percent). In my own series of vagotomy and pyloroplasty and vagotomy and antrectomy with gastroduodenal anastomoses, I have so far found no evidence of bone abnormality or elevated alkaline phosphatase levels, though only 120 patients have been followed for more than 5 years.

Radiological bone rarefaction was not found after vagotomy and drainage procedures by Morgan, Pulvertaft, and Fourman (1966), in contradistinction to their experience with elderly patients after gastrectomy.

Treatment

There is no great difficulty in formulating a policy for the treatment of the rare patient with gross osteomalacia. Oral doses of vitamin D of 50,000 units once or twice a day may be given while the patient's response is carefully checked to avoid vitamin D overdose. In all cases of postgastrectomy osteomalacia, there is probably an associated calcium deficiency, and it is advisable to give supplementary calcium therapy of up to 1 g of calcium per day.

In patients with gross osteoporosis after gastrectomy in whom there is no evidence of vitamin D deficiency, there are dangers in giving large doses of vitamin D. I have as yet to be convinced that therapy makes any difference to these patients, but in the hope that Nordin's hypothesis (1961) may prove correct I am prescribing 1 g of calcium (in the form of effervescent tablets) plus 5 mg of an anabolic steroid.

The most difficult problem is that of deciding whether to treat the much larger group of patients with no symptoms but with some biochemical or radiological deviation from normal. And if to treat them—with what? At the moment I am inclined to compromise between conscience and scientific purity and prescribe two tablets daily which contain 225 mg ferrous glycerine sulphate, 15 mg vitamin C, 200 vitamin D, and 100 mg calcium gluconate. With larger doses of vitamin D, however, the dangers of overdose are greater than those run by the untreated patient.

If some abnormality of bone metabolism is so common, universal simple prophylaxis would seem the most logical approach to the problem.

CONCLUSIONS

Serious disabling bone disease is seen after partial gastrectomy, particularly after a gastrojejunal anastomosis. Gross osteomalacia is uncommon but by the time it is detected there may be unnecessary suffering and irreparable damage. Some degree of demineralisation and biochemical abnormalities are very common but are not usually associated with any symptoms. The search for the means of detecting those patients at particular risk has not produced any one reliable simple screening test; however, the best available are the radiological detection of a low peripheral bone score or thin metacarpal cortices as an indication of osteoporosis and a raised alkaline phosphatase level as an indication of osteomalacia.

The causes of bone abnormality after gastrectomy are many, deficiencies of vitamin D and calcium playing the most important role. There is probably a combination of diminished oral intake and impaired absorption.

Prophylactic therapy with small daily supplements of calcium and vitamin D to all patients after gastrectomy may reduce the incidence and severity of bone disease, but this hypothesis lacks proof.

REFERENCES

Aub, J. C., Tibbetts, D. M., and McLean, R., J. Nutr. 13:163, 1937.
Baird, I. M., and Oleesky, S., Gastroenterology 33:284, 1957.
Barnes, A. D., and Williams, J. A., Br. J. Surg. 54:218, 1967.
Bills, C. E., Physiol. Rev. 15:1, 1935.
Brain, R. F. H., and Stammers, F. A. R., Lancet 1:1137, 1951.
Brooks, V. S., Waterhouse, J. A. H., and Thorn, P. A., Gut 1:149, 1960.
Bruusgaard, C., Acta Chir. Scand. (Suppl. 117), 1946.
Butler, T. J., Ann. R. Coll. Surg. 29:300, 1961.
Clark, C. G., Crookes, J., Dawson, A. A., and Mitchell, P. E. G., Lancet 1:734, 1964.
Cooke, W. T., Johnson, J., and Woold, W. T., Brain 89:663, 1966.
Cooke, W. T., and Smith, W. T., Brain 89:683, 1966.
Cox, A. G., Bond, M. R., Podmore, D. A., and Rose, D. P., Br. Med. J. 1:465, 1964.
Culver, P. J., Ann. N.Y. Acad. Sci. 99:213, 1962.
Deller, D. J., Begley, M. D., Edwards, R. G., and Addison, M., Gut 5:218, 1964.
Donaldson, R. M., Jr., J. Clin. Invest. 44:1815, 1954.
Ellman, P., and Irwin, D. B., Postgrad. Med. 35:358, 1959.
Everson, T. C., Int. Abstr. Surg. 95:209, 1952.
Fourman, P., Calcium Metabolism and Bone. Oxford, Blackwell, 1960.
French, J. M., and Crane, C. W., in Stammers and Williams, eds., Partial Gastrectomy, Complications and Metabolic Consequences, London, Butterworths, 1963, p. 227.
Goligher, J. C., Pulvertaft, C. N., and Watkinson, G., Br. Med. J. 1:455, 1964.
Harkins, H. N., and Nyhus, L. M., Bull. Soc. Internat. Chir. 15:111, 1956.

Harvald, B., Krogsgaard, A. R., and Louis, P., Acta Med. Scand. 172:497, 1962.

Higgins, P. McR., and Pridie, R. B., Br. J. Surg. 53:881, 1966.

Hillemand, P., Mialaret, J., and Boutelier, D., Arch. Mal. Appar. Dig. 49:489, 1960.

Irving, J. T., Calcium Metabolism. London, Methuen, 1957.

Jeans, P. C., and Stearns, G. J., J.A.M.A. 111:703, 1938.

Jones, C. T., Williams, J. A., and Nicholson, G. I., in Stammers and Williams, eds., Partial Gastrectomy, Complications and Metabolic Consequences. London, Butterworths, 1963, p. 160.

Kay, H. D., Physiol. Rev. 12:384, 1932.

Klipstein, F. A., Ann. Intern. Med. 57:133, 1962.

Knox, J. D. E., and Delamore, I. E., Br. Med. J. 2:1494, 1960.

Lagerlöf, H., Acta Med. Scand. (Suppl. 128), 1942.

LeQuesne, L. P., Hobsley, M., and Hand, B. H., Br. Med. J. 1:141, 1960.

Lightwitz, A., de Seze, S., Cachin, M., Guillaumat, M., Hioco, D., and Pergola, F., Sem. Hôp. Par. 69:3391, 1961.

Liu, S. H., Chu, H. I., Hau, H. C., Chao, H. C., and Cheu, S. H., J. Clin. Invest. 20:255, 1941.

Louyot, P., Mathieu, J., and Gaucher, A., Arch. Mal. Appar. Dig. 50:20, 1961.

Lundh, G., Acta Chir. Scand. (Suppl. 231), 1958.

Malm, O. J., J. Clin. Lab. Invest. 10 (Suppl. 36), 1958.

Malm, O. J., Nicolaysen, R., and Skjelkvale, L., CIBA Foundation Colloquium on Ageing (Vol. 1). London, Churchill, 1955, p. 109.

McCance, R. A., Widdowson, E. M., and Lehmann, H., Biochem. J. 36:686, 1942.

McCance, R. A., and Widdowson, E. M., Nature (Lond.) 153:650, 1944.

Mellick, R. A., and Benson, J. A., Jr., New Engl. J. Med. 260:976, 1959.

Morgan, D. B., Paterson, C. R., Woods, C. H., Pulvertaft, C. N., and Fourman, P., Lancet 2:1085, 1965.

Morgan, D. B., Pulvertaft, C. N., and Fourman, P., Lancet 2:772, 1966.

Nicolaysen, R., and Ragard, R., J. Clin. Lab. Invest. 7:298, 1955.

Nordin, B. E. C., Lancet 1:1011, 1961.

Nordin, B. E. C., and Frazer, R., Lancet 1:823, 1956.

Olivarius, B. de F., and Rous, D., Lancet 2:1298, 1965.

Pyrah, L. N., and Smith, I. B., Lancet 1:935, 1956.

Schachter, D., Dowdle, E. B., and Schenker, H., Am. J. Physiol. 198:275, 1960.

Schachter, D., and Rosen, S. M., Am. J. Physiol. 196:357, 1959.

Schlaeger, R., N.Y. State J. Med. 60:1780, 1960.

Schmidt, G. L. A., and Greenberg, D. M., Physiol. Rev. 15:297, 1935.

Stearns, G., and Moore, D. I. R., Am. J. Dis. Child. 42:774, 1931.

Stewart, C. P., and Percival, G. H., *Physiol. Rev.* 8:283, 1928.

Tabaqchali, S., and Booth, C. C., Lancet 2:12, 1966.

Taylor, H., Br. Med. J. 1:1133, 1959.

Thompson, G. R., Lewis, J. M., and Booth, C. C., Lancet 1:623, 1966.

Thompson, G. R., Neale, G., Watts, J. M., and Booth, C. C., Lancet 1:623, 1966.

Udaondo, C. B., and Castex, M. R., Presse Med. 73:874, 1947.

Wallensten, S., Acta Chir. Scand. (Suppl. 191), 1954.

Webling, D. D. A., and Holdsworth, E. S., Biochem. J. 100:652, 1966.

Williams, J. A., in Thompson and Gillespie, eds., Postgraduate Gastroenterology. London, Ballière, Tindall & Cassell, 1966.

Woolf, A. L., Personal communications, 1967.

28

A. AETIOLOGY, PATHOLOGY, AND DIAGNOSIS OF CARCINOMA OF THE STOMACH; PALLIATIVE OPERATIONS, INCLUDING VARIOUS TYPES OF GASTROSTOMY; RADICAL SUBTOTAL GASTRECTOMY FOR GASTRIC CARCINOMA

RODNEY MAINGOT

HISTORICAL NOTE

Avicenna (A.D. 98–1037), the famous Arab physician, gave the first account of cancer of the stomach. Avenzor (A.D. 1070–1162) described the necropsy appearances of a case of carcinoma of the stomach—*verruca ventriculi*. The first detailed memoir on malignant lesions of the stomach was written by Morgagni in 1761. Morgagni is regarded as the father of modern pathology.

An outstanding early description of the clinical picture of cancer of the stomach was that of G. L. Bayley, whose book, *Tumours of the Stomach,* was published in 1839, and contains references to the researches of Aussant, Chardel, and Laennec.

In 1810, Merrem (cited by Rydygier in 1881) successfully performed excision of the pylorus in dogs, and suggested the possible application of pylorectomy followed by end-to-end gastroduodenostomy in humans suffering from cancer of the distal end of the stomach.

Brinton, of University College Hospital, London, a superb physician, writer, and teacher, discussed the difficulty in differentiating benign from malignant ulcers in his book, *Lectures on the Diseases of the Stomach* (1858). In one of his learned articles he gave a vivid and accurate account of *linitis plastica.*

Péan (1879) performed the first gastric resection for cancer. The patient died 4 days later. Billroth (1881) carried out the first successful pyloric resection in the human for carcinoma of the pylorus. The patient died 4 months later. Connor (1884) attempted the first total gastrectomy for cancer of the stomach. The patient died on the operating table. Roentgen (1893) discovered x-rays. Schlatter (1897) performed the first successful total gastrectomy. The patient lived for 14 months.

Lange and Meltzing (1898) published the first description of an intragastric camera, which they had constructed and used with a measure of success. Dr. G. D. Hadley gives a description of *Gastrophotography* in Chapter 4B.

Cuneo (1906) and Jamieson and Dobson, following many dissections, gave the first detailed descriptions (with numerous illustrations) of the lymphatic drainage of the stomach, which influenced the extent of gastric resections for carcinoma of the organ.

Rieder (1905) and Holzknecht (1906) published a number of articles on the value of gastrointestinal studies by the employment of bismuth subnitrate meals for x-ray examinations. During 1911–12 Holzknecht and Hendrick (Vienna), Försell (Stockholm), Cole (New York), Barclay (England), and Carman (Mayo Clinic, Minnesota) demonstrated the potentials of fluoroscopy and barium-meal x-ray examinations in the diagnosis of cancer of the stomach.

During the early years of this century W. J. and C. H. Mayo and Moynihan were extending the scope of partial gastrectomy for malignant lesions of the stomach. Much credit is due to them for their teachings and example and for demonstrating that the appalling postoperative mortality for gastric resections could be considerably lowered by skill and judgment.

The Wolf-Schindler flexible gastroscope was introduced in 1932. Papanicolaou (1946) introduced the method of diagnosis of malignant growths from exfoliated cells from cancerous lesions. (See Chap. 28E.)

INTRODUCTION

Carcinoma of the stomach can be cured by gastrectomy, and by this method *alone* can the patient's life be saved. All nonsurgical methods of therapy, including deep x-rays and radium, have a mortality of 100 percent. Furthermore, cure is only possible when the disease is diagnosed early and re-section is radical.

As less than 50 percent of cancers of the stomach lend themselves to "curative resec-tion," it is obvious that no improvement is possible in the present situation until these patients are referred to the surgeon at a much earlier period in the illness than they have been hitherto.

The fight against cancer is a fight for earlier diagnosis and thus for earlier radical treatment.

After all, unless the diagnosis is made early, no technical skill will avail the patient with a carcinoma of the stomach. The fact that long-time survivors of gastrectomy for gastric cancer have usually had longer dura-tion of symptoms in no way supports the contention of MacDonald and Cotin: [16] that "the concept that early diagnosis of cancer of the stomach may improve end-results is not only fallacious but is in fact the reverse of the truth."

Blalock and Ochsner,[1] in an excellent paper, rightly state that it is fair to assume that an even higher percentage of survivors would have occurred in the group having symptoms of the longest duration if the dis-ease had been treated before so much time had elapsed. Veidenheimer and Logan [24] state that although 42 percent of their pa-tients at the Lahey Clinic had had symptoms for longer than 6 months, 82 percent of the entire group had had symptoms for less than 1 year. Again:

Contrary to what might be expected, there was no relationship between survival rate and length of delay before surgical treatment. The implica-tion resulting from these findings is that survival is basically dependent upon the type of tumor, its biologic nature, and the host resistance rather than upon the delay before surgery.

Earlier diagnosis offers the only means of treating the disease at a time when the lesion is amenable to complete extirpation and affords a "promise" of long survival.

These statements are supported and ably demonstrated by Friesen et al.[3] when, in a series of 65 cases of *superficial carcinoma of the stomach,* they showed a postoperative 5-year survival rate of 93.3 percent and a 10-year survival rate of 75 percent. In the majority of these cases, the cancer involved the entire thickness of the mucosa at some point; in other cases, although the lesion ap-peared in situ, metastases were found in the adjacent lymph nodes.

Again, it should be noted that involvement of lymph nodes indicates a considerably poorer prognosis than could be expected if no positive lymph nodes are found. Thus, ReMine and Priestley [17] found lymph node involvement in 60 percent of their patients who were subjected to radical gastrectomy. Both the operative mortality and the 5-year survival rate were materially affected by the presence of involved lymph nodes. The 5-year survival for patients with lymph node in-volvement was 15 percent, and, in contrast, it was 57 percent for those who did not have lymph node involvement. (See Prognosis in B and C, below.)

To the lay person a diagnosis of cancer of the stomach signifies impending death. There is also a widespread belief amongst doctors that carcinoma of the stomach is a hopeless condition and that only in excep-tional instances is it amenable to surgical cure. This attitude of hopelessness is a great deterrent to progress. I agree with Harold Edwards, who says that the thought engen-ders a sense of futility which blunts en-deavour and offers a ready excuse for failure. Cancer of the stomach is a curable disease. Great improvements have been made during the last decade, in both our methods of diag-nosis and surgical technique, and with the recent rapid advances in our science and art the future prospects in the management of this dread disease offer hope and encourage-ment.

That genuine progress has been made in the surgery of gastric cancer and that the chal-lenge has been taken up is reflected in the reports from the Mayo Clinic and from the Lahey Clinic. Under the title of *Prognosis,* this important subject is comprehensively dealt with by such leading authorities as William ReMine, and by Cornelius Sedgwick. Their valuable contributions carry the weight of authority and experience.

At operation it is sometimes difficult to decide whether a large, fixed, infiltrating growth is resectable, and, again, it is often difficult to decide which patients should be subjected to total or subtotal gastrectomy. In cases of cancer of the stomach, a challenge to surgical courage should always be accepted. Surely, decision is one of the duties of strength.

Aetiological Factors

INCIDENCE

The incidence of deaths from cancer of the stomach for England and Wales is given in Table 1.

Pack (1965) stated that cancer of the stomach is rapidly decreasing in the United States. A quarter of a century ago 20 to 30 percent of all cancer deaths could be attributed to malignant gastric disease. In 1970, about 5 to 8 percent of cancer deaths in America were due to gastric cancer. The ratio of males to females is 8:5 according to the American Cancer Society. During the last two decades cancers in other locations, notably the lung, colon, rectum, and pancreas, have increased in frequency. The reason for the decrease in frequency of cancer of the stomach in the United States has not been discovered. Surgeons who operate on patients with gastric cancer sometimes give the credit to their surgical efforts, but the percentage of cures is still too small to account for the improvement.

There is a wide variation in the incidence of cancer of the stomach in different races of people throughout the world. For instance, gastric cancer is particularly prevalent in such countries as Japan, Iceland, Chile, and Hawaii. Nakayama stated that about 50 percent of all persons dying of cancer in Japan have cancer of the stomach. According to the vital statistics provided by the Japan Welfare Ministry (1964), gastric cancer caused 54.2 percent of all cancer deaths in males and 39.4 percent of all cancer deaths in females. Pack believed that a possible contributing factor could be the great consumption of smoked fish and smoked meat which obtains in some of these countries, notably Iceland. Perhaps the process of smoking and curing meat and fish adds carcinogens or carcinogenic hydrocarbons to the staple foods. According to Bailey and Dungal, all food so *smoked* contains 3,4-benzpyrine.

Age and sex. Gastric cancer is rare under the age of 30, and according to Hale and Mallo [6] the incidence is 1.04 percent. Stewart and Holman [19] state that in a survey of cancer in London published by the British Empire Cancer Campaign there were 1,405 cases of gastric cancer and of these only 3 were in the age group 15 to 25, and 24 in the age group 25 to 35.

The disease is most frequently seen between the ages of 50 and 70, the peak age incidence being about 59 for both sexes. The *sex* ratio of males to females is 2:1.

Heredity. Many authorities agree that certain families show a predisposition toward the development of carcinoma of the stomach, but that such families are comparatively rare in proportion to the general population. Congenital polyposis of the stomach is a well-recognised condition. Some years ago I performed gastrectomy for malignant polyps of the stomach on brothers, aged 39 and 26, respectively; three *other* brothers had died of cancer of the stomach.

PREDISPOSING FACTORS

Chronic gastritis. Konjetzny [11] believed that cancer never developed in a previously healthy stomach and that atrophic gastritis was the most important predisposing factor. His view was supported by Hurst,[9] who maintained that achlorhydria, which is frequently observed in cases of gastric cancer, was caused by gastritis and not by the presence of the neoplasm. He believed that if a patient with a constitutional predispo-

Table 1.   DEATHS FROM GASTRIC CARCINOMA

Sex	1954		1959		1960		1964		1969	
Males	7,818	14,050	7,951	13,971	7,846	13,953	7,500	13,069	7,300	12,711
Females	6,232		5,966		6,107		5,569		5,411	

Source: Registrar-General's reviews of deaths from cancer of the stomach occurring in England and Wales for the years 1954, 1959, 1960, 1964, and 1969.

sition to cancer also had achlorhydria and gastritis, he would probably develop cancer of the stomach, but that the early diagnosis and treatment of the gastritis would diminish the frequency of gastric carcinoma.

Anacidity, atrophic gastritis and pernicious anaemia are important aetiological factors in gastric cancer. Kaplan and Rigler [10] found 36 cases of cancer of the stomach in 293 autopsy records of cases of pernicious anaemia. It is generally agreed that about 10 percent of patients suffering from pernicious anaemia will eventually develop cancer of the stomach.

The following points should be noted:

1. About 40 percent of patients with cancer of the stomach have a level of gastric acidity which is normal. The higher the gastric acidity, the better the prognosis. Most of the remaining patients do not demonstrate a *complete* anacidity.
2. Achlorhydria and hypochlorhydria is associated with an increased hospital mortality and a poor survival rate. Perhaps the degree of gastric acidity reflects the amount of destruction of the gastric mucosa and diminution of the total parietal cell mass.
3. The relationship of secretory activity of the stomach to the presence of atrophy of the gastric mucosa and the subsequent development of cancer is strong.[7]

Chronic gastric ulcer.   Most authorities are agreed that in a certain proportion of cases cancer arises in a chronic gastric ulcer. A study of statistics does not help me to state the exact percentage of gastric ulcers which turn into cancer or the number of cancers which are partially destroyed by the action of the acid gastric juice. The estimate varies considerably. An important consideration is that, whatever the percentage, some ulcers end as cancer and some *supposedly* benign ulcers are cancers from their inception.

All observers are agreed that the *position of the ulcer* in the stomach is of the greatest significance as regards its possible malignancy; thus, a chronic ulcer situated on or within half an inch (1.27 cm) or so of the *greater* curvature, even when it possesses all the radiological appearances of a benign ulcer, should be regarded and treated as malignant. Ulcers occurring in the pyloric segment should always be viewed with suspicion, as about 20 percent of these are primarily malignant ulcerating growths. The large indolent penetrating ulcer occurring on the posterior wall *away from the curvatures* should in most instances be treated by partial gastrectomy since some 10 percent of these will show malignant changes when submitted to microscopical investigation.

Innocent new growths of the stomach. This subject is discussed in B and D below.

Other possible factors.   The causes of cancer remain as yet shrouded in mystery, but constant or intermittent trauma or irritation of the mucosa, such as might be produced by unsuitable articles of food, such as *smoked* food, very hot or iced drinks, oversmoking, excessive consumption of alcohol or of certain popular beverages, ulcerogenic medication, constant nervous strain, a lack of vitamins (and especially vitamins A and C), severe chronic intoxication, malnutrition, the obscure and little detected ravages of acute specific or infectious disease, or hormonal influences have at various times been thought to predispose to cancer of the stomach.

Pathology

Of malignant tumours of the stomach 95 percent are adenocarcinomas. About 50 percent of cancers of the stomach occupy the pyloric and antral segments; approximately 20 percent involve the lesser curvature, 5 percent the greater curvature, 5 percent the fundus, and 10 percent the cardiac area, and 10 percent are diffuse.

Microscopically, the cells may be columnar, cuboidal, or round, and they may vary considerably in size. Their arrangement is either tubular or acinar—adenocarcinoma—or solid clumps—carcinoma simplex. Mucinous, gelatinous, or colloid degeneration is a common feature. Growths situated at the lower end of the oesophagus—squamous carcinoma—may also invade the stomach and project into its lumen. Squamous-cell epithelioma, as an *intrinsic* gastric lesion, is extremely uncommon. Equally rare is the gastric carcinoma that presents an admixture of glandular and squamous-cell elements, most commonly termed *adenoacanthoma*. Wood (Arch. Path. 36:177, 1943) found 19 cases of gastric adenocarcinoma showing squamous-cell elements; these had been reported in the literature. Bellegie and Dahlin (Proc. Mayo

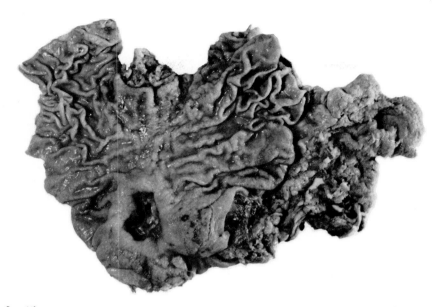

FIG. 1.   Ulcerative carcinoma of the pyloric end of the stomach. The operation performed was a radical subtotal gastrectomy combined with splenectomy. The patient made a good recovery and has remained well for over 12 years.

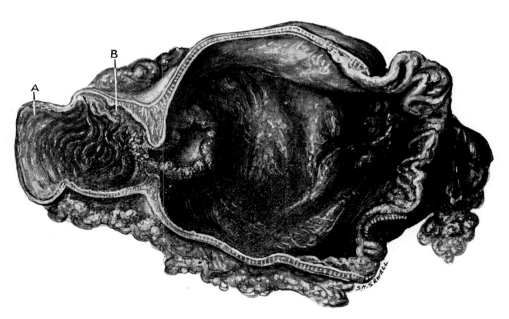

FIG. 2.   Ulcerating carcinoma of the pyloric region showing invasion of the first part of the duodenum (Hunterian Museum, Royal College of Surgeons).

Clin. 26:70, 1951) reported 2 cases of adenoacanthoma of the stomach. Pack (Ann. N. Y. Acad. Sci. **114:**717, 1964), in discussing this subject, stated that he found a case of adenoacanthoma in a stomal cancer occurring on the margin of a gastrojejunostomy performed years before for a duodenal ulcer.

A useful *pathological classification* of cancers of the stomach is as follows: 1, carcinoma in a polyp; 2, proliferative type; 3, sessile or ulcerating type; 4, atrophic or leather-bottle type; 5, mucous carcinoma; 6, adenoacanthoma; 7, carcinoid.

Macroscopically, growths of the pylorus and cardia are often densely hard and ulcerating, while some of those of the body are often of the soft, fungating, luxuriant, and polypoid type.

The naked-eye appearance of the disease may show wide variations, but three common types of growth are well recognised: 1, the malignant ulcer; 2, the fungating polypoid tumour; and 3, the leather-bottle stomach, or linitis plastica.

Mucoid or colloid cancer is merely a gelatinous degeneration of one of the above varieties.

Malignant ulcer. Ulcerative carcinoma of the stomach is the most malignant and is the commonest type seen. These growths occur most frequently in the pyloric segment or in the region of the lesser curvature, although no portion of the stomach is immune (Figs. 1 to 3). They infiltrate widely and rapidly and soon give rise to metastases of the regional lymph nodes and in the liver. The growth is scirrhous in nature, is composed of spheroidal or columnar cells in an abundant matrix of connective tissues, and is prone to undergo mucinous degeneration. The ulcer is usually oval or circular in shape and has a firm, raised, rampart-like or rolled-over edge, and a shallow crater, the floor of which is often superficially ulcerated or necrotic. At times the punched-out appearance of a benign chronic gastric ulcer may be closely mimicked, and a gastric ulcer which becomes malignant is of this variety.

When a section is made through the growth, it will often be possible to trace the muscular layers across the base of the ulcer, even in those cases where the muscle and serosa have been extensively invaded by growth. On the other hand, a section through a gastric ulcer which is undergoing malignant change will show a complete breach or obliteration of the muscular layers, the floor of the carter being composed of dense white fibrous tissue, forming an almost insurmountable barrier against invasion by cancer cells.

The growth spreads rapidly in the submucosa, but less quickly beneath the tough serosa, away from the pyloric ring toward the cardia, while outlying islets can be detected at least ½ in. (1.27 cm) in advance of the growing margin. When the growth extends to the peritoneal coat of the stomach, the overlying surface of the organ may become studded with minute, white, pearly seedlings, wrinkled or puckered, greatly thickened, oedematous, and opalescent from gelatinous degeneration, or converted into a disc-like plaque

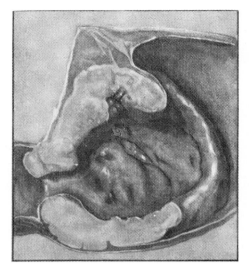

FIG. 3.   Large malignant ulcerating tumour occupying the antrum and the pylorus.

of metallic hardness, from the vicinity of which arise rigid filamentous strands or knotted cords of permeated lymphatic vessels.

Fungating and polypoid tumours. These form bulky, friable, cauliflower-like masses or rounded soft tumours with broad pedicles which project into the lumen of the stomach. They usually arise in the body of the stomach, in the region of the greater curvature, posterior wall, or fundus, and are at first of a low order of malignancy. They give rise to but few symptoms during their early stages of growth, but may by their fleshy bulk plug the outlet of the stomach and cause pyloric obstruction. They are prone to become infected, to slough, and to ulcerate; when they do so, bleeding and the effects of bleeding will be striking features.

The fungating tumours are adenocarcinomas and are composed of columnar epithelial cells. The regional lymph nodes are invaded late in the course of the disease, and infiltration is confined to a limited area of the stomach wall. A number of these growths originate in innocent tumours—polyps.

Leather-bottle stomach—linitis plastica. The *local* form of the disease starts at the pylorus, spreads *slowly* in the direction of the cardia, and is associated with much fibrosis. The pyloric canal becomes constricted by the enormous overgrowth of fibrous tissue which occurs in the submucous coat and by the accompanying congestion of the overlying mucous membrane, resulting in dilatation of the stomach in its proximal portion. When this takes place, the condition is often termed *chronic scirrhous cancer of the pylorus.*

The following conditions may be mistaken for and may, in fact, on naked-eye examination be indistinguishable from the *localised form of linitis*

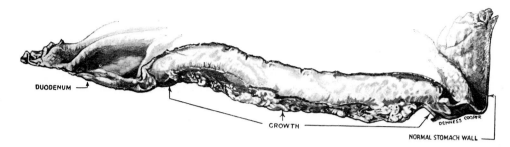

FIG. 4.   Linitis plastica.

plastica: (1) tuberculous disease of the pylorus; (2) syphilitic gummatous infiltration of the antrum and pylorus; (3) simple pyloric fibrosis caused by peptic ulceration; (4) hypertrophic pyloric stenosis of adults (benign pyloric hypertrophy).

Primary hypertrophic pyloric stenosis has been reviewed by Du Plessis (Brit. J. Surg. 53:485, 1966) who describes 6 personal cases.

The *diffuse* form of leather-bottle stomach was first described by Brinton in 1854, and is a rare type of cancer. He considered that the name "linitis plastica" was very apt and very descriptive of the thick-walled contracted organ. Like the localised type, the diffuse form starts at the pyloric ring, infiltrating the submucosa and subserosa, growing slowly around the circumference and along the longitudinal axis of the stomach toward the cardia. While the growth may end abruptly at the pylorus, it will in time advance upward toward the oesophageal opening and actually invade the lower reaches of the gullet. The stomach even-

tually becomes steer-horn in shape and is shortened and contracted by several inches. It is transformed into a leathery, rigid tube, incapable of being distended, so that its capacity is reduced to a few ounces. The mucous membrane is swollen and markedly rugose, these hypertrophied rugae appearing to be welded to the underlying submucosa (Fig. 4). A few shallow ulcers, irregular in shape, may be present, but in most cases the surface of the mucous membrane is unaffected. The pyloric and cardiac orifices become fixed and patulous, and all sphincteric control is lost. The serosal aspect of the stomach is usually of a greyish-brown colour, although occasionally it may present a normal appearance.

A section of the stomach wall shows that the thickening consists mainly of white fibrous tissue and involves chiefly the submucosa and subserosa. The walls of the stomach may be as much as an inch (2.5 cm) thick. The fragmentation of the muscular layer is strikingly apparent, being produced by fibrous septa which extend upward from

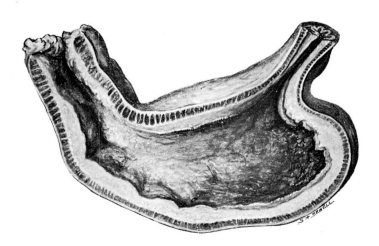

FIG. 5.   Linitis plastica.

the submucosa to the subserosa and divide up the thickened circular muscular coat into little separate bundles.

A specimen of linitis plastica may sometimes present the appearance of a stomach which has been fixed in a strong solution of formalin for a considerable period (Fig. 5). Metastases occur in the adjacent lymph nodes late in the course of the disease, and as this type of cancer is slow-growing and the growth is confined to the walls of the stomach itself for a long time, total gastrectomy is indicated whenever conditions permit of the performance of this operation. Some years ago (in 1941), I performed total gastrectomy upon a lady general practitioner who was suffering from the diffuse form of leather-bottle stomach. She was able to continue with her busy practice and remained in good health until her death (from secondary peritoneal implants) 11 years later.

Carcinoid of the stomach. Up to 1970, approximately 100 cases of carcinoid or "Kultschitzky cell carcinoma" of the stomach have been reported. Only two percent of all carcinoid tumours arise in the stomach, as compared with 70 percent in the appendix and 20 percent in the ileum and caecum. (See Chap. 63.) Thompson and Coon (Amer. J. Surg. 108:798, 1964) give an account of an interesting case; advise that an attempt should be made to remove all gross tumour (by subtotal gastrectomy) including hepatic metastases; and state that a search should always be made for multiple primaries.

MODES OF EXTENSION OF GASTRIC CARCINOMA

The eight principal routes of spread are: (1) in the stomach wall; (2) in the duodenal and oesophageal walls; (3) to neighbouring or distant lymph nodes via the lymphatic vessels; (4) to adjacent organs or to the abdominal parietes; (5) to distant organs via the blood stream; (6) by the peritoneal cavity; (7) by transplantation; (8) by transluminal implantation.

In the stomach wall. The main line of spread is upward along the lesser curvature and to a lesser extent along the greater curvature toward the cardia. The growth spreads mainly in the submucous coat, and in the high-grade infiltrating type of cancer of the stomach such spread is rapid and very diffuse. The infiltration of this coat is usually 5 cm or more in advance of the visible growing edge. The microscopical extent of the growth may therefore be extensive and some distance away from the visible and palpable margin, as Verbrugghen has so ably shown.

In the ulcerated types, outlying nodules or numerous small groups may be seen scattered in irregular arrangement just beyond the advancing edge of the tumour. The cancer involves the muscular coats lying deep to its site of origin, and splits up the muscle into pale pink blocks. This is well seen when a section is made through the growth. The segmented muscle bundles are separated by strands of white fibrous tissue and carcinoma which run at right angles to the serosa. Occasionally, the septa are arranged longitudinally, when alternating layers of pale pink muscle and white growth can be seen. When the serosa is breached, cancer cells become detached from the parent growth and profusely inseminate the whole of the peritoneal cavity with malignant cells.

In the duodenal and oesophageal walls. The oft-repeated statement that malignant growths of the pylorus very rarely invade the duodenum is, of course, not true. Paramandhan (Brit. J. Surg. 54:169, 1967) writes:

"It must be emphatically stated that gastric lesions *do* invade the duodenum, *especially if the gastric lesion abuts the pyloric ring.* The mode of spread may be either lymphatic permeation or by direct spread or a combination of the two."

Involvement of the submucosal coat occurs quite frequently, and I have specimens which clearly show pyloric growths extending through the gastric outlet and implicating at least 3 cm of the duodenum. The lower end of the oesophagus is, of course, often implicated in cases of cancer of the cardia as well as in cases of the diffuse type of linitis plastica.

When performing a radical subtotal gastrectomy for cancer of the stomach, it is most important to include the first part of the duodenum in the resection in order to make certain that the distal line of section is placed well beyond this likely avenue of invasion. This subject is discussed by Zinninger and Collins (Ann. Surg. 130: 557, 1949).

At operation a malignant growth is usually more etxensive than had been thought.

To the lymphatic nodes. Metastases in the lymph nodes are found in *about* 70 percent of subtotal gastrectomies performed for cancer of the stomach at either an early or a late stage of the disease; in some 30 percent of cases, no lymph node involvement is detectable on examination of the specimens of resected stomachs or their appendages. The statistical figures vary: some surgeons give a ratio of 60:40.

The position and extent of the nodal involvement is in part dependent upon the size, the position and the nature and grade of the malignant tumour, but a large growth may sometimes be present with little or no metastatic implants in the nodes, while a small ulcerating carcinoma may be associated with widespread metastases in the lymph nodes. Again, in diffuse leather-bottle stomach, the lymph nodes are involved at a late stage of the disease. In scirrhous growth of the pylorus, the adjacent group of nodes—i.e., the supra- the retro-, and the infrapyloric, and even the right gastric nodes situated on the lesser curvature, very soon become involved—possibly in a vigorous local peristalsis, making the prognosis in these growths poor in comparison with those situated in the body of the stomach.

Again, when a carcinoma is situated in the upper half of the lesser curvature, the nodes in this region—i.e., the upper gastric nodes, the coeliac and paracardial nodes, as well as the nodes in the splenic group, are invaded at an early date, whereas in cancer of the middle third of the lesser curvature, although the lower and upper groups may show early metastases, provided the tumour is mobile and the nodes are easily accessible, gastrectomy is followed by a high percentage of encouraging results.

As a rule, the involvement of lymph nodes is least when the growth is situated on the anterior wall of the stomach, on the greater curvature, or in the region of the fundus.

If the nodes in the portal fissure become involved with carcinoma, they may press upon and occlude the bile passages, giving rise to obstructive jaundice. Growth occasionally spreads along the ligamentum teres toward the umbilicus, where it may form a hard, knobby, bluish-red tumour. Invasion of Virchow's sentinel node in the left posterior triangle of the neck takes place via the thoracic duct in late cases, and in probably less than 1 percent of such cases the nodes in the left axilla and the groin also show evidence of metastatic deposits.

Enlarged nodes found at operation for malignant disease of the stomach are not necessarily cancerous. Inflammatory nodes are often enlarged and soft, elastic, and discrete, whereas malignant nodes may or may not be enlarged, and are often irregular in shape, hard and shotty, with whitish deposits, and sometimes matted firmly together. Permeated lymphatic vessels often stand out as small knotty cords.

To adjacent organs. Growth in the stomach may involve neighbouring viscera by direct spread. The organs most frequently invaded are those which lie near the stomach, such as the colon, pancreas, liver, gallbladder, spleen, duodenum, and upper coils of the jejunum. Spread to these viscera may also occur along *adhesions* or membranes, or through the medium of the omenta. The greater omentum, when extensively involved in growth, sometimes forms a huge, mobile, discrete abdominal tumour which may confuse the diagnosis.

To distant organs via the blood stream. When malignant cells enter the blood stream, as they are prone to do, metastases *may* occur in the liver, lungs, pleura, and bones, under the skin as hard subcutaneous nodules, or in other parts of the body. Metastases in the liver form large, white, hard, umbilicated tumours accompanied by enlargement of the organ and later by jaundice and ascites. They may closely simulate multiple gummas of the liver. It should be noted that the liver fortunately exerts a strong "filtration effect" on circulating cancer cells.

By the peritoneal cavity. When cancer has reached the peritoneal surface of the stomach, it implies that the patient is incurable, as malignant cells are soon freely discharged into the general peritoneal cavity and give rise to carcinomatosis and tumours in the pelvis. The pelvic peritoneum may become studded with growth, or large masses may form here owing to the cells gravitating downward. It is these deposits in the pelvic shelf which may be felt on rectal examination in cases of inoperable cancer of the stomach. The stomach and intestines are the commonest organs to give rise to general dissemination of growth over the peritoneum.

Ovarian Krukenberg tumours may be mistaken for primary growths of the ovary. In every case of malignant disease or cysts of the ovaries, therefore, the stomach should be carefully examined at exploratory operation for any evidence of primary growth in this organ.

By transplantation. Following exploration or the conduct of some procedure for gastric cancer, malignant cells may become implanted in the abdominal incision and later on declare their presence in the form of hard, irregular subcutaneous nodules which will grow either slowly or rapidly.

Transluminal implantation. Portions of a cancerous tumour or clumps of malignant cells may become cut adrift from the parent mass in the stomach and may be spread with the chyme into the intestine beyond where, finding root, they may survive and thrive in their new surroundings.

Signs and Symptoms

The clinical features are for the most part dependent upon the length of the history, the age of the patient, and the situation, extent, and type of the growth. In its earliest stage, cancer of the stomach gives rise to little constitutional disturbance. Cancers situated at the inlet or outlet of the stomach are associated with mild dyspeptic symptoms before they declare themselves and before they produce symptoms attributable to obstruction. Growths occurring in the body of the stomach may be clinically silent to the end or may produce vague symptoms such as anorexia or epigastric uneasiness, until a late stage in the disease has been reached. A large polypoid cancer arising on the greater curvature by a stout stalk may grow exuberantly for a long time without giving any warning of its presence until it unmasks itself with dramatic suddenness by bleeding profusely or by blocking the pylorus with its "fleshy" bulk.

There is also a lethal type of cancer of the stomach which may masquerade as a chronic peptic ulcer for many months. It may be associated with periodic bouts of indigestion and even with hunger pain. It may show a temporary satisfactory response to medical treatment; the patient may actually gain in weight and in strength for a time, the x-ray pictures may reveal evidence of healing, occult blood may disappear from the stools, and all the laboratory tests may firmly support the diagnosis of peptic ulcer. With such an ulcerating cancer it is, nevertheless, only a question of time before its true character is revealed.

The fact that one type of lesion will often produce different symptoms in different individuals and that various dissimilar lesions can cause similar symptoms adds greatly to the difficulties in diagnosis. There are no pathognomonic symptoms of *early* cancer of the stomach, although there may be dozens of "syndromes" or "triads," and the so-called classic clinical manifestations are usually those of the inoperable—or at least of the advanced—stage. The early symptoms considered individually can mean anything or nothing, and they may not point to the stomach at all, let alone to gross disease of the stomach. *The vagueness of the early symptoms may be one of the reasons for late diagnosis.* This does not imply that gastric cancer does not cause symptoms until a late, and sometimes inoperable, stage is reached.

The most common symptoms presented by patients with cancer of the stomach may be listed, in order of frequency, as follows: (1) epigastric pain and "indigestion"; (2) anorexia; (3) loss of weight; (4) vomiting and/or haematemesis, anaemia; (5) melaena; (6) dysphagia; (7) abdominal mass; and (8) diarrhoea and steatorrhoea.

While it is agreed that certain cancers of the stomach may be associated with anomalous vague and bizarre clinical phenomena, it is nevertheless possible in a number of cases to recognise three common clinical types: the insidious type, the obstructive type, and the gastric-ulcer type.

The insidious type. Cases in this group cause considerable difficulty in diagnosis on account of the vagueness of the inaugural symptoms. This is chiefly due to the position of the growth in the capacious body of the stomach or arising from the greater curvature and to the fact that there is little if any interference with gastric function in the early stages of invasion. The first manifestations of such growths may, however, be an alarming haematemesis and/or melaena which bleed the patient white, or an acute perforation which immediately threatens life.

The early symptoms in these insidious types include epigastric pain or discomfort, anorexia, nausea, loss of weight, and anaemia.

In the early stages nothing may be detected on physical examination, although the expert clinician will often pay more attention to the general appearance of the patient than to a large number of disconnected and trivial symptoms. The patient may look well or may appear a trifle pale or worn. On palpation of the abdomen there may seem to be nothing amiss or there may be a suspicion of some tenderness or rigidity in the epigastrium on firm pressure. A growth may be impalpable when the stomach lies collapsed and hidden under the cover of the liver or ribs. Hunt [8] has stressed how important it is to examine these patients in the upright position. When the patient is examined in this position the searching fingers may often palpate a small growth of the stomach which might be missed by palpating the suspected area with the patient in the horizontal position.

It should be remembered that a large growth of the body of the stomach may remain localised for a considerable period, while a small pyloric cancer, which at no time becomes palpable, may first declare itself by the presence of metastases in the liver. The size of the tumour is, of itself, no indication as to operability or of the presence of metastases; in fact, some of these large palpable tumours lend themselves very readily to resection, whereas some of the infiltrating small growths of the pylorus may be associated with widespread implants. However, a palpable mass or clinical evidence of metastatic disease is found in 25 to 30 percent of cases.

The obstructive type. Symptoms in this type vary according to whether the growth is situated at the cardia or at the pylorus. Features common to both types are associated with obstruction. If the growth occurs at or near the *cardiac orifice,* the patient complains of increasing *dysphagia,* first with solid food and later with fluids, and the condition may be exceedingly difficult to differentiate from cancer of the lower reaches of the oesophagus. Dysphagia is the first symptom experienced in 50 percent of patients with involvement of the cardiac region of the stomach. Loss of weight is excessively rapid as soon as the growth encroaches upon the narrow inlet of the stomach, but even before this channel is constricted there is a steady weekly or possibly daily reduction in weight. Pain induced by cancers of the cardia is often referred to the chest, precordium, or base of the neck. An erroneous diagnosis of angina pectoris is not infrequently made.

When the *pyloric portion of the stomach* is the seat of cancer, the late symptoms are those of pyloric stenosis, and it is often impossible to determine by the *symptoms alone* whether obstruction is due to growth or to ulcer. The early symptoms often mimic those of peptic ulceration.

The peptic-ulcer type.   About 30 percent of patients with cancer of the stomach give a history of peptic ulcer which has existed for some years prior to the discovery of the present trouble, and many of these patients are primarily treated by medical measures for chronic gastric ulcer. Swynnerton and Truelove,[20] in their series of 251 cases of cancer of the stomach, found that 26.3 percent of the patients gave a history typical of chronic peptic ulcer. Pack showed that of 155 patients who had gastrointestinal symptoms for two years or more, 53 gave a history of ulcer-pain and 102 complained of indigestion. Larson et al.[14] studied 664 patients who had been followed up for 5 to 11 years after starting medical treatment for gastric ulcers which were presumed at the time to be chronic *peptic* ulcers. Only 22 percent had complete symptomatic relief with permanent healing of the ulcer. Partial gastrectomy was later necessary in 43 percent of these 664 patients because of the lack of satisfactory response to medical therapy. A cancer of the stomach was found in 9 percent of the entire group.

The preoperative differentiation between a benign gastric ulcer and ulcerating carcinoma is impossible in certain cases, even after a trial by therapeutic tests and repeated investigations by means of radiography, gastroscopy, and gastrophotography. Even at operation it may be impossible to make any differentiation. It is necessary to emphasize that one of the important factors concerned in the mortality of gastric cancer is persistence with medical treatment for supposed gastric ulcer, particularly when, as so often happens, this treatment has afforded temporary relief.

Diagnosis

A complete and detailed history and a painstaking physical examination—i.e., clinical methods, will remain of supreme importance in the diagnosis of this disease. Apart from positive radiological findings, clinical evidence alone of the possible presence of cancer of the stomach is sufficient to warrant exploration of the abdomen. The *duration of the history* is not a criterion of the extent of the disease. There is a short history—i.e., of less than 6 months, in about 50 percent of cases of cancer of the stomach. Many patients who give a long history have had intermittent dyspeptic symptoms suggestive of, or even indistinguishable from, those of chronic peptic ulcer, and about half of these will be found on cross-examination to have received medical treatment for supposed gastric ulcer for periods often extending over many months. Lahey and Jordan [13] failed to find any correlation between the duration of symptoms and the resectability of cancer of the stomach. Malignant tumours of the stomach may become inoperable before the patient has any symptoms, but also they may be operable even when the symptoms have been present for one year or more. *La Due et al.[12] have proved that the duration of symptoms bears no relation to the resectability of the cancer.*

Hence no patient should be denied an exploratory operation simply on a basis of having had symptoms or even objective evidence of gastric cancer for many months, nor should the physician extend too much hope to a patient's family simply because the cancer had been discovered "early" so far as the duration of symptoms are concerned.

The severity of the symptoms is largely dependent upon the degree of obstruction present, and therefore more upon the part of the stomach involved than upon the actual size of the growth. Large palpable growths of the body of the stomach may be, and often are, associated with few symptoms, while, as a rule, small early growths of the prepyloric area and lesser curvature soon declare their presence by acute pain and anorexia; but in a general way the first manifestation of malignancy of the stomach is slight but definite disturbances of function.

One of the surest methods of diagnosing early cancer of the stomach is constantly to bear in mind the condition and to suspect it even when the patient gives a history of only minor gastric complaints.

The *physical examination of the patient* must be in every sense of the word *thorough,* and in every case a rectal examination must be performed in order to ascertain if there are any palpable masses in the pelvic shelf, because if these are present it denotes that the condition is beyond the reach of surgery.

It is sometimes difficult to determine whether enlarged nodes above the left clavicle are associated with gastric malignancy, and it would be permissible in doubtful cases to remove a node and have it examined microscopically so as to clarify the diagnosis. It is essential to repeat here that the mere presence of a palpable tumour in the stomach does not necessarily imply that the case is inoperable. There is no single laboratory finding upon which a positive diagnosis of

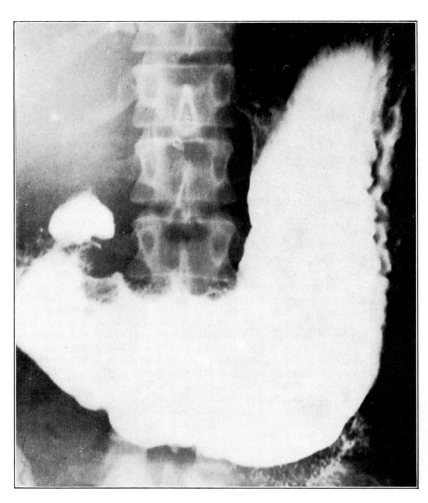

FIG. 6.   Stomach carcinoma showing "fingerprint" filling defect on the distal half of the lesser curvature.

cancer of the stomach can be based. Achlor-hydria, marked anaemia, and positive occult blood findings are suggestive but not necessarily conclusive.

Hypochlorhydria or anacidity is present in about 40 percent of patients with irremovable gastric cancer and in about 20 percent of patients with resectable lesions. *The incidence of anacidity increases in proportion to the size of the tumour.* In Marshall's series (1959), achlorhydria occurred in 36 percent and free acid of less than 20 was noted in 18 percent. Acid values were therefore normal in some 50 percent of his patients, which is a common finding in many recent series. The degree of hypochlorhydria gives no clue as to the presence or absence of cancer in elderly patients.

Other diagnostic methods include:

1. Barium-meal x-ray examination.

2. Gastroduodenal endoscopy with the fibrescope. (See Chap. 4.)
3. Gastrophotography.
4. Laparoscopy.
5. Examinations of the blood, urine, and faeces. Biochemical investigations.
6. Gastric cytology (see E, below).
7. Exploratory laparotomy.

OTHER DIAGNOSTIC METHODS

Barium-meal x-ray examination. *Barium-meal x-ray examination* is the most important single factor in the diagnosis of gastric carcinoma. (Figs. 6-11.) It would be fair to state that most of the cases which are at first misdiagnosed are of patients seen in the very early stages of the disease. The tumour may, for instance, be so small or be in such a position that even on careful screening it is invisible, and this particularly ap-

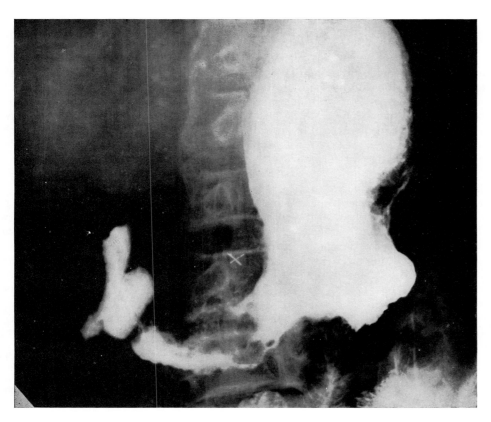

FIG. 7.   Carcinoma of the antrum of the stomach.

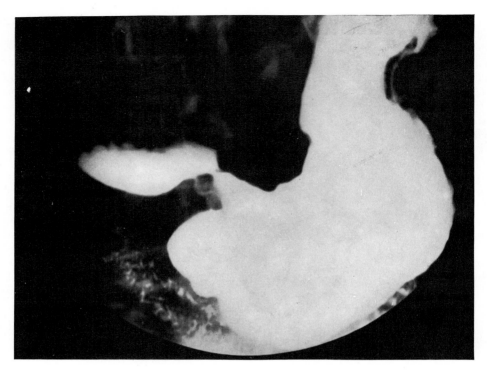

FIG. 8.   Carcinoma of the pylorus, producing obstruction. So-called pipe-stem type.

plies to growths situated on the anterior wall of the stomach, in the fundus, and in the antrum. Again, the growth may be solely confined to the mucous membrane, and the muscular coat being thus uninvolved, the typical peristaltic waves may be seen to pass unchecked across the malignant zone.

Early cases of leather-bottle stomach and growths of the greater curvature may be also elusive, and by presenting atypical and indeterminate appearances lead to misinterpretation and a delay in diagnosis. Negative x-ray findings do not prove the absence of malignant growth, nor should a decision as to operability be based solely upon the radiological findings. A large growth, which on screening appears to be fixed, may, nevertheless, prove to be resectable on exploratory operation.

The radiological signs of cancer of the stomach may be concisely summarised as follows:

1. Small or large filling defects.

2. Altered pyloric function; (a) wide gaping of the pylorus; (b) obstruction of the pylorus.
3. Absence of peristalsis from involved areas of the wall of the stomach.
4. Diminished mobility; loss of flexibility (some cases).
5. Obvious diminution of the size of the stomach.
6. Large crater in the prepyloric region within 2 to 5 cm of the pylorus which shows no sign of healing after an efficient course of medical therapy.
7. Soft-tissue densities in the cardia outlined by the gas bubble.
8. The "meniscus sign" (may cause suspicion).
9. Absence of rugal markings.
10. Niche in relief studies without radiating rugal lines.
11. Niche in the greater curvature.

Careful x-ray studies will yield a positive diagnosis of gastric cancer in some 90 percent

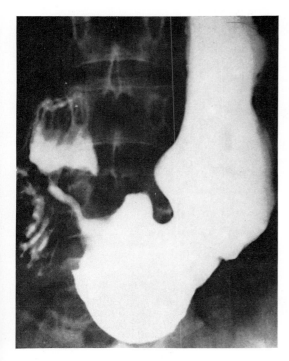

FIG. 9. Carcinoma of the pylorus in a woman 56 years of age. The original diagnosis was acquired hypertrophic pyloric stenosis. Subtotal gastrectomy was successfully performed.

of patients and a diagnosis of "highly suspicious of cancer" in 5 percent. Incorrect radiological diagnosis is made in about 5 percent in many large series.

Problems in the x-ray diagnosis of cancer of the stomach have been the subject of many instructive and valuable contributions, notably those by Templeton (*X-ray Examination of the Stomach,* 1964); Taveras and Golden (*Roentgenology of the Abdomen,* 1964); Lumsden and Truelove (*Radiology of the Digestive Tract,* 1965); and Shanks and Kerley, 1970.

Examination of the blood. A *complete examination of the blood* is made in every case, and varying degrees of anaemia are noted. The anaemia is of the secondary type, although about 10 percent of cases of pernicious anaemia may be associated with a malignant growth in the stomach. The degree of anaemia present in any given case affords no clue to the operability of gastric cancer. No correlation, as a rule, is found between the existence of anacidity and the incidence of severity of the anaemia.

Laparoscopy. See Chapter 4D.

Gastroscopic examination. A gastroscopic examination, using a fibrescope, is of the greatest value, particularly in doubtful cases or where x-rays fail to reveal the presence of a filling defect in the stomach.

Edwards [2] writes:

Gastroscopy may be invaluable, though it is not consistently reliable, and negative findings are not conclusive. Its value is probably not so much in differentiating between a simple and a malignant ulcer, but in defining the presence of a lesion missed radiologically, or in confirming the presence of a lesion when the x-ray findings are in doubt. All gastroscopists have had triumphs, to the patient's advantage, and it is idle for detractors of the method to deny its great usefulness.

Gastroduodenal endoscopy, using the fibrescope, as carried out by such experts as Dr. Kreel and Dr. Hirschowitz, is a notable advance. (See Chap. 4A and C.)

CLINICAL SIGNS OF INOPERABILITY

It is good practice to follow the rule that in cases of cancer of the stomach exploratory laparotomy should be undertaken unless recognisable, irremovable metastatic deposits can be demonstrated.

The case should be considered *inoperable* if:

1. Hard tumours or plaques of secondary growth are felt per rectum or per vaginam in the pelvic peritoneum.
2. Virchow's node in the neck is stony hard, enlarged, and adherent to the surrounding structures. In cases of doubt, biopsy of the enlarged node should be carried out to make quite sure of the diagnosis.
3. Nodules of hard, dusky-red malignant growth are present at the umbilicus.
4. Subcutaneous cancerous nodules can be detected.
5. A marked degree of ascites is present. This may occur with metastases in the liver or peritoneal carcinomatosis, or by obstruction of the portal vein by enlarged malignant nodes.
6. Both lobes of the liver are enlarged

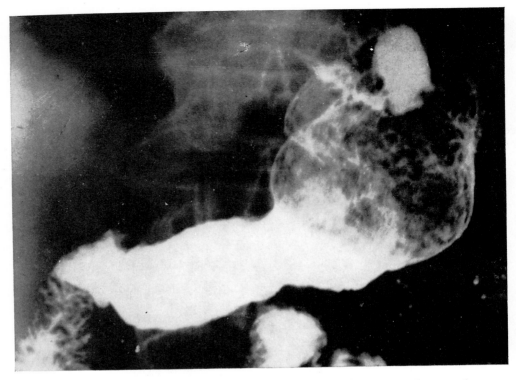

FIG. 10.   Extensive fungating carcinoma involving the proximal half of the stomach.

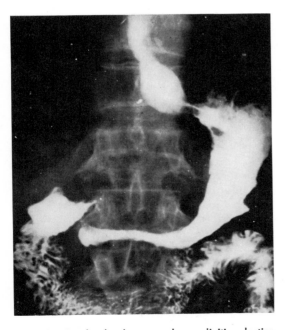

FIG. 11.   Leather-bottle stomach, or linitis plastica. Total gastrectomy was performed and the patient lived for 11 years, subsequently dying from multiple metastatic implants in the upper jejunal coils (author's patient).

and nodular from secondary metastatic implants.

7.   There is x-ray evidence of involvement of an extensive area of the stomach by an ulcerating growth and wide fixation of the organ to surrounding structures. *A large fixed growth of the stomach is usually inoperable.* However, in such cases, laparotomy may be justifiable, especially if there is no clinical proof of the existence of metastases and if the patient's general condition is tolerably satisfactory.

DIFFERENTIAL DIAGNOSIS

Cancer of the stomach has to be differentiated from other conditions which cause anorexia, debility, anaemia, loss of weight, and indigestion. Cancers of the cardia may be mistaken for peptic ulcers of the lower end of the oesophagus or of the lesser curvature close to the oesophagocardiac junction, while tumours of the pylorus may be confused with benign ulcerations. The palpable gastric cancer must be distinguished from carcinoma of the transverse colon, other forms of intra-abdominal malignant disease, cirrhosis, pancreatic tumours and cysts, tuberculous peritonitis, and ovarian cyst. The so-called nervous dyspepsias, which are so commonly associated with anorexia, nausea, exhaustion, and loss of weight, can only be correctly diagnosed after the most careful screening of the stomach. It is well to remember that nervous symptoms are often superimposed upon organic disease. In pernicious anaemia, the deathly pallor is suggestive of growth, but, in the former disease, anorexia is often absent, there is little if any loss of weight, and indigestion is, as a rule, only slight. The blood picture is, of course, conclusive, but it should be remembered that the two diseases may coexist.

Chronic gastritis from oral sepsis, alcoholism, or indiscretions in diet, or after acute illnesses such as influenza, can be diagnosed with certainty only after the exclusion of gastric carcinoma by radiology, gastric cytology, and endoscopy. A satisfactory response to medical treatment is not a valuable guide in these cases, since similar improvement may be observed for a time with cancer of the stomach. Innocent new growths of the stomach, gastric polyposis, hypertrophic gastritis, and gastric syphilis all have to be considered in the differential diagnosis.

The inaugural symptoms of chronic calculous cholecystitis in elderly patients are in many respects identical with those produced by a small malignant tumour of the stomach.

Transpyloric prolapse of the gastric mucosa. This may simulate, both clinically and radiologically, a pyloric cancer. The condition is best treated by partial gastrectomy. It is diagnosed on radiological examination when an inconstant filling defect in the base of the duodenal cap, resembling a mushroom or umbrella due to linear folds of pyloric mucosa pouting into the duodenum, can be demonstrated. The chief symptoms of this condition are those of intermittent attacks of vomiting due to temporary occlusion of the pylorus, epigastric pain, loss of weight, and indigestion. I believe that the incidence of this condition has been exaggerated.

Giant or massive hypertrophic gastritis. This is sometimes termed *Menétrier's disease* and must likewise be considered in the differential diagnosis.

This is a disease characterized by enormous enlargement of the gastric folds. Its recognition is important, for unless its distinctive features are elucidated by x-ray studies and gastroscopy, a

mistaken diagnosis of malignant disease may be made. The giant enlargement of the gastric folds may be localised or generalised; anacidity is a common feature; and a number of patients have been subjected to gastrectomy. An article by Daintree Johnson and Stansfeld (Brit. J. Surg. 46:517, 1957) contains many important points relating to pathology and treatment of this condition.

Nonspecific benign hypertrophic pyloric stenosis. This is another condition which mimics a cancer of the pylorus (Du Plessis, Brit. J. Surg. 53:485, 1966). The condition is sometimes termed *benign pyloric hypertrophy*. The symptoms are those of pyloric ulcer or obstruction of the outlet of the stomach; physical signs are absent; and the x-ray studies, although difficult to interpret, are suggestive of benign ulcer or pyloric cancer. As it is so often impossible to distinguish this lesion from pyloric cancer, the treatment advised is partial gastrectomy (with Billroth I reconstruction), followed by a meticulous microscopical investigation of the specimen to exclude carcinoma.

Phlegmonous gastritis. This in a localised form was first described by Andral in 1839. Starr and Wilson (Ann. Surg. 145:88, 1957), in an important contribution to this subject, collected 25 cases including 2 of their own occurring in the previous 10 years. This brought the total number of cases of phlegmonous gastritis reported in the literature up to 360. The death rate is high—about 30 percent. The common infecting organism is the haemolytic streptococcus, and the recognised predisposing causes, according to Horsburgh (Lancet 2:89, 1959), include gastritis, chronic peptic ulcer, cancer of the stomach, hyperacidity, and acute infections.

The *chronic form of phlegmonous gastritis* may, on x-ray examination, be mistaken for a localised carcinoma of the stomach, whereas the acute type may possibly be diagnosed as a leather-bottle stomach.

I am doubtful whether *special cancer detection clinics* (Wangensteen, 1947), the employment of *mass radiography* (Fordyce et al., Ann. Surg. 119:225, 1944), the increasing use of the *gastrocamera* (Sullivan et al., Cleveland Clin. Quart. 34:81, 1967; Hadley, 1966, 1967; Blendiss et al., Brit. Med. J. 1:656, 1967), *serological methods* (Huggins et al., Cancer Res. 9:177, 1949; Ellerbrook et al., J. Nat. Cancer Inst. 12:49, 1951), or an intensive *educational campaign of the public* concerning the monitory nature of mild abdominal symptoms in individuals of the cancer age (50 to 70) will yield any better results than obtain at the present time.

Patients with abdominal symptoms almost invariably seek advice in the first instance from their family doctor. Much therefore depends upon his skill and intuition and his knowledge of the early signs and symptoms and anomalous syndromes of this dread disease. It would help him considerably if he were in a position to have his patients investigated without delay or inconvenience and at a minimum cost at a reliable and nearby diagnostic centre.

PALLIATIVE OPERATIONS FOR CARCINOMA OF THE STOMACH, INCLUDING VARIOUS TYPES OF GASTROSTOMY

Radical Operations

The treatment of gastric cancer is best discussed under the following headings:

I. Management of the Inoperable Case
II. Operative Treatment
   A. Palliative Operations
     1. Gastrostomy by the methods of Stamm, Witzel, Marwedel, Kader, Dépage-Janeway, Spivack, and Beck-Jianu
     2. Jejunostomy by the methods of Stamm, Witzel, and Marwedel
     3. Gastrojejunostomy by the antecolic method, with or without jejunojejunostomy
     4. Exclusion of the growth followed by anastomosis of the divided (proximal) end of the stomach to the proximal jejunum—antecolic gastrojejunostomy, after the method of Devine
     5. Palliative partial or subtotal gastrectomy
   B. Radical Operations
     1. Radical subtotal gastrectomy (with or without splenectomy) followed by antecolic anastomosis (Schoemaker-Billroth II)
     2. Radical subtotal gastrectomy combined with splenectomy and with partial pancreatectomy, and/or partial colectomy (some cases) followed by an antecolic Schoemaker-Billroth II type of anastomosis.
     3. Subdiaphragmatic total gastrectomy: oesophagoduodenostomy or oesophagojejunostomy with enteroanastomosis, or with modifications in technique by Roscoe Graham, Roux, Lefèvre, Madden, Marshall, and others (see Chap. 29)
     4. Transthoracic cardiectomy, or partial oesophagogastrectomy, followed by oesophagogastrostomy or by oesophagojejunostomy by the Roux-en-Y plan.
     5. Abdominothoracic approach—oesophagogastrectomy, with gastric and oesophageal *replacement procedures,* with colon, jejunum, or ileocolic segment (see Chap. 30)

Management of the Inoperable Case

It is not death itself that the patient fears, and it is not suffering of which he is afraid. The thing that the patient with incurable cancer dreads the most is that he will be abandoned by his physician.—DR. J. E. DUNPHY

Much can be done to relieve these patients of pain, nausea, anorexia and obstruction and to treat anaemia, insomnia, and dyspeptic symptoms. Pain may be due to the pressure of the growth upon neighbouring structures, to obstruction, to gastritis, or to a combination of all three. The following measures are advocated:

Diet. In the late stages, no solid food should be given, and nutrition should be maintained by the administration of fluids and semisolids by mouth. Regular 4-hourly feedings of eggs and milk, malted milk foods, amino-acid preparations, arrowroot, vegetable cream soups, glucose, custard, jelly, junket, Ovaltine, and the like are ordered.

Medicines. Alkaline powders or mixtures may be prescribed three or four times a day. Restlessness and insomnia are combated by the administration of one of the barbituric drugs, such as butobarbitone or phenobarbital, or else by bromides in combination with chloral hydrate. Anaemia is treated by oral administration, intramuscular or intravenous injections of iron and vitamin B_{12}, and by blood transfusions. Analgesics, such as oral codeine, physeptone, nepenthe, and other such agents, should be tried, but when they prove ineffective and the patient is unable to bear the intolerable and unremitting pain with which he is tormented, the inestimable benefits of lavish doses of morphine, omnopon, heroin, or pethidine should not be denied. Pancreatic substance (such as pancreatin) may benefit the patient with dyspepsia and steatorrhoea. Massive doses of vitamin C and methyltestosterone are given as a routine measure.

Gastric lavage. This is urgently indicated in cases of pyloric stenosis in order to rid the stomach of its decomposing stagnant fluids and mucus, to relieve pain and colicky spasms, and to improve the general condition of the patient. It is also a very useful measure in relieving pain, even when no obstruction is present. A small stomach tube should be passed daily and the gastric contents aspirated. The stomach is then gently irrigated with normal saline, hydrogen peroxide (1 dram to the pint), or a weak solution (0.25 percent) of hydrochloric acid. The irriga-

tion should be continued until the contents are returned clear.

It is in these inoperable cases that the surgeon is always questioned as to the relative merits of x-rays and radium insofar as palliation is concerned. In my opinion, two-million-volt x-ray therapy or radium "bomb" therapy has no place in the treatment of carcinoma of the stomach. Antimitotic drugs have little or nothing to offer is the way of palliation (see Chaps. 109 and 111).

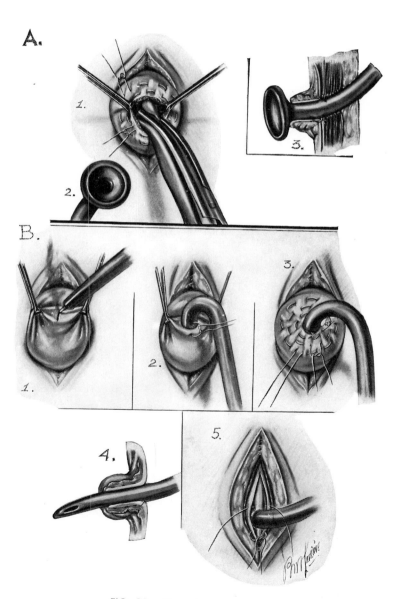

FIG. 12. Stamm's gastrostomy.

Operative Treatment

PALLIATIVE OPERATIONS

Gastrostomy. The chief *indications* for gastrostomy are:

1. Diseases of the pharynx and larynx in which swallowing becomes impossible.
2. Extensive irremovable cancer of the oesophagus.
3. Some strictures of the oesophagus which may result from corrosive poisoning (as a temporary or permanent measure).
4. Irremovable cancer of the cardiac end of the stomach in which oesophagogastrostomy or oesophagojejunostomy is not feasible.
5. Tumours of the posterior mediastinum which compress the oesophagus and for which resection is impossible.

The historical note that follows is largely based on the article by Pack and McNeer (Rev. Gastroenterol. 16:291, 1949), which contains many references.

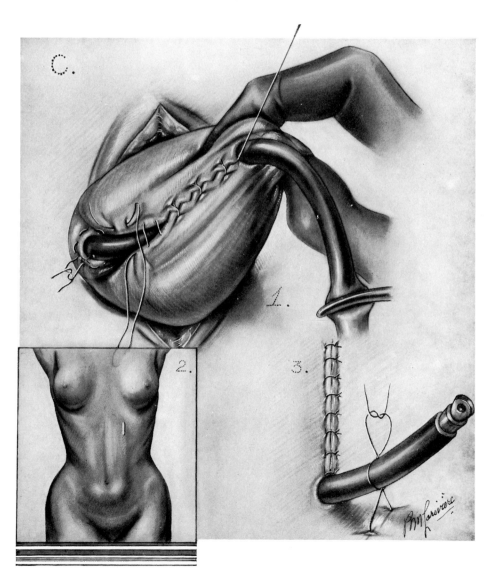

FIG. 13.   Witzel's gastrostomy.

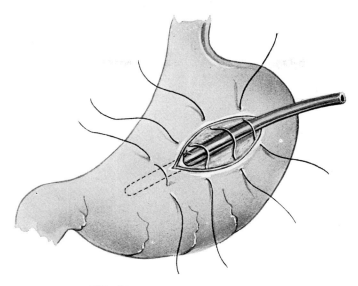

FIG. 14.   Marwedel's gastrostomy.

HISTORICAL NOTE

Gastrostomy was first suggested in 1837 by Egeberg (Norsk Mag. Laegevidensk. 97, 1841). The first operation on the human was carried out by Sédillot (Compt. Rend. Acad. Sci. 23:226, 1846) in 1839, the second in 1853; both were fatal. The first operation in Great Britain was performed by Cooper Forster, of Guy's Hospital, in 1858 (Guy's Hosp. Rep. 4:12, 1858) and the first successful operation by Sydney Jones, of St. Thomas's Hospital in 1874 (Trans. Path. Soc. London 9:101, 1860). Elevation of a simple cone from the anterior wall of the stomach and the use of the rectus muscle as a "sphincter" for the gastrostomy cone was practised by Girard (1888), von Hacker (1890), and Jaboulay (1894). Frank's operation (1893) was popular before the advent of Stamm's description of his method in 1894. The Witzel (1891) and Marwedel (1896) gastrostomies were a decided advance and overcame the bugbear of the operation, namely, leakage. In Pénier's paper (Arch. Prov. Chir. 2:284, 1893) is the first suggestion of the construction of a valve with the idea of controlling the gastric contents. It was composed of mucosa, as opposed to Fontan's valve (1896) constructed from all three layers of the gastric wall. Fontan's operation proved to be satisfactory to the surgeons of his day and it was the forerunner of the Dépage (1901) and the Janeway (1913) principle. Watsuji (Mitt. Med. Gesellsch. Tokyo 13:879, 1899) first combined the valvular principle of von Hacker and Stamm and the tubular method of Dépage-Janeway, forming a tubovalvular gastrostomy.

The Gastrostomies

The object of all gastrostomy operations is the same, namely, to establish a fistulous communication between the stomach and the surface of the abdominal wall so that the patient may be fed.

The operations may be divided into those in which the tract between the stomach and the skin is *mucus-lined* (e.g., Dépage-Janeway), and those in which the tract is *serous-lined* (e.g., Stamm, Witzel).

The former (mucus-lined) type of gastrostomy is performed when a permanent fistula is required, as for an impassable and irremovable stricture of the oesophagus; the latter (serous-lined) type is undertaken when it appears that the patient has but a short time to live, for instance, in advanced cancer of the cardiac end of the stomach, or as a palliative measure in those conditions in which the disease is capable of being corrected—e.g., in a few emaciated and elderly patients suffering from partial obstruction due to a large peptic "cardial" ulcer.

Stamm's operation. This operation is often wrongly credited to Senn (J.A.M.A. 27:1142, 1896), but there is no doubt that it was first described and practised by Stamm (Med. News 65:324, 1894). This gastrostomy is the simplest for inoperable cancer of the cardia.

The operation can be performed satisfactorily under local anaesthesia. Figure 12 illustrates the important steps of this stimple, but effective, gastrostomy.

Witzel's operation. Witzel (Zbl. Chir. 18:601,

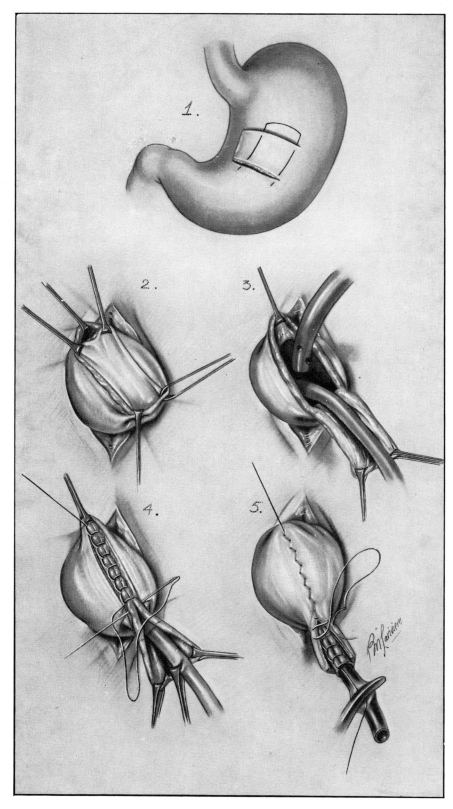

FIG. 15.　Dépage-Janeway gastrostomy.

1891) suggested this operation in 1891. This type of serous-lined gastrostomy is indicated where the stomach is unduly small and tubular and where it is difficult, or perhaps even impossible, to construct a satisfactory pedicled flap or "gooseneck" —the most reliable type of gastrostomy. The abdominal incision, the exposure of the stomach, and the method of delivering the stomach are the same as in Stamm's operation. The technique of Witzel's operation is depicted in Figure 13.

Marwedel's operation. This is a modification of Witzel's method (Marwedel, Beitr. Klin. Chir. 17:56, 1896). An incision 2 inches (5 cm) long is made through the seromuscular coat in the anterior wall of the stomach, about midway between the curvatures, down to but not through the mucous membrane. At the lower (pyloric) end of the incision, the mucous membrane is perforated and a catheter is introduced into the cavity of the stomach for 2 inches (5 cm). The catheter, being fixed to the margin of this opening by a catgut stitch, is then made to lie in a tunnel by suturing of the edges of the seromuscular incision with a series of interrupted Lembert sutures or a Cushing right-angled suture (Fig. 14).

Kader's operation. Kader (Cent. Chir. 23:665, 1896) first described this operation in 1896 and considered that his method was an improvement on the Stamm technique. The stomach is delivered through the abdominal incision and a catheter or rubber tube is inserted into the stomach, as in Stamm's gastrostomy. Two vertical and parallel seromuscular folds of the anterior wall of the stomach are then drawn together, above and below the tube, by the introduction of a few Lembert sutures. The suture line is further invaginated by the introduction of another series of sutures which pick up the stomach wall on either side of the original line of sutures. The gastrostomy tube is thus buried by a twofold pleat of stomach wall, and a cube instead of a cone, as in Stamm's operation, is made to project into the cavity of the stomach.

Dépage-Janeway operation. This operation was first described by Dépage in 1901 (J. Chir.

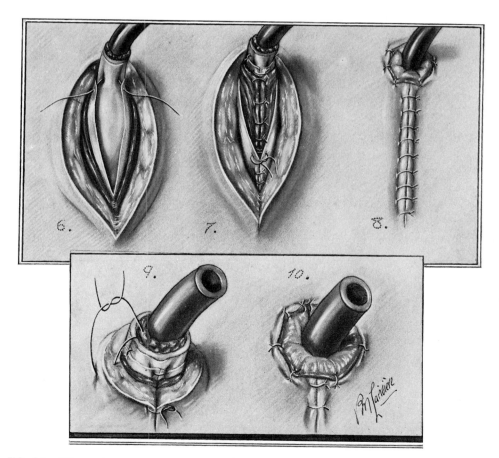

FIG. 16. Dépage-Janeway gastrostomy; method of anchoring the gastric tube to the margins of the skin.

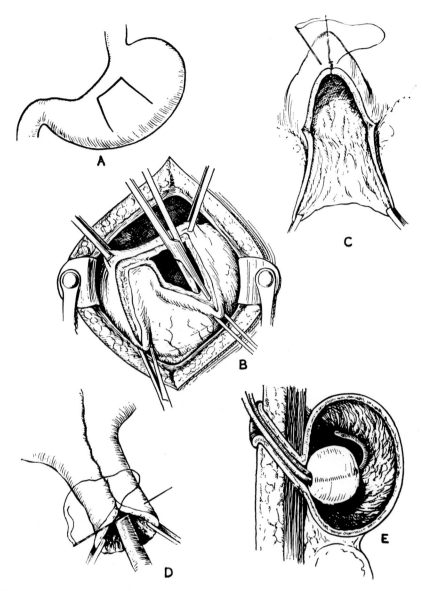

FIG. 17.   Dépage-Janeway gastrostomy. Note that a Foley balloon catheter may be used with advantage as it helps to prevent the escape of the gastric contents onto the surface of the abdominal wall.

Belge 1:715, 1901), was modified by Janeway in 1913 (J.A.M.A. 61:93, 1913), and is indicated when a permanent mucus-lined gastrocutaneous fistula is required for feeding purposes. In order to eliminate the possibility of leakage, Spivack (Beitr. Klin. Chir. 147:308, 1929) described an ingenious method, the characteristic feature of which is the formation of a valve at the base of

the tube. This valve allows the fluid nourishment to be introduced into the stomach and hermetically closes the stomach whenever the intragastric pressure is raised, thus preventing an escape of gastric contents through the tube. This valvular arrangement therefore renders the stomach watertight.

There has been controversy over the priority

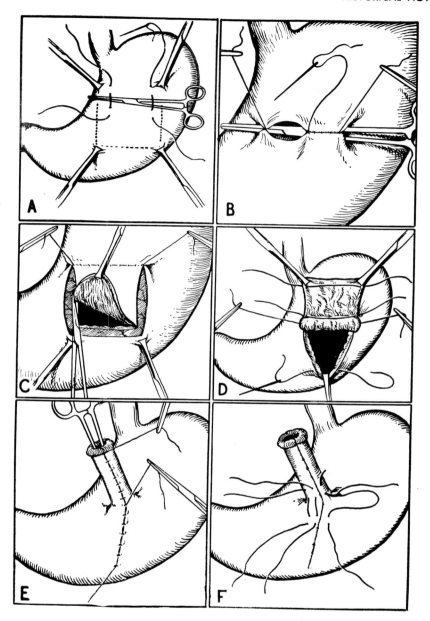

FIG. 18. Tubovalvular gastrostomy. (Courtesy of Dr. George Pack.)

of the origin of the tubovalvular gastrostomy. A careful study of the literature indicates that Watsuji (1899) was the first to combine the valvular principle of von Hacker and Stamm and the tubular gooseneck method of Dépage-Janeway, forming a tubovalvular gastrostomy. Thorek (J. Int. Coll. Surg. 6:29, 1943) gives an erudite and fascinating account of the history and development of gastrostomy, with a detailed list of references.

In my opinion, the Dépage-Janeway operation is the procedure of choice for inoperable cancers of the oesophagus and cardia, especially when these lesions (and/or the condition of the patient) do not permit the performance of a short-circuiting procedure. It can be carried out with a mortality rate of 2 percent.

The various methods of performing the Dépage-Janeway gastrostomy and its tubovalvular modifications are illustrated in Figures 15 to 18.

Tubovalvular gastrostomy by Spivack's technique. Detailed accounts of Spivack's modification of the Dépage-Janeway tubovalvular gastrostomy will be found in his The Surgical Technic of Abdominal Operations (1955). The essential steps of this operation will be readily appreciated by referring to Figure 18. With this plan a valve is created by the formation of a fold at the base of the tube pedicle. This gastrostomy is technically more difficult to execute than the others I have described.

The Beck-Jianu gastrostomy. Ropke (Zbl. Chir. 39:1569, 1912), following the researches of Beck and Carrel (Illinois Med. J. 7:463, 1905) and Jianu (Z. Chir. 118:383, 1912), was the first surgeon to perform this type of gastrostomy on a liivng patient. During the last decade, the performance of this and other types of gastrostomy has been severely curtailed by the modern concept of excision and immediate oesophagogastrostomy, oesophagojejunostomy, or replacement procedures for many carcinomas of the oesophagus and cardia. If for *any* reason, however, radical resection of highly situated cancers of the oesophagus is contemplated, not amenable to immediate union of the proximal end of the gullet to the distal segment of the stomach or proximal loop of intestine, this particular gastrostomy may comprise the *first stage* in the reconstruction (Figs. 19 and 20). (See Chap. 30.)

Postoperative duration of life. Gastrostomy, the simplest palliative operation for cancer of the cardia and oesophagus, permits the patient to live out the last few months of his life more comfortably. The average duration of life following gastrostomy for carcinoma is 5 to 7 months. Over 90 percent of these unfortunate patients are dead within 6 months.

PALLIATIVE OPERATIONS FOR CANCER OF THE STOMACH

Jejunostomy. In cases of cancer of the stomach, jejunostomy may occasionally be indicated:

1. As an alternative procedure to gastrostomy.
2. Where the invasion of the stomach wall with growth is so extensive that it renders the performance of a gastrojejunostomy or a gastrostomy impossible.
3. Where there is obstruction of the duodenojejunal flexure or proximal jejunum, due either to spread of the growth from the stomach or to the presence of malignant lymph nodes at the root of the mesentery.
4. As a method of supplying the patient with

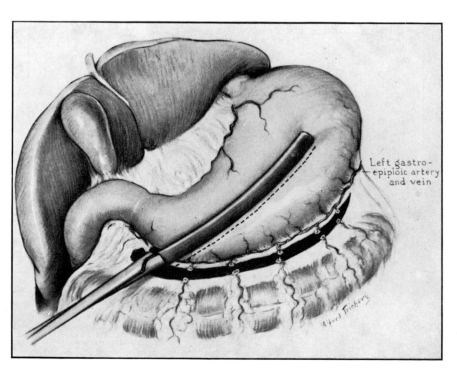

Left gastro-epiploic artery and vein

FIG. 19. Beck-Jianu gastrostomy.

much-needed nourishment in certain rare cases as a preliminary to total gastrectomy, resections of the cardia, and oesophagectomy.

Jejunostomy was first recommended by Fuhr and Wisener in 1886 (Deutsch Ztschr. Chir. 23: 315, 1886).

The best jejunostomies are those of Stamm, Marwedel, and Witzel. The complicated ones of Mayo-Robson or Travel are not recommended. The method of choice is *Marwedel's operation.*

The four essential steps of Marwedel's jejunostomy are depicted in Figure 21. At the completion of the operation, the portion of the jejunum with its contained catheter is anchored to the abdominal wall for a distance of 3 inches (7.6 cm) in order to avoid angulation of the bowel and partial obstruction (Fig. 22).

"Postoperative duration of life is not the proper measure of palliation in the case of incurable cancer. Relief of symptoms, freedom from distress and a sense of well-being far outweigh the importance of the duration of living. To live and suffer is a punishment, not the reward for undergoing such an operation."—(Pack)

Gastrojejunostomy. Palliative anterior gastrojejunostomy is yearly becoming a rarer operation. Gastrojejunostomy is now being performed upon about 5 percent of all patients with gastric cancer who are subjected to operation. The hospital mortality rate is approximately 4 percent and the average duration of life is 8 months. A few patients may survive for 12 months or more.

Anterior or antecolic gastrojejunostomy may be indicated for *irremovable* malignant lesions of the antrum and pylorus, associated with obstructive symptoms (see Fig. 23.) The anterior operation is preferred to the posterior, as cancerous invasion of the omental bursa is common in such cases; the anterior method is simpler and more rapidly performed; and as a drainage procedure, it is equally as effective as the posterior type (see Chap. 19).

Exclusion of the growth. Antral exclusion combined with antecolic gastrojejunostomy is indicated for fixed adherent irremovable growths involving the distal, antral, or pyloric portion of the stomach and for the exceptionally rare malignant lesion of the first part of the duodenum, which defies resection. The operation practised today is based on the methods described by von Eiselsberg (Arch. Klin. Chir. 50:919, 1895), Finsterer (Zbl. Chir. 45:434, 1918), Devine (Surg. Gynecol. Obstet. 40:1, 1925), and Maingot (Ann. Surg. 104:161, 1936). The operation consists of applying a Petz clamp to a healthy portion of the body of the stomach at least 5 cm proximal to the

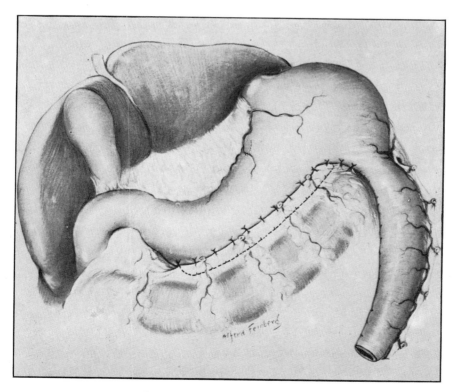

FIG. 20. Beck-Jianu gastrostomy.

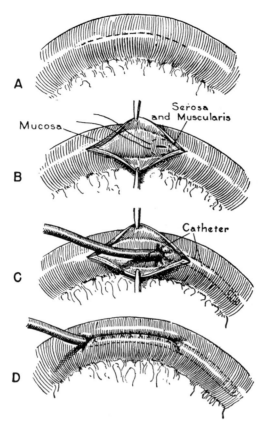

FIG. 21. Marwedel jejunostomy. (A) Longitudinal seromuscular incision of jejunum. (B) Seromuscular coat dissected free of mucosa. Purse-string suture around mucosal puncture intended for catheter. (C) Catheter inserted distally into jejunum and courses submucosally in wall fo jejunum. (D) Completed installation of catheter.

edge of the obstructing, adherent, and irremovable lesion in the pylorus; transecting the stomach with a cautery between the rows of metal clips; securely closing and inverting the distal sealed-off end; performing an antecolic gastroenteric anastomosis after the method of Balfour or Moynihan; and closing the abdominal incision securely with nylon or stainless steel wire to guard against the possibility of dehiscence of the wound (Figs. 24 to 27.)

The results in my hands have been superior to those of palliative gastrojejunostomy. There were 2 hospital deaths following 35 such operations. The *immediate results* were gratifying, as appetite was restored for some valuable months; the majority of the patients were able to return to work for short periods; none died from obstruction of the stoma; and in most the temporary

benison of well-being was a pleasing factor. The majority of the patients died within 18 months from the effects of hepatic implants or from carcinomatosis.

Palliative resection of the growth. Whenever possible, *if the malignant mass in the stomach can be resected together with a healthy margin of gastric wall, this should be undertaken,* as by gastric resection on these incurable cases the patient is rid of a foul, necrotic, sloughing mass, toxaemia is markedly diminished, obstruction is prevented, and a period of improved health and comparative freedom from pain is assured for a longer period than is afforded by anterior gastrojejunostomy.

It is necessary to emphasise that extension of cancer through the serosa of the stomach is not necessarily a proof of inoperability and that local spread—even extensive local spread—does not denote unresectability. The surgeon who operates for gastric cancer must have a very good excuse for declaring that any given case is beyond the reach of "cure" or palliation. On occasion, he must be prepared to disregard the orthodox standards of inoperability and to take a chance even when the preliminary survey is loaded with misgivings. If the surgeon is guided by the philosophy and not the technique of gastric operations, the extent of the procedure is of secondary importance. In the jejune years of gastric surgery, most surgeons performed only partial gastrectomy for palliative purposes. Today, surgeons no longer hesitate to deal radically with gastric cancer and its local extensions to neighbouring viscera whenever conditions permit and by any technical procedure that offers a reasonable chance of survival. In other words, subtotal gastrectomy is often undertaken to secure the maximum palliation and to enhance the survival rate.

Total gastrectomy should be utilised only in those patients whose obvious disease process cannot be removed completely otherwise. It should never be performed as a palliative procedure, and its uses for such a purpose cannot be too vigorously condemned.

Today some 30 percent of all resections of the stomach for cancer are palliative partial or subtotal gastrectomies, but the postoperative mortality rate is high and varies from 7 to 10 percent in expert hands. In my experience, few patients who survive palliative resection live for more than 1 to 2 years. But it is gratifying to note that there are a few patients who survive the ordeal for 5 years or more.

RADICAL OPERATIONS

An outline of Preoperative Treatment and Exploratory Laparotomy is discussed in Chapter 10.

Most surgeons agree that either the Polya-Hofmeister radical subtotal gastrectomy or

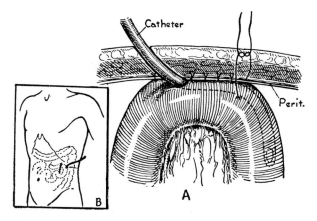

FIG. 22.   Marwedel jejunostomy. (A) Relation of jejunum to anterior abdominal wall. Anchorage for a distance of 3 inches (7.6 cm) prevents angulation of bowel and partial obstruction. (B) Anatomical exposure for jejunostomy. A 2-inch (5 cm) incision is made posterior to prolongation of anterior axilliary line beginning at tip of eleventh costal cartilage. (Courtesy of Dr. I. V. Ravdin and *Surg. Gynecol. Obstet.*)

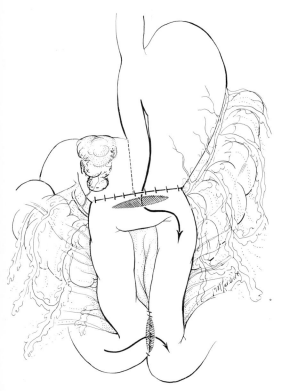

FIG. 23.   Anterior gastrojejunostomy with entero-anastomosis for an irremovable growth of the antrum.

total gastrectomy is the ideal procedure for cases of cancer of the stomach. Today, the Billroth I operation for gastric cancer is rarely performed (see *Prognosis*). In gastric cancer, however, it is essential to remove the greater and lesser omenta and all accessible lymph nodes, and to excise the lesser curvature and at least 80 to 95 percent of the stomach and the first part of the duodenum.

Radical subtotal gastrectomy for cancer of the stomach. The various radical operations for cancer of the cardia and for growths of the lower end of the oesophagus are described in Chapter 30. Tanner and Ryall's comprehensive and well-illustrated article deals with the transthoracic and abdominothoracic approaches to these regions, with the various operations they themselves, and other surgeons, employ, and with other important relative details (see Chap. 30).

This section is concerned solely with the operation of *subdiaphragmatic subtotal gastrectomy,* while the subject of *subdiaphragmatic total gastrectomy* is discussed in Chapter 29.

The essentials of all subtotal gastrectomy operations for cancer include the following:

Satisfactory exposure. The incision of choice is a long left paramedian, with liberal displacement of the belly of the left rectus

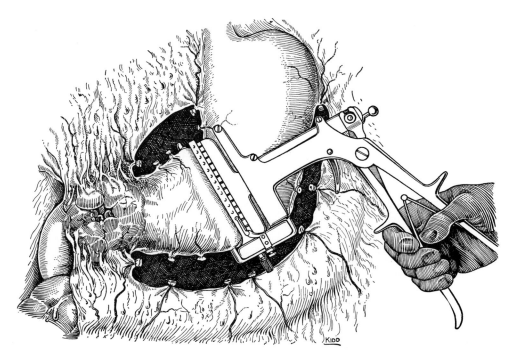

FIG. 24.   Exclusion of an irremovable growth of the pylorus.

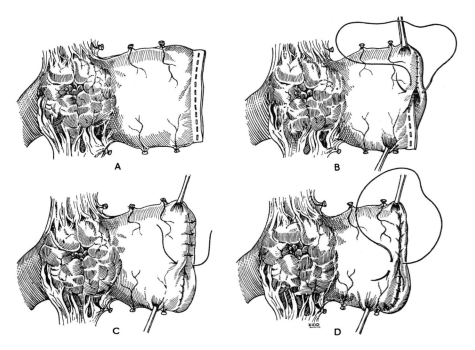

FIG. 25.   Exclusion of the growth.

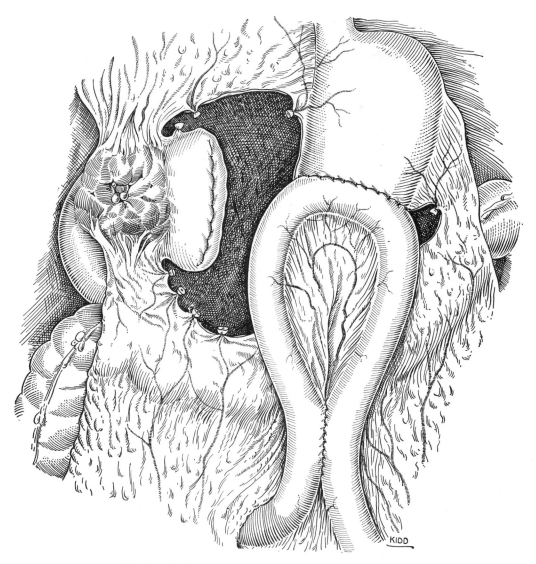

FIG. 26.   Exclusion of an irremovable growth of the pylorus.

muscle. Occasionally, particularly in obese and deep-chested individuals, it is difficult to clear the lymphatics from the cardiac region adequately by this approach. Tanner (Ann. Roy. Coll. Surg. 17:102, 1955) writes:

In such cases, removal of the xiphoid process may give a little more room, or the sternum may be split by means of a sternotome as high as and into each 4th intercostal space, the two halves of the sternum retracted, and the anterior part of the diaphragm divided up to the pericardium. In cases where at laparotomy it is found that 2 to 3 cm of oesophagus could be removed, such extensions are insufficient and it is wiser to do as much as possible through the abdominal incision, than to close it and turn the patient on to his right side and complete the operation through a left thoracotomy.

Before the operation is commenced, 3M Steri-Drapes are applied, and after the abdominal incision has been made, the opera-

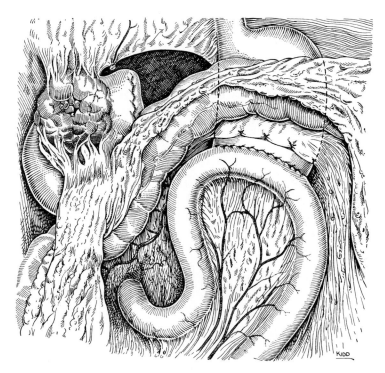

FIG. 27. Exclusion of the growth and palliative posterior gastrojejunostomy.

tive field is packed off thoroughly by the insertion of a number of abdominal packs around the margins of the wound and deep into the abdominal cavity to prevent the intrusion of unruly intestines. Haemostasis must be absolute, the minutest blood vessels being carefully tied and any large vessel doubly ligated, preferably with silk. If there is a small area of oozing, this must be attended to before proceeding with the further steps of the operation. The suture lines must likewise be carefully approximated and sufficiently reinforced with interrupted mattress sutures of silk.

Finally, the mechanics of these operations should always be sound. It is particularly important to avoid any tension at the line of anastomosis, or any drag or pull at the duodenojejunal flexure or on the afferent limb of the jejunum. The anastomosis when completed should be supple, and the afferent and efferent limbs of the jejunum should possess a moderate degree of range of movement.

Excision of the growth with a wide margin

of healthy tissue above and below the diseased area. This would also include: (1) the removal of the first portion of the duodenum; (2) the removal of all but 1 to 2 cm of the proximal portion of the lesser curvature of the stomach; (3) the removal of at least 80 to 95 percent of the greater curvature of the stomach; (4) the removal of all the regional lymph nodes, such as the suprapyloric, the retropyloric, and the infrapyloric, the nodes along the lesser curvature, the coeliac axis and hepatic artery groups of nodes, the paracardial nodes, the suprapancreatic nodes —and those along the greater curvature—the right and left gastroepiploic; (5) the removal of the greater omentum and the gastrohepatic omentum; and (6) the removal of the spleen (in most cases) and of the tail of the pancreas (in selected cases) (Fig. 30).

Radical subtotal gastrectomy for carcinoma of the stomach. The essential steps of the operation are as follows: the greater omentum is detached from the transverse colon, after the manner first described by

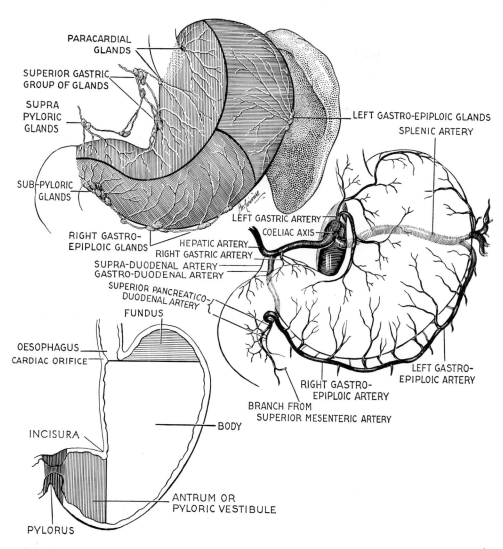

FIG. 28. Anatomical subdivisions of the stomach, blood supply, and lymphatic drainage.

Hey Groves [5] and as depicted in Figure 29. The lower half of the gastrosplenic omentum should be freed to facilitate the mobilisation of the stomach. If the posterior wall of the stomach is invaded by growth, it may be possible, and in fact desirable, to strip up the peritoneum of the posterior wall of the lesser sac from the front of the mesocolon and pancreas and to remove it with the cancerous mass.

The next step consists in liberating the duodenum and mobilising it by Kocher's method. The group of suprapyloric and sub-pyloric lymph nodes should be dissected toward the stomach to free the undersurface of the pylorus and the first portion of the duodenum, where the gastroduodenal artery will be seen lying in a deep groove in the head of the pancreas. This artery is isolated close to the upper border of the pylorus, tied in two places, and divided. This way the freeing of the duodenum, particularly at its posterior and medial aspects, becomes a comparatively bloodless undertaking. On retraction of the

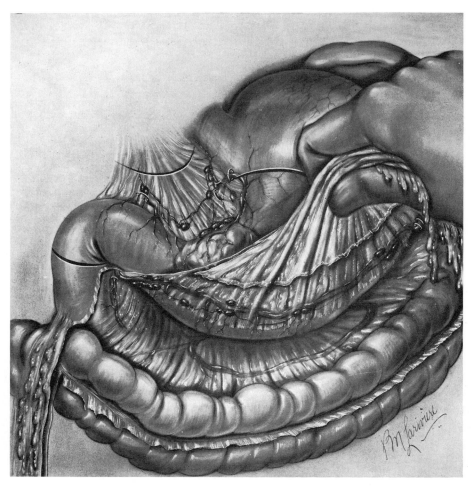

FIG. 29. Subtotal gastrectomy. The amount of duodenum, stomach, great omentum, gastrohepatic omentum, and lymph nodes which are removed en bloc in a subtotal gastrectomy is indicated in this illustration. About 80 to 95 percent of the stomach is excised, and the first part of the duodenum. Note that the greater omentum, the gastrohepatic omentum, and all the regional nodes are removed en bloc.

first portion of the duodenum firmly downward, the sheaf of right gastric vessels comes into view, and these are underrun with an aneurysm needle and tied with medium silk. When this artery is divided, the pylorus is freed and the first part of the duodenum can be mobilised more thoroughly. The right gastroepiploic and the pancreaticoduodenal arteries are then ligated and divided, and the whole of the first portion of the duodenum is isolated, doubly clamped and then transected. The duodenal stump is next oversewn, securely closed, and inverted with su-

tures of fine silk. The fan-shaped gastrohepatic omentum is snipped with scissors as high up as possible (close to the margin of the liver) and stripped downward toward the lesser curvature. Thus the nodes that lie in the region of the coeliac axis and those that cling to the hepatic artery in its course to the hilus of the liver are swept downward with their fatty envelopes and thus remain attached to the lesser curvature.

The surgeon should bear in mind that there is on occasion a large branch from the left gastric artery (an accessory hepatic artery)

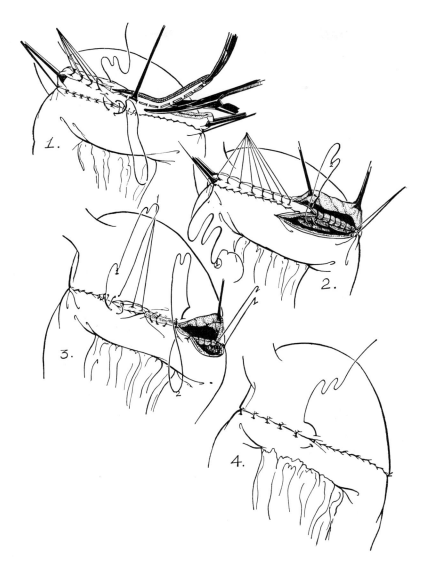

FIG. 30.   Subtotal gastrectomy for carcinoma of the stomach. The von Petz clamp technique is being employed. The stomach is being transected between two rows of von Petz clips. The proximal loop of jejunum is drawn upward to the lesser curvature of the stomach in front of the transverse colon, as in the Billroth II operation.

which runs in the gastrohepatic omentum to supply a considerable portion of the liver with blood. On no account should this important feeding blood vessel to the liver be sacrificed.

The lymph nodes in the hepatoduodenal ligament, those in the hilus of the liver, and the so-called common-duct gland are swept downwards, by gauze dissection, in the general direction of the pylorus.

The left gastric vein is cleaned, stripped of fatty tissue, ligated, and divided close to the superior border of the pancreas, after which the left gastric artery can be clearly seen, springing from the coeliac axis. This is isolated, underrun with an aneurysm needle, and tied off in two places in continuity, after which the artery is divided between the ligatures. A little dissection is needed here to lay bare the right border of the oesophagus

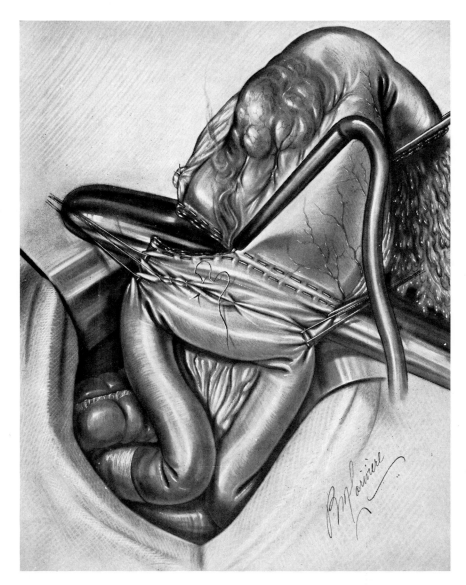

FIG. 31.   Subtotal gastrectomy based on the Polya-Hofmeister plan.

and the region of the cardia and to strip the blood vessels, fat, and lymphatic nodes down to the lesser curvature toward the eventual proposed line of transection. The raw surface high up on the lesser curvature should, where possible, be reperitonealised with a few interrupted 4-0 silk or Dexon sutures. The left gastroepiploic artery is next securely tied and divided near the lower pole of the spleen, and when this has been completed, the remainder of the gastrosplenic omentum with its contained short gastric vessels is clipped, divided, and ligated to ensure a maximum degree of mobilisation of the greater curvature. Commonly the vascular pedicle of the spleen next is clamped, ligated, and divided, and the organ removed. Sometimes splenectomy may not be carried out; especially when it is possible to restrict gastric resection to approximately 80 to 85 percent. The main trunks of the vagus nerves are divided as they course through the oesophageal foramen as this provides a greater degree of mobility to the lower end of the oesophagus and the gastric remnant itself.

It will be seen that the tube-like stomach is now very mobile and can be drawn fully through the wound. It is attached merely by the oesophagus above and by its vascular connections, such as the abdominal phrenic vessels. Ligating the vasa brevia and removing the glandular fatty tissue from the right border of the oesophagus and upper inch or more of the lesser curvature of the stomach invariably lead to the sacrifice of many blood vessels and sometimes of all the vessels feeding the lesser curvature. In such cases, the transection of the stomach must, of course, be high. It is safe to leave a stomach remnant with a diminutive greater curvature not more than 2 cm long, as the blood coming to it from the oesophagus and the phrenic blood vessels can maintain its vascular nourishment. The stomach is transected obliquely high up between small Payr clamps, or between the two rows of von Petz clips, leaving only a small pouch of the organ behind for anastomosis with the first loop of jejunum (Figs. 30 and 31).

It is often advisable to invert the short (1.5-cm) upper portion of the cut end of the stomach towards the oesophagus and to use the lower end towards the greater curvature (5 to 8 cm) for the end-to-side union with the jejunum.

When the distal portion of the pancreas is implicated or is thought to be involved in the malignant process, it should be sacrificed.

When the body of the pancreas is transected lateral to the superior mesenteric vessels, it is most important to detect, isolate, and ligate the cut end of the pancreatic duct, after which the stump of the gland should be securely sutured with a series of closely applied mattress sutures of silk.

In the average case, a fairly short loop of jejunum, rarely exceeding 6 inches (15 cm) in length, is brought up anterior to the transverse colon and applied to the posterior surface of the gastric stump. The proximal portion of the jejunum selected for the anastomosis is applied to the lesser curvature, and the distal portion to the greater curvature. The inturned portion of the new "lesser curvature" should be buttressed against the afferent limb of the jejunum. Many surgeons prefer to use the whole of the cut end of the gastric remnant for anastomosis with the jejunum and to perform the anastomosis on the lines of the Moynihan operation—i.e., with the afferent limb to the greater curvature. My own view is that the choice is immaterial.

When a von Petz or Friedrich-Petz clamp is employed, the stomach should be drawn as firmly as possible between the blades of the clamp to ensure that the correct amount of stomach may be resected (Fig. 31). After the clips have been introduced, it will be seen that they run along an oblique line stretching from a point about 1 to 2 cm below the oesophageal opening downward to a point on the greater curvature which is 6 to 10 cm distant from the oesophagogastric orifice. After the portion of jejunum selected for the anastomosis has been sutured to the posterior aspect of the stomach by a series of interrupted silk sutures, the stomach is divided between the two rows of von Petz clips. The upper third or more of the cut end of the stomach embraced by the von Petz clips is inverted by a series of interrupted mattress sutures, after which the lower half of the cut end of the stomach is prepared for anastomosis. The von Petz clips in this portion together with the crushed rim of stomach wall are trimmed away with scissors, and the anastomosis is then carried out with two posterior and two anterior rows of sutures. (See Fig. 30.)

REFERENCES

1. Blalock and Ochsner, Ann. Surg. 145:726, 1957.
2. Edwards, Br. Med. J. 1:974, 1950.
3. Friesen et al., Surgery 51:300, 1962.
4. Goldsmith and Chosh, Am. J. Surg. 120:3171, 1970.
5. Groves, H., Proc. R. Soc. Med. 3:117, 1910.
6. Hale and Mallo, Ann. Surg. 147:553, 1958.
7. Hitchcock and Scheiner, Surg. Gynecol. Obstet. 113:671, 1961.
8. Hunt, Br. Med. J. 1:650, 1936.
9. Hurst, Br. Med. J. 2:665, 1934.
10. Kaplan and Rigler, Am. J. Med. Sci. 209:339, 1945.
11. Konjetzny, Monatsh. Krebsbekämpf. 2:65, 1934.
12. La Due et al., Arch. Surg. 60:305, 1950.
13. Lahey and Jordan, N. Engl. J. Med. 210:59, 1934.
14. Larson et al., N. Engl. J. Med. 264:330, 1961.

15. Lumsden and Truelove, Radiology of the Digestive Tract, 1965.
16. MacDonald and Cotin, Surg. Gynecol. Obstet. 98:148, 1954.
17. ReMine and Priestley, Ann. Surg. 163:736, 1966.
18. Shanks and Kerley, eds. A Textbook of X-ray Diagnosis by British Authors. Parts IV and V, H. K. Lewis, Co. Ltd., London, 1970.
19. Stewart and Holman, Br. J. Surg. 31:397, 1959.
20. Swynnerton and Truelove, Br. Med. J. 1:287, 1952.
21. Tanner, Ann. R. Coll. Surg. Engl. 17:102, 1955.
22. Taveras and Golden, Roentgenology of the Abdomen, 1964.
23. Templeton, X-ray Examination of the Stomach, 1964.
24. Veidenhemer and Logan, Surg. Clin. N. Am. 47:621, 1967.

B. PROGNOSIS OF CARCINOMA OF THE STOMACH

WILLIAM H. REMINE and JAMES T. PRIESTLEY

Although it is true that progress has been made in the diagnosis and treatment of gastric cancer since Billroth first performed gastric resection for this condition in 1881, it is also true that current methods of recognition and management of patients with this condition are far less satisfactory than one would like. Despite lack of greater progress, many patients have remained free of any evidence of malignant disease for 5, 10, and 15 years, and longer, after removal of a gastric carcinoma. In our opinion, this fact alone makes the defeatist attitude toward this disease that is expressed by some quite unjustified. Although balance between aggression by tumor and resistance by host is most important, experience indicates that complete removal of the tumor may influence this balance favorably. Reduced to this consideration, the problem first resolves itself into recognition of the disease at a time when the cancer can be completely removed. For many reasons, this is a requisite which unfortunately is not fulfilled as frequently as one would like. The second requirement is for a properly planned and executed operation which the patient survives. With few exceptions this should be and can be accomplished when the diagnosis is made before extension occurs.

Some of the most intriguing observations on gastric cancer relate to the incidence of this disease in different countries. By far the highest age-adjusted death rates are found in Japan and Chile [15] and there has been no evidence of decrease in incidence in these countries during recent years. In contrast, in certain other countries, there has been a pronounced reduction in the death rate from gastric cancer during a comparable period. This decrease has been greatest in the United States and has occurred to a lesser degree in Canada, England, and Scotland (Table 2). The trend has been similar for both sexes. The incidence of diagnosis of gastric cancer in the Mayo Clinic fell from about 650 per 100,000 patients in 1935 to 150 per 100,000 in 1962.[13] It seems likely that important knowledge would be gained if the true reasons for these variations and trends could be determined. So far, explanations have been based largely on speculation and supposition.

RELATED CONDITIONS

In view of the extensive literature on gastric ulcer, its diagnosis, treatment, and possible relationship to gastric cancer, only a few comments will be made on this condition. These relate to accurate differentiation between benign and malignant ulceration. The benign nature of gastric ulceration can be determined with reasonable certainty (greater than 90 percent), if operation is not performed, only by continuing and repeated observation and study of the patient over a time so as to be certain that the ulcer disappears completely and does not return. Unfortunately, initial disappearance of a gastric ulcer does not provide complete assurance that gastric cancer will not be found subsequently. For example, gastric cancer was de-

Table 2.   TRENDS IN AGE-ADJUSTED DEATH RATES (PER 100,000 POPULATION) FOR GASTRIC NEOPLASM

Country	Males			Females		
	1950-51	1956-57	1962-63	1950-51	1956-57	1962-63
Japan	64.4	69.9	68.0	35.2	37.2	36.0
Chile	73.6	71.2	64.6	52.1	47.0	41.0
Canada	25.5	22.5	18.7	13.4	11.2	8.8
United States (white)	17.3	13.7	9.8	9.3	7.1	5.1
United States (nonwhite)	24.0	22.7	18.1	12.2	10.3	8.3
England and Wales	29.2	26.8	24.7	17.1	14.3	12.6
Scotland	31.1	28.9	26.2	22.2	19.1	15.5

Source: From Segi and Kurihara, Cancer Mortality for Selected Sites in 24 Countries. No. 4 (1962-63). Sendai, Japan. By permission of the Department of Public Health, Tohoku University School of Medicine.

tected in 43 (10.4 percent) of 413 patients who were initially treated for benign gastric ulcer.[10] In 9 of these 43 patients, cancer was diagnosed during the first month of medical management, but in 14 it was first found 4 or more years after the start of medical therapy. These data indicate the need of continuing concern for the patient who has gastric ulcer that is treated medically. This is particularly true for the patient who has no associated duodenal ulcer and in addition has hypochlorhydria.

Although much is written about the colonic polyp and the advisability of its removal, less attention seems to be given to the gastric polyp. One study of gastric polyps revealed that of 300 patients in whom this diagnosis was made roentgenologically, 60 percent were found at operation to have polyps, 20 percent benign lesions other than polyps, and 20 percent some type of malignant lesion.[9] In addition, malignant changes were found in 12 percent of the gastric polyps that were excised. The incidence of malignant changes was found to be 14 percent when multiple polyps were present and 9 percent when there was only a single polyp. This study indicates that the roentgenological diagnosis of gastric polyp should not be dismissed lightly. It is our opinion that operation should be advised, under usual circumstances, when gastric polyp is diagnosed roentgenologically.

Other findings that should arouse suspicion of gastric malignancy include any area of recurrent gastric ulceration, gastric ulceration (in contrast with gastrojejunal ulcer) after previous gastroenterostomy or gastric resection, and significant change in symptoms of a patient who has what is thought to be benign gastric ulcer. In addition, a roentgenological report of "persistent narrowing" of the gastric antrum or "obstructing duodenal ulcer" in the presence of achlorhydria or gastric ulceration associated with pronounced hypochlorhydria should always make one think of the possibility of gastric malignancy. We believe it is advisable to recommend operation if there is any significant concern about the possible presence of gastric malignancy.

CLINICAL CONSIDERATIONS

In many patients with gastric malignancy, symptoms may be nebulous, signs lacking, and results of clinical studies indefinite. The examining physician must be constantly alert to the possible existence of gastric cancer if this diagnosis is to be made in all patients as soon as opportunity presents. Unfortunately, an inoperable lesion may already exist when the patient first seeks medical attention.

It has frequently been stated that a patient who has a long preoperative history has a chance of 5-year survival after surgical removal of the lesion that is as good as or better than the chance of one who has a short preoperative history.[3, 5] This statement is contrary to the usually accepted opinion regarding the importance of "early" operation for a malignant lesion. A study made several years ago revealed that short preoperative duration of symptoms does contribute to increased survival rate for the majority of patients who are operated on for gastric cancer.[1] Thus, for patients who had a gastric cancer larger than 4.0 cm in diameter (75 percent of all patients with gastric cancer) the 5-year survival rate was 24.3 percent when preoperative symptoms had been present less than 12 months and only 11.9 percent when symptoms had been present more than 12 months prior to excision of the lesion. The opposite trend was true for those whose lesions were 4.0 cm or less in greatest diameter. Many of these patients had a long history suggestive of gastric ulcer, a diagnosis frequently made previously in this group. The issue has been confused by the fact that a disproportionately large number of those who survive for 5 years or longer after resection for gastric cancer come from this latter group.

Clinical findings such as anemia, hypochlorhydria, achlorhydria, and the presence of occult blood in the stool are noted in many patients with gastric malignancy but are not diagnostic. Varying degrees of reliability are reported from different institutions for diagnostic procedures such as roentgenological examination, gastroscopy, and cytological study of gastric washings. In our experience, roentgenological examination, including fluoroscopy, performed by one who is particularly interested and experienced in recognition of gastrointestinal lesions, is the most valuable single method of study. Some authors [4, 11, 14] have reported a high degree of accuracy in cytological study of gastric washings (90 percent and better). Our experience with this technique has been modest and less favorable. For the most part, we use it only when confronted with a difficult differential diagnosis. Perhaps a larger experience would alter our view, but until now it has been uncommon for the results of cytological studies of gastric washings to alter our plan of management for a given patient.

We employ gastroscopy with the fiberscope [8] only when the roentgenological diagnosis is negative, equivocal, or questioned by the clinician. About once in 10 times the surgeon cannot be certain whether malignancy is present in an area of gastric ulceration even when he has the lesion in his hand. This being true, it is difficult to believe that the gastroscopist can be any more accurate. This would seem to be equally true of intragastric photography, which has been used during recent years for diagnosis of various types of gastric lesions. Despite these facts, endoscopic study of the stomach may be of significant diagnostic help in some patients.

SURGICAL ASPECTS

To our knowledge, no patient has been cured of cancer of the stomach except by surgical removal of the lesion. It is important, therefore, that no patient with this lesion be denied the opportunity for surgical exploration if there is any chance that the lesion might be totally removed, assuming there is no absolute contraindication to operation because of other serious disease. It is our practice to accept only objective evidence of distant metastasis as indicative of futility of abdominal exploration. Such metastasis is found most often in a cervical lymph node, the liver, the pelvic floor, and at times the umbilicus. Biopsy may be advisable to be certain of the diagnosis. During recent years, we have performed surgical exploration in 90 percent of patients in whom the diagnosis of gastric cancer has been made.

Decision regarding the procedure of choice when gastric cancer is found at operation is based primarily on the local extent of the lesion and the presence of metastasis. If the lesion is confined to the stomach, except perhaps for involvement of regional lymph nodes, operation with hope of cure is undertaken. If it appears that the lesion can be removed completely by subtotal gastrectomy, this is performed. We prefer to term this operation *radical subtotal gastrectomy* to distinguish it from the type of gastric resection performed for benign disease, or in past years for gastric cancer. All areas of direct lymphatic drainage from the stomach are removed. Starting in the area of the celiac plexus, removal includes tissues along the entire lesser curvature of the stomach, gastrohepatic omentum, duodenohepatic area, and high on the greater curvature, in addition to the gastrohepatic omentum, subpyloric nodes, and greater omentum. In past years, splenectomy has not always been performed for lesions situated distally in the stomach, though there is evidence that this is desirable,[7] just as it is for lesions located more proximally. Histological evidence (on examination of frozen sections) that the upper and lower edges of the excised specimen are free of neoplasm is always obtained before the operation is completed.

Total gastrectomy is performed only when, in the opinion of the surgeon, a lesser operation will not remove all the neoplasm. Over the years, our associates and we have performed total gastrectomy in 15 to 20 percent of patients in whom a gastric neoplasm has been removed. No portion of the pancreas is removed unless there is evidence of extension to this structure.

Decision regarding selection of operation becomes difficult when the growth has extended beyond the stomach and perhaps has involved the colon, pancreas, liver, retroperitoneal nodes, or other nearby structures. Although it is not our belief that "ultraradical" operations will cure many patients, it has been our practice to remove the lesion en masse when in the opinion of the surgeon all the malignant growth can be removed in any reasonable manner. Unfortunately, it may be difficult or impossible at times for the surgeon to be certain that all areas of involvement can be removed until preliminary steps directed toward removal have been undertaken. It is not our practice to undertake a radical surgical procedure in the presence of hepatic metastasis. Palliative resection may be performed in the presence of distant spread for a cancer that is causing distressing symptoms such as obstruction or hemorrhage. Removal of such a growth usually affords more relief than gastrojejunostomy or any other similar procedure.

Although many different forms of anastomoses have been employed after resection for gastric cancer, the one we use most often is the Hofmeister modification of the Polya operation. This is made either anterior or posterior to the transverse colon, depending on individual circumstances. The Billroth I type of operation has not been used for cancer of the stomach during recent years, as in our opinion this does not permit adequate resection of the first portion of the duodenum and adjacent node-bearing areas.

Many different anastomoses have been employed when total gastrectomy has been performed. For some years our preference has been for end-to-side esophagojejunostomy with an enteroanastomosis between the ascending and descending jejunal limbs. The jejunum is brought anterior to the transverse colon. We do not use "pouch" operations but make a rather generous-sized stoma between the jejunal limbs. An end-to-end Roux-en-Y type of esophagojejunal anastomosis is made in the occasional patient in whom a loop of jejunum cannot be brought to the end of the esophagus without tension. When this type of operation is performed, the ascending limb of jejunum is brought through an appropriate site in the transverse mesocolon.

During the decade 1950 through 1959, 2,213 patients were operated on at the Mayo Clinic for gastric cancer.[13] The lesion was removed in 61 percent of these patients. This figure includes total gastrectomy and radical subtotal gastrectomy as well as palliative resections. Total gastrectomy was performed in 16 percent and partial gastrectomy in 84 percent of patients who had the lesion excised. Palliative (nonresective) procedures such as gastroenterostomy were performed in 7 percent, and exploration alone was performed in 32 percent. If the growth is not removed, specimens are always obtained for histological study to be certain of the true nature of the lesion. Occasionally a giant benign gastric ulcer or lymphosarcoma may be mistaken grossly for carcinoma.

RESULTS OF SURGICAL TREATMENT

Although operative risk for cancer of the stomach has been reduced over the years, it still remains significantly higher than for benign gastric lesions. During the decade 1950 through 1959, operative mortality at the Mayo Clinic was 3.0 percent for exploration alone, 4.8 percent for palliative operations, 6.7 percent for subtotal gastrectomy, and 15.4 percent for total gastrectomy (Table 3). These figures have not been significantly improved during more recent years; however, during the last several years subtotal resection of the stomach for cancer in our experience has had an operative mortality of about 4.0 percent. It has been observed that

Table 3.   HOSPITAL MORTALITY BY TYPE
OF OPERATION, 1950 THROUGH 1959

Operation	Patients	No.	Percent
	Hospital Deaths		
Partial gastrectomy, all types	1,131	76	6.7
Total gastrectomy	214	33	15.4
Resection, total	1,345	109	8.1
Palliative operation	145	7	4.8
Exploration only	723	22	3.0
Total	2,213	138	6.2

*Source: Modified from ReMine, Priestley, and Berkson,
Cancer of The Stomach, W. B. Saunders, Philadelphia,
1964.*

operative risk increases with age, size of lesion, location of lesion in cardia, involvement of lymph nodes, hypochlorhydria, achlorhydria, and anemia.[13]

Long-term (5 or more years) survival rates after resection for gastric cancer have not increased significantly with the passage of time. Perhaps this may be partially explained by the fact that operability and resectability rates have been gradually increased over the years. A follow-up study [13] made several years ago showed that for the 5-year period 1950 through 1954, resection of all types for gastric cancer was performed in 703 patients. All but 2 of these patients were traced at least 5 years. The 5-year survival rate for those who survived operation was 29.5 percent. Many different factors influenced the survival rate. The two most important findings in relationship to 5-year survival were the presence or absence of lymph node involvement and the histological grade (Broders) of the lesion. For the most recent period for which data on late results are available (1950 through 1954), it was found that 57.9 percent of 233 patients who survived resection for gastric cancer and were traced for 5 years or longer were living when there was no involvement of lymph nodes. In contrast, only 14.2 percent of 459 patients who had lymph node involvement lived 5 years or longer after removal of the lesion.[13]

Of patients who had resection for gastric cancer performed and who survived the operation during the years 1940 through 1954, 2,113 were traced for 5 years or more after operation. Of this group, 68 had grade 1

lesions; 375, grade 2; 662, grade 3; and 1,008, grade 4. The respective 5-year survival rates for these four groups were 74, 50, 32, and 21 percent. It is noted (Fig. 32) that presence or absence of lymph node involvement appears to be of paramount importance in survival rate, as patients who had grade 4 lesions without lymph node involvement had a better survival rate than those who had grade 1 lesions with lymph node involvement. During this same period 5-year survival rates for those with Type A lesions (Duke's classification) were 89.5 percent; for those with Type B, 55.6 percent; and for those with Type C, 14.7 percent.

Size of lesion also affected survival, as patients who had lesions that measured less than 4.0 cm in greatest diameter had a 5-year survival rate of 40 percent, whereas those with larger lesions had a 5-year survival rate of only 28.5 percent. Thus it is apparent that a relatively large proportion of 5-year survivals came from a comparatively small group (26 percent of total) of patients who had lesions less than 4.0 cm in greatest diameter. Those with achlorhydria had a 5-year survival rate of 29.8 percent, compared with 44 percent for those who had free acid in the gastric contents.

Patients in whom total gastrectomy was necessary to remove the lesion had a lower 5-year survival rate than did those in whom subtotal resection was performed. Thus, in a study of 275 patients who had total gastrectomy for gastric cancer and survived the operation, 14.9 percent were alive 3 years later, 9.9 percent 5 years later, and 7.9 percent 10 years later.[2]

Experience relating to incidence of exploration, excision of lesion, operative mortality, and survival of 3 and 5 years after operation is illustrated in Figure 33. Thus it is seen that of a hundred patients in whom the diagnosis of gastric cancer was made, 5 percent were living 5 or more years later in the group that was seen in the years 1907 through 1916, whereas 15 percent of those seen in the years 1950 through 1959 survived 5 or more years.

From a group of 4,586 patients with carcinoma of the stomach who underwent operation at the Mayo Clinic with hope of cure during the period 1907 through 1955, 957 patients survived 10 years or longer.[12] An

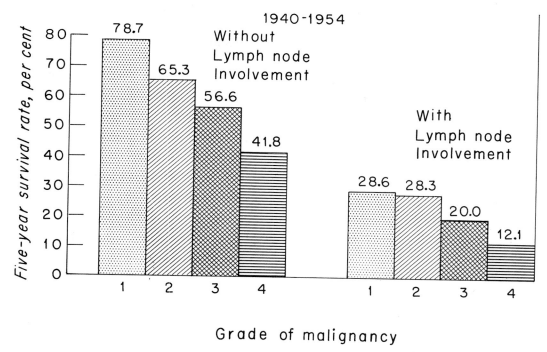

FIG. 32.   Five-year survival rate by grade of malignancy with and without lymph node involvement. (From ReMine, Priestley, and Berkson, *Cancer of the Stomach.* Courtesy of W. B. Saunders, Philadelphia, 1964, p. 225.)

additional 110 patients survived 10 years or longer but were not included in the study because their lesions were not adenocarcinomas. Follow-up studies ranged from 10 to 56 years.

Survival of these patients when compared with the survival of the normal population adjusted for age and sex indicates that if the patient lives 10 years after surgery, his life expectancy is similar to that of a comparably normal population.

These findings indicate that our previous conclusions and assumption regarding prognosis as determined by the usual criteria of location and size of the lesion, type of operation, laboratory studies, duration of symptoms, microscopic grade of the lesion, and lymph node involvement pertain primarily to the immediate years after operation and probably do not pertain to survival of 5 years or longer.

These studies indicate that an appreciable number of patients can be cured of cancer of the stomach and that they can survive for long periods. The usual morbid pessimism regarding cancer of the stomach is not necessarily justified, and greater effort should be made by physicians to offer patients with gastric malignancy an opportunity for cure.

Two hundred seventy cases of primary noncarcinomatous malignant lesions of the stomach also were reviewed.[6] Two hundred eighteen patients were diagnosed as having malignant lymphoma, manifested clinically by epigastric pain, anorexia, and loss of weight. Anemia and achlorhydria were common, and barium-meal x-ray examination usually was thought to demonstrate carcinoma. Fifty-two patients were diagnosed as having leiomyosarcoma, manifested clinically by severe, persistent bleeding and an abdominal mass. Anemia and achlorhydria were again common, and the roentgenogram usually was thought to show a benign lesion.

All patients underwent laparotomy and biopsy proof of the diagnosis was obtained.

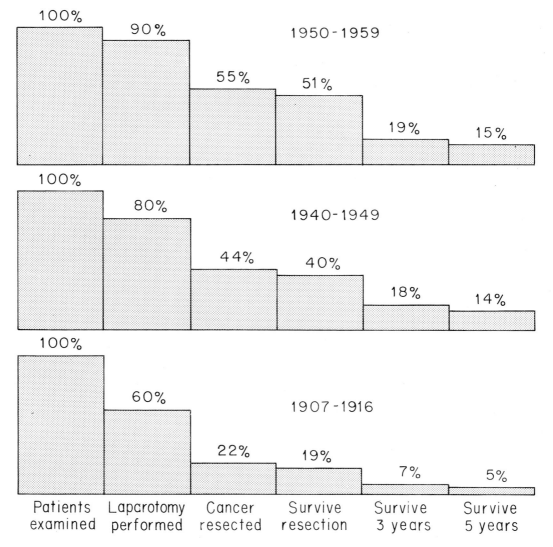

FIG. 33. Survival rates by time periods, for patients with a diagnosis of gastric cancer. (From ReMine, Priestley, and Berkson, *Cancer of the Stomach.* Courtesy of W. B. Saunders, Philadelphia, 1964, p. 235.)

The lymphosarcomatous lesions were surgically resected when possible and later the patients were given a course of radiotherapy. The crude 5-year survival rate was 50 percent and the 10-year survival rate was 32 percent. For those patients surgically treated with reasonable hope of cure, the 5- and 10-year survival rates were 64 and 44 percent, respectively. Leiomyosarcoma was resected more "locally" and did not require irradiation. The crude 5- and 10-year survival rates were 50 and 45 percent, respectively. If only those patients undergoing resection with hope of cure were included, the 5- and 10-year survival rates were 62 and 45 percent.

REFERENCES

1. Barber, K. W., Jr., Gage, R. P., and Priestley, J. T., Surg. Gynecol. Obstet. 113:673, 1961.
2. Barber, K. W., Jr., ReMine, W. H., Priestley, J. T., and Gage, R. P., Arch. Surg. 87:23, 1963.

3. Blalock, J., and Ochsner, A., Ann. Surg. 145:726, 1957.
4. Brandborg, L. L., Taniguchi, L., and Rubin, C. E., Cancer 14:1074, 1961.
5. Brown, C. H., Merlo, M., and Hazard, J. B., Gastroenterology 40:188, 1961.
6. Burgess, J. N., Dockerty, M. B., and ReMine, W. H., Ann. Surg. 173:758, 1971.
7. Fly, O. A., Jr., Waugh, J. M., and Dockerty, M. B., Cancer 9:459, 1956.
8. Hirschowitz, B. I., Lancet 1:1074, 1961.
9. Huppler, E. G., Priestley, J. T., Morlock, C. G., and Gage, R. P., Surg. Gynec. Obstet. 110:309, 1960.
10. Larson, N. E., Cain, J. C., and Bartholomew, L. G., N. Engl. J. Med. 264:119, 1961.
11. Raskin, H. F., and Pleticka, S., Cancer 10:82, 1960.
12. ReMine, W. H., Gomes, M. M. R., and Dockerty, M. B., Long-term survival (10 to 56 years) after surgery for carcinoma of the stomach. Am. J. Surg. 117:177, 1969.
13. ReMine, W. H., Priestley, J. T., and Berkson, J., Cancer of the Stomach. Philadelphia, Saunders, 1964, p. 255.
14. Schade, R. O. K., Gastric Cytology: Principles, Methods and Results. Baltimore, Williams & Wilkins, 1960, p. 83.
15. Segi, M., and Kurihara, M., Cancer for Selected Sites in 24 Countries. No. 4 (1962–1963). Sendai, Japan, Department of Public Health, Tohoku University School of Medicine, September 1966.

C. PROGNOSIS OF CARCINOMA OF THE STOMACH

CORNELIUS E. SEDGWICK

If the lymphoma group is eliminated from consideration, nothing has been added in recent years to the armamentarium of therapeutics to increase the survival rate of patients with gastric cancer. As surgical techniques improved, mortality and morbidity rates decreased. Sufficient experience with radical surgical procedures indicates that survival rates will not be improved appreciably by further advances in technique. In our experience, radical subtotal gastrectomy is as effective as total gastrectomy; removal of the omentum and adjacent organs—the spleen, colon, and pancreas—has not increased the survival rate even though such radical procedures can be performed with little increase in operative mortality. The survival rate will be further increased only with earlier diagnosis. Earlier diagnosis will increase the resectability rate and, hopefully, the survival rate. A high index of suspicion is necessary; more frequent use of gastroscopy and the study of gastric washings are now generally employed, and occasionally an early neoplasm is uncovered. Careful x-ray study should be carried out; however, routine x-ray study of the stomach of asymptomatic patients has offered little. We must look for new and better methods of detecting gastric cancer in its early stages.

At the present time, similar therapy for carcinoma simplex and adenocarcinoma has been of no value. An effective chemotherapeutic agent has not been found, although methods of regional perfusion have been perfected. Only when such an agent has been discovered can we expect improved therapy; perhaps chemotherapy combined with surgery will prove a most effective method in the future.

Fortunately, in this country, gastric cancer is on the decline. In other countries—Japan, Chile, Iceland, and Finland—it is increasing. The incidence of gastric cancer is generally high in areas of high latitude and low in countries in the lower latitudes. Studies such as that of Wynder et al. (Cancer 16:1461, 1963) on the epidemiological aspects of gastric cancer may be the key to understanding the etiological factors of this serious malignant disease. As summarized in their study, gastric cancer appears more frequently in regions where the intake of starchy foods is high and the intake of fresh fruits and vegetables is low. In some areas with a high incidence of gastric cancer, the intake of home-smoked or charcoal-broiled foods is high. Gastric cancer appears more commonly in low socioeconomic groups. It tends to be more common in edentulous individuals than in a control group, a finding probably attributable to a nutritional deficiency. Further studies in this field of investigation should prove rewarding.

CLINICAL DATA

During the 10-year period from June 1948 to May 1958, 687 patients with gastric cancer were seen in the surgical department at the Lahey Clinic. All but 5 of these patients have had careful follow-up studies— a rate of 99.3 percent. Sixty-five percent were males and 35 percent were females. The average age of this group was 59.7 years, with no age difference noted in the sexes.

The presenting symptoms of our patients varied greatly, but the most common complaints were anorexia, indigestion, and weight loss. A few of the patients had vomiting with or without gastrointestinal bleeding. Weight loss was in excess of 10 pounds in two-thirds of these patients and in excess of 20 pounds in one-third. Eighty-two percent of the patients had had symptoms for less than one year, but 42 percent had experienced symptoms for longer than 6 months.

A mass was palpable in the abdomen or clinical evidence of metastatic disease was present at the time of the initial examination in 28.4 percent of the patients. No abnormalities were found on physical examination in 71.6 percent of the entire group.

Absolute achlorhydria was not a striking feature in this group of patients. In 50 percent of the patients studied, the level of gastric acidity was either normal or above normal.

TREATMENT

Gastric resection was possible in 407 patients (59.4 percent). Judging from the surgeon's operative note and description, the gastric resection was palliative in 148 patients. Two hundred and fifty-nine patients had resections that were performed with a hope of cure. Another 278 patients had various operations for relief of symptoms or for diagnosis but without hope for cure. Two patients did not have surgical treatment.

PATHOLOGY

The various pathological types of tumors found in this series are listed in Table 4. The site of the tumor at the time of operation is described in Table 5.

Evidence of lymph node metastases was present in 355 patients (51.7 percent); 125 patients (18.2 percent) showed no evidence of lymph node involvement at the time of histological examination. In 207 patients, no definite evidence of either involvement or lack of involvement of the lymph nodes was present at the time of surgery.

RESULTS

One hundred patients in this series had total gastrectomy as the treatment of choice; the mortality rate was 9 percent. Subtotal gastrectomy was done in 307 patients with a mortality rate of 3.9 percent. The stomach was removed with a hope of cure in only 259 of the 407 patients who had resections. The 5-year survival rate for the 407 patients having gastric resection was 23.1 percent and the 10-year survival rate was 13.3 percent.

Table 4.   PATHOLOGICAL DIAGNOSIS RELATED TO SURVIVAL IN 687 PATIENTS WITH CANCER OF THE STOMACH

Pathological Diagnosis	Number of Cases	Survival (percent)	
		5 Years	10 Years
Carcinoma simplex	268	10.1	4.5
Adenocarcinoma	247	16.6	3.2
Mucinous carcinoma	31	9.1	0.0
Unclassified carcinoma	28	3.6	0.0
Malignant adenoma	1	0.0	0.0
Carcinoma in a polyp	2	50.0	0.0
Adenoacanthoma	4	0.0	0.0
Lymphoma	6	50.0	33.3
Hodgkin's disease	3	33.3	33.3
Reticulum cell sarcoma	8	50.0	25.0
Lymphosarcoma	9	66.6	22.2
Lymphocytoma	1	100.0	0.0
Leiomyosarcoma	11	36.4	9.1
Unknown	68	1.5	1.5

Table 5. SITE OF GASTRIC CARCINOMA (682 CASES)

Site	Number	Percent
Antrum	204	29.7
Lesser curvature	164	23.9
Greater curvature	56	8.2
Cardia	173	25.2
Entire stomach	62	9.0
Unspecified	23	3.3

Of the group of patients whose operation was done with a definite hope for cure, the 5-year survival rate was 36.2 percent and the 10-year survival rate was 18.5 percent.

No patient who did not have gastric resection lived for 5 years.

Of the patients who had positive lymph nodes, 7.6 percent survived for 5 years and 0.8 percent for 10 years. Of those with uninvolved nodes, 47.3 percent were alive 5 years and 18.4 percent 10 years after operation.

Of the 687 patients in this series (684 5-year survivors), 94 (13.7 percent) have survived absolutely. Four hundred and forty-five patients were available for a 10-year follow-up study; of these, 29 (6.5 percent) have survived absolutely.

COMMENT

No patient in this group who did not have gastric resection lived for 5 years. Although the *absolute* survival rates of 6.5 percent for 10 years and 13.7 percent for 5 years are not encouraging, gastric resection still remains the only hope of cure for patients with gastric cancer. The operative mortality rate of 9 percent, the postoperative morbidity, and the poor survival rate in the presence of cancers that require total gastrectomy have discouraged us from using this form of gastric resection unless forced to do so because of the extent of the tumor. The incidence of total gastrectomy at this clinic has gradually diminished in recent years. Radical subtotal gastric resection has become the most popular surgical procedure for cancer of the stomach at the Lahey Clinic Foundation. Subtotal gastrectomy for cancer includes removal of the spleen and surrounding lymph nodes and vascular channels. Radical subtotal gastrectomy eliminates many of the complications during the immediate and late postoperative course that may follow total gastrectomy.

We have not been able to demonstrate a relationship between survival time and the duration of symptoms prior to surgical treatment. Many of the patients having symptoms for the longest periods of time had the best survival rates. This implies that the biological nature of the tumor and the host resistance have played a large role in the success of surgical treatment. It is to be noted that certain tumor types have a definitely poorer prognosis than others. The survival rate of patients with certain of the lymphomatous tumors is particularly good after gastric resection.

D. GASTRIC SARCOMA AND BENIGN GROWTHS OF THE STOMACH

RODNEY MAINGOT

GASTRIC SARCOMA

Sarcoma of the stomach is not a common neoplasm, but such tumours do occur often enough that the surgeon should be aware of their frequency and their distinctive characteristics.

Aetiology

INCIDENCE

D'Aunoy and Zoeller [13] analysed 335 cases of sarcoma of the stomach up to and including the year 1929. Snoddy,[40] in presenting 34 new cases of sarcoma of the stomach, stated that up to the year 1952 a total of 474 cases of gastric sarcoma had been reported in the literature.

Marshall and Adamson [28] analysed 2,014 malignant tumours of the stomach. Of these 1,930 were carcinomas and 84 were sarcomas. The gastric sarcomas in this group included the tumours of smooth muscle (22 cases) and the malignant tumours arising from lymphoid tissue (62 cases).

In their series, 4.17 percent of all malignant growths of the stomach were sarcomatous.

Gastric sarcomas of lymphatic and reticular endothelial origin are three times more common than the leiomyosarcomas.

Leiomyosarcoma is a relatively rare tumour, as only 135 cases had been reported in the literature up to 1954 (Gilbertson et al.[20]). ReMine,[37] in 1970, in reporting a series of over 200 cases of gastric sarcoma, stated that 70 percent were lymphosarcomas and 30 percent were leiomyosarcomas. He classified these tumours as follows:

1. Lymphosarcoma:
    (a) lymphocytic lymphosarcoma
    (b) reticulum-cell sarcoma
2. Leiomyosarcoma

Leiomyosarcoma accounts for 0.25 percent of all primary gastric neoplasms.

Burgess, Dockerty, and ReMine [7] reviewed 270 cases of primary sarcoma of the stomach of which 218 were diagosed as malnignant lymphomas and 52 as leiomyosarcomas.

Today sarcomas constitute 2 to 4 percent of all malignant tumours of the stomach.

Carnazzo and Osgan [9] held the view that smooth muscle tumours comprise 2.5 percent of all gastric tumours; 40 percent are benign leiomyomas; 25 percent leiomyosarcomas of the stomach, and 60 percent of *all* gastrointestinal leiomyosarcomas.

Age. Gastric sarcomas may occur at any age, although the majority of patients are operated upon between the ages of 45 and 75, the average age being 58 for the malignant lymphoid tumours and 51 for the leiomyosarcomas.

Sex. In a large collection of cases in the literature, the sex incidence is in favour of the male sex. The ratio of females to males is approximately 1 to 1.7.

PATHOLOGY

Any classification of sarcomas based on histological characteristics is extremely difficult. Ewing [18] divided gastric sarcomas into three groups: (1) spindle-cell myosarcoma; (2) lymphomatous tumours; and (3) miscellaneous round-cell and alveolar types. Marshall and Meissner [29] and Marshall and Adamson [28] state that although sarcomas of the stomach may arise from any mesenchymal tissue component of the organ, malignant tumours arising from the fibrous tissue, fat, nerves, and blood vessels are so rare that they are merely curiosities.

For practical purposes, there are only two types of gastric sarcoma: (1) those arising from smooth muscle; and (2) those arising from lymphoid tissue.

Leiomyosarcomas. These are the malignant tumours of smooth muscle origin; they occur most frequently in the distal half of the stomach and show a predilection for the antral zone. Although most of them are well circumscribed, some are definitely lobulated, and they tend to project into the stomach rather than exogastrically. In the endogastric or intragastric types, the gastric mucosa is tightly spread over the tumour, which frequently becomes pitted with "gastric ulcers" or "central ulcerations." Invasion of the bloodstream, lymphatic vessels, and lymph nodes is rarely observed on exploration. The lesion is of a very low grade of malignancy and metastasises late.

The macroscopic types are, therefore, intragastric or endogastric, extragastric or exogastric, and diffuse infiltrating. The extragastric or exogastric types originate in the muscular wall of the organ beneath the serosa and grow away from the stomach into the general peritoneal cavity. They involve only a small portion of the stomach wall and often become pedunculated. They frequently attain a large size and form hard, circular. freely movable abdominal tumours. The pedicle by which the growth is attached to the stomach may became very attenuated, and it is even possible for such tumours to be cut adrift from their origin and to become entangled in coils of intestine or to migrate even into the pelvis, where they may be mistaken for a uterine fibroid or an ovarian cyst or tumour.

When springing from the lesser curvature. they extend in an upward direction toward the liver, often between the layers of the lesser omentum, whereas when springing from the greater curvature they may lie between the layers of the greater omentum, fill the lesser sac, and possess some of the clinical characteritics of a pseudopancreatic cyst. Growths of this type often undergo cystic degeneration, and haemorrhage into the tumour mass frequently occurs. They often cause confusion in diagnosis and have been mistaken for tumours of the liver, mucocele of the gallbladder, pancreatic cysts, hydatid cysts, and cystic swellings of the kidney. Exogastric leiomyosarcomas may grow to enormous sizes. Brodowski [6] reported a case in a 57-year-old man weighing 5,500 g and Crile and Groves [12] gave a description of a 45- × 35- × 15-cm tumour containing 4,000 ml of fluid. Carnazzo and Organ [9] gave a report of a 60-year-old female with a 10,032 g extrogastric leiomyosarcoma of the stomach, which had a long pedicle arising from the antrum and which measured 30 × 25 cm.

On exploratory operation they often appear at first sight to be irremovable owing to the numerous vascular adhesions by which they are surrounded; but *after* these adhesions have been cautiously separated, they can in fact easily be dissected out.

Leiomyosarcomas resemble the benign leiomyomas macroscopically and can be recognised only upon microscopic investigation.

As previously stated, these exogastric sarcomatous tumours are often only locally malignant, and the prognosis following their removal is good. The *crude* 5- and 10-year survival rates of patients treated by partial or subtotal gastrectomy is as high as 50 and 45 percent, respectively. If only those patients undergoing resection with hope of cure are included, the 5- and 10-year survival rates are 62 and 45 percent. The leiomyosarcomas are not sensitive to radiation therapy.

The following articles, dealing with these rare tumours of the stomach, may be studied with interest and benefit: Pack (Unusual tumours of the stomach, Ann. N. Y. Acad. Sci. 114:717, 1964); Neurogenic tumours of the stomach, by Rutten (Br. J. Surg. 52:920, 1965); Leiomyoblastoma of stomach, by Schofield and Fox (Br. J. Surg. 52:928, 1965); Reticulum cell sarcoma, by Cirolini (Chir. Triveneta 5:156, 1965); Leiomyosarcoma of the stomach, by Broders and Guerra (Postgrad. Med. 39:509, 1966); ReMine (Amer. J. Surg., 120:320, 1970), and Burgess, Dockerty and ReMine (Ann. Surg. 173:758, 1971).

Lymphoid tumours. These may occur in any portion of the stomach.

These neoplasms showed gross characteristics differing from leiomyosarcomas in that they were usually larger and more likely to grow in the same plane as the gastric wall rather than into the lumen. As a result, the typical appearance was a large flat mass, usually with extensive, shallow ulceration centrally. In some cases the tumour infiltrated under intact mucosa and smoothed it out or pushed it up into giant rugal folds. While the tumours were often partly necrotic, the non-necrotic portions typically were firm, fleshy and yellow-white. None was encapsulated, most were poorly or irregularly circumscribed. Thirteen of the 32 cases showed metastatic involvement of regional lymph nodes. Distinguishing some undifferentiated carcinomas from lymphoid tumours may give considerable difficulty and it is quite likely that some tumours classified as carcinomas are actually of lymphoid origin.

—Marshall and Meissner.

Marshall and Adamson [28] encountered 52 sarcomas arising from lymphoid tissue in a total series of 2,014 malignant gastric tumours, an incidence of 3 percent, or 1 sarcoma of lymphoid origin to 32.5 of other malignant gastric tumours. Saul Kay [25] found that the incidence in his patients was 5.3 percent, which is higher than that in most reported series.

Lymphomatous tumours of the stomach may occur as part of the generalised process or in the form of a localised sarcoma.

Hodgkin's disease of the stomach. This may likewise arise as a primary gastric lesion or as a part of a generalised process.

DIAGNOSIS

A correct preoperative diagnosis is rarely made. The cardinal symptoms are: (1) epigastric pain or discomfort; (2) indigestion, anorexia, and nausea; (3) loss of weight, usually marked; (4) haemorrhage—haematemesis and/or melaena; (5) the presence of an abdominal mass; and (6) anaemia and achlorhydria (common). It should be noted here that severe and persistent bleeding is more common in the leiomyosarcomatous group.

On x-ray examination of the stomach, the intragastric type is often diagnosed as gastric cancer or simple tumour. As previously stated, the extragastric types, which are rare, may be mistaken for cysts or tumours of the pancreas, while diffuse infiltrating sarcomas of the stomach resemble linitis plastica in its clinical, radiological, and pathological features.

Friedman,[19] in his clinical study of 75 cases of primary lymphosarcoma of the stomach, stated that pathological examination of the resected specimens revealed that the lesions could be divided grossly into five forms: (1) infiltrative, (2) ulcerative, (3) nodular, (4) polypoid, and (5) combined. These represent progressive states in the growth of the neoplasm. The ulcerative form, present in 33 cases (42 percent), was the most common type encountered. Burgess and his colleagues,[7] in a review of 218 patients (at the Mayo Clinic) treated for gastric lymphosarcoma, obtained the following results (after *gastric resection* combined with postoperative *radiotherapy*): 5-year survival rate was 50 percent, and the 10-year survival rate was 32 percent. For those patients surgically treated with a reasonable hope of cure, the 5- and 10-year survival rates were 64 and 44 percent. All patients with gastric lymphosarcomas should have radiation therapy. Irradiation gives good *palliation* for 5 years or more. (See Chap. 109.)

TREATMENT

Some 97 percent of these tumours prove to be resectable. With subserous leiomyosarcomas, extensive resections are, as a rule, unnecessary. After careful ligation and division of the surrounding adhesions, these tumours can be readily freed from their vascular bed. The area of attachment of the pedicle to the stomach is examined to determine as far as possible the amount of stomach wall invaded by the growth, and the extent of the implication will decide the amount of stomach to be removed by wedge excision or hemigastrectomy.

The resulting gap in the stomach is closed with a series of continuous sutures of chromic catgut and reinforced with interrupted silk sutures in such a manner that no appreciable narrowing results and there is no tension on the suture line. When hemigastrectomy is carried out for these exogastric tumours, the operation should be completed by the Billroth I type of anastomosis.

The intragastric leiomyosarcomas and the lymphoid gastric tumours are best treated by partial, subtotal, or total gastrectomy, depending upon the physical characteristics, the site, and extension of the growth. Marshall stated that the overall 5-year survival rate for the lymphoid tumour patients was 40 percent. The survival rate was higher. however, in the group of fibrosarcoma cases, which included 21 patients of whom 11 (52.4 percent) survived 5 years or more. Eleven patients with gastric Hodgkin's tumour were treated by gastric resection, with a 5-year survival rate of 27 percent.

Hoerr,[22] in reporting his series of 24 patients with gastric lymphosarcoma treated by local or gastric resection, found that 11 of his patients survived for 5 years (46 percent). These statistics should be compared with the recent ones submitted by ReMine[37] and Burgess et al.[7] Case[10] successfully performed total gastrectomy, with a Roux-en-Y loop, on one of his patients who harboured a huge leiomyosarcoma involving the fundus and infracardial zones of the stomach (Fig. 34).

Postoperative treatment with 2-million-volt x-ray therapy has proved most encouraging and should be advised for patients of the *malignant lymphoid* group, but such therapy is unavailing following gastric resection for leiomyosarcoma.

BENIGN GASTRIC GROWTHS

The importance of benign gastric tumours, as Kiefer[26] has rightly emphasised, does not lie in the frequency with which they occur but rather: (1) in the severity of the symptoms which they may produce; (2) in the favourableness of their surgical treatment; and (3) in their relationship to malignant disease of the stomach.

Leiomyoma is the commonest simple tumour of the stomach. Eliason and Wright[17] estimate that 60 percent of all benign gastric tumours are leiomyomas. Minnes and Ge-

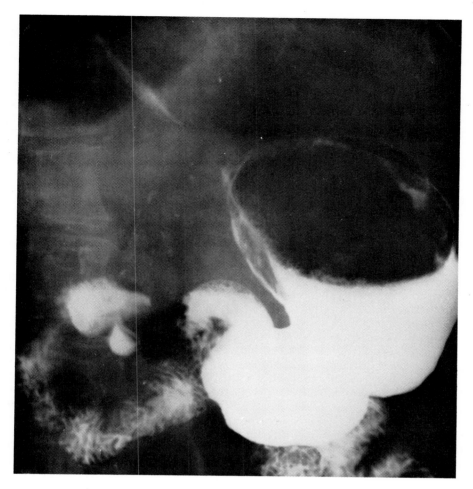

FIG. 34. Large leiomyosarcoma occupying the upper third of the stomach. The tumour was removed by partial gastric resection. The operation was performed upon this patient (aged 72) in May 1961; when examined in July 1972, he was fit and well and symptom-free (author's patient).

schickter [31] quote the following relative incidence of *simple tumours arising from mesenchyme* in 522 cases from the literature:

Leiomyomas	341	(65.3 %)
Neurofibromas	102	(19.5 %)
Fibromas	42	(8.01%)
Lipomas	32	(6.1 %)
Myomas	3	(0.57%)
Osteomas	1	(0.19%)
Osteochondromas	1	(0.19%)

Palmer,[34] in Table 6, gives an analysis of 1,660 cases of benign intramural gastric tumours reported in world literature.

Eklöf,[15] in his study of 221 patients with benign tumours of the stomach and duodenum, states that *adenomatous polyps* were present in about three-fourths of patients. *Nonepithelial tumours* and cases of *accessory pancreas* accounted for one-fifth of the cases. Their incidence increases with advancing *age;* most patients were over 40 years of age when the diagnosis was made. The *sex incidence* is slightly higher in the male.

When originating in the *body of the stomach,* innocent new growths of the stomach do not, as a rule, cause dyspeptic symptoms until they have attained a considerable size. On the other hand, benign growths situated in the pyloric segment may at quite an early stage

Table 6.   ANALYSIS OF 1,660 BENIGN INTRAMURAL GASTRIC TUMOURS REPORTED IN WORLD LITERATURE BY E. D. PALMER

Tumour	No. of Reported Cases	Total No. of Reported Cases (percent)	Probable Percentage of All Benign Intramural Tumours
Leiomyomas	610	37	54.5
Fibromas	289	17	34.5
Neurogenic tumours	263	16	7
Heterotopic pancreatic tumours	215	13	1
Fatty tumours	103	6	1
Vascular tumours	93	6	1
Cystic tumours	87	5	1
Totals	1,660	100	100.0

produce pyloric obstruction or even *intussusception* or volvulus of the stomach when the tumour is forced into the duodenum (see Fig. 35). In such cases a portion of the stomach wall may become strangulated or may even perforate and give rise to general peritonitis. Elgood [16] described an interesting case of gastroduodenal intussusception caused by a large leiomyoma of the stomach for which he performed partial gastrectomy. His patient made a splendid recovery.

All benign growths of the stomach are apt to produce epigastric pain, anorexia, occasional sharp bouts of vomiting, and haemorrhage, which at times may be very profuse. Ives,[24] in reporting a case of neuroma of the stomach which was successfully treated by partial gastrectomy, states that haematemesis and/or melaena is the presenting symptom par excellence in simple gastric neoplasms, in contrast to malignant growths in which frank loss of blood is rare (about 10 percent) (Fig. 36).

Oberhelman pointed out that haemorrhage occurs in a high percentage of cases, but it is as a rule a late manifestation of the disease because the mechanism of its production is that of central necrosis within the tumour mass with ulceration of the overlying mucosa.

These benign gastric tumours may originate in any of the layers of the stomach wall and either remain restricted to one layer or spread beyond it into some other portion of the stomach. They may be sessile or pedunculated. The majority, however, form rounded or flat tumours which project into the cavity of the stomach or into the peritoneal cavity (rare). Most benign tumours develop in the pyloric region and arise from the anterior or posterior wall, showing a predilection for the zone of the greater curvature. They vary in size from $1/4$ inch to 20 inches (6.3 mm to 50.8 cm) in diameter and are all prone to undergo malignant degeneration.

Several benign pathological varieties are discussed below: leiomyomas; tumours of neurogenic origin—e.g., neurilemmoma, ganglioneuroma, neurofibroma, plexiform neurofibroma; fibromas; adenomas; lipomas; and angiomas.

Leiomyomas. These are the most common, innocent tumours and rank third in importance among the growths of the stomach. They are usually single and variable in size, and may be sessile or pedunculated, and intragastric or extragastric. They may undergo myxomatous, colloid, or sarcomatous degeneration.

They do not cause haemorrhage until their mucus-covered surface becomes ulcerated, when haematemesis and more especially melaena may be severe.

Those of the extragastric type originate in the subserosa and spring from the greater curvature. They may form large oval or spheroidal lobulated abdominal tumours, causing the greatest difficulty in diagnosis. Chaffin [11] collected records of 363 leiomyomas of the stomach, of which 23 percent were considered malignant.

Oberhelman collected 1,105 cases of benign leiomyoma of the gastrointestinal tract reported in the literature and found the sites

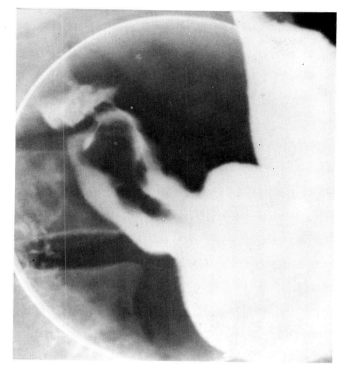

FIG. 35. Gastric polyp with stalk. (Courtesy of the Mayo Clinic.)

to be as follows: oesophagus, 66; stomach, 705; small bowel, 225; and colon, 109. No recurrence of benign leiomyoma of the stomach has been recorded where complete excision of the lesion has been accomplished.

Neurofibromas and fibromas. These arise as a rule in the pyloric or midgastric segment of the stomach. They may be sessile or pedunculated. Histologically they are difficult to differentiate from sarcomas.[39]

Adenomas. These are gastric polyps and may be single or multiple. They may form rounded, sessile, or pedunculated tumours. Stewart[42] found that 28 percent of polyps of the stomach were associated with carcinoma, but only 4.9 percent of carcinomas were associated with polyps. Benedict and Allen,[3] in a series of 17 cases of gastric polyps which were causing severe symptoms (such as melaena), found that there was microscopical evidence of malignancy in 7 cases—i.e., an incidence of 41.2 percent. They also state that Miller, Eliason, and Wright, after searching extensively

in many microscopical sections taken from adenomatous polyps, found carcinomatous change in 8 out of 23 cases—an incidence of 35 percent.

Gastroscopy and gastrophotography add to information obtained from radiographic studies. (See Chap. 4.)

Block et al.[5] state that the *size* of a gastric polyp is the major clinical factor in determining the likelihood of its being malignant.

Polyps less than 2 cm in diameter are rarely malignant; polyps larger than 2 cm are malignant often enough to justify their removal.

Ulceration or bleeding is indication enough for excision of gastric polyps, considering the possibility of malignancy and the threat to life. Block and most surgeons believe that gastric polyps *precisely shown* to be smaller than 2 cm in diameter are satisfactorily managed by periodical examinations.

Partial gastrectomy is indicated (1) for polyps *larger* than 2 cm in diameter, (2) for the rare occurrence of carcinoma in small

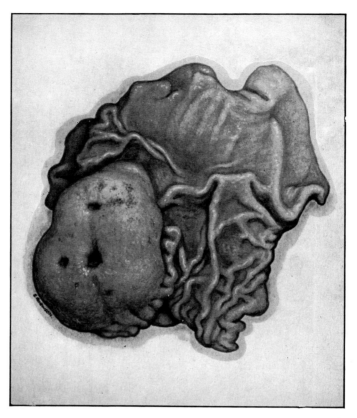

FIG. 36.   Neuroma of the stomach—operation specimen. (From Ives, *Br. J. Surg.* 37:477, 1950. Courtesy of Louis Ives.)

polyps, and (3) when it is impossible to differentiate localised areas of *polyposis* from carcinoma by sight and touch. The prognosis after local excision or partial gastric resection is better than that for other morphological varieties of gastric cancer.

When a portion or the whole of the gastric mucous membrane is studded with closely packed adenomas, the condition is termed *gastric polyposis*. The large polypoid carcinomas originate in polyps that are commonly situated in the region of the greater curvature; the tardiness of their growth, their unusual position, and the frequent absence of secondary implants in the regional lymph nodes until the disease is fairly advanced suggests this possibility.

Carlson and Ward [8] held that a gastric polyp is probably benign if, on gastroscopy, it has the same colour as the surrounding mucosa, if its surface is smooth and not nodular, and if it appears as a small dome with the margins of the base well defined. Malignancy, on the other hand, should be suspected if the tumour is paler than the surrounding mucosa, if its base is broad and merges into the adjacent thickened mucosa, and especially if it presents a cauliflower-like appearance or shows any signs of ulceration of its surface. In their series of 74 cases, malignancy was found in 16.3 percent of the solitary polyps and in 18.2 percent of the cases of multiple polyps. They again confirm that bleeding, anaemia, epigastric pain, anorexia, loss of weight, and occasional bouts of vomiting are frequent manifestations of these benign tumours of the stomach. Morson, in 1967, reported that in 160 gastrectomies for carcinoma of the stomach, polyps were found in 12 cases, while in 80 consecutive gastrec-

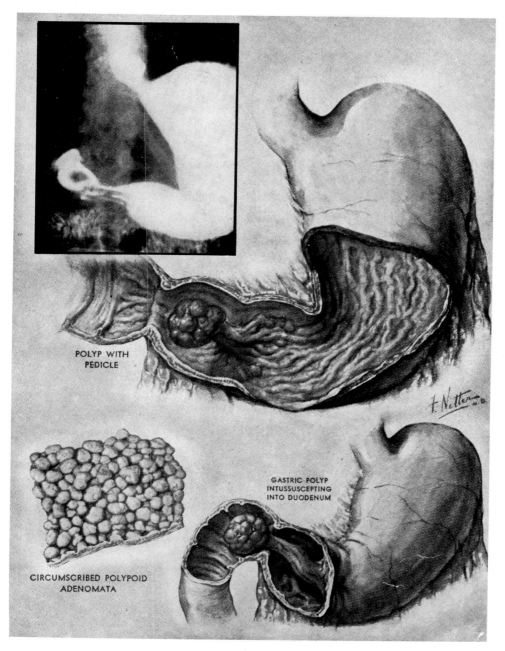

POLYP WITH
PEDICLE

CIRCUMSCRIBED POLYPOID
ADENOMATA

GASTRIC POLYP
INTUSSUSCEPTING
INTO DUODENUM

FIG. 37. Gastric polyps. (Copyright The CIBA Collection of Medical Illustrations.)

tomies for gastric ulcer, no polyps were identified (Fig. 37). According to Monaco and Tomasolo,[33] the incidence of malignancy developing in gastric polyps ranges from 0 percent (A. Monaco [32]) to 51 percent (Pearl and Brunn.[36] (See Parts B and C of this chapter.)

Lipomas. These form lobulated, yellow submucous or subserosal tumours and give rise to but few symptoms. Thompson and Oyster [45] found only 1 lipoma among 94 benign gastric neoplasms in their hospital files, an incidence of 1.1 percent.

Hart,[21] who has described a case of sub-mucous lipoma of the stomach presenting as pyloric obstruction and stated that benign tumours make up 1 to 2 percent of gastric neoplasms, and of these only 3 percent are lipomas. *Pyloric obstruction* was a complicating factor demanding immediate surgical enquiry in some 50 percent of the reported cases of gastric lipoma. According to Hart, the characteristic radiological features are a circumscribed, punched-out filling defect, with normal rugae except in the immediate vicinity of the tumour. There is little disturbance of peristalsis and no niche, incisura, or sign of spasm. If the benign nature of the tumour is recognized, a conservative resection is indicated.

Angiomas form round, spongy, sessile, sub-mucous tumours. They are dark red or mauve in colour, often undergo sarcomatous degeneration, and bleed very freely when the surface of the tumour becomes ulcerated.

Symptoms and Signs

It is rare for the symptoms produced by benign tumours of the stomach to be sufficiently characteristic to allow an accurate preoperative diagnosis. Symptoms, when present, usually suggest that the patient is suffering from chronic gastritis, peptic ulceration, or some grave form of anaemia. *Frank haematemesis is sometimes the first presenting symptom.* Intussusception is a rare complication. Occult blood tests of the stools are often positive, and a fractional test meal will not infrequently show that there is *hypoacidity or anacidity.*

On barium-meal x-ray examination of the stomach, filling defects which closely simulate those found in cases of cancer of the stomach will often be noticed; but the large rounded pedunculated tumours present no difficulty in x-ray diagnosis, as they produce filling defects which have smooth, clearly defined outlines. While on screening of large tumours of the stomach there is delay in emptying, with small tumours which produce irritability of the stomach, the peristaltic waves are vigorous and emptying is rapid.

Treatment

Large single pedunculated tumours with a narrow stalk. *Intragastric.* After the tumour is localised, an incision should be made through the anterior wall of the stomach to expose the growth. If the stalk is small and there is no induration, the tumour can be removed by *wide excision of its base;* the resulting wound being closed with a series of interrupted catgut or Dexon sutures. The large tumours and those possessing broad pedicles are best treated by hemigastrectomy, with a Billroth I type of anastomosis.

Extragastric. As these tumours are prone to undergo sarcomatous degeneration, a wedge-shaped portion of the greater curvature should be removed around the point of attachment and the opening closed with three tiers of sutures. When, however, the pedicle has a broad attachment to the gastric wall, hemigastrectomy or partial gastrectomy should be undertaken.

Diffuse sessile tumours. When these occur in the pyloric region, partial gastrectomy should be performed. When they occur in the proximal half of the stomach, total or subtotal gastrectomy is advised.

Gastric polyposis. In this disease a localised portion or the whole of the mucus surface of the stomach becomes studded with numerous closely packed polyps (see Fig. 37).

Two forms of gastric polyposis are generally recognised: (1) true benign neoplastic adenomas, and (2) "polyps" formed by hypertrophy of the mucosa. The latter are inflammatory lesions—so-called *pseudopolyps.*

Morgagni, in 1769, was the first to describe gastric polyps, and Menétrier [30] wrote a classic paper on the subject, entitled *Giant Hypertrophic Gastritis or Pseudopolyposis.*

This condition may be difficult to distinguish from true polyposis and in many cases from carcinoma. Most surgeons believe that giant hypertrophic gastritis is not a precancerous disease and does not warrant surgical measures. This subject is reviewed by Doyle et al.,[14] Patterson,[35] and Strode.[43]

Yarnis et al.[46] state:

. . . the first antemortem diagnosis of a gastric polyp was made in 1919, when Weggle discovered a piece of tissue attached to the end of a stomach tube. This, they say, was later identified as a gastric polyp. In 1922 Schindler first saw a polyp through the rigid gastroscope. Ritchie (Br. Med. J. 2:1012, 1951), however, reminds us that it was Quain (Trans. Path. Soc. 8:219, 1857) who placed on record the first instance in which the diagnosis was made during life, in the case of a girl of 19, by the presence of a tumour the size of a chestnut in the patient's vomitus.

Incidence. The general incidence ranges from 0.25 percent, as found by Spriggs and Marxer [41] in 4,400 autopsies, to 0.7 percent, as discovered in a study of 7,000 postmortem investigations by Lawrence.[27] Yarnis [46] found 30 examples in 8,735 autopsies, an incidence of 0.29 percent.

The disease is rare. Balfour [1] found 1 case of gastric polyposis in a series of 8,000 gastric operations. Pearl and Brunn [36] collected 84 cases and described an additional 6 cases of their own. Beal,[2] who described a case of *diffuse gastric polyposis,* remarks that the incidence is 1 in 200 cases of gastric polyps; 10 percent undergo malignant degeneration; 95 percent of the patients suffer from the effects of achlorhydria and 10 percent develop macrocytic anaemia. Hoffman and Goligher [23] gave an account of 3 cases of familial polyposis of the stomach in which the small bowel also contained polyps.

SEX. The incidence of gastric polyposis is greater in males than in females, in the proportion of 9 to 4.

FREQUENCY OF MALIGNANT CHANGE. Gastric polyposis is a well-recognised precancerous lesion. Ritchie,[38] and Tempest [44] have described cases of polyposis of the stomach, and consider the disease to be precancerous in character in from 12 to 28 percent of cases. Berg [4] presented histological observations on a series of 106 gastric polyps found in 45 patients. Thirteen percent of the polyps showed transition to invasive cancer.

In my view, *multiple polyps and diffuse polyposis of the stomach* should be regarded as conditions that are too dangerous to temporise with, and in the majority of cases subtotal gastrectomy is the procedure recommended.

Clinical picture. The symptoms are not as a rule typical. The patient is usually elderly, between 55 and 75 years of age. Epigastric pain, the earliest and most constant symptom, is not severe except when a large polyp obstructs the pylorus. Nausea and anorexia are common, usually in association with achlorhydria, the constancy of which has been emphasised by all observers. *Achlorhydria or hypochlorhydria is stated to be present in about 95 percent of cases.* Vomiting, loss of weight, and epigastric dis-

tress are noticed in most cases. Vomiting may be frequent when the polypoid pyloric mucous membrane prolapses into the duodenum, when an intussusception occurs as the result of a sizeable polyp dragging the mobile mucosa through the gastric outlet, and when stringy blood-tinted mucus clogs the rugae. Constitutional symptoms such as weakness are the consequence of continued bleeding from the speckled sites of ulceration on the polyps. Bleeding, which may be mild, continuous, intermittent, or massive, is a constant feature and accounts for the *anaemia* which so frequently acompanies this disease. Diarrhoea is present in 10 percent of the patients.

Radiological examination commonly shows a well-marked cobblestone or mottling effect, with numerous indentations in the outline of the stomach. These filling defects, which can be likened to fingerprint deformities, are most prominent in the prepyloric zone. Such a typical appearance has been described as that of a "bag filled with beans" (Ritchie). Air bubbles, particles of food, or foreign bodies may be a source of confusion.

Endoscopic investigation by means of the fibrescope and/or *gastrophotography* will often clinch the diagnosis. Gastric cytology may prove an invaluable method of examination and may be helpful in detecting early cancerous changes in some of the polyps. (See Part E.)

Treatment. The treatment of *pseudopolyposis* associated with hypertrophic gastritis is medical unless some grave complication is present, such as massive haemorrhage which cannot be staunched by conservative measures. True neoplastic adenomas are not associated with hypertrophic gastritis.

All large adenomatous polyps, whether single or multiple, should be removed surgically and should be considered as precursors of cancer.

If the polyps are massed in the distal half of the stomach, *partial or subtotal gastrectomy* will be the method selected. When, however, the disease appears to be diffuse, *total gastrectomy* becomes obligatory.

REFERENCES

1. Balfour, Surg. Gynecol. Obstet. 28:465, 1919.
2. Beal, Ill. Med. J. 136:242, 1969.
3. Benedict and Allen, Surg. Gynecol. Obstet. 63:79, 1934.

4. Berg, Cancer 11:1149, 1958.
5. Block et al., Bull. Soc. Int. Chir. 25:266, 1966.
6. Brodowski, Virchows. Arch. [Path. of Anat.] 67:227, 1876.
7. Burgess, Dockerty, and ReMine, Ann. Surg. 173:758, 1971.
8. Carlson and Ward, Surg. Gynecol. Obstet. 107:727, 1958.
9. Carnazzo and Organ, Nebr. State Med. J. July:415, 1970.
10. Case, J. Am. Geriatr. Soc. 19:86, 1971.
11. Chaffin, West. J. Surg. 46:513, 1938.
12. Crile and Groves, Gastroenterology 24:560, 1953.
13. D'Aunoy and Zoeller, Am. J. Surg. 9:444, 1930.
14. Doyle et al., N. Engl. J. Med. 249:477, 1953.
15. Eklöf, Acta Radiol. 58:177, 1962.
16. Elgood, Br. J. Surg. 38:388, 1951.
17. Eliason and Wright, Surg. Gynecol. Obstet. 41:401, 1925.
18. Ewing, Neoplastic Diseases, 1928.
19. Friedman, Am. J. Med. 26:783, 1959.
20. Gilbertson et al., Surg. Gynecol. Obstet. 98:186, 1954.
21. Hart, Br. J. Surg. 54:157, 1967.
22. Hoerr, Am. J. Surg. 109:14, 1965.
23. Hoffman and Goligher, Br. J. Surg. 58:126, 1971.
24. Ives, Br. J. Surg. 37:477, 1950.
25. Kay, Surg. Gynecol. Obstet. 118:1059, 1964.
26. Kiefer, Surg. Clin. North Am. June:711, 1941.
27. Lawrence, Am. J. Surg. 31:499, 1936.
28. Marshall and Adamson, Surg. Clin. North Am. 39:699, 1959.
29. Marshall and Meissner, Ann. Surg. 131:824, 1950.
30. Menétrier, Arch. Physiol. Norm. Pathol. 32:236, 1888.
31. Minnes and Geschickter, Am. J. Surg. 28:136, 1936.
32. Monaco, Cancer 15:456, 1962.
33. Monaco and Tomasolo, Cancer 27:1346, 1971.
34. Palmer, Medicine 30:81, 1951.
35. Patterson, Ann. Surg. 135:646, 1952.
36. Pearl and Brunn, Surg. Gynecol. Obstet. 76:257, 1946.
37. ReMine, Am. J. Surg. 120:320, 1970.
38. Ritchie, Br. Med. J. 2:1012, 1951.
39. Rutten, Br. J. Surg. 52:920, 1965.
40. Snoddy, Gastroenterology 20:537, 1952.
41. Spriggs and Marxer, Q. J. Med. 12:1, 1943.
42. Stewart, Lancet 2:670, 1931.
43. Strode, Surgery 41:236, 1957.
44. Tempest, Br. J. Surg. 38:525, 1951.
45. Thompson and Oyster, Gastroenterology 15:185, 1950.
46. Yarnis et al., J.A.M.A. 148:1088, 1952.

E. GASTRIC CYTOLOGY

J. G. S. CRABBE

The diagnosis of a gastric lesion is often difficult because of uncertain or even negative findings by x-ray or gastroscopy; therefore, when the lesion is suspected of being malignant, any procedure that makes it possible to detect this at an early or even at a preinvasive stage is well worth the fullest trial.

As long ago as 1882, Rosenbach[17] observed tumour particles in gastric washings, and since then a number of workers[11, 12, 19] have attempted to examine the gastric contents in order to achieve this end. In 1942, Frishman and Gorin[6] found cancer cells and fragments in gastric washings from patients suspected of having cancer of the stomach. After the successful use of exfoliative cytology as applied to gynaecological and other body fluids, Papanicolaou and Cooper[15] had some success when applying the method to specimens obtained by gastric lavage. Further trial by them and other workers, however, showed that its clinical application was limited by frequently missed diagnoses and, consequently, other techniques were introduced with a view to improving their results in this field.

TECHNIQUES FOR OBTAINING CELLULAR MATERIAL

There are several different methods of obtaining and examining cellular material from the stomach.

Lavage techniques. These techniques employ saline or Ringer's solution[21] or fluids containing mucolytic enzymes such as papain or chymotrypsin.[18, 26, 29] A Ryle or Levin tube is passed into the stomach, preferably by mouth, and with a 50-ml syringe, about 100 to 300 ml of the lavage fluid is forcibly injected and reinjected several times. When

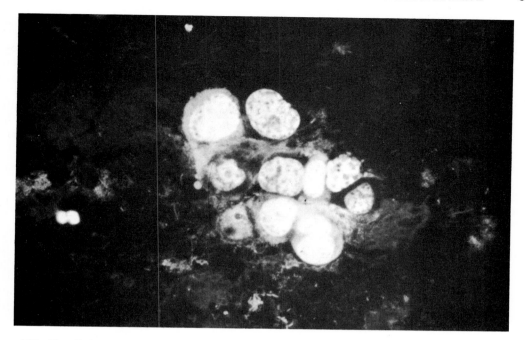

FIG. 38. Malignant cells from a gastric carcinoma. Stained wih acridine orange. (Courtesy of Dr. Chandra Grubb.)

the stomach is full of fluid, the patient is made to move around into several different positions so as to ensure thorough washing of the gastric mucosa before the fluid is finally withdrawn. The whole procedure does not take more than 10 to 15 minutes to perform, and success depends upon vigorous agitation during lavage. By the addition of mucolytic enzymes, the mucus is dissolved and it is claimed that this ensures better concentration and preservation of the cells.

Another method employed recently is by the use of forced lavage.[2, 28] Either a Levin or a modified Faucher tube is connected to a vacuum flask, which in turn is attached to an aspiration compressor motor. The apparatus forcibly injects the lavage solution and thus performs the washing. The authors claim that the procedure only takes 10 minutes. Using any of these methods, the washings are centrifuged and smears made from the deposit.

Abrasive techniques. A variety of different kinds of apparatus is used for this purpose. Panico, Papanicolaou, and Cooper [14] use an inflatable balloon which is covered with an abrasive net and attached to a gastric tube. Henning [7] uses a retractable sponge, and Ayre and Oren [1] a retractable brush. With the balloon method, the apparatus is introduced into the stomach; the balloon is inflated and left in situ for about an hour to enable it to be forced into the pyloric antrum by peristaltic movement.

The retractable sponge or brush is situated inside a plastic tube and attached to a flexible cable with a plunger and handle at the proximal end. This enables the sponge or brush to be rotated and moved about in the stomach. A syringe can also be applied to remove the washings. Smears are made from the centrifuged washings and from material obtained from the abrasive mechanism.

The advantage of the abrasive techniques over the lavage methods is that the cellular material is much better preserved and a higher degree of accuracy is attained. On the other hand, the application of the techniques of the abrasive method takes much longer to perform and also causes more discomfort to the patient. Added to this, the operation often must be performed in front of a fluorescent screen [4] to ensure that the abrasive mechanism is inserted right down into the pyloric region of the stomach. Moreover, these abrasive methods of obtaining washings are not entirely without risk.[20]

Fluorescence techniques. More recent attempts to improve on the results of gastric cytodiagnoses have been by the use of fluorescence techniques. The washings are examined after ingestion of atabrine,[8] or tetracycline,[9, 27] which produces autofluorescence of the cells, or the smears are stained with acridine orange.[3]

Takenaka, M.[24] actually stains the cells in situ by using lavage fluid containing acridine orange. All these substances fluoresce when viewed with intense blue or ultraviolet light, and malignant cells fluoresce with a higher degree of intensity than normal ones (Fig. 38).

A simple variation of this method [13] is to administer atabrine and, after a suitable interval of time, to examine the gross gastric sediment for fluorescence, which is greater when a carcinoma is present.

Fibrogastroscopic methods. The most recent development for examination of gastric cytological specimens, particularly in Japan, is by the use of the fibrogastroscope. In 1962 S. Takenaka,[25] using this instrument, was able to wash selected areas for cytological examination, to photograph them, and to take specimens for biopsy. Also, by this means the area can be brushed [10] and imprints taken from the surface.[30] A very much greater degree of accuracy is claimed by the use of this instrument.[23]

PRECAUTIONS

No matter which technique is used, the material will be unsatisfactory unless the stomach has been in a fasting state for at least 8 to 12 hours and is clean prior to the collection of the specimens. If obstruction is present, the stomach must be thoroughly emptied and washed out beforehand; otherwise the specimens will be unsatisfactory due to digestion of the cellular contents by the gastric juices or to contamination by particles of food. The washings must be performed before any barium meals are given

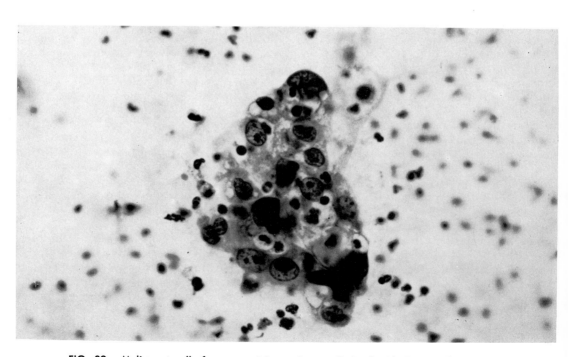

FIG. 39. Malignant cells from a gastric carcinoma. Stained with Papanicolaou stain.

or, failing that, not until at least 3 to 4 days afterwards.

It is most important that the specimens be processed immediately after collection. Indeed, Rastgeldi, Tomenius, and Williams [16] consider this to be so important that the washings are actually centrifuged at the patient's bedside. After centrifugation of a portion of the washings, smears are made from the deposit, stained, and mounted in balsam.

The slides are then scrutinized for the presence of cells showing malignant features. These apply principally to the nucleus and can be briefly summarised as: increase in size, hyperchromasia, irregularity in shape, and variation in size of the nuclei. There is a marked increase in the amount of chromatin and alteration of the chromatin pattern, while the nucleoli may be prominent and enlarged. The cells generally may be much enlarged and show very abnormal shapes (Fig. 39).

CYTOLOGICAL EXAMINATION

In washings from normal stomachs the cells most commonly seen are squamous cells carried down from the pharynx and oesophagus together with varying amounts of erythrocytes and leucocytes and histiocytes. As the stomach is lined with simple columnar epithelium of the mucus-secreting type, these cells may often be seen singly or in sheets and clusters and have a honeycomb appearance (Fig. 40). Sometimes cytolysis is very marked and nuclei without any cytoplasm

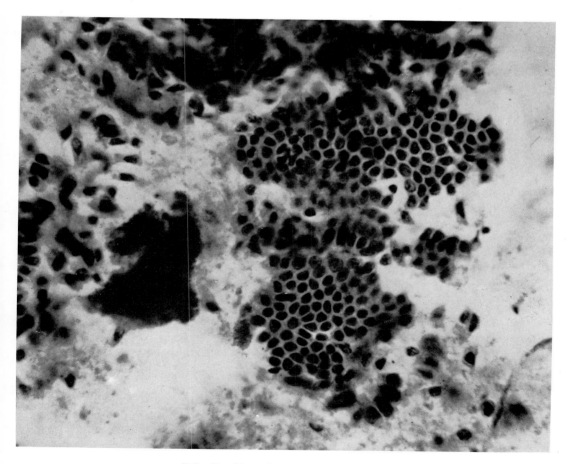

FIG. 40. Normal gastric mucosal cells.

may be present in very large numbers. It is not uncommon to see large dust-containing histiocytes in gastric washings due to sputum having been swallowed. Occasionally, partially digested food particles may be seen in the smears and these are easily recognisable by their unusual appearance. If the lavage tube is passed through the nose, cells from the nasopharynx may be present and, on occasion, such cells may simulate neoplastic ones until careful examination reveals the presence of cilia or brush borders.

Chronic irritation or gastric or duodenal ulcers cannot be distinguished with any degree of certainty from a study of the cytological picture. There may be more cytolysis than usual and there will be an increase in the number of leucocytes and histiocytes present. If an ulcer is very large and far advanced, on rare occasions, smooth muscle fibres may be seen in the smears. With achlorhydria, well-preserved squamous cells will be present in abundance. When obstruction is present, there may be diffuse bleeding and there is very marked cytolysis with the whole of the smear containing very many large rod-shaped bacilli. Characteristic cells are sometimes seen in cases of chronic hypertrophic gastritis, and these are usually present both singly and in clusters. They are of medium size, round, and often vacuolated with large eccentric nuclei.

One of the great advantages of the technique is that with cytological examination the early unsuspected carcinomas tend to show up better than the large far-advanced ones,[22] and thus a positive report can be a very great help to the clinicians. On the other hand, a negative report does not mean that a tumour is not present. Gastric mucosa cells do not readily exfoliate to any extent, and under certain conditions, they may be rapidly destroyed by the gastric juices. An advanced growth may have its entire surface ulcerated and covered with sloughs so that no cells are able to exfoliate, and indeed, a malignant leather-bottle stomach, while showing up clearly on x-ray, may contain perfectly normal looking cells in the washings. Finally, intramural or submucosal tumours may be covered with normal mucosa.

Cantrell,[5] in a paper entitled "Why Use Cytology" states that the cytological examination of gastric washings is necessary because cancer of the stomach is still a poorly diagnosed condition.

REFERENCES

1. Ayre, J. E., and Oren, B. G., Cancer 6:1177, 1963.
2. Bastos, A. L., and Madeira, F., Gut 5:192, 1964.
3. Bertalanffy, L., Masin, M., and Masin, F. Science 124:1024, 1956.
4. Bruinsma, A. H., Thesis, Leyden, 1957.
5. Cantrell, E. G., Gut 10:763, 1969.
6. Frishman, R. L., and Gorin, M. G., Klin. Med. (Mosk.) 20:59, 1942.
7. Henning, N., Dtsch. Med. Wochenschr. 77:1, 1952.
8. Henning, N., and Witte, S., Atlas of Gastroenterological Cytodiagnosis 1957, p. 39.
9. Klinger, J., and Katz, R., Gastroenterology 41:29, 1961.
10. Kobayashi, S., Prolla, J. C., and Kirsner, S. B., Acta Cytol. (Baltimore) 14:219, 1970.
11. Loeper, M., and Binet, M. E., Bull. Mem. Soc. Med. Hop. Paris 31:563, 1911.
12. Moutier, F., Arch. Mal. App. Dig. 24:1099, 1934.
13. Oria, M., and Ferrares, C. M., Minerva Chir. 19:305, 1964.
14. Panico, F. G., Papanicolaou, G. N., and Cooper, W. A., J.A.M.A. 143:1308, 1950.
15. Papanicolaou, G. N., and Cooper, W. A., J. Natl. Cancer Inst. 7:351, 1947.
16. Rastgeldi, S., Tomenius, J. H., and Williams, G., Acta Med. Scand. 163:531, 1959.
17. Rosenbach, C., Dtsch. Med. Wochenschr. 33, 1882.
18. Saburi, R., Ando, T., Kakihana, M., Tabayshi, A., and Yamada, T., Acta Cytol. (Baltimore) 11:473, 1967.
19. Sadek, O., Bratisl. Lek. Listy 5:168, 1925.
20. Sasson, L., Am. J. Dig. Dis. 9:398, 1964.
21. Schade, R. O. K., Br. Med. J. 1:743, 1958
22. Schade, R. O. K., Proc. R. Soc. Med. 63:8, 1970.
23. Shida, S., Sawada, Y., Takamura, S., Kondo, T., Takemato, T., and Tsuneoka, K., Gastroenterscopy Jap. 2:101 1967.
24. Takenaka, M., Stomach Intest (Tokyo) 5:733, 1970.
25. Takenaka, S., Gastroenterological Endosc. 4:4, 1962.
26. Ufelder, H., Graham, R. M., and Meigs, J. V., Ann. Surg. 128:422, 1942.
27. Velizaminov, Y. B., Sov. Med. 33:82, 1970.
28. Wenger, J., and Penfold, E., Gastroenterology 59:358, 1970.
29. Woyke, S., and Marliez, K., Pap. Pol. 20:49, 1969.
30. Yoshi, Y., Takahashi, J., Yamack, Y., and Kasugai, T., Acta Cytol. (Baltimore) 14:249, 1970.

29

SUBDIAPHRAGMATIC TOTAL GASTRECTOMY FOR MALIGNANT LESIONS OF THE STOMACH

RODNEY MAINGOT

In this operation, the *entire stomach is excised* and the cut end of the oesophagus is anastomosed to the cut end of the duodenum (oesophagoduodenostomy) or to a loop of proximal jejunum (oesophagojejunostomy), or a "replacement" procedure is carried out. When the resected stomach is examined, it will be seen to include at its pyloric end at least 1½ inches (3.8 cm) of the first part of the duodenum and at the cardiac end fully 1 inch (2.5 cm) of the oesophagus.

Total gastrectomy must be distinguished from subtotal gastrectomy, in which a small portion of the stomach is left behind. The distinction is important, as there are a number of cases recorded in the literature as total gastrectomies which, from the details, prove in fact to have been merely subtotal excisions of the stomach.

HISTORICAL NOTE

An able account of The Evolution of Total Gastrectomy is given by Rush and Ravitch (Int. Abst. Surg. 114:411, 1962).

Total gastrectomy was first performed by Connor in 1884 (Med. News 45:578, 1884). His patient died from shock, in the operating room, shortly after the operation. Schlatter (Beitr. Klin. Chir. 19:757, 1897) had the distinction of being the first surgeon to resect the entire stomach successfully. His patient was a woman aged 56 who lived for nearly 14 months following the operation (which was an oesophagojejunostomy), and died from secondary implants in the liver.

Brigham (Boston Med. Surg. J. 138:145, 1898) reported the second and third successful total gastrectomies, and Richardson (Boston Med. Surg. J. 139:381, 1898) the fourth. Krönlein, in 1898, coined the term *total gastrectomy*, as most descriptive of the operation for carcinoma of the stomach, and stated that it included "only those in which both the pylorus and the cardia had been removed, and which on examination showed a portion of the oesophagus at one end and the duodenum at the other." Among the early

pioneers in this field of aggressive surgery in the treatment of gastric cancer may be mentioned Harvie (1900), von Bardeleben (1901), Dollinger (1901), Herczel (1902), and Moynihan (1903).

Paterson (Hunterian Lect. 1906) collected reports of 27 cases of total gastrectomy for cancer of the stomach, in which 10 patients had died as a result of the operation and 17 recovered. Moynihan (Lancet 2:1748, 1907) gave his well-known classic account of the technical points of the operation and reported in detail a case of total gastrectomy for leather-bottle stomach. The patient upon whom he had operated was a man aged 43, who continued to live in good health until a few months before his death 3 years after the operation. This man died of pernicious anaemia, not of secondary deposits. The many readers of Moynihan's Abdominal Operations will remember his vivid description of this case and his lucid account of the various steps of his successful operation.

The first Roux-en-Y total gastrectomy was performed in 1908, and various technical improvements in the operation of total gastrectomy were submitted by Schloffer (1917), Hoffman (1922), Coenen (1930), Hilarowicz (1931), Allen (1938), Lahey (1938), Walton (1938), Joll (1938), Lahey and Marshall (1940), Lortat-Jacob (1941), Roscoe Graham (1943), Pack and McNeer (1945), Engel (1945), and Lefèvre (1946).

Finney and Rienhoff (Arch. Surg. 18:140, 1929) carefully tabulated most of the cases which had been recorded up to 1929. They were able to quote 62 cases from the literature and they added 5 of their own. In these 67 cases there was a 53.8 percent operative mortality rate, but there was a higher recovery rate with oseophagojejunostomy than with oesophagoduodenostomy.

Roeder (Ann. Surg. 98:221, 1933), in a comprehensive article, reported 88 cases, including 3 of his own, with a mortality rate of 44—i.e., 50 percent.

Waltman Walters' paper on the Physiologic and Chemical Studies Following Successful Total Gastrectomy for Cancer (J.A.M.A. 95:102, 1930) remains a classic dissertation which has had a distinct bearing upon the postoperative management of these cases. Stahnke (Zbl. Chir. 60:865, 1933) reported a case of a woman aged 39 who was living more than 8 years after total gastrectomy.

Allen (Am. J. Surg. 40:35, 1938) described 16

patients subjected to operation at the Massachusetts General Hospital, and Lahey (Surg. Gynecol. Obstet. 67:213, 1938), in an article replete with the most useful information, gave an account of his experiences with eight patients, five of whom successfully recovered from the operation and lived for varying periods of time after returning to their homes.

Morton (Surg. Gynecol. Obstet. 71:111, 1940) was one of the first to advise total gastrectomy for all resectable carcinomas of the stomach. Following this, there was considerable enthusiasm for total resection of the stomach and a number of reports were published, including those of Lahey (Surg. Gynecol. Obstet. 90:246, 1950), Pack and McNeer (Int. Abst. Surg. 77:265, 1943), and Waugh (Surg. Clin. North Am. 25:903, 1945). Subsequently, because of dissatisfaction (ReMine, Priestley, and Berkson. Surg. Gynecol. Obstet. 94: 519, 1952) relating to the high operative mortality and morbidity rates of total gastrectomy, attention was diverted to other approaches in the management of carcinoma of the stomach (e.g., high *subtotal* resection).

GENERAL PRINCIPLES

Determination of Operability

The abdomen is best explored through a lengthy left paramedian incision which commences at the costal margin and extends downward for 2 or 3 inches (5 to 7.6 cm) below the umbilicus. Some surgeons prefer a left rectus muscle-splitting incision, a transverse incision, or a large inverted U incision placed close to the costal margins. Improved exposure of the operative field may be obtained by excising the xiphoid process and/or by dividing the left costal margin and carrying the incision into the sixth or seventh space. (See Chaps. 1 and 30.)

When the abdomen is opened, the "first look" may settle the question of whether the patient is operable or inoperable. The patient is *inoperable* when the liver is studded with a large number of secondary deposits of growth; when carcinomatosis is obvious in that one can see and feel the numerous seedlings which are scattered throughout the peritoneal cavity and especially in the omenta; when malignant plaques occupy the pelvic shelf; when the cancerous stomach is welded to its bed, has invaded the vital vessels at the root of the mesentery, or is in the process of strangling the hepatic artery or portal vein; when the duodenum is hopelessly compromised; when the hilus of the liver is crowded with irremovable metastatic implants; and when, the lesser peritoneal cavity being displayed, numerous telltale nodules proclaim the futility of further enquiry.

Direct spread of the growth to the pancreas, liver, colon, and other adjacent structures does not necessarily imply that the patient is beyond the reach of aggressive surgery. In many instances, it is possible to remove the entire stomach and the spleen with portions of adjacent adherent viscera, such as the transverse colon, the tail and body of the pancreas, large segments of the liver, and so forth, without prohibitive mortality but with little hope of eventual success. Local spread to contiguous organs is not so baneful as *vascular permeation* and cellular emboli or the shedding of malignant cells into the greater or lesser peritoneal cavity—*gravity metastases.*

Extent of Operation

If total gastrectomy is to be applied to malignant lesions of the stomach, it should be *radical* in every sense of the word.

It is essential to emphasise once again that total removal of the stomach should be employed only in those cases of cancer of the stomach in which there is a reasonable possibility of removing all malignant tissue. The surgeon should always *strive* for a curative procedure. Total gastrectomy should not be carried out for palliation, since, as Marshall [12] has pointed out, such an operation will not prolong life or make the patient more comfortable and will only add to the operative morbidity and mortality. The symptoms of extensive gastric cancer with obstruction can be alleviated more readily with subtotal than with total gastrectomy. Subtotal gastrectomy does not carry the operative mortality or the postoperative nutritional and metabolic problems that are associated with total gastrectomy, and the patient will survive longer.

The *requirements of a total gastrectomy* must obviously include a block dissection of the entire stomach, the first part of the duodenum, the whole of the greater omentum, the gastrosplenic omentum, the spleen, the tail and body of the pancreas (some cases), the lesser omentum into the porta hepatis and as far to the right as where the hepatic artery gives off its feeding branches to the liver, the soft areolar tissues around the cardia, and a cuff of the distal portion of the oesophagus. The vagus nerves must be isolated and severed, and the connective tissues around them must be swept downward towards the cardia. The greater part of the dissection takes place in a plane of embryological zygosis on the dorsal abdominal wall.

All the regional lymph nodes are, of course, included in this massive and formidable en-bloc resection, with the possible exception of those lymph nodes that lurk in their hidden retreat behind the vascular bed of the head and body of the pancreas.

Total gastrectomy by the *thoracoabdominal route* is described in Chapter 30.

Following total gastrectomy by the *abdominal route,* the continuity of the alimentary canal is restored by one of many methods.

Classification of Methods of Anastomosis

Methods of anastomosis may be classified as follows:

I.   Oesophagojejunostomy

A.   Proximal jejunal loop anastomosed to the divided end of the oesophagus, end-to-side, followed by a *long jejunojejunostomy* with the object of deflecting the bile and pancreatic juices away from the oesophageal stoma and at the same time serving as a reservoir for food. The operation may be performed by the antecolic or retrocolic method, preferably the former.

B.   Roscoe Graham's technique.

C.   Lefèvre's technique.

D.   Y-shaped jejunal loop after the manner of Roux.

II. Oesophagoduodenostomy—end-to-end union (Madden's technique).

III. Replacement of the stomach by a segment of jejunum, using Kondo's "figure 6" loop jejunum, a segment of transverse colon, or the ileocolic segment.

At the present time the operation of choice is, in my opinion, total gastrectomy followed by *oesophagojejunostomy,* in which the first loop of the jejunum is drawn upward, anterior to the transverse colon, and anastomosed, to the prepared distal end of the oesophagus by the end-to-side method, the operation being completed by performing *a large entero-anastomosis between the afferent and efferent limbs of the jejunum* in order to ensure the maximum shunting of bile and pancreatic juice from the oesophagoenteric stoma, and at the same time to serve as a pouch for food. This procedure is cogently supported by many surgeons, including ReMine and Priestley.[15] This operation and its variations will be described later.

As one of the requisites of a satisfactory total gastrectomy is resection of the whole first portion of the duodenum, it would appear that the operation of *oesophagoduodenostomy* will be practised less frequently in the future. It has many appealing features, and it would seem reasonable to suspect that those surgeons who have perfected the technique of this operation will continue to apply it in cases of cancer affecting the proximal portion of the stomach. This procedure is associated with a higher mortality rate than oesophagojejunostomy, owing to the not infrequent occurrence of leakage at the suture line.

Later on in this chapter I shall deal only briefly with *replacement procedures* following subdiaphragmatic total gastrectomy for cancer, as this subject is fully discussed and illustrated in Chapter 30.

Indications for Total Gastrectomy

The indications for total gastrectomy may be listed as follows:

1.   Carcinomatous leather-bottle stomach and diffuse gastric cancer.

2.   Large infiltrating gastric sarcomas of lymphoid origin, especially when they involve the proximal half of the stomach.

3.   *Diffuse* adenomatous polyposis of the stomach.

4.   Cancers involving the proximal half of the stomach, which include those situated (but not involving) the cardia and those infiltrating the upper reaches of the lesser curvature of the stomach.

5.   Large or multiple leiomyosarcomas of the stomach, especially when the proxi-

mal half of the stomach is the seat of the lesion.

6. Suspicious "cardial" ulcers which are unsuitable for resection by Pauchet's method (rare), or when such ulcers are judged by the surgeon and his assistants to be malignant in nature.

7. In certain cases of ulcerogenic tumours.

Total gastrectomy should not, as previously emphasised, be employed as the routine procedure in the treatment of carcinoma of the stomach. Radical subtotal gastrectomy with removal of the omenta, the regional lymph nodes, and the spleen is still the most satisfactory method in the majority of cases of gastric cancer (80 percent). Owing to the position of the lesion, total excision is mandatory in about 20 percent of cases of gastric cancer. The operative mortality rate of total gastrectomy is, of course, higher than that of subtotal gastrectomy. (See *Prognosis of Malignant Lesions of the Stomach* by ReMine and Priestley in Chapter 28, Part B, and by Sedgwick in Part C.)

The all-around operative death rate for subtotal gastrectomy for gastric cancer is about 4 to 8 percent, while for total gastrectomy the figures vary from 10 to 16 percent.

The average age of patients suffering from carcinoma of the stomach has steadily increased, and the older patient, the greater the risk.

The operative mortality rate, as would be expected, is higher in total gastrectomy than in subtotal resection; likewise the mechanical aspects and the nutritional and metabolic consequences are all augmented following total ablation of the viscus (see Chaps. 27 and 106).

If only a remnant of stomach remains after gastric resection, it would appear to be sufficient to maintain a reasonable state of nutrition, to combat the grave types of anaemia, and to reduce or at least mitigate many of the evil and unpleasant postoperative sequelae which so commonly follow in the wake of total ablation of the stomach.

Once again my advice is this: Do not resort to total gastrectomy except in those patients whose gross disease can be eliminated only by this procedure.

Complications and Sequelae of Total Gastrectomy

Immediate. These complications include: (1) Chest complications—atelectasis, pneumonia, bronchopneumonia: cardiac failure; embolism (Chaps. 26 and 57). (2) Peritonitis and subphrenic abscess. (3) External fistula—due to breaking down of the anastomosis (Chap. 9). (4) wound infections and disruption of abdominal wounds (Chap. 2). (5) steatorrhoea. (6) Acute small gut obstruction. (7) Avitaminosis, especially deficiencies in Vitamin B. (8) Phlebothrombosis and thrombophlebitis.

Late. These complications include: (1) The "dumping syndrome" (Chap. 27). (2) Haematological complications (Chaps. 26 Part C). (3) Dysphagia; stenosis of the oesophagoenteric stoma. (4) Symptoms caused by nutritional, metabolic, and functional derangements—e.g., hypoproteinaemia, steatorrhoea, loss of weight, anorexia, osteomalacia, etc. (5) Intestinal obstruction. (6) Incisional hernia (Chap. 71). (7) Recurrence of growth.

Peritonitis and subphrenic abscess were the most frequent causes of death prior to 1943 —i.e., before the lavish use of the sulphonamides and antibiotics. These complications accounted for about 40 percent of the fatalities.

Cardiovascular disease, embolism, massive atelectasis, and pneumonia are now the principal complications that call for immediate attention in the postoperative phase.

Pneumonitis and cardiovascular accidents account for most of the deaths in elderly subjects, although sepsis still ranks high in the list of postoperative complications following total gastrectomy.

A grave and much-feared complication is the *formation of an external fistula* due to a defect or perforation in the suture line (Chap. 9).

Leakage at the oesophago-enteric stoma is an ominous feature, and in most cases it is a harbinger of death. Attempts to *repair the hole in the line of anastomosis* by the insertion of a number of interrupted sutures usually ends in disaster. The introduction of a moderately large stomach tube through

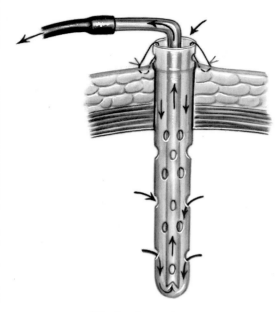

FIG. 1. Sump drain.

the oesophagus into the efferent limb of the jejunum to splint the stoma should be attempted, and if it is successfully placed in position, it may, in part, stem the flow of intestinal juices onto the skin of the abdomen. Continuous suction should be applied to a sump drain (Fig. 1) which has been introduced at the top of the abdominal incision down to the leaking area, and intravenous feeding and blood transfusions instituted without delay. If all fails and the fistulous discharge shows no sign of abating, a Stamm or Marwedhel jejunostomy will have to be performed under local anaesthesia for feeding purposes.

Severe diarrhoea may be caused by severance of the vagus nerves or by a bacterial enterocolitis. A short course of treatment with oral neomycin or colomycin will often prove beneficial in a number of these cases (Chap. 107).

Following total gastrectomy by the Roux-en-Y plan or in which the continuity of the alimentary canal has been restored by end-to-side oesophagojejunostomy combined with entero-anastomosis, *dysphagia* due to narrowing and spasm of the stoma occurs in 10 percent of the patients, and will for correction by dilatation with bougies. This symptom will require investigation by means of radiography and oesophagoscopy to exclude the possibility of a *recurrence of the growth* or a *fibrous stenosis of the stoma.*

Wangensteen [19] has advocated a *"second look"* for those patients with visceral cancer who have been subjected to some type of resection. He writes:

In cases of alimentary tract cancer and especially in patients with gastric cancer, when the lymph nodes are found to be involved, we propose to the patient that we take a "second look" after the lapse of approximately six months after the initial operation.
We have done "second looks" upon 16 patients who had metastatic cancer in the regional lymph nodes. Eleven showed residual evidence of cancer, that is, 68 percent. The cooperation of patients in this venture has not been lacking. I would like to add that I believe this is going to become an important activity of the surgeon on the management of visceral cancer.

This subject is also discussed by McNeer and co-workers.[10] It would appear to me that the "second look" has met with steadily decreasing favour in Britain.

Kirschner and Garlock [6] described their experiences with total gastrectomy:

While the increasing number of total gastrectomies reported in the literature has been accompanied by a marked reduction in the operation mortality, there has followed a rapidly increasing high morbidity in terms of impairment of digestive function, anaemia, malnutrition, stricture of the anastomosis, diarrhoea, and loss of earning power. The vast majority of these survivors become emaciated digestive cripples, difficult to manage therapeutically.

Preoperative Care

These patients are admitted to hospital about one week before operation for a complete evaluation of their physical condition and for an intensive course of preoperative treatment.

The chief aims of preoperative treatment are: (1) to correct starvation and nutritional disturbances; (2) to restore blood chemistry changes to normal; (3) to teach deep breathing and coughing exercises and improve muscle function; (4) to eliminate oral sepsis; (5) to institute gastric lavage; (6) to treat symptoms; (7) to treat anaemia by blood transfusion; and (8) to correct avitaminosis. A nasogastric tube should be passed into the stomach some two to three hours before operation and be left in place, as it will be required for suction purposes both during and after operation.

TOTAL GASTRECTOMY FOLLOWED BY OESOPHAGOJEJU-NOSTOMY

Incision

The best abdominal approach to the oesophagus and stomach is a long left paramedian incision which commences over the left lower coastal cartilages and extends downwards 2 inches (5 cm) or so below the umbilicus. The fleshy belly of the left rectus muscle must be mobilised and dislocated in an outward direction. This incision may be extended to give a better view of the cardia by removal of xiphoid process, by dividing the left costal margin, and by carrying the incision into the sixth intercostal space. Good retraction of the divided costal margin will often make division of the diaphragm unnecessary.

Before undertaking the operation, a most scrupulous examination of the stomach, the oesophagus, the regional lymph nodes, the liver, the mesenteries, the omental bursa, and the pelvic shelf should be carried out not only to determine whether there is any extragastric involvement but also to test the mobility of the stomach and the possible ease with which it can be resected, and to gauge the length of the intra-abdominal portion of the oesophagus. It is not wise to proceed with this operation if there are metastatic implants (1) in the liver, (2) in the mesocolon, or (3) where growth has involved the superior mesenteric vessels, the aorta, the inferior vena cava, the lesser peritoneal cavity, or the pelvic peritoneum.

Operation

The first step in the operation consists of lifting the greater omentum vertically upward, detaching it from the transverse colon, and gently peeling off the upper

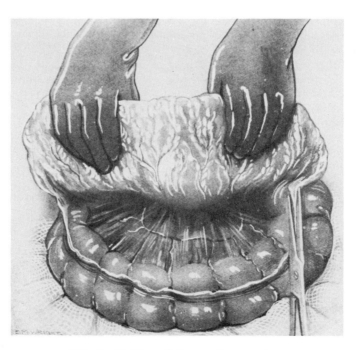

FIG. 2. Excision of the greater omentum.

leaf of the mesocolon from the fatty bed in which the right colic vessels and arching middle colic vessels lie (Fig. 2). If the superior leaf of the mesocolon has been freely stripped away, it will bare the pancreas and facilitate the clearance of the nodes below and behind the pylorus and the first portion of the duodenum. The greater omentum and superior leaf of the mesocolon will now be seen hanging from the stomach. The right gastro-epiploic artery is isolated, ligated in two places, and divided; the gastrohepatic omentum is cut adrift from its flimsy attachment to the liver, and at its right border—the hepatoduodenal pedicle—the lymph nodes extending to the hilus of the liver are stripped downward toward the pylorus; the now-naked right gastric artery is ligated and cut where it springs from the hepatic artery; and the first two portions of the duodenum are freed. After the loose cellular tissues with their contained nodes (the pyloric, subpyloric and superior retropancreatic) are pushed towards the pylorus, the bowel is transected 1 inch (2.5 cm) or so above the papilla of Vater, and the distal end closed with two rows of inverting sutures. The entire first part of the duodenum with its related nodes, the common bile duct node, and the nodes which occupy the curving portion of the head of the pancreas remain clinging to the specimen, which is about to be removed en masse.

The suspensory ligament of the left lobe of the liver is divided with scissors and the mobilised portion of the liver is retracted medially; anterior and posterior peritoneal flaps are raised from the oesophagus and drawn upward; the gullet is put on the stretch to facilitate the division of the anterior and posterior vagus nerves; the areolar tissue that covers the distal ends of the vagus nerves is swept downward toward the cardia in order to bare the oesophagus; and the connective tissue about the crura and oesophageal opening is coaxed toward the posterior aspect of the cardia.

The spleen is next firmly drawn toward the midline so as to expose the posterior leaf of the lienorenal ligament and the peritoneum overlying the left kidney. A long, curving incision is made through the peritoneum in this area which extends to the one previously made when the peritoneal flaps

were being fashioned. The right hand of the surgeon is now slipped through this incision and is insinuated behind the spleen and the tail and body of the pancreas. As I have said previously, the greater part of the dissection takes place in a plane of embryological zygosis on the dorsal abdominal wall. As the mass of spleen, greater omentum, stomach, and tail of the pancreas are lifted out of the wound and pulled upward and outward to the right, the extensive raw surface on the posterior abdominal wall is immediately covered with warm moist packs. The hepatic artery and coeliac axis are cleared of nodes and fatty tissue, after which the splenic artery, together with the splenic vein, is ligated proximal to the left gastroepiploic artery. This ligation of the splenic blood supply will permit easy removal of the spleen without multiple clamping, division, and ligation of the vasa brevia. The left gastric vein is then cleaned of fat and areolar tissue, and clipped, ligated, and divided close to the upper border of the pancreas, after which the right gastric artery is isolated for ½ inch (1.27 cm) or so and down to the point where it springs from the coeliac axis. After it has been stripped of surrounding fatty tissue and lymph nodes that are swept toward the lesser curvature, this vessel is doubly ligated with strong silk or catgut, and divided.

If the tail or body of the pancreas is involved in growth or is adherent to the stomach, the pancreas should be transected at a point that is lateral to the superior mesenteric vessels.

A sedulous search should always be made for the divided end of the pancreatic duct, and when it has been identified, it should be ligated with fine silk, after which the oozing stump of the pancreas should be securely closed with a series of mattress sutures of fine serumproof silk.

The stomach with its weighty appendages is next drawn downward and to the left of the patient, to facilitate a further dissection of the small but important area around the hepatic artery. Starting at the inferior margin of the liver, all the tissues and nodes in this vascular zone are cautiously dissected downward to the lesser curvature of the stomach. When this dissection has been completed, the entire length of the bared, throbbing, and

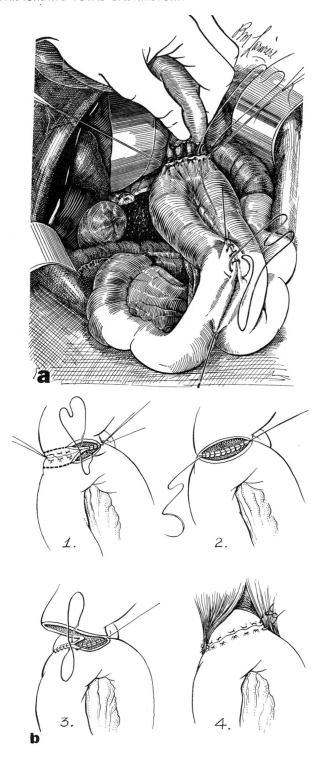

FIG. 3. (A) Subdiaphragmatic total gastrectomy. The jejunal loop selected for anastomosis is being sutured to the posterior aspect of the oesophagus by a series of interrupted mattress sutures of fine silk. The first posterior continuous suture of the entero-anastomosis is being inserted. A large stoma should be provided. (B) Oesophagojejunostomy: a simple method of performing the anastomosis.

curving hepatic artery can be clearly visu-alised.

Traction is now made on the oesophagus to facilitate further finger and gauze dissection around and above the oesophageal foramen. If the mobilisation has been well done, a segment of oesophagus measuring about 5 to 7 cm should be available for anastomosis.

The stomach and its appendages are encased in a special, spacious waterproof transparent acrylic bag, the open end of which is drawn together and then firmly tied to point just distal to the cardia. After the gastric contents have been aspirated, an indwelling Ryle or Levin tube is withdrawn for the time being into the lower end of the gullet, and a stout silk ligature or piece of linen tape is applied to the oesophagus just proximal to the cardiooesophageal junction, and tied very firmly. This prevents the contents of the stomach from spilling over into the oesophagus and possibly into the lungs.

A portion of the jejunum some 8 to 10 inches (20 to 25 cm) from the fixed duodenojejunal flexure is selected for the anasto-

mosis, brought in front of the transverse colon, and laid against the undersurface of the oesophagus, which is now well displayed by the exerting of steady traction on the stomach in an upward direction, toward the patient's chin.

The jejunum is sutured to the posterior wall of the oesophagus with a series of interrupted mattress sutures of fine silk, and at the right and left extremities of the suture line two of these sutures are left long to act as tractors (Fig. 3A). In front of these interrupted sutures a small opening is made into the oesophagus at the extreme left end of its attachment, and the suction tube in the oesophagus removes any contained secretions. A small longitudinal incision is then made through the antimesenteric border of the jejunum just distal to the first row of anchoring mattress sutures of fine silk. A posterior continuous lockstitch suture of 00 chromic catgut, mounted on a small, firm atraumatic (eyeless) needle, is introduced. Some surgeons prefer to use interrupted sutures for the outer and inner layers, and there can be no objec-

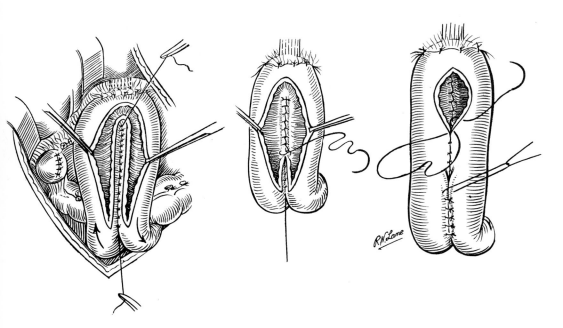

FIG. 4. Hoffman's jejunoplasty based on Finney's operation. When completed, this operation supplies a food pouch of moderate dimensions and helps diminish some unpleasant sequelae associated with the dumping syndrome.

tion to this method provided the sutures are introduced close to one another and in a watertight fashion.

These openings in the oesophagus and jejenum are enlarged little by little from left to right, and as they are enlarged, their cut edges are sutured together with a continuous *through-and-through all-coats lockstitch.* This sequence of a small incision, a few stitches, slight enlargement of the incision, and a few more stitches is continued until the whole of the posterior wall of the oesophagus has been divided and sutured to the adjacent margin of the jejunum. Around the anterior wall of the oesophagus the same sequence is continued, the stitch now being changed to the Connell type. The stomach is therefore used as a tractor, drawing up the oesophagus until the last piece is severed, at which juncture the line of anastomosis is completed, whereupon the anterior suture line is further reinforced and invaginated with a series of interrupted mattress sutures of fine silk. A few anchor sutures fixing the jejunum to the diaphragm are inserted, not only to prevent the oesophagus from slipping upward into the thoracic cavity but also to act as a sling which obviates any downward drag on the line of anastomosis.

The small posterior flap of diaphragmatic peritoneum, which was fashioned when the oesophagus was being freed posteriorly, is attached to the posterior wall of the jejunum with three or four interrupted sutures, and when this has been completed, the anterior flap of diaphragmatic peritoneum is attached to the anterior wall of the jejunum below the anastomosis to relieve the suture line from traction.

Great importance is attached to relieving as far as possible any strain on the suture line, owing to the fact that the oesophagus is very friable and leakage at the suture line is a complication to be feared.

The nasogastric tube, which was used to keep the stomach empty during the dissection and which was drawn into the lower end of the oesophagus during the performance of the anastomosis, is directed down the efferent limb of the jejunum before the anterior Connell suture is inserted. This tube is employed after operation for aspiration purposes. It is usually removed on the second or third postoperative day.

The operation is completed by making a *long entero-anastomosis between the proximal and distal loops of the jejunum* in order to divert the bile and pancreatic juices away from the oesophageal stoma and at the same time to act as a food reservoir (Figs. 4 and 5).

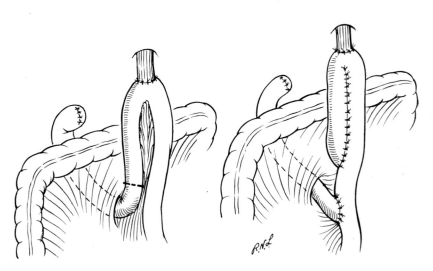

FIG. 5. A simple and effective method of forming a food pouch.

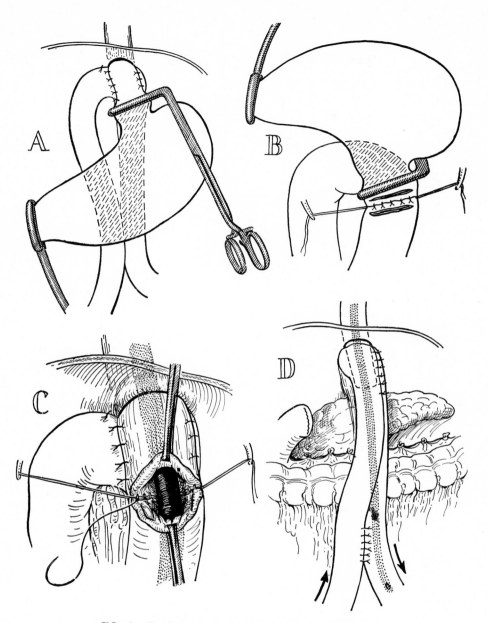

FIG. 6. Total gastrectomy. Roscoe Graham's technique.

As a precaution, two Penrose drains are inserted close to the oesophagojejunal junction and sutured to the skin, where they emerge at the top end of the incision and through a subcostal stab incision. The margins of the peritoneum and posterior rectus sheaths are approximated with a continuous lockstitch of 1 chromic catgut; the anterior rectus sheath is reconstructed with interrupted sutures of 0 or 1 nylon, or 30-gauge stainless steel wire; and the skin edges are united with vertical mattress sutures of fine black silk or Deknatel.

Hoffman and Engel preferred a Finney

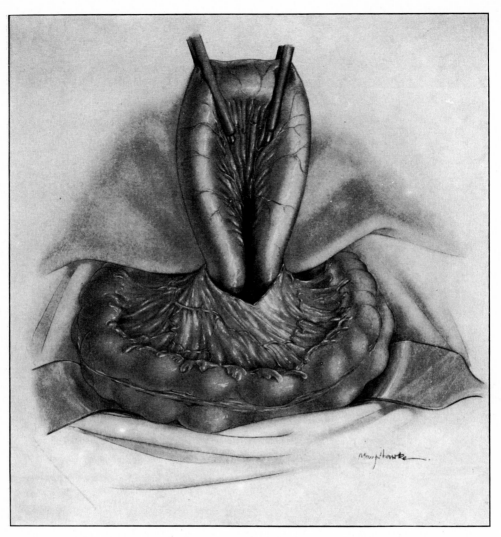

FIG. 7. Lèfevre's technique. The proximal jejunal loop is drawn into the supracolic department through an opening in the mesocolon.

type of *jejunoplasty* to the Braun entero-anastomisis (Figs. 4 and 5). The pouch that results from this type of jejunoplasty provides a miniature "stomach" for the reception of food.

This procedure of Engel's is ably described and illustrated step by step in Thorek's 1970 Atlas.[18]

Moynihan[13] was the first surgeon to suture the jejunum to the diaphgram for suspension. Hans Brun, in 1912, was the first to suggest removal of the spleen to facilitate total gas-trectomy, whilst Schmieden, in 1933, developed peritoneal flaps to cover the line of anastomosis.

Roscoe Graham's technique. The best description of this operation will be found in Archives of Surgery.[4]

After complete mobilisation of the stomach and division and closure of the duodenum, a strong, right-angled clamp is applied to the oesophagus just proximal to the cardia. This clamp aids in the downward traction of the stomach while the oesophagus is being

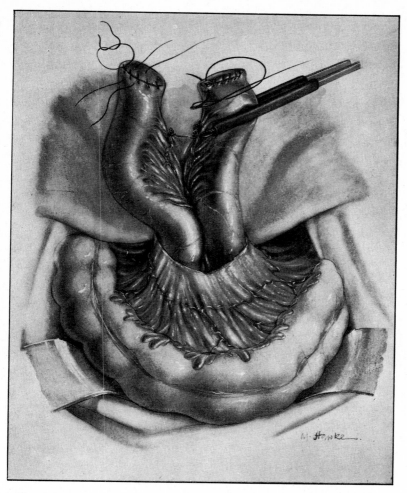

FIG. 8. Lefèvre's technique. Transection of the proximal loop of the jejunum and closure of both ends of the bowel.

sutured to the antimesenteric surface of the jejunal loop selected for anastomosis. It also prevents gastric contents from passing into the oesophagus and contaminating the stoma.

A loop of proximal jejunum some 12 to 15 inches (30 to 38 cm) from the duodenojejunal junction is brought in front of the transverse colon and sutured to the diaphragm. The apex of this loop is sutured to the oesophagus in the manner depicted in Figure 6. The most distal suture on each side is held in artery forceps to act as tractors. The oesophagus is divided and the jejunum opened, and after the posterior through-and-through all-coats lockstitch has been inserted, a Levin tube is guided down into the distal

limb of the jejunum. When the anterior suture line is completed, the proximal jejunal limb is rolled laterally across the oesophagus and sutured to the *left* lateral margin of the distal limb of the jejunum (Fig. 6D). This completely surrounds the infradiaphragmatic part of the oesophagus with jejunum and covers and supports the anastomotic line. This twisting of the proximal limb of jejunum to hide the suture line may partially obstruct the bowel, and a Braun enteroanastomosis becomes obligatory (see Fig. 6D).

Lefèvre's technique.[9] Lefèvre, who modified the operations of Hilarwociz (1931) and Roscoe Graham (1943), preferred the posterior or retrocolic approach. Figures 7 to

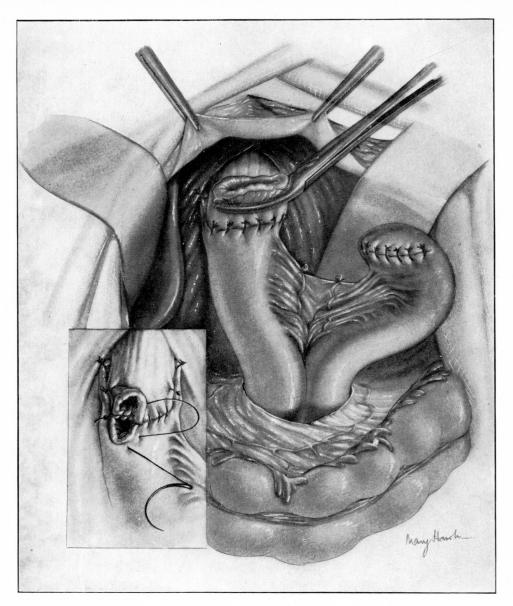

FIG. 9.   Lefèvre's technique. End-to-side anastomosis between the oesophagus and the efferent limb of the jejunum.

11 portray the essential steps and were drawn during an operation by the author at the Royal Free Hospital, London.

Roux-en-Y method. The operation of total gastrectomy proceeds along the lines already described until the stage is reached when the anastomosis should be performed. Figures 12 to 15 serve to explain the Roux-en-Y principle.

A loop of proximal jejunum, about 10 to 15 inches (25 to 38 cm) from the ligament of Treitz, is picked up and then divided between clamps. By progressive division of the arcade of vessels in the mesojejunum, the distal limb of jejunum is straightened out and elongated. The arcade closest to the bowel must not be cut at any point, since it must provide blood supply to the oesophagojejunal anastomosis.

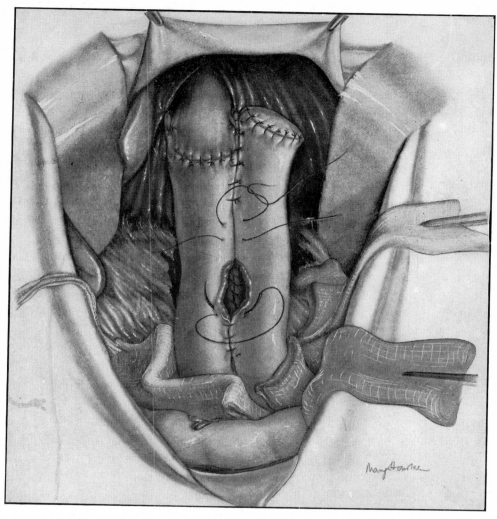

FIG. 10. Lefèvre's technique. The oesophagojejunostomy has been completed, and Braun's entero-anastomosis between the efferent and afferent jejunal limbs is being constructed to deflect bile and pancreatic juices away from the oesophagojejunal stoma.

During this liberation of the gut, ligation of individual vessels rather than the use of mass ligatures is an important point, or the cut end of the distal jejunum will remain curled or bowed toward the mesojejunum and cannot be straightened.

The anastomosis is now made between the distal ascending jejunal limb and the oesophagus by the end-to-end or end-to-side method. When this anastomosis is completed, the proximal jejunum is implanted into the distal jejunum, in the infracolic compartment, by a two-layer end-to-side anastomosis. The stoma is placed on the antimesenteric border of the distal jejunum. The jejunal limb that has been prepared for anastomosis to the oesophagus may be taken upward into the supracolic compartment in front of the colon or through an opening made in the mesacolon. My preference is for the *antecolic route* rather than the retrocolic approach. Oesophagitis and stenosis of the oesophagojejunal stoma rarely occur when the Roux-en-Y technique is employed. This operation, total gastrectomy employing a Roux-en-Y loop, has found favour with Reynolds and

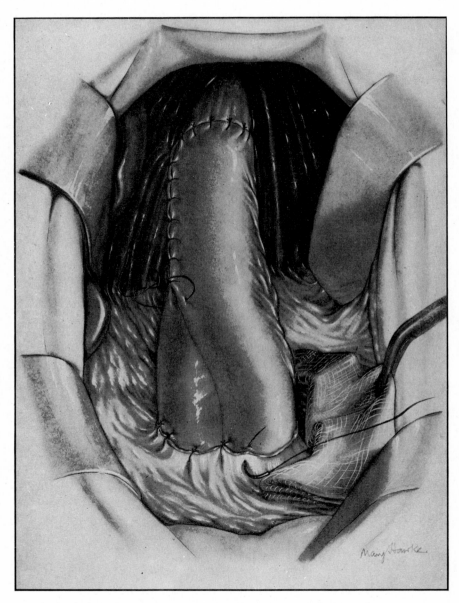

FIG. 11. Lefèvre's technique. The operation is nearly completed. Note that the afferent limb of the jejunum is sutured on top of the efferent limb and protects the stoma. Note also that the margins of the opening in the mesocolon are being sutured to the afferent and efferent limbs of the jejunum so that no gap remains. In many respects, the operation is a modification of a Roscoe Graham total gastrectomy with an oesophagojejunal anastomosis.

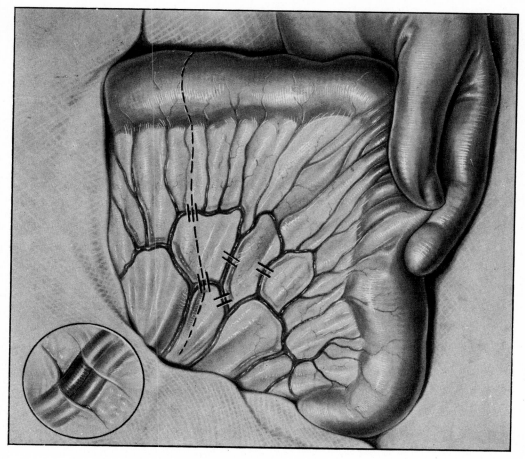

FIG. 12.   Roux-en-Y oesophagojejunostomy and end-to-side jejunojejunostomy.

Young,[16] Allison and Borrie,[9] Allison [1] (1950, and in 1969), Pack (1966), Qvist (1972), and many other surgeons.

TOTAL GASTRECTOMY WITH OESOPHAGODUODENAL ANASTOMOSIS

Doubilet [3] (1954), Madden,[11] in his *Atlas of Technics in Surgery* (1964) and others (Figs. 16–20) have advised *oesophago-duodenostomy in selected cases following total gastrectomy for carcinoma*. Although this operation after complete ablation of the stomach should be superior to oesophago-jejunostomy, on physiological grounds, clin-

ical observations tend to contradict this view. As Doubilet remarks, "This is due to the fact that the most important loss after gastrectomy is that of a storehouse for food." The use of a long jejunojejunostomy may, and in fact often does, produce sufficient storage space to compensate physiologically for the loss of duodenal function in oesophagojejunostomy. However, since admittedly oesophagoduode-nostomy can be carried out more expedi-tiously because only one anastomosis is required, the reason for avoiding this pro-cedure is the fear of tension at the anasto-mosis. When it is possible, as, for instance, in thin and visceroptotic patients, to mobilise the duodenum and head of the pancreas and to approximate the oesophagus to the divided end of the duodenum without any degree of tension, this operation will prove to be agree-

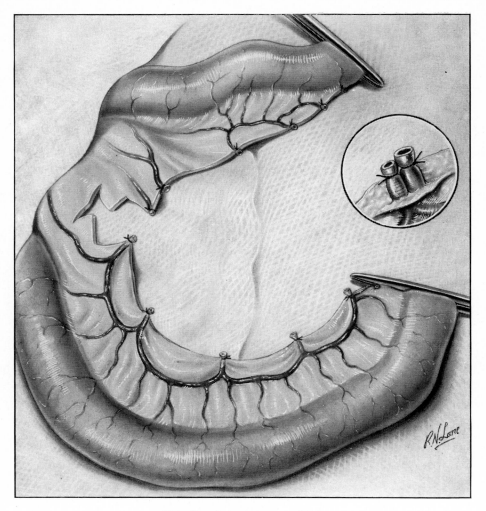

FIG. 13.   Roux-en-Y procedure.

ably straightforward and gratifying. Nevertheless, oesophagoduodenostomy has not found favour with many surgeons, mainly owing to the technical difficulties of overcoming the strain at the suture line and to the *relatively* high incidence of leakage of pancreatic juices, which leads to severe and often fatal complications. (Figs. 16–20.)

Lee [8] says that to the one who has had a total gastrectomy, the sequelae assume greater importance the longer he survives. "It is true that a good many patients make the adjustment to complete absence of a gastric reservoir astonishingly well. But the number who do not make such an adjustment is distressingly large."

Certain new procedures, which are now undergoing the acid test of trial and error and considerable experimental work, are: (1) Replacement with a segment of proximal jejunum, i.e., *oesophagojejunoduodenostomy,* or the *"figure 6" loop jejunum* procedure after total gastrectomy, as performed by Kondo and his colleagues,[7] in Japan, and which is illustrated in Figure 21. (2) Replacement with a segment of transverse colon. (3) Replacement by ileocolic segment. (Fig. 23.)

Over 50 years ago an approach to the prob-

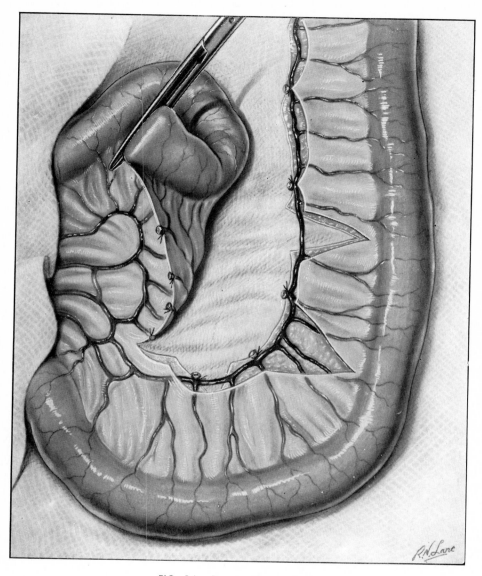

FIG. 14.   Roux-en-Y procedure.

lem was suggested by Hoffman,[5] who described an ingenious operation in which, following total gastrectomy and oesophago-jejunostomy, a gastric reservoir was constructed by uniting both arms of the jejunal loop, according to the principle of the Finney pyloroplasty. A hollow viscus with nearly twice the diameter of the jejunum was thus fashioned. The same principle has been adopted by Engel (1945) and Steinberg (1949). It was, however, Rubin's [17] work on the con-

struction of an artificial urinary bladder from a segment of sigmoid colon or ileum which stimulated Lee, Hunnicutt, Szilagyi, and Moroney to apply this principle to gastric surgery.

GASTRIC REPLACEMENT

With a segment of proximal jejunum. Henley (1952), in describing his technique,

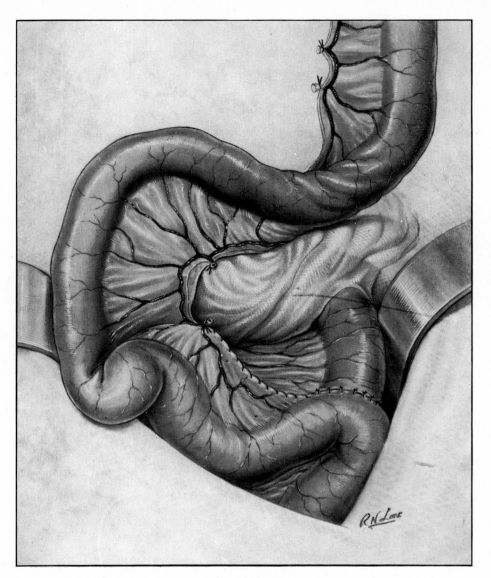

FIG. 15.   Roux-en-Y operation. The efferent limb of the jejunum is brought in front of the transverse colon to be anastomosed to the end of the oesophagus. Note the position of the end-to-side jejunojejunostomy.

states that after the stomach has been removed, a segment of proximal jejunum, 8 to 10 inches (20 to 25 cm) in length, hinged on its rich vascular pedicle, is drawn through an opening in mesocolon and anastomosed to the oesophagus at one end and to the duodenum at the other end. The jejunal continuity is restored by an axial anastomosis. At the completion of the operation, the jejunal segment lies slack in diastole and takes on the attitude of the stomach (Fig. 22). Kondo et al.[7] observe that many attempts have been made to eliminate the unpleasant sequelae of total gastrectomy but an entirely satisfactory method has not been devised. They developed a new method in which a proximal jejunal loop in the form of "figure 6" is substituted for the stomach. By this

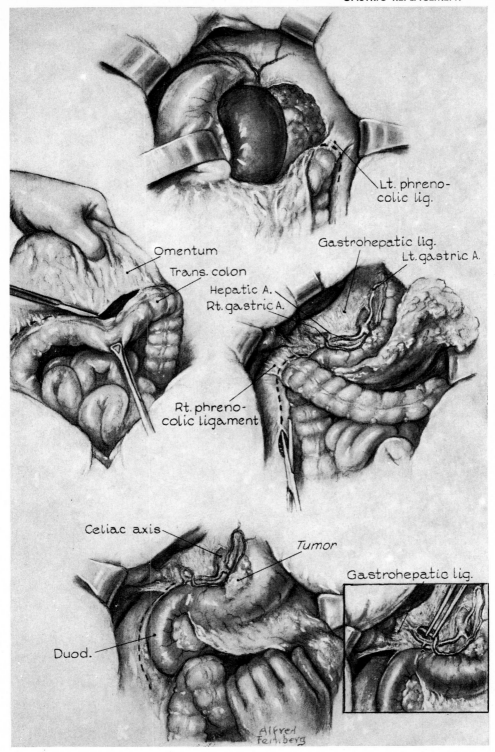

FIG. 16.   The technique of total gastrectomy as performed by Dr. John Madden. (From Madden, *Atlas of Technics in Surgery*, 2d ed., Courtesy of Appleton-Century-Crofts, New York, 1964.)

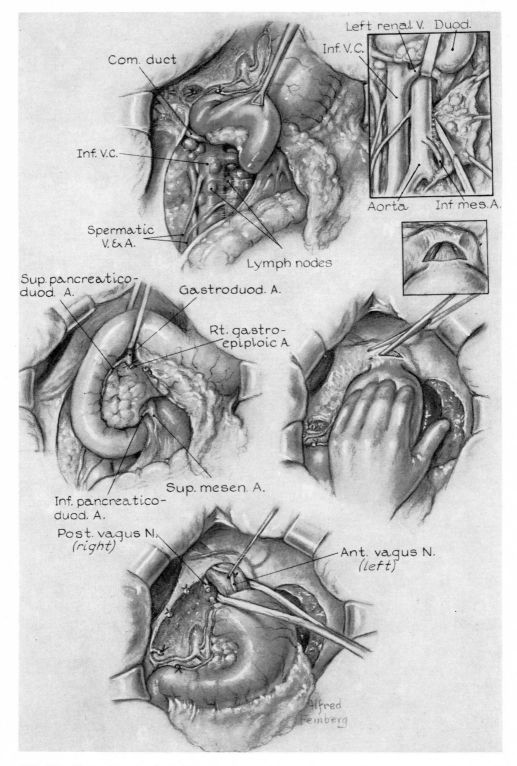

FIG. 17.   The technique of total gastrectomy. (From Madden, *Atlas of Technics in Surgery,* 2d ed., Courtesy of Appleton-Century-Crofts, New York, 1964.)

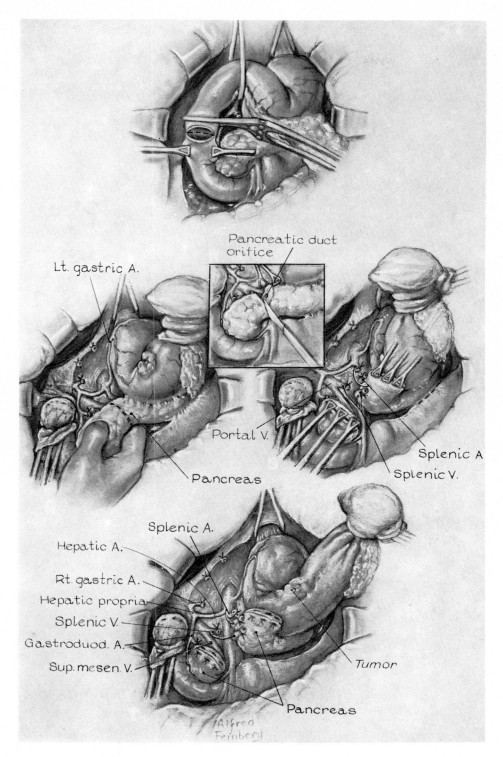

FIG. 18.   The technique of total gastrectomy. (From Madden, *Atlas of Technics in Surgery*, 2d
ed., Courtesy of Appleton-Century-Crofts, New York, 1964.)

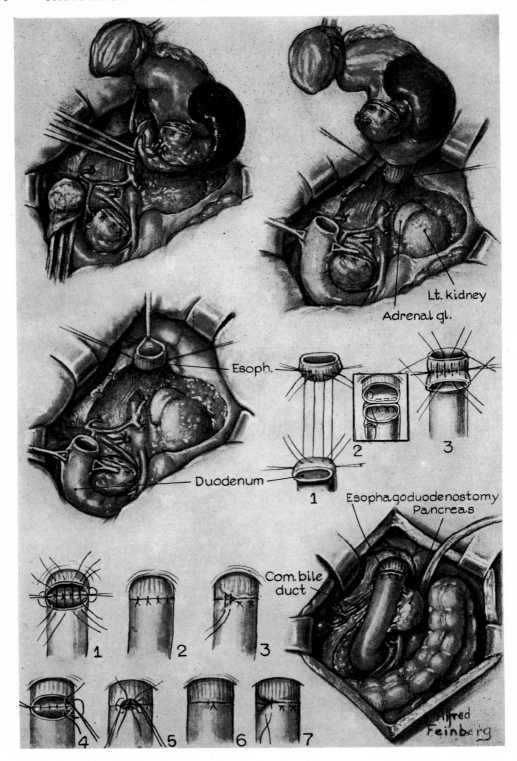

FIG. 19.   The technique of total gastrectomy followed by oesophagoduodenostomy. (From Madden, *Atlas of Technics in Surgery*, 2d ed., Courtesy of Appleton-Century-Crofts, New York, 1964.)

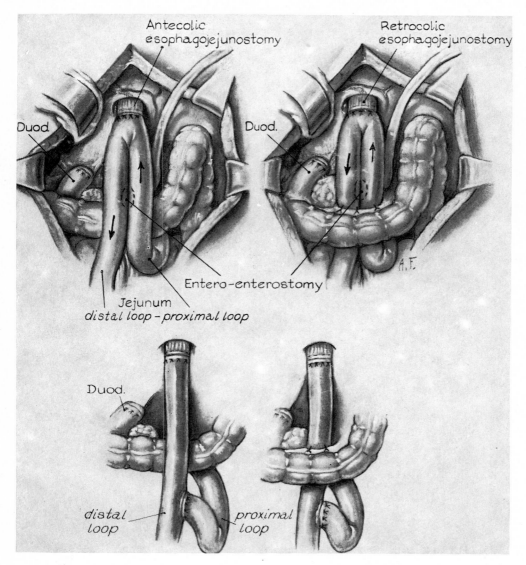

FIG. 20. Total gastrectomy, followed by oesophagojejunostomy anastomoses. (From Madden, *Atlas of Technics in Surgery*, 2d ed., Courtesy of Appleton-Century-Crofts, New York, 1964.)

method food circulates in the jejunal loop for a period of time before passing into the duodenum. The operation has not been accompanied by oesophagitis or the dumping syndrome. (Fig 21.)

They reported 16 cases of cancer of the stomach in which total gastrectomy was combined with the "figure 6" jejunal loop type of junction. There were no deaths in these 16 cases and the results were described as good. In six cases, death resulted from recurrences.

With a segment of transverse colon. Here a portion of transverse colon, 8 to 10 inches (20 to 25 cm) in length and with its blood supply intact, is drawn into the supracolic department and anastomosed at the top end to the oesophagus and at the bottom end

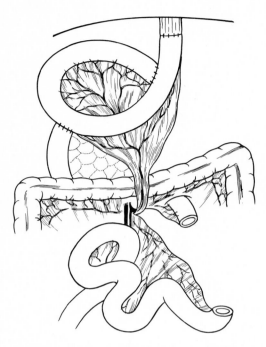

FIG. 21.   Kondo's "figure 6" loop of jejunum.

1. If a functionally adequate gastric reservoir could be devised to replace the totally removed stomach, one of the major objections to adequate surgery in gastric carcinoma would be removed.
2. The right colon is large enough, in the human subject, to act as an adequate reservoir.
3. The right colon and terminal ileum constitute an anatomical unit with respect to circulation and lymphatic drainage, the elimination of which from the intestinal tract can be accomplished without ill effect. This unit is not involved even in extensive locally invasive gastric carcinoma; it lies outside the regional lymphatic drainage of the stomach.
4. The right colon has excellent powers of water absorption and adequate peristaltic activity.
5. The ileum and esophagus are sufficiently compatible in size to make employment of a segment of terminal ileum as an extension of the esophagus feasible.
6. The ileocecal valve can function as effectively as the esophagogastric cardia in preventing the regurgitation of bile and pancreatic juice into the lower esophagus (Fig. 23).
7. Megaloblastic anemia can be controlled by substitution therapy, as has been shown in cases of total gastrectomy in which no replacement reservoir is provided.

to the open mouth of the duodenum, after which the continuity of the colon is restored by an axial anastomosis.

By an ileocolic segment.   Lee [8] stated that under favourable conditions of anaesthesia and supportive therapy gastric replacement with the ileocolic segment of bowel does not appear to be an unduly formidable procedure and should be satisfactorily withstood by a patient regarded as a suitable risk for total gastrectomy.

The operation should not be undertaken as a palliative procedure. *Its use should be reserved for those patients in whom there is definite hope of cure.* The employment of this operation in improperly selected cases would result in an inordinately high mortality and morbidity risk which might discourage its use for patients in whom the risk is justifiable.

Lee [8] writes:

The rationale for the operation is based on the following:

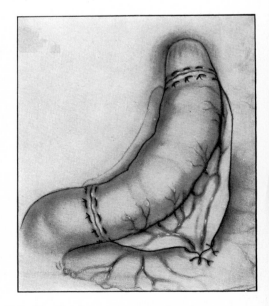

FIG. 22.   Total gastrectomy and replacement with a segment of the proximal jejunum. Henley's technique. (Courtesy of Mr. P. Henley and the British Journal of Surgery.)

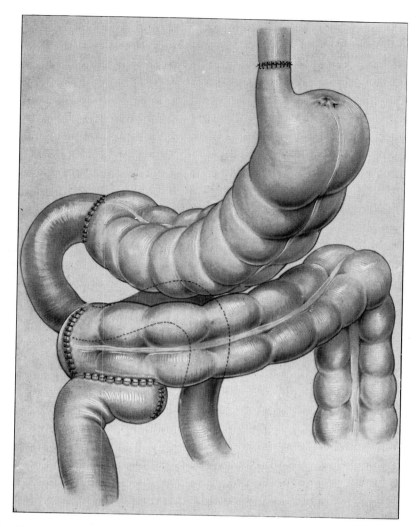

FIG. 23. Gastric replacement by ileocolic segment. Note that the ileum is anastomosed to the oesophagus (the appendix has been removed), and the lower end of the colonic segment is anastomosed end-to-end with the duodenum. Intestinal continuity is established by the performance of a side-to-side ileotransverse colostomy. (After Dr. Marshall Lee, *Surg. Gynecol. Obstet.* 92:456, 1951.)

McGlone, in discussing this operation, writes:

My experience with six cases has indicated many favorable aspects of this procedure, probably based on the fact that mechanically the digestion is more nearly normal following this procedure than after the usual gastrectomy. The x-ray photographs illustrate that the newly formed "stomach" does act as a reservoir. Also, since there is a direct continuity, the food receives the proper admixture at the proper time, with the digestive secretions from the gallbladder, pancreas and small intestine. Again, based on a limited experience, it is felt that the procedure of colon transplant is worthy of further trial. Early results suggest an improvement in the digestive function and a lessening of many side-effects of gastrectomy.

The operation is performed as follows: Total gastrectomy is carried out in the manner described, leaving the stomach attached to the oesophagus for better control during the anastomosis.

The right colon is mobilised and a point on the transverse colon distal to the hepatic flexure is then selected just to the right of the main middle colic artery; the colon is divided between clamps. The distal end of the colon is turned in and securely closed. The appendix is removed and its stump invaginated into the caecum. The ileum is picked up and a portion of the gut, some 3 inches (7.6 cm) from the ileocaecal valve, is doubly clamped and divided. The proximal end of the ileum is turned in and closed, after which the ileum is anastomosed to the transverse colon by the side-to-side method. This procedure restores the intestinal continuity. After the meso-ileum is liberated and the right colon mobilised as freely as possible, the distal end of the ileum is anastomosed to the oesophagus and the end of the colonic segment is joined to the duodenum. There are, therefore, three anastomotic junctions: (1) oesophagoileostomy, (2) coloduodenostomy, and (3) ileocolostomy (Fig. 23).

POSTOPERATIVE TREATMENT

Blood transfusions are given during and after operation; dehydration is corrected by intravenous infusions of glucose and saline; the indwelling gastric tube is aspirated every 4 hours; pain is relieved by morphine and sleep ensured by giving intramuscular injections of sodium phenobarbital. The stir-up treatment commences 12 hours after the patient has recovered from the anaesthetic and is continued for 10 days. While the intravenous drip is functioning during the first 72 hours, only small, frequent sips of clear fluids are permitted by mouth. The Levin tube is usually removed on the third day after operation, when the patient is given diluted milk and fresh fruit juice feedings. The fluid nourishment is rapidly increased until about the seventh postoperative day, when the patient is capable of taking junkets, custards, jellies, and the like. Solid food is tolerated, but rarely relished, about the tenth day following the removal of the stomach.

If there is no appreciable discharge through the Penrose drains or it is obvious that there is no leak at the line of anastomosis, these tubes may be withdrawn on the fifth postoperative day. Vitamins B and C are given as a routine measure, and hypoproteinaemia is corrected by **giving** blood transfusions and by enriching the diet with easily assimilable proteins. During convalescence it is customary to prescribe ferrous gluconate, vitamin B_{12}, and a stimulating appetiser. Antibiotic therapy (see Chap. 107) is continued for the first 3 or 4 days following operation. The average patient is discharged from hospital on the fourteenth postoperative day but will need *prolonged and careful supervision* and a special bland, nourishing diet subsequently.

REFERENCES

1. Allison, Ann. Surg. 132:563, 1950.
2. Allison and Borrie, Br. J. Surg. 37:1, 1949.
3. Doubilet, Surg. Clin. North Am. 39:441, 1954.
4. Graham, Arch. Surg. 46:907, 1943.
5. Hoffman, Zentralbl. Chir. 49:1477, 1922.
6. Kirschner and Garlock, Ann. Surg. 138:1, 1953.
7. Kondo et al., Ann. Surg. 173:529, 1971.
8. Lee, Surg. Gynecol. Obstet. 92:456, 1951.
9. Lefèvre, Mém. Acad. Chir. 22:580, 1946.
10. McNeer et al., Cancer 3:43, 1950.
11. Madden, Atlas of Technics in Surgery, 2d ed., New York, Appleton-Century-Crofts, 1964.
12. Marshall, Surg. Clin. North Am. 39:673, 1956.
13. Moynihan, Br. Med. J. 2:458, 1903.
14. Qvist, Personal communication, 1972.
15. ReMine and Priestley, Ann. Surg. 163:736, 1966.
16. Reynolds and Young, Surgery 24:246, 1948.
17. Rubin, J. Urol. 60:874, 1948.
18. Thorek, Atlas of Surgical Techniques, New York, Appleton-Century-Crofts, 1970.
19. Wangensteen, Tr. Am. SA 67:219, 1949.

30

SIMPLE AND MALIGNANT STRICTURES OF THE OESOPHAGUS AND CARDIA

NORMAN C. TANNER and ROBERT J. RYALL

It is desirable for the surgeon who deals with simple or malignant lesions of the oesophagus to be equally conversant with endoscopic procedures, transthoracic exposure of the oesophagus, and surgical manipulation of the stomach, jejunum, or colon. Under some circumstances, however, notably when the throat surgeon wishes to extirpate a malignant lesion of the laryngopharynx or cervical oesophagus widely, he may enlist the aid of an abdominal surgical colleague to work concurrently with him and mobilise a suitable length of stomach or colon, which may be drawn up to the neck and anastomosed to the pharynx to replace the whole oesophagus.[1]

TYPES OF STRICTURES

Benign Stricture of the Oesophagus

The established fibrous stricture of the oesophagus, particularly that following the swallowing of corrosives (Fig. 1) cricopharyngitis, congenital atresia, or trauma, or associated with scleroderma, lies in the first place in the province of the endoscopist, both for diagnosis and for preliminary dilatation procedures by bouginage. It may be stated in general that intermittent and forcible bouginage, which leaves a raw granulating lining to the stricture, is very likely to lead to early recurrent stenosis. The method most likely to attain success is, as reiterated by the late G. Grey-Turner,[2] daily gentle autobouginage, carried out without force and with softened and well-lubricated gum-elastic bougies.

In rare instances, the stricture may prove intractable or atresia may be complete or the patient, by reason of age or intelligence, may be unable to cooperate in treatment. Under such circumstances, surgical procedures to by-pass or replace the damaged oesophagus may be needed. For replacement of half or more of the thoracic oesophagus, the replacing organ may be the stomach itself, by the method indicated under *Cancer of the Cardiac End of the Stomach and the Lower End of the Oesophagus* (below), or better still by transverse colon, mobilised with preservation of an upper left colic artery. When only the lower half of the oesophagus is affected, either stomach or a Roux jejunal loop may be used. In these cases, a "radical" removal of the gullet is not required, the excision being confined to the oesophagus itself without the associated glands. Indeed the oesophagus may safely be left in situ and merely bypassed, though there is a risk that carcinoma may develop in lye strictures of long standing.[3]

STRICTURE OF THE OESOPHAGUS RESULTING FROM PEPTIC OESOPHAGITIS

These strictures develop as a result of fibrosis following peptic oesophagitis, and are due to reflux of gastric juice into the gullet, most commonly as a result of a sliding hiatal hernia, or from a gastric-mucosa-lined lower oesophagus, which is usually associated with hiatal incompetence (Fig. 2). They may follow operations which damage or bypass the cardia sphincteric mechanism of the lower oesophagus (cardioplasty, cardiomyotomy, oesophagogastrostomy). This type of stricture requires separate consideration, its particular feature being that dilatation by bouginage allows increased reflux to occur with exacerbation of oesophagitis followed by recurrent spasm and fibrosis. Furthermore, if the stricture is short-circuited by oesophagogastric

621

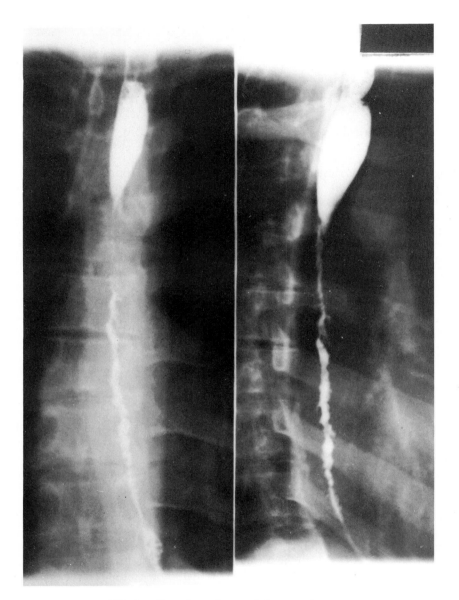

FIG. 1. Corrosive stricture of the oesophagus.

anastomosis, the elimination of the cardia mechanism may lead to reflux and rapid stricture recurrence. Therefore other methods of dealing with this type of stricture are required. Medically, methods of preventing reflux by weight reduction, avoidance of stooping, and administration of drugs to reduce gastric secretion or acidity are used with varying degrees of success.

Surgically, an indirect approach much favoured by the writers [4] is to carry out an ordinary abdominal partial gastrectomy as for a duodenal ulcer (see Chaps. 20 and 21). This, by reducing the volume and acidity of the reflux fluid, leads to a gradual improvement in the dysphagia with relief of pain, and radiographs show improvement in the narrowing of the oesophagus (Fig. 3). This

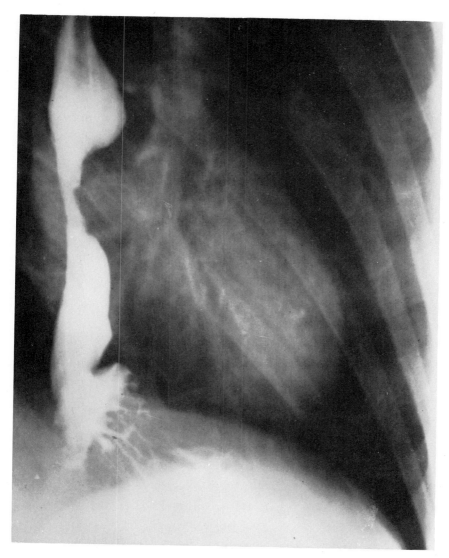

FIG. 2. Oesophageal stricture resulting from the fact that the lower oesophagus, up to the stricture level, is lined by gastric-type glandular epithelium. There is almost invariably an associated hiatal herna with reflux.

improvement is particularly marked if there is an associated duodenal ulcer, or ulcer scar, as is not infrequently the case.

Another indirect surgical method of treatment is to carry out an abdominal vagotomy, combined with repair of the hiatal hernia and a drainage operation, either pyloroplasty, gastrojejunostomy, or antrectomy.[5]

Direct surgical procedures for peptic oesophageal stricture all involve resection or bypassing the stricture, most commonly the former. The reconstruction may be by direct oesophagogastric anastomosis, but the disadvantage of this is the high incidence of recurrent peptic oesophagitis, despite the coincident vagotomy and despite resection of the upper part of the body of the stomach. To overcome this difficulty, it is recommended that a high resection of the oesophagus be undertaken, without resecting much stomach,

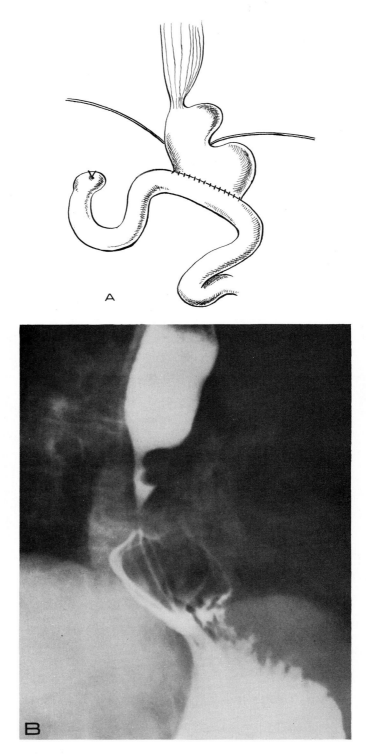

FIG. 3.   Treatment of stricture due to reflux oesophagitis by lower partial gastrectomy. (A) Diagram of operation. (B) Preoperative radiograph. (C) Postoperative radiograph (4 months later). (D) Preoperative radiograph. (E) Postoperative radiograph (6 months later).

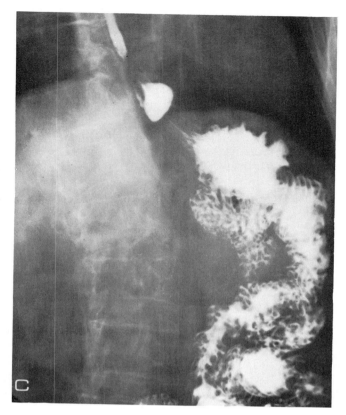

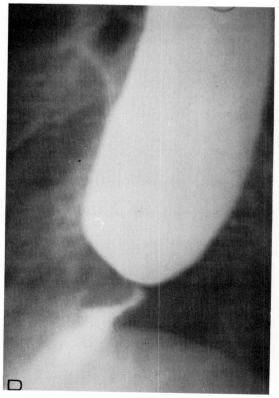

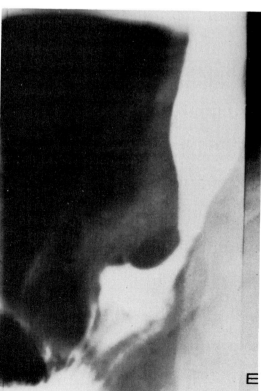

being closed at cardia level, and that an anastomosis be made between the oesophagus and gastric fundus at or about aortic arch level. Possibly because the vagotomised, atonic stomach when transposed into the thorax is not subjected to the higher intra-abdominal pressure, reflux and oesophagitis are less common after this procedure.

Despite the fact that such a high intra-thoracic resection is not "radical," however, it is a very major procedure which would have appreciable mortality and morbidity rates in the aged and infirm patients who form a large proportion of the sufferers from peptic oesophagitis following oesophageal hiatal hernia.

The variations on other methods of oesophageal replacement are manifold, but a list of some well-established replacement procedures will be considered in greater detail under *Methods of Oesophageal Replacement* (below), as they are equally applicable to replacement after oesophageal resection for simple or benign neoplasm, oesophageal trauma, congenital deformity, or fibrous stricture.

Malignant Stricture of the Oesophagus

The majority of oesophageal carcinomas are of the squamous cell type, though at cardia level an equal number are adenocarcinomas. An occasional adenocarcinoma may also be found in the mid- or upper oesophagus; the next most common malignant lesion is the leiomyosarcoma.

Generally speaking, all do best if resectable and if resected. While it is true that radiotherapy has an increasing place in the management of squamous cell cancer of the oesophagus, surgery gives the greatest chance of success except perhaps in the upper thoracic and cervical oesophagus, where the magnitude and mutilation of surgery make a preliminary attack by radiotherapy often preferable.

After a trial of preoperative radiotherapy for squamous cell oesophageal carcinomas the writer is of the opinion that primary extirpation, *followed* by radiotherapy, gives the better result.

The removal of cancer of the oesophagus is a "radical" operation insofar as an attempt

should be made to remove nonvital mediastinal structures with it, particularly the lymph nodes, and occasionally locally adherent pulmonary, pericardial, or pleural tissues. It is limited, however, because most of the surrounding structures cannot be excised without considerable risk. The late Grey-Turner expressed the opinion to the senior author that if the gullet was fixed by extra-oesophageal tumour there was little point in its excision. There is no doubt that in principle he was correct, but nevertheless, one will see an occasional long-term survivor, with the help of postoperative radiotherapy, even when tumour has breached the oesophageal wall, and so a reasonably optimistic attitude is justifiable when dealing with these tumours.

In the past, a number of oesophageal carcinomas have recurred at the site of anastomosis of oesophagus to stomach. To prevent this, an adequate length of gullet, at least 5 cm above the visible and palpable upper tumour edge, should be removed when possible. There is a great deal, in fact, to commend total thoracic oesophagectomy for middle and even lower oesophageal cancer.

METHODS OF OESOPHAGEAL REPLACEMENT

1. *Oesophagectomy and oesophagogastric anastomosis,* either in the inferior mediastinum (satisfactory for limited upper gastric tumours), subaortic (suitable for localised low oesophageal tumours, or cardia carcinoma associated with hiatal hernia), or supra-aortic (suitable for peptic oesophagitis or middle or extensive low thoracic oesophageal carcinoma).

2. *By an isolated jejunal loop,* between the oesophagus and stomach.[6, 7]

3. *By anastomosis of oesophagus to a mobilised "Roux loop"* of jejunum, either bypassing or resecting the stomach.

4. *By an isolated colonic loop* between the oesophagus above, and the stomach, duodenum, or jejunum below. The variations on this method are numerous. The loop may be isoperistaltic; for examples, ileum, caecum, and right

colon hinged on the middle colic vessel; a short length of transverse colon hinged on the middle colic vessels; a long loop of transverse colon including both flexures, hinged on the upper left colic vessels. The loop may be anti-peristaltic, a long length of the left half of the transverse, descending and sigmoid colon depending on the middle colic artery for its blood supply.

The choice of a suitable colonic loop will depend on the length of oesophagus and stomach to be replaced, on the relative size of the main colic vessels, on an intact marginal artery, and the presence or absence of degenerative vascular disease in the vessels.

Such colonic loops are most commonly intrathoracic, in the posterior madiastinum, but long loops may be placed in a prethoracic subcutaneous tunnel or in a substernal position.

Finally, it should be mentioned that autotransplantation of the sigmoid colon to replace the cervical oesophagus, taking a new venous drainage and arterial blood supply from the neck vessels, is a practicable procedure.[8]

5. *By skin tubes*[9] and plastic tubes.[10] These methods are now of historical interest only, except in the case of localised neoplasms of the upper cervical oesophagus and carcinoma of the hypopharynx and postcricoid region, which lie more in the province of the throat surgeon. There might be a *future* for the plastic tube replacement if the problem of preventing mediastinitis round the upper oesophago-prosthesis junction could be solved.

In deciding on the most suitable method of oesophageal replacement for a particular case, one must consider:

1. The nature of the disease for which replacement is needed. For example, if oesophagogastric reconstruction is considered, the very real risk of reflux oesophagitis, followed by bleeding, stenosis, or even perforation, sometimes into the pericardium or a major vessel, is to be borne in mind. If the resection or bypass is for peptic ulcer disease— e.g., peptic oesophagitis, the risk of

still further ulceration is high, whereas if the resection is for a malignant or benign oesophageal neoplasm, the risk is much less. A preoperative guide to the risk may be obtained from estimation of the patient's acid secretion after maximal histamine stimulation. If the acid secretion is 30 mEq or less in the post-histamine hour, such a means of reconstruction will be reasonably safe.

2. The length of gullet to be replaced. Colon and stomach are the most suitable organs for total oesophageal replacement.

3. The condition of the blood vessels and the relative freedom from atheroma of the jejunal as compared with the colonic vessels.

4. The condition of the colon. In particular, the presence of severe diverticulosis reduces its value.

5. Great obesity and fibrous thickening of the jejunal mesentery, which increase the difficulty of its mobilisation.

Preparation of the Colon

Before all oesophageal operations in which replacement may be required, it is advisable to have the colon as empty as possible and sterilised by intestinal antiseptics, in case it proves to be the organ of choice for replacement. A further advantage of this preparation is that the oesophagus too is sterilised, particularly if there has been stagnation and infection above an obstruction.

The simplest method is merely to give the patient 1 g of phthalylsulphthiazole (Sulphathalidine) every 4 hours for 5 days before operation.

A method we have found very effective and which is a routine in the Middlesex Hospital, London, is as follows.

The patient is given only fluids for 48 hours before operation. Two days before operation, starting at 8 A.M., he is given Mist. Mag. Sulph, 8 ml every 2 hours until diarrhoea occurs, and two more doses are given thereafter. Neomycin, 0.5 g, is given every 6 hours for 48 hours. Two nights prior to the operation the patient is given two tablets of bisacodyl (Dulcolax), and on the evening prior to operation a Veripaque enema is given.

A third method used by the senior writer

is first to give nonabsorbable sulfonamide for 5 days. Then the following technique is used in order to empty the colon:

It is confirmed that the patient has no history of coronary or advanced vascular disease. On the morning of operation a medical officer prepares a syringe with 1 ml of pituitrin. After the patient is seated on a bedpan, and while the stomach is empty, the pituitrin is given intravenously, not more than 0.1 ml every 10 to 15 seconds. Colic and pallor occur at about 0.6 ml, and micturition and defaecation usually take place shortly afterwards. Not more than 1 ml should be given and it should not be repeated.

Gastric Replacement of the Oesophagus

The technique of replacement of the lower oesophagus is considered later (see *Cancer of the Cardiac End of the Stomach and the Lower End of the Oesophagus*).

For any cancer of the middle oesophagus, an anastomosis above the aortic arch will be necessary if an adequate length of healthy oesophagus above the growth is to be removed. This may be most easily effected in one of two ways: by an extension of the left abdominothoracic approach via the eighth rib bed; or by the abdominal and right thoracic approach.

EXTENSION OF LEFT ABDOMINOTHORACIC APPROACH

An abdominothoracotomy via the eighth rib bed is made, with limited incision into the abdomen, and wide division of the diaphragm. Through this it is relatively easy to mobilise the whole stomach, carefully preserving the right gastric and right gastroepiploic vessels, but sacrificing the left gastric vessels, the left gastroepiploic vessels, and the vasa brevia (the spleen and pancreas are left in situ). The lower oesophagus, vagus nerves, mediastinal fat, and lymphatics, as well as the paracardial lymph nodes, are freed en bloc as high as the aortic arch. Above this level, the exposure will be found inadequate. One can get a higher exposure either by dividing and resecting about 3 cm each of the posterior ends of the fifth, sixth, and seventh ribs, or better still, the "two-rib" approach is used. For the latter, the retractor

is removed from the abdominothoracic opening, and the posterior part of the incision is extended upwards to the level of the third rib, deepening the incision to divide the trapezius and rhomboideus muscles. The scapula, aided by the anaesthetist exerting traction on the left arm, is drawn upwards to expose the fourth and fifth ribs. A generous length of the fourth rib is then excised subperiosteally, and the upper thorax reentered after division of the periosteum and pleura.

After a retractor of the Finochietto type is inserted, and the lung drawn forward with an Allison retractor, excellent views of the superior mediastinum may be obtained. An incision is made in the mediastinal pleura over the oesophagus, and the oesophagus dissected free. Dissection of the oesophagus at the aortic arch level will be "blind," though it usually presents little difficulty. Nevertheless, this dissection would be hazardous if the tumor itself lay at aortic arch level or if there were dense adhesions present, for the aorta or vena azygos major may be damaged. Visualisation may be improved, however, by dividing enough intercostal arteries to mobilise the upper descending aorta, though the writers have only once found this necessary.

Once the supra-aortic oesophagus is thus mobilised and freed, a Stevenson or similar slim clamp is placed across it just above the desired level of transection, preferably at least 5 to 6 cm above the palpable tumour; a firm silk ligature is placed below this, and the oesophagus is transected between them. The oesophagus and tumour can now be withdrawn and resected, the lower point of transection being just below the cardiac orifice of the stomach, with removal of the paracardial and left gastric lymph nodes, which have already been mobilised.

The opening in the stomach is closed in two layers, for which the writer uses continuous chromic 00 catgut, though interrupted nonabsorbable sutures may be used if preferred.

The fundus of the stomach is now drawn up into the superior mediastinum to the left of the aortic arch, and an anastomosis made between the cut end of the oesophagus and an incision which has been made in the highest part of the gastric fundus. The method of anastomosis will be described later (see *The Oesophagogastric Anastomosis,* below). The technique preferred is to make the "all-coats" layer first, and then the second layer is so inserted that a fold of gastric seromuscularis is drawn upwards to surround the first layer.

Any possible tension on the anastomosis may be relieved by a few interrupted stitches between the upward-drawn stomach and the cut edge of the mediastinal pleura. The mediastinum and site of anastomosis are lightly powdered with antibiotic (penicillin). The intercostal muscles and other layers are then repaired in the usual way, leaving a generous intercostal tube drain to the pleural cavity.

ABDOMINAL AND RIGHT THORACIC APPROACH

This is a simpler method of dealing with midoesophageal resections, particularly for the experienced abdominal surgeon. With the patient supine, a high midepigastric incision is made. After a general exploration to exclude irremovable metastases, the epiploic vessels in the gastrocolic omentum are ligated and divided from the duodenum to the spleen, carefully preserving the gastroepiploic arch of vessels. The gastrosplenic ligament is similarly divided until the left margin of the oesophagus is reached, dividing not only the vasa brevia but also the left gastroepiploic artery. The lesser omentum is next exposed and divided above the stomach from above the pyloric antrum to the right margin of the oesophagus. In this division, the hepatic branches of the anterior vagus nerve will be divided, and in addition an accessory hepatic artery coming from the left gastric artery to the liver, or an accessory gastric vein draining directly into the liver may be present, needing ligation and division.

The stomach is drawn forward and adhesions of the posterior wall to the pancreas are freed. The left gastric pedicle is now visible; it is dissected free and divided between secure ligatures.

An incision is now made in front of the oesophagus, through peritoneum and phreno-oesophageal ligaments to expose the oesophagus and vagus nerves. This incision is continued behind to free the cardia region completely from the diaphragm. One or two incisions may now be made in the margins

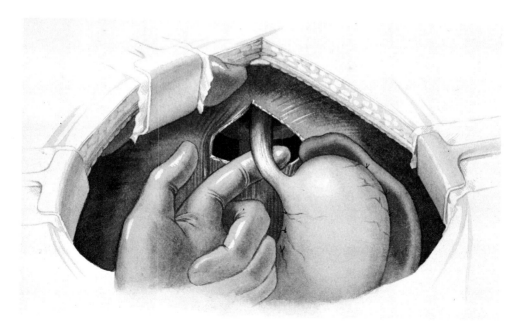

FIG. 4.   Abdominal mobilisation of the stomach and lower esophagus; diaphragm incised to expose the base of the pericardium; liver retracted.

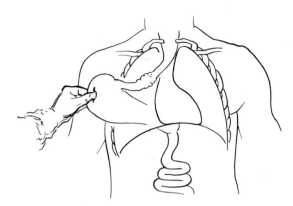

FIG. 5. Stomach and lower oesophagus mobilised into the right side of the chest.

of the oesophageal hiatus, with either formal ligation or care to avoid damage to the inferior phrenic vessels, until the hiatus is wide enough to take the palm of the hand. Through this incision, the lower gullet is mobilised (Fig. 4), and usually the midoesophageal tumour can be felt and its resectability assessed.

The stomach will now be mobile and the fundus could be pushed easily into the posterior mediastinum. It is helpful to mobilise

the duodenum by Kocher's method so that the pylorus can later be drawn up to the level of the oesophageal hiatus.

A very short (3 cm) pyloroplasty [11] is now made, to counteract the impaired gastric emptying that will follow the vagal resection. The wound is next closed in layers.

The patient is then turned on to his left side. An incision is made from behind the posterior border of the right scapula, through the trapezius and rhomboideus muscles, and then forwards, skirting below the angle of the scapula. The scapula, aided by traction on the right arm, is drawn forwards and upwards to expose the fourth right rib. A subperiosteal resection of the rib is made and the upper pleural cavity entered. After the inserting and opening of a Finochietto retractor, the lung is drawn forward with an Allison retractor.

The vena azygos major is seen passing forwards under the pleura. It is ligated in two places and divided between them. The mediastinal pleura is incised above and below this point, encircling any pleura which appears to be invaded by or adherent to tumour. The boundaries of the mediastinum are dissected out, the aorta behind, the pericardium in front, and the left pleura and aorta to the left; the contents, with oesophagus and glands, are thus freed to a point

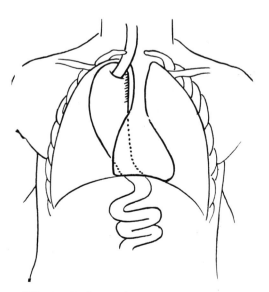

FIG. 6. High oesophagogastric anastomosis.

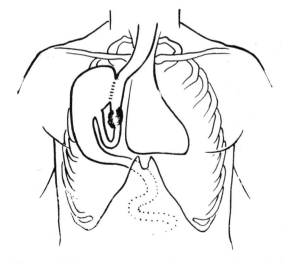

FIG. 7. Palliative short circuit for irremovable high carcinoma of the oesophagus.

just below the pleural apex. By gentle pulling on the lower oesophagus, the mobilised stomach is drawn into the right thorax. It is now an easy matter to resect the oesophagus from just below the cardia (and including the paracardial and left gastric lymph nodes) to a point fixed to 6 cm from the upper limit of the thoracic oesophagus (Figs. 5 and 6). After closing of the cardia, the oesophago-fundic anastomosis is carried out as described for the left thoracic approach, but with greater facility. The thorax is closed with wide intercostal underwater tube drainage.

Unresectability of middle oesophageal tumour. If it is found that the tumour of the middle oesophagus is unresectable *after* the right thorax is opened, the stomach should be brought up in the usual way, the upper oesophagus mobilised, and a side-to-side anastomosis made between the oesophagus above tumour level and the gastric fundus, without disturbing the integrity of the diseased oesophagus (Fig. 7). This gives complete relief of dysphagia, and can be followed by radiotherapy if the tumour is squamous cell in origin.

Total Oesophageal Replacement by the Pull-through Method

Recently, the use of stomach has been recommended again as a total oesophageal replacement after pharyngo-oesophagectomy. LeQuesne and Ranger have pointed out that following adequate gastric mobilisation by an abdominal surgeon as described above, and concurrent resection of the pharynx and cervical oesophagus by the throat surgeon, it is possible by the "pull-through" method to draw the fundus of the stomach up through the posterior mediastinum, into the neck, to anastomose the gastric fundus to the pharynx, without opening either thoracic cavity. The writer has confirmed this observation, despite failures in the past when the stomach was drawn up in the subcutaneous route.

Reversed Gastric Tube Method

Another method which has much to commend it, though not widely used, is the Heimlich-Gavriliu reversed gastric tube.[12, 13]

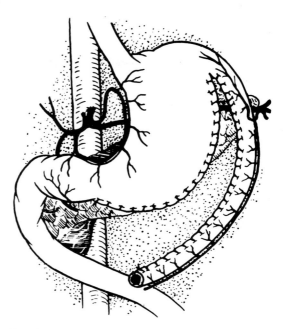

FIG. 8. Completed gastric tube after staples have been inverted into the stomach with continuous seromuscular silk suture.

A tube 2 cm wide is made from the greater curvature of the stomach, based at the cardiac end, and terminating 5 cm proximal to the pylorus (Fig. 8). The spleen is removed, with great care to preserve the splenic vessels and the left gastroepiploic vessels. The pancreatic tail is mobilised, and the pyloric end of the tube can then be brought up subcutaneously, retrosternally, or through the posterior mediastinum as high as the pharynx. Heimlich has designed a clamp with which a row of metal clips can be introduced, so facilitating making of the tube and reducing the time required for it.

Jejunal Replacement of the Oesophagus

JEJUNAL INTERPOSITION BETWEEN OESOPHAGUS AND STOMACH

This method has been found satisfactory, and is strongly commended by Brain. Jejunal segments were used as far back as 1904 by Wullstein [14] to bridge gaps between the antethoracic (usually skin tube) oesophagus and stomach, and it appears to have been first used in the posterior mediastinum by Harrison.[15] This method is mainly suitable following resection of the lower oesophagus and cardia.

   The operation. The part to be resected is exposed by a generous left abdominothoracic incision, through the bed of the seventh or eighth ribs, with wide division of the diaphragm and the use of a Price-Thomas rib spreader.

  After excision of the affected part of the oesophagus, the upper jejunal mesentery is exposed, and a Roux loop is prepared. The jejunum and adjacent arcade of vessels are divided, and then one or two main branches from the superior mesenteric artery supplying the distal part are carefully divided between ligatures in such a way as to mobilise the distal jejunum enough for it to reach the oesophagus.[16] The cut end of the Roux loop is now closed and an anastomosis

made between the end of the oesophagus and the side of this jejunal loop. Then the jejunum is transected at a convenient place lower down, opposite the stomach and preserving the marginal vessels. The proximal part of this is anastomosed end-in-side to the stomach (Fig. 9), thus restoring continuity between the oesophagus and stomach, and the distal part is closed. The operation is completed by end-in-side anastomosis between the proximal jejunum and the side of the Roux loop some 12 to 18 inches (30 to 45 cm) from its end, thus directing the gastric, biliary, and pancreatic juices back into the jejunum.

Replacement by a Roux Jejunal Loop

  This is suitable after resection of the whole stomach with up to a third of the gullet. It is possible to use this method following high oesophageal resection, particularly in young people, but for such higher resections the use of stomach or colon is easier and preferable.

  The approach is by the left abdominothoracic route as just described, and the procedure is the same as far as the formation of the Roux loop and its anastomosis to the oesophagus. The Roux loop is left intact and completed by anastomosis of the proximal

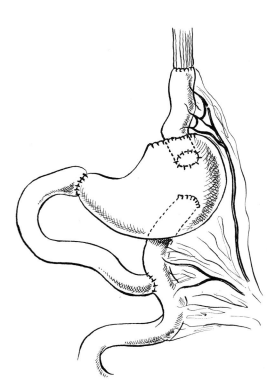

FIG. 9. Method of jejunal interposition recommended by R. H. F. Brain. The oesophagojejunal anastomosis may be end-to-end, as illustrated, or end-to-side. Brain prefers the latter.

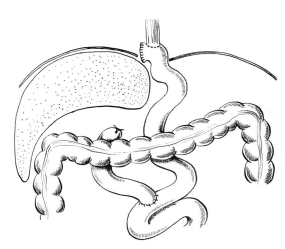

FIG. 10. Replacement of resected stomach and lower oesophagus by the "Roux loop" of jejunum.

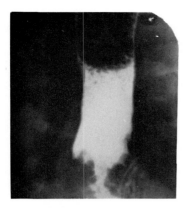

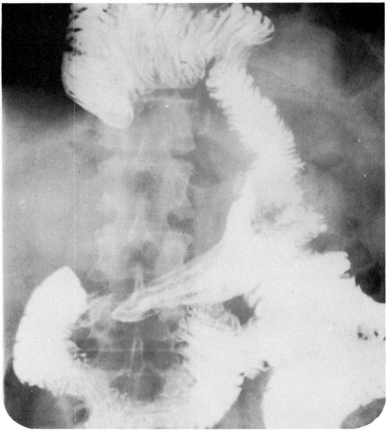

FIG. 11. X-ray after replacement of excised cardia by the Roux loop, followed by side-to-side anastomosis between the stomach and the Roux loop, thus partially restoring gastric function.

jejunum, carrying the biliary and pancreatic secretions into the side of the Roux loop some 18 to 24 inches (45 to 60 cm) beyond the oesophagojejunal anastomosis (Fig. 10). This results in an extremely comfortable and satisfactory end-result. Dumping symptoms are no more frequent than after partial gastrectomy, there is no biliary regurgitation or heartburn, and the patients are, in our experience, all able to return to their normal work.

However, a vitamin B_{12} deficiency is inevitable whether the stomach is retained or removed. There is also a tendency to iron and sometimes calcium deficiency. Therefore, after this operation, vitamin B_{12} should be given routinely. Iron and calcium supplements to the diet are also helpful, though the latter can be omitted if the patient takes milk or milk products.

A variant of this procedure is much favoured by Tanner [4] in cases in which the stomach is retained and only the cardia is removed (e.g., after oesophagojejunal anastomosis carried out for peptic oesophagitis following an unsuccessful Heller operation or cardioplasty). In this variant, after resection of the cardia, a Roux loop is made as described above and anastomosed to the oesophagus. A side-to-side anastomosis is then made between the Roux jejunal loop and the stomach, so that some of the swallowed food passes directly down the jejunum, and some enters into the stomach (Fig. 11). Restoring

some gastric function in this way diminishes dumping and so far seems to have eliminated B_{12} deficiency.

Colonic Replacement of the Oesophagus

The colon is a very adequate substitute for the oesophagus, either isoperistaltic or as an antiperistaltic loop. The former is preferable, as the latter may lead to a period of regurgitation and bloating, which may, however, be helped by the use of anticholinergic drugs.

For a short loop—e.g., after resection of a bulky cancer of the stomach invading the oesophagus, a length of transverse colon with intact marginal artery, hinged on the middle colic artery, will easily bridge the gap between the subaortic oesophagus and the duodenum (Fig. 12).

For a longer loop—e.g., for total oeso-

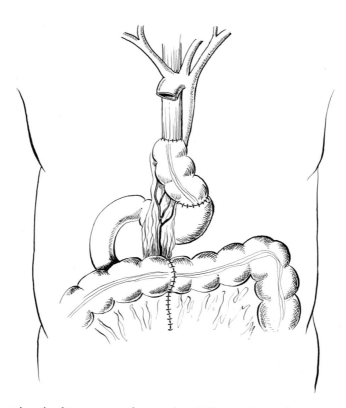

FIG. 12. Short length of transverse colon, used to bridge a defect after resection of the lower oesophagus and half of the stomach. It replaces the whole stomach equally well, in which case the lower end is anastomosed to the duodenum.

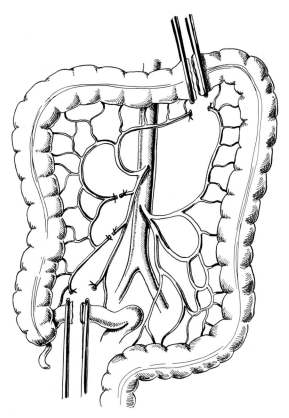

FIG. 13.   Preparation of the right colon and ileum for isoperistaltic replacement of the whole thoracic oesophagus or part of it. This method may also be used to replace the stomach.

phageal replacement, there are three alternatives:

1. The ileum, caecum, right colon, and hepatic flexure, supplied by the middle colic artery, and isoperistaltic (Fig. 13). This was previously regarded as ideal, as the oesophagus could be anastomosed to the ileum, the ileocaecal valve prevented reflux, and the inverted caecum radiologically simulated the gastric fundus. Alternatively, the caecum can be joined to the oesophagus and the ileum brought out in the neck as an ileostomy. A decompressing and feeding tube can be passed through this into the stomach (Fig. 14). There is, however, an uncertain venous circulation between the caecum and the ascending colon which may jeopardise the blood supply of the caecum. Furthermore, the caecum is bulky, and if brought up to the cervical oesophagus in the substernal region, its volume may embarrass respiration; if brought up subcutaneously, it is very unsightly.

2. The transverse colon is an ideal substitute if the upper or ascending left colic artery is well developed. In such a case, the middle colic vessels may be sacrificed, and the upper left colic artery will supply the transverse colon and the splenic and hepatic flexures of the colon via the marginal artery (Fig. 15). The ascending colon can thus after transection be taken high into the neck, even to the pharynx, and the transected descending colon anastomosed to the stomach or proximal jejunum. Anastomosis between the ascending and de-

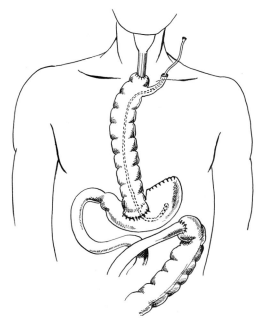

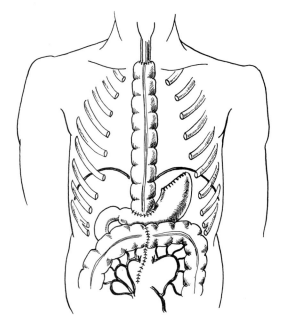

FIG. 14.   Replacement of the whole thoracic oesophagus and the cardiac end of the stomach by the right colon. Cervical ileostomy is useful for decompressing or feeding into the stomach; this is completed by ileocolic anastomosis.

FIG. 16.   Transverse colon replacing the whole thoracic oesophagus; it may replace the stomach equally well.

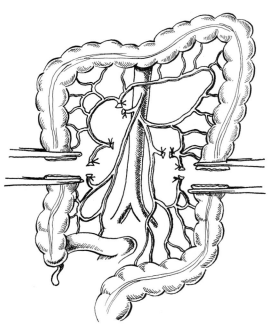

FIG. 15.   Preparation of the transverse colon and flexures for isoperistaltic total oesophageal replacement.

scending colon restores colonic continuity (Fig. 16).

3. Should the left colic artery be poor, a long colonic loop may be constructed from the left transverse colon, splenic flexure, and descending colon as low as the sigmoid, fed by the middle colic vessels via the marginal artery. This too will provide a long length of substitute oesophagus (as in one patient in whom, when she opened her mouth, the anastomosis between the base of the tongue and the sigmoid colon could be seen). As already indicated, in such cases there may be reflux of gastric juice for a time, or if the anastomosis is made to the jejunum, reflux of bile, which gradually diminishes.

The route the colonic replacement takes is governed by its length and by the operative approach.

For limited oesophageal resections, less than total thoracic oesophageal replacement, the oesophagus will follow the oesophageal route, the posterior mediastinum. For

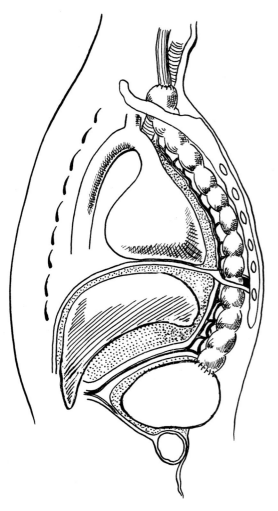

FIG. 17. Substernal replacement of the oesophagus. The oesophagus may be left in situ (in which case the cervical oesophagus must be transected and the lower end ligatured) or the oesophagus may be removed.

lengthier replacements, the colon may be drawn up through the posterior mediastinum to the neck. Alternatively, a substernal route may be made, after removal of the xiphoid process and after making a cervical incision to approach the retromanubrial region (Fig. 17). By digital dissection with both hands, aided if necessary by spade-like blunt dissectors, the whole retrosternal area is opened to produce a tunnel through which the mobilised colon may be drawn up from the abdomen into the neck, where it is anastomosed to the oesophageal stump. Difficul-

ties here lie in the occasional opening of the pleura, or in cases of portal hypertension, of producing mediastinal haemorrhage.

The simplest route is digitally, aided by the spade dissector, making a subcutaneous tunnel from the abdomen to the neck by the presternal route. This is a little longer and is somewhat unsightly. On the other hand, if leakage occurs, or necrosis of the colon, which is an occasional catastrophe, it is less likely to be lethal. There is also some incidence of stenosis at the oesophagocolonic junction which may be difficult to deal with endoscopically if the colon is presternal.

CANCER OF CARDIAC END OF STOMACH AND LOWER END OF OESOPHAGUS

This subject will be dealt with in greater detail, as it is very definitely the province of the abdominal surgeon. Although the cardiac orifice normally lies in the abdomen, diseases in this region come within the realm of both the abdominal and the thoracic surgeon. In practice, this means that the abdominal surgeon must be prepared to perform a transthoracic approach whenever an anastomosis above the level of the cardia is contemplated. This is no new venture for the abdominal surgeon, as thoracotomy may be required in dealing with lesions of the diaphragm, liver, or even spleen.

HISTORICAL NOTE

Because the peritoneal cavity was invaded by the surgeon before the pleural cavity, it is not surprising to find that the earliest successful resections of the cardia were by a transperitoneal route. The first was by Voelcker in 1908, followed by Kummell in 1910 and Bircher in 1918.

The advantages of a thoracic approach were well known, for in 1895 Biondie, and later Sauerbruch in his early work, had experimentally worked out transthoracic operations for resection of the cardia and restoration of alimentary continuity. Hedblom [17] and Muir [18] recorded cases of recovery after resection of the cardia by an abdominal and thoracic approach, each patient being left with oesophagostomy and gastrostomy. Ohsawa,[19] in his remarkable record in 1936, was able to cite eight successful resections of the cardia with restoration of alimentary continuity either by high laparotomy or by combining the laparotomy with a free thoracotomy by extending the incision into the seventh left intercostal space. In 1938 Adams and Phemister [20] successfully resected the cardia with intrathoracic anastomosis using a formal thoracotomy, and this case was the first of many which have since been reported from all parts of the world.

Other landmarks in the history may be briefly mentioned: Sauerbruch's "Einstulpung," invagination of the cardia with the tumour into the stomach and strangulating it to make it slough off and pass per anum. Cattell introduced a two-stage operation which was later successful, the first stage being the freeing of the stomach and pushing it into the posterior mediastinum, the second the transthoracic resection of the fundus. Several British surgeons, led by Grey-Turner and including Tanner,[21] performed abdominal mobilisation of cardiac tumours followed by a "pull through" or collo-abdominal resection of the oesophagus, but found that the subsequent attempts to construct an antethoracic oesophagus from small bowel or skin were rarely successful.

Aetiology

Tumours of the cardia may be gastric in origin, in which case they have the same aetiological and pathological characters as tumours of the body of the stomach. The malignant tumours of the lower oesophagus are usually squamous cell carcinomas and occur predominantly in the male sex. Some 50 percent of the carcinomas of the oesophagus appear in the lower third. The average age of onset of the disease is between 55 and

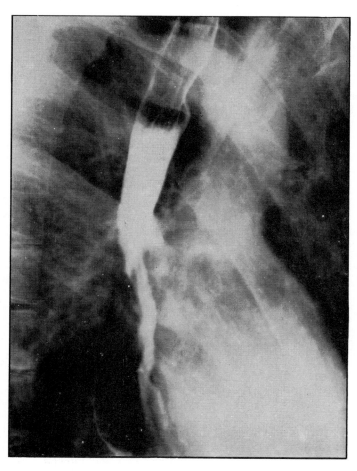

FIG. 18.   Barium-meal x-ray, adenocarcinoma of the cardia region associated with oesophageal hiatal hernia. (Confirmed at operation.)

60, and fewer young people are attacked by carcinoma in this situation than in any other part of the alimentary canal.

Pathological Anatomy

The squamous cell tumour of the oesophagus usually conforms to one of three types: the polypoidal, slightly ulcerated tumour; the more deeply ulcerative lesion; and the scirrhous type, which tends to cause thickening with contraction and obstruction of the passage. The adenocarcinomas do not differ in their characteristics from those seen in other parts of the stomach. The squamous cell carcinomas of the oesophagus have a reputation for slow growth, which is probably unjustified, as about a third disseminate rapidly and many of the others prove to be unresectable on exploration.

Tumours of the oesophagus may infiltrate or project into the stomach. Tumours of the

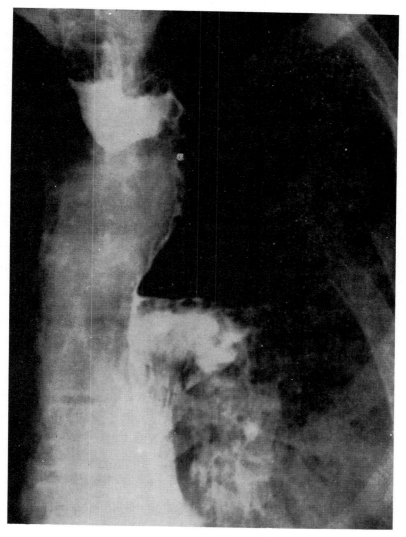

FIG. 19.   Same case as shown in Figure 18, 5 weeks after resection of the lower three-fifths of the oesophagus and the cardiac end of the stomach. The oesophagogastric anastomosis is at the clavicular level; the upper stomach is gas-filled.

upper stomach may infiltrate the lower oesophagus, producing a constrictive effect difficult to distinguish from cardiospasm. It is not uncommon to find a sliding diaphragmatic hiatal hernia associated with carcinoma in this region, though after a time extension of the growth will fix the cardia to the hernial sac within the lower mediastinum (Figs. 18 and 19). Whether the association is merely fortuitous, whether carcinoma may cause oesophageal shortening, or whether the reflux oesophagitis caused by a sliding hernia is a cancer-provoking condition is unknown.

The lymphatic drainage of the cardiac end of the stomach and the lower oesophagus is of particular importance in considering radical extirpation of this area. The lymphatic vessels of the stomach and oesophagus are in continuity across the cardia, so that it provides no barrier to the spread of malignant disease. In the stomach, a submucous plexus of vessels drains into the subserous plexus. In the oesophagus the latter is represented by a plexus around the gullet.

In the stomach, the lymphatic vessels follow the course of the blood supply closely as far as the first set of glands. From the upper lesser curvature of the stomach vessels pass: (1) to the inferior gastric glands which are in proximity to the descending branch of the left gastric artery; (2) direct to the superior gastric glands along the main trunk of the left gastric artery; and (3) to the paracardial glands which lie like a necklace around the cardia. The vessels from the greater curvature side of the upper stomach—that is, those from the left of a line dropped vertically downward from the cardia, pass with the vasa brevia and the left gastroepiploic artery either directly over the roof of the lesser sac to the left suprapancreatic lymph nodes or to the glands in the splenic hilum, which lie just above and occasionally below the tail of the pancreas, and from there they pass to the left suprapancreatic glands and then to the middle suprapancreatic glands which surround the origin of the left gastric artery and also drain the superior gastric glands.

From the oesophageal plexus, lymphatic vessels run to the glands which lie in close relation to it in the posterior mediastinum. From these glands, efferents run directly to the thoracic duct, upward to the tracheobronchial group, and downward to the paracardial and superior gastric glands. Churchill and Sweet [22] found malignant glands under the diaphragm in 8 out of 16 cases of carcinoma of the lower third of the oesophagus.

Symptomatology

The patient who develops a nonobstructive tumour of the cardiac end of the stomach is particularly unfortunate. because it may grow beyond the limits of possible resection before symptoms bring him to consult a physician. The symptoms, when they do appear, may be due to chronic anaemia or sudden blood loss, or may be of dyspepsia or vague ill health. I have seen patients whose only complaint was of persistent pain in the left hypochondrium, which proved to be caused by local hepatic invasion from fundic carcinoma. The first symptom may even be of abdominal distention resulting from peritoneal carcinomatosis and ascites, or it may be of distant glandular or blood-borne metastases.

In the cardiac orifice or lower oesophagus, however, obstructive symptoms usually bring the patient to seek advice at an earlier stage, although considerable narrowing must occur before such symptoms become urgent. The classic order is first of difficulty in swallowing solids, later of semisolids; finally even liquids cannot be retained. In the earliest stages, the symptoms may be indefinite—excessive "slime" (saliva and oesophageal mucus) in the mouth, foul eructations, or a dull, deep-seated discomfort in the chest, which probably results from distention and inflammation of the oesophagus with increased peristalsis above an obstruction. Later on, vomiting or regurgitation of undigested food mixed with saliva and mucus occurs shortly after swallowing. Pain in the back suggests pancreatic or spinal invasion; hiccough or pain in the shoulder, diaphragmatic or phrenic nerve irritation. The rare appearance of a patient with a carcinoma low in the oesophagus or cardia with a bolus or foreign body impacted above it shows the wisdom of bearing this disease in mind when one is called upon to remove such obstructions.

Diagnosis

Clinical examination is negative until a late stage of the disease, apart perhaps from signs of loss of weight or of anaemia. The bulkier tumours of the stomach eventually become palpable under the left costal margin. A pleural or peritoneal effusion, a pelvic mass felt on rectal examination, tumours in the liver, or hard glands in the supraclavicular region show that the disease has become inoperable by any standard.

Radiological examination of the oesophagus and stomach should never be omitted when there is suspicion of a carcinoma. Examination in the Trendelenburg position is particularly valuable in the investigation of the cardia and the lower limits of oesophageal tumours. Some dilatation of the oesophagus is usually present in carcinoma, but it is not so marked as in the simple lesions. There may be a filling defect, and perhaps a central crater. A soft-tissue opacity may give an indication of the bulk of the tumour.

If the tumour is at the cardiac orifice, the opaque meal may be seen to enter the stomach in a thin, steady trickle instead of in spurts as is normal, and the intra-abdominal part of the oesophagus may be deformed or its stream duplicated. With the patient upright, the shape of the fundic air bubble may be deformed, or there may be an increase in the soft-tissue shadow between air bubble and diaphragm.

An oesophagoscopic examination should be performed on all sufferers from dysphagia whether radiology findings be positive or negative. It gives an opportunity to confirm the x-ray diagnosis, it may bring into view a nonobstructive lesion missed by the radiological examination, and a small portion of any suspected tissue may be taken for histological examination. If doubt remains as to the innocence of oesophageal ulceration, then reexamination and removal of a further portion for microscopical study should be made after 10 days' rest in bed and use of the medical regimen for ulcer. A further advantage of oesophagoscopy is that it gives an opportunity to remove food debris from the gullet with consequent improvement in the patient's power of swallowing. This is important for nutritive purposes and as a preoperative measure. The introduction of the flexible fibre-optic oesophagoscope makes diagnostic oesophagoscopy a very safe procedure. The biopsy forceps is very small, however, and the volume of biopsy material is frequently too small for accurate diagnosis by the histopathologist. A further disadvantage of the modern instrument is that strictures cannot be dilated.

Gastroscopy and gastrophotography are of undoubted value in the diagnosis of lesions at the cardiac end of the stomach. It may of course be impossible to introduce the instrument—and this information is of some value—but if it does enter, the lower end of a cardiac tumour may be seen and its nature discovered.

Exfoliative cytological studies of oesophageal secretions may be helpful, particularly in cases in which oesophagoscopy is contraindicated, or in doubtful cases of carcinoma supervening on corrosive or peptic oesophagitis strictures or of recurrent carcinoma following oesophagectomy. Any gross food debris must first be removed with gentle saline lavage and then the gullet washed with Ringer's solution. These washings are centrifuged and examined microscopically (Bruinsma [65]). The value of cytology in the early diagnosis of carcinoma of the oesophagus and stomach was reported by Messelt in a thesis issued by Kemink en Zoon, N.V., Domplein 2, Utrecht.[23]

It is disappointing to perform a transthoracic exposure of the stomach only to find that there is widespread peritoneal carcinomatosis. Peritoneoscopy, while it will not give much indication of the extent of local infiltration by growth, may show the presence of peritoneal or hepatic metastases, and it can be added to the list of routine investigations of carcinoma of the upper stomach. Finally, where carcinoma cannot be disproved and there is strong suspicion of its presence, an exploratory operation is justified.

Treatment

Treatment may be palliative or it may be aimed at curing the disease.

PALLIATIVE TREATMENT

This treatment may be designed to improve the patient's abilities of normal eating, and in the first place simply means giving frequent semisolid or fluid feedings, and giving advice on methods of improving mastication. Further relief may follow oesophageal lavage or gentle dilatation of the passage through the tumour, carried out under vision through an oesophagoscope. In suitable cases, such as with smaller and more accessible infiltrative lesions, the insertion of a tube such as Symond's, Souttar's, or that of Mousseau-Barbin [24] or one of its modifications, into the lumen after dilatation may give ease in swallowing fluids and semisolids.

If these measures fail to enable the patient to take adequate nourishment, a feeding gastrostomy or jejunostomy may become necessary.

Finally, short-circuiting operations may be performed in suitable cases, but in practice such patients are those who undergo exploratory operations to determine whether resections can be performed but in whom the tumours are found to be unresectable. This will be considered later.

CURATIVE TREATMENT

In view of the resistance of gastric adenocarcinoma to irradiation, no hope of cure can be held out by this means, although lymphosarcoma may react well to it.

The squamous cell carcinomas of the oesophagus are more radiosensitive, but the depth and the difficulty of localisation of tumours of the lower oesophagus have prevented any great success in this region. Consequently deep x-ray treatment is rarely curative though recent work reveals more 5-year survival rates,[25] and attempts to irradiate the tumour by means of radium or intra-oesophageal carriers has had little success. A method which is perhaps more rational is the insertion of radon seeds after transthoracic or oesophagoscopic exposure of the growth. The former entails a major operation and the latter is uncertain, particularly in introducing the seeds to the lower part of the growth. High-voltage or cobalt radiotherapy, given preoperatively or postoperatively, is of value in some cases of squamous cell carcinoma of the cardia region.

SURGICAL EXTIRPATION

In our experience, this has produced the greatest proportion of long survivals and should be aimed at whenever possible.

Preoperative management. The outstanding feature of this disease is a process of starvation; thus, the preparation for operation is chiefly directed to restoring lost nutritional reserves. The patient who can take semisolids presents a simple problem and should be given a high-calorie and high-protein diet with adequate vitamin value. Frequent feeding should be insisted upon, and if a fine tube can be passed to the stomach, drip feeds may be given at night. Oral alimentation may be assisted by occasional oesophageal cleansing, and water or saline should be given after each feeding as a means of lavage. Such foods as egg, milk (or skimmed condensed milk), minced meat, soya, and protein digests if the patient can tolerate them, are valuable. Protein is essential not only because its lack slows wound-healing, but also because hypoproteinaemia produces tissue oedema. If swallowing is very difficult, added protein may be given by the intravenous infusion of blood, plasma, amino acid preparations, and fat solutions. Dehydrated patients will also require intravenous saline, or saline and glucose. Specific vitamin deficiencies occasionally manifest themselves in these patients, particularly after major surgery, and so vitamins of the B complex and C should be given in large doses. Anaemia may be masked by haemoconcentration, but if it is present and unresponsive to iron therapy, repeated blood transfusions may be required. If the patient is unable to gain weight and vitality by these means, however, a feeding jejunostomy must be made and nutrition improved by this route before operation can be considered. Gastrostomy should be avoided because the stomach must be mobilised during the resection of tumours near the cardia or in the lower oesophagus. If a gastrostomy has been made already, however, it can be excised with the stomach or repaired during the subsequent resection.

An attempt should be made to diminish

the bacterial content of the upper respiratory and alimentary tracts. If there is any sputum, the bacteria should be examined for their sensitivity to antibiotics and the appropriate antibiotic used just prior to and after operation. The teeth and gums should be cleaned but multiple extractions avoided if there is much dysphagia. For 12 hours of the day prior to operation, antibacterial lozenges (e.g., phthalylsulfathiazole, 0.5 g every 4 hr) should be taken by mouth to help sterilise the oesophagus. A full bowel sterilisation is necessary if there is any likelihood of a colonic replacement of the stomach and oesophagus (see above). Smoking should be avoided.

The risks of respiratory infection and of venous thrombosis may be diminished by encouraging active limb and respiratory exercises both before and after operation.

Immediately prior to operation, an oesophageal cleansing should be given and an intravenous saline infusion set up near the wrist or ankle where it will not intrude during the operative procedures. When the thoracotomy commences, the infusion should be replaced by blood.

Anaesthesia. The operation is performed under general anaesthesia. The use of relaxant drugs and an endotracheal tube gives absolute control of pulmonary ventilation, an immobile diaphragm, and a quiet lung at critical points of the operation. Halothane, which is noninflammable, can be used in high-oxygen concentration and is relatively nonirritant, so that the postoperative cough and pain are diminished.

During the operation, should cardiac irregularities develop, or work in the vicinity of the heart become necessary, anaesthetic agents are stopped and pure oxygen is administered. If this does not restore normal cardiac rhythm, practolol 2 to 5 mg or 50 to 100 mg of lignocaine can be given intravenously.

At the end of the operation, any intercostal nerve likely to be damaged during resuturing should be exposed at the posterior end of the intercostal space, and 2 to 3 cm of the nerve resected to diminish postoperative pain.

Operative technique. The optimum approach to the cardia region is by a combined abdominal and thoracic approach. Many satisfactory varieties of the incision have been described, all of which have as their basis a transverse, oblique, or vertical abdominal incision extended across the left costal margin either into an intercostal space or over a rib, which is resected and the rib bed incised. It is an advantage to make the abdominal part of the incision first, and if conditions are found to be favourable for resection, it may be continued into the thorax and through the diaphragm.

For the abdominothoracic approach, the patient lies carefully fixed in the right lateral position and hips and knees flexed, the left upper arm drawn forward and upward, the back near and parallel to the left side of the operating table. It is useful to have an operating table which will tilt laterally, there being a slight dorsal tilt in the beginning or abdominal part of the operation, and a slight ventral tilt for the latter part. When the patient is secure, the operation area is painted with antiseptic and drapings are clipped round it. It is helpful, particularly in the more robust patients, to infiltrate the line of incision with a local anaesthetic solution containing epinephrine, in order to diminish the vascularity of the tissue. The incision used by the writer will be described.

The abdominothoracic approach. After fixing a Steridrape or similar adherent drape over the skin, a transverse incision is made from a point between the xiphisternum and the umbilicus to cross the left costal margin. This is deepened through the anterior rectus sheath, the rectus muscle and posterior sheath, and the peritoneum to make an opening wide enough to introduce the hand into the peritoneal cavity with ease (Fig. 20). The cardia and the stomach can now be examined in order to confirm the diagnosis and determine whether the tumour is removable. If necessary, the lesser sac may be opened through the gastrocolic omentum in order to discover the posterior extensions of the growth. If the primary tumour appears to be removable, the liver, pelvic peritoneum, and other parts of the peritoneal cavity are examined for the presence of peritoneal, glandular, or other metastases, and to discover any associated lesion. If no contraindication to resection is found, the thoracic part of the incision is made.

It is convenient to identify the correct rib with the left hand in the abdomen. The incision is then prolonged over the desired inter-

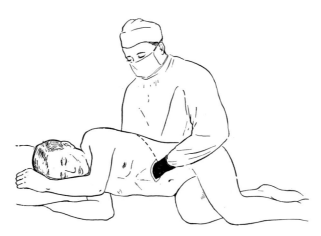

FIG. 20. Abdominal viscera are carefully palpated and may be inspected through the preliminary incision.

costal space or rib, as far back as the lateral edge of the erector spinae muscle. The intercostal incision is adequate, particularly in the young, and is somewhat less time-consuming, but the removal of a rib and incision through the rib bed is generally more satisfactory, as it gives a little more room, less firm retraction is needed, and the wound is more easily repaired. According to the height at which it is judged that the oesophageal section will be made, the decision will be made to remove the seventh, eighth, or ninth rib. The serratus anterior, latissimus dorsi, and trapezius muscles are divided down to the periosteum, which is incised as far back as the neck of the rib, the erector spinae being retracted medially. Every vessel must be carefully caught in artery forceps as soon as it is divided or much blood may be lost from the incision. Each bleeding point is then ligated or coagulated by diathermy. The periosteum is separated from the rib well medial to its angle with Farabeuf's rougine and Doyen's raspatory, and the rib removed from behind the angle to its costal end together with the costal cartilage and enough of the costal margin to prevent subsequent overriding. Bránches of the musculophrenic vessels will require ligation. At this point, the writer routinely excises a few centimetres of the posterior part of the intercostal nerve below the resected rib. This diminishes post-

operative chest pains considerably. The pleural cavity is now opened near the costophrenic sulcus, below the lung level, and when the lung drops away, the incision is widely opened. Next the diaphragm is divided from the point where the costal margin was divided almost to the oesophageal hiatus (Fig. 21), the cut being made in the line of the phrenic muscle fibres. Many vessels are encountered and require ligation, the largest, near the diaphragmatic hiatus, being branches of the inferior phrenic artery. It is then convenient to attach each cut edge of the diaphragm temporarily to a superficial muscle on the corresponding side of the parietal incision, for example, the external oblique or serratus anterior, with one or more stitches.[26] This saves retracting it separately and improves the view of the upper abdomen (Fig. 22). After protecting the wound edges with sterile towels, a large rib spreader is introduced (Price-Thomas's or Finochietto's are very suitable) and opened widely. The lung is partially collapsed, but the anaesthetist should reinflate it at intervals during the operation.

Any adhesions of the base of the lung which interfere with exposure are freed, but adhesions affecting the upper lobe should not be divided. The lower part of the pulmonary ligament is divided to enable the lung to be retracted and expose the left side of the

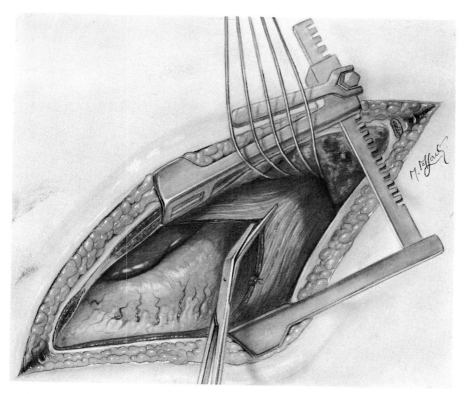

FIG. 21.   Parietal part of the abdominal incision completed. A rib, together with a short length of costal margin, has been removed. With scissors, the diaphragm is being incised in the direction of the oesophageal hiatus.

posterior mediastinum. Further palpation is made to discover the ramification of the tumour and the extent of glandular invasion. At times unsuspected intrathoracic extensions of the growth may be found which render curative resection impossible, though palliative measures may still be undertaken.

Extent of the resection. At this stage, when oesophagus and stomach are viewed in continuity, the pattern of the operation will have to be finally decided. The most important decision concerns the level of visceral section. The oesophageal transection should be made a minimum of 5 to 6 cm above the level of obvious growth. The lower level should be 6 cm or more below its lower edges. In the bulkier cardia growths, this usually means that the lower transection is so near to the duodenum that it is advisable to perform total gastrectomy and anastomose the oesophagus to jejunum—the writer for many years has preferred an end-to-end or

end-to-side anastomosis to a mobilised Roux loop of jejunum.[27] In the more localised cardia growths and in the squamous cell tumours of the lowest oesophagus, the pyloric antrum or anything up to half of the stomach may be retained.

Now a resection for carcinoma must be radical, that is to say, the adjacent lymphatic fields and structures most liable to be invaded by growth must also be removed. This entails removal of the greater and lesser omenta to a large extent, the paracardial, inferior mediastinal, left gastroepiploic, and left gastric glands, and glands along the gastroepiploic arch. In a total gastrectomy, the right gastric and subpyloric glands must also be excised.

At times the growth may not have spread diffusely and yet it has invaded a neighbouring organ. In such cases it is often possible to remove totally or in part the locally invaded structures or organ. For example, the

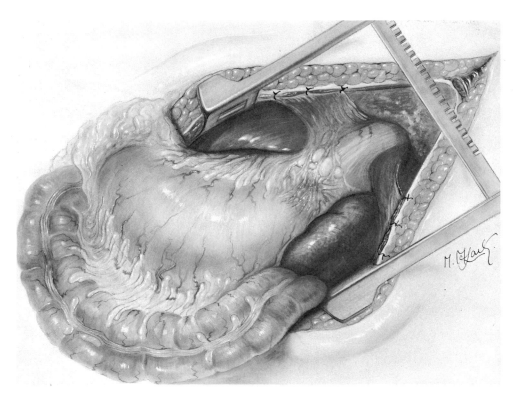

FIG. 22. The diaphragm has been divided to expose the cardia region. The intercostal incision has been retracted. To eliminate the need for separate retraction of the diaphragm, the cut edges of the diaphragm are sutured to suitable muscle on the corresponding side of the parietal incision.

diaphragm, anterior abdominal wall, lung, liver, spleen, or body or tail of the pancreas may be so invaded and may be readily amenable to inclusion in the resection.

The resection. Resectability being confirmed, it is convenient to commence by freeing the cardia region, as this brings the organ nearer to the surface. A longitudinal incision is made in the inferior mediastinal pleura between the aorta and pericardium, and the pleura is finely dissected off the underlying posterior mediastinal contents. A small moist swab is useful for this. With the swab, the front of the aorta is separated from the oesophagus, mediastinal glands and fatty tissue, and vagus nerves. Usually two small arteries to the oesophagus, which pass obliquely forward and downward from the anterior surface of the aorta, will require division. Next, the right boundary of the mediastinum is cleared until the right mediastinal pleura is seen, the right lung being faintly visible through it. Next, the mediastinal contents are freed anteriorly—as high as the inferior pulmonary vein. Here, as throughout the whole operation, the most careful attention must be paid to haemostasis. A tape is then passed round the oesophagus with its attached mediastinal contents to steady it during subsequent manipulation. The tendency to steady the parts being dissected by grasping or pressing on the tumour should be avoided, for such manipulations may favour dissemination of tumour cells into the blood stream.

The incision in the diaphragm is now continued into the oesophageal hiatus, branches of the inferior phrenic vessels being ligated prior to division. If the growth extends into the oesophageal hiatus, it is preferable to remove a ring of diaphragmatic tissue with the oesophagus. Medially the lesser (hepatogastric) omentum tethers the stomach to the liver. This should be divided close to the liver, a vessel near its upper margin requiring careful ligation. Prior to this division, a careful inspection should be made to ensure that the left or even the main hepatic artery does not take an anomalous origin from the left gastric artery and run to the liver behind the upper part of the lesser omentum. Needless to say, such an anomalous vessel, if of large size, should be spared unless adjacent to tumour tissue. The division of the lesser omentum continues until the right gastric vessels are met.

The greater curvature of the stomach is next freed. The decision of whether to remove the spleen must be made. If it is infiltrated by growth or there are glandular metastases near its hilum, splenectomy is imperative. There is some danger of splenic vein thrombosis and hepatic embolism if the spleen is removed.[28] The author usually removes it en bloc with the stomach. An incision is made in the lienorenal ligament and the splenic vessels are exposed. After the splenic vessels are very carefully ligated in

continuity, they are divided just above the pancreatic tail, and the glands from this region are freed with the spleen. Most of the vasa brevia and the left gastroepiploic artery will have been dealt with if the splenic vessels are ligated, but if the spleen is not to be removed, the former vessels will require to be ligated and divided in the gastrolienal ligament. Usually one or two accessory vasa brevia are found running from the trunk of the splenic artery, taking origin some distance before its termination and passing behind the lesser sac toward the incisura cardiaca. These vessels, too, should be carefully ligated and divided near their origin, as lymphatic vessels accompany them. The presence of these latter vessels is not emphasised in the standard books of anatomy, but they are prominent in this operation. The epiploic vessels in the gastrocolic omentum are now divided as far as the duodenum, leaving the gastroepiploic arch and glands attached to the stomach. After freeing of the posterior wall of the pyloric antrum of any adhesions to the pancreas and mesocolon, the stomach should be very mobile in its distal half.

The left gastric vessels and lymph nodes

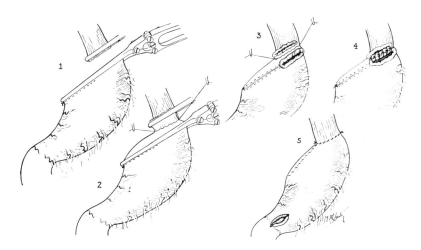

FIG. 23. (1 and 2) If more stomach is retained, an anastomosis of the oesophagus to the greater curve side of the cut end is least likely to lead to tension. (3 and 4) After closing the lesser curve side of the cut end of the stomach, the oesophagus is united to the open greater curve side. (5) Finally, a seromuscular row of stitching covers the closed part of the stomach and oesophagogastric suture line, and the pyloric muscle is divided. The final result resembles an upside-down Billroth I (Péan) anastomosis.

will now be very clearly displayed as they pass in the gastropancreatic ligament (falx coronarium) from the upper border of the pancreas to the lesser curvature of the stomach. These may be doubly ligated and divided en masse at the upper border of the pancreas. Better still, the lymphatics, left gastric vein, and artery may be separately dissected from the upper border of the pancreas and then tied and divided separately, with removal of the superior gastric lymph glands and perhaps some suspicious suprapancreatic glands with the stomach. The stomach and spleen can now be easily lifted out of the wound.

The transection level of the stomach is now precisely defined. The omenta on the greater and lesser curvatures are divided distal to the level of gastric section, and the omenta and glands are dissected up proximally in order both to demonstrate the exact limits of the stomach wall and to include as many glands as possible with the part to be resected. Two Payr clamps are applied across the stomach and the stomach is divided between them.

Next, the level of oesophagus section is demarcated. The areolar tissue and glands attached to the oesophagus are brushed down to below this level and the vagal nerve fibres are divided at the level. Suitable fine clamps are then applied across the oesophagus, the gullet divided between them, and the specimen removed. (It is unnecessary to retain the specimen as a retractor for the gullet.)

The Oesophagogastric Anastomosis. In the past, it has been the rule to close the cut end of the stomach and then anastomose the end of the oesophagus to an incision or to a rounded opening made in the anterior wall of the stomach. For 25 years now Tanner has abandoned this method and instead made end-to-end anastomosis between the oesophagus and part of the cut end of the stomach.[29]

The details of the anastomosis technique may vary, but the basic principle must be to obtain a tension-free union with exact mucosa-to-mucosa apposition. The steps, as carried out by Tanner, are as follows: After the area has been surrounded with protective towels, the wide cut end of the stomach is narrowed by one layer of suturing until the open gastric and oesophageal diameters are nearly equal. It is an advantage to have the gastric opening slightly the wider. The lesser-curvature half of the cut end of the stomach should be closed in order to retain the advantage of greater length of stomach on its greater curve side (Fig. 23, *1*). The posterior surface of the open part of the stomach and the oesophagus are now united by a continuous chromic catgut suture. This may conveniently be inserted as a loose, continuous stitch which is pulled tight when the row is complete (Fig. 23, *2*). The clamps are now removed and an all-coats suturing of the posterior and then the anterior margins is made, with either interrupted fine nonabsorbable sutures or a continuous suture of 00 chromic catgut on an eyeless (atraumatic) needle. In inserting this row, great care should be taken that the oesophageal mucosa, which tends to slip upward, is included in the suturing. When this is complete, the posterior seromuscular stitching is continued round to the front. The sutured lesser curve should now be buried by a second or seromuscular row, and in this case the anastomosis will resemble an upside-down Billroth I (Péan) union with the oesophagus taking the place of duodenum (Fig. 23, *3, 4,* and *5*).

In view of the fact that the all-coats layer is the stronger of the two layers used in this anastomosis, the writer has of late years varied the method of anastomosis. Provided that the two parts are well mobilised and can be rotated, the stronger inner or all-coats suture is inserted first, with careful inversion of the mucosa. The second layer is then introduced, with rotation of the anastomosis first of all to commence the outer row. This newer method is illustrated in Figure 24A, where an end-to-side anastomosis is being made between the oesophagus and a mobilised Roux loop of jejunum. In making the outer continuous suture, it is to be borne in mind that the seromuscularis of the stomach or jejunum is brought up around the oesophagus, thus invaginating the more fragile oesophageal muscularis (Fig. 24B). Some surgeons obtain good results by using one row only of interrupted fine stainless-steel wire sutures.

The packs which were inserted are removed and clean gloves put on. Penicillin is powdered round the anastomosis and into the mediastinum.

Now it must be remembered that the portion of the stomach retained is completely deprived of its vagal nerve supply and so tends to evacuate slowly, particularly during the first postoperative year. Thus it has been the writer's habit to perform a simple Heineke-Mikulicz pyloroplasty to overcome this tendency.[11] Tanner has also modified this during the last 8 years by performing a simple myotomy of the pyloric sphincter (a procedure similar to the Ramstedt operation) with satisfactory results (Fig. 23, 5).

Next the stomach must be so fixed as to remove gravitational or other forms of tension from the suture line. The remaining stomach and first and second parts of the duodenum will have been freed of any ad-

hesions and if necessary the second part of the duodenum may be mobilised by an incision in the peritoneum to its right side. It will usually then be possible to attach the pyloric part of the stomach to the diaphragm near its crural origin. Next, with a few interrupted sutures, the seromuscular coat of the well-elevated gastric remnant is sutured to the cut posterior edge of the mediastinal pleura, and when completed it will be confirmed that there is no tension on the anastomosis. The mediastinum should not be completely closed off from the pleural cavity, for it is desirable that mediastinal exudates should drain freely into the latter.

The diaphragm is closed with a continuous stitch of No. 60 linen, and reinforced with a few interrupted sutures, leaving just enough room posteriorly for the stomach to pass through, and one or two additional fine sutures may be placed to approximate the diaphragm to the pyloric antrum. These sutures also prevent subsequent herniation of the abdominal contents into the chest (Fig. 25). When completed, it should be confirmed that even, full contraction of the diaphragm (which may be simulated by pushing it downward) will not cause tension on the anastomosis. If this freedom from tension on contracting the diaphragm cannot be obtained, there is no alternative but to crush the phrenic nerve. The author has always been able to avoid this step, and believes that an active diaphragm is an added insurance against retention of bronchial secretions.

Pleural drainage. No dogmatic statement can be made on this subject. It is most important that any pleural exudates should be removed from the chest, and this may best be effected by the insertion of an intercostal drainage catheter at a convenient point, projecting 1 to 2 inches (2.5 to 5 cm) into the chest.

At the end of the operation, the anaesthetist inflates the lung and the abdomino-thoracic wound is closed, first the posterior rectus sheath and peritoneum, then the pleura and intercostal muscles, and finally the anterior rectus sheath, thoracic muscles, and skin. Additional security may be obtained by passing two or three stout sutures through opposing drill holes made in the ribs on either side of the thoracotomy incision. If an intercostal catheter is used, it

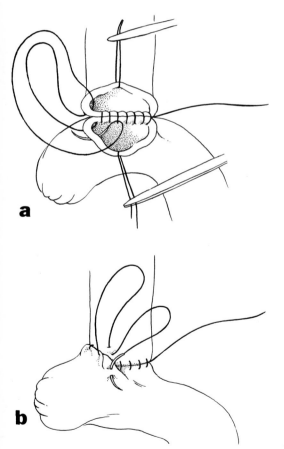

a

b

FIG. 24. (A) Insertion of the all-coats layer with complete inversion of the jejunum. (B) Technique of insertion of the seromuscular layer bringing the jejunum up around the oesophagus.

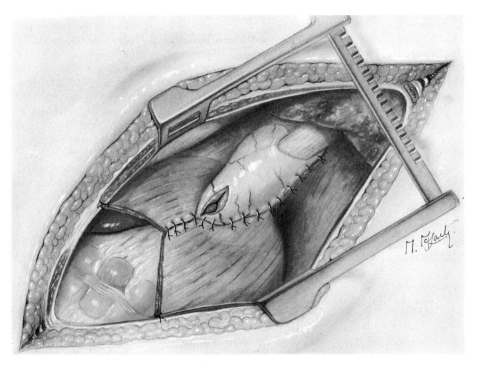

FIG. 25. Tension is removed from the suture line by fixing the well-elevated stomach and pyloric region to the edges of the opening left in the diaphragm and the mediastinal pleura.

should be spigotted pending the setting-up of an underwater seal drainage on the patient's arrival in the ward.

Before the patient leaves the operation table, any bronchial or pharyngeal secretions should be aspirated.

Variations of the standard operation. In the surgery of malignant disease, one must be prepared to adapt the operation to suit any of the vagaries of the lesion. A few adaptations of this operation of which the author has experience may be mentioned.

If the peritoneum of the lesser sac has been invaded, it may be stripped away and removed with the stomach. If the pancreas has been invaded or the suprapancreatic lymph nodes are carcinomatous, a block resection of the peritoneum of the posterior wall of the lesser sac, spleen, and body and tail of the pancreas may be performed, with ligation of the splenic and left gastric arteries at their origins from the coeliac axis. Indeed, for almost all malignant diseases of the cardiac end of the stomach the writer now performs

this extension of the standard operation routinely, for there is a very direct lymphatic drainage from the cardia region and upper greater curvature of the stomach to the suprapancreatic lymph nodes—which cannot with safety be stripped from the left half of the pancreas. This variation is readily carried out by omitting to divide the gastrosplenic omentum and instead making an incision in the parietal peritoneum lateral to the spleen and reflecting the spleen, pancreas, and posterior lesser-sac peritoneum forward and to the right. The left gastric and splenic vessels are doubly ligated and divided (Fig. 26). Rarely the tumour or malignant lymph nodes may invade the coeliac artery itself. If by ligating the coeliac artery flush with the aorta a satisfactory operation can be carried out, this step should be taken. The hepatic branch will require ligation above the neck of the pancreas and proximal to its gastro-duodenal branch, and a length of the hepatic artery removed. Before carrying out this step, it is essential to make certain that the supe-

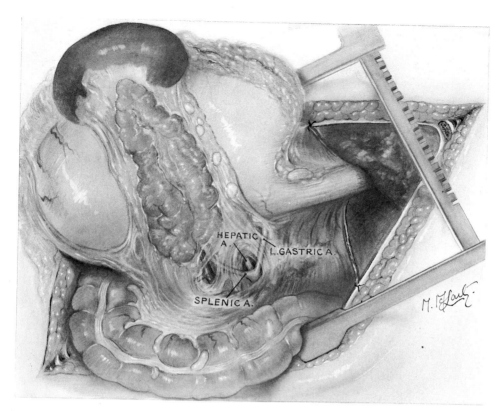

FIG. 26.   En-bloc removal of the body and tail of the pancreas, spleen, and posterior peritoneum of the lesser sac, with the stomach and lower oesophagus. These structures are dissected forward to expose the main branches of the coeliac artery. The left gastric and splenic arteries are divided near their point of origin. (To clarify the diagram, the posterior part of the gastric fundus is shown. Normally, it is not in view, being obscured by the posterior peritoneum.)

rior mesenteric artery does not take origin from the coeliac. The splenic vein will be divided near the level of transection of the pancreas. In view of the risks attendant on splenic vein thrombosis, it is best whenever feasible to divide the vein to the left of the entry of the inferior mesenteric vein, as the venous current produced by retaining this vessel will diminish the tendency to clotting. The transected neck of the pancreas must be carefully repaired. Haemostasis must be secured at the cut end, and if the pancreatic duct is seen, it should be carefully ligatured. The writer finds it helpful to transect the pancreas with a V-shaped cut, so that the remaining part resembles a fish tail. The two limbs of the V may be sutured together with chromic catgut sutures so as to leave no raw surface exposed—a great help in preventing

leakage. At the end of the operation, a small tube drain should be placed down to this point in case there is postoperative escape of pancreatic secretion; and because the pleural and peritoneal cavities are in communication at the end of the operation, it is wise to use underwater seal drainage to this tube for 48 to 72 hours.

In the event of local invasion of the liver by carcinoma, it is justifiable to remove part of the left lobe after transfixing it with mattress sutures, or the liver can be transected by piecemeal clamping with artery forceps and ligating bit by bit. The author has a patient with this complication of the operation who is alive and working 19 years after the resection.

In many cases, if not in most, carcinoma involving the cardiac end of the stomach will

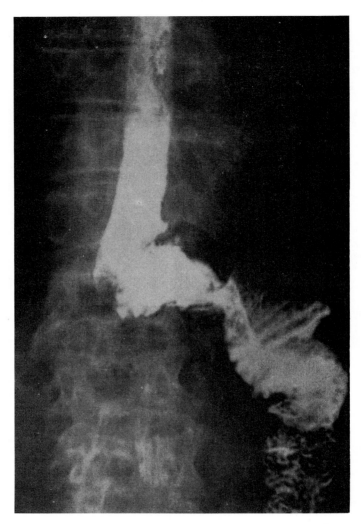

FIG. 27.   X-ray 7 years after gastrectomy, splenectomy, and hemipancreatectomy and end-to-end oesophagojejunal anastomosis. The patient is well, takes normal meals, and is working.

require total gastrectomy because of the extensive invasion of the stomach itself or because the subpyloric glands are invaded, for the latter cannot be removed without sacrifice of the right gastroepiploic vessels, which in turn requires sacrifice of the pyloric antrum. In such a case, the greatest comfort will undoubtedly be obtained by making an anastomosis between the oesophagus and a mobilised Roux loop of jejunum, which is brought up into the pleural cavity through an opening in the mesocolon (Fig. 27).

A *palliative short circuit* may be considered advisable in order to ameliorate the symptoms if the growth is found to be irremovable. In such cases, the author finds that the most satisfactory procedure is as follows: The proximal jejunum is transected and the distal segment mobilised by dividing the main mesenteric vessels until such mobility is obtained that the jejunum can reach the oesophagus above the growth without mesenteric tension. This mobilised loop is then drawn up through a short channel made through the mesocolon into the retroperitoneal tissues *behind* the pancreas and lesser

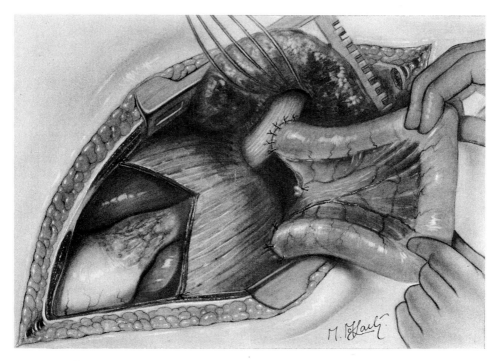

FIG. 28. Palliative side-to-end oesophagojejunostomy for irremovable cancer of the cardiac end of the stomach. A Roux loop of jejunum was brought up through the transverse mesocolon and behind the pancreas into the pleural cavity through the small posterior diaphragmatic incision.

sac and then through an opening made in the diaphragm into the pleural cavity. Its end is then anastomosed to the side of the dilated oesophagus (Figs. 28 and 29). (This retroperitoneal route is chosen because it is short and is practically never invaded by the primary growth.) The free proximal cut end of the jejunum is, of course, implanted end-in-side to the jejunum lower down, thus completing the Roux type of anastomosis (Fig. 30).

Postoperative Management

On the patient's return to the ward, water-sealed drainage is instituted if there is an intercostal or abdominal drainage tube, or a Heimlich-type tube may be used. In most hospitals, it will be helpful for the patient to spend the first few days in an intensive care ward.

Any blood loss must be completely replaced, though cardiac embarrassment due to overloading of the circulation should be avoided. The blood transfusion should be followed by a slow continuous saline and glucose infusion, with about half a litre of plasma daily. To ensure that the lungs are expanded, the chest should be x-rayed on or just before the patient's return to the ward.

Adequate doses of penicillin and streptomycin should be continued until the fifth day and until any postoperative pulmonary or wound infection has subsided. If jejunostomy feedings were being given before operation, they should be recommenced about 20 hours later. On the fifth postoperative day, a routine barium swallow using gastrografin is carried out to ensure that the oesophageal anastomosis has healed. The nasogastric tube is then removed and oral feeding with fluids is commenced with small meals of fruit juices, sugar, and skimmed milk. Egg may be introduced on the sixth day, by which time the patient should be able to take enough nour-

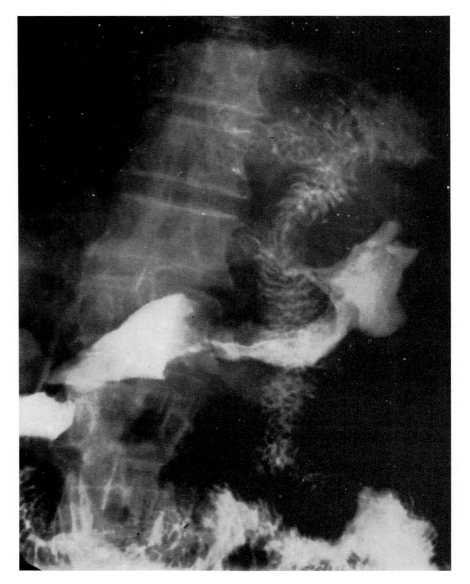

FIG. 29. Barium-meal x-ray film after palliative side-to-side oesophagojejunal anastomosis.

ishment by mouth to dispense with intra-venous feeding.

If cyanosis occurs after the patient's return to the ward, one should suspect excessive bronchial secretion, bronchial obstruction, haemothorax, or pneumothorax.

The intercostal drainage tube drains bloody secretion for 2 to 3 days, after which it may be removed. It is wise to radiograph the chest and if necessary carry out a pleural aspiration after removal of the tube; then take a further radiograph and, if necessary, aspirate again 48 hours later.

The performance of such transthoracic op-erations is not infrequently complicated by the collection of excessive quantities of tena-cious bronchial mucus. This should be antici-pated and the patient be told to cough vigorously at frequent intervals after the operation. It is helpful if the patient has had

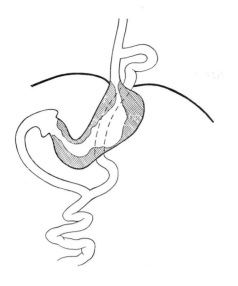

FIG. 30. Diagrammatic representation of growth and short circuit shown in Figure 29.

preoperative lessons in correct breathing and coughing. If these coughing exercises are done shortly after the administration of morphine, the dulling of the wound pains may result in a more effective cough. Changes of posture—lying on one side or the other without pillows or with the head lower than the feet—also aid the expulsion of fluid. Inhalations of tincture of benzoin compound cum menthol in steam, or one of the aerosol detergents—e.g., Alevaire, may help to render the mucus less tenacious. Injections of full doses of nikethamide intravenuosly also help to stimulate coughing.

Some patients are too ill, too lethargic, or too uncooperative to clear their passages adequately. The result of this may be pulmonary atelectasis from obstruction of a bronchus, or the secretion may become infected or the very volume of secretion may prevent adequate pulmonary ventilation. In such cases, three courses are open: Either pass a bronchoscope and aspirate the secretion under vision, or pass a rubber catheter, size 16 French, blindly through the nose and on into the trachea during deep inspiration (holding out the tongue may help to prevent the tube from being swallowed). Through this tube, aspiration of the main bronchi may

be effected.[30] The third course is to perform tracheotomy and carry out repeated bronchial aspiration through the tracheostome.

Cardiac arrhythmia may occur, usually about the second day, and the rapid irregularities are often improved with digoxin therapy. Some physicians use quinidine as a prophylactic against arrhythmia, but its value is doubtful. In shock states, cortisone may tide the patient over a difficult period.

There is no objection to—in fact there is much to be said for—early ambulation in these cases, the more robust patients being allowed out of bed on the third or fourth day, and to walk when they feel so inclined.

The incidence of postoperative empyema has almost vanished since the routine use of penicillin and pleural drainage, though the possibility of this complication must be borne in mind if any postoperative pyrexia occurs.

Late Complications and Prognosis

Stricture at the site of anastomosis is almost invariable if methods of oesophagogastric implantation similar to the introduction of a gastrostomy tube in the stomach are used, but with careful mucosa-to-mucosa apposition, it is much less common, and prolonged and comfortable deglutition may be anticipated (Fig. 31). Stenosis of the lumen may occur if the mucosal sutures tear apart or were inadequately inserted, if there is recurrence of growth around or in the anastomosis, or if there is development of peptic ulceration of the oesophagus.[26] In view of the usually extensive gastric resection, the vagotomy, and the generally diminished likelihood of peptic ulceration in gastric cancer, the latter cause of stricture is, in the writer's opinion and experience, rare.

Despite a division of the pyloric muscle, some patients suffer much from regurgitation of gastric juice into the gullet after oesophagogastric anastomosis, leading to anorexia, wasting, and depression. In four such cases, Tanner[31] has effected a considerable improvement by making a gastrojejunostomy between the proximal jejunum and pyloric antrum (Fig. 32).

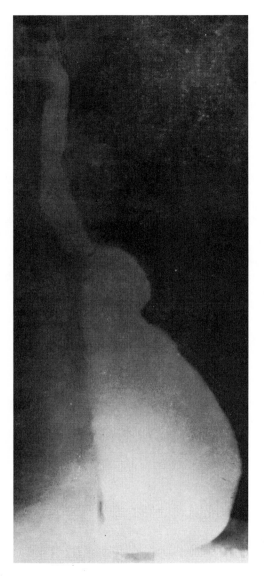

FIG. 31. Film showing an oesophagogastric anasto-mosis following resection of the upper stomach and lower half of the oesophagus. Deglutition is com-fortable.

The operative mortality depends on the patient's age and general condition, and on the extent of the growth. The mortality rate mounts with increasing age.[32] The more ad-vanced the growth the poorer the general condition usually is. Advanced growths in the middle or upper gullet are usually ir-removable because of the contiguity of vital structures, but they may be removable in the cardiac region because so much more of the surrounding tissue is resectable. As the au-thor has seen the most feeble patients survive this operation, many survivors being septua-genarians and 3 over 80 years of age, 1 of whom made over a 5-year survival, it is diffi-cult to be dogmatic as to when a patient should be refused operation simply on ac-count of age or poor general condition, par-ticularly in view of the great symptomatic relief derived from surgery.

Of a total of 353 patients with carcinomas in this region coming to the writer's clinic between 1940 and 1959, 76 had squamous cell tumours and 141 adenocarcinomas local-ised to the cardia region, and 136 had exten-sive adenocarcinomas of the stomach invad-ing the lower oesophagus. Of these, 41 (53.9 percent) of the squamous cell tumours and 154 (55.6 percent) of the adenocarcinomas were resected. Sweet records a resectability rate of 65 percent.

The mortality rate of oesophagectomy di-minishes from the upper oesophagus down-ward. The mortality rate will depend on when the operation was carried out (being lower during recent years), and on the per-centage of patients who required multiple or complicated resections. For carcinoma in the cardiac region, De Amneste and Otaiza[33] record an operation mortality rate of 57 per-cent and Pack and McNeer,[34] 33 percent; for a series including more recent cases, Sweet[35] records a mortality rate of only 11.6 percent (compared with 24.3 percent for the midoesophagus). Of 43 operative deaths (in Sweet's series), 22 were attributed to cardiac failure and only 5 to infection.

LONG-TERM SURVIVAL RATES

These cannot be clearly defined yet, but they appear to be comparable with those of cancer of the stomach. Sweet found little difference between survival rates in the adenocarcinoma and in epidermoid carci-noma of the cardiac region, though he thought the results were, if anything, better in the adenocarcinomas. Of the survivors of resections carried out over 5 years before, 17.5 percent were still alive in 1951 (5-year survival rate with affected lymph nodes, 13.5

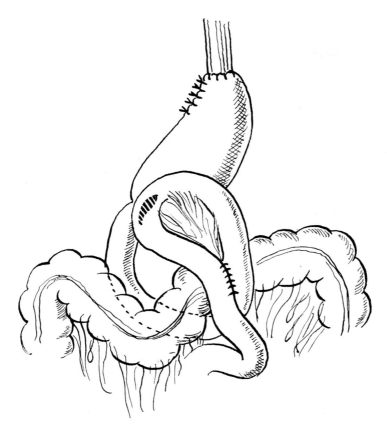

FIG. 32. In the event of there being much reflux, or inability to take adequate diet after oesophagogastric anastomosis following upper gastric resection, a great improvement may follow gastrojejunostomy made across the pylorus and the antrum.

percent; without affected nodes, 40 percent). Garlock [36] had nine patients with adenocarcinoma of the cardia alive 5 years or more after resection, one having survived for 10 years, two for 9 years, two for 8 years, and two for 7 years. Tanner,[3] in his series, has 6.8 percent of all patients with squamous cell cancer of the oesophagus surviving 5 years or more. Of those who survived resection, 33.3 percent were alive 5 years later. Of the adenocarcinomas affecting the cardiac region, 7.7 percent were alive 5 years later. There were 24.7 percent alive, however, of those who survived resection. These results are despite the fact that several of the nonsurvivors had died of other diseases, pulmonary tuberculosis, accidents, etc., and many of those successfully resected had really palliative resections. Several of the 5-year survivors also had a pan-

createctomy and splenectomy, and 1 (a 19-year survivor) had a partial hepatectomy and splenectomy added to the cardia resection. This confirms the view held by some that extensive local infiltration without distant metastases is of good prognostic import if all the locally invaded tissues can be excised. Pearson [25] has compared the results of surgery and radiotherapy in the treatment of squamous cell carcinoma of the oesophagus in Edinburgh between the years 1956 and 1964. Of 227 patients treated by resection or short circuit, 8 percent lived for 5 years. Of 88 patients who had no treatment, gastrostomy or intubation only, none lived for 5 years. Of 260 patients treated by radical or palliative radiotherapy, 8.5 percent lived for 5 years.

In our clinic, between the years 1957 and

1963, 111 cases of squamous cell and adeno-carcinoma of midoesophagus and cardia were treated. This represents every case seen during this time; 78 were resected (70 percent resectability rate). There were 13 overall survivors, or 11 percent were alive at 5 years. This figure includes those patients with squamous cell carcinoma who were given post-operative radiotherapy. Out of a total of 575 cases of carcinoma of the oesophagus, including adenocarcinomas treated to date at our clinic, 8 percent had lived for 5 years.

The overall survival figures will continue to improve as the operative mortality rate continues to diminish from the high levels suffered a decade ago. The writer's operative mortality rate for extended resections of the whole stomach or cardia is now under 10 percent.

In view of the 100 percent mortality rate of patients who do not undergo operation or radiotherapy, as well as the discomforts of artificial methods of feeding and the loss of the pleasure of living which is so obvious in these sufferers, the operations are justified even if a permanent cure cannot be anticipated. At the very least, they provide sufferers from carcinoma of the cardiac end of the stomach and lower oesophagus the most satisfactory palliation and the most certain means of restoring comfort and the capacity to work.

OESOPHAGEAL ACHALASIA (CARDIOSPASM)

It is now generally accepted that *achalasia* is the correct term for this condition, although the term *cardiospasm* is still widely used.

HISTORICAL NOTE

Thomas Willis (1674), writing in *Pharmaceutica Rationalis,* was the first to treat achalasia of the cardia by dilatation ". . . *with a rod of whale bone with a little round button of sponge fitted to the top of it."* Luck was on the side of Thomas Willis as he did not perforate the gullet and his patient was able subsequently to pass the "bougie" himself as well as "to take his sustenance for 16 years." [37]

The attention of early writers was directed towards the dilatation of the upper oesophagus. Zenker and von Ziemssen [38] believed that the condition was a simple ectasia, whilst Rosenheim [39] thought it was caused by primary muscular atony.

When radiology was used increasingly in diagnosis, attention was directed to the lower narrow segment of the oesophagus. Mikulicz [40] suggested that the condition was due to spasm of the cardiac sphincter. Einhorn [41] gave a good description of cardiospasm and suggested that the oesophageal dilatation was produced by a failure of reflex opening of the cardia during the act of swallowing. Hurst [42] propounded the same theory and coined the term *achalasia,* which means failure of relaxation. Hurst and Rake [43] described pathological changes in Auerbach's plexus in the region of the epicardia. Rake's microscopical investigations were carried out on autopsy specimens of gullets of patients who had died as a result of the disease. Wooler,[44] however, opined that the degeneration of Auerbach's plexus was secondary to dilatation of the oesophagus and was not the cause of achalasia.

The term *mega-oesophagus* was first used by von Hacker because he considered that the pathogenesis was similar to that of Hirschsprung's disease. Knight (1934) submitted experimental evidence supporting the theory of spasm due to overaction of sympathetic nerve supply to the cardia. The few patients he operated upon by sympathectomy did not yield the results he anticipated, and this operation has in consequence been abandoned.

On April 14, 1913, Heller [45] in Leipzig set out to do a cardioplasty with oesophagogastric anastomosis on a patient with cardiospasm, but after he had mobilised the oesophagus and drawn it into the abdomen, he lost heart. The anastomosis looked too difficult and the oesophagus, uncovered with peritoneum, looked unreliable. So he decided to do a myotomy because of the good results which followed such an operation at the pylorus. He made 8-cm-long incisions through the muscle layers down to the mucosa, anterior and posterior to the oesophagus and stomach. The immediate success of this operation impressed Heller, but it took a long time in Great Britain for the value of the operation to be recognised. Barlow [46] was the first British surgeon to publish reports of four patients treated successfully by submucous oesophagocardiomyotomy. The rival operations of cardioplasty and oesophagogastric anastomosis were finally abandoned in this country when Barrett and Franklin [47] revealed the frequency with which they were followed by oesophageal ulceration.

Aetiology

The aetiology of this condition has never been convincingly explained, although all writers are agreed that there is either a degeneration or congenital absence of ganglion cells in Auerbach's plexus in the oesophagus.

Johnstone,[48] on radiological study at a stage before any dilatation or hypertrophy had occurred, noted completely dissociate movements of the oesophagus without any propulsive action.

Adams et al.[49] maintain that the four cardinal changes that typify achalasia are (1) a failure of the cardia to relax; (2) the disappearance of normal oesophageal peristalsis, and its replacement by segmental and tertiary contractions; (3) dilatation and hypertrophy of the oesophagus above the cardia; and (4) an increased sensitivity of the oesophagus to cholinergic drugs. These workers proved that there is a disturbance in the innervation of the *whole* oesophagus and that ganglion cells are completely absent in the dilated part of the gullet and almost absent in the narrow segment. Certainly these findings explain the pathological changes, signs, symptoms, and clinical course of the disease.

Further advances in our knowledge have been made as a result of intraoesophageal pressure records and motility studies made by many investigators, particularly in America, such as those by Anderson et al.[50] True peristalsis can now be differentiated from the uncoordinated and ineffective oesophageal movements that persist after peristalsis has disappeared.

Cassella et al.[51] reinvestigated 88 of their patients with the electron microscope and found that in only 19 was there any degeneration in Auerbach's plexus. They found a reduction, however, in the number of cells in the dorsal motor nucleus of the vagus and Wallerian degeneration in the thoracic portion of every vagus nerve they examined. They believe the primary cause lies in one of these two findings. Further support for this concept of an extra-oesophageal vagal lesion is provided by the animal experiments of Higgs et al.,[52] who produced a condition closely resembling human oesophageal achalasia by focal destruction of the nucleus ambiguus in dogs and of the dorsal motor nucleus in cats.

Ellis and co-workers [53] maintained that it was important to distinguish achalasia from a disturbance of oesophageal motility known as diffuse oesophageal spasm, in which the patient experiences generalised oesophageal pain on swallowing and radiologically is seen to have both peristaltic and uncoordinated oesophageal movements. However, evidence that these two conditions may be related has been produced by many workers, particularly Kramer et al.,[54] who recorded by serial motility studies and balloon kymography the transition from diffuse spasm to achalasia.

Mega-oesophagus has been considered by some authorities to be a separate disease entity, but more sophisticated methods of investigation make it probable that it represents an advanced form of achalasia.

Achalasia of the cardia has been compared to Chagas' disease (Brazilian trypanosomiasis) by Brazilian workers who found the canine counterpart of oesophageal achalasia when dogs were infested with the parasite *Trypanosoma cruzi*.[55] Degeneration of the cells of the nerve plexuses in the dogs' oesophageal wall, caused by the toxin of *T. cruzi*, certainly indicates the basic pathological change, but has not advanced our knowledge about achalasia.

Transient achalasia may occur following vagotomy. Clinically and radiologically it simulates true achalasia, but it responds rapidly to conservative measures.

Pathology

The chief pathological features are: (1) dilatation, (2) hypertrophy, and (3) lengthening of the oesophagus.

A study of the fine structure of oesophageal smooth muscle in achalasia was made by Cassella et al.[56] Myofilament detachment, ribosomal activity, and changes in cell size were the major morphological changes noted. The area most involved was the junctional zone between the narrowed and dilated segments of the oesophagus. It is suggested that the smooth-muscle changes result from oesophageal denervation.

At operation, the cardiac orifice itself is normal in appearance and in diameter, while immediately above the cardia the terminal 3 to 6 cm of the oesophagus are pale, thin, atrophic, and narrowed, often having a diameter of not more than 1 to 1.5 cm. There are no signs of adhesions and mediastinal adenitis is not a feature as it is with stenosing peptic oesophagitis. The hiatal mechanism is

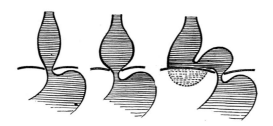

FIG. 33. Dilatation of the oesophagus varies in shape according to the stage of the disease. In an early case, it is fusiform; later, it becomes flask-shaped; a sigmoid or S-shaped variety represents an advanced stage. (After Maingot.)

usually intact. The culpable area of the gullet feels soft and yielding and no signs of diffuse or localised fibrosis can be detected. Above the narrowed segment, the thick-walled, dilated, funnel-shaped oesophagus can be seen disappearing into the chest.

The dilatation of the oesophagus varies in shape according to the stage of the disease (Fig. 33). Thus, in an early case it is fusiform and later on it becomes flask-shaped, while the lengthened, tortuous, sigmoid or S-shaped variety represent an advanced stage. Adams and Trounce from Guy's Hospital, writing in 1961, stated that the sigmoid shape or third stage takes about 15 years to develop. Barrett [57] maintains that the disease does not necessarily pass through these stages, for he has patients he has followed for 30 years, in whom the fusiform dilatation or "cucumber oesophagus," as he calls it, remains static.

A final stage is reached when the oesophagus, filled to capacity with retained putrefying food, is a huge, distended, flabby, atonic tube sagging downward and resting on the right cupola of the diaphragm. Peristalsis now ceases as the muscular coats are in part replaced by fibrous tissue, and the reaction to a low-grade infection waterlogs the entire gullet.

Owing to the marked sagging that occurs, the cardiac orifice now comes to lie at a higher level than the most dependent portion of the sigmoid loop, so that gravity can no longer aid the process of emptying.

Complications

Complications may be listed as those occurring in association with the disease per se, those associated with investigation, and those of operation. These last (operative complications) will be dealt with under *Treatment*.

In Association With Disease Per Se

Pulmonary complications ranging from transient episodes of pneumonitis to pneumonia, abscess, etc., are well known and are due to oesophageal contents spilling from the oesophagus into the trachea when the patient lies down. Sometimes areas of pneumonitis resembling a bronchial carcinoma occur. Barrett [57] reports the presence of atypical mycobacteria which resemble acid-fast bacilli and are usually nonpathogenic but when coated with oils such as liquid paraffin and butter or milk fats can produce lung lesions that simulate pulmonary tuberculosis.

Oesophagitis from stagnation of food in the gullet may occur when decompensation occurs. Occasionally it may lead to ulceration and severe or even fatal haemorrhage.

Malnutrition may lead to vitamin deficiency. Electrolyte imbalance may occur rapidly, especially when food has become impacted.

Spontaneous rupture of the oesophagus in achalasia was reported for the first time by Benedict and Grillo.[58] Hill quoted by Bates,[59] recently recorded 2 such cases, 1 occurring in late pregnancy.

There is an appreciably higher incidence of carcinoma of the oesophagus occurring in patients with achalasia than in the general population. In the Guy's Hospital series [49] 29 percent of the patients developed a carcinoma. This is supported by Belsey,[60] who reported 9 carcinomas out of 94 cases of achalasia. Camera-Lopez [61] found approximately 70 cases reported in the world literature. These carcinomas are generally squamous cell in origin and appear in the dilated portion of the oesophagus.

In Association With Investigation

Instrumental perforation of the oesophagus is the chief hazard. The oesophagoscope is a dangerous weapon in untrained hands. Plummer or Negus bag dilatation and bougies of various kinds, unless used with skill and circumspection, are all potentially dangerous.

Diagnosis

The onset of clinical symptoms is remarkably varied. Often the disease starts vaguely and with troubles that seem to be unconnected with the oesophagus. In the well-established case, however, 70 percent of patients will complain of one or more of the following: a choking feeling on attempting to swallow, difficulty in swallowing, regurgitation of food and saliva, vomiting, praecordial pain, or hunger.

Radiology. The classic picture is well known. The lower end of the oesophagus is narrowed and ends in a smooth, cigar-shaped, symmetrical cone (Figs. 34 and 35). In mega-oesophagus, the gullet is a huge, distorted, patulous sac showing purposeless writhing movements on the screen. Two further radiological features are important: (1) The normal gas bubble in the fundus of the stomach is generally absent. (2) No patient suffering from achalasia can swallow in the head-downward position.

Oesophagoscopy. Although the diagnosis of cardiospasm may appear to be obvious, there are several pitfalls. Conditions affecting the lower oesophagus or cardiac end of the stomach may produce a secondary spasm which is indistinguishable radiologically from a true idiopathic achalasia. Reflux oesophagitis, a high gastric ulcer, or carcinoma of the cardia may all simulate achalasia. A mistake in the other direction may occur if solid food collects at the lower end of the oesophagus, giving rise to an x-ray appearance of carcinoma. For these reasons, it is advisable to confirm the diagnosis in every case by oesophagoscopy, unless there is a strong contraindication.

Clinical Course

The disease can present at any age but commonly in the third and fourth decade. The sex incidence varies. Below the age

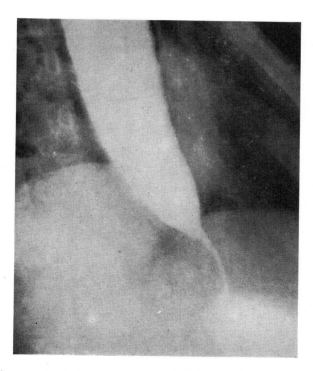

FIG. 34. An early case of achalasia. The lower end of the oesophagus is narrowed and ends in a smooth cigar-shaped symmetrical cone.

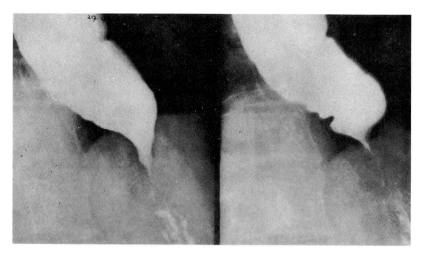

FIG. 35. Radiographs showing a moderate degree of achalasia (R. Maingot's patient).

of 50 males predominate but after that females predominate.

The course of the disease is unpredictable as regards length of life, severity of incapacity, and complications that may occur. In the beginning, symptoms may be intermittent and consist of a mild dysphagia with a sensation of food sticking in the lower chest. Patients become "oesophagus conscious" and an acute attack of dysphagia may coincide with an emotional upset, a sudden excitement, or an acute infection. Later, difficulty in swallowing and retrosternal aching are accentuated and these patients learn to avoid certain foods, to eat infrequently or slowly, and to wash down solids with copious fluid drinks. One patient claimed that she blew her gullet content into the stomach by rapidly taking an aerated drink, and then squeezing her nose and clapping her hand on her mouth!

Adams and Trounce [49] divided the condition into three clinical groups. In the first there is marked dysphagia with frequent regurgitation and weight loss. There is little oesophageal dilatation.

In the second stage of oesophageal dilatation there is no pain or regurgitation, weight loss improves, and the appetite returns. An adequate quantity of food is forced through into the stomach purely by the weight of food which lies above it.

In the third stage the patient has a mega-oesophagus, suffers severe weight loss, and may die from inanition.

Although it is believed that these three stages are slowly progressive, it is possible for the oesophagus to remain fusiform for 20 or more years and carcinoma may develop in this type of gullet as in mega-oesophagus.[57]

Treatment

Achalasia never resolves spontaneously after peristalsis has disappeared. The objective of treatment is to alleviate symptoms. In the past, medical therapy, psychiatry, high spinal anaesthesia, the use of antispasmodic drugs, and bouginage were in vogue for the early case. Today it is realised that bouginage and inhalations of amyl nitrate rarely influence the course of the disease, although some patients find them beneficial. The two effective forms of treatment are forceful dilatation under direct vision and Heller's operation. Patients with achalasia should avoid oil aperients for fear of developing "oil pneumonia" or paraffinoma.

DILATATION

Hydrostatic dilatation differs from bouginage in that the dilating bag is expanded to a transverse diameter of about

5 cm—i.e., wider than the cricopharyngeus can accommodate, and this ruptures the circular muscle fibres in the narrow segment. There are obvious dangers and drawbacks to this method, and even more to certain other mechanical devices used for dilatation:

1. Dilatation that is too forceful may rupture the esophagus.
2. The dilating bag cannot always be engaged in the narrow segment.
3. Relief is usually transitory and requires repetition.
4. Dilatation is hazardous and may be impossible in the late stages of megaoesophagus.

Tanner believes that a transabdominal cardiomyotomy is safer than repeated dilatations. Nevertheless, there are many records of early cases in which the symptoms have been relieved by dilatation for a long period of time.

Operation. This is indicated (1) when dilatation is not feasible; (2) when dilatation fails to relieve symptoms, or symptoms return after temporary relief; (3) in infancy and childhood, when stretching of the lower end of the oesophagus is fraught with danger; and (4) when carcinoma cannot be excluded.

Operative procedures. The following operations are now no longer practiced

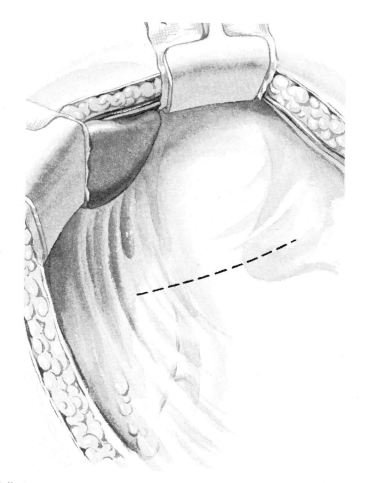

FIG. 36. Heller's operation. Exposure showing the cardia and the line of incision in the phreno-oesophageal ligament.

owing to the high incidence of oesophageal rupture, or of reflux oesophagitis with ulceration, stenosis, or bleeding.

1. Mikulicz transgastric digital dilatation of the lower end of the oesophagus.
2. Oesophagogastrostomy by the methods advocated by Heyrovsky (1912), Grondall (1916), Grey-Turner (1945), and Sweet (1947).
3. Oesophagocardioplasty after the fashion of the Heineke-Mikulicz pyloroplasty.

THE MODIFIED HELLER OPERATION

Today the operation of choice is oesophagocardiomyotomy, which is based on Heller's procedure.

A modified Heller's operation, as at present carried out by the authors, is as follows.

Preoperative preparation. The patient is admitted to hospital 1 week before the operation for a course of oesophageal wash-outs. This is especially important in a

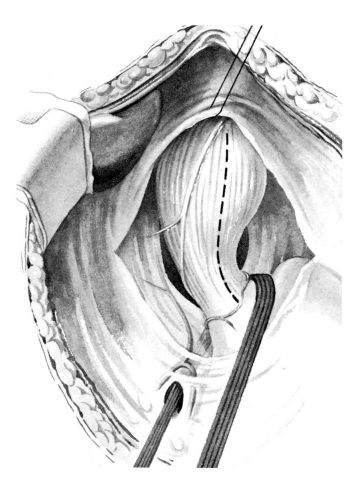

FIG. 37. Heller's operation, showing a view of the posterior mediastinum and the lower oesophagus. The anterior vagus nerve is shown and the line of the oesophageal incision is indicated. (Note that the myotomy stops inferiorly precisely at the cardia.)

patient who has considerable retention and pyrexia. During this time, he is kept on a fluid diet, anaemia and electrolyte disturbances are corrected, and pulmonary infections are treated. If oesophagoscopy has not previously been carried out, it is wise to do this before operation. A Ryle's tube is passed through the nostril into the stomach on the morning of the operation.

Operation. The abdomen is opened through a right upper paramedian incision, and the ligamentum teres is divided between ligatures. A general examination is carried out to exclude a stenosing lesion in the pylorus or duodenum, a high gastric ulcer, or a neoplasm. An associated hiatal hernia is found occasionally.

The left lobe of the liver is drawn down and the left triangular ligament divided under direct vision. The left lobe is drawn to the right and held there with a Deaver retractor and then a good exposure of the cardia is obtained (Fig. 36).

The peritoneum and phreno-oesophageal ligament overlying the cardia are incised transversely as two definite structures. It is important not to damage the phreno-oesophageal ligament unnecessarily. The posterior mediastinum and lower oesophagus now come into view. One or two stay sutures are placed in the anterior margin of the hiatus and held by an assistant (Fig. 37).

An opening is made lower down in the gastrohepatic ligament, through which the

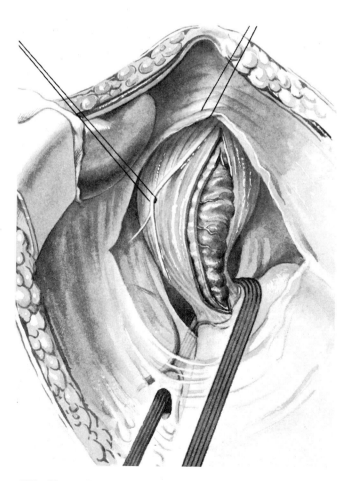

FIG. 38. Heller's operation, showing the myotomy completed.

left thumb is placed. If the left index finger is now placed through the opening made into the mediastinum to the left and behind the oesophagus, the two digits are separated only by the layer of peritoneum in the roof of the lesser sac. With the left thumb as a guide, a forceps is thrust through this layer to emerge at the left of the oesophagus. A rubber band can now be grasped and drawn through. This acts as a sling for traction on the oesophagus, which can now be pulled down after gentle mobilisation. The anterior vagus nerve is identified and drawn out of harm's way to the right.

A longitudinal incision is made through the muscular coats of the narrowed part of the oesophagus and slowly and very carefully deepened through the somewhat adherent circular muscle, dividing the fibres until the oesophageal mucosa bulges outwards without restraint (Fig. 38).

The mucosa can be recognised from the fine submucosal vessels coursing over it; also, if the anaesthetist blows a little air into the oesophagus or stomach, bubbles may be recognised through the mucosa.

Once this level has been reached, it is easy to extend the myotomy upwards. A long, blunt-ended, closed dissecting forceps may be easily insinuated upwards under the muscle coat and then allowed to open gently. With a long curved scissors, the overlying muscle

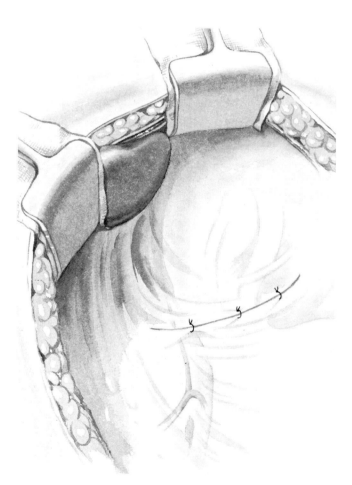

FIG. 39. Completed Heller's operation, showing accurate repair of the phreno-oesophageal ligament.

is incised between the blades of the dissecting forceps.

This incision must be extended upwards well on to the dilated part, usually some 6 to 8 cm. It is also recommended that the incision extend downwards into the stomach for 1 to 2 cm, although we have for some time given up this gastric myotomy and stop inferiorly at the cardia, in the hope that preservation of the oblique gastric fibres near the cardia may help to prevent gastro-oesophageal reflux. The anaesthetist is again asked to insufflate the oesophagus with air via the Ryle's tube. In this way the integrity of the exposed mucous membrane is checked, and it is confirmed that no strands of circular fibres are left. If the mucous membrane be opened inadvertently it can be closed with fine catgut sutures upon atraumatic (eyeless) needles, but this should be a rarity.

Strict attention is paid to repairing the phreno-oesophageal ligament accurately with interrupted sutures of fine nylon (Fig. 39).

The operation should be completed by doing a pyloromyotomy or Heineke-Mikulicz pyloroplasty if there is any suggestion of muscular hypertrophy or mucosal stenosis at the pylorus. If an associated peptic ulcer is present, the appropriate treatment should be carried out, usually a Billroth I gastrectomy for a gastric ulcer, or a vagotomy with drainage for a duodenal ulcer. A hiatal hernia, if present, may be repaired.

Postoperative care. Parenteral nutrition is usually maintained for 48 hours. Intermittent aspiration via the Ryle's tube is maintained until there is evidence that there is no gastric retention, when it may be withdrawn. Fluids only are given by mouth for the first 3 days, and it is wise to maintain the patient on a semisolid diet for 10 days, as late perforations of the oesophagus have been recorded, particularly in the elderly and in those who presented with considerable retention.

Results. Our total series is some 70 patients. One was seen only at autopsy, with an "oesophagolith," inspissated food blocking the cardia, leading to starvation. A second, a nurse seen at the earliest stages, with a fusiform gullet, was dealt with by a high spinal anaesthetic during a crisis and then had regular dilatations with a mercury-filled

large stomach tube ("Hurst bougie"), at first daily, then weekly, and then monthly. She finally regained a normal-shaped oesophagus and when last seen had been symptom-free and without bouginage for 6 years. Three other patients with mega-oesophagus declined surgery and were treated by occasional oesophageal lavage.

In our series of 65 surgically treated patients, 80 percent were operated on more than 5 years ago; it was necessary to reoperate for recurrent dysphagia in 3. The first was a 67-year-old woman who developed recurrent dysphagia due to stricture following cardiomyotomy in 1949. Her cardia was resected and end-to-end oesophagogastrostomy was carried out. One month later she suffered a fatal haematemesis from anastomotic ulceration. This form of reconstitution is no longer favoured by us. The second was a 64-year-old man who developed dysphagia within 2 years of his cardiomyotomy. Barium studies revealed a large hiatal hernia, which was repaired with relief of symptoms. The third was an 80-year-old man who developed reflux oesophagitis and persisting oesophageal retention following cardiomyotomy, selective vagotomy, and gastroenterostomy for oesophageal achalasia and duodenal ulcer. Because of his frail condition, only dilatation of the cardia was carried out.

Our immediate results for mega-oesophagus are satisfactory. One patient, the first to be diagnosed in England by Sir Arthur Hurst, nearly 40 years ago, swallowed bougies for 30 years. She presented in 1966 with complete dysphagia and severe oesophageal retention. A transabdominal Heller's operation was carried out 1 year ago and up to the present time she swallows without difficulty and has gained 14 pounds.

There was 1 operative death—a 70-year-old woman who suffered a cerebrovascular postoperative accident and died from a massive pulmonary embolus.

There were 6 late deaths in the series; 3 of these patients had developed carcinoma of the midoesophagus. The other causes of death were pseudomyxoma peritonei, diagnosed at the original Heller's operation; bronchiectasis and cor pulmonale, and haemorrhage from anastomotic ulcer following resection of the cardia (the case mentioned above). In only 2 of these cases can death be attributed directly to achalasia of the cardia.

Froebese et al.[62] reported 58 good results from 60 cases of transabdominal Heller's operation, combined with pyloroplasty in 30 of the cases.

Complications. The chief complications of cardiomyotomy are (1) reflux and (2) persisting obstruction or stenosis.

Reflux. Reflux may occur, and according to Ellis,[63] the main factors responsible for its occurrence are (1) errors in preoperative diagnosis, (2) hiatal herniation, (3) delayed gastric emptying, and (4) loss of the physiological gastro-oesophageal sphincter.

Errors in preoperative diagnosis can be avoided if oesophageal pressure tracings and motility studies are carried out in atypical cases, and oesophagoscopy in every case.

Excessive mobilisation of the oesophagus, stretching the hiatus at operation, and failure to repair the phreno-oesophageal ligament may contribute to postoperative incompe-

tence of the cardia. Any manoeuvre that weakens the hiatus must be avoided.

Delayed gastric emptying may result from coincidental duodenal ulceration or from damage to the vagus at operation. *Pyloroplasty should be carried out in all such cases.*

Loss of the physiological gastro-oesophageal sphincter seems inevitable when the myotomy is extended to the stomach. It is for this reason that the cardia is not transgressed in the operation described above. McVay et al.[64] have shown that radical incision into the gastric side does not lower the sphincter pressure barrier any more than does a myotomy stopping short at the cardia, and does predispose to reflux oesophagitis.

The wearing of tight corsets or spinal belts that press on the abdomen may also cause postoperative reflux, particularly in the obese.

Restenosis. The factors responsible for restenosis are (1) incomplete myotomy at the first operation, and (2) peptic oesophagitis following reflux.

Repetition of Heller's operation is indi-

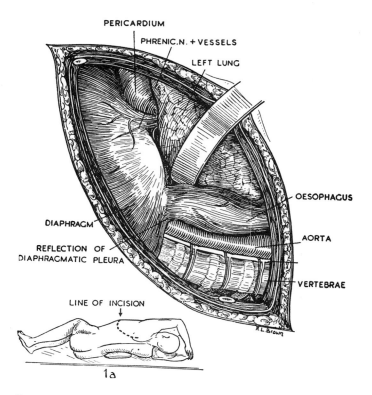

FIG. 40. Heller's operation by transthoracic approach. (From Maingot, *The Management of Abdominal Operations*, 2d. ed., 1950. Courtesy of Mr. John Borrie and H. K. Lewis & Co., Ltd., London.)

cated if it is probable that the first myotomy was inadequate—e.g., in inexperienced hands. In all other cases, second myotomies only afford temporary benefit.

In the majority of cases, recurrent obstruction is due to peptic oesophagitis.

Several procedures are available for this complication:

1. The cardia may be resected and the stomach brought up into the chest. This may lead to recurrent ulceration with repeated stenosis, bleeding, or perforation.

2. The most satisfactory method of reconstruction following resection is an end-to-side oesophagojejunal anastomosis utilising a Roux loop and closing the cardiac end of the stomach. Macrocytic anaemia will eventually develop if the stomach is completely bypassed. This may be prevented by carrying

out a side-to-side anastomosis between the vagotomised stomach and Roux loop above the mesocolon. In the rare event of an anastomotic ulcer's developing, it would be relatively easy to dismantle. The majority of thoracic surgeons perform cardiomyotomy through a left transthoracic approach (Figs. 40 and 41). Although a satisfactory myotomy can be made by this approach, it is more often followed by pleural effusion, collapse of the left lung, and intercostal aching, and it requires a longer convalescence. Again, it is more difficult to carry out pyloroplasty or diagnose intra-abdominal lesions predisposing to postoperative reflux. The abdominal approach has these advantages: It is simple, the exposure is excellent, it is safer for elderly patients, pyloroplasty can be carried out, and other intra-abdominal lesions

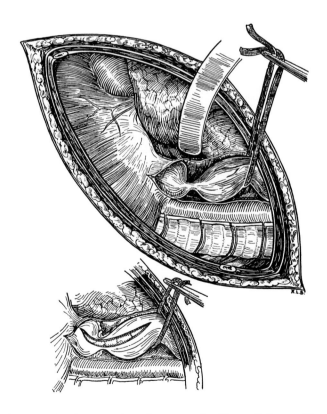

FIG. 41. Heller's operation by transthoracic approach. (From Maingot, *The Management of Abdominal Operations*, 2d. ed., 1950. Courtesy of Mr. John Borrie and H. K. Lewis & Co., Ltd., London.)

can be corrected. In spite of the manifest imperfections of Heller's operation, it remains the best available procedure for achalasia.

Follow-up.   Long-term follow-up is essential after surgery. Cardiomyotomy does not remedy the underlying neurological defect and the gullet never returns to normal however well the patient claims to be clinically. It is probable, therefore, that the long-term results will be less satisfactory than the early postoperative assessments suggest.

References

1. Le-Quesne and Ranger, Br. J. Surg. 53:105, 1966.
2. G. Grey-Turner, Injuries and Diseases of the Oesophagus, London, Cassell, 1946, p. 53.
3. Gowing, Tumours of the Oesophagus, Tanner and Smithers, eds., Edinburgh, Livingstone, 1961, p. 82.
4. Tanner, Lond. Clin. Med. J. 1:27, 1966.
5. Tanner, Lancet 2:1050, 1955.
6. Merendino and Dillard, Ann. Surg. 142:486, 1955.
7. Brain, Ann. R. Coll. Surg. 40:100, 1967.
8. Chrysospathis, Br. J. Surg. 53:122, 1966.
9. Grey-Turner, Injuries and Diseases of the Oesophagus, London, Cassell, 1946, p. 91.
10. Berman, J. Int. Coll. Surg. 18:695, 1952.
11. Tanner, Langenbecks Arch. Klin. Chir. 267:369, 1951.
12. Heimlich, Surgery 42:693, 1957.
13. Heimlich, Br. J. Surg. 53:913, 1966.
14. Wullstein, Dtsch. Med. Wochenschr. 30:734, 1904.
15. Harrison, J. Thorac. Surg. 18:316, 1949.
16. Allison and da Silva, Br. J. Surg. 41:173, 1953.
17. Hedblom, Surg. Gynecol. Obstet. 35:284, 1922.
18. Muir, Lancet 2:75, 1936.
19. Ohsawa, Arch. Jap. Chir. 10:605, 1933.
20. Adams and Phemister, J. Thorac. Surg. 7:621, 1938.
21. Tanner, Proc. R. Soc. Med. 39:411, 1946.
22. Churchill and Sweet, Ann. Surg. 115:897, 1942.
23. Kemink en Zoon N.V. Domplein 2, Utrecht Acta. Chir. Scand. 103:440, 1952.
24. Mousseau-Barbin et al., Arch. Mal. Appar. Dig. 45:208, 1956.
25. Pearson, Clin. Radiol. 17:242, 1966.
26. Allison and Borrie, Br. J. Surg. 37:1, 1949.
27. Tanner, Postgrad. Med. J. 23:109, 1947.
28. Quan and Castleman, N. Engl. J. Med. 240:835, 1949.
29. Tanner, Proc. R. Soc. Med. 42:662, 1949.
30. Haight, Ann. Surg. 107:218, 1938.
31. Tanner, Gastroenterologia 92:146, 1959.
32. Sweet, Surg. Gynecol. Obstet. 94:46, 1952.
33. De Amneste and Otaiza, Surgery 23:921, 1948.
34. Pack and McNeer, Surgery 23:976, 1948.
35. Sweet, Surg. Gynecol. Obstet. 94:46, 1952.
36. Garlock, Modern Trends in Gastroenterology, 1952, p. 220.
37. Franklin, Surgery of the Oesophagus, 1952.
38. Zenker and von Ziemssen, Cyclopaedia of the Practice of Medicine, 3:204, 1876.
39. Rosenheim, Dtsch. Med. Wochenschr. 24:53, 1899.
40. Mikulicz, Wien Med. Presse 22:1537, 1881.
41. Einhorn, Med. Rec. 34:751, 1888.
42. Hurst, Proc. R. Soc. Med. 8 Clin. Sec. 22, 1914.
43. Hurst and Rake, Q. J. Med. 23:491, 1930.
44. Wooler, Thorax 3:53, 1948.
45. Heller, Mitt. Grenzeb Med. Chir. 27:141, 1914.
46. Barlow, Br. J. Surg. 29:415, 1942.
47. Barrett and Franklin, Br. J. Surg. 37:194, 1949–50.
48. Johnstone, Br. J. Radiol. 33:723, 1960.
49. Adams et al., Guys Hosp. Rep. 110:191, 1961.
50. Anderson et al., An Atlas of Oesophageal Motility in Health and Disease, 1958.
51. Casella et al., Ann. Surg. 160:474, 1964.
52. Higgs et al., J. Thorac. Cardiovasc. Surg. 50:613, 1965.
53. Ellis et al., J.A.M.A. 166:29, 1958.
54. Kramer et al., Gut 8:115, 1967.
55. Koberle, Gastroenterology 34:460, 1958.
56. Casella et al., Am. J. Pathol. 46:467, 1965.
57. Barrett, Br. Med. J. 1:1135, 1964.
58. Benedict and Grillo, J. Thorac. Cardiovasc. Surg. 44:272, 1962.
59. Bates, Postgrad. Med. J. 41:781, 1965.
60. Belsey, Postgrad. Med. J. 39:290, 1963.
61. Camera-Lopez, Am. J. Dig. Dis. 6:742, 1961.
62. Froebese et al., Am. J. Surg. 107:249, 1964.
63. Ellis, Ann. R. Coll. Surg. 30:155, 1962.
64. McVay et al., Br. Soc. Internat. Chir. 22:419, 1963.
65. **Bruinsma, Belgisch Tijdschrift Voor Geneeskunde, 12:(14) 754–755, July, 1956.**

Spleen

31

INDICATIONS FOR SPLENECTOMY AND THE TECHNIQUE OF SPLENECTOMY

RODNEY MAINGOT

During the last two decades, many important advances have been made in the management of patients with conditions that call for surgery of the spleen. The surgeon is the first to admit that these significant advances have been mainly due to the excellent work of the haematologist, who has improved and enlarged the methods of diagnosis, expanded and rationalised the indications for splenectomy, and can now forecast with a considerable degree of accuracy the results following the removal of the spleen for splenopathy.

It can be said that the results of splenectomy depend largely on teamwork and on the selection of cases by the haematologists.

Whitby [52] considered the haematologist the arbiter and the dictator of surgery of the spleen. "Save for rupture of the organ, it is not often that a spleen is removed without the haematologist having, not a finger in the pie, but a needle in a vein, the sternum, or the spleen itself." He stated that it is obvious from all the reports in the literature that excision of the spleen has come to be a relatively common operation, providing effective, sometimes dramatic, treatment for a number of conditions for which there neither was nor is any efficient medical therapy.

Experience has now shown that, with the exception of a few fairly well-defined risks and contraindications, splenectomy per se has a low death rate; and that, even if the removal of the spleen does no good, at least it appears to do no harm, except, perhaps, in infancy and childhood.

It is this last fact which has led to the extension of splenectomy to the treatment of a number of diseases in which its rationale is difficult to establish and its chance of clinical success, according to previous experience, may be quite small. One is inclined to take the chance if nothing else can be done to relieve perhaps an intolerable situation.[52]

It is interesting to read a number of articles written 30 or more years ago and dealing with the surgery of the spleen. The main indications for splenectomy at that time were rupture of the spleen and splenomegaly of known or, more frequently, unknown origin.

Thanks to the excellent work of many authorities in this country and abroad, the indications for splenectomy are rapidly becoming clarified and to some extent stereotyped.

It is obvious to anyone who has made a special study of splenic diseases that some of them are strictly medical in their therapy, whilst others are surgical, and that there is still a fairly definite group in which treatment is difficult to advise with confidence. The degree of danger in any given case in which injury or disease of the spleen demands splenectomy is dependent upon individual peculiarities and cannot in all fairness be rightly estimated on the mortality percentage basis of any of the statistics which have so far been compiled. We do, however, know that the operative mortality rate in cases of familial haemolytic anaemia, idiopathic thrombocytopenic purpura, and the primary hypersplenisms is low (less than 3 percent), and that the results are most encouraging. The mortality rate of splenectomy for secondary hypersplenism is about 8 percent.

The reduction in the operative mortality rate is undoubtedly due to our increasing knowledge of splenic diseases, to more clear-cut opinions as to the indications for operative intervention, and to improvements in our methods of preoperative investigation combined with an ever-increasing understanding of the basic principles of preoperative and postoperative treatment and better anaesthesia, and surgical judgment and technique.

PHYSIOLOGICAL EFFECTS

Congenital absence of the spleen is extremely rare and is invariably associated with other, and frequently multiple, anomalies of the cardiovascular and gastrointestinal systems. Aguilar et al.[1] collected 27 cases from the literature and recorded 3 additional cases of their own. All these cases were carefully reviewed from the anatomical and pathological standpoint.

Although the spleen has many functions, it is not essential to life and its removal is not, as a rule, followed by any marked or permanent disturbances.

The main *functions of the spleen* are as follows:

1. It acts as a reservoir for erythrocytes. It yields increased quantities of blood during periods of stress and exercise.
2. It is capable of destroying erythrocytes, especially when they are aged, damaged, or effete, probably during stasis in the venous sinusoids. In hypersplenism, the organ may possess a voracious appetite for the cellular elements of the blood. One would expect blood destruction to occur in the spleen as in all reticuloendothelial tissue.
3. It has a haematopoietic function, and also exerts a hormonal influence that regulates the maturation and release of the cellular elements of the blood from the bone marrow.
4. It has a definite phagocytic and reticuloendothelial activity. By tagging the patient's erythrocytes with ^{51}Cr, it is possible not only to measure the rate of erythrocyte destruction, but also to determine the main sites of erythrocyte sequestration and destruction.[23]

The physiological effects of splenectomy may be summarised as follows:

1. *Changes in the blood*
   (a) *Erythrocytes.* Following splenectomy there is a transient erythrocytosis, the erythrocytes tend to be thinner, and some of them contain nuclear remnants described as Cabot or Howell-Jolly bodies.
   (b) *Platelets.* The number of platelets is increased temporarily—thrombocytosis.
   (c) *Leucocytes.* There is an increase in the total number of leucocytes, this being almost entirely owing to an increase in the number of polymorphonuclear leucocytes. The leucocyte count slowly returns to normal, there may be a slight oesinophilia, and with this there is often an increase in the number of mast cells.
2. *Enlargement of the lymph nodes.* There is a slight general enlargement of all the lymph nodes in the body, due to compensatory increased haematopoietic activity.
3. *Changes in the bone marrow.* The yellow marrow in the long bones is gradually replaced by red marrow, this change usually being complete within 6 months.
4. *Changes in the reticuloendothelial system.* As the spleen contains a large collection of lymphoid tissue and a considerable amount of reticuloendothelial elements, the specialised cells of the remaining portions of this system undergo marked proliferation.
5. *Hypertrophy of accessory spleens.* Accessory spleens, found in 18 to 20 percent of all patients at autopsy, hypertrophy after splenectomy. When splenectomy is carried out for hypersplenism, the surgeon should search for and remove all accessory spleens, since they may be the cause for continuation or recurrence of the disease.
6. *An increase of iron in the liver* (Hill and Flack), *and copper in the tissues.*[14]
7. *Diminished resistance to infection.* Excision of the spleen is not detrimental to the general well-being of patients who are over the age of 15.

This statement has the support of Pedersen

and Videback,[35] who followed 40 otherwise healthy persons who underwent splenectomy for traumatic rupture during 1920–57. The average follow-up interval was almost 20 years.

It is concluded that no lasting sequelae of any severity follow splenectomy. There is no reason why loss of the spleen should be given any significance from the standpoint of compensation or insurance.

It should be remembered that the spleen, as the largest member of the reticuloendothelial system, plays an important role in phagocytosis. This is one of the ways in which the spleen is involved in the control of infection. Swenson reminds us that attention has been recently focussed on the susceptibility to infection that some children exhibit following removal of the spleen. For instance, King and Shumaker [24] reported the occurrence of meningococcal meningitis following splenectomy in a number of small infants. It was found that this complication was more common in infants than in children. Gofstein and Gellis [17] found that about 5 percent of a large series of splenectomies in children resulted in repeated bouts of infection, primarily with pneumococci. In Swenson's review of 50 infants and children after splenectomy, this complication of infection had appeared in 2 patients (4 percent).

Lowdon et al.[26] state that pneumococcal septicaemia and other fulminating infections sometimes occur within 2 or 3 years after splenectomy, particularly in children, in patients with underlying disease predisposing to infection, and in patients receiving corticosteroids. Splenectomy should be avoided whenever possible during the *first 4 years of life* and postoperative antibiotic therapy should probably be given for long periods in young children and patients in the high-risk groups. Carl Smith [45] points out that the increased susceptibility to infection after splenectomy in infancy emphasizes the need for close observation for at least 2 years postoperatively.

These reports support the view that the spleen plays an important role in the production of antibodies, and thus in the defence mechanism of the body.

8. *Diminished metabolic activity of the liver.* As about 25 percent of the total amount of portal blood passing through the liver comes from the spleen, the result of splenectomy will be to relieve the liver of some of its burden, especially when it is cirrhotic.

9. *Splenosis.* There is a danger during an expeditious, rough-and-ready splenectomy of autoplastic transplantation of particles of spleen torn loose from the main splenic tissue. In certain diseases, such as idiopathic thrombocytopenic purpura and familial spherocytosis, these autoplastic transplants are quick to luxuriate in the peritoneal cavity and to assume the sinister characteristics of their forbear.[27]

INVESTIGATION OF SPLENIC DISORDERS

The following are some of the more important investigations required in the diagnosis of splenopathy.

1. *History of the case.*
2. *Physical examination of the patient.* The examination of the patient must be thorough and complete.

   The normal spleen, which weighs approximately 250 g, does not extend further forward than the midaxillary line, so that when it can be palpated below the left costal margin, it is already markedly enlarged and its normal weight at least doubled. The enlarged spleen moves on respiration, has a sharp anterior border with a notch in it, is of firm consistency and is therefore dull to percussion. It will be seen that this dullness to percussion is continuous over the lower ribs and extends to the margin of the erector spinae muscle.
3. *Peripheral blood studies.* These will include erythrocyte count, haemoglobin estimation, mean corpuscular volume, volume index, colour index, fragility (*initial* haemolysis and *complete* haemolysis), haematocrit, reticulocyte count, sedimentation rate, total and differential leucocyte counts, estimation of the number of platelets,

and report on the bleeding time, clotting time, and prothrombin index and concentration. The majority of these haematological investigations can be carried out on only 5 ml of blood if placed in a special container.

4. *Bone marrow studies.* Bone marrow samples may be obtained by puncture or trephine. Puncture or needle biopsy, using a Vim-Silverman needle, is the usual method adopted, and the sternum, iliac crest, or upper end of the shaft of the tibia (especially in children) are the sites that are most frequently tapped. Trephining will, of course, be indicated when the bones are unduly sclerotic.

Dameshek and Welch [7] have emphasised that whenever splenectomy is considered for patients with blood dyscrasias, the bone marrow should be shown either by needle or trephine biopsy to exhibit a degree of haematopoiesis that is at least normal. The main exception to this is in the hypoplastic anaemias, which are usually congenital in type.

In the majority of cases in which removal of the spleen is indicated, the bone marrow is actually hyperplastic, and, indeed, it is seldom possible otherwise to expect good results from splenectomy.

5. *Radiology.* Barium-meal x-ray examination of the stomach and barium enema may help to exclude tumour of the stomach or colon. The enlarged spleen usually displaces the stomach medially, and indents the greater curvature and pushes the splenic flexure downward. Plain x-ray pictures may reveal areas of calcification in the wall of a simple intrasplenic cyst or a hydatid cyst, whilst in certain cases an *intravenous pyelogram* may be called for to clinch the diagnosis between a renal swelling and an enlarged tethered spleen. Radiology of the long bones will help in the diagnosis of Gaucher's disease and of Albers-Schönberg disease.

6. *Splenic puncture.* The most outstanding and learned contribution to this subject will be found in an article by Chatterjea, Arrau, and Dameshek.[3]

Excellent accounts of splenic puncture will also be found in the following papers: Ferris and Hargraves,[15] Watson et al.,[50] and Shields et al.[43] Splenic aspirate is usually obtained by the puncture method of Moeschlin (1951). Splenic puncture may be very useful in the diagnosis of certain atypical or cryptic types of leukaemia and clinical hypersplenism and is particularly valuable in the diagnosis of myleofibrosis associated with myeloid metaplasia of the spleen and in certain neoplastic processes that involve that organ.

7. *Portal angiography.* The diagnosis of the site of obstruction, whether this be intrahepatic or extrahepatic, in cases of congestive splenomegaly has been rendered much easier by portal angiography after injection of an opaque fluid into the spleen through the parietes. As Walker et al.[49] and a number of other authors have shown, a good visualisation of the portal system (splenoportogram) can be obtained by this method. For further details of this method of investigation, including its advantages and inherent dangers, the reader is referred to Chapters 58 and 108.

8. *Liver biopsy.* This may be performed either by puncture, using a Vim-Silverman needle or some modification of it, or through a peritoneoscope. It may prove of some help in suspected cases of portal hypertension and in the reticuloses.

9. *Lymph node biopsy.* This should be undertaken if adenopathy is present.

10. *Radiology by barium swallow and endoscopic examination of the oesophagus.* These investigations are indicated in patients suspected of suffering from portal hypertension. Varices that do not show on barium swallow may be detected by endoscopy.

11. *Liver function studies.* These include: (a) prothrombin time, (b) serum bilirubin and the bromsulphalein dye retention test, (c) serum proteins: albumin, globulin, total electrophoresis, (d) cholesterol, total and esters, (e) alkaline phosphatase, (f) thymol turbidity, (g) zinc sulphate turbidity, (h)

blood urea, and (i) G.P.-transaminase. (See Chap. 45.)

12. *Immunological studies* (Coombs' test and other antibody studies). Coombs' test for haemolysin in the blood, which is often negative in familial haemolytic anaemia, but usually positive in acquired haemolytic anaemia owing to overactivity of the spleen, may be helpful, but more studies of this test are required.

13. *Angiography* (see Chap. 108). According to an editorial comment in *World Medicine*,[12] Dr. Leon Love, Director of Diagnostic Radiology at Cook County Hospital, Chicago, cogently recommends *splenic arteriography* as a method for evaluating suspected injuries of the spleen, blunt abdominal trauma, cryptic splenic tumours, etc. He uses retrograde aortography via the percutaneous femoral approach. He inserts a catheter to one inch above the level of the coeliac axis and injects 40 ml of sodium iothalamate at the rate of 30 ml a second. Serial x-ray films of the vessels are then made for a short period of time afterward.

14. The role of [75]*Selenomethionine Se* uptake in the diagnosis of lymphoma. The reader is referred to the articles by Herrera et al.[21] and Meeker et al.[28]

INDICATIONS FOR SPLENECTOMY

The indications for splenectomy are constantly undergoing a process of revision. From time to time additions are made to the list of well-established reasons for surgical removal of the spleen and occasionally new forms of treatment tend to lessen the advisability of this procedure in some diseases. Thus, the list is never static and what may be an indication today may not be tomorrow.[31]

The indications for splenectomy may be listed as follows:

Injuries of the Spleen

1. Penetrating or open wounds—e.g., gunshot wounds, stabs, etc.
2. Nonpenetrating (subcutaneous, blunt, or closed) wounds due to blunt trauma to the left chest, abdomen, or left kidney region—e.g., as in motor car accidents.
3. Spontaneous rupture of a normal or of a pathological spleen.
4. Operative (or iatrogenic) injury—e.g., during partial gastrectomy.[37]

Ptosis of the Spleen

Ptosis of the spleen (wandering, mobile, or ectopic spleen), with or without torsion of the pedicle of the spleen.

Local Diseases

1. Infections—e.g., intrasplenic abscess.
2. Primary neoplasms—e.g., lymphosarcoma and haemangiosarcoma.[28, 39]
3. Cysts
   (a) True—epithelial or endothelial lined—e.g., cystic haematoma of the spleen caused by blunt trauma.
   (b) False.
   (c) Parasitic—e.g., hydatid cyst of the spleen.
4. Aneurysm of the splenic artery.

Adjunct to Other Surgery

In combination with total gastrectomy for carcinoma of the stomach; oesophagogastrectomy for cancer of the cardia or lower end of the oesophagus; cancer of the tail and/or body of the pancreas; certain cases of hyperinsulinism combined with distal pancreatectomy; cancer of the splenic flexure of the colon (some cases); large hiatal hernia (some cases), etc.

Functional Disorders and Selected Cases of Splenomegaly

It is generally agreed that excision of the spleen for the idiopathic types of hypersplenism, effects good results when medical measures have failed or are definitely contraindicated. Primary hypersplenism: (a) idiopathic thrombocytopenic purpura; (b) familial haemolytic anaemia (familial spherocytosis); (c) primary splenic neutropenia; (d) idiopathic pancytopenia (panhaematocytopenia). The *indication for splenectomy* in diseases associated with hypersplenism is discussed by Sir Ronald Bodley Scott in Chapter 32, Part B. The reader is also referred to the contributions by Doan et al.,[10] Sandusky et al.,[40] and Egal et al.[13]

TECHNIQUE OF SPLENECTOMY

There are many ways of performing the operation of splenectomy, varying according to the technique favoured by the individual surgeon and the particular conditions that characterise each case. Special emphasis will here be laid upon the difficulties and dangers that so frequently arise at certain stages of the operation.

Before the operation is commenced, it is important to pass a nasogastric tube and to aspirate the contents so as to ensure that the stomach is empty and flaccid throughout the operation. If the stomach is distended with gas and fluid, it will push the spleen into an even more inaccessible position, in addition to rendering all intra-abdominal manipulations more difficult and not free from danger, inasmuch as the stomach itself may receive some injury when the uppermost portion of the gastrosplenic omentum is being ligated. Therefore this tube, which has been introduced prior to the operation, is left in situ until the operation is completed, thus ensuring an empty stomach and simplifying the various steps of the procedure.

There are four important stages in the operation:

1. The *abdominal incision,* involving the question of choice of incision and the exposure of the spleen.
2. *Exploration of the abdomen,* the freeing of adhesions, and the mobilisation of the spleen and its delivery through the abdominal wound.
3. *The methods of securely ligaturing the vascular pedicles of the spleen.*
4. *Closure of the wound* and the steps taken to prevent disruption of the wound or the subsequent formation of ventral hernia.

The *incision of choice* depends upon the nature of the disease. Thus, in idiopathic thrombocytopenic purpura, in primary hypersplenism, and in rupture, a lengthy left paramedian incision, with outward dislocation of the rectus muscle, is adequate; in familial haemolytic anaemia, a transverse epigastric incision which permits exploration of the biliary tract affords excellent exposure; and in certain cases of congestive splenomegaly, a combined abdominothoracic incision with partial division of the diaphragm is indicated, owing to the tethering adhesions which are so often encountered.

A large number of incisions has been devised. In practice six are in common use today: (1) midline, (2) paramedian, (3) left vertical muscle-split, (4) oblique subcostal, (5) transverse epigastric, and (6) combined abdominothoracic approach.

The *midline incision* is the one chosen for cases of suspected rupture of the spleen, liver, or stomach, as it is easy to make and can be readily closed, besides affording satisfactory access to the spleen and permitting inspection of the liver, stomach, duodenum, and other viscera of the upper abdomen which may or may not be implicated. If any difficulties are encountered during the operation, the spleen can be more easily approached by dividing the left rectus muscle transversely through one of its tendinous intersections. On no account should this transverse incision be carried beyond the tip of the ninth rib, as *extensive* transverse slashes are difficult to suture at the completion of the operation; they usually cut across two or more of the motor nerves to the abdominal muscles, and unless suturing is meticulous an incisional hernia may develop at some future date.

The *left paramedian incision* is the one preferred by most surgeons, and is the one which I have used in the majority of my cases, as it does not in any way damage the rectus muscle, and provided the muscle is well dislocated outward the exposure afforded is excellent. This incision must reach to or extend beyond the costal margin in every case, and extend about 2 inches (5 cm) below the umbilicus.

The *left vertical muscle-splitting* incision divides the inner portion of the left rectus muscle in a vertical plane from a point starting at the costal margin itself and ex-

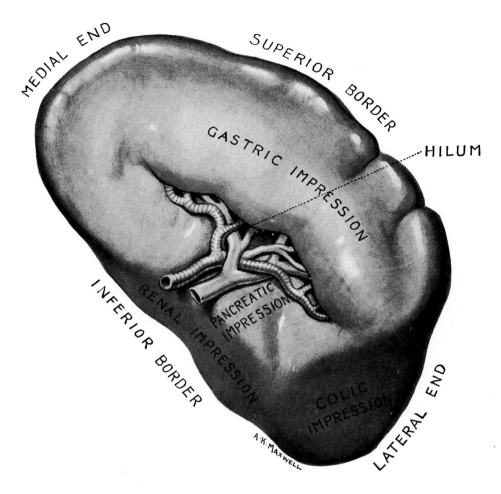

FIG. 1. Gross anatomy of the spleen.

tending downward to the level of the umbilicus or slightly below. It is of course readily made and is simple to suture, while the exposure is as good as that afforded by the paramedian incision.

The *left oblique subcostal incision* begins at the tip of the xiphoid process and proceeds obliquely outward and downward about one fingerbreadth below the costal margin, the left rectus muscle and the medial portion of the flat muscles of the lateral abdominal wall being divided in line with the incision. It is, in fact, similar to Kocher's gallbladder incision on the opposite side and should be employed whenever splenectomy is called for in obese patients or where it is

thought that the spleen may be unduly adherent to the diaphragm and surrounding structures. This incision invariably divides the seventh and eighth dorsal nerves, but every endeavour should be made to preserve the important ninth intercostal nerve. If skilfully sutured, it is rarely followed by ventral hernia, and in the majority of cases it leaves a very fine and neat scar. In some instances a *transverse incision* starting at the tip of the left ninth costal cartilage and curving upward across the epigastrium to the tip of the right eighth costal cartilage and completely dividing the rectus muscles affords excellent exposure to the spleen and to the biliary tract and may be employed with advantage in cases of familial haemolytic anaemia, associated with gallstones.

There are four salient features which should characterise all these incisions:

1. They should be large and generous so that there is no hampering of the intra-abdominal manipulations.
2. Special care should be taken to see that wound haemostasis is complete; ne-glect of this, owing to the condition of the blood in such patients, may lead to subsequent haemorrhage or a dangerous oozing.
3. Precautions should be taken to prevent infection of the wound and suitable-sized Steri-Drape is applied to the skin before the incision is made.
4. Closure of the wound should be per-formed accurately, and after closing

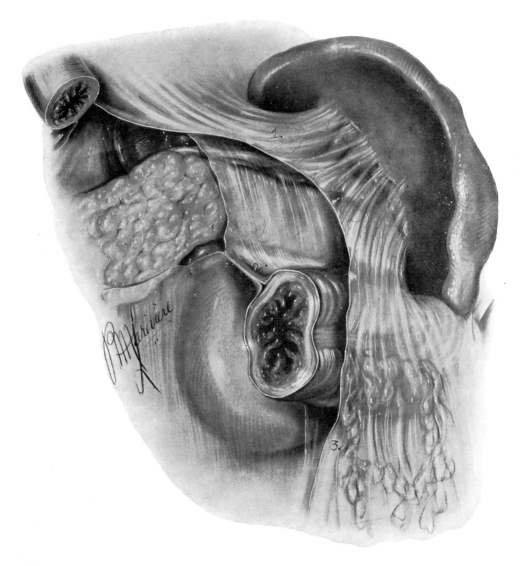

FIG. 2. Anatomy of the spleen, showing complicated peritoneal reflections in the region of the hilus.

the posterior sheath of the rectus muscle and peritoneum with a continuous suture of 0 chromic catgut or Dexon, reinforced with interrupted mattress sutures of silk or cotton, the anterior sheath of this muscle should be accurately approximated with interrupted sutures of silk, cotton, tycron, nylon, or 33-gauge stainless steel wire. Where speed is imperative, all the layers of the wound may be closed with a series of figure-of-eight sutures, Ethilon, or stainless steel wire, after which the edges of the skin are closed with interrupted vertical mattress sutures of fine black silk or Deknatel (see Chap. 1).

A good acount of the *combined thoraco-abdominal approach* is given by Carter.[2] I should like to express my indebtedness to Dr. B. Noland Carter and to the editor of *Surgery, Gynecology and Obstetrics* for their kind permission to reproduce here the instructive pictures of the combined thoraco-abdominal approach, which is illustrated in Figures 14 to 23 at the end of this chapter.

Exploration of the Abdomen, Freeing of Adhesions, and Mobilisation of the Spleen and Its Delivery Through the Abdominal Wound

As soon as the abdomen is opened, the first step should be a rapid and thorough exploration of the liver, the gallbladder, the bile ducts, the pancreas, the stomach, the duodenum, and other abdominal viscera if conditions permit. If this routine is not conducted prior to the examination of the spleen, some concomitant pathological lesion may be overlooked, thus detracting from the ultimate benefits of the operation. For example, in hereditary spherocytosis, a fair proportion of cases show the presence of gallstones or biliary mud in the bile passages as an added complication, and cholecystectomy (combined, if necessary, with choledochostomy) may be required. Whether the combined operation—i.e., removal of the spleen plus

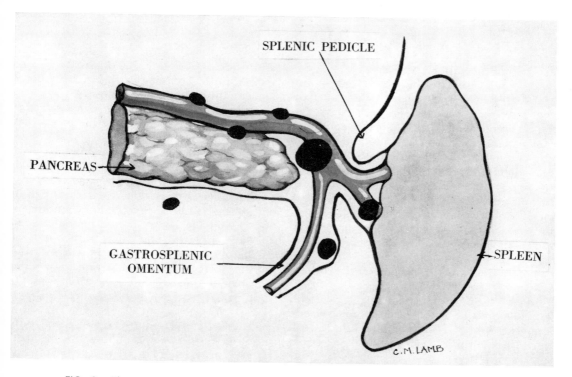

FIG. 3.   The more common locations of accessory spleens. (Modified from Hollinshead.)

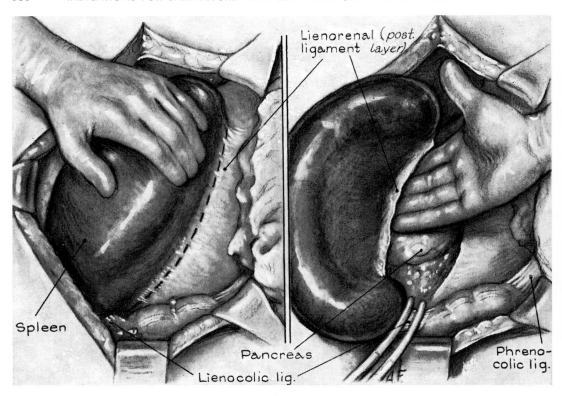

FIG. 4.   Splenectomy. Division of the lienorenal ligament and mobilisation of the spleen. (From Madden, *Atlas of Technics in Surgery*, 2d ed. Courtesy of Appleton-Century-Crofts, New York, 1964.)

excision of the gallbladder—should be undertaken in the first instance is a moot point, and the decision will of course depend upon the ease with which the splenectomy can be performed and on the general condition of the patient. In *severe* cases, and particularly when *jaundice* is pronounced, I advise that splenectomy be undertaken first in order to remove the excessive strain which is thrown upon the bone marrow, this being the most urgent need of the moment. When the patient has sufficiently recovered from the splenectomy, the gallbladder is removed, stones—if present—are extracted from the common duct and drainage of the biliary passages is instituted.

In performing splenectomy, a careful search should be made for *accessory spleens.* These accessory tissues with blood sinuses fall into three groups: (1) the true accessory spleen with blood sinuses and malpighian bodies, (2) haemal gland with blood sinuses,

and (3) haemal lymph gland with blood and lymph sinuses communicating with the blood and lymph systems, respectively.

Milroy Paul[34] classified true accessory spleen into two types: In the first, the accessory spleen is a constricted part of the main spleen, to which it is bound by a band of fibrous tissue, while in the second type it is a distinct and separate tissue mass.

The splenuli are found near the hilus of the spleen, in the gastrosplenic omentum, in the greater omentum, in the mesenteries of the small intestine and colon; rarely, near or in the left ovary or the left testicle,[32, 47] and in the pancreaticosplenic ligament—i.e., in that part of the dorsal mesogastrium which is supplied by branches of the coeliac axis (Fig. 1–3).

Putschar and Manion[36] reviewed all published cases of splenic-gonadal fusion (aberrant splenic tissue in the reproductive organs) and added 4 cases of their own. There were

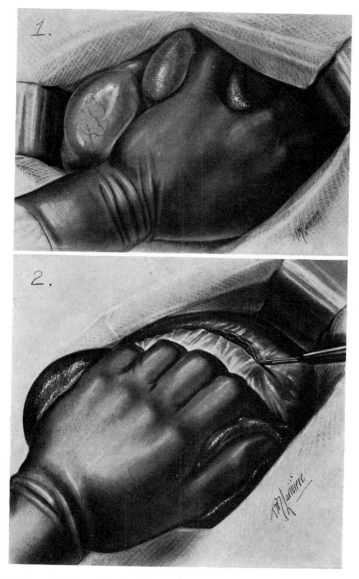

FIG. 5. Splenectomy. (1) The right hand is passed between the diaphragm and the spleen to ascertain the size of the spleen, to gauge the consistency, and to determine the degree of mobility. (2) Division of the posterior leaf of the lienorenal ligament.

30 cases that could be divided into two distinct groups: (1) in 18 cases a cord-like structure connected the spleen and the ectopic tissue, and (2) in 12 cases there was no continuity between the two. Another case of Type 1 was later described by Daniel.[8] Horovitz and Griffel[22] have reported an interesting case belonging to Type 2.

Settle[42] stated that in children an accessory spleen may become twisted on its pedicle and give rise to an acute abdominal emergency.

It is commonly stated that an accessory spleen is present in 18 to 30 percent of patients undergoing splenectomy. Jolly (1895), however, found 20 cases of accessory spleens in 80 postmortem examinations in children under 16 years of age and suggests that they are more common in early life and that possibly they atrophy with increasing years. There is no doubt that in certain splenic diseases they are encountered quite frequently.

Curtis and White,[6] in the course of 35 splenectomies, observed accessory spleens in 7 instances (20 percent). Morrison and his associates [29] made a special search for accessory spleens at necropsies and as a result were able to report an incidence of 35 percent. In 200 consecutive elective operations upon the gallbladder and stomach (1967), I found accessory spleens in 19 patients. This subject receives the expert consideration of Settle,[42] Curtis and Movitz,[5] De Weese and Coller,[9] and Gomes, Silverstein, and Re-Mine.[18]

According to Learmonth: [25]

Splenosis is a different condition, in which numerous (up to 300 have been counted) small

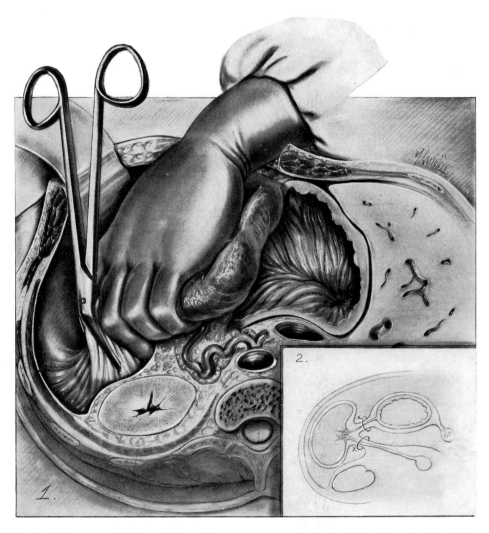

FIG. 6.   Splenectomy. Division of the peritoneum over the upper pole of the kidney to aid mobilisation of the spleen. The inset shows the gastrosplenic omentum—first pedicle; lienorenal ligament —second pedicle of the spleen.

masses of splenic tissue are found widely scattered over the peritoneum in situations other than those to be expected on embryological grounds. It results from the implantation of fragments of spleen which are freed by injury, either ruptured by violence or incomplete operative removal, and possibly distributed throughout the peritoneal cavity by bleeding from the torn vessels of the organ. This autografting of splenic tissue occurs most readily in young patients.

Very good accounts of *splenosis* are given by Hamrick and Bush,[19] by Storseen and ReMine,[46] by Garamella and Hay,[16] and by Cotlar and Cerise.[4]

Except when operating for rupture, I have always made a point of searching for an accessory spleen in all cases in which I have performed splenectomy. In a series of 32 cases of splenectomy for idiopathic thrombocytopenic purpura, I have found one or more accessory spleens in 10 cases. Where sple-

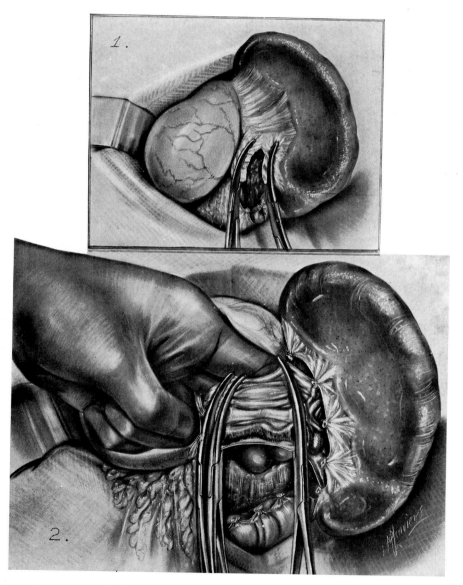

FIG. 7.   Splenectomy. (1) Division of the gastrosplenic omentum. (2) Three-clamp method. Note the position of the fingers guarding the pancreas while the clamps are being applied.

nectomy is indicated and an accessory spleen is discovered at operation, it should be excised in *all* cases except when the spleen is being removed on account of rupture, because these tissues undergo a further maleficent hypertrophy and cause a continuance of the morbid condition for which the splenectomy was undertaken, and cases are on record in which after splenectomy an unremoved splenculus has grown as large as a normal spleen [11] (Fig. 3).

It will be noticed that as a result of passing the stomach tube the stomach lies high up, tucked beneath the liver, empty and contracted. Both edges of the wound should be widely retracted and any adhesions that are

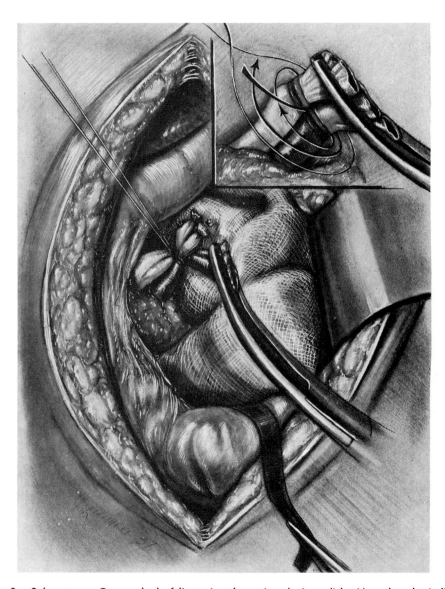

FIG. 8.   Splenectomy. One method of ligaturing the main splenic pedicle. Note that the individual vessels beyond the main ligature on the pedicle are ligated with silk, cotton, or chromic catgut.

found between the spleen and the anterior abdominal wall or between this organ and the diaphragm or colon should be carefully divided.

The further steps of the operation will be governed by the following factors: (1) the size of the spleen, (2) the presence of ad-

hesions between the spleen and the diaphragm, and (3) the length and mobility of the lienorenal ligament.

The right hand should be passed between the diaphragm and the spleen to ascertain the size of the spleen, to gauge its consistency, and to determine its degree of mobility. In

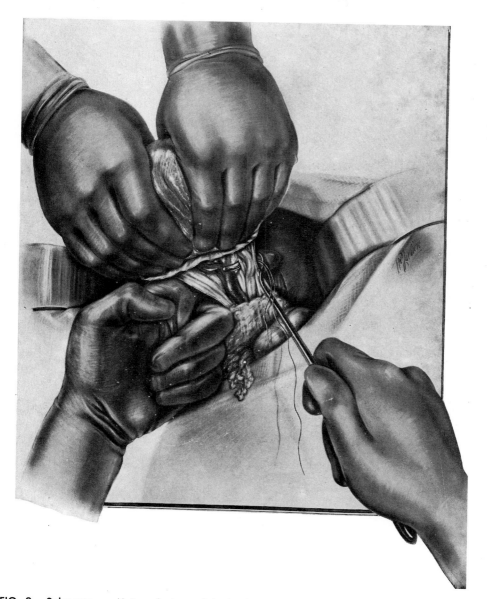

FIG. 9.   Splenectomy. Main splenic pedicle is displayed and splenic artery is underrun with aneurysm needle. By this method artery and vein are individually isolated and ligatured before spleen is cut adrift. In some cases, it may be wise to ligate and divide splenic artery and then to wait a few minutes before isolating, ligating, and dividing splenic vein, thus restoring considerable quantity of splenic blood to circulation.

cases where the spleen is of *normal size* or where, if enlarged, it is *freely mobile* and does not appear to be anchored to the diaphragm by adhesions, the fingers should be swept right round the inferior border to the renal impression and the organ retracted medially or even hooked through the abdominal incision.

If at this stage there is any difficulty in delivering the spleen through the incision, the splenocolic ligament and the lower portion of the gastrosplenic omentum should be divided between ligatures, the remaining upper portion being severed at a later stage in the operation.

Firm retraction on the wound is necessary

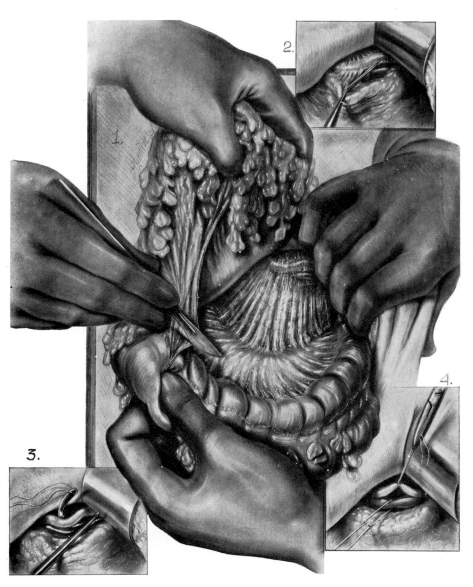

FIG. 10. Ligature of splenic artery in cases in which, although splenectomy is indicated, removal of organ is impossible. Splenic vein is, of course, not ligatured. In inset *4* it is shown surrounded by ligature, but after artery has been tied this loose ligature is removed. In some cases of splenomegaly it is advisable to ligate splenic artery at upper border of pancreas before proceeding with splenectomy.

in addition to levering the spleen medial-ward in an attempt to bring the posterior aspect of the lienorenal ligament into view.

With a long knife, the posterior sheath of the lienorenal ligament, which in essence is the posterior parietal peritoneum as it goes medially and anteriorly over the spleen, is carefully divided longitudinally, thus render-ing further mobilisation of the organ pos-sible (Fig. 4). The underlying areolar tissue and fascia propria are then incised, and with the finger and gauze dissection the tissues are cautiously separated, permitting an even wider freeing of the spleen (Figs. 5 and 6).

In certain cases, the peritoneum over the upper pole of the kidney may be divided with scissors. A finger is then inserted into this aperture, and by working this finger in an inward and upward direction the main splenic pedicle can be mobilised. This is a most important step and was first suggested and practised by Wilkie [53] and may be re-garded as the key to the whole operation, as it is the lienorenal ligament which binds the spleen down in its hidden retreat in the abdominal cavity. When the lienorenal liga-ment is very mobile and adhesions are mini-mal, it is of course possible to draw the spleen through the abdominal wound with-out employing this method.

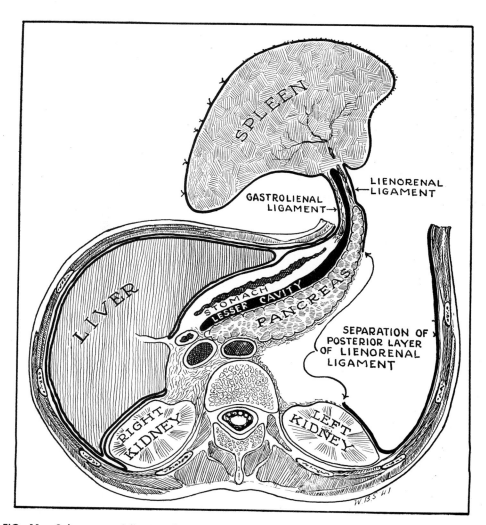

FIG. 11. Splenectomy following division of the posterior leaf of the lienorenal ligament. (Ives.)

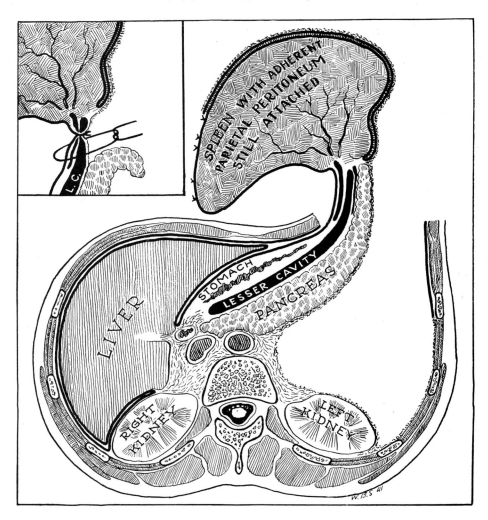

FIG. 12.   Splenectomy. Delivery of the spleen by the method suggested by Rives.

When the spleen is fully delivered—and not until then—the remaining portion of the gastrosplenic omentum and the phrenico-splenic ligament are divided, great pains being taken when clamping the blood vessels not to include a portion of the greater curvature of the stomach, as this would predispose to troublesome oozing of blood, to subsequent haematemesis, or even to perforation of the viscus itself.

Methods of Securely Ligaturing the Vascular Pedicles

The spleen is now quite free and can be drawn even more fully through the ab-dominal wound, as it is attached only by its main blood vessels—i.e., the splenic artery and vein. After carefully identifying and dissecting the blood vessels away from the tail of the pancreas, the main vascular pedicle is ready to be ligatured. If the pedicle is very small, as in cases of idiopathic thrombo-cytopenic purpura, it may be transfixed with an aneurysm needle and tied off in two places with strong silk; after clamping distal to the ligature, the spleen is removed. If the pedicle is moderately broad, the three-clamp method of Fédoroff should be employed (Fig. 7). Before applying these clamps, the index and middle fingers of the left hand are insinuated between the vascular pedicle and the tail of the pancreas in order to protect it while three large haemostats are applied, side by side, to the pedicle. These fingers lift the pedicle forward to ensure that the forceps are applied by sight and that in their application no damage is done to the pancreas, stomach, or colon.

The spleen is then cut adrift by severing the pedicle with a knife between the middle and distal haemostats. The inner or medial haemostat is then removed, thus leaving a groove or crushed area in the pedicle. Two stout catgut ligatures or two strong silk ligatures are applied to this groove and tied firmly side by side, after which each individual vessel distal to this is picked up and ligatured off seriatum (Fig. 8).

After making sure that there is no bleeding point to be seen anywhere, a portion of the adjacent gastrosplenic omentum, or better yet the greater omentum, is drawn over the raw surface of the pedicle and stitched to this area so that none of its surface remains exposed at the completion of the operation.

In cases of *marked splenomegaly,* the procedure will be different. The gastric surface of the spleen and the gastrosplenic omentum

covered by the presplenic fold at once come into view when the peritoneal cavity is opened. The spleen in these cases lies very closely applied to the greater curvature of the stomach, the gastrosplenic omentum is vertically lengthened and horizontally shortened, and the blood vessels are enlarged, tortuous, and increased in number. This enlargement is particularly prominent near the upper pole of the spleen, and is especially noticeable in cases of congestive splenomegaly. Each of these blood vessels in the gastrosplenic omentum must be cautiously and individually underrun with an aneurysm needle and ligatured with silk in two places, proximal and distal to the line of section.

Henry [20] stated that the presplenic fold, which is often present, springs from in front of the greater omentum and overlies the gastrosplenic ligament. Normally free at its lateral border, it forms attachments to large pathological spleens, especially at the lower pole, and carries vessels of the left gastroepiploic group.

After the blood vessels in the presplenic fold and gastrosplenic omentum have been dealt with, the right hand should be passed

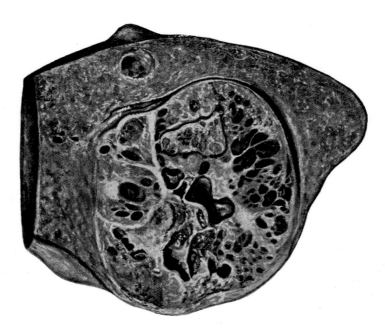

FIG. 13. Portion of haemangiosarcoma removed by splenectomy. (Courtesy of the Museum, University College Hospital, London.)

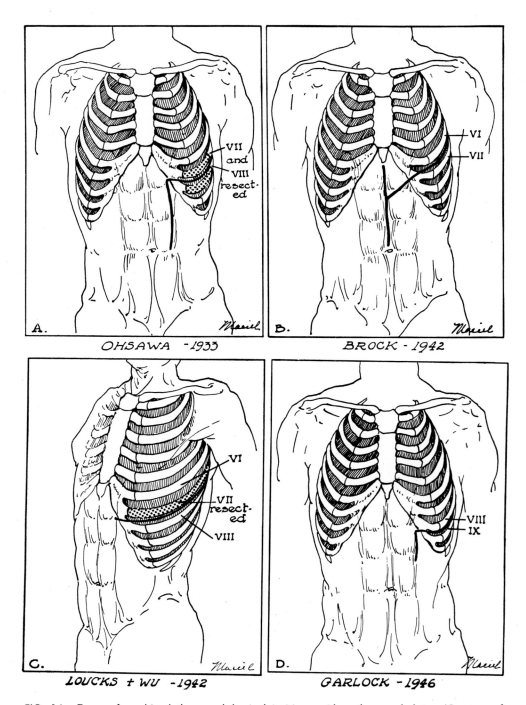

FIG. 14. Types of combined thoraco-abdominal incisions, with authors and dates. (Courtesy of B. Noland Carter; and Surgery, Gynecology and Obstetrics.)

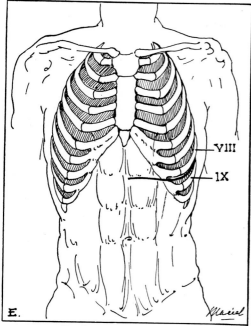

B.N. CARTER -1946

FIG. 14.E.

to the back of the spleen. Adhesions in this remote area are investigated, and must in the majority of cases be separated by blunt dissection with the fingers. Bleeding may be sharp and troublesome at this stage of the stripping, but the breaking down of the adhesions will have to be proceeded with, as it is essential to free the organ posteriorly so that it can be drawn over to the right to display the peritoneum, which forms the posterior leaf of the lienorenal ligament. Firm retraction is exerted on the spleen to render the ligament taut so that it can be widely divided to produce greater mobility of the organ, as already described.

A gauze pad soaked in warm saline solution is crammed against the diaphragm to control bleeding for the time being. The spleen is turned well over on to the abdomen toward the right side to display the posterior aspect of its pedicle and to permit the tail of the pancreas to be isolated from the enlarged and sacculated blood vessels which comprise the pedicle of the spleen. Each individual vessel is separated, and with meticu-

lous care an aneurysm needle carrying a ligature of strong silk is passed round it and the vessel is ligatured in two places fully ½ inch (1.27 cm) apart (Fig. 9).

It is advantageous to tie off the artery first so that some of the blood from the spleen may be drawn back into the circulation. Each vessel that is doubly ligated is then cut between the two ligatures, and this procedure is repeated step by step until the whole vascular sheath has been dealt with. When the splenic veins are the seat of endophlebitis, they are particularly soft, and if the ligatures are applied too forcefully, they may cut through these veins and initiate a very troublesome haemorrhage. In these cases, it is obvious that on account of the great size of the pedicle the three-clamp method, which has already been described, is unsuitable.

After the vascular pedicle has been dealt with, the abdominal pack that has been placed against the diaphragm is removed and any oozing surfaces on the diaphragm are picked up, underrun with a "snaking" suture, and tied off; or they may be coagulated with a diathermy button. Drainage is unnecessary, and in fact may be harmful, as it may initiate infection in the wound or left subphrenic space, as pointed out by Olsen and Beaudoin.[33] "Prolonged prophylactic drainage of the left subphrenic space increases the incidence of subphrenic abscesses and significant drain tract infections, without offering evident advantages. Drainage of the splenic bed after splenectomy is not advised unless the pancreas or stomach has been injured."

In a few cases of splenomegaly, a state of cohesion rather than of adhesion may exist between the opposing surfaces of the spleen and diaphragm, and this fixation may be so strong and dense that any attempt at splenectomy is quite out of the question. In such circumstances, therefore, where splenectomy, although indicated, is impossible, it may be wise to ligature the splenic artery behind the stomach at the upper border of the pancreas and at a point medial to where it gives off the left gastroepiploic artery. The splenic artery is best approached through the omental bursa by detaching the greater omentum from the transverse colon and by retracting the stomach upward, when the artery will be seen and can be isolated some

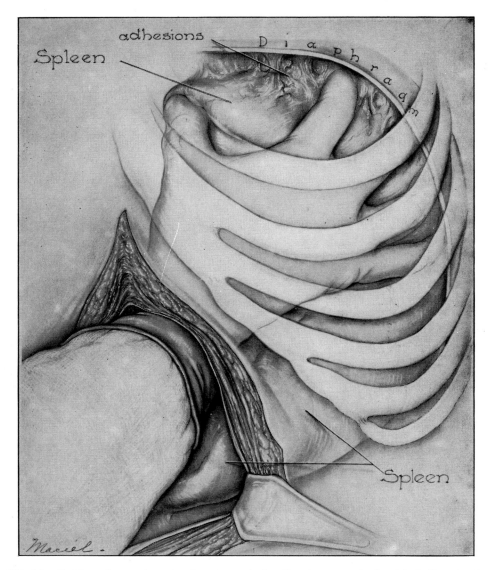

FIG. 15. Position of an enlarged spleen beneath the rib edge, necessitating blind dissection in order to mobilise it for delivery through the abdominal incision. (Courtesy of B. Noland Carter; and Surgery, Gynecology and Obstetrics.)

distance away from the hilus of the spleen (Fig. 10).

Some surgeons, however, prefer to divide the gastrocolic or the gastrohepatic ligament and ligate the splenic vessels before attempting removal of the spleen, as a routine measure, and in those cases where the spleen is almost felted to the diaphragm they prefer this approach to the one I have just described. Henry advocated dividing multiple and dense adhesions between the convex surface of the spleen and diaphragm with the high frequency current, and maintains that most "irremovable" spleens can be cut adrift from their moorings, bloodlessly and safely, by this method.

Rives [38] divided the peritoneum lateral to the spleen and mobilised the organ by stripping away the peritoneum from its posterior and lateral attachments. The spleen is then

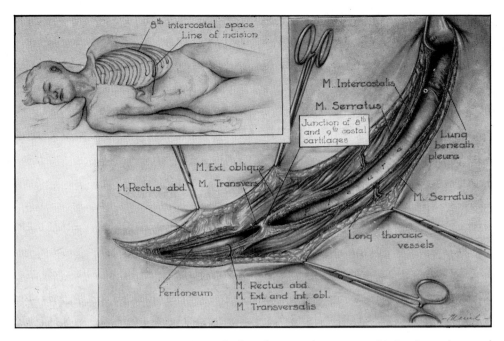

FIG. 16.   An incision has been made on the line shown in the insert, and it has been deepened through muscles down to the pleura and peritoneum. The eighth costal cartilage has not been divided. (Courtesy of B. Noland Carter; and Surgery, Gynecology and Obstetrics.)

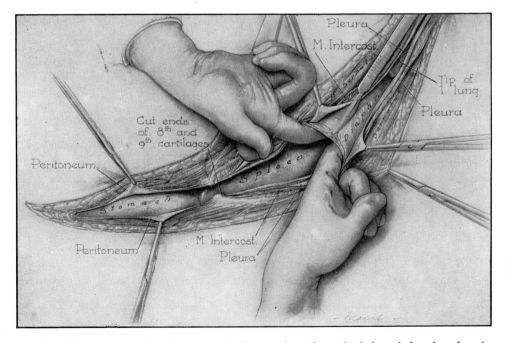

FIG. 17.   The peritoneum has been opened, the costal cartilage divided, and the pleural cavity entered. The diaphragm is now being divided, thus throwing the peritoneal and pleural cavities into one. (Courtesy of B. Noland Carter; and Surgery, Gynecology and Obstetrics.)

delivered through the wound together with its parietal peritoneal coat, to which it is inextricably bound. Reference to Figs. 11 and 12 will clarify this point.

A number of cases of combined abdominothoracic splenectomies with splenorenal shunts for congestive splenomegaly have now been reported (Chap. 58).

COMPLICATIONS FOLLOWING SPLENECTOMY

These are to some extent dependent upon the disease for which the operation is performed. The main complications are: (1) *haemorrhage,* which may be external (oozing from the wound) or internal, from a splenic blood vessel; (2) *shock;* (3) subphrenitis (localized peritonitis); *subphrenic abscess;* (4) *thrombosis of the splenic vein;* (5) *infection*

of the wound; haematoma, dehiscence, and/or "burst abdomen"; (6) *atelectasis* of the left lower lobe; pneumonitis, etc.; (7) *fistulas,* pancreatic or gastric; (8) splenic, gastric, and colonic injuries;[41] and (9) *cerebrovascular accidents.*

Haemorrhage may occur during operation when the capsule is torn accidentally or when strong vascular adhesions between the diaphragm and liver are severed and retract out of view. Generalised oozing, too, occurs when hypoprothrombinaemia is present. Severe haemorrhage, of course, occurs and may soon prove fatal when the ligatures on the main vascular pedicle give way in the postoperative period.

Infection sometimes settles in the subdiaphragmatic space, causing abscess and requiring drainage. It is the most common cause of continuous and intermittent pyrexia following removal of the spleen. Torraca,[48] however, considers that in certain cases a

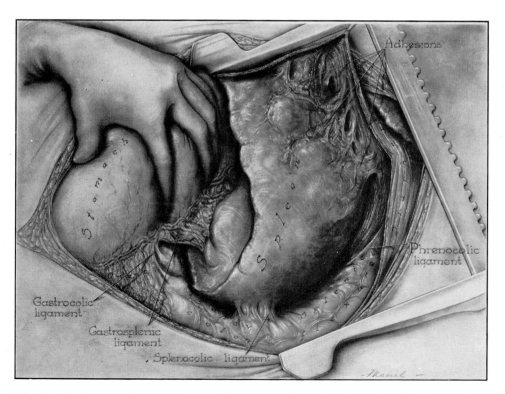

FIG. 18.   The extent of exposure obtained in a case of grossly enlarged and adherent spleen. Note the free access obtained to the diaphragmatic surface of the spleen with its many vascular adhesions. (Courtesy of B. Noland Carter; and Surgery, Gynecology and Obstetrics.)

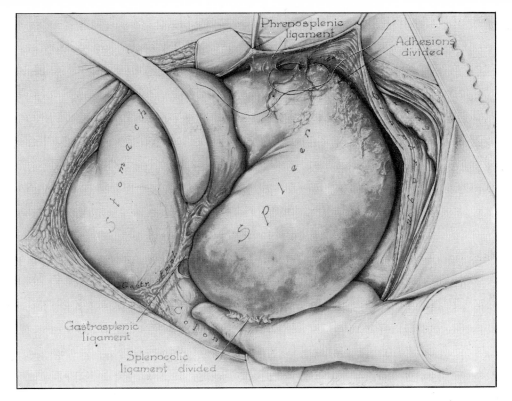

FIG. 19. The splenocolic and splenorenal ligaments have been divided. Vascular adhesions between the spleen and the undersurface of the diaphragm are being ligated prior to division. (Courtesy of B. Noland Carter; and Surgery, Gynecology and Obstetrics.)

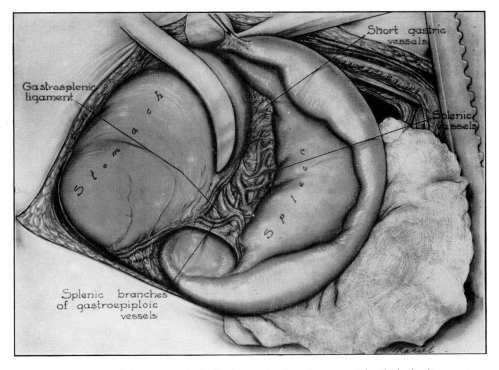

FIG. 20. Exposure of the gastrosplenic ligament, showing the ease with which the ligament can be isolated into segments and divided. The splenic vessels are likewise shown. (Courtesy of B. Noland Carter; and Surgery, Gynecology and Obstetrics.)

mild fever, which cannot be explained on the basis of infection or absorption, is present for several weeks. Among the theories that are discussed as to the cause of the pyrexia are the following: (1) ligation of the tail of the pancreas, (2) formation of exudate in the operative area, and (3) collection of blood in the splenic bed.

Infection of the wound occurs in 2 to 5 percent of the cases.

Fistula formation is a rare event and may result from injury to the tail of the pancreas, or to the greater curvature of the stomach during ligation of the vasa brevia.

Thrombosis of the splenic vein has occasionally been reported following splenectomy.[44] In my experience, this complication is rare.

Anticoagulant therapy is not ordinarily instituted unless the platelet counts exceed 1 million per cubic millimeter.

Norcross [30] considers that once thrombosis has spread down the splenic vein and into the rest of the portal system, all therapy is without avail. Sudden fever, abdominal pain, ascites, and leucocytosis followed by jaundice and abdominal distention indicate disaster.

Pulmonary complications are common after splenectomy and may prove serious if treatment is not instituted at an early stage. The danger of atelectasis and pneumonitis may be minimised by the prevention of gastric contents gaining access to the upper respiratory tract, by the guarded use of such drugs as morphine, which is a respiratory depressant, and by avoiding compression from intra-abdominal distention.

SPLENECTOMY EMPLOYING THE LEFT ABDOMINOTHORACIC APPROACH

In certain cases for which splenectomy is indicated, where the spleen is tethered to the diaphragm, splenectomy should be carried out through a left abdominothoracic

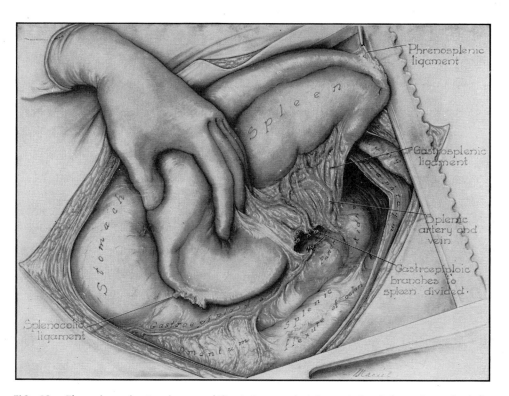

FIG. 21. The spleen, having been mobilised, is turned right and freed from the tail of the pancreas. (Courtesy of B. Noland Carter; and Surgery, Gynecology and Obstetrics.)

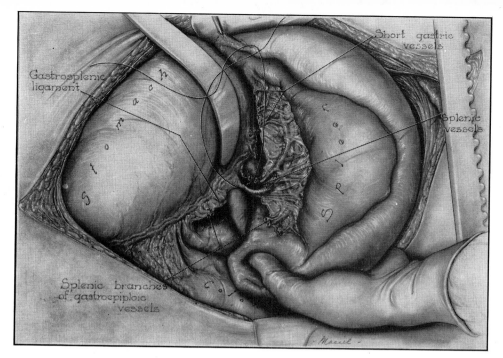

FIG. 22. Exposure of the pedicle. The arteries have been ligated and divided. A vein is being ligated. (Courtesy of B. Noland Carter; and Surgery, Gynecology and Obstetrics.)

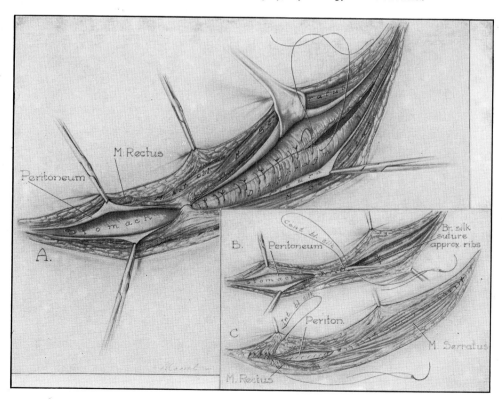

FIG. 23. (A) The diaphragm is being closed with figure-of-eight sutures. (B) One pericostal suture of braided silk has been tied and has approximated ribs. Muscles of the chest wall are being closed with continuous silk suture. (C) The chest wall closure has been completed. The peritoneum has been closed with continuous suture of silk; the sheath of rectus muscles is being sutured with figure-of-eight stitches of silk. (Courtesy of B. Noland Carter; and Surgery, Gynecology and Obstetrics.)

incision, as is well illustrated in Figures 14 to 23.

SUMMARY

The basic operation in surgical disorders of the spleen is splenectomy.

Splenopexy for simple ptosis, which was originally performed by Tuffier in 1882, is nowadays never performed and is only of historical interest.

The incisions of choice are left paramedian, left subcostal, transverse epigastric, and combined abdominothoracic.

A search should always be made for accessory spleens, which should be removed whenever they are found. In primary hypersplenism, an overlooked accessory spleen may grow in stature and reproduce the disease for which the primary splenectomy was undertaken.

The operative mortality rate of splenectomy is low, and the results are excellent in ptosis, idiopathic thrombocytopenic purpura, familial haemolytic anaemia, primary splenic neutropenia, and idiopathic pancytopenia, in cases of cysts of the spleen, and in nonpenetrating injuries limited to the organ.

In secondary hypersplenism associated with any form of splenomegaly, the operative mortality rate is relatively low, being about 8 percent, but the late results are, on the whole, disappointing.

Finally, it may be justly said that in splenopathy, surgery will always be an important weapon of research and inquiry, and that the haematologist and the surgeon working in the closest union can solve many of the problems associated with splenic disorders.

REFERENCES

1. Aguilar et al., Circulation 14:520, 1956.
2. Carter, B. N., Surg. Gynecol. Obstet. 84:1019, 1947.
3. Chatterjea, Arrau, and Dameshek, Br. Med. J. 1:987, 1952.
4. Cotlar and Cerise, Ann. Surg. 149:402, 1959.
5. Curtis and Movitz, Ann. Surg. 123:276, 1946.
6. Curtis and White, Tr. W. Surg. Ass. p. 346, 1936.
7. Dameshek and Welch, Hypersplenism and Surgery of the Spleen, New York, Grune & Stratton, 1952.
8. Daniel, Ann. Surg. 145:960, 1957.
9. De Weese and Coller, in Abdominal Surgery, Allen and Barrow, eds., New York, Hoeber, 1961.
10. Doan et al., Proc. Internatl. Soc. Haematol. 1:429, 1956.
11. Eccles and Freer, Br. Med. J. 2:515, 1921.
12. Editorial Comment, World Med. 3:40, 1968.
13. Egal et al., J.A.M.A. 186:745, 1963.
14. Elvehjem, Physiol. Rev. 15:471, 1935.
15. Ferris and Hargraves, Arch. Surg. 67:402, 1953.
16. Garamella and Hay, Ann. Surg. 140:107, 1954.
17. Gofstein and Gellis, Am. J. Dis. Child. 91:566, 1956.
18. Gomes, Silverstein, and ReMine, Surg. Gynecol. Obstet. 129:129, 1969.
19. Hamrick and Bush, Ann. Surg. 115:84, 1942.
20. Henry, Br. J. Surg. 27:464, 1940.
21. Herrera et al., Lahey Clin. Found. Bull. 17:43, 1968.
22. Horovitz and Griffel, Lancet 2:442, 1959.
23. Jones and Szur, Br. J. Haemat. 3:320, 1957.
24. King and Shumaker, Ann. Surg. 136:239, 1952.
25. Learmonth, Br. Med. J. 2:67, 1951.
26. Lowdon et al., Br. Med. J. 1:446, 1966.
27. McCann, Br. Med. J. 1:1271, 1956.
28. Meeker et al., Surg. Clin. North Am. 47:1163, 1967.
29. Morrison et al., Am. J. Med. Sci. 176:672, 1928.
30. Norcross, Surg. Clin. North Am. 39:583, 1944.
31. Norcross, Surg. Clin. North Am. 39:831, 1958.
32. Olken, Am. J. Pathol. 21:81, 1945.
33. Olsen and Beaudoin, Am. J. Surg. 117:615, 1969.
34. Paul, Lancet 2:74, 1937.
35. Pedersen and Videback, Acta Chir. Scand. 131:89, 1966.
36. Putschar and Manion, Am. J. Pathol. 188:15, 1956.
37. Rich et al., Am. J. Surg. 110:209, 1965.
38. Rives, Surgery 11:223, 1942.
39. Rousselot, Surg. Clin. North Am. 33:493, 1953.
40. Sandusky et al., Ann. Surg. 159:695, 1964.
41. Schwegman and Miller, Surg. Clin. North Am. 42:1509, 1962.
42. Settle, Am. J. Surg. 50:22, 1940.
43. Shields et al., Proc. Mayo Clin. 31:440, 1956.
44. Siderius, Surg. Clin. North Am. 41:173, 1961.
45. Smith, C., Am. J. Surg. 107:523, 1964.
46. Storseen and ReMine, Ann. Surg. 137:551, 1953.
47. Tate and Goforth, Texas J. Med. 45:570, 1949.
48. Torraca, Gior. Ital. Chir. 4:675, 1948.
49. Walker et al., Br. J. Surg. 40:392, 1953.
50. Watson et al., Blood 10:259, 1955.
51. Welch and Dameshek, N. Engl. J. Med. 242:601, 1950.
52. Whitby, Lancet 1:625, 1952.
53. Wilkie, Am. J. Surg. 14:340, 1931.

32

A. SPLENIC DISEASES OF SURGICAL IMPORTANCE

RODNEY MAINGOT

ANEURYSM OF THE SPLENIC ARTERY

An aneurysm of the splenic artery was first mentioned by Baussier (*J. Méd. Toulouse 32:* 157, 1770). Winckler (*Zbl. Chir. 32:257,* 1905) recognised the condition in the living. Högler (*Wien Arch. Inn. Med. 1:*543, 1920) made the diagnosis prior to operation 10 years before St. Leger Brockman described his much-quoted case (*Br. J. Surg. 17:*692, 1930). Lindboe (*Acta Chir. Scand. 72:*108, 1932) was the first to make a radiological diagnosis of the condition.

Sherlock and Learmonth [28] reported that they were able to collect 125 cases up to 1942. They stated that the average diameter of the aneurysmal sac was 3.4 cm and the largest 15 cm. The main splenic artery was involved in 81 percent, a branch artery or both the main artery and a branch artery in the remainder. In no fewer than 26 percent, there were multiple aneurysms; 64 percent occurred in women, their average age being 48 years. The aneurysm was attributed to arteriosclerosis (46 percent), embolism (23 percent), trauma, syphilis, splenomegaly, destructive lesions of the stomach, and Banti's disease. In 6 patients, the aneurysm was apparently congenital. Owens and Coffey [22] reported 204 cases, and Hill and Inglis [15] found 35 survivors after surgery, including only 9 after rupture of the aneurysm. Sheps et al.[27] gave a clinicopathological analysis of 47 aneurysms of the splenic artery noted during necropsy. Up to 1970, 350 cases of aneurysm of the splenic artery had been recorded in the world's literature.

Bedford and Lodge,[4] in their valuable contribution, state that far from being rare, aneurysm of the splenic artery is in fact a common condition, and many cases are being brought to light by the more recent use of *contrast arteriography.* They studied a consecutive series of 250 routine necropsies on patients dying at the Geriatric Unit, Cowley Road Hospital, Oxford. There were 108 male and 142 female cadavers in their series, with an age range from 31 to 100 years. Aneurysm of the splenic artery was found in 26 of the 250 specimens, an incidence of 10.4 percent— 7.4 percent of males and 12.9 percent of females. All the lesions were asymptomatic and unsuspected. The average age of patients in their series, 76.4 years, was undoubtedly due to the selection exercised in admitting patients to this particular hospital. The average age reported by others has been around 48 years. According to Bedford and Lodge, many of the diseases which have been described as associated with aneurysm of the splenic artery are probably coincidental.

Degeneration of the media on the vessel wall would appear to be the most consistent finding; mycotic endocarditis, congenital defect in the vessel wall, syphilis, arteriosclerosis, and trauma are considered as aetiological factors.[4]

Pregnancy is a predisposing factor in the rupture of such aneurysms.

Under ordinary circumstances, almost 50 percent of the patients in whom this diagnosis was made were seen as a result of rupture of the aneurysm. Treatment by splenectomy before rupture is therefore considered advisable in view of the excessive mortality rate when this complication occurs. A strong argument against this concept, however, is found in the fact that over 10 percent of all elderly patients who die of other causes have an unsuspected asymptomatic splenic artery aneurysm. This type of aneurysm is the second most common within the abdomen. (See Chap. 56.)

Clinical picture. In Sherlock and Learmonth's series, the signs and symptoms included epigastric pain, bouts of colic, vomiting, anorexia, wasting, splenic enlargement, and even intestinal obstruction. In 10 percent of the cases, the aneurysm could be felt on examination, and in 6 percent, the tumour was pulsatile or had a distinct bruit. A shadow with peripheral density calcification and possibly pulsation was observed on straight x-ray examination in 14 cases. Rupture into the colon, stomach, intestine, or general peritoneal cavity occurred in 53 percent. In 12.5 percent, a warning haemorrhage took place and was characterized by sharp pain in the left upper quadrant of the abdomen, vomiting, Kehr's sign, and rigidity and tenderness below the left costal margin, being followed in from 1 to 55 days by fatal bleeding. About 8 percent of cases were correctly diagnosed. Kreel, working at the Royal Free Hospital, London, however demonstrated a considerable number of cases of splenic aneurysm (some of which were asymptomatic) by means of coeliac angiography. He noticed the presence of calcification in the walls of such aneurysms, in a few elderly patients, on preliminary radiological investigation. (See Chap. 108.)

Treatment. In 38 of the 135 cases described by Sherlock and Learmonth,[28] operation was carried out, with recovery in 20. The procedure of choice was splenectomy with removal of the segment of the splenic artery from which the aneurysm has arisen. If the aneurysm is near the origin of the artery, proximal ligation or proximal and distal ligation may be successful. The authors note that of the 19 patients operated upon *before* rupture had occurred, 18 were cured, and that of 19 patients operated upon *after* rupture only 4 survived operation.

In Ward-McQuaid's series [31] of 5 patients, 4 survived. In 2 the aneurysm had ruptured; 1, a pregnant woman with a portacaval shunt, recovered. The other 3 were diagnosed on radiological grounds before operation.

In his series, resection of the artery and splenectomy formed the treatment of choice. Double ligation of the artery or resection of the sac been successful in a few cases. I would advise excision of the aneurysm if possible, or proximal and distal ligation when excision is unsafe. Splenectomy need not necessarily follow ligation of the splenic artery.

Many calcified aneurysms have been treated conservatively, apparently without disaster. Ronnen [26] stated that he could find no case of rupture of calcified splenic aneurysm in the literature.

SPLENIC ABSCESS

Abscess of the spleen is rarely seen in cold and temperate climates. Chaffee and Lasher (*Ann. Surg. 148*:979, 1958) reported 4 cases of splenic abscess which were observed within 1½ years. They consider that this is unique, as only 10 such cases have been recorded in the United States since 1942. Parrish and Sherman (*Am. Surg. 30*:712, 1964) reported 2 cases and reviewed the literature. They found that 15 percent of splenic abscesses were secondary to trauma, 10 percent were due to direct extension fom a neighbouring pathological process, and about 75 percent were caused by metastatic spread of infection from elsewhere. Asopa and Elhence (*Indian J. Med. Sci. 19*:618, 1965) reported a rare case of ruptured splenic abscess which presented as a case of peritonitis.

Frankel et al. (*J. Mount Sinai Hosp. 33*:404, 1966) recorded 2 patients who, although critically ill, were successfully treated by splenectomy.

An authoritative article by DeSmet (*Acta Chir. Belg. 55*:729, 1956), of Yangambi in the Congo, should be consulted, as he has had occasion to treat 16 patients with acute splenic abscess and 1 with tuberculous abscess of the spleen among 3,750 major operations performed between 1947 and 1956. None of his cases was associated with an epidemic.

The frequency with which the spleen escapes abscess formation in infections in general is probably linked up with its abundant content of phagocytic cells and its normal function as the scavenger of stray organisms entering the blood stream. An abscess may, nevertheless, develop during the course of any chronic or acute blood infection and in certain parasitic diseases, notably hydatid disease of the spleen.

It may thus occur: (1) in acute specific infectious diseases, the most common being typhoid fever; (2) in pyaemia; here mutiple abscesses are usually present; (3) in ulcerative endocarditis; here the breaking down of a septic infarct leads to abscess formation; (4) in pneumococcal septicaemia; (5) in certain staphylococcal infections, such as carbuncle and furunculosis; (6) in such diseases as malaria, dysentery, and relapsing fever, and in spirochaetosis; (7) following injuries; and (8) by direct extension from carcinoma or diverticulitis of the colon, from cancer or ulcer of the stomach, and from suppuration in the left kidney.

DeSmet states that in a series of 107 transparietal splenoportographies 3 cases of abscess due to direct inoculation were discovered, and more will appear as the practice of injecting opaque substances into the spleen increases. In his cases cure was effected with irrigations of 1 percent acriflavine, without splenotomy.

The possibility of a splenic abscess must not

be overlooked in cases of septicaemia and in diseases peculiar to tropical and subtropical climates; it is accompanied by high temperatures, frequent rigors, localised left hypogastric pain and tenderness, weight loss, splenomegaly, and signs suggestive of suppuration in the left hypochondriac region and in the base of the left lung.

In the early stages of splenic abscess, the symptoms are somewhat mild and obscure, there being no characteristic feature until the abscess has attained a considerable size and has started to stretch the capsule of the spleen or has actually burst and produced a localised peritonitis in the region of the splenic bed.

In all well-established cases, the patient looks gravely ill and there is often anorexia, occasional bouts of vomiting, diarrhoea, asthenia, rapid loss of weight, rigors, and high temperature. Pain, localised to the upper left quadrant of the abdomen, is constant and severe, and respiratory excursions on the left side of the chest are restricted and painful. When the abscess is situated in the *upper pole of the spleen* (as it is in 60 percent of the cases) the infection may spread through the diaphragm and give rise to pleurisy or empyema. The clinical manifestations in such cases at once suggest subphrenic suppuration or empyema. When the *lower pole* is involved, tenderness below the costal margin may be exquisite, guarding of the muscles in the left half of the abdomen may be marked, but especially so in the left hypochondrium and left postrenal angle, and there may be oedema and pitting on pressure in this area.

A splenic abscess may burst between the convex surface of the spleen and diaphragm and become localised as one form of subphrenic abscess; into the general peritoneal cavity, giving rise to acute peritonitis; into the left pleural cavity, producing empyema; through the abdominal wall; or into the stomach, colon, or small intestine. Ochsner and Graves (*Ann. Surg. 98:*961, 1938) reported a 2.4 percent incidence of this association in 3,000 subphrenic abscesses.

Treatment. *Splenectomy is the best treatment if it can be performed with safety.* If, however, the spleen is firmly bound down by dense adhesions and suppuration is extensive, as is often the case, the technical difficulties alone will preclude removal of the organ, and splenotomy combined with drainage will have to be substituted. Again, if there are localising signs, such as redness of the skin and oedema over the lower chest, excision of the twelfth rib overlying the abscess should be performed in order to give free vent to the pus. A counterincision in the lumbar region is a wise procedure, especially for some of these *large gaseous tropical abscesses* which are so often adherent to the abdominal wall and diaphragm. In some instances, it may be wise to ligate the splenic pedicles first, and then to remove the pus-laden necrotic splenic tissue piecemeal!

In DeSmet's series, splenectomy was performed in 4 cases of splenic abscess with 1 death, and splenotomy with drainage in 11 cases with 1 death.

Blood transfusions and modern supportive therapy should be instituted as soon as possible and, following sensitivity tests, suitable antibiotic agents should be given in large doses by the intravenous or oral route. Antibiotic therapy has markedly reduced the incidence and mortality of splenic abscess. Before the advent of the antibiotic agents, the mortality rate in surgically treated patients with splenic abscess was 25 percent.

CYSTS OF THE SPLEEN

Andral (1829) described the first splenic cyst, which was found at postmortem examination and proved to be a dermoid. Twelve dermoid cysts of the spleen have now been reported. Weinstein and his coworkers [33] give an account of an interesting case of *dermoid cyst of the spleen* which occurred in their practice. In recent years, Bolot [5] has recorded a case.

Péan (1880) performed the first splenectomy for a solitary cyst of the spleen, and Powers (1906) collected 36 cases from the literature.

The most important article dealing with nonparasitic splenic cysts of the spleen was published by Fowler,[11] who collected 265 cases from the world literature and considered both pathogenesis and classification. Since 1953, an additional 170 cases have been reported. Qureshi et al.[23] reported 14 of their cases, and made a special study of 75 consecutive cases recorded in the English language over the past 12 years. The article by Qureshi and Hafner [24] on the *clinical manifestations of splenic cysts* (study of 75 cases) is a valuable contribution to this subject.

Classification of Splenic Cysts

Splenic cysts are classified as outlined below (after Qureshi and Hafner [24]):

Extended Fowler's Pathogenic Classification of Nonparasitic Benign Splenic Cysts
A. Primary, with cellular lining, component endothelium
    1. Congenital
       a. Serous

  b. Transitional cell-lined; noncomponent epithelium
2. Traumatic
3. Inflammatory
  a. Infoliation cysts
  b. Dilatation cysts; lymphangiectatic, polycystic disease
4. Neoplastic cysts (also congenital)
  a. Epidermoid) noncomponent,
  b. Dermoid   } epithelium
  c. Lymphangioma
  d. Benign, cavernous, and capillary haemangioma
B. Secondary, no cellular lining
  1. Traumatic (blood and serous types)
  2. Degenerative (liquefaction)
  3. Inflammatory (necrosis, tuberculosis)

Since Fowler's report,[11] the total number of documented calcified cysts has increased to 50, and of epidermoid to 43.

It is important to distinguish between parasitic and nonparasitic cysts, as the former are relatively common. Arce [3] stated that the spleen is affected by hydatid cysts in 3 percent of cases; Dew (1956) in 4 percent; and Larghero (1961) at 6 percent (see Chap. 55, Part A). The ratio of incidence is four parasitic cysts to one nonparasitic cyst, whilst the ratio of true cysts to false cysts of the spleen is 1 to 4.

True cysts include: (1) dermoids, (2) epidermoids, and (3) those lined with endothelium.

Although it is difficult to explain the presence of ectoderm in the spleen, this is the only source of these tumours. A possible explanation is that they are derived from a primitive totipotential cell capable of producing any of the three layers, such as is postulated to explain the ovarian and testicular dermoids.

Endothelium-lined cysts are easier to explain and can be accounted for as haemangiomata, lymphangiomata, and serous cysts arising possibly from inclusion of peritoneal cells, together with the multiple cysts associated with polycystic disease of other organs. Lubarsch considers that some of the serous cysts may be neoplasms arising from anlagen of lymphatic endothelium (Harmer and Chalmers, *Br. Med. J.* 1:531, 1946).

PSEUDOCYSTS

Pseudocysts are usually single and fairly large, and they contain blood or serous fluid and often cholesterol crystals. They are usually situated at either pole of the spleen, with normal splenic tissue elsewhere, and part of the cyst wall may be formed by fibrous tissue or compressed splenic tissue. Fowler describes smooth muscle and cartilage occurring in the walls. Hongisto,[16] in reporting his case, stated that calcified cysts of the spleen are rare; only 31 cases had been reported in the literature up to 1950 (Fig. 1).

The cause of false cysts is considered to be trauma, infection, or degeneration in an infarcted area. Malaria, syphilis, and splenomegaly from any cause are mentioned as predisposing factors.

Approximately 60 percent of the splenic cysts occur in females, and 60 percent of these lesions are found in patients less than 40 years of age.

Ferris, Dockerty, and Helden [9] made a careful study of 19 at the Mayo Clinic over a period of 46 years. The nonparasitic cysts of the spleen were divided into capsular types (5 cases) and parenchymatous types (14 cases). The capsular types are multicentric, small, and clinically of no importance; they are derived from lymphatic spaces or peritoneal mesothelium. The parenchymatous types include epidermoid cysts, cystic haemangiomas, and sizeable unilocular cysts of uncertain origin. These authors maintain that to label the latter "true" or "false," depending upon the presence or absence of an "endothelial lining," is impractical, since many of the cysts would be labelled "true-false" by this criterion. About 500 nonparasitic splenic cysts have been reported since the condition was first described in 1929 by Andral. The first splenectomy for a nonparasitic cyst was performed in Paris, by Péan in 1880.

Diagnosis. The findings on physical examination of the abdomen with the characteristic x-ray appearance of these cysts should enable the surgeon to make a diagnosis in cases of *large cysts of the spleen.* An intravenous pyelogram will often show the left kidney displaced downward, whilst barium-meal studies will show the stomach to be pushed across to the right and compressed backward, and the splenic flexure of the colon to be displaced downward and to the right according to the size of the tumour (Fig. 2). Coeliac angiography and scanning the spleen may prove of value in diagnosis.

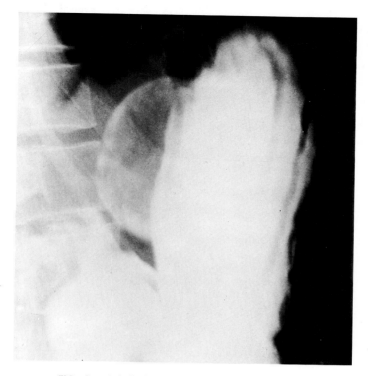

FIG. 1. Calcified splenic cyst (author's patient).

It should be noted that nearly 50 percent of patients suffering from splenic cyst have a palpable mass; 32 percent are asymptomatic; 40 percent complain of pain and a dragging sensation in the epigastrium, and 10 percent have a weight loss ranging from 10 to 30 pounds. Preoperatively, a number of splenic cysts closely resemble tumours of the tail of the pancreas.

Large cysts arising in the splenic parenchyma cause pressure symptoms and localised pain, but they are not a cause of hypersplenism.

Treatment. Splenectomy is the operation of choice and should be performed in all cases. The removal of the spleen is sometimes facilitated by aspirating the cyst, provided of course that infection and hydatid disease are excluded. There is no place nowadays for such operations as marsupialisation, incision and drainage, or enucleation of the cyst.

TUMOURS OF THE SPLEEN

In classifying splenic tumours, Smith and Rusk [29] and Hausmann and Gaarde [14] divided them into the following five groups: I. Capsular and trabecular framework; II. Lymphoid elements; III. Vascular and sinusoidal elements; IV. Reticuloendothelial system; and V. Nerve elements. The only important innocent tumour is haemangioma, and the most important malignant tumour is sarcoma.

Benign new growths of the spleen are strikingly uncommon and are of little surgical importance. Reports of series of cases are to be found in the papers by Krumbhaar,[17] Matas,[19] and Grove [13]. Abrahamson and Hughes [1] state that benign tumours sometimes show a transition to malignant types.

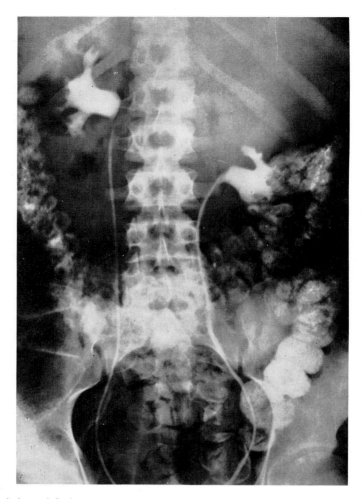

FIG. 2.   Radiological findings in a case of large unilocular cyst of the upper pole of the spleen. Note that the splenic flexure of the colon and the left kidney are displaced downward. Splenectomy was performed; the cyst was lined throughout with endothelium (author's patient).

They described an interesting case of hae-mangioendothelioma of the spleen.

Primary carcinoma of the spleen does not occur.

It has been taught that unlike the liver the spleen is very rarely the seat of *secondary carcinomatous deposits,* but such teaching is fallacious, as has been pointed out by Mc-Menemey,[20] who made statistical enquiries on this subject, and Shields Warren and Davis,[32] who in a series of 1,140 consecutive cases of carcinoma of all types found macroscopic metastases in the spleen in 1.9 percent. These metastases occurred most frequently when the primary growth was in the lung (23 percent of 13 cases) or in the breast (15 percent of 193 cases).

Tasker Howard[30] was able to collect 116 cases of primary sarcoma of the spleen. Bostick[6] reported a total of 157 primary splenic neoplasms, of which the most frequent were lymphomas or reticulum-cell sarcomas. Gordon and Paley[12] reported on 2 patients with primary lymphosarcoma of the spleen and collected a total of 189 instances in the world literature; 42 of these were diagnosed as lymphosarcomas. Das Gupta et al.[7] stated that from 1951 to 1962, 10 additional cases could be found in the literature. They give a learned account of 9 tumours arising from the lymphoid elements and 1 from vascular sinus endothelium. There were 5 patients with reticulum-cell sarcoma, 4 with lymphosarcoma, and 1 with angiosarcoma.

Clinical features. These may be summarised as follows:

1. Splenomegaly associated with mechanical discomfort.
2. Persistent or intermittent pain occasionally radiating to the centre of the abdomen or between the scapulae.
3. Nausea, anorexia, loss of weight, and indigestion.
4. Medial displacement of the stomach and splenic flexure on x-ray pictures and medial and/or downward displacement of the left kidney by the tumour on retrograde pyelography.
5. Secondary anaemia, often associated with thrombocytopenia.

Clinical, biochemical, haematological, and radiological investigations, and bone marrow studies should be carried out to exclude any evidence of disease elsewhere.

Pyrexia and leucocytosis are inconstant features. Spontaneous rupture was reported in 4 patients. Splenic sarcomas are highly malignant, they metastasise rapidly, and they frequently involve the liver, and less frequently the lungs, lymph nodes, and pancreas.

The only treatment which offers any hope is early splenectomy.

Results of splenectomy. Hausmann and Gaarde [14] wrote that of the 45 splenic growths reviewed between 1923 and 1943, the spleen had been excised in 18 cases. Four patients died within 30 hours of operation. Of the remaining 14, 2 died within 1 year, and 12 were alive for 3 to 8 years.

Ahmann et al.[2] reviewed information on 29 males and 20 females (average age, 56 years) *who underwent splenectomy and had no previous histological evidence of lymphoma.*

These patients represented about 1 percent of all patients with lymphoma seen during 1946–63 at the Mayo Clinic.

Some 50 percent of the patients reported pain in the upper abdomen or the left costal margin.

The spleen was enlarged in 84 percent and the edge of the liver was palpable in 30 percent. Lymphadenopathy was observed in 12 percent.

Eleven patients had pancytopoenia and 4 had haemolytic anaemia, and in none of 30 having bone marrow study preoperatively was a definite diagnosis of lymphoma made.

The bone marrow was hyperplastic in 15 patients and hypocellular in 3. Splenic calcification was observed preoperatively in 2 patients.

All patients but 6 received radiotherapy or alkylating agents shortly after excision of the spleen.

Two patients died within 1 month of operation, 1 of lymphoma, and 15 patients are still alive, 10 after more than 5 years. The 5-year survival rate is 31 percent.

Patients with follicular distribution of disease had a slightly better prognosis than those with a diffuse distribution.

Of the patients with lymphocytic lymphosarcoma, 75 percent survived for 3 years and 60 percent for 5 years. Only 20 percent of those with lymphoblastic lymphosarcoma or reticulum-cell sarcoma survived 3 years.

Those with Hodgkin's disease also had a poor outlook. *The Role of Splenectomy in Malignant Lymphoma and Leukaemia* by Meeker and colleagues [21] may be consulted with profit.

MALARIAL SPLENOMEGALY

In certain tropical countries, malaria is the most common cause of splenic enlargement. It was customary in the past to advocate splenectomy in certain cases of malarial splenomegaly, as the enlarged spleen which obtained in these cases was very prone to injury, torsion of the pedicle was said to be a common occurrence, and the removal of the organ permitted the resumption of active work in cases in which medicinal measures had failed to produce any improvement. We now know that many "malarial spleens" which had failed to respond to antimalaria treatment were due to kala-azar. It is now exceedingly rare to have recourse to excision of the spleen for malaria alone, for, except in cases of rupture which demand immediate surgery, medicinal treatment with such drugs as Camoquin, Avloclor, Paludrine, Camoprima, or Daraprim (pynimethamine), combined if necessary with radiation therapy, often proves successful.

WANDERING SPLEEN

Wandering spleen (*syn.*: ptosis of the spleen or splenic ectopia) is a rare condition, as shown by the reports that of 1,003 splenectomies performed at the Mayo Clinic up to 1944 only 2 were for wandering spleen (Pemberton). According to Adkins (*Ann. Surg. 107*:832, 1938), Irvin Abell (1933) analysed 97 cases collected from the literature. Emmett and Dreyfuss (*Ann. Surg. 117*:754, 1943) reported 25 cases which were recorded in the literature between 1933 and 1943, and Hall (*Br. Med. J. 1*:957, 1952) has given an account of a wandering spleen in a female child aged 10, for whom splenectomy was successfully performed. Balestra (*Radiol. Med. Milano 44*:1026, 1958) reviewed the literature on the subject and presented an analysis with reproductions of radiological findings in 13 cases of splenic ectopia. In Balestra's opinion, the stomach is the organ most commonly involved and its normal x-ray appearances may be changed considerably by an ectopic spleen. In his series, deformity of the greater curvature, at times suggesting an intrinsic gastric lesion, and interposition of the spleen between the stomach and diaphragm were observed in association with dyspepsia, nausea, belching, regurgitation, and other symptoms of upper gastrointestinal tract disorders.

Ptosis of the spleen is indeed a rare abnormality. Maingot (*Lancet 1*:625, 1952), in recording a case with torsion of the splenic pedicle, remarks that few surgeons have operated on wandering spleens, and Chamberlain (*Ann. R. Coll. Surg. 30*:8, 1962) agreed with this view. Binns (*Br. J. Surg. 54*:79, 1967), in describing a case of wandering spleen in association with enlargement of the left kidney, states that approximately 150 cases of wandering spleen (and its complications) have been recorded. A study of statistics, however, reveals that the figure today is about 175. Since 1958, a number of cases have been reported by Chamberlain (1962), Pearson (*Br. J. Surg. 5*:393, 1964), Anand and Davey (*Br. J. Surg. 52*:335, 1965), Simpson and Ashby (*Br. J. Surg. 52*:344, 1965), and a number of other surgeons. Anand and Davey's series of 4 cases is of particular interest.

The causes of this condition may be:

1. *Congenital.* Here the ectopic position of the spleen is due to absence of the supporting phrenicocolic ligament and an unusually lax lienorenal ligament.
2. *Acquired.* This type is a result of either trauma—as a result of direct or indirect injury, the suspensory ligaments of the spleen may give way or become stretched and elongated—or splenomegaly—here the weight of the spleen may stretch the supporting peritoneal folds and the organ become unduly mobile.

The wandering spleen may be found in the thorax in cases of diaphragmatic hernia; it may wander into any part of the abdominal cavity, showing a predilection for the midepigastric region abutting upon the diaphragm above and the lesser curvature of the stomach; the left iliac fossa; the hollow of the pelvis; or even a large inguinal hernial sac.

In the migrations of the spleen, the following *complications* may occur: torsion of the pedicle; engorgement and consequent enlargement; haemorrhagic cystic formations; atrophy; or dislocation. The movable spleen is said to be dislocated when as a result of localised chronic peritonitis it becomes fixed in an abnormal position and remains so.

Clinically, there is usually no difficulty in recognising the condition, as the wandering spleen has a characteristic shape and generally lies in a superficial position. It may often be replaced into its former bed in the abdominal cavity. Occasionally, however, it may be mistaken for a uterine fibroid with a long pedicle, an ovarian cyst or growth of the ovary, a pregnant uterus, a polycystic kidney, a hydronephrotic kidney, or even carcinoma of the stomach or of the splenic flexure.

The symptoms are usually mild and may include a dull ache in the epigastrium from engorgement, flatulent dyspepsia from the dragging on the stomach, nausea, pressure effects, and a variety of symptoms akin to those caused by movable kidney.

When *torsion of the pedicle* occurs, the symptoms are acute and may resemble those of a severe abdominal catastrophe. There is a sudden agonising abdominal pain, prostration, vomiting and distention, in fact a combination of symptoms frequently seen in twisted ovarian cyst. Often there is an acute pain in the left shoulder (Kehr's sign) and in the left loin, with a degree of shock, both reflex and as the result of blood loss into the general peritoneal cavity. Vomiting may be copious and, according to Sheppard (*Br. J. Surg. 31*:97, 1943), the signs and symptoms may resemble those of acute intestinal obstruction or acute pancreatitis.

Fiore (1956) presented a case of a patient who had torsion of the spleen with the unusual symptomatology of haematemesis and melaena.

Christeas et al. (*Grece Med. 25*:1077, 1956) reported a case of *torsion of the pedicle of an accessory spleen* which was successfully operated upon by them.

A diagnosis *may* be impossible until the abdomen has been opened, as Michaels (*Lancet 2*:23, 1954) and Chamberlain (1962) have emphasised. Coeliac angiography may help to clinch the diagnosis.

The acute symptoms are due to thrombosis of the blood vessels of the pedicle, which have long been twisted, rather than to rotation of the pedicle itself, which as a rule is a slow process. As soon as the blood vessels in the pedicle thrombose, the spleen becomes a massive infarct and localised peritonitis ensues. It may in addition become gangrenous, slough, or produce a localised abscess or generalised peritonitis.

Treatment. Splenectomy is the operation recommended for *all* cases of wandering spleen, whether complications are present or not. Torsion of the spleen, of course, demands immediate operation to relieve the intense pain associated with infarction and to prevent the onset of serious intra-abdominal complications. The operative mortality for splenectomy for ptosis of the spleen, with or without torsion of its pedicle, is less than 1 percent.

GAUCHER'S DISEASE

In the present state of our knowledge, there appear to be three primary disorders of lipoid metabolism which are intimately associated with one another. According to the *type of lipoid* involved, they may conveniently be grouped as: (1) Gaucher's disease, a cerebroside (kerasin) disturbance; (2) Hand-Schüller-Christian disease, a cholesterol disturbance (generalised xanthomatosis), and (3) Niemann-Pick disease.

Gaucher's disease is a rare, congenital, familial disturbance of cerebroside metabolism, characterised by abnormal storage of cerebrosides in the reticuloendothelial cells, splenomegaly, hepatomegaly, marked chronicity, haematological changes of hypersplenism, pigmentation of the skin, and changes in the bones. In the majority of cases, the disease is due to a gene which is transmitted as an autosomal recessive.

It was originally described in 1882 by Gaucher, who regarded the condition as a primitive endothelioma of the spleen. Mandlebaum (*Am. J. Med. Sci.* 157:366, 1919), Lieb (*Z. Physiol. Chem.* 140:305, 1924), Epstein (*Biochem. Z.* 145:398, 1924), Pick (*Am. J. Med. Sci.* 185:453, 1933), and Thannhauser (*Lipoidoses: Diseases of the Intracellular Lipid Metabolism,* 3d ed., 1958), as a result of extensive research work, founded the present conception of the disease, which is now regarded as a disturbance of lipoid metabolism in which the Gaucher substance—kerasin—is deposited in certain cells of the reticuloendothelial system.

The onset is insidious, there being no sign of the disease at birth. The first indication of its presence may be the accidental discovery of an enlargement of the spleen, osseous or neurological complications, or symptoms referable to the haemorrhagic diathesis.

According to Pack and Silverstone (*Am. J. Surg.* 41:77, 1938) and Hsia et al. (*N. Eng. J. Med.* 261:164, 1959), the disease affects mainly children and young adults. In a review by Hoffman and Makler (*Am. J. Dis. Child.* 38:775, 1929), 51 percent of the 89 reported cases were in patients under 25 years of age, 30 percent under 5 years, and 16 percent under 1 year. The youngest patient recorded was 1 week old, and the oldest was 60.

There is an acute infantile form which begins in the first weeks of life and pursues a rapid and highly virulent course. In the average case, the condition is slowly progressive. The disease is more common in females than in males in the proportion of 2 or 3 to 1, and is congenital and familial. In about one-third of the cases examined by Pick, several members of one generation were affected, but the disease was limited to this generation only. As many as 4 cases in one family have been reported. It should be noted that Niemann-Pick disease occurs *only in infants.* Females predominate in a ratio of 5 to 1, and the ratio of Jewish to non-Jewish infants is 3 to 1 (Crocker and Farber, *Medicine* (Baltimore) 37:1, 1958).

Splenomegaly is the most characteristic feature of Gaucher's disease. The spleen undergoes a slowly progressive enlargement and in the late stage may fill the greater part of the abdominal cavity. Some of the largest spleens ever seen belong to this group.

As a rule, the liver slowly enlarges as the disease progresses. Nevertheless in the more chronic varieties, and especially in elderly patients, following splenectomy the swollen impregnated liver may remain stationary for several months or years; but in children the tendency is for it to grow slowly and relentlessly until eventually it occupies the greater portion of the abdominal cavity. There is little or no ascites.

The blood changes are fairly constant; there is usually moderate haemolytic anaemia, thrombocytopenia, and leucopenia. These changes are present in the majority of cases, but not in all (Stefanini and Dameshek, *The Hemorrhage Disorders,* 2d ed., 1962, New York). After splenectomy, there is frequently a temporary leucocytosis. Thrombocytopenia is present in cases in which splenectomy is not performed. After removal of the spleen, the platelet count mounts rapidly, often to a normal figure. This preoperative platelet deficiency may in part account for the haemorrhages from the gums, petechiae, and haematuria so frequently seen. After splenectomy, such bleeding is very rare and the blood picture shows an all-around improvement.

The characteristic Gaucher cells have never been demonstrated in the blood stream at any time, although they have been obtained from the spleen by puncture, from the marrow by sternal puncture, and from the sputum.

Pigmentation of the skin is an expression of general haemochromatosis, which becomes more marked as the disease progresses. The peculiar diffuse or blotchy pigmentation, limited principally to the face, neck and hands, imparts a greyish or yellow-brown to ochre tone.

There may be brownish-yellow, wedge-shaped, pinguecula-like thickenings of the ocular conjunctivae, but this is present in only some 20 percent of all cases.

The osseous changes observed in the primary disorders of lipoid metabolism are usually of three varieties:

1. Flask-like expansion of the lower ends of

the long bones, and especially of the femora, accompanied by a dull ache or even sharp pain.
2. Localised swellings over the bones, suggestive of a localised periostitis or abscess.
3. Pathological fracture.

Infants suffering from the disease are prone to spastic irritative contraction and tremors of the central type.

Disturbances of the organs of internal secretion, as noted by Norbertenzer, are by no means infrequent. Cases of dwarfism, infantilism, and general dystrophy have been seen in association with this disease.

The outstanding feature is the presence of Gaucher cells, which are found in the malpighian bodies, in the venous sinuses of the spleen, in the bone marrow, in the sinusoids of the liver, and in the lymph nodes. They are in all probability modified reticular cells—histiocytes. Collections of these peculiar, large (about 20 to 80 μ in diameter), clear, vesicular cells with their small nuclei will be seen in the sections, grouped together and often, in alveolar arrangement. The cytoplasm under a high magnification appears wrinkled. This wrinkling is due to a mass of minute threads woven together in an irregular network. The wrinkles are the remains of the spongioplasm in the interstices of which kerasin is stored. It is important to note that the Gaucher cells do not take the Smith-Dietrich stain as do the lipoid-filled foamy-appearing cells of Niemann-Pick disease.

A diagnosis is made when an enlarged spleen is discovered in a patient who has a peculiar ochre-like tint of the skin and in whom there is usually hepatomegaly without ascites, flask-like expansion of the lower ends of the femora, a degree of pyrexia, leucopenia, haemolytic anaemia, and thrombocytopenia, and on sternal puncture the finding of Gaucher cells. Death usually results from cachexia, rapidly progressing anaemia, severe haemorrhages, nephritis, bronchopneumonia, or phthisis.

Treatment. From the very nature of the disease, which is a congenital anomalous defect of constitution, it will be evident that there can be no specific treatment for Gaucher's disease. There is no evidence that ACTH, corticosteroids, or salicylates modify the course of the disease.

Acute nephritis occurs in about 40 percent of cases, and it is commonly a diffuse glomerulonephritis. This, when present, should be treated on the usual lines.

The haemolytic anaemia, which is invariably present, does not respond to iron and liver therapy; blood transfusions have no influence on the course of the disease; while deep x-ray therapy or radium, although given a trial in many cases, has produced little or no effect.

Splenectomy offers the only hope of palliation. It prolongs life, it improves the patient's general health, it is associated with very marked changes in the haemorrhagic diathesis, as there is a return of the erythrocytes, leucocytes, and blood platelets to normal for some time, and there is in addition a greatly diminished tendency to spontaneous haemorrhages; the pigmentation of the skin decreases, and the patient is rid of the discomfort arising from the presence of a large intra-abdominal tumour.

I have said that life may be prolonged by removal of the spleen in this disease. This is especially true for patients in the fourth and fifth decades of life, when the disease tends to be lethargic, and many instances have been recorded of operations performed during this period after which the patients have survived for many years. In *infants and young children,* the prognosis following splenectomy, so far as duration of life is concerned, is of course less promising, and the majority of these subjects die from an extension of the disease to such vital organs as the liver and, as Myers (*Br. Med. J.* 2:8, 1937) has shown, to the lungs. The best that can be hoped is that the adult patient may live for 5 to 10 years following splenectomy.

In the *phosphatid* lipoidoses, no success has followed the use of splenectomy or irradiation.

SPLENECTOMY AS AN ADJUNCT TO OTHER PROCEDURES AND INCIDENTAL TO IATROGENIC TRAUMA

In operations for cancer involving organs in close proximity to the spleen, it is often necessary to perform splenectomy.

For instance, in many cases of subtotal or total gastrectomy for malignant lesions of the stomach, the cardiac orifice, or the lower end of the oesophagus, excision of the spleen simplifies the operation, reduces haemorrhage, and at the same time renders the operation more radical, thus offering greater prospects of cure.

Infiltrative carcinomas of the splenic flexure of the colon and of the tail or body of the pancreas require splenectomy along with removal of the primary growth.

During caudal pancreatic resection for hyperinsulinism, the spleen is nearly always sacrificed.

Splenectomy is also called for in cases of total pancreatectomy, in *some* cases of diaphragmatic hernia, and where haemorrhage from the splenic pulp owing to accidental injury during a partial or subtotal gastrectomy cannot be staunched.[18]

The subject of splenectomy incidental to

iatrogenic trauma is fully discussed by Rich et al.[25]

Trendelenburg, in 1882, tore the capsule of the spleen during the removal of a retroperitoneal sarcoma and had to remove the organ to arrest a brisk haemorrhage. Quan and Castleman (*N. Engl. J. Med. 240*:885, 1949) were amongst the first to discuss the frequency of *incidental splenectomy*. They reported 70 splenectomies, 13 of which were performed as a result of iatrogenic injury to the spleen during some other intra-abdominal procedure.

Zollinger et al.[35] reported 748 splenectomies and only 23 (3 percent) of these were classified as iatrogenic in origin.

Finney and Sumner [10] list 13 cases of operative injury in 116 splenectomies at Johns Hopkins Hospital, an incidence of 11 percent.

Rich and his colleagues [25] write:

Our interest in this not infrequent complication has been stimulated by an exhaustive study of 925 splenectomies taken from the hospital records of five major hospitals in the San Francisco metropolitan area. It is significant that in this series of 925 splenectomies, 26 percent of spleens were removed secondary to *iatrogenic trauma*.

Exploration of the left upper quadrant, partial gastrectomy, vagotomy, hiatus hernia repair, left adrenalectomy, pancreatic surgery, and left colectomy are always mentioned amongst the causes of iatrogenic trauma.

An analysis of our records reveals that at least 20 different surgical procedures have contributed to splenic injury.

Zollinger [34] remarked that 2 to 3 percent of patients undergoing partial gastrectomy for duodenal or gastric ulcers underwent splenectomy necessitated by inadvertent splenic capsular laceration.

Dunphy [8] whose opinion carries the weight of authority, in discussing Rich's paper makes these cogent remarks:

It is very important to call attention to this *avoidable accident*. The statistics put things a little out of focus, because one gets the impression that in San Francisco, spleens are injured 26 percent of the time which, of course, is wrong. If one considers Zollinger's figures, only 3 percent of all splenectomies are for surgical injury. This places the few for trauma in their proper perspective.

This is an avoidable accident, and I think we should stress that, as the authors have. But I think we should also make clear that the meaningful figures are, how many laparotomies were carried out? There were 240 splenectomies for trauma, but how many thousand upper abdominal laparotomies were performed, especially gastrectomies? *Those are the important figures to know.*

The *treatment* of choice for this "avoidable accident" is splenectomy.

Tamponade or suture of the laceration cannot be relied upon to staunch the bleeding.

REFERENCES

1. Abrahamson and Hughes, Br. J. Surg. 40:68, 1952.
2. Ahmann et al., Cancer 19:461, 1966.
3. Arce, Arch. Surg. 43:789, 1941.
4. Bedford and Lodge, Gut 1:312, 1960.
5. Bolot, Lyon Chir. 56:548, 1960.
6. Bostick, Am. J. Pathol. 21:1143, 1945.
7. Das Gupta et al., Surg. Gynecol. Obstet. 120:947, 1965.
8. Dunphy, Am. J. Surg. 110:216, 1965.
9. Ferris, Dockerty, and Helden, Minn. Med. 41:614, 1958.
10. Finney and Sumner, Virginia Med. Month. 90:4, 1963.
11. Fowler, Surg. Gynecol. Obstet. 96:209, 1953.
12. Gordon and Paley, Surgery 29:907, 1951.
13. Grove, Ann. Surg. 105:969, 1937.
14. Hausmann and Gaarde, Surgery 14:246, 1943.
15. Hill and Inglis, Br. J. Surg. 42:408, 1955.
16. Hongisto, Ann. Chir. Gynaecol. Fenn. 39:270, 1950.
17. Krumbhaar, Ann. Clin. Med. 5:833, 1927.
18. Maingot, Lancet, 1:625, 1952.
19. Matas, Encycl. Med. 12:834, 1933.
20. McMenemey, Lancet 1:69, 1937.
21. Meeker et al., Surg. Clin. North Am. 47:1163, 1967.
22. Owens and Coffey, Int. Abst. Surg. 97:313, 1953.
23. Qureshi et al., Arch. Surg. 89:570, 1961.
24. Qureshi and Hafner, Am. Surg. 31:605, 1965.
25. Rich et al., Am. J. Surg. 110:209, 1965.
26. Ronnen, Acta Radiol. (Stockh.) 39:385, 1953.
27. Sheps et al., Proc. Mayo Clin. 33:381, 1958.
28. Sherlock and Learmonth, Br. J. Surg. 30:151, 1942.
29. Smith and Rusk, Arch. Surg. 7:371, 1923.
30. Tasker Howard, J. Lab. Clin. Med. 14:1157, 1929.
31. Ward-McQuaid, Br. Med. J. 1:1448, 1958.
32. Warren, Shields, and Davis, Am. J. Cancer 21:517, 1934.
33. Weinstein et al., Ann. Surg. 148:851, 1951.
34. Zollinger, Am. J. Surg. 105:413, 1963.
35. Zollinger et al., Postgrad. Med. 27:148, 1960.

B. HYPERSPLENISM

SIR RONALD BODLEY SCOTT

We owe the term *hypersplenism* to Chauffard (1907), but, apart from its use by Eppinger (1920), in his well-known book *Die hepatolienal Erkrankungen,* it did not establish itself in the medical vocabulary until the publications of Doan (1949) and Dameshek (1955). The observed facts upon which these two writers erected their several hypotheses are simple. It had long been known that in various diseases in which splenomegaly was a feature, anaemia with leucopenia and thrombocytopenia was common and that when the spleen was removed, the blood picture was restored to normal. This clearly pointed to a connection between the spleen and the changes in the peripheral blood. It was suggested that cause of the changes lay in an exaggeration of the spleen's normal functions. In Doan's (1949) view, the cytopenia was due to increased sequestration of erythrocytes, leucocytes, and platelets. He claimed, in support of his contention, that smears from the pulp of the excised spleen showed an excess of leucocytes and platelets. Dameshek (1955) took the view that the bone marrow was under the influence of a splenic hormone, which either inhibited haematopoiesis or delivery of cells from the bone marrow.

It has been recognized for some years that neither of these hypotheses stands up to criticism. The functions of the spleen are ill-understood, and thus the very notion of "hypersplenism" has a shaky foundation. No hormone has ever been demonstrated. There is no evidence that leucocytes or platelets undergo pooling in the splenic pulp. Effete erythrocytes and those that are damaged or abnormal are certainly trapped and detroyed in the organ; there is no evidence that healthy, normal erythrocytes are liable to destruction there. The spleen has been called the graveyard, but not the slaughterhouse of the erythrocyte. Nevertheless, it is possible that when it is enlarged and its structure is abnormal, it may assume a more active haemolytic role; it is known that erythrocytes emerge from its pulp thicker and thus more vulnerable than they are on entry.

Although hypersplenism is a vague concept, the facts are not in question and the term is usefully descriptive. Its diagnosis requires, first, the characteristic changes in the blood; second, a hypercellular, but not otherwise abnormal, bone marrow; third, splenomegaly; and fourth, a return to a normal blood picture after splenectomy. The changes in the blood include a variable degree of anaemia, which is almost always haemolytic. It may require an isotopic estimation of erythrocyte life to demonstrate this point. The leucocytes are reduced in number and the leucopenia which mainly affects the neutrophils may be profound. The leucocyte count is most frequently between 2,000 and 3,000 per cubic millimeter, but it is sometimes below 1,000 per cubic millimeter. Thrombocytopenia is the rule; the platelets commonly range about the 50,000 per cubic millimeter level, but may be lower. Frequently the changes in the blood do not affect all the formed elements equally: anaemia is often mild and perhaps thrombocytopenia is the most constant finding.

The bone marrow, while qualitatively normal, shows increased activity. There is erythroblastic hyperplasia proportional to the degree of haemolysis: there is often an increased number of less mature granulocytes. This finding has been interpreted as indicating "maturation arrest," but increased peripheral destruction would explain it equally well.

Adult megakaryocytes are increased in number; there is no increase in less mature forms. A normal proportion of the cells is actively engaged in platelet formation (Dameshek and Miller, 1946).

Splenomegaly is clearly a sine qua non, and the final proof that the diagnosis was correct is given by restoration of a normal blood picture by splenectomy.

Diagnosis is largely by a process of exclusion; from this description, it will be clear that many infiltrative and neoplastic diseases can cause splenomegaly and pancytopenia. Although this may be by a "hypersplenic mechanism," it can also be due to bone-marrow infiltration.

Hypersplenism has been divided into primary and secondary varieties. It is said to be secondary when the splenomegaly is due to some recognised cause. If the concept of hypersplenism is ill-defined, that of "primary hypersplenism" is even more vague. It envisages a spleen which has become enlarged for no recognisable reason, which is the seat of no recognised morbid anatomical change, and which is associated with cytopenia. The diagnosis was not uncommonly made 25 years ago and descriptions of "primary splenic neutropenia" and "primary splenic pancytopenia" were published by Doan and Wright (1946). Dameshek and Miller (1946) suggested that idiopathic thrombocytopenic purpura was a form of hypersplenism and thus that hereditary spherocytosis could be explained in the same way. Gradually reports of such cases have ceased to appear, and although textbooks grudgingly admit that primary hypersplenism may exist, few modern haematologists can recall seeing an example. It has been suggested that acquired hypogammaglobulinaemia with splenomegaly is one of the disorders formerly regarded as "primary splenic pancytopenia" (Prasad, Reiner, and Watson, 1957). It is possible too that the various forms of tropical splenomegaly (Basu and Aikit, 1963), then little understood, as well as nontropical idiopathic splenomegaly (Dacie, Brain, Harrison, Lewis and Worlledge, 1969), could also have received this label.

The causes of secondary hypersplenism are numerous and may be listed as follows:

1. *Chronic infections:* tuberculosis; syphilis; brucellosis; subacute bacterial endocarditis; histoplasmosis.
2. *Reactive hyperplasias:* Felty's syndrome; acquired hypogammaglobulinaemia.
3. *Tropical splenomegaly and related disorders:* Kala-azar, chronic malarial splenomegaly; cryptogenetic splenomegaly of Hong Kong (McFadzean, Todd, and Tsang, 1958); Indian splenomegaly (Basu and Aikit, 1963); Uganda "big spleen disease" (Marsden et al. 1965); tropical splenomegaly of Uganda (Pryor, 1967); Nontropical idiopathic splenomegaly (Dacie, Brain, Harrison, Lewis and Worlledge, 1969).
4. *Neoplastic splenomegaly:* Lymphoma; chronic lymphatic leukaemia; myelosclerosis.
5. *Storage and infiltrative diseases:* Gaucher's disease; amyloidosis.
6. *Portal hypertension:* Congestive splenomegaly.
7. *Sarcoidosis.*
8. *Thalassaemia.*

Diagnosis

The diagnosis of hypersplenism is made by exclusion. When splenomegaly and pancytopenia are associated, it is important first to determine whether a marrow infiltration is responsible. If the marrow is qualitatively normal but overactive, the diagnosis of hypersplenism is likely. In some cases, marrow infiltration and hypersplenism may coexist, and assessment of these is particularly difficult. If the total number of megakaryocytes and immature granular cells seems adequate in spite of leucopenia and thrombocytopenia, a hypersplenic element is probably present. This is made even more likely when the anaemia can be shown to be haemolytic. The second step in diagnosis is to determine the cause of the splenomegaly; in most instances, this is easy enough, but in some it is impossible until the spleen has been removed.

Indication for Splenectomy

The mere existence of a hypersplenic syndrome is no justification for splenectomy. This operation should be contemplated only when there is anaemia, repeated severe infection due to neutropenia, or a significant haemorrhagic state resulting from thrombocytopenia. When marrow infiltration is also present, as in Gaucher's disease or chronic lymphatic leukaemia, assessment is particularly difficult. Isotope studies are especially helpful in such situations and, in the presence of haemolytic anaemia, the accumulation of excessive radioactivity over the spleen would encourage splenectomy. If the main problem is neutropenia or thrombocytopenia, the outlook depends upon the marrow's content of immature granulocytes and megakaryocytes.

REFERENCES

Basu, A. K., and Aikit, B. K., Tropical Splenomegaly, London, 1963.

Black, M. M., Preston, J. A., and Speer, F. D., Blood, 10:145, 1955.

Chauffard, A., Sem. méd. 27:25, 1907.

Dacie, J. V., Brain, M. C., Harrison, C. V., Lewis, S. M., and Worlledge, S. M. Br. J. Haemat. 17:317, 1969.

Dameshek, W., Bull. N.Y. Acad. Med. 31:133, 1955.

Dameshek, W., and Miller, E. B., Blood, 1:27, 1946.

Doan, C. A., Bull. N.Y. Acad. Med. 25:625, 1949.

Doan, C. A., and Wright, C. S., Blood, 1:10, 1946.

Eppinger, H., Die hepatolienalen Erkrankungen, Berlin, 1920.

Marsden, P. D., Hutt, M. S. R., Wilks, N. E., Voller, A., Blackman, V., Shah, K. K., Connor, D. H., Hamilton, P. J. S., Banwell, J. G., and Lunn, H. F., Brit. Med. J. 1:89, 1965.

McFadzean, A. J. S., Todd, D., and Tsang, K. C., Blood, 13:513, 1958.

Prasad, A. S., Reiner, E., and Watson, C. J., Blood 12:926, 1957.

Pryor, D. S., Quart. J. Med. (NS) 36:321, 337, 1967.

C. IDIOPATHIC THROMBOCYTOPENIC PURPURA

SIR RONALD BODLEY SCOTT

HISTORICAL

Purpura haemorrhagica was first described in a brief report by Werlhof in 1735, and his name has, perhaps overgenerously, been attached to the disease. Its association with thrombocytopenia was recognised by Krauss (1883) and by Denys (1887), and only in the last 40 years has it been distinguished clearly from the various types of secondary thrombocytopenic purpura. Indeed, it is likely that the idiopathic group still contains a number of syndromes of different causation.

AETIOLOGY

Idiopathic thrombocytopenic purpura is of necessity defined in negative terms as thrombocytopenic purpura not due to any recognisable cause. Clinically, the patients are readily separated in those with an acute self-limiting disease and those whose illness has an insidious onset and a chronic relapsing course. Infrequently, the acute variety passes into the chronic form.

The acute form is more common than the chronic and is essentially a disease of children—thus of the entire group, 45 percent occur below the age of 15 years; 65 percent below 21 years, and only 10 percent over the age of 40 years. In the younger, males and females are equally affected, above the age of 12 years it is 2 to 4 times more common in females.

In most cases, the cause of thrombocytopenia is the formation of autoantibodies directed against platelets. The importance of immunological mechanisms in this connection was first suggested by Ackroyd's (1949) work on thrombocytopenia due to apronal (Sedormid) sensitivity. He showed that in sensitive persons apronal after absorption became attached to platelets, to form a loose complex which was antigenic. The first dose of the drug sensitised the patient, and when a second was taken, the antibodies that had been raised reacted with the drug-platelet complex to cause a sudden and profound thrombocytopenia. The association of autoimmune haemolytic anaemia with thrombocytopenia and a positive antiglobulin test had been described in 1949 (Evans and Duane, 1949). This disorder, known as the Evans' syndrome, again pointed to the importance of immunological causes. Proof of its relevance to idiopathic thrombocytopenic purpura awaited the demonstration by Harrington, Minnich, and Arimuro, (1951, 1953) that when plasma from a patient with this disease was transfused into a healthy recipient of compatible ABO group, transient purpura and thrombocytopenia resulted, indicating the presence of an antiplatelet factor in the patient's plasma. The existence of such a factor, and of its ability to cross the placenta, was supported by observations that infants born of mothers with idiopathic thrombocytopenic purpura frequently showed short-lived thrombocytopenia immediately after birth. Additional evidence came from the finding that normal platelets of compatible groups have a greatly reduced survival when transfused into patients with idiopathic thrombocytopenic purpura (Cohen, Gardner, and Barnett, 1961). With recent techniques, it has been possible to show that antibodies to platelets exist in 85 percent of patients with this disease, and these have proved to be IgG immunoglobulins (Colombani, 1966; Karpatkin and Siskind, 1969).

As in most diseases in which auto-immunity plays a part, the cause of the antibody production is purely conjectural. Many of the acute cases of idiopathic thrombocytopenic purpura follow viral infections. It is known that some viruses can become attached to platelets, and it is quite possible that cells thus modified become antigenic.

THE CLINICAL PICTURE

The hallmark of idiopathic thrombocytopenic purpura is bleeding into the skin. The lesions may take the form of minute capillary haemorrhages or petechiae or of ecchymoses, larger extravasations of blood into the deeper layers of the dermis. They are often spontaneous but when occasioned by trauma they are of an extent out of proportion to the severity of the injury. Spontaneous petechiae tend to be most frequent about the lower third of the shin, presumably because the upright position leads to a high local intracapillary pressure.

Bleeding from mucosal surfaces is less common, although the buccal cavity and the endometrium provide exceptions. Submucous haemorrhages are common in the first, and in one clinical variant—described in Africa and known as "onyalai"—large bullae filled with blood are seen in the mucosae of the oral cavity (Strangway and Strangway, 1949). Oozing from the gums when the teeth are cleaned and persistent epistaxis are common. In some adult women, menorrhagia is the outstanding complaint.

Haemorrhage from the urinary tract is not rare, but from the gastrointestinal tract it is less common. Internal haemorrhages are unusual; the only exception is bleeding into the central nervous system, which is a recognised and serious hazard, but it occurs almost exclusively in the acute, severe forms of the disease. Haemarthrosis is so rare that its occurrence casts doubt on the diagnosis.

Idiopathic thrombocytopenic purpura is a risk to the parturient woman and to the neonate. Haemorrhage in the second stage of labour can be serious, and the perinatal mortality of the offspring of such women is as high as 17 percent (Heys, 1966).

Physical examination reveals the petechiae and ecchymoses described above. Any anaemia is due to loss of blood. There are no enlarged lymph nodes, and while the spleen may be palpable in 10 percent of children, if it is felt in an adult, the diagnosis should be reconsidered.

COURSE

The acute form of the disease is seen most commonly in children. It frequently occurs 2 to 3 weeks after a virus infection such as rubella or varicella. Its onset is usually abrupt and the severity of the haemorrhagic state varies from the trivial to the life-threatening. It is usually a self-limiting disorder. It often remits within 3 or 4 weeks and almost always within 6 months. It occasionally passes into a chronic stage. The acute fulminating varieties alone present a threat to life,, and it is in such cases that haemorrhage into the central nervous system is likely to occur.

The chronic form occurs most frequently in adults. The onset is insidious and it is preceded by no infection or prodromes. The haemorrhagic state is usually mild, often limited to recurrent crops of petechiae and ecchymoses, and sometimes shown only by menorrhagia. The course is commonly one of relapses and remissions, and there is rarely serious disability unless as a result of anaemia from menorrhagia or uncontrollable epistaxis.

THE BLOOD

Anaemia, if present, is solely the result of blood loss. There are no characteristic changes in the leucocytes; the total number is normal or occasionally slightly raised; sometimes in children there is an increase in lymphocytes. The platelets are reduced in number. In the acute form, they may be absent and they rarely exceed 10,000 per cubic millimeter. In the chronic variety the reduction is less profound, perhaps most frequently to about 40,000 per cubic millimeter. It is rare for haemorrhagic phenomena to occur with a platelet count above 60,000 per cubic millimeter. Morphological changes are common in the platelets; giant forms are often seen, and they frequently stain more intensely than usual.

The bleeding time is prolonged and may exceed 30 minutes. Clot-retraction is impaired, but the clotting time and other tests of the coagulation process are normal. The tourniquet test is positive. To carry out this, the armlet of the sphygomanometer is applied and the pressure within it raised to 100 mm Hg and kept at this level for 5 minutes. A positive test is shown by the presence of petechiae distal to the armlet when it is removed. It is assumed that the venous obstruction raises the intracapillary pressure, and the test is thus one of capillary "fragility"; it seems likely that one of the platelet's functions is to repair breaches in the capillary wall and thus the test indirectly becomes one of platelet function or deficiency.

THE BONE MARROW

Erythropoiesis is normal unless there is an erythroblastic reaction to loss of blood or iron deficiency. Leucopoiesis likewise shows no characteristic changes, although an increase in eosinophils is common but unexplained. Megakaryocytes are increased in number, often strikingly. Frequently, there is a higher proportion of immature forms than normal, and granularity is less evident. There are few platelets, and the drifts of these cells that surround the megokaryocytes in normal marrow are not seen. This has been interpreted as indicating defective thrombopoiesis, but it could be as well explained by increased peripheral destruction of platelets.

DIFFERENTIAL DIAGNOSIS

The diagnosis of idiopathic thrombocytopenic purpura is largely determined by the exclusion of diseases to which thrombocytopenia might be secondary. Viewed more positively, the essential features of the idiopathic form are thrombocytopenia with no other changes in the blood apart from possible posthaemorrhagic anaemia, a normal erythrocyte sedimentation rate (E.S.R.), plentiful megakaryocytes in the bone marrow, and an absence of splenomegaly, lymphadenopathy, and hepatic enlargement.

The possible causes of thrombocytopenia are numerous. They may be classified as those due to defective platelet formation and those due to excessive destruction or consumption. Into the first group, come such disorders as leukaemia, aplastic anaemia, myelomatosis, myelosclerosis, lymphoma, carcinoma metastasising to the bone marrow, megaloblastic anaemia, myelotoxic drugs, fulminant infections, and perhaps hypersplenism; examples of the second are systemic lupus erythematosus (L.E.), massive blood transfusion, the defibrination syndrome, giant haemangioma, sensitivity reactions to drugs, microangiopathic haemolytic anaemia, and thrombotic thrombocytopenic purpura. Most of these causes are easily excluded by competent haematological study and present little difficulty. Occasionally the earliest evidence of acute leukaemia is a thrombocytopenic purpura with no demonstrable abnormality other than a marked reduction of megakaryocytes in the bone marrow (amegakaryocytic thrombocytopenic purpura). There are two others deserving note. Sometimes thrombocytopenic purpura is the first manifestation of systemic lupus erythematosus, and it may remain the only one for several years. In every case, the E.S.R. should be measured and an L.E. cell preparation examined. It is quite exceptional for the E.S.R. to be raised in idiopathic thrombocytopenic purpura. Drug sensitivity may be overlooked unless particular enquiry is made. Although apronal was the first recognised cause of an auto-immune thrombocytopenia, it has since been recorded with quinine, quinidine, digitoxin, chlorothiazide, chlorpropamide, meprobramate, sulphonamides, phenylbutazone, and antazoline.

TREATMENT

The aims of treatment are two: to restore the platelet count to normal and thus control the haemorrhagic state, and to repair anaemia, avoid trauma, and support the patient until cure has been effected. There are two methods by which the first aim may be achieved: administration of corticosteroid hormones and splenectomy.

Supportive treatment includes blood transfusion when haemorrhage is important, or prescription of iron when chronic blood loss has caused anaemia. Platelet transfusions are of little value for the donor platelets are so rapidly destroyed; occasionally they may raise the count for a short while and make splenectomy less hazardous in a fulminating case. The avoidance of trauma, surgical or incidental, is particularly important in the fulminating variety when sneezing, coughing, or straining may precipitate a cerebral haemorrhage.

Management depends upon the form the disease takes. In the acute variant commonly seen in children, spontaneous recovery is the rule, and thus treatment should be expectant. If the haemorrhagic state is anything more than trivial, corticosteroids should be given. In the adult, there is no point in exceeding 60 mg of prednisolone daily, and the dose should be reduced as the platelet count rises. An adequate dose in children is 4 to 5 mg per kilogramme body weight. In the great majority, the disease remits and the drug can be withdrawn; if after 6 months there has been no remission, splenectomy must be considered.

In the chronic type usually seen in the adult, remission is rare after 3 months have elapsed. Nevertheless, corticosteroids should always be given; in 60 percent, there is some improvement, but it is seldom maintained once the drug has been withdrawn.

Splenectomy was first suggested as a means of treating idiopathic thrombocytopenic purpura by Kaznelson in 1916, when he was still a medical student. The indications are three: first, in the chronic form when there has been no response to corticosteroids, when there has been a relapse on their withdrawal, or when they are for some reason contraindicated. These indications also apply when the disease has been of sudden onset but has passed into a chronic phase, and in all instances the assumption is made that the haemorrhagic state is causing sufficient disability to justify surgery. An occasional crop of petechiae on the legs is not an adequate reason for operation. The second indication is the acute fulminant type when control by corticosteroids proves impossible and there appears to be a threat to life. Third, splenectomy should be recommended in the fourth or fifth month of pregnancy if no complete remission can be obtained with corticosteroids. This is justified by the risk to the mother and the child.

In some 70 percent of cases, splenectomy is followed by a rise in the platelet count, which reaches a maximum about the tenth day, often far exceeding the upper limit of normal. Thereafter, it usually declines until it reaches the normal range. The results of splenectomy are more favourable in younger patients and in those in whom the onset has been acute. The majority of patients who have shown a response to corticosteroids respond also to splenectomy, but in 50 percent failing to improve with corticosteroids, splenectomy will be followed by remission.

At least 10 percent of patients in whom splenectomy has led to remission later relapse. This will usually occur within a few months, but occasional relapses continue for years after operation and thus the longer the follow-up, the higher the relapse rate. It is most unlikely that splenunculi overlooked at operation are the cause of relapse. Sometimes corticosteroids will prove effective in patients who have relapsed after operation, or in whom splenectomy has failed. It is in this situation too that the immunosuppressive drugs have been used. Reports of their efficacy are conflicting. Azathioprine is that most frequently prescribed. It is given in doses of 50 to 150 mg daily, and careful control by regular blood counts is essential.

Cyclophosphamide 150 to 200 mg daily and chlorambucil 5 to 10 mg daily have also been used, and the same precautions must be observed. It is doubtful whether any one of these drugs is more effective than any other.

REFERENCES

Ackroyd, J. F., Clin. Sci. 7:249, 1949.
Baldini, M., N. Engl. J. Med. 274:1245, 1301, 1360, 1966.
Cohen, P., Gardner, F. H., and Barnett, G. O., J. Clin. Invest. 264:1294, 1350, 1961.
Colombani, J., Seminars in Hematol. 3:74, 1966.
Denys, J., Cellule, 3:445 1887.

Duke, W. W., J.A.M.A. 55:1185, 1910.
Evans, R. S., and Duane, R. T., Blood 4:1196, 1949.
Harrington, W. J., Minnich, V., and Arimuro, G., J. Lab. Clin. Med. 38:1, 1951.
Harrington, W. J., Minnich, V., and Arimuro, G., Ann. Intern. Med. 38:433, 1953.
Heys, R. F., J. Obstet. Gynecol. Br. Commonwealth 73:205, 1966.
Karpatkin, S., and Siskind, G. W., Blood 33:795, 1969.
Kaznelson, P., Wien. Klin. Wschr. 29:1451, 1916.
Krauss, E., Keber Purpura Mang. Dissert, Heidelburg, 1883.
Najaen, Y., and Andaillon, N., Br. J. Haematol. 21: 153, 1971.
Robson, H. N., Quart. J. Med. (NS) 18:279, 1949.
Strangway, W. E., and Strangway, A. K., Arch. Intern. Med. 83:372, 1949.
Sussman, L. N., J.A.M.A. 202:259, 1967.
Werlhof, P. G., Opera omnia, Hannover, 1775.

D. HAEMOLYTIC ANAEMIA

SIR RONALD BODLEY SCOTT

When the mean life span of the erythrocytes is reduced to such an extent that the bone marrow is unable to maintain their normal level, the resulting anaemia is said to be haemolytic. Provided bone-marrow function is unimpaired, the enhanced rate of haemolysis stimulates erythropoiesis to a degree that may be sufficient to compensate for a moderate shortening of erythrocyte survival. This situation is described as a "compensated haemolytic state."

In this section, haemolytic anaemia is discussed from the standpoint of the therapeutic efficacy of splenectomy, and only certain chronic varieties for which it is the definitive treatment are considered in detail. The subject is exhaustively treated by Dacie (1960–1967).

GENERAL FEATURES OF HAEMOLYTIC ANEMIA

The features that distinguish haemolytic from other forms of anaemia are, first, those of an increased rate of blood destruction and, second, the cause of the particular haemolytic state. The first can be further subdivided into increased haemoglobin breakdown and the haemopoietic reaction.

Normal haemolysis is almost entirely an intracellular process. Effete erythrocytes are removed by reticuloendothelial phagocytes within which haemoglobin is set free and split into haem and globin moieties. Iron is removed from the haem and the resulting porphyrin broken down and returned to the plasma as bilirubin, where it is loosely attached to albumen. In the liver it is separated from the albumen, conjugated with glucuronic acid, and excreted in the bile. In the bowel, the bilirubin-glucuronide is reduced to stercobilinogen (urobilinogen), a proportion of which is absorbed and re-excreted by the liver, although a small quantity, not exceeding 4.0 mg daily, escapes in the urine. In health, the daily faecal excretion is usually 100 to 200 mg, with limits of 50 to 300 mg.

In chronic haemolytic anaemia, the disposal of haemoglobin breakdown products follows the normal route. Thus the level of unconjugated bilirubin in the serum, which gives an indirect van den Bergh's reaction, is usually above the normal upper limit of 1.0 mg per 100 ml, causing clinically recognisable jaundice. In this form, bilirubin cannot pass the renal filter, and none is found in the urine (acholuric jaundice). The quantity reaching the liver is increased and thus also the faecal stercobilinogen output, which may rise to 1,500 mg daily; increased absorption from the bowel results, and thus an increased urinary excretion often sufficient to darken the urine and to give positive Schlesinger and Ehrlich tests.

The second feature is the group of changes due to stimulation of the bone marrow by anaemia. There is extreme erythropoietic activity with proliferation of normoblasts and macronormoblasts. The depth of anaemia varies with the intensity of the haemolysis and the adequacy of the compensatory process; it is usually normochromic, but may be macrocytic. Reticulocytosis may exceed 50 percent, and the greater size of reticulocytes explains the macrocytosis. Normoblasts are often found in the peripheral blood when anaemia is severe, and particularly in children. With intense haemolysis, leucocytosis may occur, and in extreme examples a "leukaemoid" reaction.

The diagnosis of haemolytic anaemia is made in two stages. The first task is to establish the haemolytic nature of the anaemia, and the second to demonstrate the cause of the excessive haemolysis. The first depends upon finding the abnormalities already described: jaundice due to unconjugated hyperbilirubinaemia, acholuria with urobilinogenuria, anaemia, reticulocytosis and erythroblastic hyperplasia of the bone marrow. Estimations of faecal stercobilinogen excretion are seldom undertaken nowadays.

Ultimate proof is given by showing that the erythrocyte survival is reduced by following the rate at which autologous erythrocytes labelled with radioactive chromium (^{51}Cr) disappear from the circulation (Veall and Vetter, 1958). The normal half-life of the erythrocytes (^{51}Cr/T$\frac{1}{2}$) by this method is about 25 days. Surface-counting over the liver and spleen can give an indication of where the erythrocytes are being sequestrated and destroyed (Hughes Jones and Szur, 1957).

THE CAUSES OF HAEMOLYTIC ANAEMIA

The causes of a shortened erythrocyte life fall into two broad groups: those within the erythrocyte itself and those which are extracellular. The abnormalities of the erythrocyte that reduce its longevity and that concern us here are all congenital: they are hereditary spherocytosis, hereditary elliptocytosis, the hereditary types of enzymopathy, and the various types of haemoglobinopathy. Extracorpuscular causes are per contra all acquired. The list is extensive, but in only two does splenectomy play a part in management: they are acquired auto-immune haemolytic anaemia and hypersplenism, which has already been discussed.

THE SPLEEN IN HAEMOLYTIC ANAEMIA

The dictum that the spleen is the graveyard of the erythrocyte, but not the slaughterhouse, even if trite, is partially true. In health it probably plays an important part in removing effete erythrocytes from the circulation. The peculiar anatomical arrangement of its pulp constitutes a trap for erythrocytes misshapen by age or intrinsic disease, and its large concentration of phagocytes removes those irreparably damaged. It is thus a fine grade filter for aged and pathological cells, a function well-illustrated in hereditary spherocytosis where the spherocytes are sequestrated in the splenic pulp and undergo phagocytosis. Splenomegaly in this instance is due to reticuloendothelial hyperplasia in response to increased work load.

When anaemia with shortened erythrocyte life and splenomegaly are associated, other circulatory changes take place. There is often a considerable expansion of plasma volume, which contributes to the anaemia by haemodilution (Pryor, 1967; Blendis, Clarke, and Williams, 1969). Its degree is directly related to spleen size; it occurs most markedly in proliferative splenomegaly such as that of lymphoma and in the tropical types of splenomegaly; it is seldom seen with haemolytic anaemia due to intrinsic erythrocyte defect. Splenectomy is followed by a gradual fall in plasma volume.

There is, too, an increase in the size of the splenic erythrocyte pool. This is seen particularly when erythrocyte defect increases trapping. It is of importance because these cells, being excluded from the general circulation, are not functionally effective.

Finally, the spleen contains the largest localised aggregation of antibody-forming cells in the body, and is, therefore, an important source of antibody.

An indication of the importance of some of these various aspects of splenic function in the individual patient can be obtained by isotope studies (Jandl, Greenberg, Yonemoto, and Castle, 1956; Bowdler, 1969). Erythrocyte life and erythrocyte mass can be estimated with radioactive chromium. The importance of the spleen as a site of haemolysis can be determined by counts over its surface compared with those over the liver; the plasma volume can be measured by a technique using ^{131}I, labelled human albumen (Veall, Pearson, and Hanley, 1955).

Nightingale and his colleagues (Nightingale, Prankerd, Richards, and Thompson, 1972) regard splenectomy as indicated first, when the ^{51}Cr/T$\frac{1}{2}$ is less than 10 days, the splenic uptake shows a climbing curve, and counts over the spleen exceed those over the liver by a factor of two; and second, when there is anaemia with splenomegaly extending more than 4 cm below the ribs and a plasma volume 50 percent above the expected normal. The benefit to be anticipated from splenectomy is not related to the size of the erythrocyte pool. Specific indications are discussed later.

HEREDITARY SPHEROCYTOSIS

Hereditary spherocytosis, or familial acholuric jaundice, is the most common type of congenital haemolytic anaemia of those of European descent. It is rare in blacks. It is transmitted as a mendelian dominant and affects both sexes equally.

The syndrome depends upon an inherited intrinsic abnormality of the erythrocytes, which causes them to assume a spherical shape (spherocytes). The nature of this abnormality is unknown, but it is associated with increased permeability of the cell membrane to sodium and with loss of surface lipid (Jacob, 1968). The spherocytes are selectively trapped in the splenic pulp.

CLINICAL PICTURE

Symptoms of anaemia or jaundice or both commonly bring the patient under observation. The age at which this occurs varies, with the severity of the haemolytic state; it may be in infancy or it may be deferred until old age; frequently the finding of one case in a family leads to the discovery of many others.

The anaemia is seldom severe and the jaundice is usually mild. Splenomegaly of moderate degree is almost invariable. In many patients, the grade of anaemia remains curiously constant, but in some, crises occur in which the level of haemoglobin drops abruptly. These sometimes follow infection, but are often inexplicable; several members of a family may be affected at the same time. Some crises are due to a sudden increase in the intensity of haemolysis, others to a transient hypoplasia of the marrow (Dameshek and Bloom, 1948; Gasser, 1951).

At least 50 percent of patients develop gallstones, which may lead to cholecystitis, cholangitis, or biliary obstruction, when this element is added to the haemolytic jaundice. Biliary disease may be the presenting feature.

Ulceration of the lower third of the leg is a rare but well-authenticated complication. It heals rapidly after splenectomy.

THE BLOOD PICTURE

The features common to all types of chronic haemolytic anaemia are evident, but certain additional changes indicate the diagnosis. Many small, densely staining erythrocytes are to be seen. These are the characteristic spherocytes. Spherocytosis explains the increased osmotic fragility of the erythrocytes, which is further increased after incubation at 37°C for 24 hours. Spontaneous haemolysis after incubation is also increased. Erythrocyte life is much reduced; plasma volume is normal; splenic haemolysis and splenic pooling are both excessive.

To arrive at a *diagnosis*, the clinical and haematological features are required, and a family history of the disease must be available. When this last is lacking, it is usually possible to demonstrate characteristic changes in the blood of relatives, although in mild cases, an increase in "incubated fragility" may be the only abnormality.

TREATMENT

The definitive treatment for hereditary spherocytosis is splenectomy. It should be advised in all afflicted with the disease unless there is a completely asymptomatic and fully compensated haemolytic state, although even then there is an increased risk of developing gallstones. It should be forcibly urged upon those who have persistent anaemia with a haemoglobin level below 11.0 G per 100 ml or a history of aplastic crisis. It is probably advisable to wait until the patient has reached the age of 7 years; there is evidence that below this age children are unduly susceptible to serious infection after splenectomy (Ellis and Smith, 1966; Whitaker, 1969). It is likely that this point has been laboured and overriding indications are anaemia requiring transfusion, and failure to thrive.

Splenectomy abolishes hyperhaemolysis and cures the anaemia, but it does not affect the spherocytosis. The erythrocyte survival is not always restored to normal. Failure almost always indicates an incorrect diagnosis, although a few incontestable examples are recorded (Brain, Beilin, and Dacie, 1968). Exceptionally, a splenunculus has been overlooked, of which the existence and location can be established by surface-counting after administration of autologous ^{51}Cr labelled erythrocytes.

At operation the gallbladder should be removed if it contains stones.

HEREDITARY ELLIPTOCYTOSIS

Hereditary elliptocytosis is inherited as a mendelian dominant with equal sex incidence. In these patients, 25 to 50 percent of the cells are elliptical. In an occasional instance, there is splenomegaly and significant haemolytic anaemia. Diagnosis is based on the study of the blood film: the osmotic fragility is often slightly increased. Splenectomy cures the anaemia, but leaves the elliptocytosis unchanged (de Gruchy, Loder, and Hennessy, 1962).

HEREDITARY TYPES OF ENZYMOPATHY

Of recent years, a number of types of nonspherocytic congenital haemolytic anaemia have been shown to be due to deficiency of one or other of the many intraerythrocytic enzymes (Valentine, 1968). There are three main types: glucose-6-phosphate dehydrogenase (G-6-PD) deficiency, pyruvate kinase (PK) deficiency (Tanaka, Valentine, and Miwa, 1962; Keitt, 1966), and a much rarer miscellaneous group of defects. Only the second is of relevance in this chapter.

PK deficiency is transmitted as an autosomal recessive trait; heterozygotes are clinically and haematologically normal. It is most frequently seen in those of European stock and it affects both sexes equally.

Symptoms usually appear in childhood. There are the usual features of anaemia, jaundice, splenomegaly, and a liability to cholelithiasis. The blood picture is that of chronic haemolytic anaemia often with a uniform macrocytosis. Osmotic fragility of fresh erythrocytes is normal, but often increased after incubation. Autohaemolysis is increased, and this is not corrected by the addition of glucose. The antiglobulin (Coombs') and acid lysis (Ham) test results are negative, and haemoglobin electrophoresis results are normal. Confirmation is given by finding the erythrocyte PK activity reduced, usually to less than 40 percent of normal.

Blood transfusion may be sufficient to maintain a reasonable haemoglobin level, but splenectomy is indicated when the ^{51}Cr/T$\frac{1}{2}$ is less than 10 days and there is evidence of excessive splenic haemolysis. The operation is followed by an increase of erythrocyte survival and haematocrit, although neither is restored to normal; after operation there is also a lessening of transfusion requirements (Necheles, Finkel, Sheehan, and Allen, 1966).

HEREDITARY TYPES OF HAEMOGLOBINOPATHY

These consist of the thalassaemic syndromes and what de Gruchy (1970) has called qualitative haemoglobinopathy. In both the globin moiety of the haemoglobin molecule is abnormal, haemoglobin synthesis is impaired, and erythrocytes are less durable. In the thalassaemic syndromes, there is defective production of one or other of the two polypeptide chains, pairs of which go to make up globin. The only variant which concerns us here is β-thalassaemia where compensation for a defect of β-chain synthesis is by production of γ-chains of Hb-F and δ-chains of Hb-A$_2$. A full review can be found in the monographs by Weatherall (1965) and by Lehmann and Huntsman (1966).

The homozygous form of β-thalassaemia is usually fatal within the first year, but occasional patients reach adult life. The heterozygous forms vary in severity from a profound anaemia with massive splenomegaly to a virtually symptomless disorder with minimal reduction of haemoglobin.

The blood picture varies with the severity of the anaemia. Hypochromia, polychromasia, basophilic stippling, and reticulocytosis are the rule, with many target cells and sometimes normoblasts. Osmotic fragility is notably reduced. The serum bilirubin level is slightly raised: the serum iron content is usually above normal and the iron-binding capacity fully saturated. Proof is given by electrophoresis of the haemoglobin, which will show an increase of Hb-F in severe and of Hb-A$_2$ in mild cases. Erythrocyte survival is usually moderately reduced, but plasma volume is commonly raised and the erythrocyte pool increased.

Splenectomy does not affect the course of the disease but is valuable in patients whose transfusion requirements show progressive increase, and in those in whom massive splenomegaly is causing discomfort and retarding physical development (Smith, Erlandson, Stern, and Schulman, 1960).

AUTO-IMMUNE HAEMOLYTIC ANAEMIA

Auto-immune haemolytic anaemia is due to the formation by the patient of antibodies which react with antigens on the surface of his own erythrocytes. These antibodies fall into two broad groups, depending upon whether they associate with the antigen at body temperature, or only in the cold. The subject is reviewed by Dacie and Worlledge (1969), but the only variety relevant to this discussion is the chronic warm antibody type. This presents either as an idiopathic disorder, or as one secondary to some other disease of which the more common are lymphoma, chronic lymphatic leukaemia, and systemic lupus erythematosus.

In the idiopathic variety, the onset is gradual; all ages are affected and it occurs rather more often in women than in men. The picture is of a chronic haemolytic state, but the patient is frequently more ill than in hereditary spherocytosis with a comparable degree of anaemia. Splenomegaly is usual. The distinction between idiopathic and secondary types is usually easy, but is sometimes only revealed by histological study of the excised spleen.

The blood shows the usual features of haemolytic anaemia, and the presence of antibody can be demonstrated by the antiglobulin (Coombs') test. Indeed, the diagnosis cannot be sustained if this test is negative.

The majority of patients respond well to treatment with corticosteroids. Doses of 60 to 80 mg of prednisolone daily are often required to establish control. Prognosis is uncertain and the mortality rate is considerable, probably 10 to 15 percent. A proportion recover after 2 or 3 years of treatment, but in most, the haemolytic process continues for many years. In one series, recovery was reported in 27 percent. Secondary cases often respond well to corticosteroids, but the ultimate prognosis depends upon the causative disease.

Splenectomy is indicated when anaemia

cannot be controlled by a daily dose of 60 mg of prednisolone, when there is some strong contraindication to corticosteroid treatment, or when it has given rise to serious complications. In this situation, some favour the use of immunosuppressive drugs (Schwartz and Dameshek, 1962; Hitzig and Massimo, 1966), but at present, majority opinion is on the side of splenectomy as the second line of defense.

It is difficult to assess the likelihood of a good response to splenectomy. It is likely that phagocytosis by reticuloendothelial cells is a major cause of haemolysis in this disease, and in this connection the liver and bone marrow are even more important than the spleen (Jandl, 1965). Even good evidence of splenic sequestration of erythrocytes is not an infallible guide. Operation is more likely to be successful when the cells are coated with incomplete IgG antibody than when they carry complement-fixing IgM. The possible benefits of splenectomy, however, should not be denied to the patient because the laboratory portents are unfavourable, if the clinical indications are present. The removal of such a large agglomeration of antibody-producing cells may be an important effect of splenectomy.

Remission is claimed in 50 percent of idiopathic and in 30 percent of secondary cases.

REFERENCES

Blendis, L. M., Clarke, M. B., and Williams, R., Lancet 1:795, 1969.

Bowdler, A. J., Br. J. Haemat. 16:557, 1969.

Brain, M. C., Beilin, L. J., and Dacie, J. V., Br. J. Haemat. 15:373, 1968.

Dacie, J. V., The Haemolytic Anaemias, Parts I to IV, 2d ed., London, 1960–67.

Dacie, J. V., and Worlledge, S. M., Progress in Hemat. 6:82, 1969.

Dameshek, W., and Bloom, M. L., Blood 3:1381, 1948.

de Gruchy, G. C., Clinical Haematology in Medical Practice, 3d ed., Oxford, 1970.

de Gruchy, W., Loder, P. D., and Hennessy, I. V., Br. J. Haemat. 8:168, 1962.

Ellis, E. F., and Smith, R. T., Pediatrics 37:111, 1966.

Gasser, C., Sang 21:237, 1950.

Hitzig, W. H., and Massimo, L., Blood 28:840, 1966.

Hughes Jones, N. C., and Szur, L., Br. J. Haemat. 3:320, 1957.

Jacob, H., Br. J. Haemat. 14:99, 1968.

Jandl, J. H., Series Haemat. 9:35, 1965.

Jandl, J. H., Greenberg, M. S., Yonemoto, R. H., and Castle, W. B., J. Clin. Invest. 35:842, 1956.

Keitt, A. S., Am. J. Med. 41:762, 1966.

Lehmann, H., and Huntsman, R. G., Man's Haemoglobins, Amsterdam, North-Holland, 1966.

Necheles, T. F., Finkel, H. E., Sheehan, R. G., and Allen, D. M., Arch. Intern. Med. 118:75, 1966.

Nightingale, D., Prankerd, T. A. J., Richards, J. D. M., and Thompson, D., Quart. J. Med. (NS) 41:261, 1972.

Pryor, D. S., Br. Med. J. 3:825, 1967.

Schwartz, R., and Dameshek, W., Blood 19:483, 1962.

Smith, C. H., Erlandson, M. E., Stern, G., and Schulman, I., Blood 15:197, 1960.

Tanaka, K. R., Valentine, W. N., and Miwa, S., Br. J. Haemat. 8:168, 1962.

Valentine, W. H., Calif. Med. 108:280, 1968.

Veall, N., Pearson, J. D., and Hanley, T., Br. J. Radiol. 28:633, 1955.

Veall, N., and Vetter, H., Radioisotope Techniques in Clinical Research and Diagnosis, London, 1958.

Weatherall, D. J., The Thalassaemia Syndromes, Oxford, 1965.

Whitaker, A. N., Med. J. Austral. 1:1213, 1969.

33

SPONTANEOUS AND TRAUMATIC RUPTURE OF THE SPLEEN

RODNEY MAINGOT

Orloff and Peskin,[15] in an authoritative and learned collective review entitled Spontaneous Rupture of the Normal Spleen—a Surgical Enigma, state:

Several excellent reports have appeared in recent years describing the experiences at various hospitals with traumatic rupture of the normal spleen, a condition which has become particularly common in this age when emphasis is placed on speed in transportation. Similarly, cases of traumatic and spontaneous rupture of the pathologic spleen involved by a great variety of diseases are not infrequently encountered, especially in the tropics. However, rupture of the spleen in the absence of either trauma or disease, so-called spontaneous rupture, is a rare occurrence.

Since Atkinson's first description in 1874 [*Br. Med. J.* 2:403, 1874], reports of cases of spontaneous rupture of the *normal spleen* have appeared periodically. As in Atkinson's case, the diagnosis frequently has been erroneous or open to serious question. As a result, one author states, "There is no such clinical entity as spontaneous rupture of the normal spleen," and another writes, "Careful enough questioning will always reveal a story of injury." Nevertheless, analysis of all of the reports reveals a small number of cases which, when subjected to careful scrutiny, defy any conclusion other than that they represent instances of spontaneous rupture of the normal spleen.

Parsons and Thompson [16] also believe that many of these ruptures are caused by relatively minor injuries. It does seem probable that most of these cases of spontaneous rupture of a normal spleen fit into the category of delayed rupture, where the injury was so trivial or the latent period so long that the responsible accident was forgotten. Nevertheless, an analysis of all the reports reveals a small number (28 cases) which, when subjected to careful scrutiny, defies any conclusion other than that they represent instances of spontaneous rupture of the normal spleen.

So excellent an account is given by Orloff and Peskin of this condition that I cannot do better than quote their conclusions in full:

Spontaneous rupture of the normal spleen is a condition of unknown etiology which does not show a predilection for any age group and occurs more frequently in males than in females. There is no evidence that forgotten or unrecognized trauma plays a role in the etiology, although such is possible. According to our criteria, which include failure to obtain a history of trauma upon thorough questioning and evidence that the spleen and its environs were normal prior to rupture, only 28 cases of this condition have been reported in the English literature, including a case of our own. Analysis of these cases reveals that both the pathologic and clinical features of spontaneous rupture of the normal spleen are identical to those of traumatic splenic rupture. Upper abdominal pain, usually in the left hypochondrium, pain in the left shoulder, nausea, vomiting, dizziness, and syncope are the characteristic symptoms. The physical findings include abdominal tenderness and rigidity, either in the left hypochondrium or throughout the abdomen, tachycardia, and in advanced cases frank shock. Anemia and leucocytosis are usually associated features, and abdominal roentgenography and needle paracentesis are ancillary studies which may be of considerable aid in the diagnosis. The treatment of this disorder is splenectomy. The mortality rate in the reported cases was low, although it probably did not represent the true mortality rate because of the manner in which the cases were selected.

Spontaneous rupture of the normal spleen represents a problem in diagnosis rather than in therapy. Although the clinical features clearly indicate the true nature of this disorder, the diagnosis usually fails to receive consideration because of the absence of a history of injury. In all but one of the cases on record some other disease was believed to be responsible for the symptoms and signs, most commonly perforated peptic ulcer. As a result, valuable time was often wasted in observation of the patient, and once operation was undertaken the initial abdominal incision was usually one through which splenectomy was difficult or impossible. It is our belief that in the majority of instances the surgeon who encounters a case of spontaneous rupture of the normal spleen will make the correct diagnosis if he is familiar with this disorder.

For a further study of this subject the following contributions should be consulted: Durban and Langley,[4] Johnson,[9] Fultz and Altmeier,[6] and Shirkey et al.[18]

SPONTANEOUS RUPTURE OF A PATHOLOGICAL SPLEEN

This condition is not often seen in temperate climates, but it is by no means infrequent in subtropical and tropical countries.

Spontaneous rupture of the pathological spleen may occur in cases of malaria, kala-azar, Cooley's anaemia, typhoid fever, typhus, acute general infections, infectious mononucleosis,[19] during pregnancy,[2, 7, 12] parturition and the puerperium, during defaecation,[3] and in patients with splenomegaly from any cause.[8]

In all these conditions, the spontaneous rupture is probably dependent upon some slight unnoticed trauma to the softened and congested spleen. Again, the vascular endothelium of the spleen may be damaged by the circulating toxins that are present in some of these conditions. These toxins cause increased permeability and softening of the smaller radicles of the splenic blood vessels which disrupt when the intrasplenic pressure is unduly raised from any cause, leading to extravasation of the blood under the capsule of the organ. This subcapsular haematoma will, by the increase of tension, produce a pressure necrosis and secondary softening of the splenic pulp, and fresh blood vessels will eventually be eroded until bleeding of such a severe nature is produced that the capsule yields and bursts and the peritoneal cavity becomes flooded with blood.

A correct preoperative diagnosis is often difficult to make in cases of spontaneous rupture of a pathological spleen. More often than not, an exploratory operation is advised on account of an unexplained intraperitoneal haemorrhage, the cause of which is not revealed until the abdomen has been opened.

The operation to be advised in all cases is splenectomy.

TRAUMATIC RUPTURE OF THE SPLEEN FROM NONPENETRATING INJURIES

It is generally thought that in civilian practice the incidence of blunt trauma to the spleen far exceeds that of penetrating injury.

However, Shirkey and his colleagues from Houston, Texas,[18] in analysing 189 consecutive cases of patients with injury to the spleen, found that 70 percent of the patients had received their injuries as a result of a *penetrating wound.*

Even though a greater number of associated intra-abdominal organ injuries were seen after penetrating wounds, the overall mortality rate was lower than that after injuries sustained as a result of blunt trauma— 18 to 30 percent, respectively.

Shotgun wounds were associated with the highest mortality rate—50 percent.

Blunt trauma, resulting from an automobile accident, a fall, or blows to the abdomen, was the mechanism in 30 percent of the cases.

Automobile accidents were responsible for the greatest number of injuries. This mechanism of injury was responsible for 42 percent of all accidental deaths in the United States in 1961. Splenic injury as a result of blunt trauma resulted in a high mortality rate related to the greater frequency of overall associated injuries, such as trauma to the head and chest.

The mortality rate of injury to the spleen *alone* is about 9 percent, rising to 65 percent when five or more organs are injured.

They sum up as follows:

In 189 consecutive patients with splenic injuries sustained during the seventeen years from 1946 through 1962, there were forty-two deaths, an overall mortality of 22 percent, comparing favorably with other reported series. Injury to the spleen alone was associated with a mortality rate of 9 percent, while simple stab wounds were associated with a mortality rate of only 5 percent. No deaths occurred in patients with delayed rupture. The mortality rate for the total group whose injury was a result of blunt trauma was 30 percent compared with 18 percent for the group with penetrating injuries. This difference in mortality rates was due primarily to the large number of associated injuries in patients with blunt trauma. Twenty-four percent of the deaths occurred pre-operatively, the majority as a result of intra-cranial injury from blunt trauma. Excluding the ten deaths occurring preoperatively, the operative mortality rate for the entire series would be 18 percent.

Welch and Giddings,[22] on the other hand, found 86 percent of nonpenetrating and 14 percent of penetrating injuries of the spleen in civilian practice. Their incidence of splenic injury was 19 percent of all abdominal injuries.

Pontius et al.[17] found an incidence of 36 percent of ruptured spleens in a series of 42 closed abdominal injuries. Parsons and Thompson [16] reported that 22 percent of 119

patients with nonpenetrating abdominal injuries had injury to the spleen. The most frequently associated injury of other organs is that of the *left kidney* (about 15 percent). Fracture of the left lower ribs is also a frequent concomitant finding—about 8 percent. With penetrating wounds of the abdomen, the jejuno-ileum and the liver are the organs most commonly injured; the stomach, kidney, and spleen are next in frequency, although only about one-third as common (Fig. 1).

One hundred cases of traumatic rupture of the spleen among the 308 splenectomies performed over 8 years are reported by State, Getzen, and Laning,[20] of the Naval Hospital, San Diego. Among 22 patients *under* the age of 16, falls caused 9 of the splenic injuries,

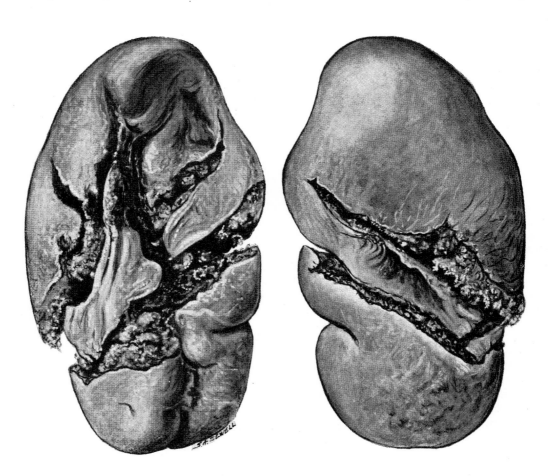

FIG. 1. Rupture of the spleen caused by blunt trauma. (Courtesy of the Hunterian Museum, Royal College of Surgeons.)

automobile accidents 8, and other blunt trauma 5. Among 78 patients *over* 16, automobiles caused 37 of the injuries, fights 19, falls 9, contact sports 2, other blunt trauma 6, and penetrating trauma 5.

The adult male between the ages of 20 and 30 is most commonly predisposed to this injury. The ratio of male to female is about 3 to 1.

SIGNS AND SYMPTOMS

The clinical picture is that of intra-abdominal haemorrhage and shock, with signs of diffuse or localised peritonitis associated with facial pallor. In some instances, an ill-defined enlarging mass may be palpated in the left flank. Pain referred to the left shoulder region (Kehr's sign) is present in about 30 to 40 percent of these cases. O'Connell [13] suggested that before announcing that Kehr's sign is negative in suspicious cases, and as a method of diagnosis, the patient should be asked to lie down flat, with the foot of the bed raised on blocks. If there is free blood in the abdominal cavity, the patient will complain of shoulder tip pain within a few minutes.

When admitted to hospital it will be found that some 70 percent of the patients are suffering from mild to severe hypovolaemic shock. During the first 6 hours or so following injury to the spleen, *anaemia* is not a notable feature, owing to its masking by haemoconcentration, and leucocytosis is an inconstant finding. Serial blood counts are unreliable, and this especially relates to haematocrit readings during the first 24 hours following trauma.

Mansfield [10] and Meschan [11] consider the following *radiological signs* to be of material help in localising the injured organ:

1. Increase in density of the left upper quadrant of the abdomen.
2. Elevation of the left cupola of the diaphragm with diminished movement.
3. Downward displacement of the gastric bubble and of the splenic flexure of the colon.
4. Serration of the greater curvature of the stomach.
5. Reflex gastric dilatation.

Leon Love (1968) states:

We have evaluated a number of suspected splenic injuries with *arteriography*. In all 17 cases of rupture which were treated surgically we made the correct preoperative diagnosis. A break in the margin of the spleen outline can indicate the site of a fracture, and intrasplenic "shadows" are suggestive of haematomas.

Fracture of a rib or ribs is, of course, a significant finding, but it may on occasion be misleading.

Peritoneal tapping to determine the presence of free blood in the abdominal cavity has proved of value in certain cases, as has *intravenous pyelography* in cases of possible renal damage.

OPERATIVE MORTALITY AND POSTOPERATIVE COMPLICATIONS

The operative mortality rate of splenectomy for rupture of the spleen alone due to nonpenetrating injury varies from 0 to 20 percent. Thus, Estes [5] reported 12 cases without fatality, Mansfield [10] 16 cases with no deaths, Parsons and Thompson [16] 23 cases with no deaths, and Larghero and Giuria (1951) 18 cases with 1 death (5 percent).

In Shirkey's series the overall mortality rate was 22 percent, whereas the mortality rate for isolated splenic injuries was only 9 percent. *Mortality was directly proportional to the number of associated injuries.* Stivelman et al. [21] had an overall mortality rate of 22 percent for laceration of the spleen due to nonpenetrating trauma. This figure included 13 patients who died without surgery.

The mortality rate is, of course, greatly increased when splenic rupture is associated with injuries to other organs such as the kidney, the liver, the fixed duodenojejunal flexure, the lung, or the head, or with fractures. Contusion of the left kidney does not appreciably affect the morbidity or mortality rates, but when the liver or small gut is concomitantly involved, the death rate rises sharply and is at least doubled.

The following complications frequently follow splenectomy for splenic rupture:

1. Atelectasis and pneumonitis.
2. Infection of the wound: dehiscence and/or eventration.

3. Thrombophlebitis.
4. Infection below the left cupola of the diaphragm. Subphrenic abscess (see Chap. 67).
5. Incisional hernia.

Splenosis is a possible, but rare, late complication, and has been discussed in Chapter 31.

TREATMENT

Preoperative treatment consists of blood transfusion to replace blood lost, and other measures directed to combating shock. Shock, even when proving stubborn to efficient treatment, should not—and does not—constitute a contraindication to splenectomy. Nearly 50 percent of these patients have multiple injuries which mask the abdominal injury and thus lead to delay in diagnosis.

As soon as the condition is suspected or recognised, laparotomy should be carried out. As there is a possibility of other intra-abdominal injuries, it is best to open the abdomen through a left paramedian epigastric incision which can be extended downward if desired.

The ruptured spleen will often be found to be mobile and can usually be drawn easily through the wound. If the spleen is fixed by adhesions or has a short pedicle, it should be mobilised by division of the gastrosplenic and lienorenal ligaments. The spleen should be delivered through the wound, the vascular pedicles being controlled with the fingers, after which the splenic blood vessels are secured and tied and the spleen is cut adrift.[14] Any blood clots which are present in the peritoneal cavity should be removed, and any free blood aspirated with a sucker. In most cases, splenectomy should be performed by the *posterior approach* to the splenic pedicle, as is well illustrated in Figure 2.

A rapid search should always be made for other injuries to such organs as the liver, the left kidney, the small intestine, the pancreas, and so forth.

The bared splenic bed which remains after splenectomy should be cloaked with omentum to prevent coils of small gut from forming any attachment there.

Where speed is essential, the abdominal incision should be closed with a series of figure-of-eight sutures of wire, but as a rule the

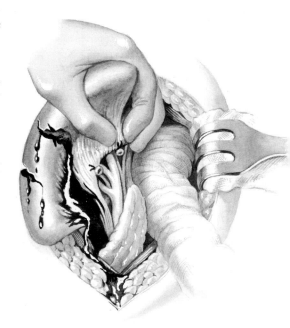

FIG. 2. Splenectomy for rupture of the spleen. The recommended posterior approach to the blood vessels in the splenic pedicle is depicted.

routine methods of closure are employed.

Drainage is usually unnecessary, except where subdiaphragmatic oozing is persistent or a hollow viscus or the pancreas has been damaged in the accident and has required some type of repair.

DELAYED RUPTURE OF THE SPLEEN

In delayed rupture of the spleen, acute symptoms associated with internal haemorrhage (collapse and shock, pallor, abdominal rigidity, etc.) do not occur until an arbitrarily selected period of 48 hours has elapsed since the time of injury.

In these cases, then, the patient will have sustained an injury to the trunk, this being followed by the usual signs of a ruptured spleen—shock, recovery from shock, and then a latent period of apparent well-being. Following this latent period, which may last from 48 hours to 21 days (or even longer), there is a dramatic return of the signs and symptoms of severe intra-abdominal haemorrhage. According to Harkins and Zabinski, the latent period is less than 7 days in 50 percent of the cases, and less than 25 days in a further 25 percent of cases. Attenborough [1] reported 2 cases of delayed splenic rupture in which the latent periods were 22 and 26 days, respectively. Zabinski reviewed 171 cases of delayed rupture and found them to constitute an incidence of 14 percent of all splenic ruptures. McIndoe, in 1932, was the first to suggest that the formation and later rupture of a subcapsular splenic haematoma accounted for many of these cases.

The rupture may in some instances be a result of an exacerbation of bleeding which was initially controlled by tamponade.

McIndoe classified these injuries as follows:

1. Minor capsular rupture or parenchymal laceration.
2. Subcapsular haematoma.
3. Capsular haemorrhage with perisplenic haematoma.

Operative Mortality

The operative mortality rate of delayed splenic rupture does not exceed 3 percent. The writer has operated on 5 patients without a postoperative death.

Splenectomy is, of course, the treatment in all cases.

PENETRATING INJURIES OF THE SPLEEN

As would be expected, in war penetrating wounds predominate, and the abdominal organs most commonly injured, in order of frequency, are: liver, colon, small gut, stomach, rectum, kidney, bladder, spleen, and pancreas.

Penetrating wounds which involve the spleen may be abdominal or abdominothoracic. The injuries are commonly multiple and extensive. The symptoms are those of rapidly progressive shock; the signs are those of peritonitis. The operative mortality rate is high, about 30 percent.

The treatment is splenectomy combined with control of haemorrhage from any other source within the abdomen and dealing *se-*

cundum artem with any other injured organ or organs.

ACCIDENTAL INJURIES TO THE SPLEEN DURING ABDOMINAL OPERATIONS (IATROGENIC INJURIES)

Accidental splenic trauma has occurred most frequently during the isolation, clamping, and ligation of the vasa brevia; the gastrosplenic omentum may be dragged upon or retracted too firmly during partial gastrectomy, with the result that the splenic capsule tears and bleeding ensues.

Again, when the spleen is anchored to its bed by adhesions, traction on the stomach—or even on the greater omentum—may produce posterior tears of the splenic capsule which are not readily seen. I have witnessed cases in which the spleen was severely lacerated by the firm outward pull of large abdominal retractors.

The spleen may be accidentally torn during the course of left colectomy for carcinoma or diverticulitis, adrenalectomy, and repair of a diaphragmatic hernia.

There are a number of recorded cases of severe haemorrhage from the splenic pulp following percutaneous splenoportal venography.

Splenectomy is the only means of arresting haemorrhage from accidental trauma of the organ. Darning the injured site with catgut, the use of omental plugs and grafts, and tamponade are unreliable methods of dealing with the situation.

References

1. Attenborough, Br. Med. J. 1:380, 1953.
2. Barnett, J. Obstet. Gynaecol. Br. Emp. 59:795, 1952.
3. Druitt, Lancet 2:662, 1947.
4. Durban and Langley, Br. Med. J. 1:183, 1944.
5. Estes, Jr. Bull. Am. Coll. Surg. 39:11, 1954.
6. Fultz and Altmeier, Surgery 33:414, 1955.
7. Gorman and Rowe, Am. J. Obstet. 62:1361, 1951.
8. Harwell Wilson, Surg. Clin. North Am. 46:1311, 1964.
9. Johnson, Aust. New Zeal. J. Surg. 24:114, 1954.
10. Mansfield, Am. J. Surg. 89:759, 1953.
11. Meschan, Roentgen Signs in Clinical Diagnosis, W. B. Saunders Company, 1956.
12. Moore, West. J. Surg. 64:306, 1956.
13. O'Connell, Br. Med. J. 2:1404, 1951.

14. Olsen, Surg. Gynecol. Obstet. 123:351, 1966.
15. Orloff and Peskin, Int. Abst. Surg. 106:1, 1958.
16. Parsons and Thompson, Ann. Surg. 147:214, 1958.
17. Pontius et al., Arch. Surg. 72:800, 1956.
18. Shirkey et al., Am. J. Surg. 108:630, 1964.
19. Smith and Custer, Blood 1:317, 1946.
20. State, Getzen, and Laning, Arch. Surg. 99:498, 1969.
21. Stivelman et al., Am. J. Surg. 106:888, 1963.
22. Welch and Giddings, Am. J. Surg. 79:252, 1950.

Pancreas

34

A. ANOMALIES OF THE PANCREAS AND ITS DUCTS

RODNEY MAINGOT

The pancreas originates from a ventral and a dorsal bud which lie in relation to that portion of the primitive alimentary canal that will later form the duodenum. The ventral bud is bifid and, as the result of a rotation of the primitive gut, comes to lie behind the dorsal bud and ultimately to coalesce with it. The dorsal bud gives rise to the major portion of the gland, i.e., the tail, body, neck, and ventral part of the head. The left half of the ventral bud is thought by most authorities to atrophy and disappear, while the right half produces the rest of the head and the uncinate process.

No account here will be given of the embryology or physiology of the pancreas, as all details relating to these subjects are described in current textbooks. In Figures 1 and 2, however, some of the more important anatomical relations of the pancreas and of its arterial supply and venous drainage are clearly illustrated.

I am indebted to Dr. William Silen [16] and to W. B. Saunders Company for allowing me to reproduce Figure 2 in this chapter. One thing that can be said of the arterial supply and venous drainage of the pancreas is that it is *remarkably constant.*

This chapter is concerned with pancreatic anomalies: (1) *pancreas divisum* and bifid tail of the pancreas; (2) annular pancreas; (3) heterotopic (aberrant or accessory) pancreatic tumours; and (4) anomalies of the pancreatic ducts. Chapter 35 deals with *pancreatic injuries* and the consequences and treatment of such injuries.

PANCREAS DIVISUM AND BIFID TAIL OF THE PANCREAS

Pancreas divisum takes place when the vertical and dorsal buds fail to coalesce. Each portion functions normally and independently and has its own separate ductal system. This anomaly is commonly confused with an accessory pancreas. *Bifid tail* denotes partial division of the tail of the gland. When scanning the pancreas becomes more popular, it seems obvious that these anomalies will be discovered more frequently.

ANNULAR PANCREAS

In the condition known as annular pancreas, an interesting but rare anomaly of the pancreas, a band or a ring of pancreatic tissue continuous with the head of the gland completely or almost completely surrounds the second part of the duodenum. Originally described by Tiedmann in 1818, it was Ecker [4] who first suggested the name *annular pancreas.* Vidal (1905), recognising the condition during an exploratory operation for "duodenal atresia," performed the first successful operation for this condition, gastrojejunostomy on a 3-day-old girl. Whelan and Hamilton [22] stated that from 1905 to 1949, 26 additional patients were operated upon, and that from 1950 through 1955, 67 further

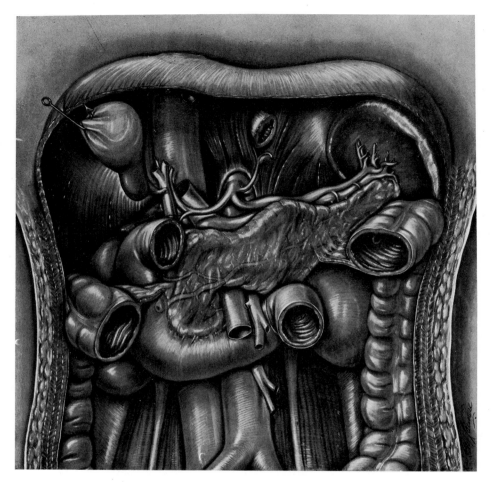

FIG. 1.   Some of the more important anatomical relations of the pancreas.

cases, including 3 of their own, were recorded, bringing the total number of patients operated upon to 93. Boothroyd[3] stated that there have been about 100 patients who have now been subjected to operation, and that 50 percent of these were during the last 15 years or so. Most of the early reports dealt with autopsy findings, but since Lehman's classic paper,[9] several cases have been correctly diagnosed before operation.

Cases of interest have been recorded by Bickford and Williamson,[2] Wakeley,[20] MacPhee,[10] Swynnerton and Tanner,[18] and Mast et al.[12] One hundred and one reported cases of patients requiring operation were reviewed by Reemtsma.[15] In his series, males were affected more frequently than females. Thirty-one of his patients developed symptoms before the age of 1 year, and a second peak was found to occur in the fourth decade; in 47 patients the condition was recognized between the ages of 20 and 50 years.

In children, in 70 percent of the cases there are other anomalies, such as duodenal atresia, malrotation of the intestine, congenital heart disease, and mongolism, while associated anomalies occur in 14 percent of adults.

About 70 percent of the patients are males. Sir Cecil Wakeley[20] considered that the most likely explanation of this abnormality is a failure of the ventral anlage of the pancreas

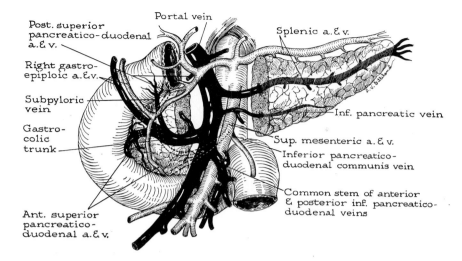

FIG. 2. Arterial supply and venous drainage of the pancreas. Note particularly the anatomical importance of the gastrocolic venous trunk in defining the interior portion of the neck. (Courtesy of Dr. William Silen and W. B. Saunders Company, Philadelphia.[16])

to rotate with the duodenum. As the outlet of the duct rotates to the right and posteriorly, a band of pancreatic tissue is left encircling the anterior portion of the second part of the duodenum.

Pathology

The annulus is usually healthy pancreatic tissue, and frequently contains a cen-

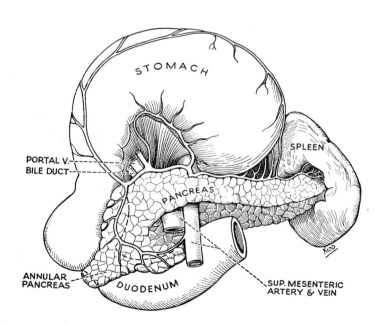

FIG. 3. Annular pancreas. (Courtesy of Mr. John Wakeley.)

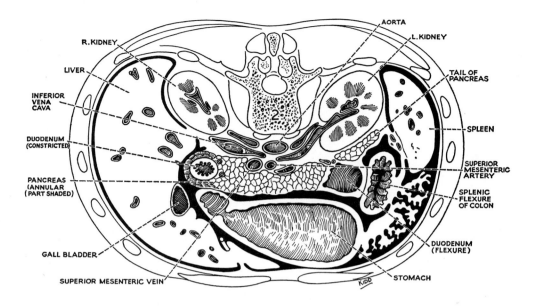

FIG. 4.   Annular pancreas. (Courtesy of Mr. John Wakeley.)

tral duct opening into the posterior aspect of the main pancreatic duct or even into the ampulla of Vater. In a number of cases, chronic pancreatitis has been reported in the annulus in adults. Underlying atresia or stenosis of the second portion of the duodenum accounts for some of the failures which were reported to follow excision of the ring of pancreatic tissue. Distention and hypertrophy of the duodenal wall and stomach proximal to the blockage is often striking, and this seldom diminishes to any marked extent even after successful surgical procedures.

Complications

These include the following:

1. *Duodenal obstruction.* The obstruction varies in degree, being complete or almost complete in infants, and more chronic and less marked in adults.[22]
2. *Peptic ulceration of the stomach or duodenum.* The prolonged stasis of ingested food and acid gastric chyme in the first portion of the duodenum and antrum predisposes this group of patients to peptic ulceration. According to Whelan and Hamilton, this complication arose in 18 of 56 reported cases (32 percent).
3. *Acute or chronic pancreatitis.* This complication was observed in 16 percent of adult patients with annular pancreas.
4. *Secondary involvement of the biliary tree with obstructive jaundice.* Three cases of obstructive jaundice have been reported by the following authors: Vasconcelos et al.,[19] Anderson and Wapshaw,[1] and Pincus in Bockus,[13] who wrote: *"Jaundice may be the most obvious clinical feature in a few patients, usually in infants in whom the common duct is involved in the annular pancreas."*

Diagnosis

It should be noted that many individuals with annular pancreas may live to old age without ever having any symptoms. Incidental annular pancreas has been observed in postmortem material on many occasions.

There are two *clinical types:* acute duodenal obstruction and chronic duodenal obstruction.

Acute duodenal obstruction is the common

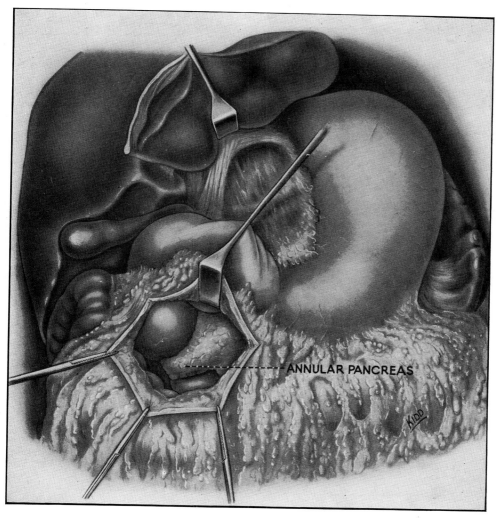

ANNULAR PANCREAS

KIDD

FIG. 5. Exposure of the annular pancreas. (Courtesy of Mr. John Wakeley.)

type in *infants,* and frequently demands an emergency operation such as duodenoduodenostomy (see Fig. 6).

The anomaly is characterised by feeding problems from birth, jaundice, severe bouts of vomiting, dehydration, alkalosis, and rapid weight loss. Abdominal distention is absent, owing to spontaneous decompression of the stomach by vomiting. These infants are gravely ill and require correction of fluid and electrolyte imbalances before an emergency operation.

On *barium-meal x-ray examination,* the stomach and first portion of the duodenum are usually markedly dilated, and the "double-bubble-of-gas" sign of Kiesewetter and Koop [7] may be present. The double bubble of gas in the duodenal bulb and in the stomach resembles a transparent hourglass.

In the second type, observed in *adults,* the signs and symptoms are those of chronic low-grade duodenal obstruction, which include epigastric pain, gastric flatulence, intermittent vomiting, and a sensation of fullness after meals. Weight loss is often observed, and pancreatitis and peptic ulceration are common sequelae. Haemorrhage from a chronic peptic ulcer has been described in many of the recorded cases as the presenting symptom.

Gonzalez Ayala, of Mexico, was among the first to describe cases of *obstruction of the*

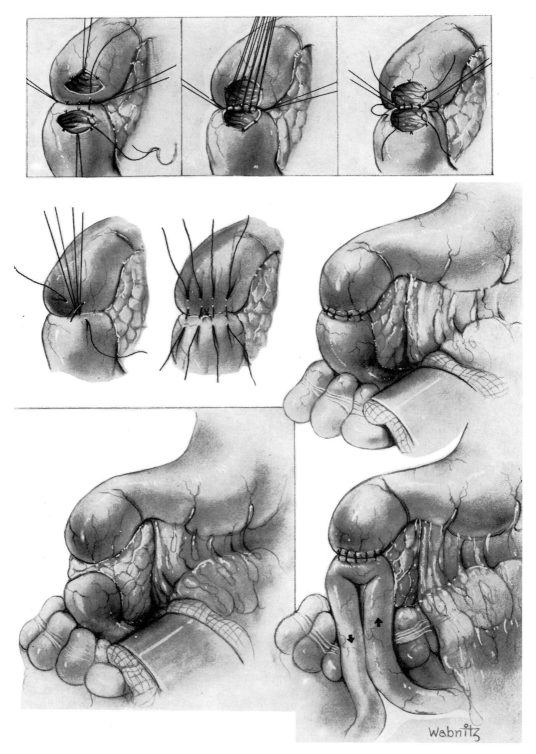

FIG. 6.   Annular pancreas, showing the operations of duodenoduodenostomy and duodenojejunostomy. When loop-duodenojejunostomy is performed, it is advisable to complete the operation by carrying out a short-circuiting side-to-side jejunojejunostomy. (From Madden, *Atlas of
Technics in Surgery*, 2d ed., Courtesy of Appleton-Century-Crofts, New York, 1964.)

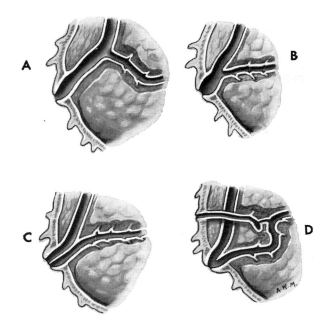

FIG. 7. Various ways in which the common bile duct and pancreatic duct open into duodenum. (A) Pancreatic duct opening into common bile duct considerable distance from duodenal opening. (B) Pancreatic duct opening into the upper part of the papilla of Vater. (C) Common bile duct and pancreatic duct opening into the duodenum by two separate openings. (D) Normal condition of the papilla of Vater. The accessory pancreatic duct or the duct of Santorini, can be seen opening high up in the duodenum, and its communication with the main pancreatic duct can also be seen. (Courtesy of Sir Cecil Wakeley.)

choledochus associated with jaundice caused by repeated bouts of subacute or chronic pancreatitis involving the annulus.

The diagnosis of the lesion in the adult form, or second type, is dependent upon barium-meal x-ray studies. Here the usual findings consist of a dilated first portion of the duodenum (with or without gastric distention) and a narrowed second portion of the bowel. K. W. Warren,[21] a shrewd diagnostician, has pointed out that the duodenal bulb may not be distended if it is the site of contraction secondary to peptic ulceration.

Differential Diagnosis

1. *In infants:* hypertrophic pyloric stenosis; duodenal atresia or stenosis; and congenital bands, e.g., malrotation of the gut.
2. *In adults:* duodenal diverticula; aberrant pancreas; tumours and ulcers of the duodenum, e.g., postbulbar ulcer; arteriomesenteric ileus; and pericholecystitis.

Operative Treatment

Obstruction of the duodenum sufficient to produce symptoms can be remedied only by operation. This may take the form of (1) division or partial resection of the annalus; (2) some form of bypass operation, such as duodenojejunostomy or duodenoduodenostomy; or (3) partial gastrectomy followed by the Billroth II procedure (in the presence of chronic peptic ulceration).

If the annulus is thin, avascular, and easily removable, resection may be performed, but this operation is seldom feasible or advisable. If the ring is thickened as the result of acute or chronic pancreatitis or in any way difficult to remove, a bypass operation such as side-to-side duodenoduodenostomy or antecolic or retrocolic duodenojejunostomy combined with entero-anastomosis should be carried out (see Fig. 6).

When massive enlargement of the annulus is present, as it is in the infantile cases, duodenoduodenostomy should *always* be performed.

When obstructive jaundice is present, I would advise duodenoduodenostomy combined with exploration of the common bile duct, dilatation of the ampulla of Vater, and T tube choledochostomy.

The danger in division or partial resection of the ring of pancreatic tissue lies in the possible early development of acute pancreatitis, as well as in the formation of a pancreatic fistula, an inflammatory pseudo-pancreatic cyst, a duodenal fistula, or a recurrence of obstructive symptoms owing to incomplete removal of the anterior and lateral portion of the constricting arm of the annulus and the subsequent formation of a fibrotic ring constriction of the second portion of the duodenum (Figs. 3 to 6).

HETEROTOPIC (ABERRANT OR ACCESSORY) PANCREATIC TUMOURS

Pancreatic heterotopia (syn: pancreatic dystopia, heterotopic pancreatic tissue, aberrant pancreatic tissue, or pancreatic rest) is defined as the presence of pancreatic tissue outside its usual position and without anatomical relation either of continuity or of vascularisation with the pancreas proper (Fig. 9).

Historical Note

The occurrence of *aberrant or accessory pancreatic tissue*, discovered either at operation or at postmortem examination, has been reported on various occasions since the first case was discovered by Klob (*Z. Ges. Aerztl. Wien* 15:732, 1859). Van Gieson (*Proc. N.Y. Path. Soc.* p. 93, 1888) gave an account of a case of accessory pancreas in the wall of the duodenum simulating a tumour. Warthin (*Phys. Surg.* 26:337, 1904) investigated and analysed 49 cases, which led to a widespread interest being created in ectopic remnants; later, Hunt and Bonesteel (*Arch. Surg.* 38: 425, 1934) studied all the cases, and these numbered 186, reported up to the time of the publication of their article. The most exhaustive treatise on this subject is that by Branch and Gross (*Arch. Surg. 31*:200, 1935), who recorded 200 cases including 24 of their own. Kreig (*Ann. Surg. 113*: 364, 1941) collected 340 cases, and Barbosa, Dockerty, and Waugh (*Surg. Gynecol. Obstet.*

82:527, 1946) carefully analysed 471 cases including 41 from the Mayo Clinic.

Fernald [6] reviewed 720 reported cases of heterotopic pancreatic tissue. The condition is usually explained by abnormal embryological development of the pancreas. The incidence in nine autopsy series was 1 percent. The highest incidence of surgically significant lesions in heterotopic tissue occurs at 30 to 60 years of age. *Cases in infants are rare.* Fernald encountered 12 male and 9 female patients and observed a male-female ratio of 1.9:1 in a collected series of 105 cases.

Aberrant pancreatic tissue, which is usually 1 cm in diameter, has been found in the stomach (25 percent), duodenum (28 percent), jejunum (15 percent), and ileum (3 percent); in the wall of a Meckel's diverticulum (5 percent), and in diverticula of the stomach and jejuno-ileum (3 percent); in the hilus of the spleen and in the splenic capsule, in the omentum, in the wall of the gallbladder, and rarely, in the retroperitoneal tissues. Thus, at least 68 percent of accessory pancreases are found in the stomach, duodenum, and jejunum.

This ectopic tissue may persist throughout life without giving rise to any clinical symptoms or pathological changes, but occasionally it may cause pyloric or intestinal obstruction, or intussusception, it may block the ampulla of Vater and produce pancreatitis or obstructive jaundice, it may ulcerate, it may give rise to haematemesis or melaena, or it may simulate the signs and symptoms of peptic ulcer. It may undergo inflammatory changes, and when occurring in the walls of a Meckel's diverticulum, it may give rise to symptoms closely simulating those of appendicitis. Rarely, it may undergo cancerous transformation, in which case it is of a high order of malignancy. Silver and Lublin [17] have reported instances of carcinoma of pancreatic acini and islet-cell cancer occurring in aberrant tissue in the hilus of the liver and duodenal wall. About 10 to 15 percent of pancreatic rests, especially those in the stomach and duodenum, have a central duct opening into the lumen. This usually occurs at the summit of the tumour, and an umbilicated area is seen in the region of the orifice of the duct. Radiating folds may be seen as well. Rarely, opaque medium may penetrate

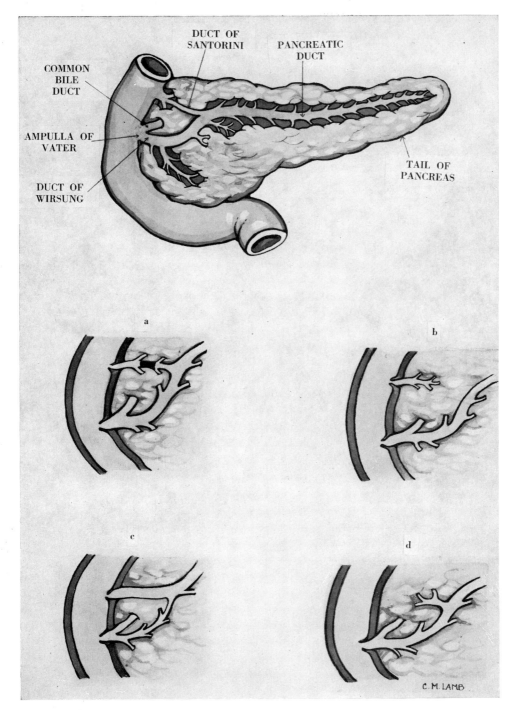

FIG. 8.   Top, common arrangement of the pancreatic ducts. Below, some variations in the duct system of the pancreas: (A) 24 percent; (B) 15 percent; (C) 7 percent; (D) 2 percent. Percentages for A, B, and C are provided by Reinhoff and Pickrell and for D, by Baldwin. (Adapted from Hollinshead's *Anatomy for Surgeons*, 2d ed., Courtesy of Hoeber Division, Harper & Row, New York, 1967.)

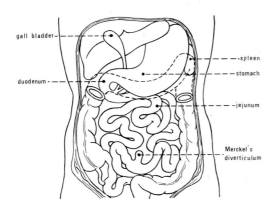

FIG. 9.   Sites of heterotopic pancreatic tissue.

into the ductal system. A radiological diagnosis of benign or malignant tumour or simple peptic ulcer is often made. Fibre-endoscopy may clinch the diagnosis in certain cases, especially when the rest is large.

According to Braasch and Gross, these lesions in aberrant pancreatic tissue are of interest to those dealing with the surgery and pathologic conditions of the gastrointestinal tract, and it is important to recognise the nature of this anomalous tissue and to appreciate that it may occur without giving rise to any important changes. Mistaking the tissue for a carcinomatous lesion of the stomach or intestine has been an unfortunate experience in several cases. The prolongation of the operation while removing benign pancreatic nodules and the danger of unnecessarily opening the intestine in these instances might have been obviated had the true nature of the ectopic pancreatic tissue been recognised at the time of the operation.

The subject of heterotopic pancreatic tissue which may be benign or malignant, functioning or nonfunctioning, is discussed by Kreig,[8] Ravitch and Woods,[14] Feldman and Weinberg,[5] Marshall and Curtiss,[11] Reemtsma,[15] and Fernald.[6]

ANOMALIES OF THE PANCREATIC DUCTS

The normal anatomical arrangement (see Fig. 8) of the common bile duct and the duct of Wirsung, uniting to form the ampulla of Vater, may be altered so that:

1. The duct of Wirsung joins the common bile duct some distance away from the duodenum.
2. The two ducts open separately into the duodenum.
3. The two ducts open separately at the apex of the papilla, the ampulla being absent.
4. Rarely, the common bile duct unites with the duct of Santorini. (See Chap. 43.)

With regard to the two pancreatic ducts, the rule is that both are present and they anastomose with one another near the neck of the gland in some 90 percent of individuals. The duct of Santorini opens into the second portion of the duodenum, within 3.5 cm of the pylorus, at a higher level than the duct of Wirsung (within 5 to 6 cm of the pylorus), which is usually (in over 85 percent of subjects) the larger of the two. Occasionally, however, the duct of Santorini may be quite separate and larger (in 6 to 10 percent of cases) while, in exceptional cases, the duct of Wirsung may be obliterated near its termination, in which event the common bile duct and the duct of Santorini open by separate orifices into the duodenum.

Opie (1910), in 100 bodies studied at autopsy, found that the choledochus and the duct of Wirsung usually enter the duodenum through a common orifice, and this was true in 65 percent of 200 subjects dissected by Mann and Giordano (*Arch. Surg.* 6:1, 1923). Rienhoff and Pickrell (*Arch. Surg.* 51:205, 1945) examined the pancreas of 250 adults, both fresh and fixed specimens. The main and accessory pancreatic ducts were dissected out. In 73 specimens (29 percent), there was no junction of the pancreatic and the common bile duct. In 92 (36 percent) instances, the pancreatic duct and choledochus were continuous and the dividing septum ended 1 to 2 mm from the apex of their common orifice. *In this group a true ampulla was not considered to be present.* In 81 instances (32 percent), a true ampulla was present. In 47 specimens (18 percent), the length of the ampulla exceeded the average diameter of the duodenal orifice, and a complete block at the papilla would convert the two ducts into a communicating system. The average diameter of the papilla was 3 mm.

Concerning the accessory pancreatic duct, in only 89 of 100 specimens studied for this purpose could any intraglandular communication between the ducts be demonstrated. In 4 instances the duct of Santorini carried the greater part of the secretion, while the main duct was fibrosed; 85 specimens had a normal duct arrangement.

There were 23 instances in which the accessory duct did not communicate with the duodenum, regardless of the duct arrangement. This, then, made a total of 34 percent in which fluid could not pass from the main pancreatic duct to the duodenum via the duct of Santorini.

These findings have a significant bearing on the subject of acute pancreatitis.

Howard and Jones (*Am. J. Med. Sci. 214*:617, 1947), in Anatomy of the Pancreatic Ducts and the Etiology of Acute Pancreatitis, state that in 81 of 150 fresh, unfixed specimens consisting of pancreas, duodenum, and common bile duct, a common channel was found to be present (54 percent). In 69 cases (46 percent), no reflux could be demonstrated. A patent duct of Santorini connecting the duct of Wirsung with the duodenum was demonstrated in 36 percent of 150 cases. In 44 percent of the 81 cases in which reflux at the ampulla occurred, a patent duct of Santorini connecting the duct of Wirsung with the duodenum was demonstrated. Howard and Jones concluded their valuable work by confirming the finding of Cameron and Noble (*J.A.M.A. 82*:1410, 1924) that in at least 50 percent of individuals there is an anatomical possibility for the formation of a common channel at the ampulla of Vater.

According to Birnstingl (*Br. J. Surg. 47*:128, 1959), the diameter of the distal portion of the pancreatic duct ranges from 1.8 to 9.2 mm. Hand (*Br. J. Surg. 50*:486, 1963), in a brilliantly illustrated, interesting, and authoritative account of the anatomy of the lower end of the choledochus, has clearly demonstrated that the narrowest part of the common bile duct is at its junction with the pancreatic duct.

The common channel, usually 4 to 7 mm long, when present, is wider than either the common or pancreatic ducts at their junction, but evidence of a true ampullary dilatation was not found. The common channel was demonstrated in 80 percent of Hand's specimens. He noted separate openings of the two ducts in the papilla of Vater in 18 percent, and no main pancreatic duct in 2 percent of his carefully dissected specimens. (See Le Quesne's observations in Chapter 43, Part A.)

The pancreatic duct is narrowed at two points: (1) at the junction of the duct of Santorini and duct of Wirsung, and (2) in the area where the pancreas (at or about its neck) is crossed by the superior mesenteric artery and vein.

The accessory duct or the main duct may be injured during gastroduodenal resection for peptic ulcer or growth, leading to such grave complications as acute pancreatitis, fistula, pseudocyst, subphrenic abscess, etc. The optimal time for the "correction" of such a gross surgical misdemeanour is during the primary operation.

REFERENCES

1. Anderson and Wapshaw, Br. J. Surg. 39:43, 1951.
2. Bickford and Williamson, Br. J. Surg. 39:49, 1951.
3. Boothroyd, Ann. Surg. 146:139, 1957.
4. Ecker, Z. Nat. Med. 16:354, 1862.
5. Feldman and Weinberg, J.A.M.A. 48:893, 1952.
6. Fernald, Int. Surg. 52:44, 1969.
7. Kiesewetter and Koop, Surgery 36:146, 1954.
8. Kreig, Ann. Surg. 113:304, 1941.
9. Lehman, Ann. Surg. 115:574, 1942.
10. MacPhee, Br. J. Surg. 40:510, 1953.
11. Marshall and Curtiss, Surg. Clin. North Am. June:867, 1952.
12. Mast et al., Am. J. Surg. 94:80, 1957.
13. Pincus, in Bockus, ed., Gastroenterology, 2d ed., Philadelphia, Saunders, 1966, Vol. 3, Chap. 122.
14. Ravitch and Woods, Ann. Surg. 132:116, 1950.
15. Reemtsma, in Howard and Jordan, eds., Surgical Diseases of Pancreas, Philadelphia, Lippincott, 1960.
16. Silen, Surg. Clin. North Am. 44:1253, 1964.
17. Silver and Lublin, Surg. Gynecol. Obstet. 86:703, 1948.
18. Swynnerton and Tanner, Br. Med. J. 1:1028, 1953.
19. Vasconcelos et al., Brazil Gastroenterology 1:535, 1949.
20. Wakeley, C., Lancet 2:811, 1951.
21. Warren, K., Surg. Clin. North Am. 39:877, 1952.
22. Whelan and Hamilton, Ann. Surg. 146:252, 1957.

B. FIBRE-OPTIC DUODENOSCOPY WITH CANNULATION OF THE SPHINCTER OF ODDI (ENDOSCOPIC PANCREATOCHOLANGIOGRAPHY)

LOUIS KREEL

Cannulation of the sphincter of Oddi with subsequent visualisation of the pancreatic and common bile ducts has now been shown to be a practical and safe procedure. This is due largely to the efforts of Japanese workers who benefited from the rapid development of flexible fibre-optic instruments in their country. The stimulus for this, however, came initially from America, where direct cannulation using fluoroscopic control was later followed by duodenoscopy. Due recognition must also be given to the many surgeons who have insisted that operative pancreatography can give much worthwhile information in both chronic pancreatitis and pancreatic carcinoma. At present there is a considerable body of knowledge in respect to the normal and abnormal radiological appearances that may be found after retrograde intubation of the sphincter of Oddi and the subsequent contrast demonstration of the pancreatic and bile ducts.

THE METHOD

To date, the instruments that have been successfuly employed are the Olympus Fibreduodenoscope JF, Type B, and the Machida FDS, Type L. The essential features are: the instrument must be at least 100 cm in length, with a side-viewing lens, a flexible tip that can be remotely controlled, and a channel through which a cannula can be passed.

The patient is prepared in the usual way as for endoscopy with a 6-hour fast, atropine 0.5 mg and diazepam (Valium) 10 mg intramuscularly. Topical anaesthesia to the pharynx by the use of an amethocaine lozenge followed by a 4 percent lidocaine (Xylocaine) spray is carried out immediately before passage of the instrument, with the patient lying in the left lateral position on a fluoroscopy table.

After negotiating the pyloric canal, duodenal juice is aspirated and the duodenal loop is rendered atonic with an injection of hyoscine-N-butyl bromide (Buscopan) 40 mg, which is given intravenously. The papilla of Vater is identified. A Teflon catheter with a small metal tip, which has been fully loaded with contrast medium, is then passed down the biopsy channel. Care must be taken not to spill any of this contrast medium onto the duodenal mucosa, as this stimulates peristalsis.

With the papilla of Vater seen en face, the tip of the catheter is inserted 5 to 20 mm into the orifice and 50 percent meglumine diatrizoate (Angiografin) is slowly injected. The catheter tends to enter the pancreatic duct when it is inserted perpendicularly to the duodenal wall; an upward insertion tends to lead the tip into the common bile duct.

For the demonstration of the pancreatic duct, 2 to 8 ml of contrast medium is required; for the common bile duct, biliary ducts, and gallbladder 15 to 30 ml is needed. Films are taken in the lateral, supine, and oblique positions, and subsequently after removal of the catheter to show drainage from the duct system. It is important not to have the outside diameter of the catheter greater than 2 mm so that it cannot completely occlude the pancreatic duct, allowing a relatively free egress of contrast medium in order

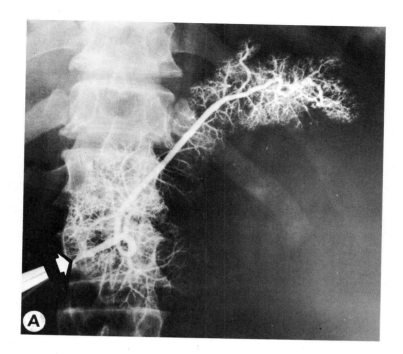

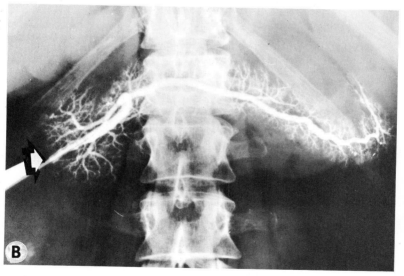

FIG. 10. Various shapes of the pancreas and main pancreatic duct. (A) The pancreas runs obliquely upwards across the bodies of L2/3 to the hilum of the spleen. Arrowhead at sphincter of Oddi. (B) Horizontal lie of the pancreas running across the body of L1.

to avoid excessive pressure in the pancreatic duct.

A transient rise in amylase levels frequently occurs in the 48 hours following this procedure, but this rise is minimised by avoiding sodium salts of iodine contrast agents and using diatrizoates or iothalomates. Prophylactic penicillin and Trasylol have also been used to counteract the possible development of acute pancreatitis. A success

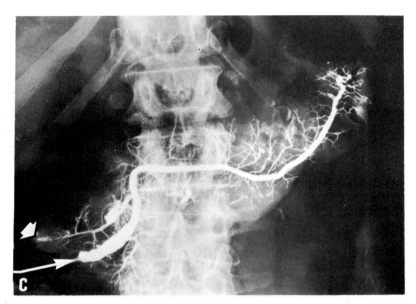

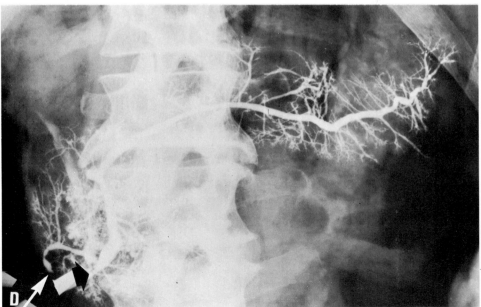

FIG. 10. (cont.) (C) Sigmoid configuration of the pancreas. An accessory duct (Santorini) is shown (arrow); it is considerably smaller than the main duct (Wirsung), indicated by arrow. (D) L-shaped pancreas with a small accessory duct (arrow). Arrow at sphincter of Oddi.

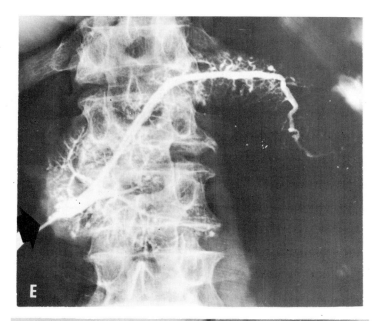

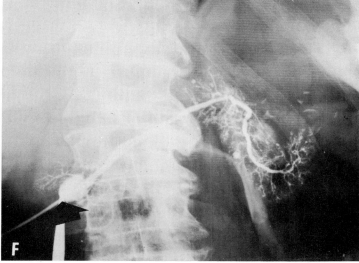

FIG. 10. (cont.) (E) Inverted U-shaped pancreas. Note that the tail of the pancreas is well below the spleen in the region of the splenic flexture of the colon. (F) Inverted V-shaped pancreas. Splenic artery calcification is present.

rate of over 80 percent has now been claimed by some workers in this field.

NORMAL RADIOGRAPHIC ANATOMY

There is a wide variation in the size, shape, and position of the pancreas and its ducts as well as in the biliary system. Many of these variations are congenital but some are age-dependent and occur most frequently in individuals over 65 years of age.

In an excellent study of the mucosal surface of the duodenum, Poppel indicated that a minor papilla was present in all cases. If the ducts are examined, however, an accessory duct (Fig. 10C) will only be found in a quarter to a third of all cases. In the majority of these, this accessory duct lies above the main duct, but rarely it may open onto the duodenal mucosa below the sphincter of Oddi.

The papilla of Vater—that is, the papilla of the main duct—lies on the posteromedial aspect of the duodenum, usually about two-thirds of the way down on the second part of the duodenal loop. In some it is in the proximal second part, while in others it may lie in the third part. Moreover, its position with regard to the spine is also very variable and it can lie as high as the body of the first lumbar vertebra or as low as the second sacral vertebra, though it is usually in the region of the second and third lumbar vertebral bodies. The lower positions occur in elderly patients.

Just as the position of the papilla is variable, so is the actual position of the head of the pancreas. In most patients, it lies on and to the right of the spine, but in a significant proportion, it will be found to be entirely on the spine and in a small number even to the left of the spine (Fig. 11).

The shape of the pancreas and the direction of the main duct is often obliquely upwards and to the left (Fig. 10A) but not infrequently it is horizontal (Fig. 10B) or has a sigmoid shape (Fig. 10C). In many cases it is more of an L-shape (Fig. 10D), with the short limb running up the spine and the long limb lying horizontally to the left. Inverted U- and V-shapes also occur (Figs. 10E and F), and in one case a double tail was found (Fig. 12).

Besides the variations in the direction of

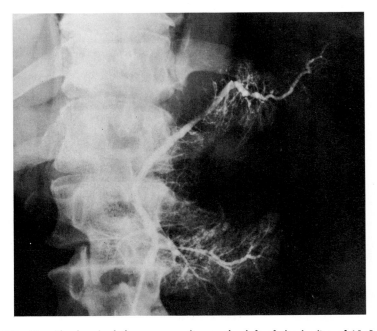

FIG. 11.   The head of the pancreas lies to the left of the bodies of L1/2.

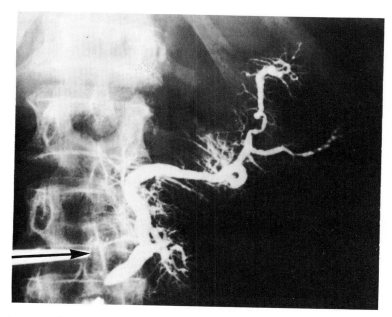

FIG. 12.   An unusual pancreatic shape. There is a reduplication of the tail of the pancreas as well as an accessory duct (*arrow*).

the duct and in the presence of an accessory duct, a complete loop in the major duct will be found in approximately 12 percent of cases (Fig. 10A). This loop may be large or small. It is also worth noting that the actual calibre of the duct in the head varies from

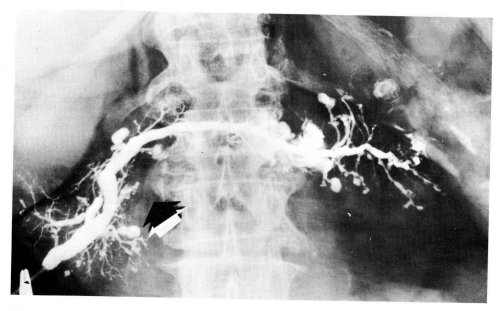

FIG. 13.   Multiple acinar dilatations in an elderly subject. No filling of part of the duct system (*arrowhead*) due to pressure from a large lateral osteophyte at L1/2.

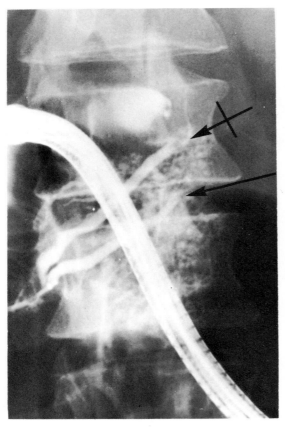

FIG. 14. Fibre-optic endoscope in position in stomach and duodenum. The main pancreatic duct is blocked with an abrupt termination (*arrow*) due to a pancreatic carcinoma, and there is overfilling of the pancreatic acini. The common bile duct is displaced to the left and downwards and is almost completely blocked (*crossed arrow*). Some contrast medium is getting into the dilated common bile duct proximal to the tumour. These appearances indicate late stage pancreatic carcinoma involving both the pancreatic and common bile ducts. (By kind permission of Dr. P. B. Cotton and Dr. J. M. Beales of St. Thomas's Hospital, London.)

2 to 4 mm in the adult, but rarely may reach a calibre of 9 mm in the normal elderly patient. This senile dilatation may extend along the whole length of the duct or be confined to the head. Normally the calibre of the duct gradually tapers towards the tail, where it is 1 to 2 mm in diameter. The calibre of the main pancreatic duct is invariably greater than that of the accessory duct, but very occasionally this relationship is reversed. The

width of the pancreas itself tends to be about 6 cm at the head, 4 cm at the body, and 3 cm at the tail.

These variations in size, shape, and position of the pancreas and its ducts will need to be borne in mind when undertaking radiographic examinations of the pancreas, but more important is the fact that extrinsic compression by the superior mesenteric artery and to a lesser extent by the splenic artery also occurs. In the elderly, with the development of arteriosclerotic changes in these vessels, linear and curvilinear filling defects can be produced in the pancreas. This has already been noted as a cause of nonuptake of radioisotope in the body of the pancreas, producing a bare area on the scan. It can produce a similar defect on injection of the pancreatic ducts. Compression-filling defects of the head of the pancreas may also be due to pressure from an aortic aneurysm and even from larger anterolateral osteophytes arising from the lumbar vertebral bodies.

The other important change that has been noted in elderly patients is the formation of ductular and acinar dilatations. These produce a spotty or nodular appearance of contrast medium (Fig. 13), and sometimes even small cystic spaces. These appearances in many respects resemble the "sialectasis" patterns which occur in the salivary glands, but in the pancreas their significance, if any, is as yet not known.

Variations in relationship to the common bile duct also occur. In most cases, the pancreatic and common bile ducts join to form a common channel, but this junction is of variable length. In a small minority of cases, about 5 percent, the pancreatic and common bile duct orifices are separate. The calibre of the common bile duct varies from 4 to 8 mm, but it may be up to 14 mm in diameter in the normal individual, the larger normal diameters being found in the elderly.

Besides the actual anatomical variations that may occur, variable appearances may also be due to different degrees of filling of the duct systems. At present, the tendency is to underfill the pancreatic ducts so as to minimise the possible production of chemical pancreatitis. Thus, not infrequently only the main pancreatic duct is shown; however, with further filling, the main pancreatic duct

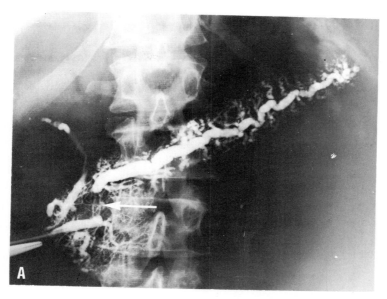

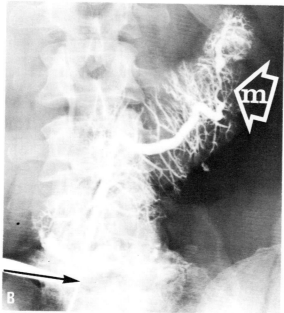

FIG. 15(A). Small filling defect in the head of the pancreas with marked narrowing of the duct (arrow). There is marked proximal dilatation with a corkscrew appearance of the main pancreatic duct in a case of primary pancreatic carcinoma. (B) Filling defect and narrowed duct in the tail of the pancreas due to a metastatic deposit.

and branches become filled, and in a significant number there is even filling of the acini. In the last situation, the whole gland is visualised. On withdrawal of the cannula, the contrast medium flows back into the duodenum within a few minutes in most cases; however, in the elderly, it may remain in the pancreatic duct for up to 10 minutes.

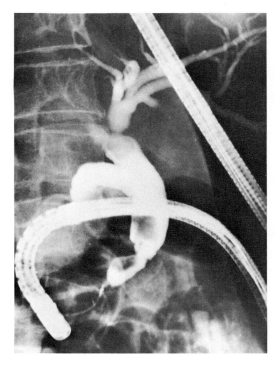

FIG. 16. Multiple gallstones in a dilated common bile duct. Fibre-optic duodenoscope in position. (By kind permission of Dr. P. B. Cotton and Dr. J. M. Beales of St. Thomas's Hospital, London.)

Contrast material can frequently remain in the common bile duct for half to one hour (see Fig. 17).

ABNORMAL RADIOLOGICAL APPEARANCES

The Pancreas

In carcinoma of the pancreas, the radiological signs are very much as were to be expected from malignant infiltration in any organ, namely narrowing of the duct, later leading to complete obstruction (Fig. 13), proximal dilatation of the main duct and branch ducts, displacement of ducts, and an area of nonfilling or nonvisualisation. In fact, similar appearances occur in metastases in the pancreas as well as in primary pancreatic carcinoma (Fig. 14B). While the well-advanced case presents no difficulty in diagnosis, the object of fibre-optic duodenoscopy with retrograde pancreatography is to detect early lesions so as to produce a significant cure rate for surgery in pancreatic carcinoma. These signs must therefore be considered in some detail.

A localised filling defect with an area of nonvisualisation is likely to produce the most difficulty in arriving at an accurate diagnosis. The neighbouring branch ducts show displacement if this is a true filling defect and this displacement of the ducts is curvilinear. In the absence of irregularity and narrowing of the main duct indicating infiltration or encasement, the lesions may be an adenoma, a small primary carcinoma, a metastasis in the pancreas or in an adjacent lymph node, or even a normal anatomical structure such as a ganglion of the autonomic nervous system.

Slight localised narrowing of the duct without evidence of a filling defect or displacement of ducts has been noted in an otherwise normal pancreas. Marked main pancreatic duct narrowing, however, is the hallmark of malignant infiltration, especially pancreatic carcinoma (Fig. 15A), but may also occur from secondary carcinoma deposits in the pancreas (Fig. 15B). This malignant duct stricture is associated with marked dilatation of the proximal duct system, which takes on a beaded appearance. The duct occlusion may become complete and then there is nonfilling of the duct system beyond with a danger of overdistention of the gland (Fig. 14).

Areas of nonfilling will also have to be distinguished from the pressure effects of the superior mesenteric and splenic arteries, as has been previously mentioned. On the other hand, where there is a very large filling defect associated with marked displacement of the main pancreatic duct, this could be due either to a pseudocyst or a cystadenocarcinoma of the pancreas. Duodenography and arteriography will distinguish between these conditions, however.

In chronic pancreatitis, the distribution of duct branching becomes irregular, with multiple fine strictures and intervening dilatation of ducts. Cyst formation and calculi

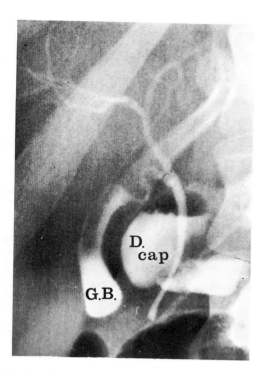

FIG. 17. Normal biliary duct system still visible half an hour after removal of endoscope and cannula in a case of obstructive jaundice. These appearances indicate the presence of hepatocellular jaundice and not a "surgical" cause. Contrast medium is also present in the gallbladder. (G.B.) and duodenal cap (D.cap). (By kind permission of Dr. P. B. Cotton and Dr. J. M. Beales of St. Thomas's Hospital, London.)

may also be seen. The real difficulty lies in distinguishing milder forms of chronic pancreatitis from the changes that occur in the elderly, and occasionally an inflammatory stricture may resemble a malignant condition, particularly when the common bile duct is involved.

The Biliary System and Gallbladder

Carcinoma of the pancreas also causes narrowing and obstruction of the common bile duct. The changes in the pancreatic duct, however, will indicate the primary diagnosis (Fig. 14). Stones in the common bile duct and in the gallbladder can also be shown (Fig. 16), as can the abrupt obstruc-

tion caused by a primary carcinoma of the biliary system.

As well as these conditions, it has become possible to diagnose a primary carcinoma of the gallbladder by the demonstration of an irregular filling defect within it. Metastases in the liver have been shown as producing multiple curvilinear displacements of the intrahepatic bile ducts.

A most important observation is the finding of a perfectly normal biliary system in a patient suspected of having obstructive jaundice (Fig. 17). This indicates that surgery is contraindicated, and that the cause of the jaundice is in fact due to intracellular "obstruction."

COMMENT

As with all newer investigations, there is bound to be overwhelming enthusiasm initially, with many successes claimed. The failures and mistakes tend to be glossed over. In spite of this, it has already become clear that fibre-optic duodenoscopy with retrograde pancreatocholangiography is a safe procedure with a definite place in the diagnosis of pancreatic and biliary disease. It is particularly valuable in cases of obstructive jaundice and suspected pancreatic carcinoma. The greatest contribution to date has been in the former.

In the case of pancreatic carcinoma, however, the merits of any investigation will ultimately be judged by whether the endeavor has increased the chances of survival. If a significant number of pancreatic carcinomas can be diagnosed while they are still curable as a result of this procedure, it will be greatly welcomed. Preliminary studies, however, suggest that this is unlikely to occur. Nevertheless, this method must be fully explored in patients with pancreatic disease, as at present it is the most reliable method of direct examination of the pancreas.

The purely endoscopic aspects of this procedure will of course remain an important part of it. It is possible with a side-viewing instrument to see enough of the lower oesophagus to diagnose varices. The gastric mucosa can be seen but cannot be examined in detail during the procedure. Direct visualisation of the duodenum, however, enables the examiner to diagnose lesions of the ampulla of Vater and duodenal mucosa, especially carcinoma and ulceration. Furthermore, biopsy specimens of these lesions can be taken.

It is clear that fibre-optic duodenoscopy has a very real place in the diagnosis of duodenal lesions, and, when combined with retrograde cannulation of the sphincter of Oddi, is invaluable in the diagnosis of suspected obstructive jaundice. In malignant lesions of the pancreas, it is unlikely to alter the ultimate prognosis greatly, but in chronic pancreatitis, it may well prove to be a most significant contribution. A positive nonoperative diagnosis becomes possible, and where stones or strictures in the pancreatic duct are demonstrated, it will indicate a possible line of treatment. As this method of diagnosis gains wider acceptance, a more thorough knowledge of many aspects of chronic pancreatitis will emerge.

ACKNOWLEDGMENTS

I am greatly indebted to Dr. P. B. Cotton and Dr. J. M. Beales of St. Thomas's Hospital, London, for the contribution of Figures 14, 16, and 17. I would also like to thank Mr. Richard Bowlby of the Department of Medical Illustration, Clinical Research Centre, Northwick Park, for his assistance in preparation of the other illustrations.

REFERENCES

Cotton, P. B., Gut, 13:1014, 1972.

Cotton, P. B., Blumgart, L. H., Davies, G. T., Pierce, J. W., Salmon, P. R., Burwood, R. J., Lawrie B. W., and Read, A. E., Lancet 1:53, 1972.

Doubilet, H., and Mulholland, J. H., Surg. Clin. North Am. 36:385, 1956.

Gregg, J. A., and Garabedian, M., Surg. Clin. North Am. 51:657, 1971.

Howard, J. M., and Short, W. F., Surg. Gynecol. Obstet. 129:319, 1969.

Kasugai, T., Kuno, N., Kizu, M., Kobayashi, S., and Hattori, K., Gastroenterology 63:227, 1972.

Kreel, L., Sandin, B., and Slavin, G., Clin. Radiol., 24:154, 1973.

McCune, W. S., Shorb, P. E., and Moscovitz, H., Ann. Surg. 167:752, 1968.

Millbourn, E., Acta Chir. Scand. 118:286, 1959/1960.

O'Beirn, S. F., Gut, 10:323, 1969.

Oi, I., Takemoto, T., and Kondo, T., Endoscopy 3:101, 1969.

Oi, I., Takemoto, T., and Nakayama, K., Surgery 67:561, 1970.

Rabinov, K. R., and Simon, M., Radiology 85:693, 1965.

Sandin, B., Kreel, L., and Slavin, G., Radiography 39:151, 1973.

Shearman, D. J. C., Warwick, R. R. G., MacLeod, I. B., and Dean, A. C. B., Lancet 1:726, 1971.

Takagi, K., Ikeda, S., Nakagawa, Y., Sakaguchi, N., Takahashi, T., Kumakura, K., Maruyama, M., Someya, N., Nakano, H., Takada, T., Takekoshi, T., and Kin, T., Gastroenterology 59:445, 1970.

Trapnell, J. E., Howard, J. M., and Brewster, J., Surgery 60:1112, 1966.

Trapnell, J., Br. J. Surg. 58:849, 1971.

Waldron, R. L., II., Am. J. Roentgenol. 104:632, 1968.

Waldron, R. L., Seaman, W. B., and Foster, S., Radiology 104:295, 1972.

35

PENETRATING AND BLUNT INJURIES OF THE PANCREAS; PANCREATIC INJURIES RESULTING FROM UPPER ABDOMINAL OPERATIONS

RODNEY MAINGOT

I agree with Lee Strohl [39] that pancreatic trauma has long been a neglected realm in abdominal surgery, largely because the pancreas has been considered a friable, relatively inaccessible, and highly hazardous structure with which to work. The pancreas occupies an unfortunate position for the patient and for the surgeon, being centrally placed, buffered by the stomach and transverse colon, and overlying the rigid aorta and vertical column.

Pancreatic injuries may occur as a result of (1) nonpenerating or blunt trauma, (2) penetrating wounds, or (3) upper abdominal operations.

It is difficult to assess the ratio of penetrating to nonpenetrating injuries of the pancreas. For instance, Thompson and Hinshaw [42] reviewed 87 patients who had sustained pancreatic injury due to external trauma during 1948–1963, and found that the injury was due to nonpentrating or blunt trauma in 55.2 percent. Penetrating wounds accounted for 44.8 percent of the cases.

Dippel et al. [11] reviewed 82 cases in which the diagnosis of pancreatic injury was confirmed by early operation. Of these, 59 had penetrating wounds and 23 had blunt or nonpenetrating injuries.

Werschky and Jordan, Jr., [51] reviewed data on 140 consecutive patients who had external trauma with injury to the pancreas. The 23 patients with blunt trauma injury had contusions, lacerations, and partial or complete transections. The mortality rate was 4 percent. Of 117 patients who had penetrating injury, 71 had gunshot wounds, usually from a low-velocity missile. The 71 patients injured by shotgun blasts had the most serious wounds. Thirty-nine patients sustained stab wounds. The liver was injured in 63 patients, the stomach in 61, the kidney in 27, the duodenum in 31, the spleen in 29, the colon in 24, and the small bowel in 21. A total of 25 patients died— 18 percent.

Bach and Fry [2] reported 44 cases of which 39 were males and 5 females. The average age was 30. Penetrating wounds accounted for 10 of the cases whilst 34 of the injuries were caused by blunt trauma. A considerable number of the patients had combined injuries of the pancreas, bile ducts, and duodenum. The mortality rate in this series was 20 percent.

NONPENETRATING (BLUNT OR SUBCUTANEOUS) INJURIES OF THE PANCREAS

Traumatic subcutaneous injuries of the pancreas are relatively rare. The first case of rupture of the pancreas due to blunt trauma was reported by Travers, of St. Thomas's Hospital, London. [43]

In 1876, Otis collected 7 reports of pancreatic injury and added 5 cases that occurred during the American Civil War.

Pancreatic injuries with pseudocyst formation—the most common complication— were reviewed by Lloyd. [26]

The expectant or conservative treatment

of pancreatic injury ended in 1903: "It is only in the last 10 years that surgical treatment has been seriously considered." [28] Fogelman and Robinson [16] estimate the total number of wounds of the pancreas reported in the world literature prior to 1961 to be 300 cases Sturim,[40] in one of the most important contributions to the surgical management of pancreatic injuries, writes: *"In the last 5 years almost 500 cases of pancreatic injuries have been reported."*

Blandy et al.,[4] in reporting their 2 cases of transverse fracture of the pancreas, state that the first example of *complete rupture* as an isolated lesion occurring after nonpenetrating trauma was reported by Jaun.[21] Garré [17] was the second surgeon to report the successful treatment of a patient with a totally transected pancreas. He was able to collect 30 cases of pancreatic injury, and in 8 cases the pancreas was the sole organ injured.

In 1965 only 56 cases of *complete transection of the pancreatic duct* could be collected in the world literature. Three years later Weitzman and Rothschild [50] reported 8 cases of caudal pancreatectomy for *complete pancreatic section.* All patients recovered without any complication and were discharged, fit and well, on the eleventh or twelfth postoperative day.

Martin et al.[27] described 4 cases which were successfully treated by end-to-end suture of the pancreas with repair of the duct of Wirsung.

In *nonpenetrating lesions,* other adjacent viscera are commonly involved at the same time; however, many reports in recent years indicate that isolated injury is not so uncommon. In *penetrating lesions,* multiple injuries involving neighbouring or distant organs are constant findings at operation or autopsy.

The pancreas may be bruised, lacerated, or torn completely across by a sudden severe force which drives the organ against the unyielding bony spine and crushes it. The pancreas may be damaged owing to an automobile accident, and contusion or fracture of the gland by steering-wheel injury is a common aetiological factor. Again, the patient may receive a pancreatic injury while employed in heavy factory work, during fights, or during strenuous games, e.g., foot-

ball, or he may be crushed by buffers, run over, kicked in the abdomen by a horse or steer,[9] fall face forwards against the edge of a table or chair, or fall from a height (*contre-coup*).[9]

Falconer and Griffith [14] considered that rupture is not complete unless the duct of Wirsung is torn, together with some sizeable pancreatic blood vessels. In some cases, bleeding causes death within a few hours, while in others there is no significant haemorrhage.

During World War II, a number of cases of severe contusion of the pancreas resulting from *blast injuries in the field or undersea explosions* were recorded by Keynes,[24] Gaston and Mulholland,[18] Roscoe Clark,[7] and others.

Letton and Wilson (1959) have reminded us that damage to the pancreas may be the result of a *contre-coup* type of mechanism.

It should be noted again that the number of reported cases of blunt injury to the pancreas published in the literature is relatively *small.* Mikulicz [28] collected 24 instances of such injuries that were caused by external violence. Thirteen of the patients were not operated upon, and all died. Of 11 who were operated upon, 7 recovered. Here the operation consisted of exposure of the pancreas and drainage of the lesser peritoneal sac. Mocquot and Constantini [30] collected from the literature 30 examples of injury by violence to the pancreas alone. Of these, 21 patients were treated surgically with 16 survivors; of 9 who were not operated on, all died.

Stuart (1921) reviewed 46 cases; Volkman (1928) reported that he had operated on 32 patients with only 1 death; Venable [45] gave his experience of 6 patients, 5 of whom he was able to save by timely operative interference, and since his publication there have been reports of a number of similar cases. One of the most interesting of these is the case of complete rupture of the pancreas recorded by Curr,[10] in which the patient survived suturing and later closure of a pancreatic fistula. Aldis [1] was one of the first to point out that if the abdominal muscles happen to be flaccid at the time of injury, or the patient is asleep, the pancreas may be crushed against the vertebrae, even by *mild force.*

Philips and Seybold,[34] Estes and co-workers,[13] Sturim,[40] and Strohl [39] have reported a number of cases and have emphasised the value of *determination of serum amylase* for patients suffering from upper abdominal injuries, especially if evidence of injury is slight or uncertain. In any case, a high value of serum amylase indicates the urgency of careful examination of the pancreas and neighbouring structures. The concentration of serum amylase usually rises and falls rapidly, as in acute pancreatitis. Pinkham,[35] in a review and analysis of 10 cases of pseudocysts of the pancreas, has suggested that a sustained high level is indicative of the formation of a pseudocyst.

Considerable credit is due to Elman [12] for showing the correlation between the blood amylase concentration and the presence of disease of the pancreas.

Keith et al.[23] observed that the peritoneal fluid in cases of pancreatic injuries is often tinted with blood and contains high amounts of amylase, and suggested the use of diagnostic paracentesis.

Wright and his colleagues [52] have emphasised that significant injury to the organ may occur in the absence of dramatic symptoms. A notable feature of grave pancreatic injuries in many instances is the delayed appearance of severe symptoms.

PENETRATING INJURIES

Penetrating injuries are caused by stabs, gunshot wounds, and the like, and although they may involve solely the pancreas, it is more common to find that other organs, such as the stomach, liver, spleen, kidney, intestines, and mesocolon, are implicated also. In a study of 965 cases of gunshot wounds of the abdomen, Wallace [46] found that the pancreas was injured 5 times. In World War I gunshot wounds of the pancreas were less frequent—or at any rate less often recognised—than injuries of any other abdominal organ.

Culotta et al.[9] stated that injuries of the pancreas resulting from penetrating injuries occur in 1 to 2 percent of abdominal wounds. These injuries, rare in civilian practice, are seen infrequently even in wartime. They collected the records of 31 patients of this type who were seen in civilian hospitals during a 15-year period. Twenty-six patients had penetrating wounds caused by a knife or bullet, and the remaining 5 had blunt injuries. Five of the 31 patients died, all within 3 days after injury and usually within 24 hours. In 35 percent of the survivors, pancreatic fistulas developed; in 8 percent, pseudocysts; and in 4 percent, abscess of the head of the pancreas. Death was primarily due to *associated injuries,* whereas nonfatal complications were due to pancreatic injury alone.

In World War II, pancreatic injury was found at laparotomy in 2 percent of abdominal wounds. Additional organs were almost invariably involved, and the mortality rate was 56 percent, with shock and haemorrhage as the causes of death in 74 percent of these. This mortality rate was reduced to about 20 percent in the Korean conflict. In a review by Poole (1955) of 3,154 abdominal injuries treated by the U.S. Army Second Auxiliary Surgical Group in 1944–45, the pancreas was wounded less frequently than any other abdominal organ, with only 62 cases reported, or an incidence of 2 percent. The mortality rate was 56 percent.

From the Korean conflict, 9 cases of pancreatic injury were collected, with 7 survivors.[36]

Culotta [9] emphasised that prompt surgical intervention, improved preoperative and postoperative care, and the use of antibiotic agents played a major part in this creditable reduction, although deaths were still numerous when multiple organs were involved.

Complications

The complications of pancreatic injuries may be enumerated as follows :

Early complications: (1) pulmonary–pleural effusion, etc.; (2) immediate or delayed "shock"; (3) immediate or delayed haemorrhage; (4) acute pancreatitis; (5) inflammatory pseudocyst; (6) peritonitis, subphrenic or subhepatic abscess; (7) fistula; and (8) abscess.

Late complications: (1) pseudocyst; (2) fistula; (3) recurrent chronic pancreatitis; (4) intestinal obstruction; (5) fibrosis of the sphincter of Oddi; (6) duodenal ulcer; (7) diabetes mellitus; (8) steatorrhoea; (9) pancreatolithiasis; and 10) retention cyst.

Diagnosis

There are no classic *symptoms* or *signs* indicative of injury of the pancreas. In cases of *penetrating wounds,* the likely course of a bullet or dagger and the position of the wound of entrance and exit are usually the best guides. Penetrating injuries of the abdomen demand *early* exploratory laparotomy. In cases of blunt injury, there may be bruising, haematoma, or superficial laceration of the skin of the abdominal wall, but these, even when present, are not of themselves of special diagnostic importance.

In the initial stages, the *clinical picture* is that of *shock,* while later on it is often that of severe internal *haemorrhage,* peritonial irritation, or spreading peritonitis. On recovery from the shock, the patient will often complain of intense epigastric pain or of a sensation of increasing constriction in the pit of the stomach. Pain may be referred to the shoulder or scapula if there is leakage into the omental bursa.[1] *Localised rigidity and tenderness* are usually present, and there may be shifting dullness in the flanks owing to the presence of blood, pancreatic or peritoneal exudates. Nausea occurs, and vomiting is often most distressing. When there has been bruising or a small tear of the pancreas, without outpouring of fluid into the lesser sac, the patient may complain of but few and insignificant symptoms, but days or weeks later a cystic swelling may develop in the epigastrium—*pseudopancreatic cyst.*

It is well known that diagnosis, as to both the existence and the extent of injuries of the pancreas, is difficult and hazardous. It is seldom correctly made before operation, and may even be unrecognised during a scrupulous surgical exploration. Nevertheless, in all cases of injury to the epigastrium, the possibility of pancreatic injury should be kept in mind. *A plain x-ray picture* of the abdomen will aid in ruling out the possibility of spinal injury or rupture of a hollow viscus—pneumoperitoneum. Occasionally the first loop of the jejunum may appear to be unduly dilated in the x-ray films. Blood investigations are of paramount importance, as leucocytosis is noted in many cases of pancreatic injury, and *serum enzyme values* may mount precipitously when this organ is traumatised, as Naffziger and McCorkle [31] have so convincingly demonstrated. Again, the erythrocyte count, haemoglobin estimation, and haematocrit reading will determine fairly accurately the degree of haemorrhage.

In cases diagnosed some days or weeks after the injury, irregular mottling of the skin in the epigastrium or in the flanks has been observed, as have Cullen's and Grey Turner's signs. The presence of a gradually *expanding* mass in the epigastrium or flank following an upper abdominal injury is strongly suggestive of pancreatic involvement. Such a mass may represent: (1) a large haematoma, (2) a pseudopancreatic cyst, or (3) a pancreatic abscess.[48]

Waugh and Lynn [49] attributed 6 of their 58 cases of pseudocysts to blunt trauma, while Connolly and Lempka [8] believed that 15 to 30 percent of such cysts are due to trauma. Hannon and Sprafka [19] have emphasised that most reports of blunt injury to the pancreas have indicated a *high incidence of pseudocyst formation together with pancreatic fistula.*

The Long-Term Results of Nonpenetrating Pancreatic Trauma, by Warren and Wagner [48] and Thal and Wilson's Pattern of Severe Trauma to the Region of the Pancreas,[41] should be consulted, as they are notable contributions to this subject. *"It should be noted that 14 of the 20 patients underwent three or more procedures and that 9 patients required surgery for a complication of pancreatic trauma more than one year after the original injury. Each patient experienced at least one major complication and the development of an inflammatory pseudocyst or a fistula was the most common."* [48] To date, some 100 cases of *complete severance of the pancreas* have been recorded.

Letton and Wilson (1959) have given a detailed account of 14 cases of complete traumatic rupture of the pancreas, and have recorded 2 cases that occurred in their practice. These authors have also submitted the operative details (and two excellent illustrations) of a previously unreported technique employing the Roux-en-Y anastomosis. Their procedure, which ensures preservation of the entire gland when it has been "fractured," is worthy of trial in suitable cases.

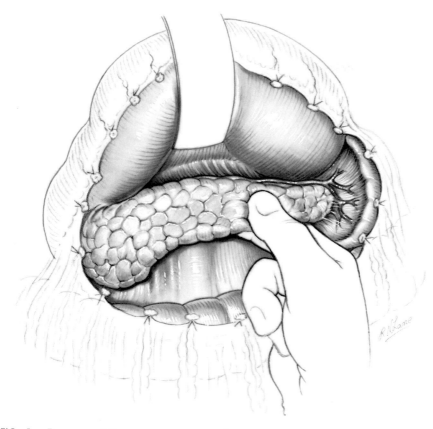

FIG. 1. Exposure of the pancreas in cases of penetrating and nonpenetrating wounds.

Operative Treatment of Pancreatic Injuries

There is a choice of three incisions: (1) vertical midline epigastric, (2) right or left epigastric paramedian, or (3) transverse. In most instances, the second of these is chosen.

When the abdominal cavity has been opened, it may be evident that there is some injury to the pancreas, as fat necrosis can be made out and there may be a quantity of blood-stained fluid lying free in the abdominal cavity or shut up in the lesser sac.

The abdominal viscera should be examined seriatim, starting with the liver and then proceeding to the stomach and duodenum, the spleen, the duodenojejunal flexure, the biliary system, the kidneys, and lastly, the intestines. If there is a large quan-

tity of free fluid in the peritoneal cavity, it should be removed by suction. The pancreas is then meticulously inspected and palpated, and in all cases in which one or more of the upper abdominal organs has sustained some injury, the surgeon should make a practice of always scrutinising the pancreas before closing the abdominal wound; otherwise injuries to this organ may frequently be overlooked.

There are various *routes for approaching the pancreas.* These are:

1. *Through the gastrohepatic omentum.* In visceroptotic patients, this affords the most ready access, as the central portion of the gastrohepatic omentum is very thin and diaphanous and can be widely divided without producing any bleeding. On retracting the stomach downward and the liver upward,

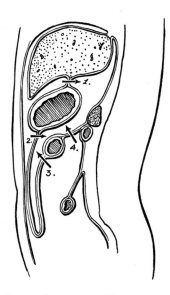

FIG. 2. Routes for approaching the pancreas: (1) through the gastrohepatic omentum; (2) through the gastrocolic omentum; (3) by detaching the great omentum from the transverse colon; and (4) through the mesocolon.

the whole of the superior and inferior aspects of the pancreas can be visualised.

2. *Through the gastrocolic omentum.* This is the route chosen by most surgeons. The gastrocolic omentum is snipped below the stomach through avascular portions, after which this structure is completely freed from the pylorus to the hilus of the spleen in order to afford the maximum view of the anterior face of the pancreas (Figs. 1 and 2). The stomach is then drawn upwards and the transverse colon downwards.

3. *By detaching the greater omentum from the transverse colon.* This is a good approach to the organ, as on separating the omentum from its slender attachment to the transverse colon, the whole of the lesser sac can be explored.

4. *Through the mesocolon.* This approach has little to commend it. The mesocolon is snipped in an avascular spot below one of the arches of the middle colic artery, and after retract-

ing the edges of this incision the body and tail of the organ can be examined. It does not permit easy inspection of the head of the gland, and there is danger of wounding the middle colic artery or one of its important branches. Again, should drainage be required, the tube will have to traverse the general peritoneal cavity, unless, of course, a fresh opening is made through the gastrocolic ligament.

5. *By Kocher's method.* This provides an approach to the posterior aspect of the head of the gland.

6. *Through an incision in the anterior wall of the second portion of the duodenum.* Through this route the papilla of Vater and the opening of the accessory duct into the gut can be revealed.

7. *By the posterior route.* This affords poor exposure of the tail of the pancreas. Here a left kidney incision or one which is placed just below the lower costal margin is chosen. This is the retroperitoneal route, which is rarely used when posterior drainage is required, as for an abscess of the tail of the pancreas.

The *measures advocated* depend upon the extent and position of the lesion or lesions, thus:

1. If there is no obvious laceration of the organ but it is *contused,* a drainage tube is led down near to the site and brought out through a laterally placed stab incision.

2. *A clean laceration should be carefully sutured* with a series of interrupted sutures of Mersilk or Merselene on half-curved atraumatic (eyeless) needles. Penrose drains are used in the adjacent site. Catgut should not be used.

3. If the *tail of the gland is pulped or has been cut or torn adrift from the body of the pancreas, immediate distal pancreatectomy (with splenectomy) should be carried out.* The proximal end of the duct of Wirsung should be transfixed and tied or doubly ligated with silk sutures, after which the anterior and posterior margins of the gland are approximated, with inter-

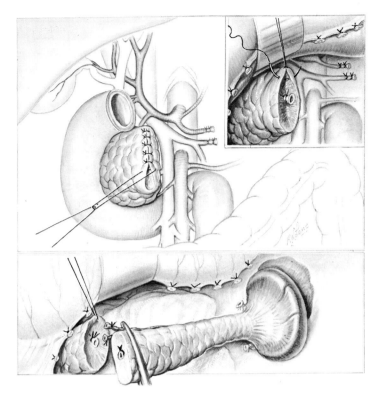

FIG. 3.   A buffer accident causing transection of the neck of the pancreas. Subtotal resection
of the pancreas with splenectomy; and methods of dealing with the duct of Wirsung and the
margins of the head of the pancreas.

rupted silk sutures, as illustrated in
Figure 3. *Drainage of the lesser peri-*
toneal sac is always instituted after
such an operation, and in fact after
any operation, on the pancreas for
contusion, laceration, or fracture.

Hannon and Sprafka [19] reported 4 cases
of rupture of the pancreas owing to blunt
trauma to the epigastrium, and advised resection of the pancreas distal to the rupture,
combined with splenectomy. The dangers
and discomforts that attend a fistula are
thus eliminated, and the speedy and complete recovery in 3 cases following excision
of 20 to 80 percent of the pancreas supports
the view that distal resection (with splenectomy) is better treatment than simple drainage. There were no symptoms of pancreatic
insufficiency in their 3 patients subjected to
immediate distal pancreatectomy.

4. In certain instances following resection of the tail or body and tail of
the pancreas, it may be wise to carry
out *pancreatogastrostomy* on the lines
depicted in Figure 4. This particularly
applies to those cases where the head
of the gland appears to be moderately
contused.

Therefore, when complete rupture of the
pancreas occurs, distal pancreatectomy with
splenectomy is the correct procedure, provided the general condition of the patient is
satisfactory.

5. If the main duct has been torn across,
it *may* be possible, as Waugh and
Hallenbeck (1956) have suggested, to
reconstruct it over a T tube or an in-
dwelling latex tube and approximate

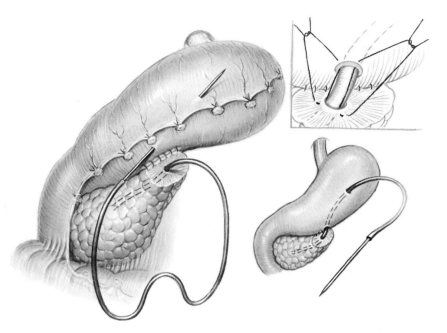

FIG. 4.   Pancreatogastrostomy (Rodney Smith's technique). With half of the anastomosis completed, a long latex tube is inserted into the pancreatic duct and the other end is brought out through the stomach and then the abdominal wall.

the ends of the gland with fine silk sutures.

6.   *Transduodenal splintage of a repaired duct of Wirsung.* In this operation, the

second portion of the duodenum is opened, sphincterotomy is performed and a ureteral catheter or a latex tube is passed through the proximal end of

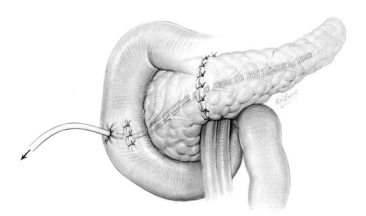

FIG. 5.   Transection of the pancreas treated by duodenotomy and insertion of a ureteric catheter into the duct of Wirsung and then onwards into the distal pancreatic duct. The two portions of the gland are then drawn together and approximated with a series of interrupted sutures.

the duct. The distal portion of the pancreas is coaxed toward the proximal end and an end-to-end duct anastomosis is carried out with interrupted sutures of 0000 Dexon silk or Deknatel after which the catheter or tube is guided through the anastomotic junction and then onwards toward the tail of the gland.

The anterior and posterior margins of the pancreas are approximated with fine Mersilk sutures; the duodenotomy incision is closed, and the catheter or tube is led to the exterior for drainage purposes through a small puncture in the lateral wall of the duodenum. The subhepatic space is drained with corrugated sheets of latex (Fig. 5).

7.   In some cases of complete severance of the neck or body of the pancreas, the Roux-en-Y method of anastomosis, as practiced by Letton and Wilson, may be performed (Figs 9 and 10). The appealing feature of this operation is that the maximum amount of pancreatic tissue is preserved.

Werschky and Jordan, Jr.,[51] after performing caudal pancreatectomy, have advised anastomosing the face of the proximal end of the pancreas to the ascending loop of a Roux-en-Y end-to-side pancreatojejunostomy. At the present time, however, most surgeons would prefer to close the proximal end *securely* after caudal pancreatectomy for cases of complete amputation of the gland. The pancreas continues to function normally even when 75 percent of the gland is removed.

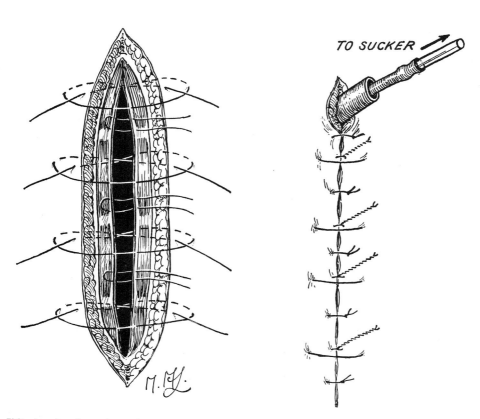

TO SUCKER

FIG. 6.   A safe and rapid method of closure of the abdominal wound in *some cases of grave injury* to the pancreas. This is done with through-and-through "near-far, far-near" sutures of stainless steel wire. Sump drains are best led through a stab incision placed *lateral* to the incision. Following operations upon the pancreas, the majority of abdominal incisions are closed with silk and also nylon sutures.

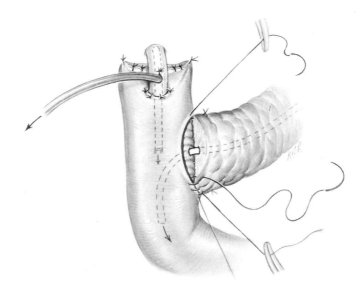

FIG. 7.   Pancreatoduodenectomy.

The abdominal incision may be closed with interrupted sutures of stainless steel wire, in the manner shown in Figure 6.

8. *Pancreatoduodenectomy.* This operation should be performed when there is extensive damage or avulsion of the

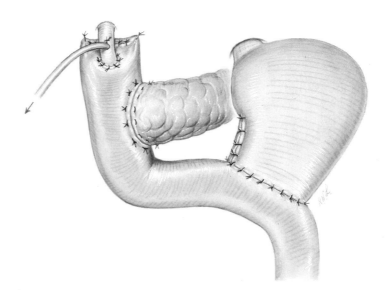

FIG. 8.   Pancreatoduodenectomy for severe blunt trauma to the second portion of the duodenum and the head of the pancreas. Completion of the operation.

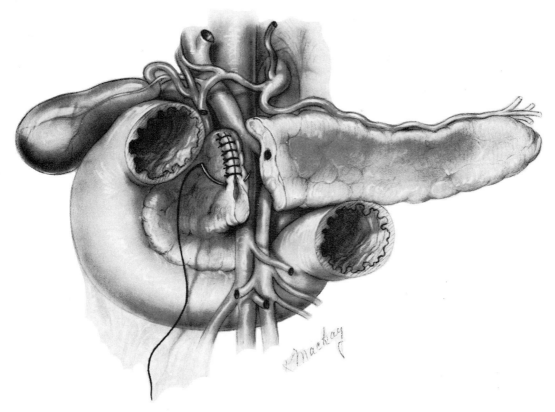

FIG. 9. Complete rupture of pancreas. Illustrates almost identical findings in two patients operated upon by Dr. Letton and Dr. Wilson. It shows pancreas completely divided and ends retracted, with exposure of superior mesenteric vein and splenic vessels intact. (Courtesy of Dr. A. H. Letton and Dr. J. P. Wilson, and of *Surgery, Gynecology & Obstetrics.*)

head of the pancreas associated with compromise of the blood supply to the duodenum, and in combined injuries involving the head of the pancreas, duodenum, and common bile duct.

Figure 7 illustrates the stage in the operation when the pancreatic duct is being anastomosed to the lateral wall of the jejunum. Note that the gallbladder is excised, that the common hepatic duct is drained with a guttered T tube, and that the final stage in the operation will consist of anastomosing the gastric pouch to the jejunum a few inches below the pancreatojejunostomy (Fig. 8). Details of the operation of pan-

creatoduodenectomy will be found in Chapters 38C and 39.

George Gordon, Jr., a leading authority on pancreatic injuries, operated upon 10 patients with transection of the pancreas, with no mortality. His operative mortality rate for blunt trauma involving the pancreas is low—9 percent, whereas the mortality rate following gunshot wounds involving the pancreas and other organs is 29 percent.

The mortality rate of pancreatic injuries is, of course, greatly increased when the chest, head, limbs, or other abdominal organs are concomitantly involved.

As a large section of this work is concerned with the management of trauma to the abdominal viscera, the reader is referred to the appropriate chapters.

PANCREATIC INJURIES RESULTING FROM UPPER ABDOMINAL OPERATIONS

This subject is discussed by Schmieden and Sebening,[37] Stern,[38] Warren,[47] Hollender et al.,[20] and Millbourn.[29] Schmieden and Sebening collected 145 cases of pancreatic injuries attending various operations on the upper abdominal viscera. The relative incidence which they found is shown below:

Operation	Injuries to Pancreas
Stomach	91
Biliary tract	38
Spleen	7
Diagnostic biopsy	4
Other	5
Total	145

Peterson et al.[33] stated that acute pancreatitis remains an infrequent, but potentially disastrous, postoperative complication. In their series, 8 out of 22 patients, or 36 percent, with postoperative pancreatitis died compared with a mortality rate of 18 percent for patients with other types of pancreatitis.

Operations upon the stomach, duodenum, gallbladder, spleen, and colon may in certain instances result in injury to the pancreatic tissue, sometimes without any ill effect, but occasionally with pseudocyst or fistula formation, subphrenic abscess, acute pancreatitis, or even necrosis of the gland.

It is exceedingly difficult in some cases to determine whether a hard craggy mass in the head of the pancreas is a growth or a localised patch of chronic pancreatitis, and the temptation to excise a small portion of the gland for *biopsy* is a very real one. It should be resisted, however, as cutting into the gland for purposes of taking a biopsy specimen is sometimes followed by injury to the major and minor pancreatic ducts or by the subsequent development of pancreatitis or peritonitis. Biopsy with the aid of a Vim-Silverman needle, however, is safe, speedy, and bloodless, and *may even be helpful.*

Pancreatitis, too, may sometimes follow *transduodenal sphincterotomy or exploration of the common bile duct or the duct of Wirsung, or pancreatography* (Birnstingl,

1959). Following Kocher's mobilisation, a too-vigorous manipulation of the terminal portion of the common bile duct in palpating a stone or a suspected stone has been known to be followed by severe inflammatory reaction of the head of the gland (Fig. 11). A number of cases of acute pancreatitis have been reported following the use of *a long-limb T tube* (originally designed by Cattell) for biliary tract diseases—e.g., choledocholithiasis, sphincterotomy for fibrosis of the sphincter of Oddi, etc. Postoperative pancreatitis has not been observed when the author's long guttered T tube has been employed, as the orifice of the duct of Wirsung is in no way compressed and, in fact, faces and empties its contents into the "gutter" itself.

Gastric and duodenal ulcers which deeply penetrate the pancreas and which are often associated with a marked degree of surrounding fibrosis may not be capable of excision without serious injury to the glandular tissue. It is safer in such cases to cut around the ulcer so as to leave its base intact in the pancreas rather than to cut out the ulcer from its indurated bed together with a portion of pancreatic tissue. Even cauterisation or the application of carbolic acid to the ulcer bed has been known to be followed by pancreatitis, peritonitis, fistula formation, or an inflammatory pseudocyst.

Perhaps the pancreas is most frequently injured in connection with the *Billroth II types of operation* for a chronic duodenal ulcer that has deeply pitted the pancreatic substance. Here, in removing the ulcer together with a generous portion of the first part of the duodenum, a portion of the gland may be excised, with disastrous consequences. Again, in *transfixing and ligating the pancreatoduodenal artery,* a portion of the gland containing a small segment of the duct of Santorini may be included in a ligature and this may give rise to subsequent trouble.

Following wide excision of the first portion of the duodenum and inversion of the stump, *a suture may pick up and occlude the duct of Santorini* or strangle a portion of pancreatic tissue, producing pancreatitis, localised necrosis, or an external pancreatic fistula.

Reflux of duodenal contents may be an ex-

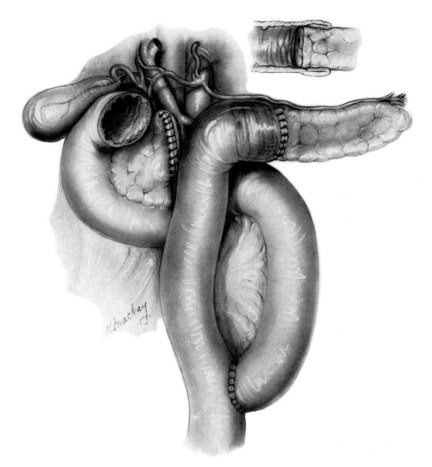

FIG. 10.   Complete rupture of body of pancreas, and technique adopted by Dr. Letton and Dr. Wilson. Roux-en-Y type of pancreatojejunostomy has been made with caudal portion of pancreas and defunctionalised jejunum. The raw surface in the head of pancreas has been closed with interrupted sutures. Inset shows technique of anastomosis. (Courtesy of Dr. A. H. Letton and Dr. John P. Wilson, and of *Surgery, Gynecology & Obstetrics.*)

citing cause of postgastrectomy pancreatitis.

Attempts at radical excisions of *gastric carcinoma* provide more possible sources of danger. In attempting to carry the dissection well beyond a suspicious infiltrating area, it may be necessary and it is, in fact, desirable, to include a portion of the gland in the resected mass. It can be appreciated how in doing this the main duct itself may be laid bare. Kraft[25] stated that *pancreatic fistula* complicating partial gastrectomy is not a common occurrence and that Triska[44] gives an incidence of 0.25 percent in 2,343 resections. According to these authors, only 61 recorded cases can be traced since 1881.

In a series of 1,689 partial or subtotal gastrectomies (mostly of the Billroth II types) reported by Burton et al.[5] there were 94 deaths, 12 of which were due to acute pancreatitis (12.7 percent, or 0.7 percent of the total). According to Pendower and Tanner,[32] collected figures from various authors show that in 128 cases of postgastrectomy pancreatitis the mortality was 55.5 percent. The true incidence of this complication is difficult to ascertain because the less severe cases are probably not diagnosed, and many who die from inadvertent surgical accidents are

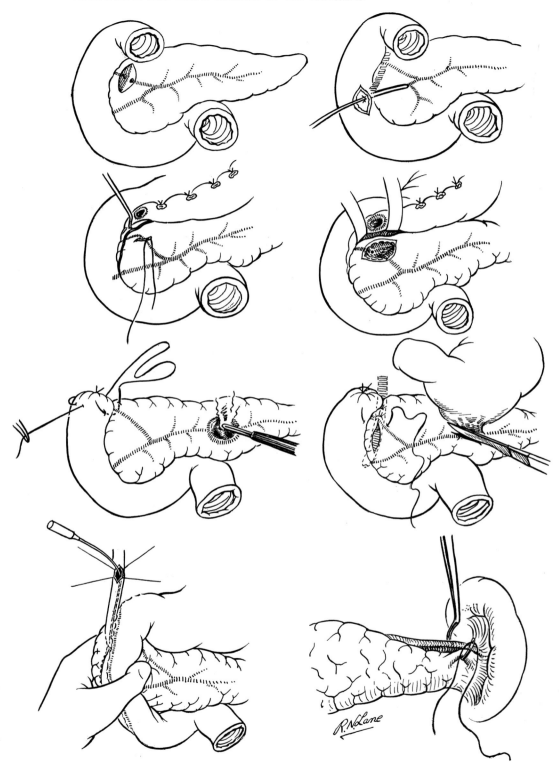

FIG. 11. Operative injuries of the pancreas. (Adapted from Mr. A. Dickson Wright)

not reported. They record 9 cases following gastrectomy, with 2 deaths.

Splenectomy is another operation in which the pancreas may be injured.[3] The tail of the gland may be clamped with haemostats or ligated as the pedicle is being secured, and as a result a fistula or pseudocyst formation may subsequently occur.

To mention involvement of the pancreas during the performance of *nephrectomy* does not appear to indicate fortunate surgery, but since instances have been quoted in the literature, the possibility must be recognised.

Postoperative pancreatitis may occur after excision of a *diverticulum* involving the second position of the duodenum and following *operations upon the pancreas itself.*

Cases have been reported following pancreatojejunostomy, pancreatogastrostomy, and pancreatoduodenectomy for chronic or relapsing pancreatitis.

The *signs and symptoms* of acute postoperative pancreatitis are often baffling, nonspecific, and atypical, and its clinical forms are varied and unexpected. According to Hollender et al.,[20] the disease usually occurs between the second and the fifth day after operation; the earlier it appears, the more serious it is likely to be. The clinical diagnosis rests primarily on circulatory collapse, with fall in the arterial blood pressure and acceleration of the pulse rate, and urinary disturbances, oliguria or anuria being seen in about 50 percent of the cases. Elevation of amylase and lipase levels in the blood and urine classically accompanies this grave condition. Severe hypocalcaemia, if present, indicates a poor prognosis.

The *treatment of operative injuries of the main pancreatic ducts* following partial gastrectomy for penetrating duodenal ulcer depends to some extent upon whether the injuries are detected at the time of operation or subsequently.

Division of the duct of Santorini is best treated by ligation with fine silk or cotton. If the duct appears to be large, the surgeon should assume that the *duct of Santorini* constitutes the main duct, in which case the divided end must be anastomosed to the duodenum. According to Warren,[47] division of the *main pancreatic duct* should be treated by direct end-to-side anastomosis to the adjacent duodenum. When the division of the duct of Wirsung is associated with injury to the common bile duct, *both* structures should be anastomosed to the duodenum. The divided ducts should be united to the duodenum end-to-side by the mucosa-to-mucosa method, employing interrupted through-and-through sutures of 0000 silk or Deknatel. Sometimes T tubes are employed to act as a mould or splint to the anastomotic junction.

When injury to the duct of Santorini or Wirsung occurs and is unrecognised, the grave complications of peritonitis, pancreatic abscess, subphrenic abscess, external pancreatic fistula, or pseudocyst may follow.[15] The prompt recognition of these serious complications will depend upon the surgeon's being alert to the possibility of such an injury and upon the demonstration of elevated serum amylase values. The immediate treatment will include: sump drainage of the operative field, continuous suction to collect the escaping pancreatic juice and to prevent digestion of the wound, parenteral replacement therapy, blood transfusions, withholding of oral fluids or food, administration of propantheline bromide (Pro-Banthine), and antibiotic therapy.

When the fistula stubbornly refuses to heal after an intensive course of medical management, surgical measures will become obligatory. Carpenter and Crandell[6] collected and tabulated 16 cases of injury of the common bile duct or the duct of Wirsung, alone or in combination, which occurred during gastric operations. They state that the suspicion exists that such injuries may be more common than is generally appreciated.

In certain cases, exeresis of the most severely affected pancreatic tissue should be followed by alimentary jejunostomy-en-Y.

Prompt surgical treatment should improve the prognosis of acute postoperative pancreatitis, which up to now has been very poor.

REFERENCES

1. Aldis, Br. J. Surg. 33:323, 1946.
2. Bach and Fry, Am. J. Surg. 121:20, 1971.
3. Baronofsky et al., Surgery 29:852, 1951.
4. Blandy et al., Br. J. Surg. 47:150, 1959.
5. Burton et al., Am. J. Surg. 94:70, 1957.
6. Carpenter and Crandell, Ann. Surg. 148:66, 1958.
7. Clark, R., Lancet 2:877, 1954.

8. Connolly and Lampka, Am. J. Surg. 74:805, 1947.
9. Culotta et al., Surgery 40:320, 1956.
10. Curr, Br. J. Surg. 32:386, 1945.
11. Dippel et al., Arch. Surg. 86:1088, 1963.
12. Elman, Arch. Surg. 19:943, 1929.
13. Estes et al., Am. J. Surg. 83:434, 1952.
14. Falconer and Griffith, Br. J. Surg. 37:334, 1950.
15. Farringer et al., Surgery 60:964, 1966.
16. Fogelman and Robinson, Am. J. Surg. 101:698, 1961.
17. Garré, Beitr. Klin. Chir. 46:233, 1905.
18. Gaston and Mullholland, Surg. Clin. North Am. April:463, 1955.
19. Hannon and Sprafka, Ann. Surg. 146:136, 1957.
20. Hollender et al., J. Chir. (Paris) 97:177, 1969.
21. Jaun, Indian Ann. Med. Sci. 3:721, 1856.
22. Jordan, G., Jr., Am. J. Surg. 119:200, 1970.
23. Keith et al., Arch. Surg. 61:85, 1950.
24. Keynes, Br. J. Surg. 32:300, 1944.
25. Kraft, Br. J. Surg. 41:546, 1954.
26. Lloyd, Br. Med. J. 2:1051, 1892.
27. Martin et al., Surgery 63:697, 1968.
28. Mikulicz, Ann. Surg. 38:1, 1903.
29. Millbourn, Acta Chir. Scand. 98:1, 1949.
30. Mocquot and Constantini, Rev. Chir. Paris 61: 289, 1923.
31. Naffziger and McCorkle, Ann. Surg. 118:594, 1943.
32. Pendower and Tanner, Br. J. Surg. 47:145, 1959.
33. Peterson et al., Surg. Gynecol. Obstet. 127:23, 1968.
34. Philips and Seybold, Proc. Mayo Clin. 23:254, 1949.
35. Pinkham, Surg. Gynecol. Obstet. 80:225, 1945.
36. Sako et al., Surgery 37:602, 1955.
37. Schmieden and Sebening, Surg. Gynecol. Obstet. 46:735, 1928.
38. Stern, Am. J. Surg. 8:58, 1930.
39. Strohl, L., Surg. Gynecol. Obstet. 124:115, 1967.
40. Sturim, Surg. Gynecol. Obstet. 122:133, 1966.
41. Thal and Wilson, Surg. Gynecol. Obstet. 119: 773, 1964.
42. Thompson and Hinshaw, Ann. Surg. 163:153, 1966.
43. Travers, Lancet 12:384, 1827.
44. Triska, Wien Med. Wochenschr. 100:597, 1950.
45. Venable, Surg. Gynecol. Obstet. 55:652, 1932.
46. Wallace, War Surgery of the Abdomen, 1917.
47. Warren, Surgery 26:643, 1951.
48. Warren and Wagner, Lahey Clin. Found. Bull. 16:217, 1967.
49. Waugh and Lynn, Arch. Surg. 77:47, 1958.
50. Weitzman and Rothschild, Surg. Clin. North Am. 48:1347, 1968.
51. Werschky and Jordan, Jr., Am. J. Surg. 116:768, 1968.
52. Wright et al., Am. J. Surg. 80:170, 1950.

36

ACUTE PANCREATITIS

IAN A. D. BOUCHIER

The term *acute pancreatitis* implies an acute inflammation of the pancreas following which there is clinical and biological restitution of the pancreas if the primary cause is eliminated. The differentiation between acute oedematous pancreatitis and the clinically more severe acute haemorrhagic pancreatitis remains arbitrary and probably represents one end of the spectrum of inflammation. Thus all grades of oedema, necrosis, and inflammatory response are seen in pancreatitis, and in the present state of uncertainty regarding the pathogenesis of pancreatitis it is best to group all forms of acute pancreatic inflammation and necrosis under the broad term of acute pancreatitis.

AETIOLOGY

The most important causes of acute pancreatitis are listed below:

Biliary tract disease
Excessive intake of alcohol
Unknown causes
Obstruction of the pancreatic duct or ampulla of Vater
Mumps
Corticosteroid therapy
Postoperative causes

Of these, by far the most important are

the first three. In a recent review of the aetiology of pancreatitis in over 1,000 patients, Creutzfeldt and Schmidt (1970) found that in approximately one-third of the patients the cause was biliary tract disease; in another third, the cause was alcoholism; and in the remainder, either no cause could be identified or the inflammation was caused by very uncommon agents. There are marked geographic variations in the distribution of the recognised causes of acute pancreatitis. In surveys of patients in the United States of America, France, and South Africa, alcoholism features prominently in the list of causes; in Great Britain, biliary tract disease appears to be more important and alcohol abuse less common. The association between biliary tract disease and pancreatitis includes acute cholecystitis, cholelithiasis, and choledocholithiasis.

A large number of other aetiological factors have been implicated in acute pancreatitis, including hereditary factors and familial pancreatitis; infections (bacterial, viral, and parasitic); endocrine (particularly hyperparathyroidism); metabolic (such as hyperlipaemia and diabetes mellitus); nutritional; connective tissue diseases (such as systemic lupus erythematosus) (polyarteritis nodosa) and vascular disease (such as malignant hypertension, arteriosclerosis, and arteritis). Drugs which have been implicated include ethionine, chlorothiazide, salicylazosulphapyridine, and methyltestosterone. Pancreatitis has also been reported after renal homotransplantation (Tilney et al., 1966) and scorpion stings (Bartholomew, 1970).

PATHOGENESIS

In the present state of knowledge, it is best to regard acute pancreatitis as originating from the digestive action of activated pancreatic enzymes on the gland. It is probable that a variety of agents or factors are responsible for the enzyme activation, but the fundamental pathogenic mechanism is one of autodigestion. Acute pancreatitis can be produced experimentally by many methods, and it is likely that different techniques produce different morphological changes.

Effect of pancreatic enzymes. The question is frequently raised whether an acutely inflamed pancreas contains activated trypsin. The available evidence suggests that active trypsin cannot be detected in the pancreas of either humans or experimental animals with acute pancreatitis. The activation of trypsinogen to trypsin is directly related to the amount of calcium ion present, but at the concentrations present in normal human pancreatic juice, little or no activation can occur on this account. Furthermore, there are large quantities of trypsin inhibitor, which would inactivate any trypsin that might be released. Thus, the role of trypsin is uncertain, as is the part played by other proteolytic enzymes such as chymotrypsin and elastase. The evidence is contradictory regarding the role of lipase (Anderson, et al., 1969). Schmidt and Creutzfeldt (1969) suggested that phospholipase A might be implicated in the pathogenesis of the acute inflammation. Although the pure enzyme does not cause damage, the enzyme exerts marked cytotoxic and necrotic effects in the presence of bile salts. This is thought to be mediated via the formation of lysolecithin. Creutzfeldt and Schmidt (1970) believe that "the typical effect of pancreatitis occurring in man is best explained by the effect of phospholipase A." It must be recalled that trypsin is necessary in order for the phospholipase A to be activated.

Bile reflux. In 1901, Opie first proposed that reflux of bile into the pancreas could cause acute pancreatitis. This concept implies that the bile duct and the pancreatic duct must form a common channel and that this common channel becomes blocked, thus enabling bile to enter the pancreatic duct system. A common channel is found in about 85 percent of normal subjects (Hand, 1968). Much of the experimental work in inducing pancreatitis by the injection of bile into the pancreatic duct is nonspecific and only reflects the destructive effect of a marked elevation of the intrapancreatic pressure. Reflux of bile can be shown to occur normally in dogs, particularly during digestion (Hansson, 1967). On the whole, the evidence incriminating bile reflux is unconvincing.

1. It is possible to demonstrate reflux into the pancreatic duct at the time of biliary radiology in patients who have no evidence of pancreatitis.

2. Impaction of a gallstone at the ampulla of Vater can only be demonstrated in about 5 percent of patients with acute pancreatitis found at postmortem.

3. It is probable that the secretory pressure of the pancreas is sufficiently great to protect against bile reflux.

The subject remains controversial, however, and there are many experiments that suggest that under some circumstances bile, which has refluxed into the pancreas, may be modified, or may modify pancreatic enzymes, in such a way as to cause acute inflammation of the gland.

Reflux of Duodenal Contents

Experimental work suggests that if the intraduodenal pressure is elevated, reflux of the duodenal contents occurs into the pancreatic duct, and this may initiate pancreatitis. There are a few clinical situations in which this mechanism can be seen to operate, such as in afferent loop obstruction and intraluminal obstruction in the duodenum. It is probably an uncommon cause of acute pancreatitis; nonetheless this mechanism does have strong support from some authorities (McCutcheon, 1968).

Alcohol and Pancreatitis

Alcohol has been implicated in the genesis of both acute and chronic pancreatitis. It is possible that the acute administration of alcohol causes spasm of the sphincter of Oddi and obstruction to the pancreatic duct. Since alcohol also acts to stimulate the pancreatic secretions, it has been suggested that the high intraduct pressures that would result could rupture the acini and release enzymes into the pancreatic tissues. Obstruction to or ligation of the pancreatic duct in animals, does not cause pancreatitis but rather pancreatic atrophy. Thus, other factors must be operating, and it is possible that some degree of vascular insufficiency may convert atrophy or oedema into necrosis.

Pancreatitis may be associated with a tumour of the gland or with a penetrating peptic ulcer. Bacterial infection is not a primary factor but viral disease, such as the mumps virus, may initiate pancreatitis via direct injury to the cell. The relationship of hyperparathyroidism and pancreatitis is believed to be through the abnormality of calcium metabolism rather than any direct effect of parathyroid hormone on the gland (Leeson and Fourman, 1966). The relationship between pancreatitis and hyperlipidaemia is complex. Disturbances in the circulating lipids are recognised with increasing frequency in patients with acute pancreatitis, but it is probable that this is usually secondary to the pancreatic inflammation in the majority of patients, and it would seem that the primary hyperlipidaemic states are rarely complicated by pancreatitis.

In summary, it is clear that the pancreatic enzymes, which are normally enveloped by the membrane of the zymogen granules, become activated once the membrane has ruptured. While it seems reasonable to suggest that the damage in pancreatitis is due to the activities of trypsin, chymotrypsin, phospholipase A, elastase, and lipase, it is difficult to demonstrate their causative role with certainty. It remains to be explained how the enzymes become activated.

PATHOLOGY

The gland is oedematous with varying degrees of inflammation, necrosis, and haemorrhage, which can be seen macroscopically and histologically (Fig. 1). The oedema may produce a rather glassy appearance and the damage may be localised or generalised. Areas of fat necrosis are recognised as yellow waxy areas usually present in the gland or the lesser sac and the omentum, but occasionally the fat necrosis is widespread and is found on the parietal and visceral peritoneum. Fat necrosis may also be demonstrated in the bone marrow, where it has been related to the release of lipase into the systemic circulation. The presence of fat necrosis is the traditional explanation for the low serum calcium levels which are such a feature of acute pancreatitis. The calcium is believed to be taken up by free fatty acids which are released by the action of lipase with the consequent formation of calcium soaps (Storck, 1971). The release of trypsin

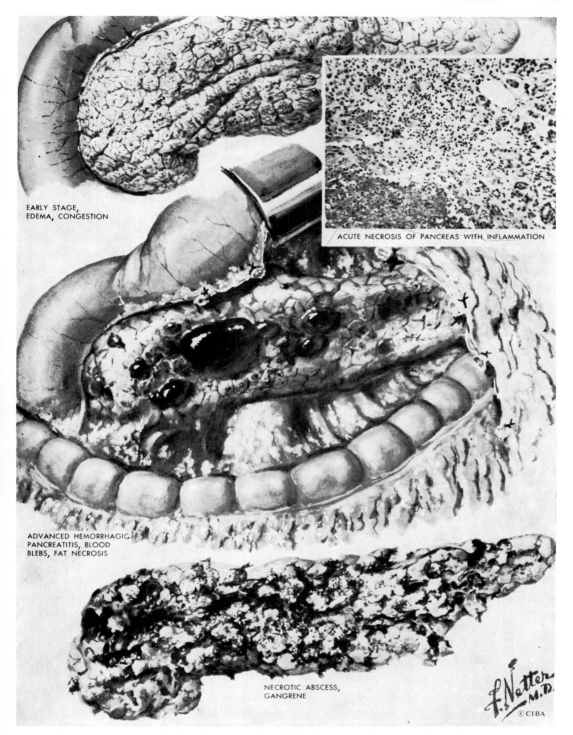

EARLY STAGE,
EDEMA, CONGESTION

ACUTE NECROSIS OF PANCREAS WITH INFLAMMATION

ADVANCED HEMORRHAGIC
PANCREATITIS, BLOOD
BLEBS, FAT NECROSIS

NECROTIC ABSCESS,
GANGRENE

FIG. 1. Acute pancreatitis. (Copyright, The CIBA Collection of Medical Illustrations, by Frank H. Netter, M.D.)

into the bloodstream might explain the necrosis and inflammation that can be demonstrated in skeletal muscle. Other features of the disease include ascites, pleural effusions, and myocardial damage. Release of bradykinin, kallikrein, kallidin, and other vasoactive polypeptides is responsible for the pain, increased capillary permeability, local oedema, vasodilatation, hypotension, and leucocyte accumulation.

By definition, acute pancreatitis does not proceed to chronic pancreatic damage or insufficiency, and those patients who recover from the acute episode have normal pancreatic function. There is sound experimental work that supports this clinical observation (Fitzgerald et al., 1966). Regeneration appears to commence in the pancreatic ductules, following which there is restoration of acinar tissue and the islets of Langerhans (Tiscornia, 1966).

CLINICAL FEATURES

Acute pancreatitis can occur at any age. In younger patients, when a cause can be identified, the aetiology may be mumps, or round worm infestation (Stein, 1963), or corticosteroid therapy (Riemenschneider et al., 1968). The sex distribution appears to depend on the recognisable aetiology: biliary tract pancreatitis is more common in women; alcoholic pancreatitis is more common in men.

The classic presentation of acute pancreatitis is acute abdominal pain, vomiting, shock, and collapse. Pain is severe, steady, and boring in nature, and at times it is excruciatingly severe. Rarely, the pain is described as a colic. The pain is usually felt in the epigastrium or to the right or left of the midline in the upper abdomen. Characteristically, it radiates through the abdomen to be felt in midline posteriorly in the region of T 6-12. The pain may be relieved by sitting upright and leaning forward, although it is frequently so profound that the patient is unable to obtain relief by any mechanism other than large doses of potent analgesics. There may be diffuse generalised abdominal discomfort. In the moderately severe episode, the pain will last for a few days and then gradually subside within

a week. Marks and Bank (1963) have stressed that the relationship of the pain to alcohol may be somewhat obscured by a delay of 12 to 48 hours from the time of ending a bout of drinking to the onset of the pain: "the afternoon after the night before."

Accompanying the pain are nausea and vomiting, which may be marked; hiccough; and constipation.

Physical examination reveals varying degrees of shock, with cold clammy extremities, tachycardia, and hypotension. In more severe inflammation, there is peripheral circulatory collapse and cyanosis. The patient is usually febrile, although a temperature greater than 39°C is uncommon. Marked retroperitoneal haemorrhage may manifest as a yellow-brown ecchymosis in the flanks (Grey Turner's sign) or around the umbilicus (Cullen's sign), and this is generally seen within the first week of the illness. Jaundice occurs in about 10 percent of patients and is related to oedema in the head of the pancreas which compresses the bile duct. Other reasons may be an excess bilirubin load on the liver because of the breakdown of the extravasated blood or hepatic dysfunction which is related to hypotension and hypoxia.

On abdominal examination, there is rebound tenderness which may be localised to the upper abdomen or more generally demonstrated. Signs of an ileus are usually present. Board-like rigidity is uncommon, so that in up to 20 percent of patients it may be possible to detect a vague pancreatic mass. Ascites, which may or may not be blood-stained, may develop. Pulmonary signs are relatively common and include atelectasis and a small pleural effusion at the left lung base. T wave changes will be found on the electrocardiogram in about a quarter of the patients (Pollock, 1959).

Trapnell (1972) has stressed that there may be a disparity between the severity of the pain and the character of the physical signs so that the symptoms are out of proportion to the degree of the signs. The presentation may vary according to duration of the illness: initially, there is mainly upper abdominal pain, but after a few days this becomes generalised and there will be abdominal distention and vomiting. In 5 percent of patients, the course of the disease is painless and the presentation is mainly one of profound shock and a paralytic ileus (Dooner and Aliaga, 1965).

The frequency of the various clinical features of acute pancreatitis in 90 patients who were reviewed in a French series (Sarles et al., 1965) is given below:

Features	Frequency (percent)
Pain	100
Pain referred to the back	54
Vomiting	67
Paralytic ileus	58
Dyspnoea	10
Shock	44
Transient hypertension	13
Temperature exceeding 38°C	60
Meteorism	72
Moderate guarding	49
Rigidity	15
Jaundice	17

LABORATORY DIAGNOSIS

Serum amylase. The demonstration of an elevation in the serum amylase concentration is the test that is most widely used in the diagnosis of acute pancreatitis. The rise occurs within 2 to 12 hours of the onset of the inflammation and returns to normal by the end of the first week. Normal values will depend on the laboratory, but values up to 400 Somogyi units per 100 ml are normal for many laboratories, and concentrations greater than 1,000 units per 100 ml suggest the diagnosis of pancreatitis (Mc-Gowan and Wills, 1964). The serum amylase can be elevated from nonpancreatic disorders (see below), and therefore it is only when the values are fivefold elevated that they can be regarded as strongly supportive of a diagnosis of acute pancreatitis. The amylase reaches the bloodstream via the lymphatics and the enzyme is cleared in the kidneys. Although the circulating amylase in pancreatitis arises from the pancreas, it is probable that under normal conditions the serum and urinary amylase is of hepatic origin (Nothman and Callow, 1971). Significant quantities of amylase are also found in the salivary glands, liver, kidney, heart, intestines, muscle, and adipose tissue.

Prolonged elevation of the serum amylase beyond the first week of the illness suggests that the inflammation is persisting, or that a pseudocyst has developed. Renal failure is another cause for persistently raised serum amylase concentrations (Ebbesen and Schönebeck, 1967; Adams et al., 1968). The binding of amylase in the serum to a 7S globulin forms a macromolecular complex which is too large to be excreted in the urine. Such "macroamylase" molecules are a rare cause of hyperamylasaemia and may be recognised by the association of elevated serum amylase levels which are unaccompanied by amylasuria (Wilding et al., 1969).

The serum amylase concentrations may be elevated in a great number of clinical states other than pancreatitis, and this is a cause of much confusion. As a general rule, the higher the amylase level the greater the probability of pancreatitis. Serum amylase elevations have been recorded in mumps, viral hepatitis, ectopic pregnancy, renal failure, perforation of an abdominal viscus, and acute mesenteric thrombosis. Drugs such as morphine and its derivatives, which produce spasm of the sphincter of Oddi, may be responsible for mild and transient enzyme elevations.

Urinary amylase excretion. Elevated urinary amylase levels may be used to make the diagnosis of acute pancreatitis, but this investigation has never found favour. The rapid clearance of amylase into the urine may cause an elevated urinary concentration at a time when the serum concentration is normal, and for this reason the estimation of urinary amylase has been recommended in the diagnosis of pancreatitis. The difficulty of collecting urine samples from sick patients, the accurate timing of such samples, and the problem of impaired renal function in the acutely ill patient all serve to reduce the clinical value of this test. It is possible to measure the hourly rate of amylase excretion in the urine, but this is elevated in gastrointestinal disorders other than pancreatitis. It is therefore unlikely that, taken on its own, the urinary amylase estimation has any advantage over serum amylase measurements except in the diagnosis of very mild pancreatitis when the serum levels may be normal, and in the diagnosis of macroamylasaemia (Waller and Ralston, 1971).

Amylase in other body fluids. Raised levels of amylase can be demonstrated in the pleural effusion or ascites, which may accompany pancreatitis. This is often of much diagnostic value, particularly as the elevated concentrations of the enzyme may persist for longer in the effusion than in the serum.

Serum lipase. The highest lipolytic activity in the body is to be found in the pancreas and therefore the determination of the serum lipase concentration has been used in the diagnosis of acute pancreatitis. Up to now, the routine estimation of the serum lipase activity has been laborious, but a newer continuous method for the determination of serum levels of the enzyme offers a simpler alternative, and experience with the test has been encouraging (Rick, 1972). In acute pancreatitis, the serum lipase concentration may be elevated more consistently and for longer periods than either the serum or the urinary amylase values. The enzyme also has the advantage that it does not have extrapancreatic causes for its elevation.

Other serum enzymes. A great variety of pancreatic enzymes may be detected in the blood of patients with acute pancreatitis. These include phospholipase, elastase, ribonuclease, deoxyribonuclease, and carboxypeptidase, but they have little diagnostic advantage over amylase and trypsin. It is usually not possible to find circulating activated trypsin or chymotrypsin in the blood of patients with pancreatitis.

Other biochemical changes. A variety of haematological and biochemical changes may be demonstrated in acute pancreatitis. No single test is of itself diagnostic, but taken together with the other alterations, the biochemical features amount to a recognisable syndrome. Mild leucocytosis and anaemia are frequent. Serum bilirubin levels are minimally elevated in up to 50 percent of patients, as is the serum alkaline phosphatase. Increased concentrations are more likely when there is a biliary cause for the pancreatitis. The serum calcium values are usually reduced, and this has been related to presence of fat necrosis and the formation of calcium soaps in the tissues. Hypocalcaemia is such a constant feature of the acute inflammatory episode that it has been claimed that if the serum calcium values remain within the normal range in a patient with acute pancreatitis, associated hyperparathyroidism must be suspected. Hyperglycaemia

occurs in about one-third of patients. The presence of methaemalbumin in the serum suggests that the pancreatitis is of the haemorrhagic variety.

RADIOLOGICAL DIAGNOSIS

There are a variety of signs which may be seen singly or in combination on the plain film of the abdomen, which is frequently of help in making the diagnosis (Guien, 1972). Thus, a local ileus may be demonstrated in a loop of small bowel overlying the pancreas ("sentinel loop"), or less commonly the ileus is seen in the transverse colon ("colon cut-off sign"); a more generalised ileus may be present. There may be loss of the psoas shadow. None of these signs is specific for the diagnosis of acute pancreatic inflammation, but it is claimed that a mottled radiotranslucent appearance in the abdomen is characteristic of fat necrosis and is due to normal fat being intermingled with areas of water density (Berenson et al., 1971). Calcification may be seen in and around the pancreas. The presence of gallstones may be noted on the plain x-ray.

A chest radiograph is suggestive of pancreatitis in about 25 percent of patients. There is linear basal atelectasis, elevation of the diaphragm, and a left-sided pleural effusion. The bones may show the radiological features of fat necrosis such as osteolytic lesions, which later become sclerotic and calcified. The changes are most commonly encountered in the femur and tibia.

Barium studies are not always possible in the acutely ill patient. If the patient can tolerate a barium meal, it may be possible to demonstrate an expanded duodenal loop, a deformed duodenal, cap, and an oedematous medial wall of the duodenum. Unfortunately the conventional barium study is notoriously inaccurate. The introduction of hypotonic duodenography has enabled a more accurate assessment to be made of disease in the head of the pancreas. The technique may be performed if the clinical state of the patient is satisfactory. The radiological signs are oedema, stiffening, straightening, and rigidity of the medial wall of the duodenum (Bilbao et al., 1967). Angiography is of little diagnostic value in acute pancreatitis (Aakhus et al., 1969).

There is seldom an indication for performing tests of pancreatic function in patients with acute pancreatitis. Either direct or indirect stimulation of the acutely inflamed gland is potentially hazardous and such tests should not be contemplated. Pancreatic scanning using ^{75}Se selenomethionine is of limited value in the diagnosis, although the pancreatic scan may be used to obtain an indication that synthetic and excretory capacity of the gland have returned to normal once the acute inflammatory process has subsided (Bouchier et al., 1972).

CLINICAL VARIANTS

Acute pancreatitis may present with a number of unusual clinical features.

Extrapancreatic Fat Necrosis

Areas of necrosis in the subcutaneous adipose tissue may occur in the legs and less frequently over the arms and trunk. There are tender red nodules which are adherent over the skin with the characteristic histology of necrotic fat rimmed by haemophilic material. The areas of fat necrosis must be distinguished clinically from nodular panniculitis (Weber-Christian disease), erythema nodosum, periarteritis nodosa, and allergic vasculitis. Periarticular fat necrosis may cause polyarthritis; fat necrosis in the bone marrow may be painless, or present as acutely painful osteolytic lesions or chronic intramedullary calcification (Banks and Janowitz, 1969).

Gastrointestinal Bleeding

Occasionally gastrointestinal haemorrhage may be the major symptom of acute pancreatitis while the pain is only moderate or minimal. Bleeding may be a manifestation of an associated chronic peptic ulcer but the other causes include alcoholic gastritis, salicylate erosions, and the Mallory-Weiss syndrome (Marks et al., 1967).

Profound hypocalcaemia causes marked *tetany*. The pancreas may be so severely damaged that *diabetic ketotic coma* domi-

nates the clinical picture. *Hyperlipidaemia* may be prominent and the hyperlipaemic serum may interfere with the estimation of the serum amylase so that apparently normal serum levels are obtained. The hyperlipidaemia is usually of the Type V variety. It is generally accepted that the increased blood lipid values are a secondary phenomenon and may reflect damage to the α-cells of the islets of Langerhans. Another explanation is that there is inhibition of lipoprotein lipase activity. *Abnormalities of coagulation* occur with prolongation of the whole-blood clotting time and prothrombin time, and a decrease of fibrinogen and factors II, VII, and IX. This may be a reflection of the proteolytic activities of circulating enzymes (Greipp et al., 1972). These changes rarely give rise to clinical problems of haemostasis. A rare complication is *acute renal failure*.

DIFFERENTIAL DIAGNOSIS

It will be apparent from the foregoing that it is necessary to consider a large number of abdominal and extra-abdominal conditions in the differential diagnosis of acute pancreatitis. Other important causes of acute abdominal pain include perforation of a peptic ulcer, acute cholecystitis, mesenteric vascular disease, acute appendicitis, intestinal obstruction, and a ruptured abdominal viscus. Extra-abdominal diseases that can cause diagnostic confusion are myocardial infarction, basal pneumonia, porphyria, and primary hyperlipidaemic syndromes, particularly of the Type I variety.

Once the diagnosis has been established, it is necessary to determine the underlying cause for the pancreatitis. The patient is questioned about alcohol intake, and radiology of the biliary tract is performed once the clinical condition is satisfactory. The patient must be assessed for abnormalities of calcium and lipid metabolism.

THERAPY

It is generally agreed that the management of a patient in whom a reasonably certain diagnosis of acute pancreatitis has been made will be nonsurgical.

Fluid Replacement

The first step is to restore the blood volume and attend to any imbalance of the body electrolytes. Most patients require intravenous fluid, and normal saline is the most appropriate. In hypovolaemia and shock, 6 to 8 litres may be required within the first 24 hours; the rapid administration of large volumes of fluid is made much safer if the central venous pressure is monitored by an appropriately sited catheter. Dextran and plasma are recommended as plasma volume expanders if the hypovolaemia is severe. A blood transfusion is indicated when there is anaemia, and this may only become apparent once the patient has been rehydrated and any haemoconcentration reversed. Potassium and calcium supplements are administered in doses according to the severity of the depletion. Disturbances of glucose metabolism will require soluble insulin, which is administered on a sliding scale according to the urinary or blood sugar. Acute renal failure or diabetic ketosis will require appropriate therapeutic measures.

Relief of Pain

Adequate analgesia is provided once the diagnosis has been established. Morphine and its derivatives are contraindicated because of the hazard of inducing spasm of the sphincter of Oddi. Meperidine hydrochloride is of much value, in doses of 50 to 100 mg by intramuscular injection; pentazocine hydrochloride 30 to 60 mg by intramuscular injection is another potent analgesic. The pain may be controlled by including a small dose of a sedative or tranquilising agent.

Suppression of Pancreatic Function

It seems reasonable to attempt to rest the inflamed gland, and the pancreatic metabolic activity can be reduced by gastric suction and by the administration of anticholinergic agents. Oral feeding is withheld and gastric suction instituted; the appropriate replacements are made in the fluid and electrolytes. Not only does this reduce the amount of pancreatic stimulation and secretion, but nasogastric suction is also required should there be an ileus. Most authors recommend the use of atropine or atropine-like agents to reduce the secretory activity, but Trapnell (1972) has argued against this practice. Drugs frequently used include atropine sulphate 0.25 to 2.00 mg by intramuscular injection or propantheline bromide 30.0 mg by intramuscular injection. Oral anticholinergic agents are introduced once the patient is taking food by mouth.

After the attack has subsided and there is minimal pain, the patient is given a light diet.

Antibiotics

Many authorities recommend the use of a broad-spectrum antibiotic in order to reduce the risk of developing a pancreatic abscess or pseudopancreatic cyst.

Enzyme Inhibitors

An antienzyme preparation, Trasylol, which is effective against typsin, chymotrypsin, and kallikrein, has been assessed in the management of acute pancreatitis. The initial reports, which were based on experimental work, were promising, but clinical experience with the agent has been disappointing and its use is not recommended (Baden et al., 1969).

Other Agents

The observation that carbonic anhydrase inhibitors reduce pancreatic secretion suggested their use in acute pancreatitis. Anderson and Copass (1966) recommended *acetazolamide,* 1 g daily in divided doses for 2 weeks, to be followed by a gradual reduction in the dose so that therapy is discontinued after 3 to 4 weeks. *Antacids* are often advised once the patient is being fed orally, but there is no good evidence that they have any beneficial effect. *Radiation therapy* has been recommended but is not in general use. The doses are determined by the severity of the inflammation. Single daily doses of 50, 100, and 150 R are given to a total of 300 to 550 R. If the signs persist, a further brief course of radiation may be given (Wachtfeidl and Vitez, 1968). *Hypo-thermia* has also found favour with some authors Rodenberg and Conger, 1967). *Peritoneal dialysis* has been recommended. Recently, the observation has been made that *glucagon* therapy may benefit patients with acute pancreatitis. The physiological justification for its use is the known depressant effect which this hormone has on the rate, flow, and enzyme concentration of pancreatic secretions. Glucagon is infused intravenously at the rate of 1 mg over six hours, and preliminary observations suggest that this is accompanied by marked relief of pain (Knight et al., 1971). Further work is required to assess the value of glucagon in acute pancreatitis.

Once the patient has recovered from the acute episode, an assessment is made of the probable cause of the inflammation. Biliary tract radiology and barium studies of the upper gastrointestinal tract are performed; the appropriate biochemical tests are undertaken to exclude a metabolic abnormality. Alcohol is prohibited for 3 to 6 months, but total abstinence is advised if the cause of the pancreatitis is thought to be alcohol. The patient who has recovered does not require any dietary restrictions.

SURGERY

Surgical intervention may be required at any early stage of the disease or once the acute inflammation has subsided. During the acute phase of the illness, it may be necessary to operate for two reasons: if the diagnosis is in doubt or to treat complications. Ideally, the acute inflammatory episode is managed without the need for a laparotomy. The diagnosis, however, is not always apparent, and if there is any doubt, a laparotomy is performed. If the operation is limited and of short duration, there is little extra hazard to the patient. No further procedure is undertaken if the biliary tract is found to be normal (Trapnell, 1972), although drainage of the normal gallbladder has been recommended for severe pancreatitis (Diaco et al., 1969). If gallstones are present in the gallbladder and the patient is not severely ill, a cholecystectomy is performed; if the patient is icteric and gallstones are palpated in the common bile duct, it is necessary to perform a choledochostomy and drainage. If circumstances are unfavourable, a cholecystostomy is probably the safest procedure. There is no indication for any surgical manipulations to the ampulla of Vater in the acute phase of the illness unless a gallstone is present. The place of total pancreatectomy is controversial. Decisions regarding the nature of the operation in acute pancreatitis will depend upon the clinical condition of the patient and the skill and facilities of the surgeon.

The formation of an abscess, haematoma, or pseudocyst during the acute inflammatory phase will necessitate an operation. The procedure should be limited to opening and draining abscesses and haematomas while a pseudocyst is anastomosed to the small intestine.

The ideal time to deal with any disease in the biliary tract or stomach and duodenum is once the patient has fully recovered from the acute episode. Sphincterotomy and sphincteroplasty are not recommended if the patient has experienced only one attack of pancreatitis, particularly if the cause can be recognised and remedied.

COMPLICATIONS

By definition, acute pancreatitis does not lead to a state of chronic pancreatic insufficiency. The patient will be liable to recurrent inflammatory episodes if an underlying cause such as biliary tract disease, alcoholism, or hyperparathyroidism is not corrected. About 20 percent of patients in whom no cause can be recognised will go on to have *relapsing acute pancreatitis*.

Complications occurring during the acute stage include abscesses, pseudocyst, haematemesis, duodenal ileus, burst abdomen, and toxic psychosis (Trapnell, 1971). Some patients have more than one complication, and this adds to the diagnostic difficulties and increases the mortality rate. *Pancreatic abscess* is the most common and serious complication, and it usually develops during the first 21 days after the onset of the illness. The diagnosis is suggested by abdominal and back pain, tenderness, and abdominal mass, swinging fever, leucocytosis, prolonged elevation of the serum amylase level, and the radiological sign of gas in the abscess cavity. A *pancreatic pseudocyst* is also a relatively frequent complication and represents the collection of fluid in the lesser sac. This manifests during the second to fourth weeks of the illness as abdominal pain, a mass, and persistent hyperamylasaemia. The barium meal will show elevation of the stomach with anterior displacement and a widened duodenal loop, and angiography demonstrates stretching of the pancreatic vessels over an avascular mass. *Duodenal obstruction* is recognised by severe vomiting during the 10- to 15-day period. It is usually associated with persistent inflammation or a pancreatic abscess. The patient requires nasogastric suction and intravenous feeding. *Toxic psychosis* occurs within 1 to 3 days of the onset of the illness, and in some patients it may represent acute alcohol withdrawal syndromes. Persistent *diabetes mellitus* is surprisingly uncommon after an acute inflammatory episode and no doubt reflects the capacity of the gland to regenerate. Acute renal failure, prolonged tetany, and widespread panniculitis and other complications.

PROGNOSIS

Acute pancreatitis is associated with a mortality rate of 23 to 26 percent (Pollock, 1959; Trapnell, 1972). The mortality rate in a mild attack is less than 5 percent, whereas in severe fulminating acute haemorrhagic pancreatitis the mortality rate may rise to 33 percent or greater. An indication that the prognosis may be unfavourable is given by the following:

1. The presence of methaemalbuminaemia
2. Severe shock and cyanosis
3. Marked and persistent reduction in the serum calcium concentration to below 8.0 mg per 100 ml
4. The presence of Grey Turner's or Cullen's sign
5. Acute painless pancreatitis

The mortality rate is greater in the aged, and may be as high as 68 percent when there is associated cardiovascular disease. Pancreatitis in the diabetic patient is a grave disease. The presence during the first few weeks of the illness of any of the complications outlined above increases the mortality rate to between 40 and 50 percent.

Acute pancreatitis is an important cause of morbidity and mortality in many parts of the world. In the present inadequate state of our knowledge regarding the aetiology and pathogenesis of the condition, treatment remains unsatisfactory and there are a number of areas of uncertainty and controversy which remain to be resolved.

REFERENCES

Aakhus, T., Hofsli, M., and Vestad, E., Acta Radiol. 8:119, 1969.
Adams, J. T., Libertino, J. A., and Schwartz, S. I., Surgery 63:877, 1968.
Anderson, M. C., and Copass, M. K., Am. J. Dig. Dis. 11:367, 1966.
Anderson, M. C., Needleman, S. B., Gramatica, L., Toranto, I. R., and Briggs, D. R., Arch. Surg. 99:185, 1969.
Baden, H., Jordal, K., Lund, F., and Zachariae, F., Scand. J. Gastroenterol. 4:291, 1969.
Bank, P. A., and Janowitz, H. D., Gastroenterology 56:601, 1969.
Bartholomew, C., Br. Med. J. 1:666, 1970.
Berenson, J., Spitz, H. B., and Felson, B., Radiology 100:567, 1971.
Bilbao, M. K., Frische, L. H., Dotter, C. T., and Rösch, J., Radiology 89:438, 1967.
Bouchier, I. A. D., Youngs, G. R., and Agnew, J. E., Clin. Gastroenterol. 1:105, 1972.
Creutzfeldt, W., and Schmidt, H., Scand. J. Gastroenterol. (Suppl. 6):47, 1970.
Diaco, J. F., Miller, L. D., and Copeland, E. M., Surg. Gynecol. Obstet. 129:263, 1969.
Dooner, H. P., and Aliaga, C., Arch. Int. Med. 116:828, 1965.
Ebbesen, K. E., and Schönbeck, Acta Chir. Scand. 133:61, 1967.
Fitzgerald, P. J., Carol, B. M., and Rosenstock, L., Nature (Lond.) 212:594, 1966.
Greipp, P. R., Brown, J. A., and Gralnick, H. R., Ann. Int. Med. 76:73, 1972.
Guien, C., Clin. Gastroenterol. 1:61, 1972.
Hand, B., Br. J. Hosp. Med. October, 8, 1968.
Hansson, K., Acta Chir. Scand. Suppl. 375, 1967.
Knight, M. J., Condon, J. R., and Smith, R., Br. Med. J. 2:440, 1971.
Leeson, P. M., and Fourman, P., Lancet 1:1185, 1966.
Marks, I. N., and Banks, S., S. Afr. Med. J. 37:1039, 1963.
Marks, I. N., Bank, S., Louw, J. H., and Farman, J., Gut 8:253, 1967.
McCutcheon, A. D., Gut 9:296, 1968.
McGowan, G. K., and Wills, M. R., Br. Med. J. 1:160, 1964.

Nothman, M. M., and Callow, A. D., Gastroenterology 60:82, 1971.

Pollock, A. V., Br. Med. J. 1:6, 1959.

Rick, W., Clin. Gastroenterol. 1:3, 1972.

Riemenschneider, T. A., Wilson, J. F., and Verner, R. H., Paediatrics 41:428, 1968.

Roodenberg, S. A., and Conger, A. B., J.A.M.A. 201: 825, 1967.

Sarles, H., Sarles, J. C., Camatte, R., Muratore, R., Gaini, M., Guien, C., Pastor G., and Leroy, F., Gut 6:545, 1965.

Schmidt, H., and Cruetzfeldt, W., Scand. J. Gastroenterol. 4:39, 1969.

Stein, D., S. Afr. Med. J. 37:1066, 1963.

Storck, G., Acta Chir. Scand. Suppl. 417, 1971.

Tilney, N. L., Collins, J. J., Jr., and Wilson, R. E., N. Engl. J. Med. 274:1051, 1966.

Tiscornia, O. M., Gastroenterology 51:267, 1966.

Trapnell, J., Ann. R. Coll. Surg. 49:361, 1971.

Trapnell, J., Clin. Gastroenterol. 1:147, 1972.

Wachtfeidl, V., and Vitez, M., Am. J. Surg. 116:853, 1968.

Waller, S. L., and Ralston, A. J., Gut 12:878, 1971.

Wilding, P., Geokus, M. C., Haverback, B. J., and Stanworth, D. R., Am. J. Med. 47:492, 1969.

37

PANCREATIC CYSTS AND FISTULAS

RODNEY MAINGOT

HISTORICAL NOTE

Morgagni, in 1761, was the first to describe pancreatic cysts observed at autopsy. Cleason (1842) gave a good account of the pathology of these tumours.

The first operation for pancreatic cyst was carried out by Le Dentu (*Bull. Soc. Anat. Paris* 40:197, 1865). He performed *external drainage* of a large pseudocyst. His patient died of peritonitis. Lucke and Klebs (*Arch. Path. Anat. 41*:1, 1867) likewise drained a cyst, with fatal results. The first successful operation for pancreatic cyst was recorded by Bozeman (*Med. Rec. 21*:46, 1882), who *excised* the cyst.

Gussenbauer (*Arch. Klin. Chir. 29*:355, 1883) suggested and practised the operation of *marsupialization* which, subsequently, had few supporters. Umberdan (1911) was the first to report the procedure on *internal drainage*. In his case he anastomosed a cyst of the head of the pancreas to the duodenum. The patient died a few days later. Jedlicka (*Zbl. Chir. 50*:132, 1923) was the first surgeon to perform *cystogastrostomy;* Hahn, shortly afterwards, carried out and popularised the operation of *cystojejunostomy.*

The transgastric technique of *pancreatocysto-gastrostomy* was first described by Jurasz (*Arch. Klin. Chir. 164*:272, 1931). The passing years have proved that Jurasz's operation is a safe and effective surgical remedy for the majority of clinically encountered pancreatic cysts.

Warren and Baker [26] write:

When one takes into account the facts that pancreatic cysts vary in etiology, in size, in location and anatomical relationships, that inflammatory reaction may or may not be associated, that cysts may be solitary or multiple, benign or malignant, and that they afflict individuals who vary in their capacity to withstand complicated surgical procedures, it does not seem reasonable that all pancreatic cysts, or even the majority of them can best be treated by any single procedure.

PANCREATIC CYSTS

Classification

Pancreatic cysts may be classified as follows:

1. True Cysts
   a. Congenital
      Single or multiple cysts confined solely to the pancreas.
      Simple cysts of the pancreas associated with multiple cysts in other organs—polycystic disease.
      Fibrocystic disease (mucoviscidosis).
      Dermoid cysts.
   b. Acquired
      Retention cysts.
      Parasitic cysts.
      Neoplastic cysts: cystadenoma, cystadenocarcinoma, cystic teratoma, and unusual tumours.
2. Pseudocyst
   Postinflammatory.
   Post-traumatic: following penetrating and nonpenetrating wounds of the abdomen;

operative injuries to the pancreas during the performance of certain abdominal operations, such as splenectomy, partial or subtotal gastrectomy, exploration of the bile ducts or pancreatic duct, etc.
3. Secondary to obstructing carcinoma
4. Idiopathic

True Cysts

Congenital cysts of the pancreas.
Inclusion cysts. These arise from faulty fusion of ductal elements. They are encountered rarely and are usually small and symptomless.
Dermoid cysts.[5]
Cysts associated with polycystic disease of the kidney and other organs.
Fibrocystic disease of the pancreas. This is a familial disorder of the exocrine glands usually appearing in infancy and childhood, with signs and symptoms predominantly gastrointestinal and respiratory in nature.

Great credit is due to the pioneer work of Dorothy Anderson who, in 1938, reported a series of 49 cases of fibrocystic disease of the pancreas, collected from the literature and from the autopsy files of the Babies Hospital in New York (*Am. J. Dis. Child.* 56:344, 1938). Her classic contributions to this subject (*Am. J. Dis. Child.* 69:221, 1945; *Proc. R. Soc. Med.* 42:25, 1949; *Ann. N.Y. Acad. Sci.* 93:500, 1962) should be carefully studied by those who are called upon to treat such cases.
She wrote: Our knowledge of cystic fibrosis of the pancreas has progressed to a point where a clinical diagnosis can be made early in the disease. *Response to a combination of dietary therapy and chemotherapy depends on the sensitivity of the infecting bacteria to available chemotherapeutic agents and on the stage of the pulmonary lesion when therapy is begun.* Early diagnosis and therapy lead to an improved prognosis, and may result in freedom from respiratory infection, at least for the span of years over which observation has been possible. The urgent unsolved problem is the discovery of the cause of the respiratory infection. There is strong presumptive evidence that it is due to specific nutritional deficiency (1949).
Matheson (*Br. Med. J.* 2:206, 1949) described seven cases seen in one hospital between June 1947 and September 1948. This amounted to 2 percent of the medical admissions to the children's ward during that period. The evidence strongly suggests that the disease is inherited and Matheson considers that inheritance may be explained by incomplete dominance. Priestley and ReMine (*Surg. Clin. North Am.* 38:1313, 1958) stated that the fundamental changes responsible for this condition have not been clearly estab-

lished, but currently it is considered to be evidence of *"generalised mucoviscidosis,"* which also involves other exocrine glands. The reader is referred to two excellent editorial articles (*J.A.M.A.* 135:717, 1947; and *Br. Med. J.* 2:1462, 1949); to the monograph *Fibrocystic Disease of the Pancreas* by Martin Bodian (1953); to the instructive survey in the *Lancet* (2:955, 1959); and to the contribution by Thomaidis and Arey (*Am. J. Path.* 43:42a, 1963); and to that most learned and fully documented paper on *Cystic Fibrosis of the Pancreas: A Generalised Disturbance of Water and Electrolyte Movement in Exocrine Tissues,* which was published in *Lancet* 1:445, 1968.
Taken as a whole, *congenital cysts* of the pancreas occur only infrequently. They may be small, and be single or multiple. They do not ordinarily cause any symptoms or disturbance of the function of the pancreas, but they may on occasion give rise to a painless, tense, and circumscribed swelling in the epigastrium.

Frequency

Pancreatic cysts are rare. Piper et al.[16] reported that only 298 cases were seen at the Mayo Clinic over a 51-year period (1907 to 1958). Howard and Jordan [11] collected 151 cases of pancreatic cysts from a total of over 2 million hospital admissions in the United States—a frequency of 0.007 percent!
Approximately 2 percent of abdominal wounds involve some type of injury to the pancreas and inflammatory pseudocysts follow in about 15 percent of such injuries. Nonpenetrating wounds and acute pancreatitis are the commonest causes of pseudocysts, and such cysts comprise the great majority of pancreatic cysts.
Warren et al.[27] reported cysts in 25 percent of patients (at the Lahey Clinic) requiring operation for pancreatitis. In Piper's Mayo Clinic series of 298 patients, there were 36 with cystadenocarcinoma and 20 with cystadenoma. Neoplastic cysts account for about 15 percent of all cysts of the organ. Rarely, a teratomatous cyst or a cystic haemangioendothelioma will be encountered at operation.
Acquired cysts. *Retention cysts.* These may be unilocular or multilocular, they have a communication with the duct, and they are caused by any condition which obstructs the pancreatic ducts, such as chronic relapsing pancreatitis, stone, or tumour.
According to Priestley and ReMine,[18] they do not as a rule form acute or complete

obstruction of the duct of Wirsung, but more likely arise in association with a gradually developing partial obstruction.

They may be small and circumscribed (rare), or they may form a baggy cystic mass which distends the whole gland and eventually produces a fibrotic degenerative process in the encasing parenchymal tissues.

Starting within the pancreas, they may extend beyond the gland and present in a variety of positions depending upon their original site of origin and upon local anatomical relationships. In the majority of cases, these retention cysts contain relatively clear pancreatic juice in which all the pancreatic enzymes are found.

They possess a lining of epithelial cells, unless protracted intracystic pressure has resulted in flattening out these cells so that they are no longer recognisable on serial microscopic sections. The wall of the cyst (which often contains a jejune encrustation of pancreatic substance) is usually well defined from adjacent structures.

Pseudocysts of the Pancreas

Aetiology. *These cysts are unquestionably the most common type of cystic lesion that the surgeon finds associated with the pancreas.*

A *false cyst* is caused by the encapsulation of extravasated blood and pancreatic fluid in the peripancreatic cellular tissues or, rarely, in the lesser peritoneal sac. About 30 percent of the cases are due to injury and follow a severe blow to the epigastrium which causes contusion, fracture, or laceration of the pancreas and of the posterior peritoneal layer of the lesser sac. The pancreatic secretions and blood escape into the retroperitoneal tissues around and sometimes above or below the pancreas. The foramen of Winslow may be sealed by inflammatory exudates, and the peritoneum become thickened around the effusion, encapsulation thus being produced.

Cases of pseudocyst not infrequently complicate an attack or repeated attacks of acute pancreatitis. They are also observed following a number of operations, which include drainage of the omental bursa in cases of acute pancreatic necrosis, drainage of a localised pancreatic abscess, pancreatolithotomy, caudal pancreatectomy plus splenectomy

(alone or combined with pancreatojejunostomy), pancreatoduodenectomy (for cancer of the periampullary area and of the head of the pancreas, and, also, for relapsing pancreatitis), and gastroduodenal resection for destructive lesions which penetrate or are found firmly adherent to the gland, e.g., gastric and duodenal ulcer and malignant gastric lesions.

The role of acute and chronic relapsing pancreatitis as an aetiological agent has been emphasised by Waugh and Lynn.[30]

Warren et al.[28] stated that of 148 patients undergoing surgery for cysts of the pancreas, approximately 50 percent had pseudocysts. The operative mortality rate was 2.7 percent.

In a more recent contribution, Warren et al.[29] write:

The pancreatic cysts are classified etiologically as: (1) inflammatory, 140—79 pseudocysts and 61 retention cysts; (2) traumatic, 15; (3) neoplastic, 18—8 cystadenomas and 10 cystadenocarcinomas; (4) retention cyst secondary to malignant tumors of pancreas, 10; and (5) miscellaneous cysts, 2—1 in aberrant pancreas and 1 angiocyst.
Pseudocysts are often associated with an attack of acute pancreatitis, while *retention cysts are often associated with chronic pancreatitis.*

In the series of 58 cases reported by Waugh and Lynn, 37 patients presented histories compatible with recurrent episodes of acute pancreatitis; 12 were found to have pathological conditions of the biliary tract at the time of operation; 11 were chronic alcoholics; 6 related the onset of their symptoms to an episode of severe nonpenetrating trauma to the abdomen; and there was nothing significant in the histories of 3 patients to suggest a cause for the development of a pancreatic pseudocyst.

The condition is more common in men than in women, the ratio being 2:1; the majority of patients are between the ages of 30 and 70 at the time of operation. In Waugh's series of 58 cases of pseudocyst, 35 of the patients were men and 23 were women, and nearly 50 percent of the patients were between 30 and 60 years of age. It should be noted here that in cases of cystadenoma the female-to-male ratio is 9:1.

The incidence of pancreatic pseudocyst in childhood is low. Beltex et al.[3] found 44 instances reported in the literature and added 2 of their own. Except for the 2 reported patients, no others were seen during a 16-year period at the pediatric hospitals at Zurich and Bern. The most common causes of pseudocyst in childhood are blunt trauma and acute haemorrhagic pancreatitis.

A swelling or mass may form within a few days or it may be weeks or even months before a noticeable tumour appears. Pseudocysts vary considerably in size. They may be small, measuring not more than 2 inches (5 cm) in diameter, or they may be as large as a football or as a human head. The wall may be thin or thick, its lining may be smooth, and septa may be present. Rarely is the cyst multilocular.

The fluid contained in these cysts is alkaline in reaction, of medium or low specific gravity, and when analysed is found to contain albumen, mucin, cholesterin, blood cells, and a little necrotic tissue. It may be clear or may be light brown or pale green in colour, or, again, it may be cloudy with pus cells (abscess). One or more ferments may be present, but in long-standing cysts ferments are not found, or, if present, they are inert. The absence of ferments appears to be of relatively little value in confirming or excluding the diagnosis of pancreatic cyst.

Pseudocysts are most frequently found in the region of the body or tail of the gland, and nearly all of them occupy the retroperitoneal space in the vicinity of the pancreas itself or farther afield.

A pseudocyst may bulge between the stomach and liver, protrude between the transverse colon and the stomach, below the transverse colon, or be lodged in one of the left subphrenic spaces or in the left flank. At times it will either merely push the stomach forward, or else strip the leaves of the mesocolon as it expands, or again it may insinuate itself into the root of the mesentery of the small intestine.

Diagnosis. The taking of a careful history is of great value, as a record of trauma may be obtained in about 30 percent of the cases or the survey may reveal one or more *severe attacks of epigastric pain* suggestive of recurrent pancreatitis or repeated attacks of biliary colic. Kehr's sign may be positive, indicating irritation of the diaphragm or pleura. There may also be a history of a previous operation upon the pancreas or of an exploratory laparotomy

for some acute upper-abdominal catastrophe. While the cyst is slowly expanding, the symptoms may be vague. There is usually a sensation of fullness after meals, or a dull ache may be felt above the umbilicus, while flatulence, anorexia, dyspepsia, nausea, and vomiting are commonly noted. *Epigastric pain is the most common symptom of pancreatic pseudocyst.* The *pain* is more often referred to the left hypochondrium or to the upper dorsal region—backache—than to the right subcostal region. It is rarely experienced in the lower one-half of the abdomen.

Later on, the expanded cyst may compress the bile duct and lead to *jaundice.* Diabetes mellitus and loss of weight and of strength are frequent symptoms. Diabetes is found in 10 to 15 percent of patients who develop a false pancreatic cyst. Eventually a rounded or oval, nontender tumour is felt in the epigastrium, either in the midline or toward the left side, although sometimes it may extend lower than this. The mass seldom extends below the umbilicus.

Mattson and Mahorner [15] stated that in fully 95 percent of the cases of pseudocyst, the swelling is confined to the epigastrium and that a mass is readily felt in about 75 percent of the cases. Fluctuation may be elicited, but if the cyst is very tense, it may feel like a solid tumour. In the majority of cases the cystic tumour does not move on respiration, although there may be some lateral or vertical movement on palpation.

A diagnosis is often reached following x-ray examinations of the stomach, colon, gallbladder, and kidneys. On *barium-meal x-ray examination* the presence of a widened C-shaped duodenal loop, or a filling defect, distortion, or indentation of the stomach, duodenum, or transverse colon produced by an extrinsic cystic mass in the epigastrium is evidence in support of a presumptive diagnosis of pancreatic cyst (Figs. 1 and 2). Pyelograms may reveal displacement of the kidneys and ureters. On occasion a plain x-ray film may show calcification of the wall of the cyst. Calcification is, however, more frequently observed in cases of cystadenoma of the pancreas. Haukohl and Melamed [9] have reported 2 cases showing calcification, while in Waugh's series, 9 patients had x-ray evidence of calcification.

Briefly, other diagnostic tests include *co-*

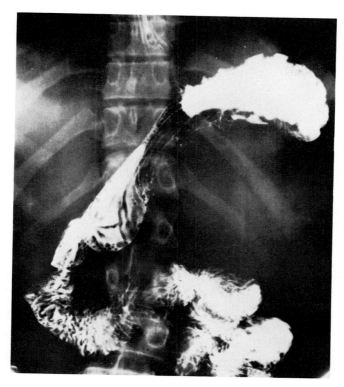

FIG. 1.   Pancreatic cyst. The body of the stomach is displaced upwards and to the right by a large round soft tissue tumour that compresses the greater curve. The duodenojejunal flexure is displaced downwards. (Courtesy of Dr. William Young, Radiology Department, Royal Free Hospital.)

eliac and superior mesenteric arterial angiography (see Chap. 108), duodenography (see Chap. 4C), and the *routine laboratory tests,* especially serum amylase and lipase estimations. *Radioisotope scanning of the pancreas* is discussed later in this chapter. Hyperamylasaemia is observed in about 50 percent of all cases.

Pseudopancreatic cysts may be confused with parasitic and nonparasitic (simple) cysts of the liver, mucocele of the gallbladder, hydronephrosis, mesenteric cysts, omental cysts, cysts of the spleen, cystadenomas or cystadenosarcomas of the pancreas, retroperitoneal cysts and sarcomas, and even ovarian cysts.

The *prognosis* is dependent upon early diagosis and treatment. The clinical course is steadily progressive, and unless the compression and degenerative changes in the gland produced by the cyst are relieved by surgical measures, a fatal outcome owing to rupture of the cyst, peritonitis, or haemorrhage ensues in almost every case.

Types. *Neoplastic cysts.* Neoplastic cysts comprise: (1) cystadenoma; (2) cystadenocarcinoma; (3) cystic haemangioendothelioma; (4) cystic adenocarcinoma of the islets of Langerhans; and (5) cystic non-beta, noninsulin-producing adenoma of pancreatic islet cells (so-called ulcerogenic adenoma of the pancreas).

Neoplastic cysts of the pancreas account for 15 percent of all cysts of the gland. They are cysts—degenerative cysts—associated with benign or malignant tumours of the pancreas. Lichtenstein [14] has given a clear account of the pathology of these cysts and has suggested a useful classification. Kennard,[13] who has done a considerable amount of research work on this subject, collected from the literature 25 cases of malignant pancreatic cysts. He described an interesting case which occurred in his practice. Kennard

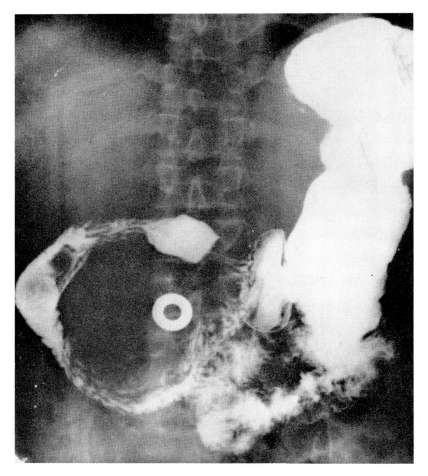

FIG. 2.   Barium-meal x-ray showing a cystadenoma in the head of the pancreas. A metal ring has been placed on the abdomen to mark the site of the palpable abdominal tumour. (From *The London Clinic Medical Journal,* 2:32, 1961. Courtesy of R. Smith.)

considers that true papillary cystadenocarcinoma of the pancreas is an extremely rare pathological lesion. Abeshouse [1] states that neoplastic pancreatic cysts are of the proliferative type. They are usually multilocular and are situated most frequently in the body or tail of the gland. They possess a thick fibrous capsule. The contents are mucoid, occasionally blood-stained, and the irregular papillary projections from the cyst lining are often seen.

Sawyer and his collaborators [20] collected 47 cases of benign cystic adenoma and 29 of malignant cystic adenocarcinoma from the literature. Piper, ReMine, and Priestley,[17] in reporting 20 cases of cystadenoma of the

pancreas, found 100 cases in the literature. Adenocarcinomas of the pancreas (with or without cystic degeneration) are discussed in Chapter 39.

In the absence of a history of trauma, of recurrent attacks of pancreatitis, or of an operative procedure on the gland, neoplasm should be considered as a possible cause of pancreatic cyst.

Rarely do the cystadenomas interfere with either the exocrine or endocrine functions of the gland. Epigastric pain is a rare feature; backache may be present in the late cases; indigestion and loss of weight may be noted; and the tumour is tardy in its growth.

The first sign of neoplastic cysts is frequently a palpable mass in the epigastric area. A barium-meal x-ray examination may prove of some help in diagnosis, as it often indicates the size and position of the cyst by visualising the distorted stomach or colon (Fig. 2). Aortography, selective angiography (Swanson [23]), and scintiscanning (Bouchier [4]) are useful aids in diagnosis.

The *treatment* is wide excision, as for removable malignant disease of the pancreas. In a few cases of cystadenocarcinoma of the *tail* or *body* of the pancreas, an attempt to eradicate the disease should comprise splenectomy, distal pancreatectomy, and partial resection of the stomach when it is adherent to the growth. This radical operation may be completed by: (1) secure closure of the pancreatic duct and stump of the gland or (2) by performing pancreatogastrostomy by the transluminal method of Rodney Smith.[22] In many cases of benign neoplastic cyst, however, splenectomy plus distal (partial) pancreatectomy have been performed with success. (Fig. 3.) When the malignant cystic growth occupies the *head* of the gland and is resectable, pancreatoduodenectomy is the treatment advocated. Radiotherapy and chemotherapy may, however, offer some palliation. (See Chaps. 109 and 111.)

Hydatid cysts of the pancreas. Solitary hydatid cysts of the pancreas are very rare, and few British or American surgeons have ever seen a case.

Anderson and Peebles Brown [2] reported an interesting case in which the cyst communicated with the main pancreatic duct and leaked along it during operation. The cyst was excised and the patient made an excellent recovery. Fitzpatrick (1958) could find only 2 instances of involvement of the pancreas out of 1,802 cases of hydatid disease.

In Greece, during the period 1920 to 1950, among 14,662 cases, Procos et al.[19] were not able to find more than 15 cases in the literature.

Most of the few recorded cases were treated by enucleation, but when the cyst is large and involves the tail or body of the pancreas, distal pancreatectomy (with splenectomy) should be preferred. This subject is discussed by Dr. Kourias, of Athens, in Chapter 55A.

Surgical treatment of pseudopancreatic cysts. Ellison and Carey [7] state that the management of pseudocyst includes a period of close observation and palliative medical measures as the cyst may resolve spontaneously. This allows for the development of a well-defined wall which aids surgical treatment when required.

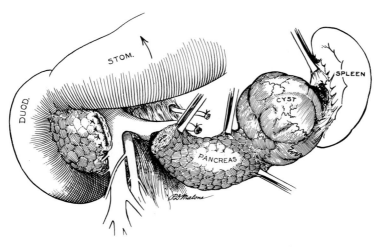

FIG. 3. Splenectomy and distal pancreatectomy with splenectomy for cystadenoma of the tail of the pancreas. (Courtesy of K. W. Warren.)

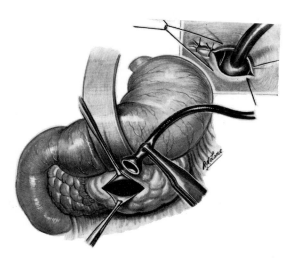

FIG. 4. Simple drainage of a pseudopancreatic cyst with a de Pezzer catheter. (After Cattell and Warren.)

The choice of operation depends upon the size, the nature, the situation, and the type of cyst, as well as upon the general condition of the patient.

Seven types of treatment are available:

1. Simple external drainage.
2. Marsupialization.
3. Internal drainage: cystogastrostomy, cystojejunostomy, and cystoduodenostomy.
4. Excision of the cyst.
5. Resection of the tail and/or body of the pancreas plus splenectomy—to include the entire cyst in the resected specimen. This operation may be completed by *meticulous closure of the pancreatic duct* and surrounding glandular tissue, or by performing pancreatojejunostomy or preferably pancreatogastrostomy.
6. Pancreatoduodenal resection.
7. Transduodenal sphincterotomy combined with the passage of a polyethylene tube or catheter via the pancreatic duct into the cystic cavity. The contents of the cyst are aspirated, after which the distal end of the plastic tube is led into the third portion of the duodenum or to the exterior. The tube acts as an efficient splint and affords free drainage into the bowel.

Simple external drainage. Simple drainage is an effective method of treatment, especially for those pseudocysts which follow nonpenetrating injuries of the pancreas and operative trauma, and also for those which occur after one or more attacks of acute pancreatitis. Again, external tube drainage is advocated for the *inflammatory cyst of recent origin with a poorly developed cyst wall,* when marked infection or an abscess is present and the patient's general condition is poor. Although the recurrence rate is low, a pancreatic fistula may result which may require a further operation.

This method is particularly applicable to cysts situated in the head of the gland or connected with the uncinate process. Cysts in these situations may, however, be treated by transduodenal cystoduodenostomy (see Fig. 7).

I believe that the classic operation of Gussenbauer [8]—pseudocyst *marsupialization*—should rarely be employed. External drainage can be speedily and successfully carried out by aspirating the fluid in the cyst with an Ochsner-Mayo trocar and cannula, after which the cystic cavity is inspected and curetted for the possible presence of new growth. If the cavity does not contain any neoplastic elements, a de Pezzer catheter, a Malecot or Foley catheter is passed through the opening in the cyst wall, which is then securely closed around the catheter, with a

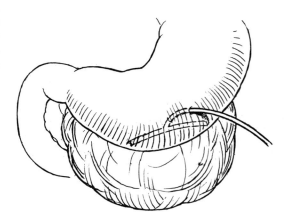

FIG. 5. Transgastric T tube drainage of an infected pancreatic cyst. (From *Lancet*, 2:1063, 1965. Courtesy of R. Smith.)

series of interrupted silk sutures (Fig. 4).

The catheter is next brought through the abdominal wall lateral to the incision and anchored there with an encircling suture of silk. Continuous suction is then applied to the catheter. This procedure obviates the chief objection to marsupialization, i.e., the irritation and erosion of the skin by escaping pancreatic ferments.

Simple drainage yields good results in poor-risk patients and for the types of cases recommended above. In approximately 60 percent of cases, the fistulous tract closes within 1 to 6 months; a further 15 percent persist for 1 to 2 years before "drying up." About 25 percent of the cases treated by simple drainage or marsupialization require further operative procedures.

R. Smith's technique [22] may be employed for the *recently infected pseudocyst* which is attached to the posterior wall of the stomach. In such a case, through a suitably placed gastrotomy incision, a Mayo-Ochsner trocar and cannula are plunged through the posterior wall of the stomach and the cyst contents are removed by suction. The aperture in the posterior wall of the stomach and cyst is slightly enlarged by introducing a finger into the cavity of the cyst, after which a Maingot's guttered T tube is inserted into the cystic cavity and led to the exterior through small stab wounds in the stomach and anterior abdominal wall. The gastrotomy incision is closed by two or three layers of fine silk; the stab wound in the stomach is invaginated with a purse string suture; the puncture spot is securely anchored to the adjacent peritoneum; and the distal end of the tube is fastened to the abdominal wall. Suction should be continued for a few days until no further fluid can be withdrawn. Cystograms can now be taken, at suitable intervals, to ascertain the fate of the cyst. The late results of this simple procedure are gratifying as in some 60 percent of these cases "obliteration" can be demonstrated (Fig. 5).

The operation of *marsupialization* is performed as follows:

Access to the cyst is obtained through a vertical epigastric incision or through an oblique incision which is made over the most prominent portion of the tumour. When the abdomen is opened, it will at once be obvious whether the cyst should be approached through an incision in the gastrohepatic omentum, through the gas-

trocolic ligament, or through the mesocolon. The most prominent portion of the dome of the cyst is brought clearly into view, preferably above the transverse colon, and after the abdominal incision and the area around have been packed off to prevent soiling, two pairs of Allis forceps grasp the cyst wall and steady it to allow a trocar and cannula to be plunged into the cavity. The trocar is withdrawn and the cannula connected to a suction apparatus so that the contents of the cyst can be quickly evacuated with the minimum amount of leakage. The puncture hole made by the trocar is next enlarged with scissors for an inch or so (about 2.5 cm), the margins of the cyst wall are picked up with a number of Allis forceps in order to elevate the cyst; then gauze swabs are introduced into the cavity to mop up any remaining fluid, to break down any multilocular compartments, and to remove any necrotic tissue.

The margins of the cyst wall are then stitched to the peritoneal edges at the lower end of the abdominal incision, after which the edges of the cyst are sutured to the skin itself. Continuous suction is applied to a tube inserted into the sac and precautions are taken to prevent digestion around the lowest portion of the incision in the abdominal wall. According to Ellison and Carey,[7] this operation is especially useful in pseudocysts with thin friable walls, and in patients in whom expedient surgery is necessary. It would be unwise to anastomose a pseudocyst with thin and friable walls to the adjacent stomach or jejunum, as leakage at the site of the anastomosis is a common postoperative sequel.

Internal drainage. During the last 20 years, internal drainage of pseudocysts into

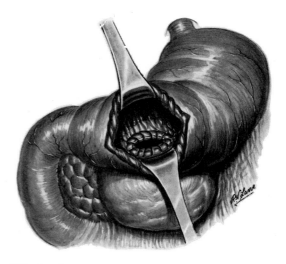

FIG. 6. Transgastric cystogastrostomy. (After Cattell and Warren.)

the proximal gastrointestinal tract (stomach, duodenum, and proximal jejunum) has become increasingly popular.

Cystogastrostomy was employed first by Jedlicka (*Zbl. Chir. 50*:132, 1923); Jurasz (*Arch. Klin. Chir. 164*:272, 1931) was the first to report the technique of transgastric cystogastrostomy; Kirschner (*Beitr. Klin. Chir. 147*:28, 1929) originally drained a cyst of the head of the pancreas by the transduodenal route; Hahn first employed the proximal jejunum for the drainage of pseudocysts (*Zbl. Chir. 54*:585, 1927); while Neuffer (*Arch. Klin. Chir. 170*:488, 1932) performed the first cholecystocystostomy.

Internal drainage by *transgastric cystogastrostomy* is by far the most favoured procedure, and has the weighty support of Judd,[12] Hillis,[10] Warren,[24] and other authorities. It is especially indicated in cases of large thick-walled cysts with little associated pancreatitis.

If internal drainage is to be employed, it can often be performed by *transgastric cystogastrostomy,* as the posterior wall of the stomach is frequently firmly adherent to the pseudocyst. The cyst is approached through a vertical or transverse epigastric incision. An opening is made in the anterior wall of the body of the stomach overlying the dome of the cyst; a trocar and cannula are thrust into the cyst through the adherent posterior wall of the stomach, and the contents of the cyst are evacuated; the puncture hole is enlarged sufficiently to permit a good inspection of the cystic cavity, to break down any septa, and to make sure that no neoplastic tissue is overlooked; the opposing margins of the stomach and cyst wall are sutured together with a continuous lockstitch of 0 silk or cotton in order to keep the stoma widely patent and to control any haemorrhage; the aperture in the anterior wall of the stomach is closed with a continuous (inverting) Connell suture of catgut, followed by a series of interrupted sutures of fine silk; and the abdominal incision is then securely closed by one of the approved methods (Fig. 6). A *large opening* of at least 3 to 4 cm between the posterior wall of the stomach and anterior wall of the cyst should always be constructed.

The immediate and late results are excellent in 80 percent of patients; the postoperative mortality rate is around 3 percent, and convalescence is short—about 10 days. "One might expect the cyst to fill with food and continue to cause difficulty, but most often the cysts have closed down within a few weeks." [12]

Large pseudocysts which occupy the region

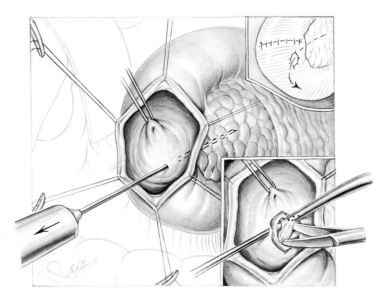

FIG. 7.   Transduodenal cystoduodenostomy for a pseudocyst of the head of the pancreas.

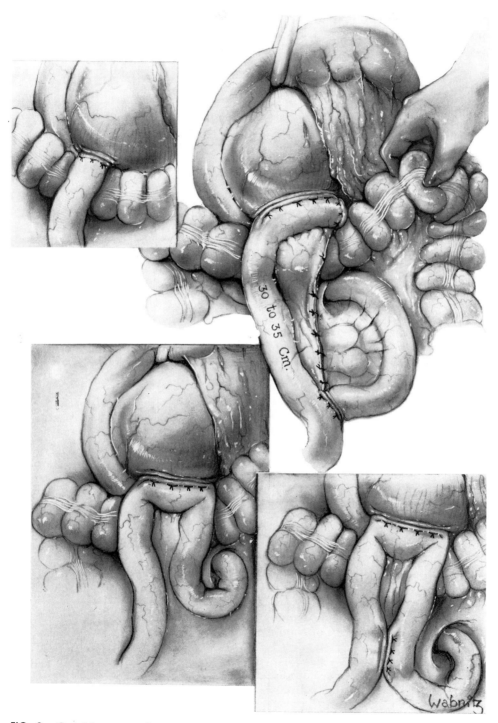

FIG. 8.   Cystojejunostomy for a pseudopancreatic cyst, illustrating Roux-en-Y method and the simple loop method with or without enteroanastomosis. (From Madden, *Atlas of Technics in Surgery*, 2d ed. Courtesy of Appleton-Century-Crofts, New York, 1964.)

of the head of the pancreas are, likewise, best treated by performing *transduodenal cysto-duodenostomy*. The duodenotomy incision is securely sutured and in such a fashion that any narrowing of the duodenal lumen is avoided (Fig. 7).

Cystojejunostomy may be performed by the antecolic or retrocolic route, employing the Roux-en-Y plan, or by anastomosing the cyst to a loop of proximal jejunum, followed by enteroanastomosis.

The Roux-en-Y method consists in transecting the jejunum between clamps some 6 to 8 inches (15 to 20 cm) below the ligament of Treitz; the distal jejunal limb is anastomosed to the *most dependent portion of the cyst* by the side-to-side or end-to-side method; the end of the proximal jejunum (the portion near the ligament of Treitz) is then anastomosed end-to-side to the ascending (afferent) limb of the jejunum (Fig. 8).

Anastomosis of the pseudocyst to a defunctionalised loop of jejunum (Roux-en-Y plan) has proved a useful method of treatment of these cysts when they are situated *away* from the stomach and yet are not suitable for excision. For this purpose, an anastomosis similar to that of transgastric cysto-gastrostomy can be carried out between the cyst and the ascending limb of jejunum. I prefer to bring a loop of proximal jejunum upward towards the cyst and to perform a side-to-side anastomosis (with a wide stoma) and to complete the operation with a side-to-side jejunojejunostomy. The results of transgastric cystogastrostomy are, in every respect, superior to those of cystojejunostomy.

Zaoussis [31] analysed 105 cases of pseudocysts which were treated by internal drainage. He stated that *total excision* remains the ideal procedure to be performed whenever possible; that external drainage should be limited to cases of pseudocysts which cannot be excised or which have a wall unsuitable for anastomosis; and that, in his opinion, *transgastric cystogastrostomy,* is the operation of choice for the majority of cases.

Excision of pancreatic cysts. Although in theory excision of pancreatic cysts is an ideal operation, the mortality rate of the collected series and the technical difficulties of accomplishment limit its practical application unless the cyst is located in the distal part of the pancreas and is unattached to vital adjacent structures.[27] Warren and Baker [26] are of the opinion that some of the large cysts encountered are susceptible to total excision by enucleation. This, they say, is possible because *cysts* are usually devoid of pancreatitis or peripancreatitis. When these large cysts are encountered and no inflammatory reaction is evident on their exposed surface, every effort should be made to remove them in toto. It is generally agreed, however, that excision of the pseudocyst may occasionally be indicated, especially if the cyst is small. In my opinion, if a pseudocyst, situated in the body or tail of the pancreas, proves recalcitrant to external or internal drainage, distal pancreatectomy should be performed.

Warren et al.[28] state:

Of the 71 patients with *pseudocysts, external drainage* was used in 32 patients and internal drainage in 14. *Sphincterotomy* was performed in 3 cases, the *cyst was totally excised* in 8, and distal pancreatectomy was performed in 9 cases. Three patients required pancreato-duodenal resection. For the 51 patients with *retention cysts* who were operated on, external drainage was used in 5, internal drainage in 4, and sphincterotomy in 12. In 10 patients the cysts were excised, 9 patients required *distal pancreatectomy*, 10 patients pancreatoduodenectomy, and in one patient, a total pancreatectomy was necessary. Of the 6 patients with *cystadenomas*, 2 were treated by excision, 2 by distal pancreatectomy and 2 by pancreatoduodenal resection.
Following these procedures, pancreatic fistulas occurred in 23.6 percent, and pancreatic abscess or peripancreatic infection in 8.1 percent. There were 4 postoperative deaths, an operative mortality of 2.7 percent. (See also Table 1.)

Table 1. RESULTS OF 70 PROCEDURES ON CYSTS AND CHRONIC ABSCESSES OF THE PANCREAS TREATED BETWEEN 1940 AND JUNE 1965

Procedure	Number of Patients	Satisfactory Result	
		Number	Percent
Internal drainage of cyst	29	23	79
External drainage of cyst	23	14	61
Drainage of abscesses	14	10	71
Cyst excision	4	3	75
Total	70	50	71.4

Source: From Warren, Am. J. Surg. 117:28, 1969.

Resection of the tail or of the tail and body of the pancreas. As previously stated resection of the tail or of the tail and body is an effective and radical method of treatment of cysts in these locations. The spleen is mobilised with the pancreas and also removed. (See Fig. 3.)

Cysts of traumatic origin, which are sometimes associated with complete division of the duct of Wirsung, are best dealt with by distal pancreatectomy, as they have a tendency to persist or recur following drainage procedures.

Pancreatoduodenal resection. Pancreatoduodenal resection is an extensive operative undertaking, and, in my opinion, *it should not be employed as a primary procedure;* but in certain instances (at a *secondary* operation), it may be resorted to for complicated recurrent cases associated with chronic relapsing pancreatitis. In cases of cystadenoma, cystadenocarcinoma, or multiple cysts, involving the head of the pancreas, it is the operation of choice. In certain cases of unduly large cystadenocarcinomas, *total pancreatectomy* may be in order.

Sphincterotomy. Transduodenal sphincterotomy may be indicated in certain cases when it is possible to pass a polyethylene tube or catheter along the main pancreatic duct in order to puncture and drain the pseudocyst. If a quantity of fluid is removed by suction, the tube should be left in situ in the cystic cavity and its distal end should be directed downward into the third part of the duodenum. The splint is secured by one stitch which pierces the tube and then a lip of the papilla of Vater.

PANCREATIC FISTULAS

The majority of pancreatic fistulas result from the draining of pseudopancreatic cysts. Doubilet and Mulholland [6] have advised sphincterotomy with drainage of the pancreatic duct for the treatment of certain types of pseudocysts, stating that this operation reduces intraductal pressure and allows the cyst to collapse. Bringing the drainage tube to the exterior enables pancreatography to be carried out to follow the course of the cyst.

A *pancreatic fistula* may occur after:

1. External drainage of pseudocysts.
2. Penetrating and nonpenetrating epigastric wounds which involve the pancreas (contusion, laceration, or fracture of the gland).
3. Removal of stone or stones from the pancreatic ducts.
4. Excision of pancreatic cysts.
5. When an ulcerating lesion of the stomach or duodenum, embedded in the pancreas, is excised during partial gastrectomy, energetic fulguration of the base of a gastric or duodenal ulcer.
6. Splenectomy, with ligature of the tail of the pancreas.
7. Pancreatoduodenectomy.
8. Following an injudicious biopsy of a portion of the gland.

Fistulas arising from the tail or body of the gland are best treated by distal pancreatectomy combined with splenectomy. A fistula following drainage of a retention or false cyst will close if a pancreatogram shows that the dye passes into the duodenum–duct continuity. If, on the other hand, a pancreatogram reveals duct obstruction between the cyst and the duodenum, spontaneous closure of the fistula is a most unlikely event (Fig. 9). In such cases, the fistulous tract should be dissected down to the pancreas itself and excised. An anastomosis is then constructed, with two layers of interrupted 000 or 0000 silk sutures, between the main pancreatic duct and the stomach, or jejunum (Fig. 10). When the fistula involves the head of the pancreas and this portion of the gland is the seat of chronic pancreatitis, a chronic abscess, or pancreatolithiasis, the procedure of choice is pancreatoduodenectomy.

Local Treatment Following External Drainage

It is, I think, important to emphasise the fact that some 50 percent of such fistulas *close spontaneously* in due course, and such closure has been observed up to two years or even longer after the fistula has been established (Priestley). Treatment should therefore in the first instance be conservative and should be directed toward: (1) the restoration and maintenance of fluid requirements and normal blood chemistry; (2) the protection of the wound when digestive activity is a feature of the condition; and (3) diminution in the volume of the secretion to encourage closure.

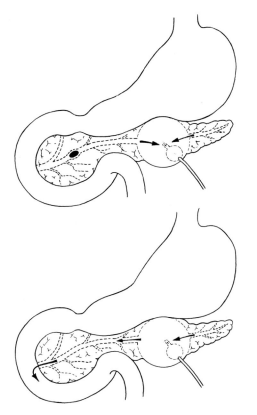

FIG. 9. External drainage of a pseudopancreatic cyst. Closure of the fistula is unlikely if there is an obstruction in the proximal portion of the duct of Wirsung.

Protection of the skin. Simple external drainage, employing the de Pezzer catheter technique, has eliminated the need for protecting the skin and ensures adequate drainage for weeks or even many months without any inconvenience to the patient.

At first the tube should be attached to a continuous suction apparatus, and when the secretion diminishes the tube can be clamped for a few hours every day.

During convalescence, Hypaque, diodone, or biligrafin should be injected into the catheter to ascertain whether the duct of Wirsung, which originally communicated with the cyst, is blocked proximally, i.e., in the region of the head of the pancreas. If the radiopaque solution flows without hindrance into the main pancreatic duct and then onward into the duodenum, and if drainage of pancreatic juice is slight, it is safe to remove the de Pezzer catheter. The chances of subsequent complete healing of the fistula in such circumstances are great. (Fig. 9.)

The principal fear that arises from the presence of a pancreatic fistula following marsupialization is that the skin and superficial tissues will become digested, will be excoriated and inflamed, and that the abdominal incision will gape and finally disrupt. With care and skillful handling in the early stages, however, the extreme pain of a self-digested abdominal wall, the raw skin, and the anguish associated with the numer-

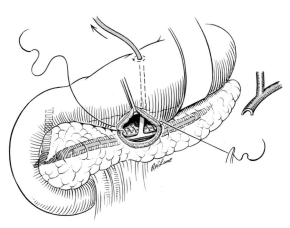

FIG. 10. Pancreatogastrostomy, with T tube drainage, for a chronic pancreatic fistula involving the duct of Wirsung. *Inset:* guttered T tube.

ous applications and constant change of dressings can largely be avoided by adopting the following measures: A rubber tube, a Foley catheter, or a balloon catheter fitting closely into the fistulous tract should be connected with a small noiseless electric suction apparatus and suction should be carried out day and night. The pancreatic secretion should be preserved for measurement and also for reintroduction into the alimentary tract through an indwelling intestinal tube. Vaseline, zinc and castor oil paste, kaolin, aluminum paste, bronze powder, or liquid plastic substances are packed thickly around the tube and on to any part of the skin to which leaking juices can obtain access. It is important to see that the rubber drainage tube fits the fistulous opening tight, and as the tract dilates, a larger tube should be substituted.

Measures for lessening the secretion. Atropine, belladonna, and anticholinergic drugs are worthy of a trial in each case. In early stages, oral feedings should be strictly supervised.

Summary of Operative Treatment

If, following the injection of the radiopaque substance and x-ray studies, the radiographs reveal proximal ductal obstruction, at reoperation the surgeon should core out and then excise the fistulous tract down to its point of communication with the duct of Wirsung. The opening in the duct should be enlarged by careful knife dissection, after which this portion of duct should be anastomosed to the posterior wall of the stomach or to a loop of proximal jejunum. (See Fig. 10.)

If the opening in the duct of Wirsung is anastomosed to the apex of a loop of proximal jejunum, it is imperative to perform a complementary jejunojeunostomy. Every effort should be directed toward relieving any strain on the suture line.

Operations in which the fistulous tract is cored away from surrounding and adherent structures and then implanted into the stomach or jejunum (usually based on Coffrey's method), although yielding good temporary results, in most instances prove disappointing owing to fibrotic contraction of the stoma after the lapse of some weeks or months.

If the fistula communicates with the main pancreatic duct in the tail, or caudal part of the gland, distal pancreatectomy should be carried out rather than anastomosing the duct to the stomach or jejunum.

In those cases in which the duct of Wirsung is inadvertently transected during partial gastrectomy for a penetrating callous duodenal ulcer and this is followed by a persistent pancreatic fistula, at the secondary operation the open mouth of the duct should be anastomosed to the lateral aspect of the second portion of the duodenum. If these procedures are not feasible undertakings, the duct should be recovered by "splitting" the head of the pancreas, after which it should be splinted with a short T tube and then anastomosed to a loop of proximal jejunum or to the ascending limb of jejunum fashioned on the Roux-en-Y plan.

If the tract of a pancreatic fistula communicates with the main duct in the head of the gland and there are in addition multiple strictures, calculi, or the manifestations of severe, long-standing chronic pancreatitis, pancreatoduodenectomy may eventually provide the benison of good health.

REFERENCES

1. Abeshouse, Int. Abst. Surg. 96:1, 1953.
2. Anderson, and Peebles Brown, Br. J. Surg. 47: 147, 1959.
3. Beltex et al., Schweiz. Med. Wochenschr. 96:342, 1966.
4. Bouchier, Lond. Clin. Med. J. 8:13, 1967.
5. De Courcy, Ann. Surg. 118:394, 1943.
6. Doublet, and Mulholland, Am. J. Surg. 105: 741, 1963.
7. Ellison and Carey, in L. Davis, ed., Christopher's Textbook of Surgery, 9th ed., Philadelphia, Saunders, 1968, Chap. 28.
8. Gussenbauer, Arch. Klin. Chir. 29:355, 1885.
9. Haukohl, and Melamed, Am. J. Roentgenol. 63: 234, 1950.
10. Hillis, Am. J. Surg. 105:651, 1963.
11. Howard, and Jordan, Jr., Surgical Diseases of the Pancreas, Philadelphia, Lippincott, 1960.
12. Judd, Mayo Clin. Proc. 39:927, 1964.
13. Kennard, Surgery 7:65, 1941.
14. Lichtenstein, Am. J. Cancer 21:542, 1934.
15. Mattson, and Mahorner, Arch. Surg. 22:838, 1931.
16. Piper et al., J.A.M.A. 180:648, 1962.
17. Piper, ReMine, and Priestley, J.A.M.A. 180:80, 1962.
18. Priestley, and ReMine, Surg. Clin. North Am. 38:1313, 1958.
19. Procos et al., Acta Chir. Hell. 11:79, 1964.
20. Sawyer et al., Ann. Surg. 135:549, 1952.

21. Smith, Rodney, London Clin. Med. J. 2:32, 1961.
22. Smith, Rodney, Lancet 2:1063, 1965.
23. Swanson, Radiology 81:592, 1963.
24. Warren, Surg. Clin. North Am. 45:599, 1965.
25. Warren, Am. J. Surg. 117:28, 1969.
26. Warren, and Baker, Surg. Clin. North Am. 38: 815, 1958.

27. Warren et al., Ann. Surg. 147:903, 1958.
28. Warren et al., Surg. Clin. North Am. 44:743, 1964.
29. Warren et al., Ann. Surg. 163:886, 1966.
30. Waugh and Lynn, Arch. Surg. 77:47, 1958.
31. Zaoussis, Ann. Surg. 138:13, 1953.

38

CHRONIC RELAPSING PANCREATITIS
A. The Recognition of and Operations for Chronic Relapsing Pancreatitis

RODNEY MAINGOT

In most cases, pancreatitis is an expression of disease elsewhere. As I have previously emphasised, most clinicians now regard pancreatitis as a *secondary disease* in which the pancreatic "features" are so overwhelming as to obscure the primary disease.[43] This is especially the case in relapsing or recurrent pancreatitis associated with acute or subacute exacerbations.

By recognizing the *form* that pancreatitis takes, deductions can be made as to the most likely reason for the appearance of the disease, as DuVal [23] has so cogently stressed. In a general way, pancreatitis may assume one of three forms: (1) an acute condition, (2) a recurring disease, and (3) a chronic disorder.

Form 1—*acute pancreatitis*—is by far the most common; this type may be of the oedematous or haemorrhagic type, and it is commonly caused by (a) cholecystitis and gallstones, (b) abdominal trauma, (c) acute alcoholic poisoning, or (d) systemic infection, e.g., mumps (see Chap. 36).

Form 2—*relapsing pancreatitis*—that is, chronic pancreatitis associated with recurrent episodes of acute pancreatitis is *usually* related to infections of the gallbladder, to choledocholithiasis, to sclerosing papillitis, or to stenosis or dysfunction of the sphincter of Oddi occasioned by stone, fibrosis, or

spasm. In Form 2, alcoholism does not appear to be an impressive aetiological factor.

Form 3—*chronic pancreatitis*—is a crippling progressive disorder leading to sclerosis of the gland and many distressing complications; it is commonly caused by alcoholism, hyperparathyroidism, familial hyperlipaemia, severe protein-deficiency states, and metabolic disturbances. Alcoholic poisoning, hyperparathyroidism, and the hereditary forms of pancreatitis are significant factors in pancreatolithiasis and calcification of the gland.

A *diagnosis* between acute pancreatitis and chronic pancreatitis can be made with assurance, but the *distinction* between the recurrently acute (Form 2) and chronic pancreatitis may be, and often is, very difficult. Nevertheless, it should be possible in most instances to distinguish between these two types of chronic pancreatitis provided the clinician is prepared to undertake an elaborate and searching study of the clinical findings, laboratory investigations, and radiological studies. For instance, during the period of *remission,* patients with relapsing pancreatitis regain their health and strength, appetite and weight are restored, and they are able to resume their normal occupation after a brief convalescence.

Those patients who suffer from chronic pancreatitis (Form 3) present a different picture. They continue to complain of indigestion, nausea, anorexia, flatulence, loss of weight, loss of courage, steatorrhoea, sullen and sometimes severe epigastric pain, backache, and they may display objective evidence of pancreatic insufficiency. They usually do not respond to medical measures aimed at improving their appetite or digestive functions. According to DuVal,[23] most of them seek solace in alcohol and/or narcotic drugs, and show little if any keenness to return to a normal mode of life. As the disease "drags on," weight loss becomes pronounced, and they become lethargic and apathetic. These unfortunate patients are prone to develop a recalcitrant type of diabetes mellitus, severe steatorrhoea, obstructive lesions of the duct of Wirsung, intraglandular cystic collections, pancreatolithiasis, duodenal ulceration, and (rarely) pulmonary tuberculosis.

It is a remarkable fact, however, that in rare instances of *primary inflammatory fibrosis of the pancreas* the patient may be symptomless.

Sarles et al.[54] have pointed out that repeated attacks of acute pancreatitis do *not* invariably result in chronic pancreatitis; in fact, advanced chronic pancreatitis may, and often does, occur in the absence of a clinical history of acute pancreatitis.

CAUSES OF PANCREATITIS

The causes of pancreatitis may be briefly summarised as follows: (1) alcoholism; (2) biliary tract diseases, including gallstones and lesions of the ampulla of Vater; (3) trauma: nonpenetrating, penetrating, and operative injuries; (4) hyperparathyroidism; (5) certain systemic diseases such as mumps, scarlet fever, and viral infections; (6) familial hyperlipaemia and certain other hereditary conditions; (7) protein-deficiency states such as malnutrition; (8) association with the following lesions such as benign and malignant tumours of the pancreas, pseudocysts, parasitic infection, duodenal and gastric ulceration, vascular disease; (9) metabolic disturbances such as chemotoxic agents; (10) hyperplasia and metaplasia of the pancreatic ductal epithelium; and (11) idiopathic factors, e.g., *primary* sclerosis of the pancreas.

In 35 to 40 percent of patients, there are no aetiological antecedents to explain the presence of chronic relapsing pancreatitis.

A number of noteworthy general reviews of clinical and surgical experience with chronic pancreatitis and relapsing pancreatitis are available and include the following: Warren (*Surg. Clin. North Am. 39*:799, 1958); Warren and Veidenheimer (*N. Engl. J. Med. 266*:323, 1962); Warren (in *Modern Trends in Gastroenterology*, Third Series, Avery Jones, ed., Butterworths, London, 1961, p. 277); Warren (*Am. J. Surg. 117*:25, 1969); Warren and Mountain (*Surg. Clin. North Am. 51*:693, 1971); DuVal and Enquist (*Surgery 50*: 965, 1961; *Am. J. Surg. 109*:113, 1965); Nardi (*New Engl. J. Med. 268*:1065, 1963); Egdahl (*Surgery 55*:604, 1964); Thistlethwaite and Smith (*Ann. Surg. 158*:226, 1963); Goulston and Gallagher (*Gut 3*:252, 1962); Fitzgerald (*Rev. Surg. 21*:77, 1964); and Bockus (in *Gastroenterology*, Vol. 3, Saunders, Philadelphia, 1966, Chap. 127); Fleming (*Br. Med. J. 1*:813, 1968); Dean, Scott, and Law (*Ann. Surg. 173*:443, 1971); Vernon, Steningand, and R. Smith (*Br. J. Surg. 57*:906, 1970); Strum and Spiro (*Ann. Int. Med. 74*:264, 1971); Child, Frey, and Fay (*Surg. Gynec. Obstet. 129*:49, 1969); and personal communications from Charles Frey (1972) and Rodney Smith (1973).

Aetiology and Pathogenesis

INCIDENCE

Acute pancreatitis accounts for less than 1 to 2 percent of cases of acute abdominal disease, and must therefore be regarded as a rare disease in Britain. Chronic pancreatitis accounts for about 0.5 percent of all cases admitted to our large hospitals.

SEX

In young children one would suspect that a systemic infection is an aetiological factor or perhaps an hereditary pancreatitis. Most of the pseudocysts encountered in infancy and childhood result from trauma.

According to Bockus[3] the sex distribution depends upon the relative number of cases attributed to alcohol versus biliary tract disease. He writes: "In our series of 44 males and 34 females, there was a preponderance of "alcohol pancreatitis" among males and of "biliary pancreatitis" in females." The preponderance of "biliary pancreatitis" evidently explains the high ratio of females to males in the series of Siler and Wulsin (59 percent females) and Pollock (71 percent females, three-fourths of whom had abnormal gallbladders).

AGE

Chronic relapsing pancreatitis may occur at any age. In the hereditary form, the attacks begin in most cases in childhood or early adult life. The majority of patients, however, are admitted to hospital between the ages of 40 and 60; the average age of onset is 45 years.

The chronicity of the disease is indicated by the period that elapses between the onset of symptoms and abdominal exploration.

Gross, Comfort, and Ulrich[32] discussed the subject of chronic relapsing pancreatitis occurring in *infancy and childhood.*

Hendren, Greep, and Patton[34] reported that 12 of 15 children who underwent surgery for chronic recurrent or chronic progressive pancreatitis were greatly improved, though one had minor symptoms.

Dean, Scott, and Law[16] recorded one of their own cases and reviewed 7 others found in the literature.

Vernon et al.,[58] in discussing the incidence of chronic relapsing pancreatitis in childhood, reported 4 cases that were successfully treated by surgery. They confirmed that this disease is rare in infancy and childhood, but must be considered in young patients suffering from recurrent attacks of abdominal pain, nausea, vomiting, weight loss, and steatorrhoea. Most of these patients enjoyed long periods of complete freedom from any symptoms.

ALCOHOL

I would estimate the incidence in the British Isles of alcoholic pancreatitis to be about 30 percent, and in the United States, 40 percent. Owens and Howard[50] reported 32 patients suffering from chronic relapsing pancreatitis, all of whom were chronic alcoholics. Cattell and Warren, in their *Surgery of the Pancreas,*[9] stated that 46 percent of the patients operated upon at the Lahey Clinic for recurrent pancreatitis imbibed alcohol to excess. The relationship between the consumption of alcohol and the development of pancreatitis is discussed in consid-

erable detail by Strum and Spiro[55] and by T. T. White in his *Pancreatitis.*[63] In their opinion, alcohol is associated with approximately 75 percent of all cases of chronic pancreatitis in the United States. Strum and Spiro[55] state that *chronic relapsing pancreatitis* can be defined as chronic pancreatitis with acute symptomatic exacerbations characterized primarily by abdominal pain, in contrast to *chronic pancreatitis,* which is irreversible pancreatic destruction with its associated complications and without significant abdominal pain.

Calcification of the pancreas is present in over 60 percent of patients suffering from "alcoholic" pancreatitis; while steatorrhoea is observed in some 30 percent, and chronic peptic ulceration is an added complication in about 20 percent of these patients.

BILIARY TRACT DISEASE

Cholecystitis, calculous cholecystitis, choledocholithiasis, stricture of the lower end of the choledochus, papillitis, dysfunction or fibrosis of the sphincter of Oddi, or benign and malignant growths of the ampulla of Vater or periampullary region are important aetiological factors; they are responsible for fully 50 percent of cases of acute and chronic relapsing pancreatitis. The presence of gallstones is a more impressive aetiological factor in acute pancreatitis than it is in the chronic varieties.

TRAUMA

Penetrating and nonpenetrating wounds and operative trauma account for an appreciable number of cases (see Chap. 35).

The combination of three specific aetiological factors: (1) trauma, (2) alcoholism, and (3) gallstones accounts for more than 90 percent of cases of acute and chronic pancreatitis.

HYPERPARATHYROIDISM

On occasion, pancreatitis may be a secondary manifestation of adenoma, carcinoma, or hyperplasia of a parathyroid gland or glands.[46, 52]

Hereditary Pancreatitis: Hyperlipaemia

Gross [30] stated that Comfort and Steinberg [15] reported an occurrence of relapsing pancreatitis affecting *four members of a single family, with two other members probably affected.* Gross himself has reported on two well-documented families with a high incidence of pancreatitis while Gross, Gambill, and Ulrich [31] have reported subsequent studies on five kindreds from the Mayo Clinic. Several similar familial occurrences have been reported by Poulsen [51] and Beall et al.[2]; one of these cases was associated with familial parathyroid adenomas.

Wollaeger pointed out that the hereditary form of chronic pancreatitis is being recognised with increasing frequency. A few cases have been reported in association with hyperlipaemia or with hyperparathyroidism, but the significance of these associations is not clear (Fig. 1).

According to Strum and Spiro [55] *"hereditary pancreatitis* appears to be inherited as a non-sex linked Mendelian dominant, but incomplete recessiveness and poor penetrance of the gene have not been excluded." The disorder is not associated with gallstones, alcohol, or any other specific cause of pancreatitis in any more than the usual frequency. The operative and necropsy findings suggest that the inherited defect might well be muscular hypertrophy of the sphincter of Oddi. Calcification of the gland was noted in most patients before operation. The operation of choice for this disease in its early stages, is sphincterotomy or sphincteroplasty, combined with short-T-tube choledochostomy.

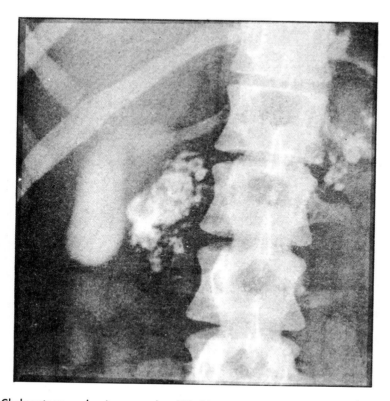

FIG. 1. Cholecystogram showing normal gallbladder. Advanced calcification of the pancreas is present. The patient was a 14-year-old girl suffering from *congenital hyperlipaemia.* Her main symptoms were severe epigastric pain and bouts of steatorrhoea. Transabdominal coeliac and superior mesenteric ganglionectomy failed to relieve her symptoms. (R. Maingot's patient.)

The Common Channel Theory

Opie [48] stressed the importance of the "common channel," which is present in some 50 percent of human subjects. At autopsy on a patient with acute haemorrhagic pancreatitis, Opie found an impacted stone at the ampulla of Vater and was able to express bile into the main pancreatic duct by applying pressure to the gallbladder. From this observation arose the concept, which has many supporters, of the *"common channel" mechanism* for the development of acute pancreatitis, that is, the existence of an anatomical arrangement in which these ducts form a common intercommunicating channel, permitting regurgitation of bile into the pancreatic ducts. But in the absence of disease of the lower reaches of the choledochus, it is unlikely that any bile enters the pancreatic ducts. When, however, the ampulla of Vater is obstructed by stone, fibrosis, tumour, or prolonged spasm, the pent-up stagnant enzyme-laden fluids are capable of initiating an attack of acute pancreatitis.

Archibald [1, 1a] of Montreal was one of the first to make original fundamental and clinical observations on the importance of spasm of the sphincter of Oddi as the prime cause of pancreatitis, and he performed transduodenal sphincterotomy in the treatment of the recurrent lesion.

Doubilet and Mulholland [18] continued the work of Archibald and have been enthusiastic about transduodenal choledochal sphincterotomy in the relief of relapsing pancreatitis.

Doubilet [17] stated that a common passageway exists in all cases of recurrent pancreatitis.

Obstruction to the Outflow of Pancreatic Juice

Intrapancreatic obstruction, partial or complete, involving the duct of Wirsung or the duct of Santorini, or both, is often responsible for continuing or recurrent attacks of pancreatitis. In many patients with chronic relapsing pancreatitis, multiple points of obstruction have been demonstrated at operation or autopsy (Figs. 2 and 3). Consequently, surgeons have attempted to detect and to eliminate the intrapancreatic obstruction. Partial or complete obstruction to the outflow of pancreatic juice may be caused by hyperplasia of the mucosa of

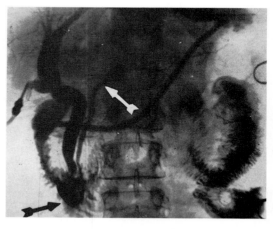

FIG. 3. Operative cholangiogram demonstrating common passageway. While radiopaque solution was being injected, spasm of the sphincter of Oddi was produced by injection of N/10 hydrochloric acid through a Rehfuss tube with a metal tip positioned against the papilla (*black arrow*). Consequent reflux resulted in visualisation of the whole duct of Wirsung (*white arrow*). (Courtesy of Dr. H. Doubilet; and The Royal Society of Medicine.)

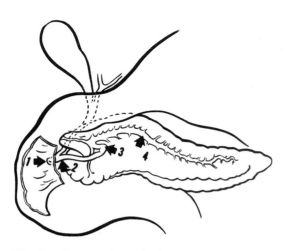

FIG. 2. Common sites of obstruction of the main pancreatic duct. (Courtesy of Dr. Alan Thal; and *Annals of Surgery.*)

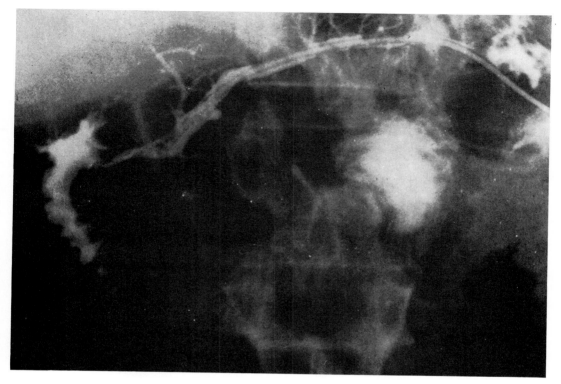

FIG. 4. Pancreatogram showing partial obstruction of the duct of Wirsung in the head of the pancreas. The patient was a young man who had previously had *low inversion of the duodenal stump following Billroth II gastrectomy.* An inflammatory reaction around the inverted stump has produced a narrowing of the terminal duct of Wirsung. The main duct is moderately dilated. The catheter is inserted through the tail of the gland at the site of the retrograde pancreatojejunostomy. (Courtesy of Dr. Alan Thal; and *Annals of Surgery.*)

the duct of Wirsung, by oedema or inflammatory stricture, a benign polyp,[65] annular pancreas, and fibrosis of the sphincter of Oddi.

K. W. Warren has reminded us that the recognition of intrapancreatic obstruction as an important aetiological factor in recurrent pancreatitis is not new, as reference to the works of Prisell (1921), Rich and Duff (1936), and Appleby (1951) will readily prove. Berens (1954) made postmortem studies in 16 cases of chronic pancreatitis and found various evidences of intrapancreatic obstruction in all (Fig. 4). Most of these cases were caused by hyperplasia or metaplasia of the ductal epithelium. In cases of pancreatolithiasis, the pancreatic ducts are almost invariably obstructed. It may, of course, be argued that the stones cause the blockage, but it is more plausible that fibrotic obstruction of the duct precedes and gives rise to the calculi.

PEPTIC ULCER AND OTHER FACTORS

Peptic ulcer may be a cause of, or the result of, chronic pancreatitis, in some 10 to 20 percent of cases.

Strum and Spiro [55] found 10 patients suffering from chronic peptic ulceration in their series of 50 patients with chronic pancreatitis.

Recurrent peptic ulcer is a relatively common complication following operative procedures on the pancreas. Trauma to the gland and previous pancreatic surgery are aetiological antecedents in 3 percent and 0.4 percent, respectively.

Frey [25] believes that in 10 to 25 percent of patients with chronic relapsing pancreatitis no clear cause can be formed. Warren and Mountain,[60] on the other hand, found no aetiological antecedent in 196 of their 530 patients with chronic relapsing pancreatitis—an incidence of 37 percent.

DIAGNOSIS

Clinical Picture

Clinical experience has taught that the patient who has had one attack of pancreatitis will usually have other frequent and similar attacks. The clinical syndrome may be divided into two stages: (1) an early stage characterised by repeated attacks of acute or subacute pancreatitis without obvious evidence of permanent damage to the pancreas and (2) a late state during which, in addition to the painful seizures, permanent functional impairment of the gland (diabetes mellitus, steatorrhoea, etc.) occurs, and pancreatolithi-

asis or calcinosis is evident on x-ray studies.

The painful episodes in both stages are identical with those that occur in acute pancreatitis and may last for a few days or even weeks. Between these acute attacks the patient may be symptom-free. The attacks recur at varying intervals, with remissions that may, on occasion, persist for some years. During the second stage of the disease, the frequency of the acute exacerbations increases and the attacks may occur weekly or monthly. It is important, however, to point out that there are a number of patients suffering from the effects of pancreatic insufficiency—steatorrhoea, loss of weight, etc.—due to the chronic type of pancreatitis, and who do not suffer any epigastric pain or discomfort of any kind.

With some patients in Group 3, pain may be constant and unrelenting; in fact, its devastating effects frequently lead to narcotic

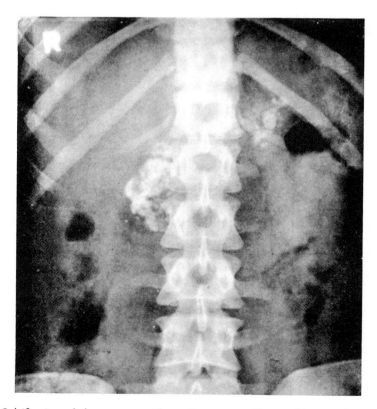

FIG. 5.   Calcification of the pancreas. The patient was a 53-year-old man who was a chronic alcoholic. Considerable relief of his symptoms was afforded by the performance of total pancreatectomy. (R. Maingot's patient.)

addiction. Some 20 percent of patients give a history of transient obstructive jaundice.

During the early phase of the disease, the diagnosis is usually "clinched" if the patient is examined during one of the painful seizures when determinations of serum amylase, lipase, and blood sugar show temporary significant elevations. It should be noted, however, that low serum amylase levels do not exclude acute pancreatitis. Intravenous cholangiography, scout films of the abdomen, and *x-ray studies* of the stomach, duodenum, and pancreas often prove of considerable help in diagnosis.

When a late stage has been reached, the development of diabetes mellitus or steatorrhoea, the demonstration of pancreatolithiasis on x-ray examination, and a careful clinical study of the patient make it possible to establish a clear-cut diagnosis, even in the intervals between the acute attacks.

Pancreatic calculi or calcification of the parenchyma of the gland was present in 40 percent of the cases studied by Birnstingl (1959), which is in accord with the 48 percent reported by Comfort (1946) in a series of 29 cases. Today, as cases of relapsing pancreatitis are diagnosed at an earlier stage in the disease, the incidence of calcinosis is certainly not higher than 30 percent (Fig. 5). Calcification is almost never seen in pancreatitis owing to biliary tract disease (see Part D of this chapter—Pancreatolithiasis).

The disease has to be *differentiated* from biliary colic; calculous cholecystitis; choledocholithiasis; periampullary carcinoma; cancer of the head, body, or tail of the pancreas; malignant disease of the stomach; penetrating gastric and duodenal ulcer; aortic aneurysm; retroperitoneal sarcoma; subacute attacks of high-gut obstruction; disease of the coronary arteries; nontropical sprue; and Whipple's disease.

Diagnostic Procedures

Important *aids to diagnosis* include:

ROUTINE LABORATORY TESTS

A complete blood count; liver function tests; an estimation of serum bilirubin and serum lipase; blood calcium; blood sugar; the serum pancreozymin–secretin test; and stool examination, including the amount of proteolytic enzyme in the stools (see Chap. 45).

RADIOLOGICAL INVESTIGATIONS

(a) Plain x-ray films of the abdomen may display radiopaque gallstones, pancreatic calculi, or calcinosis of the gland. (b) Barium-meal x-ray examination may prove useful in displaying or excluding concomitant peptic ulceration or in demonstrating the presence of an unresolved pancreatic mass or pseudocyst. Irregularity of the duodenal curve may suggest involvement of the head of the pancreas. (c) *Duodenography,* the value of which method of investigation for chronic pancreatitis and periampullary cancer is fully discussed in Chapter 4, Part C by Dr. Louis Kreel (Fig. 6).

CHOLECYSTOGRAPHY AND INTRAVENOUS CHOLANGIOGRAPHY

These tests are of the greatest value and should be carried out as a routine mea-

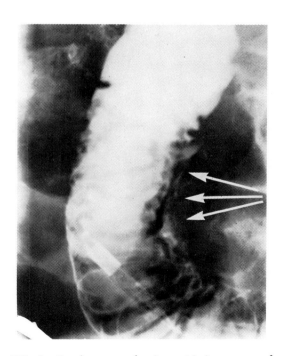

FIG. 6. Duodenogram showing extrinsic pressure effect caused by chronic pancreatitis with a smooth inner margin (arrows). (Dr. L. Kreel's patient.)

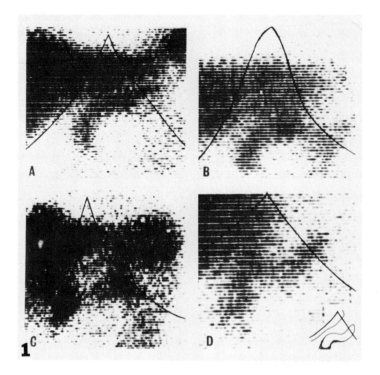

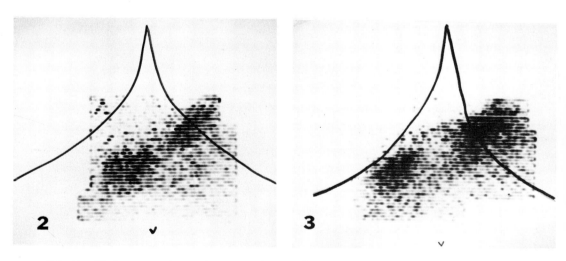

FIG. 7. (1) Conventional pancreatic scan showing the variation in the shape and position of the gland. (2) Normal subtraction scan. (3) Pancreatic scan by the subtraction technique in a patient with pancreatitis. There is a filling defect in the body of the gland.

sure. *Repeated* negative cholecystograms suggest chronic disease of the gallbladder, with or without gallstones. Any pathological state involving the gallbladder (cholecystitis, gallstones, etc.) or biliary ducts (choledocholithiasis, partial simple stricture, fibrosis of

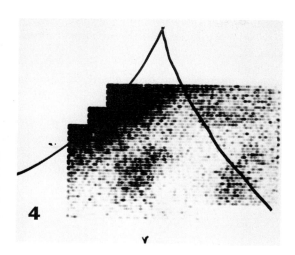

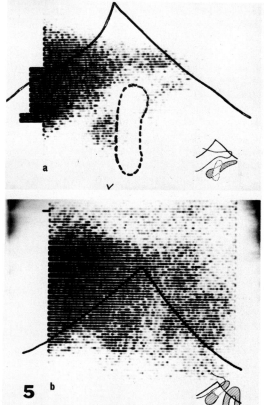

FIG. 7. (Cont.) (4) Conventional pancreatic scan in a patient with a cancer of the body of the gland which shows a large filling defect. (5) Difficulties in the interpretation of the pancreatic scan. (A) Filling defect in the body of the gland. This was diagnosed on the scan as a cancer, but at operation an aneurysm of the aorta was found and the gland was normal. (B) A scan which was interpreted as having the normal "thin" area of the body but at operation a large cancer of the body of the gland was found.

the sphincter of Oddi, etc.) should receive appropriate surgical treatment as soon as conditions permit.

Retrograde Pancreatography and Cholangiography by Fibreduodenoscopy

This is discussed by Dr. Louis Kreel in Chapter 34, Part B. The reader is referred to this relatively new and important method of investigation of pancreatic disease.

Scintiscanning of the Pancreas (Fig. 7)

This method of radioisotope scanning of the pancreas is described by Professor Ian Bouchier of Dundee University, Scotland as follows:

Pancreatic Scanning

Ian Bouchier

^{75}Se-selenomethionine is a γ-emitting compound which can be used to scan the pancreas. The isotope has a physical half-life of 120 days and in man a biological half-life of 77 to 87 days. The total-body radiation dose is about 1.6 rad for a 70-kg man given the usual dose for scanning.

No special preparation is required for the scan, and a dose of 3μ Ci ^{75}Se-selenomethionine per kilogram of body weight is given intravenously. The scan is commenced immediately thereafter. High-quality scanning equipment is necessary and careful attention to technique is required. The selenomethionine is taken up by both the pancreas and the liver, and therefore it is necessary to follow the selenomethionine scan with a ^{198}Au colloid gold scan. The liver outline and the pancreatic outline may be separated visually: the conventional pancreatic scan, or electronic techniques can be used to obliterate the liver image so that only the pancreas is visible on the print-out: the subtraction scan. Although the addition of a subtraction scan to the conventional scan makes the procedure rather long, our observations indicate that diagnostic accuracy is improved.[4] More recently gamma cameras have been used for pancreatic scanning.[33]

Normal scan. The shape and position of the normal pancreas varies (Fig. 7, *1* and *2*). The gland usually takes an oblique position in the epigastric region, but horizontal and sigmoid shapes are also encountered. There is normally an area of decreased uptake in the body of the gland, which probably represents thinning from compression by adjacent vessels.

Pancreatitis. An abnormality can be seen in 75 to 80 percent of patients with established disease. There is usually diffuse failure of the gland to take up the isotope, but filling defects also occur (Fig. 7, *3*).

Cancer. The pancreatic scan is effective in screening for cancer of the gland, and false negative results (i.e., a tumour is missed) are uncommon. A normal scan excludes cancer with a probability of greater than 95 percent. The appearance is either that of a filling defect (Fig. 7, *4*), or of diffuse failure of uptake.[42]

Pancreatic scanning is now well established as a technique in the diagnosis of pancreatic disease, but it must be appreciated that a high degree of training and skill is required in order to perform and interpret a pancreatic scan. The scan is of particular value in indicating that the gland is normal, and a normal scan is strong evidence against the presence of disease in the pancreas. Unfortunately there is an appreciable number of false positive scans (i.e., the scan appears abnormal when no disease is demonstrable). The cause for this remains uncertain; factors such as obesity, ascites, previous surgery to the stomach, diabetes mellitus, and cirrhosis of the liver must be considered, for these all tend to give rise to an abnormal pancreatic scan in the presence of normal exocrine pancreatic function.

An area of much diagnostic difficulty is the "thin" area of the body. It is easy to overlook lesions in this region and to misdiagnose the reduced isotope uptake as a filling defect (Fig. 7, *5*). The scan is not particularly accurate in distinguishing between pancreatitis and cancer. In our experience, most patients present for scanning at an advanced stage of their disease, and the finding of a cancer on the scan is associated with a poor prognosis; less than 10 percent of the tumours are resectable and 50 percent have spread by the time of surgery.[42]

LUNDH TEST OF PANCREATIC FUNCTION

Sir Francis Avery Jones

The trypsin concentration in the duodenum after a test meal is measured.[40] The meal is made up of corn or soya bean oil, 18 g; Casilan (dried milk protein powder), 15 g; glucose, 40 g; Crusha syrup (for flavouring), 15 g; and hot water to 300 ml.

A radiopaque, number 12 French gauge, rubber tube with a finger cot containing mercury attached to its tip is passed through the nose or mouth in the fasting subject. The tube is gradually advanced with the patient lying on his right side until the tip is 80 to 100 cm from the nostril.

The position of the tube is checked radiologically and it should be adjusted until it lies in the third part of the duodenum.

Duodenal juice is collected by siphonage into a measuring cylinder placed below the level of the patient and surrounded with ice. Gentle suction may be required to start the flow.

The test meal is given and juice is collected for 2 hours thereafter. Attention is needed to maintain a continuous flow. The volume of the specimen and its pH are noted. An aliquot is stored at $-20\,°C$ until the chemical estimation [64] is performed.

INTERPRETATION

The tryptic activity in the 2-hour collection is normally greater than 9 μ Eq per minute per milliliter. Slightly lower values may be found in nonpancreatic steatorrhoea but not as low as in pancreatic steatorrhoea, where values less than 2 μ Eq per minute per milliliter are obtained. In chronic pancreatitis or pancreatic carcinoma without steatorrhoea values, between 2 and 9 μ Eq per minute per milliliter are common.

The test is particularly valuable in the diagnosis of pancreatic steatorrhoea.

ANGIOGRAPHY AND SELECTIVE ARTERIOGRAPHIC TECHNIQUES

These methods are described in Chapter 108 by Dr. Louis Kreel.

ATYPICAL PANCREATITIS

Atypical pancreatitis has been ably described by Morlock.[47]

Recurring attacks of acute pancreatitis lead to disturbances in function of the acinar and islet cells of the gland, and certain sequelae—such as diabetes mellitus, steatorrhoea, creatorrhhoea, jaundice, wasting, intractable abdominal pain, and backache—almost inevitably ensue, either singly or in combination.

Chronic Painless Pancreatitis

This condition was recognised by Opie[49] many years ago. Readers who are interested in this subject should refer to two valuable and learned contributions by Bartholomew and Comfort[14] and by Goulston and Gallagher.[28]

PATHOLOGY

The subject of *acute pancreatitis* is discussed in Chapter 36; *pancreatolithiasis* in Part D of this chapter; and *pancreatic cysts, fistulas, and abscesses*, in Chapter 37.

According to Warren and Veidenheimer,[61] variability of pathology is extreme: oedema, induration, fibrosis, atrophy, necrosis, cysts (true and false), stones, calcification, and partial or complete ductal obstruction.

Diabetes is present in about 15 to 20 percent of patients, and jaundice in 15 percent. Pancreatolithiasis is observed in 20 to 25 percent of the advanced cases and, as previously noted, calcification of a portion or of most of the gland is evident on radiologi-

cal examination in some 30 percent or more of the chronic cases.[38]

Medical Treatment

Treatment for acute pancreatitis is discussed in Chapter 36.

The medical measures directed towards the *prevention* of acute attacks and towards halting the progression of the disease are indeed few and of limited value. Briefly, medical therapy consists of ordering a bland, low-fat and high-protein diet, and *advising and entreating* the patient to avoid alcohol, caffeine in any form, and overeating. Control of diabetes mellitus is important, and usually requires the administration of insulin. Steatorrhoea is best treated with pancreatic enzyme preparations of which pancrex-V Forte, Panteric and Viokase tablets, 4 to 5 *with* each meal or 4 times a day 2 hours *after* meals, have proved useful in absorption of fat and nitrogen.

Codein phosphate tablets of 120 mg should be taken twice a day, morning and night, to alleviate or control diarrhoea and flatulence. The diet should be low in fat and high in protein.[45] *Alcohol should be eschewed!* Anticholinergic drugs may be prescribed at the onset of discomfort preceding an attack, but I have found tincture of belladonna more helpful. Gastric acidity must be depressed.

Instructive accounts of medical management of this disease are given by McDonough,[41] Morlock,[47] Gordon and Grossman,[27] and Fleming.[24]

Operative Treatment of Relapsing Chronic Pancreatitis

The *surgical principles* entailed are:

1. Eradication of biliary tract disease.
2. Ensuring a free flow of bile and pancreatic juice into the duodenum, stomach, or proximal jejunum.
3. Overcoming any point of obstruction in the pancreatic ducts.

The *surgical procedures* may be classified as follows:

1. Correction of the pathological changes

in the biliary system, e.g., cholecystectomy for gallstones.

2. Miscellaneous procedures, including diversionary choledochojejunostomy [45]; lateral choledochoduodenostomy; and nerve interruption to the pancreas.

3. Transduodenal sphincterotomy or sphincteroplasty, with or without dilatation and drainage of the main pancreatic duct, but combined with short T tube choledochostomy.

4. Distal pancreatectomy alone, when the disease is limited to the tail of the gland.

5. Distal pancratectomy followed by anastomosis of the pancreatic duct to the proximal jejunum, employing the Roux-en-Y plan (DuVal and Leger), or by using the simple loop method combined with entero-anastomosis.

6. Distal pancreatectomy followed by pancreatogastrostomy.

7. Longitudinal pancreatojejunostomy by the method advocated by Puestow.

8. Pancreatoduodenal resection, as practised by Warren.

9. Subtotal (Frey) or total pancreatectomy.

INDIRECT OPERATIONS UPON THE PANCREAS

Correction of pathological changes in the biliary system. "The key to successful operative treatment of chronic relapsing and chronic pancreatitis is the evaluation of the nature and extent of the pathological changes that involve the gland and adjacent anatomical structures, and the individualization in the application of one or more operative procedures aimed at overcoming intrapancreatic obstruction and other pathological conditions present." (Kenneth Warren, 1972.)

Operations fall into 2 major groups: (1) those having an *indirect* effect on the pancreas and (2) those dealing *directly* with the pancreas.

As I have previously stated, the best results are obtained when pancreatitis is a secondary manifestation of biliary tract disease.

When gallstones are present, the gallbladder should be removed and the common bile

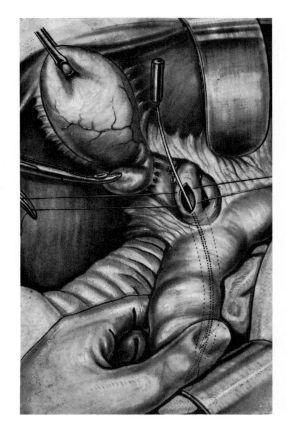

FIG. 8. Gallstones in association with chronic relapsing pancreatitis. Exploration of bile ducts; cholecystectomy combined with choledochostomy. Incision in the common bile duct is made through its anterior wall, just below the ligated stump of the cystic duct. After removing any stones that lie in duct and after thoroughly irrigating the whole ductal system with normal saline solution, graduated Bakes' dilators are passed into the duodenum to dilate the ampulla of Vater and the sphincter of Oddi. If no sounds can be passed into the duodenum, transduodenal sphincterotomy must be performed. These sounds must be passed gently and cautiously, otherwise considerable damage may be done to the lower reaches of the bile duct or false passages produced. Following exploration of the bile passages, T tube drainage is instituted. Maingot's guttered T tube, which is made of latex, should be used.

duct explored as a routine measure. After removing any ductal stones, the ampulla should be carefully dilated with graduated Bakes' dilators. T tube choledochostomy completes the operation (Fig. 8).

In some instances a 3- to 4-mm Bakes' dilator cannot be passed through the am-

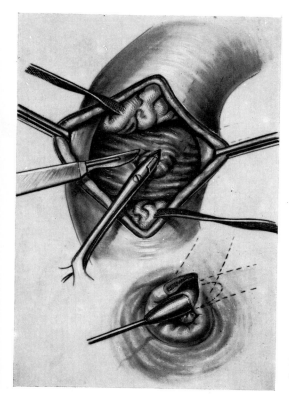

FIG. 9. Transduodenal choledochal sphincterotomy, as practised by many surgeons. *Inset:* The duct of Wirsung is being dilated with a Bakes' dilator. (After Cattell and Warren.)

pulla into the duodenum owing to the presence of stenosis of the sphincter of Oddi or an impacted stone. The dilator should be held in situ, as it will act as a useful guide to the position of the papilla. Transduodenal sphincterotomy should then be performed after one of the many approved methods, and a search should be made for the orifice of the duct of Wirsung. The pancreatic duct should be gently probed and dilated using a small-bore polyethylene tube or ureteric catheter (numbers 3 to 5 French). A pancreatogram is usually performed, with the customary precautions. *If no obstruction is encountered or visualised,* the duodenotomy incision should be closed obliquely or transversely, using a *single* layer of closely applied Gambee sutures of fine silk.

Short T tube choledochostomy completes the operation. Cattell's long T tube should not be used because the "duodenal" portion of the tube *may,* in certain instances, block the mouth of the pancreatic duct and thus give rise to a grave type of postoperative pancreatitis (Figs. 8-13).

The subhepatic area should always be drained with sheets of corrugated latex or a Penrose tube.

As would be expected, the results of this operation are highly satisfactory; many surgeons claim a cure rate as high as 80 percent.

Keddie [37] has advocated *pancreatography* for all patients undergoing operation for recurrent pancreatitis, and the adopted surgical procedure should be based on the radiological findings.

Following transduodenal sphincterotomy, the orifice of the pancreatic duct is sought for below the orifice of the common bile duct. If it is difficult to find, *secretin* (2 units per kg of body weight) can be given intravenously, and the orifice recognised as pancreatic juice freely flows out of it. "When secretin has been administered, the dye solution should not be injected for about 15 minutes, during the phase of most active secretion. A ureteric catheter (Numbers 3

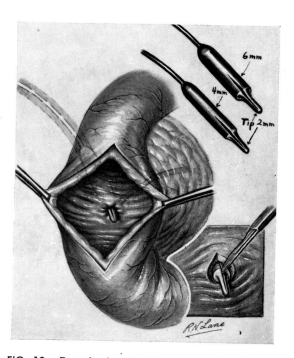

FIG. 10. Transduodenal sphincterotomy—R. Smith's technique.

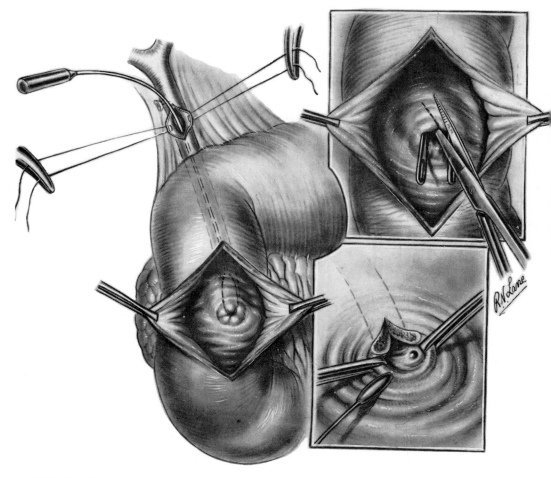

FIG. 11.   Maingot's method of performing a transduodenal sphincterotomy after exploration of the common bile duct.

to 5 Fr.) is inserted into the orifice for about 3 cm. A syringe containing 2–3 ml. 40 percent hypaque solution is attached to the catheter and the dye injected—*slowly and gently.*" [37]

Acute pancreatitis has occurred after pancreatography, especially when too much dye had been used and the opaque solution had been injected hurriedly and forcefully.

Retrograde pancreatography is commonly employed after distal pancreatectomy followed by pancreatojejunostomy or pancreaticogastrostomy. (See Fig. 4.)

Transduodenal sphincterotomy. This operation was originally sponsored by Archibald,[1a] but during the last 25 years it has

been cogently advocated by Doubilet and Mulholland.[18, 20] (See Figs. 9-13.)

These surgeons have recommended sphincterotomy as a definitive treatment of chronic pancreatitis and have claimed good results in 89 percent of their cases (500 cases of chronic pancreatitis were treated by sphincterotomy up to May 1, 1957).

Doubilet, in Treatment of Recurrent Pancreatitis by Sphincterotomy (*Current Surgical Management*, Philadelphia, Saunders, 1957) stated that the concept that pancreatitis results from the reflux of bile into the pancreatic duct must be based on three premises: (1) that the bile and pancreatic ducts join above the papilla of Vater; (2)

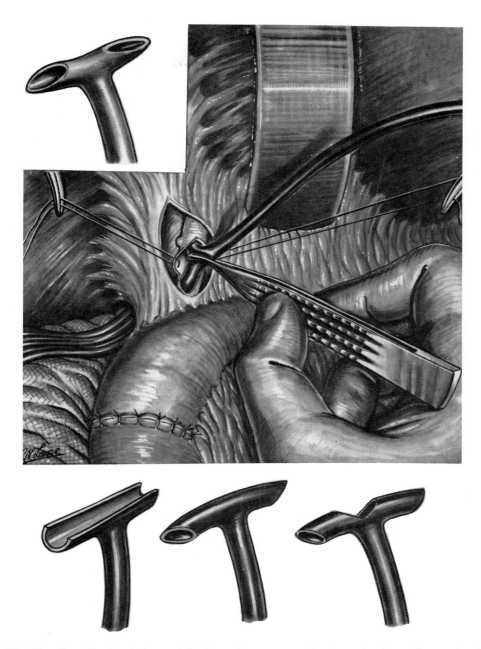

FIG. 12.   Short T tube drainage following sphincterotomy. The operation is nearly completed. A short T tube is being inserted into the choledochus, and the incision will be sutured around the issuing limb of the T tube. *Inset:* Various types of T tubes in common use are depicted. Maingot's guttered T tube has proved invaluable.

that increased tonicity of the sphincter of Oddi converts these ducts into a common passageway, allowing bile to be retrojected into the pancreatic duct; and (3) that section of the sphincter of Oddi, by preventing further entry of bile into the pancreatic duct,

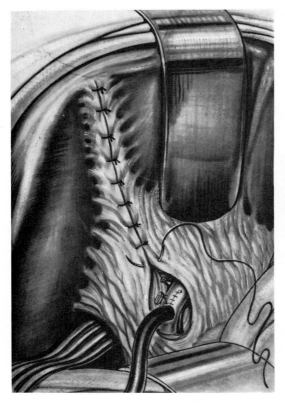

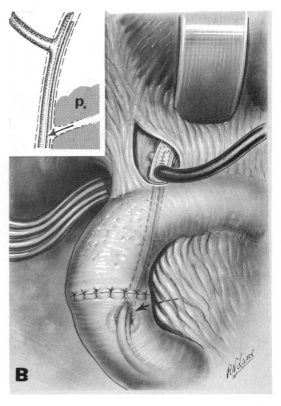

FIG. 13. (A) Cholecystectomy, exploration of the bile ducts, dilatation of the ampulla of Vater with graduated Bakes' dilators, and T tube choledochostomy.

FIG. 13. (B) Chronic pancreatitis associated with fibrosis of the sphincter of Oddi. Transduodenal sphincterotomy combined with cholecystectomy and long-T-tube choledochostomy and duodenostomy, employing Maingot's guttered T tube.

will halt the progress of the disease.

Jones et al.[36] reported that after sphincterotomy in 25 patients, 76 percent experienced no further attacks of pancreatitis. According to Waugh (1958), the operations of sphincterotomy and sphincteroplasty had not appeared to be effective in more than 65 percent of patients.

Warren and his associates performed sphincterotomy as a definitive procedure in 39 cases. This operation was carried out in patients with moderate degrees of pancreatitis, although the disease was severe in two instances. The results were good in 49 percent of cases, although 3 of 39 patients died of postoperative pancreatitis.

Thistlethwaite and Smith[57] collected 23 cases in which sphincterotomy was performed for chronic pancreatitis. All were caused by

alcoholism. More than 70 percent of the patients failed to be relieved of their symptoms (Fig. 10).

Sphincterotomy or sphincteroplasty is also indicated in cases of fibrosis or stenosis of the sphincter of Oddi, for stones impacted in the ampulla of Vater or the distal reaches of the common bile duct (Fig. 11), and for overlooked or recurrent stones in the biliary passages (see Chap. 43, Parts A and B).

The following observations are worth emphasising: (a) Sphincterotomy as a definitive procedure (combined with cholecystectomy—when the gallbladder is present and normal—and T tube choledochostomy) will relieve about 40 percent of patients suffering from the milder forms of relapsing pancreatitis. (b) When sphincterotomy is combined with direct procedures upon the pancreatic

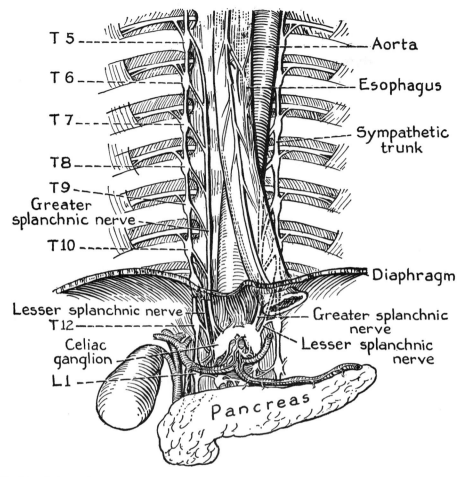

FIG. 14. Pain pathways from the pancreas. (Courtesy of Dr. Charles Puestow; and The Year Book Medical Publishers, Chicago.)

ducts (such as retrograde dilatation of the duct of Wirsung or the duct of Santorini, or both), good results may be expected if the obstructing agent (e.g., stone) is removed or a proximal stricture is adequately dilated or divided. (c) Following routine transduodenal exploration of the ducts of Wirsung and Santorini with Bakes' and other dilators, varying degrees of intrapancreatic obstruction have often been demonstrated. It is unusual to find an obstruction at the mouth of the duct of Wirsung. The most common sites of obstruction, in order of frequency, are: the junction of the two pancreatic ducts in the head of the gland, then the body and tail. When, on the other hand, the duct of Santorini is involved, the point of obstruction is at the ostium of the minor papilla itself or a few millimeters further on. The duct of Santorini is the major pancreatic duct in some 10 percent of cases. The ostium of the duct of Wirsung is situated at the *summit* of the papilla of Vater in about 12 percent of cases. (d) Retrograde dilatation of the main duct should be performed in selected cases, and this, when combined with pancreatography, will frequently confirm the fact that partial or complete ductal obstruction is a common event. It is exactly in these types of cases—with multiple ductal obstructions—that Puestow's operation should be entertained. (See Part B.)

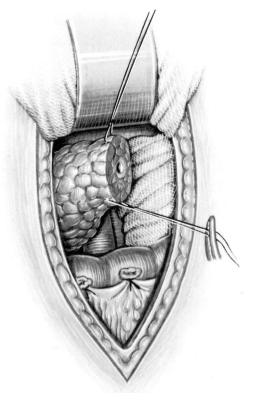

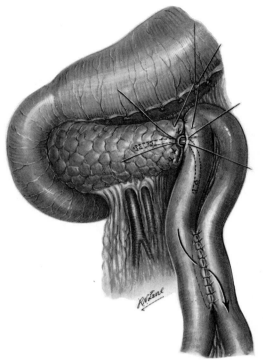

FIG. 16. Pancreatojejunostomy and entero-anastomosis. DuVal usually performs this operation employing a Roux-en-Y loop of proximal jejunum.

FIG. 15. Distal pancreatectomy with pancreatojejunostomy or pancreatogastrostomy. The pancreas has been transected at its neck, and the body and the tail of the gland have been removed. The duct of Wirsung is cleared of stones and debris. At this stage, a pancreatogram may be taken. (From Smith and Sherlock, *Surgery of the Gallbladder and Bile Ducts,* 1964. Courtesy of Rodney Smith and Butterworths, London.)

A pancreatogram is preferable to *transpancreatic* exploration of the main duct. It can be performed by inserting a needle into a dilated portion of the duct, aspirating pancreatic juice, and then by injecting about 2 ml of 35 to 40 percent telepaque. The "immediate" pancreatograms will serve as a useful guide to the surgeon in his selection of the most appropriate procedure in the circumstances.

Nerve interruption. There are a number of operations that have been directed toward the interruption of portions of the sympathetic nervous system; they include the following: (a) Unilateral or bi-lateral thoracolumbar sympathectomy and splanchnicectomy (Guy and de Beaujeu).[44] (b) Transabdominal coeliac and superior mesenteric ganglionectomy or transthoracic splanchnicectomy.[29] (c) Total neurectomy of the head of the pancreas.[66]

It is claimed that such nerve interruption procedures may not only relieve pain, which is the most prominent symptom in chronic pancreatitis, but may also have a beneficial effect on the diseased gland by markedly increasing its blood supply (See Fig. 14). Warren sums up the views held by most surgeons regarding nerve interruption in the treatment of chronic relapsing pancreatitis as follows: "Our experience with thoracolumbar sympathectomy and splanchnicectomy has not justified continuing its use."

Biliary-intestinal diversionary anastomosis. Bowers and Greenfield[6] have long championed biliary-intestinal diversionary anastomosis, and they claim good results in

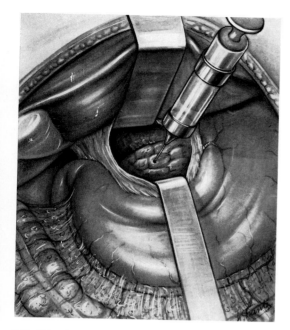

FIG. 17. Leger's technique. (From Leger, J. Chir.
76:93, 1958. Courtesy of Dr. Lucien Leger; and
Journal de Chirurgie.)

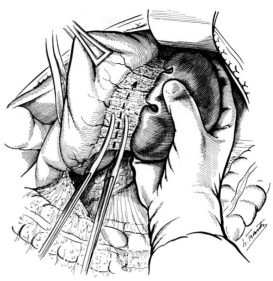

FIG. 19. Leger's technique. (From Leger, J. Chir.
76:93, 1958. Courtesy of Dr. Lucien Leger; and
Journal de Chirurgie.)

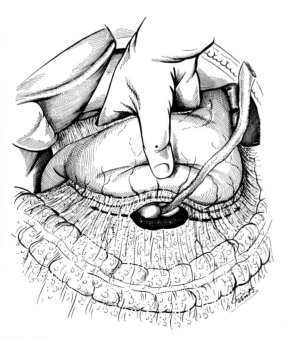

FIG. 18. Leger's technique. (From Leger, J. Chir.
76:93, 1958. Courtesy of Dr. Lucien Leger; and
Journal de Chirurgie.)

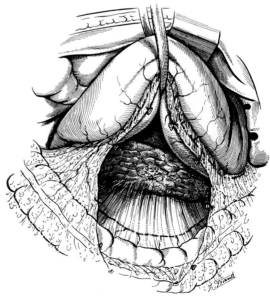

FIG. 20. Leger's technique. (From Leger, J. Chir.
76:93, 1958. Courtesy of Dr. Lucien Leger; and
Journal de Chirurgie.)

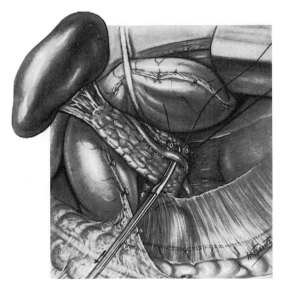

FIG. 21. Leger's technique. (From Leger, J. Chir. 76:93, 1958. Courtesy of Dr. Lucien Leger; and Journal de Chirurgie.)

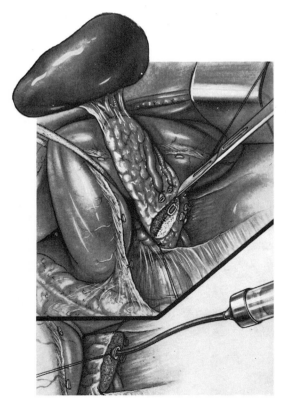

FIG. 22. Leger's technique. (From Leger, J. Chir. 76:93, 1958. Courtesy of Dr. Lucien Leger; and Journal de Chirurgie.)

chronic relapsing pancreatitis with chole-dochojejunal anastomosis on the Roux-en-Y plan. The common bile duct is transected well below the orifice of the cystic duct and the ascending Roux-en-Y limb of jejunum is anastomosed to the cut end of the chole-dochus while the other limb is joined end-to-side and as low as possible to the com-mencement of the ascending limb of jejunum.

The simple loop method is equally effica-cious and less complicated. Here, the apex of a lengthy loop of proximal jejunum is brought over the transverse colon and anasto-mosed (end-to-side) to the cut end of the common bile duct. When this is completed, a 3-inch (7.6-cm) entero-anastomosis between the afferent and efferent limbs of jejunum is constructed to deflect gastric contents away from the biliary-enteric anastomosis.

In some instances, the common bile duct has been anastomosed (side-to-side) to the first portion of the duodenum, and especially in cases of chronic pancreatitis, associated with severe obstructive jaundice. (Chole-dochoduodenostomy.)

On the whole, these operations have proved disappointing, except in the hands of Bow-ers[5] and Bowers and Sensenig.[7] They per-formed 31 of these operations: 26 of the patients had good results, 5 had poor re-sults, and 3 had developed ulcers of the stomach or duodenum. One patient devel-oped a stricture at the biliary-intestinal anas-tomosis.

Rousselot et al.[53] reported poor results in 4 of 5 patients treated by the Roux-en-Y technique.

Burgess and Kidd[8] have claimed good re-sults following *choledochoduodenostomy* for chronic pancreatitis: "Of 22 cases of chronic pancreatitis, 20 were completely relieved of their symptoms." In my opinion, the best biliary-intestinal diversional anastomosis is choledochoduodenostomy, side-to-side and with a large stoma.

DIRECT OPERATIONS UPON THE PANCREAS

Distal pancreatectomy alone. Distal or caudal pancreatectomy alone is indicated *when chronic pancreatitis is limited to the tail of the pancreas*, the remainder of the organ being, in every respect, normal. This type of pancreatitis is rare, but it is prone to

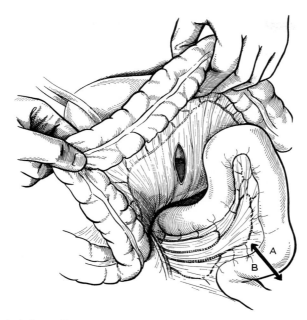

FIG. 23.   Leger's technique. (From Leger, J. Chir. 76:93, 1958. Courtesy of Dr. Lucien Leger; and Journal de Chirugie.)

occur after nonpenetrating abdominal injuries. Following the transection, the proximal end of the pancreatic duct is found, transfixed at two sites, and then elevated with two stay sutures, after which a number 3 or 4 French ureteric catheter is cautiously passed along its lumen and directed toward the pancreatic mouth and the lumen of the duodenum. If any obstacle (such as a fibrous stricture) is encountered, pancreatography becomes a mandatory procedure. When the catheter passes without restraint into the duodenum, the end of the duct is elevated and carefully sutured with a series of closely applied sutures of fine silk. This method is more secure than transfixion-ligation of the ductal stump. The operation is completed by snugly suturing the anterior and posterior margins of the gland together—without tension. If, on the other hand, there is definite evidence that the main duct is obstructed, say at a point where it traverses the head of the pancreas, *retrograde drainage*—pancreatojejunostomy or pancreatogastrostomy—will have to be carried out (Fig. 15).

Pancreatojejunostomy by the methods of Duval and Leger.   Cattell[9] was the first to suggest the performance of *lateral or*

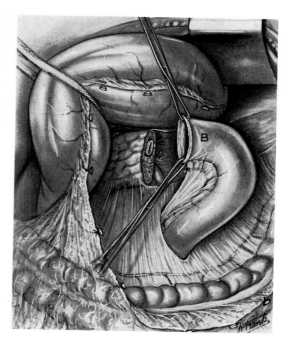

FIG. 24.   Leger's technique. (From Leger, J. Chir. 76:93, 1958. Courtesy of Dr. Lucien Leger; and Journal de Chirurgie.)

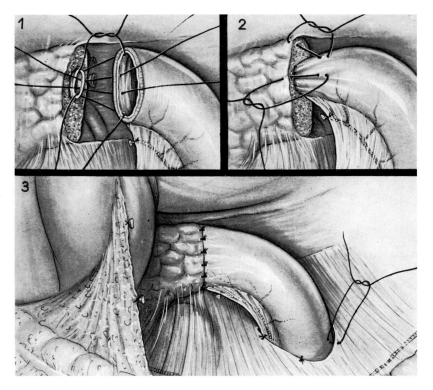

FIG. 25.   Leger's technique. (From Leger, J. Chir. 76:93, 1958. Courtesy of Dr. Lucien Leger; and Journal de Chirugie.)

side-to-side anastomosis of the duct of Wirsung to an antecolic loop of proximal jejunum to relieve the proximal obstruction of the main pancreatic duct in cases of irremovable carcinoma of the head of the pancreas or of the periampullary zone. The additional operative procedures included cholecystojejunostomy combined with anastomosis of the afferent and efferent limbs of the jejunum to shunt the pent-up bile in the gallbladder and biliary tree into the intestine and thereby overcome (for a few months at least) jaundice and its teasing effects.

By his method, pancreatic juice and bile were therefore restored to the alimentary tract with the result that icterus was allayed and weight-gain assured for a period of about 5 to 7 months. Again, should the diagnosis perchance prove to be wrong, the combined procedures would afford considerable mitigation of some of the manifestations of chronic pancreatitis.

Pancreatojejunostomy may be carried out by the Roux-en-Y plan or by uniting the duct of Wirsung to the apex of a loop of proximal jejunum.

When the latter operation is selected, a *supplementary entero-anastomosis* should be performed to divert the irritating gastrointestinal contents away from the pancreatojejunal stoma (Fig. 16).

In certain instances, and especially where the main pancreatic duct is small, the stoma may with advantage be splinted with an inlying radiopaque latex tube.

DuVal [22] advocated caudal pancreatectomy with end-to-side pancreatojejunostomy, based on the Roux-en-Y plan, for certain cases of chronic relapsing pancreatitis associated with irremovable ductal obstruction in the head of the gland. The primary point of stricturing almost invariably occurs at a point approximately 4 cm above the sphincter of Oddi in the pancreatic duct, that is, in the neck of the gland where it crosses the vertebral bodies.

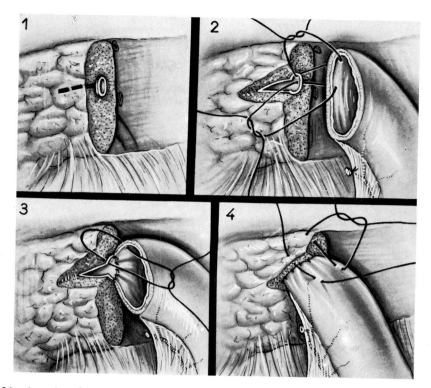

FIG. 26.   Leger's technique. (From Leger, J. Chir. 76:93, 1958. Courtesy of Dr. Lucien Leger; and Journal de Chirugie.)

The object of this operation is to procure relief of this blockage by permitting retrograde flow of the pancreatic secretions into a loop of proximal jejunum.

The technical steps include splenectomy with resection of the tail (and, on occasion, a portion of the body) of the pancreas; end-to-side anastomosis of the duct of Wirsung to a loop of proximal jejunum, and an adequate side-to-side anastomosis between the afferent and efferent limbs of the jejunum.

It should be noted that the pancreato-jejunal anastomosis is accomplished with a series of all-coats interrupted sutures of fine silk, that the mucosa of the duct is approximated to the musoca of the jejunum, and that the stoma is splinted with a polyethylene or latex tube which is subsequently passed into the small intestine by means of jejunal peristalsis.

Leger [39] *gives a good account of this operation based on the Roux-en-Y principle.* He submits a number of well-executed illustrations depicting the important steps in his technique (Figs. 17 to 27).

On the whole, the results of this operation are good when there is a localized proximal point of obstruction in the head of the gland. Where, however, there are *multiple* points of struction in the duct of Wirsung (a not uncommon finding), the operations of DuVal and Leger will often fail to decompress the ductal system.

Where there is an irremovable obstruction in the proximal portion of the main pancreatic duct, better results may be anticipated by anastomosing the duct in the proximal end of the tail of the divided pancreas to the posterior wall of the stomach—pancreatogastrostomy by R. Smith's technique.

Pancreatogastrostomy — Rodney Smith's technique. (Figs. 28-32.) The initial steps of this operation include: liberation of the gastrocolic ligament from the entire length of the greater curvature of the stomach in order to obtain an excellent view of the

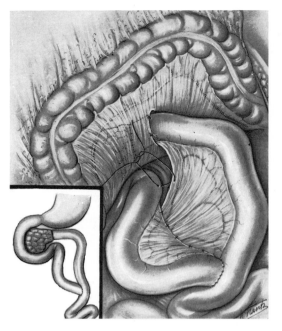

FIG. 27. Leger's technique. (From Leger, J. Chir. 76:93, 1958. Courtesy of Dr. Lucien Leger; and Journal de Chirurgie.)

anterior face of the pancreas; ligating and dividing the vasa brevia; mobilizing the tail of the pancreas together with the spleen; isolation, ligation, and division of the splenic blood vessels in the hilus of the spleen; transection of the neck of the pancreas; and removal of the spleen together with the body and tail of the pancreas. Two transfixion sutures are inserted and tied in the substance of the superior and inferior surfaces of the pancreas to control bleeding and also to act as tractors during the early stages of the pancreatogastrostomy. After the transection of the gland, the proximal end of the duct is gently dilated, irrigated with warm saline solution, and any debris or stones are removed. A number 3 or 4 French catheter is passed down the duct toward the duodenum and a pancreatogram is taken to illuminate the ductal system. If any obstruction is detected in the head of the gland, the surgeon should proceed with the performance of intraluminal pancreatogastrostomy.

The technical steps of this procedure are illustrated in Figures 28 to 32. Note that the

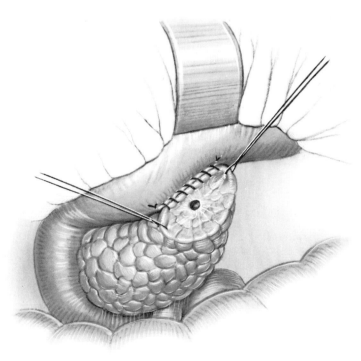

FIG. 28. Pancreatogastrostomy. An anastomosis of the main duct in the transected pancreas to the posterior aspect of the stomach is begun using silk sutures. (From Smith and Sherlock. *Surgery of the Gallbladder and Bile Ducts,* 1964. Courtesy of Rodney Smith and Butterworths, London.)

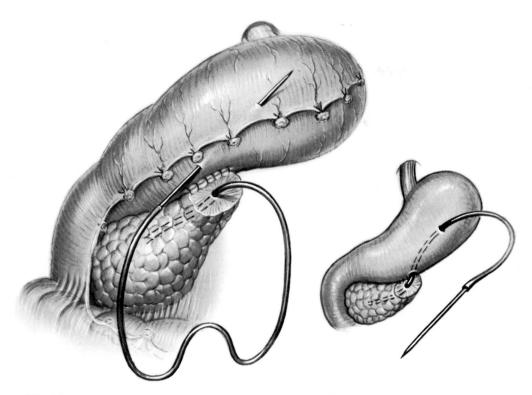

FIG. 29. Pancreatogastrostomy—Rodney Smith's technique. With half of the anastomosis completed, long polyethylene tube is inserted into pancreatic duct and other end brought out through stomach as illustrated. (From Smith and Sherlock. *Surgery of the Gallbladder and Bile Ducts,* 1964. Courtesy of Rodney Smith and Butterworths, London.)

mucosa of the pancreatic duct is sutured to the mucosa of the stomach with a few interrupted sutures of 0000 silk or merselene. This ensures a mucosa-to-mucosa approximation which mitigates the tendency to stricture formation at the small stoma.

The polyethylene tube is brought through the abdominal wall to the exterior and the gap between the anterior wall of the stomach and the parietes is closed with two interrupted sutures of catgut. The end of the tube is fastened to the abdominal wall with strips of Micropore and the excess of the tubing is cut away. The tube drains pancreatic juice into a Uri-bag or bottle for 7 to 10 days and then, after a final pancreatogram, it is removed.

Pancreatogastrostomy is, unquestionably, one of the most efficient retrograde duct drainage procedures practised at the present time. It yields about 75 percent good results.

Subtotal and total pancreatectomy. *Subtotal Pancreatectomy* (95 percent pancreatectomy) entails removal of the spleen and 95 percent of the distal pancreas (Figs. 33, 34 and 35). At the completion of the operation, all that remains is a small cuff of pancreas lying within the lesser curvature of the duodenum. The duct of Wirsung is ligated; haemostasis of the raw surface of the pancreas is obtained by means of transfixion sutures; and the normal choledochoduodenal relationships are maintained. In most cases exocrine substitution therapy is required.

Good accounts of the operation are given by Child and Fry.[12] Fry and Child III,[20] and Child, Frey, and Fry.[11] I am indebted to Dr. Charles F. Frey, Associate Professor of Surgery, University Hospital, Ann Arbor, Michigan, for supplying me with his important and valuable contribution on *95 percent pancreatectomy for chronic pancreatitis.*

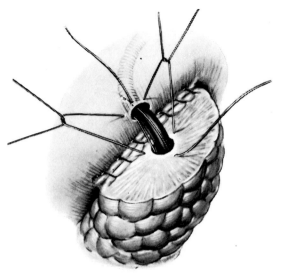

FIG. 30. Distal pancreatectomy. The posterior half of the anastomosis between the pancreas and the back of the stomach has been completed. Note the insertion of fine silk sutures to obtain an approximation of the mucosa of the stomach to the mucosa of the pancreatic duct. (From Rob, Smith, Morgan. *Operative Surgery*, 2d ed., 1964. Courtesy of the editors and Butterworths, London.)

95 PERCENT PANCREATECTOMY FOR CHRONIC PANCREATITIS

Charles F. Frey

The 95 percent pancreatectomy has been performed on 54 patients with chronic pancreatitis (Fig. 35). There was one operative death. The patient had portal hypertension and, in retrospect, should have undergone portal decompression prior to pancreatoduodenectomy. We have had 13 late deaths, all in alcoholic patients, a year or more following operation. Ten of the 13 patients who died were free of pain following operation, until death. Six of the 13 patients who died following 95 percent resection, gave a history of continued alcoholism, inadequate nutrition, mismanagement of insulin replacement, and narcotic addiction. Pneumonia, delerium tremens, hepatic failure and diabetic coma were often terminal events. These poor results represent a failure in proper patient selection.

Seven of the 13 late deaths following 95 percent pancreatic resection were either unre-

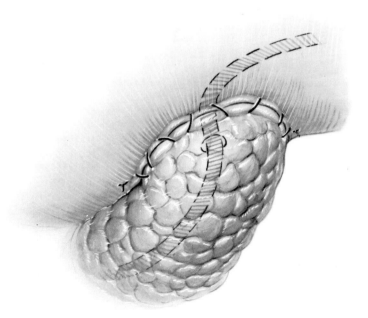

FIG. 31. Pancreatogastrostomy. An indwelling tube anastomosis of the pancreas to the stomach is completed. (From Smith and Sherlock. *Surgery of the Gallbladder and Bile Ducts*, 1964. Courtesy of Rodney Smith and Butterworths, London.)

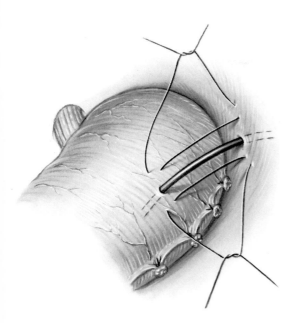

FIG. 32. Pancreatogastrostomy. A polyethylene tube is brought through the abdominal wall to the exterior, and the gap between the anterior wall of the stomach and the parietes is closed with two interrupted sutures of catgut. The tube will drain into the bottle for 7 to 10 days; then after the final pancreatogram, it will be removed. (From Smith and Sherlock, *Surgery of the Gallbladder and Bile Ducts,* 1964. Courtesy of Rodney Smith and Butterworths, London.)

lated or only indirectly related to the nutritional and metabolic effects of the operation. Alcoholism, pancreatitis, and the exocrine and endocrine insufficiency resulting from 95 percent distal resection of the pancreas probably contributed in part to the death of three patients. Death occurred in one patient from suicide, in one from gastrointestinal hemorrhage followed by myocardial infarction, and in one from pneumonia. Continued alcoholism and exocrine or endocrine insufficiency did not seem important in the deaths of 4 patients one from carcinoma of the breast, one from peritonitis following dilatation and curettage, one from myocardial infarction, and one from unrelieved intestinal obstruction.

Thirty-five patients (66 percent), all alive and free of pain following 95 percent distal

resection of the pancreas. In addition, 10 of the 13 patients who died late were free of pain. Thus, relief of pain was achieved in 85 percent of all patients subjected to 95 percent distal resection of the pancreas.

Five of 54 (9.4 percent) patients with 95 percent distal resection of the pancreas had a poor result. These five patients are still alive. Three patients (5.6 percent) had a recurrence of pain following 95 percent distal resection of the pancreas, and later died.

Preoperatively, 24 of 54 patients (44.4 percent) were diabetic, 9 (16.6 percent) of the patients were insulin-dependent diabetics, and 15 (27.8 percent) were diet-controlled prior to 95 percent pancreatectomy. After 95 percent pancreatectomy, 38 (71.7 percent) of the patients were insulin-dependent diabetic, 4 (7.54 percent) required oral hyperglycemic agents, and in 11 (20.75 percent), diabetes was controlled by diet.

We have found excision of the proximal or distal pancreas a useful procedure in the relief of pain associated with pancreatitis, but it should be reserved for individuals responsible enough to manage the exocrine and endocrine deficiencies that may result.

Total pancreatectomy has been carried out when the whole gland and ductal systems have been hopelessly compromised and the pancreas is a useless organ riddled with cysts, calculi, and chalk.

In an article by Warren et al.,[59] *Life after Total Pancreatectomy for Chronic Pancreatitis: Clinical Study of Eight Cases,* it is stated that total pancreatectomy is a feasible operation, as evidenced by more than 150 successful cases reported in the literature. These authors describe the management of 8 cases. Long-term follow-up study was possible in all the patients (satisfactory results in 80 percent), in whom they were able to observe the course of the physiological derangements this extensive operation produces. The main complications are: (1) diabetes and steatorrhea, (2) loss of weight, and (3) jejunal ulceration. The postoperative management was, in many respects, similar to that of the four successful cases reported some 20 years previously by Waugh and his colleagues.[62]

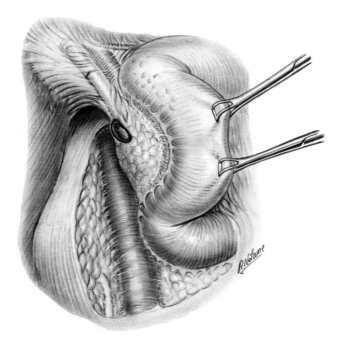

FIG. 33. Exposure of the head of the pancreas and the choledochus by Kocher's method. The common duct lymph node, the inferior vena cava, and the right ureter are also displayed. A good view of the posterolateral aspects of the duodenum (second part) and the head of the pancreas is obtained.

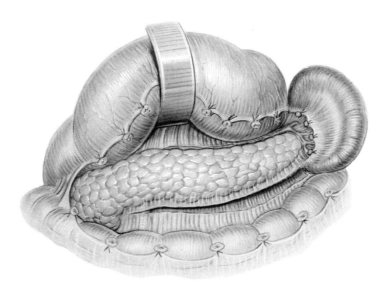

FIG. 34. Exposure of the pancreas and the hilus of the spleen. The peritoneum on the posterior wall just inferior and superior to the pancreas is incised to allow a ready manipulation of the organ prior to the performance of 95 percent pancreatectomy.

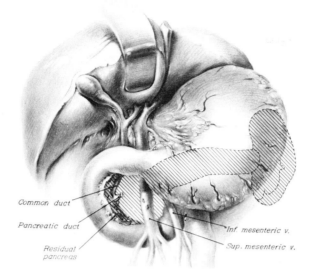

FIG. 35. A 95 percent pancreatectomy for relapsing or chronic progressive pancreatitis. (Courtesy of Charles F. Frey; and *Surgery, Gynecology and Obstetrics.*)

REFERENCES

1. Archibald, Surg. Gynecol. Obstet. 28:529, 1919.
1a. Archibald, Ann. Surg. 74:426, 1921.
2. Beall et al., Gastroenterology 39:215, 1960.
3. Bockus, ed., Gastroenterology, Vol. III, Philadelphia, Saunders, 1966.
4. Bouchier, Youngs, and Agnew, Clin. Gastroenterology 1:105, 1972.
5. Bowers, Surgery 30:116, 1951.
6. Bowers and Greenfield, Ann. Surg. 134:99, 1951.
7. Bowers and Senning, Surgery 38:113, 1955.
8. Burgess and Kidd, Br. Med. J. 1:607, 1967.
9. Cattell, Surg. Clin. North Am. 6:636, 1947.
10. Cattell and Warren, eds., Surgery of the Pancreas, Philadelphia, Saunders, 1953.
11. Child, Frey, and Fry, Surg. Gynecol. Obstet. 129:49, 1969.
12. Child and Fry, Surg. Clin. North Am. 42:1352, 1962.
13. Comfort and Steinberg, Gastroenterology 21:54, 1952.
14. Comfort, Gastroenterology 31:727, 1956.
15. Cook, Lennard-Jones, Sherif, and Wiggins, Gut 8:408, 1967.
16. Dean, Scott, and Law, Ann. Surg. 173:443, 1971.
17. Doubilet, Proc. R. Soc. Med. 50:629, 1957.
18. Doubilet and Mulholland, Ann. Surg. 128:609, 1948.
19. Doubilet and Mulholland, Surg. Gynecol. Obstet. 86:295, 1948.
20. Doubilet and Mulholland, Am. J. Surg. 105:741, 1963.
21. Dreiling and Janowitz, The Measurement of Pancreatic Secretory Function, in de Reuck and Cameron, eds., The Exocrine Pancreas, Boston, Little, Brown, 1961.
22. DuVal, Ann. Surg. 140:775, 1954.
23. DuVal, Am. J. Surg. 109:541, 1965.
24. Fleming, Pancreatitis, In Diseases of the Digestive System, Br. Med. J. 1:165, 1969.
25. Frey, Arch. Surg. 98:466, 1969.
26. Fry and Child, III, Ann. Surg. 162:543, 1965.
27. Gordon and Grossman, Gastroenterology 36:447, 1959.
28. Goulston and Gallagher, Gut 3:252, 1962.
29. Grimson et al., Surgery 22:230, 1947.
30. Gross, Ann. Intern. Med. 49:796, 1958.
31. Gross, Gambill, and Ulrich, Am. J. Med. 21:54, 1962.
32. Gross, Comfort, and Ulrich, Trans. Assoc. Physicians 70:127, 1957.
33. Hatchette, Shuler, and Murison, J. Nucl. Med. 13:51, 1971.
34. Hendren, Greep, and Patton, Arch. Dis. Child. 40:132, 1965.
35. Howard and Jordan, eds., Surgical Diseases of the Pancreas, Montreal, Lippincott, 1960.
36. Jones et al., Ann. Surg. 147:180, 1958.
37. Keddie, Br. J. Surg. 54:106, 1967.
38. Kelley et al., N.Y. State J. Med. 57:721, 1951.
39. Leger, J. Chir. (Paris) 76:93, 1958.
40. Lundh, Gastroenterology 42:275, 1962.
41. McCarthy, Brown, Melmed, and Bouchier, Gut 13:75, 1972.
42. McDonough, Surg. Clin. North Am. 35:775, 1955.
43. Maingot, R. Free Hosp. J. 29:169, 1966.
44. Mallet-Guy and de Beaujeu, Arch. Surg. 60:233, 1950.
45. Marks et al., Gut 4:217, 1963.
46. Mixter et al., N. Engl. J. Med. 266:265, 1962.
47. Morlock, Proc. Mayo Clin. 49:80, 1957.

48. Opie, Am. J. Med. Sci. 121:27, 1901.
49. Opie, Diseases of the Pancreas, 2d ed., Philadelphia, Lippincott, 1910.
50. Owens and Howard, Ann. Surg. 147:326, 1958.
51. Poulsen, Acta Med. Scand. 138:413, 1950.
52. Pyrah et al., Br. J. Surg. 53:245, 1966.
53. Rousselot et al., New Engl. J. Med. 250:267, 1954.
54. Sarles et al., Am. J. Dig. Dis. 6:688, 1961.
55. Strum and Spiro, Ann. Int. Med. 74:264, 1971.
56. Svoboda et al., Gastroenterology 44:855, 1963.
57. Thistlethwaite and Smith, Ann. Surg. 158:226, 1963.
58. Vernon et al., Br. J. Surg. 57:906, 1970.
59. Warren et al., Ann. Surg. 164:830, 1966.
60. Warren and Mountain, Surg. Clin. North Am. 51:693, 1971.
61. Warren and Veidenheimer, New Engl. Med. J. 266:323, 1962.
62. Waugh et al., Proc. Mayo Clin. 21:25, 1946.
63. White, ed., Pancreatitis, Baltimore, Williams & Wilkins, 1966.
64. Wiggins, Gut 8:415, 1967.
65. Wright, Br. J. Surg. 45:394, 1958.
66. Yoshioka and Wakabayashi, Arch. Surg. 76:546, 1958.

B. Longitudinal Pancreatojejunostomy

CHARLES B. PUESTOW

Chronic pancreatitis may be a primary disease of the organ itself or may be secondary to disease of adjacent structures such as the biliary tract or peptic ulcer disease of the duodenum or stomach. If it is a secondary disease, correction of the primary disease, particularly of the biliary tract, will usually result in recession of pancreatitis. Primary chronic pancreatitis may result from a number of etiological factors including alcoholism, inflammation often caused by infection, dietary indiscretion, intraductal tumors, and trauma. In most of our patients with primary chronic pancreatitis, we have found multiple strictures of the pancreatic ducts with dilated pockets creating a "chain of lakes" effect. Continuous pancreatic secretion into these pockets builds up a considerable pressure which we believe is responsible for the pain of this disease. Long proximal strictures of the ducts of Wirsung and Santorini—extending from the duodenum for a distance of 2 to 4 or more cm—are almost invariaby found (Fig. 36). Throughout the remainder of the duct of Wirsung, multiple strictures are encountered. To treat this disease properly, it is essential to open and drain all pockets and incise all strictures except the long proximal ones. It is not feasible to approach these strictures transduodenally and through the papilla of Vater. Adequate drainage can be established by incising the anterior wall of the pancreas and the duct of Wirsung from the tail through the body and head until the final and generally largest pocket is opened close to the duodenal wall. It is not necessary to incise the long proximal strictures if no pockets are overlooked. A defunctionalized limb of jejunum is then anastomosed to the pancreas and intestinal continuity is reestablished by a Roux-en-Y jejunojejunostomy. We utilize two techniques: one in which the pancreas is inserted into the divided end of the jejunum; the other in which a side-to-side longitudinal pancreatojejunostomy is performed.

PANCREATO-JEJUNOSTOMY WITH SPLENECTOMY

The abdomen is opened through a long high left paramedian incision. If the surgeon so desires a long transverse incision may be made about 2 inches (5 cm) above the umbilicus. The anterior surface of the pancreas is exposed by division of the gastrocolic omentum (Fig. 37). The pancreas may be aspirated with a syringe and needle in an effort to locate pockets, although this is not essential if the disease is manifest. The pancreas is then mobilized from its bed, beginning at its inferior margin. Because of mini-

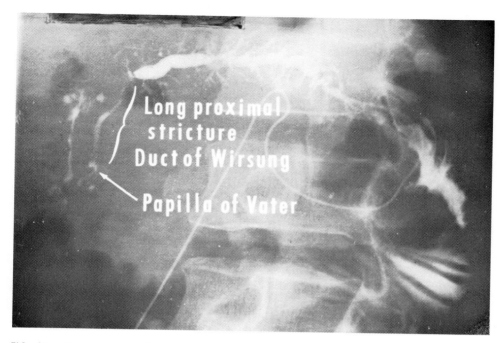

FIG. 36. Pancreatogram demonstrating long proximal strictures of the ducts of Wirsung and Santorini, with multiple strictures in the remainder of the duct of Wirsung.

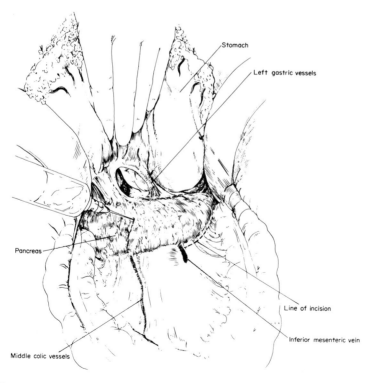

FIG. 37. Exposure of the anterior surface of the pancreas by division of the gastrocolic omentum. Aspiration of the pancreas to locate a pocket.

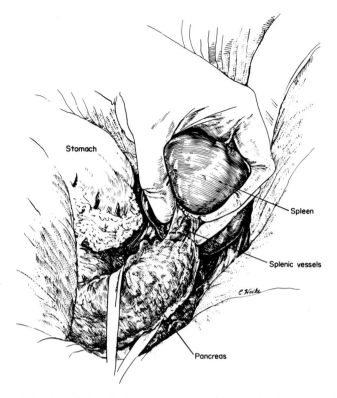

Stomach

Spleen

Splenic vessels

C Nocke

Pancreas

FIG. 38.   Mobilization of the distal pancreas and spleen, and subsequent splenectomy.

mal vascularity in this anatomical region, little bleeding is encountered. The main blood supply to the pancreas comes from the splenic vessels, which are on its superior margin. In chronic pancreatitis, however, the splenic vessels are densely adherent to or incorporated within the pancreas. For this reason, it is usually necessary to remove the spleen. The spleen is mobilized by dividing the splenorenal and splenophrenic ligaments and dividing the gastrosplenic ligament with its vasa breva and the splenocolic ligament. This permits the spleen and left portion of the pancreas to be elevated from the abdominal cavity. The splenic vessels are then divided and ligated (Fig. 38). Mobilization of the posterior surface of the pancreas is continued to the right until the superior mesenteric vessels are reached. It is well to re-ligate the splenic vessels at this level.

The pancreas is vertically transected about $\frac{1}{2}$ cm from its tip until the duct of Wirsung is divided (Fig. 39). A probe is inserted into the duct and passed to the right. The probe usually encounters a stricture in from 2 to 3 cm from its introduction (Fig. 40). By sharp dissection, the anterior portion of the pancreas and the anterior wall of the duct of Wirsung are divided, the dissection continu-

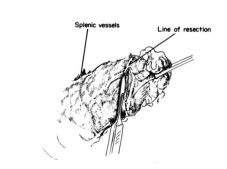

Splenic vessels

Line of resection

FIG. 39.   Transection of the tip of the pancreatic tail to locate the duct of Wirsung.

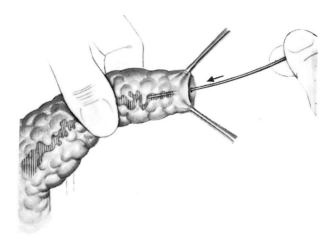

FIG. 40. Probing of the pancreatic duct to locate the most distal stricture. (From Rob, Smith and Morgan. *Operative Surgery*, 2d ed., 1969. Courtesy of the editors and Butterworths, London.)

ing to and through the first stricture. Beyond this stricture, the duct is usually considerably dilated, permitting further section of the pancreas and anterior duct wall to be performed with scissors—one blade being within the duct and the other outside the pancreas (Fig. 41). The dissection is carried toward the duodenum well into the head of the pancreas. A large pocket is usually encountered in the head of the gland and is of sufficient size to admit the surgeon's finger (Fig. 42). This pocket must not be overlooked. It is usually necessary to carry the incision to within 1/2 to 1 cm of the duodenum. In a fibrotic pancreas, very little bleeding is encountered and it can be controlled by clamping with Allis forceps. It is seldom necessary to ligate such vessels, as bleeding is usually under control when the surgeon is ready to remove the forceps. During dissection of the pancreas, bleeding can be minimized if the surgeon will place his index finger behind the gland and his thumb anterior to apply pressure. This completes the operation upon the pancreas itself.

The jejunum is then divided about 25 cm below the ligament of Treitz, the site being selected by the vascular arcades to permit free mobility of the distal limb. The distal limb of the jejunum is brought through a rent in the transverse mesocolon. The jejunum is placed beside the pancreas to measure the site at which the transfixion sutures will be brought through the bowel wall (Fig. 43). One or two traction sutures are placed through the tail of the pancreas and tied (Fig. 44). With the needle reversed in the needle holder, it is passed into the lumen of the bowel for the desired distance and then brought through the bowel wall (Fig. 45). These sutures aid in pulling the pancreas into the bowel. When the pancreas is properly positioned, the traction sutures are tied. They hold the pancreas in position and also take tension off the suture line between the end of the bowel and the outer surface of the pancreas. A single row of nonabsorbable sutures is placed between the serosa at the end of the bowel and the outer surface of the pancreas. Anteriorly the anastomosis must go to the right of the incision in the pancreas. Posteriorly the suture line cannot go beyond the superior mesenteric vessels (Fig. 46).

The opening in the transverse mesocolon is closed snugly around the jejunal limb. The proximal limb of the divided jejunum is anastomosed to the distal limb by a Roux-en-Y anastomosis approximately 25 cm below the pancreatojejunostomy (Fig. 47).

Occasionally a portion of the duct of Wir-

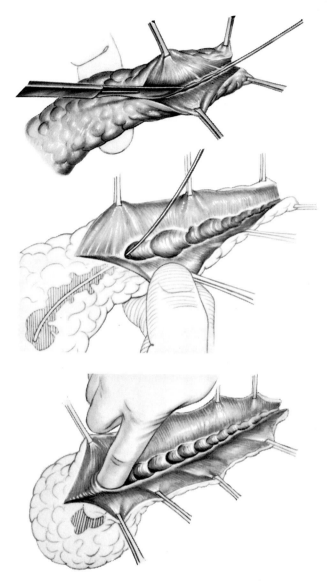

FIG. 41.   Using the probe as an indication of the site of the anterior surface of the duct, the pancreas is split in order to open up the pancreatic duct. This proceeds from the tail end of the gland right up into the neck and head, every pocket being opened, in the manner shown. (From Rob, Smith, and Morgan. *Operative Surgery,* 2d. ed., 1969. Courtesy of the editors and Butterworths, London.)

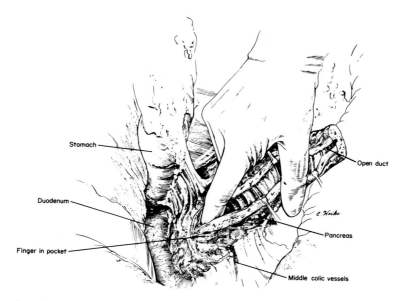

FIG. 42. Completion of dissection of the pancreas to open all pockets including the final one in the head of the gland.

sung will be totally obliterated. When this condition is encountered, one should make two to four longitudinal incisions approximately two-thirds of the way through the pancreas and about 3 mm apart throughout the length of the stricture. This will divide tributary ducts and permit them to drain into the jejunum.

PANCREATO-JEJUNOSTOMY WITHOUT SPLENECTOMY

This technique exposes the anterior surface of the pancreas in a manner similar to the preceding operation. The pancreas, however, is not mobilized from its bed. After completely exposing its anterior wall, the pancreas is aspirated to identify a pocket (Fig. 48). When a pocket is encountered, the needle is left in place as a guide, and an incision is made into the pocket by sharp dissection (Fig. 49). The duct is then incised to the right and to the left until all pockets have been opened. Any calculi within the ducts are removed (Fig. 50).

The jejunum is divided about 25 cm below the ligament of Treitz and the distal end brought through an opening in the transverse mesocolon. The antimesenteric border is crushed and incised for a sufficient distance to give a lumen somewhat larger than the opening in the pancreas. The serosa of the bowel is sutured to the anterior surface of the pancreas around the opening (Figs. 51–53). The sutures should be placed at least 5 mm beyond the cut edges of the pancreas. One should not attempt a mucosa-to-ductal anastomosis nor should one place sutures in the cut surface of the gland. By placing the sutures well beyond the margin, all divided ducts will drain freely into the bowel. Intestinal continuity is then reestablished by performing a Roux-en-Y jejunojejunostomy about 25 cm below the pancreatojejunostomy.

This technique is of value when the size of the pancreas prevents it from being introduced into the lumen of the bowel. It also obviates the need for splenectomy. Both techniques yield equally good results and the selection depends upon the desires of the surgeon.

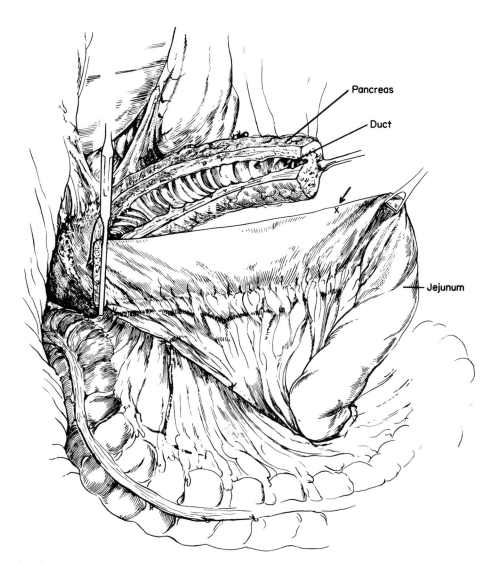

FIG. 43. Measurement of the distal limb of the jejunum to determine the length necessary to cover the incised portion of the pancreas completely.

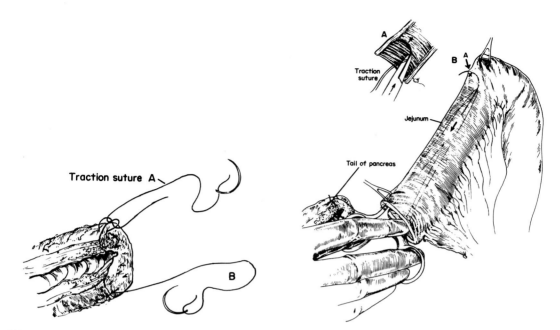

FIG. 44.   Traction sutures placed in the tail of the pancreas.

FIG. 45.   Traction sutures inserted in the lumen distal of the jejunum and brought out through the serosa surface.

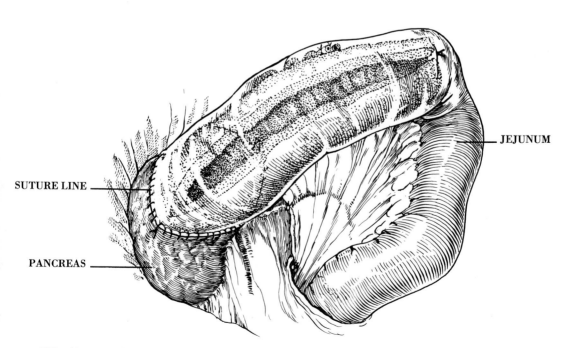

FIG. 46.   Completion of an anastomosis between the distal limb of the jejunum and the outer surface of the pancreas.

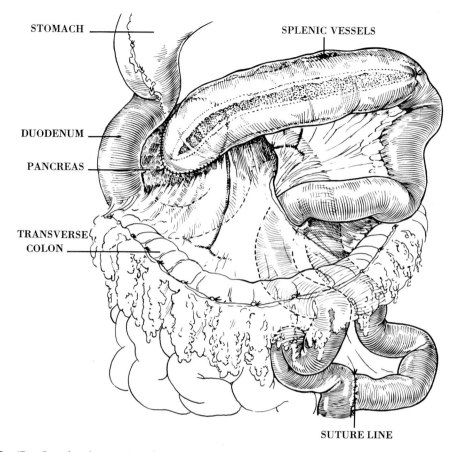

STOMACH

SPLENIC VESSELS

DUODENUM

PANCREAS

TRANSVERSE
COLON

SUTURE LINE

FIG. 47. Completed operation showing pancreatojejunostomy and entero-anastomosis. (Warner-Chilcott)

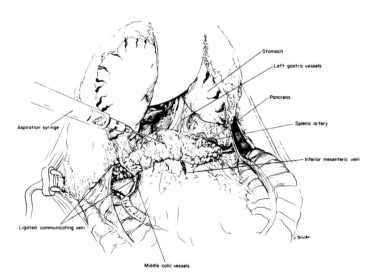

Stomach

Left gastric vessels

Pancreas

Splenic artery

Aspiration syringe

Inferior mesenteric vein

Ligated communicating vein

Middle colic vessels

FIG. 48. Aspiration of the exposed anterior surface of the pancreas with the spleen intact.

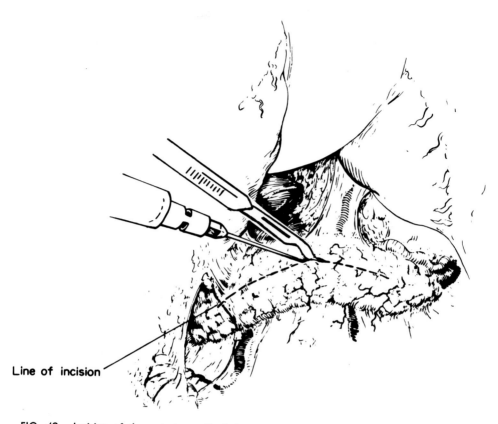

Line of incision

FIG. 49.   Incision of the anterior wall of the pancreas using a needle as a guide. (Hines)

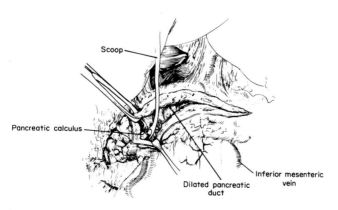

Scoop

Pancreatic calculus

Dilated pancreatic
duct

Inferior mesenteric
vein

FIG. 50.   Completed incision of the anterior wall of the pancreas and duct. Removal of calculi.

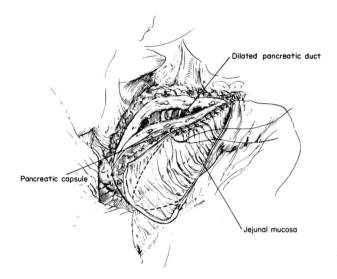

FIG. 51. Posterior row of sutures for pancreatojejunostomy. Suturing the serosa of the jejunum to the anterior wall of the pancreas. (Warner-Chilcott)

There are a few cardinal principles in the performance of longitudinal pancreatojejunostomy that are essential to its success:

1. All pockets within the pancreas must be opened and drained.
2. One should not attempt a mucosa-to-ductal anastomosis.

3. A defunctionalized limb of the jejunum should always be used. This prevents activation of pancreatic enzymes in proximity to the pancreas and digestion of the organ. Therefore, the pancreas should not be anastomosed to the small bowel in continuity.
4. The distal jejunal limb should be

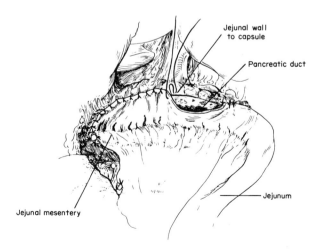

FIG. 52. Continuation of pancreatojejunostomy inserting anterior superior row of sutures. (Warner-Chilcott)

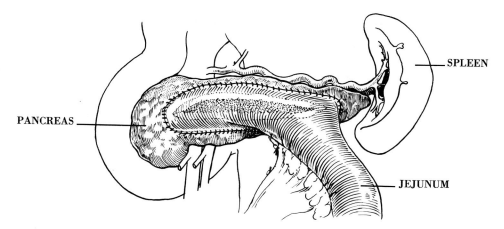

FIG. 53. Completed pancreatojejunostomy with spleen intact. (Warner-Chilcott)

brought to the pancreas retrocolically. If the jejunum is anastomosed to the pancreas antecolically, distension of the bowel may cause a disruption of the anastomosis.

RESULTS

Chronic pancreatitis has been a discouraging disease to treat. Few medical or surgical techniques have given good results. We have performed approximately 120 longitudinal pancreatojejunostomies. There have been 3 hospital deaths. Many of these patients have been poor-risk cases who have had from one to five previous operations of various kinds for pancreatitis. Seventy-five percent of the patients have been relieved of pain, have regained their normal weight, and have had a return to normal pancreatic digestion. Ten percent of the patients have not been benefited; most of these people were severe alcoholics and narcotic addicts who returned to their drinking and drug habit and generally had an inadequate diet. The remainder were benefited but had an occasional recurrence of pancreatic pain, usually associated with alcoholic excesses.

Longitudinal pancreatojejunostomy sacrifices little if any of an organ that has been destroyed to a point when it cannot carry on its normal physiological function. The operation has returned these patients to a normal digestion without the need of pancreatic supplements. If the patient has become diabetic, the operation will not cure this disease but it may allay it. We believe it should be tried before resort to the more radical pancreatic resections which carry a high mortality and may leave the patient a pancreatic invalid.

REFERENCES

1. Beattie, E. J., and Economou, S. G., An Atlas of Advanced Surgical Techniques, Philadelphia, Saunders, 1968, pp. 256-285.
2. Gillesby, W. J., and Puestow, C. B., Surg. Clin. North Am. 41:83, 1961.
3. Gillesby, W. J., and Puestow, C. B., Surgery 50:859, 1961.
4. Higgins, G. A., Pancreatojejunostomy, in C. B. Puestow and W. J. Gillesby, eds., Orr's Operations of General Surgery, Philadelphia, Saunders, 1968, pp. 475-478.
5. Puestow, C. B., Chronic Pancreatitis: Technique and Results of Longitudinal Pancreatojejunostomy, Comptes Rendus XXI Congres de la Societe Internationale de Chirurgie, Bruxelles, 1965.
6. Puestow, C. B., Hospital Practice 5:60, 1970.
7. Puestow, C. B., Surgery of the Biliary Tract, Pancreas and Spleen, 4th ed., Chicago, Year Book, 1970, pp. 257-345.
8. Puestow, C. B., and Gillesby, W. J., Longitudinal Pancreatojejunostomy, in E. Ellison, S. Friesen, and J. Mulholland, eds., Current Surgical Management, Vol. III, Philadelphia, Saunders, 1965, pp. 183-187.

9. Puestow, C. B., and Gillesby, W. J., Surg. Procedures, 1966.
10. Rob, C., and Smith, R., Operative Surgery, Vol. 4, 2d ed., London, Butterworth, 1969.
11. Zollinger, R. M., and Zollinger, R. M., Jr., Atlas of Surgical Operations, Vol. 2, New York, Macmillan, 1967, pp. 102-113.

C. Pancreatoduodenectomy for Chronic Relapsing Pancreatitis

KENNETH W. WARREN

While there are innumerable theories about the cause of pancreatitis, there are few established facts despite the volume of experimental projects and clinical reviews. There is also a tendency to classify patients with chronic pancreatitis into precise categories based upon theoretical etiological factors and to treat them accordingly. Our experience does not justify this approach because the clinical features and course of the disease are often unrelated to these factors.

Approximately one-third of our patients are alcoholics, one-third have gallstones, and one-third have no obvious clinical antecedent. More significantly, 18 percent of patients with chronic relapsing pancreatitis have gallstones and are addicted to alcohol. Equally striking is the usual mildness of so-called gallstone pancreatitis and the infrequency (6 to 9 percent) of common duct stones in patients with gallstones and pancreatitis. Furthermore, if gallstones were a precise etiological factor in pancreatitis, the disease would be common; its incidence would increase with increasing age. The opposite occurs. The incidence of gallstones increases dramatically after the age of 65 years, while the incidence of pancreatitis diminishes significantly. It is evident that there must be another factor contributing to the cause of pancreatitis when gallstones are present.

GENERAL PRINCIPLES

Relation of Pathological Changes to the Choice of Operation

Pancreatitis produces such a wide variety of progressive and irreversible structural changes that we choose the method of treatment on the basis of these changes in each patient rather than on any etiological classification.

The pathological changes of chronic relapsing pancreatitis range from swelling and mild induration of the gland to fibrosis, atrophy, patchy or widespread necrosis, cystic change, and pancreatolithiasis. Several of these alterations may be seen in the same gland, and different phases in the progression of the disease may be observed in the same patient. The head of the pancreas, for example, may be normal macroscopically, while its body and tail are involved by far-advanced disease. The core of these observations is that partial or complete intrapancreatic obstruction is apparently responsible for recurrent attacks of pancreatitis, and the treatment, therefore, depends upon relief of this obstruction.

Our increased understanding of these obstructive features has shown the futility of dealing with pancreatitis by procedures directed to the biliary tract, stomach, or pancreatic autonomic nerves. There is no question but that associated biliary tract disease should be corrected; however, our extensive experience in the surgical management of patients with severe pathological alterations proves that the most effective methods of treatment involve direct pancreatic ductal decompression or resection.[1, 7] The method of decompression or the extent of resection is dictated by the specific pathological changes found at laparotomy.[3-6, 8] Our choice is pancreatoduodenectomy if there are many points of obstruction in the head of the pancreas, long-standing advanced pancreatic disease, pancreatolithiasis, where the distribution of the pancreatic stones is associated with complete anatomical disorganization of the head of the pancreas, or failure of lesser operations. It is a technically difficult procedure, involving the sacrifice of a considerable portion of the pancreas; thus we employ it only if we feel that the pathological alterations are too advanced to be dealt with by less radical measures. Approximately 1 in 8 surgical patients with chronic relapsing pancreatitis seen at the Lahey Clinic has a sufficient number of indications for pancreatoduodenectomy.

Regardless of whether the pathological changes are minimal or advanced, caution should be the watchword in surgical manipulation of an inflamed and edematous pancreas because of the risk of postoperative acute pancreatitis. In contrast, the pancreas, which is fibrotic and calcific, tolerates surgical manipulation with less postoperative reaction.

Clinical Features

Table 1, showing the clinical features of our patients who have had pancreatoduodenectomy, indicates the chronicity and severity of the disease in this group. Of these patients, 81 percent have had one or more operations for pancreatitis and 33 percent have had sphincterotomy before registering at the Lahey Clinic. Intractable pain was the principal reason for operation. Almost 80 percent had a marked weight loss. Alcoholism and narcotic addiction were prominent features, although the exact incidence is difficult to determine because many persons deny having these problems.

Pancreatic calculi, which were present in two-thirds of our patients who had pancreatoduodenectomy, are probably a phase in the natural course of chronic pancreatitis. Usually they are associated with far-advanced disease. The precise mode of formation of these calculi is unknown, but we have observed repeatedly that the first calculus usually forms just distal to the most proximal intraductal stricture and that subsequent stones, which are usually smaller, appear distal to this point.[8] We have called this large proximal stone the sentinel stone, because it indicates the most proximal site of intraductal obstruction. When two or more major points of obstruction are present, pancreatolithiasis is often extensive, involving the primary and secondary pancreatic ducts throughout the gland.

Geevarghese[2] has reported 400 patients with pancreatolithiasis observed in India; only 2 percent were alcoholics. Dietary habits, unknown genetic factors, and other metabolic aberrations must play a definite, if subtle, role in the onset or progression of pancreatitis and pancreatolithiasis.

PREOPERATIVE CARE

Because of the variety and severity of nutritional and metabolic changes associated with far-advanced pancreatitis, particular attention must be directed toward assessment and correction of such deficiencies. Restoration of blood volume by appropriate transfusions of whole blood and by administration of albumin is urgent. Severe protein deficiency may require forced feeding using the Barron pump. If the patient can ingest an adequate amount, we prescribe a high-carbohydrate, high-protein, and low-fat diet—supplemented with vitamins. If the patient is diabetic, the dose of insulin is increased to cover the increased amount of food.

Diabetes mellitus is common in advanced chronic relapsing pancreatitis, although it may be so mild that a fasting blood sugar determination will fail to detect it. A blood sugar value determined 2 hours after a meal is much more reliable.

The status of calcium metabolism must be determined, since hypocalcemia or, more

Table 1.   CLINICAL FEATURES IN 148 PATIENTS WHO HAD PANCREATODUODENECTOMY FOR CHRONIC RELAPSING PANCREATITIS

Clinical Features	Number	Percent
Pain	148	100
Weight loss	117	79
Previous operation	120	81
Pancreatolithiasis	98	66
Alcoholism	90	61
Narcotic addiction	64	43
Cysts	58	39
Diabetes	74	50
Jaundice	43	29
Peptic ulcer	25	17

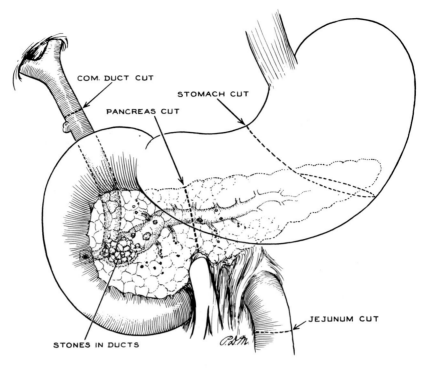

FIG. 54. The extent of the resection is indicated. Note that approximately 65 percent of the stomach is removed. The common duct is divided above its junction with the cystic duct. The jejunum is divided approximately 5 cm distal to the ligament of Treitz. The pancreas is divided at its neck, where it crosses the superior mesenteric and portal veins.

rarely, hypercalcemia secondary to a parathyroid adenoma may be present. Adequate replacement therapy when hypocalcemia is detected is most efficiently managed by intravenous administration of appropriate amounts of calcium gluconate. If a parathyroid adenoma is present, it should be removed before pancreatic surgery is attempted.

In addition to the previously mentioned studies, we routinely perform liver- and pancreatic-function tests. Barium contrast studies of the stomach and duodenum and intravenous cholangiograms are also helpful in the evaluation of patients for whom pancreatic resection is planned.

Selective celiac angiography is giving increasing information regarding the pancreas, and it outlines the origin and course of the major and even the smaller arteries to the pancreas and the liver. An understanding of these may be helpful during the operation. Pancreatic scans have been less revealing.

The increasing experience with the flexible fiber-optic duodenoscope has provided many useful data when the pancreatic duct and bile ducts has been cannulated and studied by radiographic contrast techniques. The Department of Gastroenterology at the Lahey Clinic can intubate the duct of Wirsung in approximately 90 percent of patients selected for this study.

SURGICAL TECHNIQUE

The operation is usually performed through a long right paramedian incision extending superiorly to the costal margin near the xiphoid. If the patient is obese, a transverse incision may be preferred. Lysis of extensive adhesions is usually necessary. The extent of the operation and the structures to be removed are indicated in Figure 54.

It is important to perform the operation in the following order: (1) mobilization of the head of the pancreas and duodenum; (2) elevation of the neck of the pancreas from the superior mesenteric and portal veins; (3) mobilization of the distal segment of the common bile duct; (4) division of the stomach; (5) mobilization and division of the proximal jejunum; (6) division of the neck of the pancreas and common bile duct; (7) removal of the specimen by division of the blood supply to the uncinate process of the pancreas and duodenum, and division of the uncinate process; and (8) reconstruction of the digestive tract by anastomosis of the pancreatic duct, common bile duct, and stomach to the jejunum.

Mobilization of the head of the pancreas and duodenum. After thorough examination of the pancreas and the abdominal and pelvic structures, the peritoneum is in-cised along the lateral aspect of the descending duodenum (Fig. 55). With Babcock forceps elevating the duodenum, the head of the pancreas is dissected from the posterior abdominal wall. This will expose, in turn, the right spermatic or ovarian vein, the inferior vena cava, the aorta, and approximately 2 inches of the *left* renal vein.

Elevation of the neck of the pancreas from the superior mesenteric and portal veins. The lesser omental sac is entered through the anterior layers of the gastrocolic omentum at the extreme right margin of this bursa. The ventral peritoneal leaflet of the transverse mesocolon is then displaced downward, displaying the middle colic vessels in the transverse mesocolon. The peritoneal incision is continued to the right, freeing the hepatic flexure and right half of the trans-

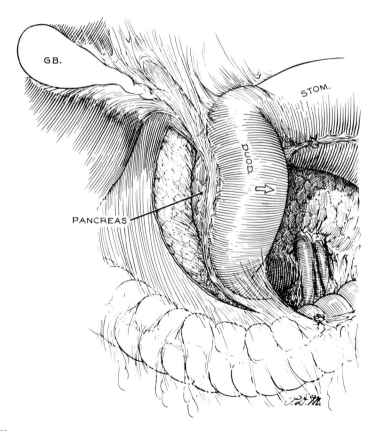

FIG. 55. The peritoneum lateral to the descending portion of the duodenum has been incised. A hepatic flexure of the colon has been displaced downward. The duodenum and head of the pancreas have been completely mobilized. This mobilization is extended from right to left beyond the inferior vena cava and the abdominal aorta. Superiorly, the dissection extends to the common bile duct.

verse colon. A moist abdominal pad is placed over the hepatic flexure of the colon and retracted downward.

The peritoneum is incised along the inferior border of the pancreatic neck and body, exposing the superior mesenteric vein inferior to the neck of the pancreas. The superior pancreatic lymph node will be used as a guide to the cleavage plane where the portal vein emerges from beneath the neck of the pancreas. The superior mesenteric artery can then be palpated and identified and the inferior pancreatoduodenal artery ligated and divided.

Using a small wad of gauze in a right-angle clamp, and beginning from below, the neck of the pancreas is elevated from the anterior surface of the superior mesenteric vein (Fig. 56). A small Penrose drain is then

passed around the neck of the gland (Fig. 57). It is used for subsequent manipulation and provides a helpful anatomical landmark throughout the operation.

Mobilization of the distal segment of the common bile duct. The common bile duct is usually only slightly distended in advanced chronic pancreatitis, but it is thickened and pale. It is freed from the portal vein medially and posteriorly, preferably at a site above the entrance of the cystic duct. The segment of mobilized duct is encircled with a Penrose drain to facilitate future mobilization (Fig. 58).

Division of the stomach. Once resectability has been determined, the right lateral half of the gastrohepatic omentum is incised, and the right gastric artery is divided and ligated. The course of the hepatic

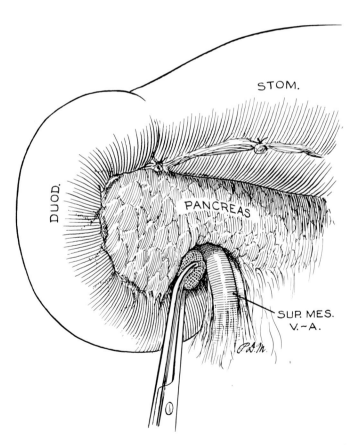

FIG. 56.   The neck of the pancreas is being elevated from the superior mesenteric vein following incision of the peritoneum. A small pledget of gauze, secured by a right-angle clamp, is used for this delicate dissection, which will be carried completely under the neck of the pancreas.

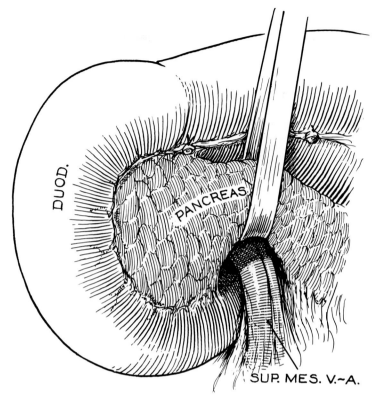

FIG. 57. The neck of the pancreas has been completely mobilized from the superior mesenteric and portal veins, and a small Penrose drain has been passed beneath it. The drain will be used subsequently for manipulation of this structure.

artery is then determined (Fig. 59). It is important to know whether this artery arises from the celiac axis (as usual) or from the superior mesenteric artery. The gastroduodenal artery is identified where it joins the hepatic artery. It has a very short trunk and then divides into four branches, allowing about 1 cm to be dissected and divided between ligatures. The stomach is then pulled downward and to the right to allow the main trunk of the left gastric artery to be identified, divided, and ligated.

A von Petz clamp is applied along the line of division for a 65 percent gastrectomy. If less of the stomach is resected, a bilateral subdiaphragmatic vagotomy is performed to prevent jejunal ulceration. The stomach is divided between the rows of von Petz clips by electrocautery, and the lesser curvature

segment of the transected stomach is closed in preparation for a Hofmeister gastrojejunostomy.

Mobilization and division of the proximal jejunum. With the Penrose drain encircling the neck of the pancreas and serving as a landmark, the ligament of Treitz is incised *to the right* of the superior mesenteric vessels, exposing the fourth portion of the duodenum and the proximal jejunum. The mesentery of the proximal jejunum is then divided and the vessels are ligated. The proximal jejunum is drawn to the right and beneath the superior mesenteric vessels and divided between two Kocher's clamps (Fig. 60). The stump of the proximal jejunum is inverted by an inner row of continuous chromic catgut sutures reinforced by a row of interrupted fine silk sutures. The peri-

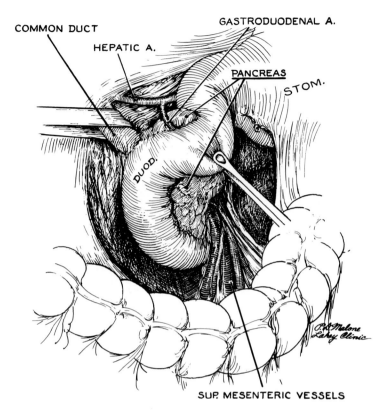

FIG. 58. Completed mobilization of the distal portion of the common bile duct, the course of the hepatic artery, and a segment of the gastroduodenal artery. The gastroduodenal artery will be divided approximately 1 or 2 cm from its junction with the hepatic artery.

toneum is closed at the ligament of Treitz.

Division of the neck of the pancreas and common bile duct. Four nonabsorbable hemostatic ligatures are placed, two superiorly and two inferiorly, into the neck of the pancreas, about 1 cm deep, to control the longitudinal pancreatic arteries (Fig. 61A). A right-angle arterial clamp is placed for protection beneath the neck of the pancreas on the anterior surface of the superior mesenteric and portal veins. The neck of the pancreas is divided with a scalpel. During this procedure, the duct of Wirsung is identified and left to project from the cut surface of the distal pancreas. As the duct is divided, a fine silk suture is placed in each quadrant. Bleeding from the proximal neck is controlled by a series of silk mattress sutures (Fig. 61B).

After scooping any small calculi from the duct of Wirsung, the distal pancreas is closed with interrupted mattress sutures of silk, leaving the duct open for the pancreatojejunostomy (Fig. 61C). Following division of the neck of the pancreas, the portal vein and the junction of its tributaries (the superior mesenteric and splenic veins) are exposed.

The gallbladder is removed after careful identification of the common bile duct, common hepatic duct, origin of the cystic artery, and the approximate junction of the cystic duct with the common bile duct. The common bile duct is then divided between paired clamps above its junction with the cystic duct.

Division of the blood supply to the uncinate process of the pancreas and duo-

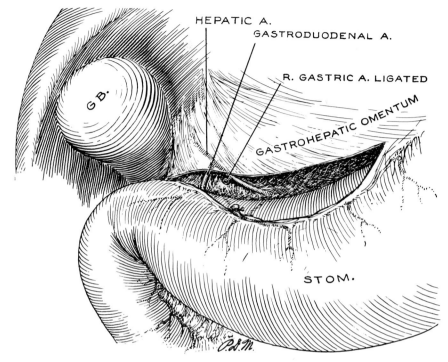

HEPATIC A.

GASTRODUODENAL A.

R. GASTRIC A. LIGATED

GASTROHEPATIC OMENTUM

G.B.

STOM.

FIG. 59. The distal 60 percent of the gastrohepatic omentum has been divided. The right gastric artery has been divided and ligated, exposing the courses of the hepatic and gastroduodenal arteries.

denum. Elevation of the duodenum and head of the pancreas allows the uncinate process to be freed posteriorly. This dissection permits visualization of the mesial aspect of the uncinate process. Following the plane between the right lateral wall of the portal vein superior to the neck of the pancreas, the areolar tissue between the portal vein and the common duct is divided. This division permits further mobilization of the neck of the pancreas as it is apposed to the right lateral wall of the superior mesenteric and portal veins. One major and several small venous branches emerge from the posterior aspect of the neck of the pancreas and enter the portal or superior mesenteric vein. These veins are carefully isolated, divided between clamps, and ligated. This dissection facilitates visualization of the mesial aspect of the uncinate process.

By applying gentle traction to the divided segment of the distal common duct superiorly and the divided jejunum inferiorly, the uncinate process is further elevated and separated from the superior mesenteric and portal veins. The uncinate process is then divided between paired clamps near the superior mesenteric artery (Fig. 62). The entire specimen is then removed. This can be the most difficult part of the procedure. The tributaries of the superior mesenteric artery and vein are so short that great care must be exercised while they are being clamped, divided, and ligated.

Reconstruction of the digestive tract. *Pancreatojejunostomy.* Using interrupted silk sutures, the dorsal surface of the neck of the pancreas is sutured to the proximal jejunum. A small opening is made in the jejunum to permit precise mucosa-to-mucosa anastomosis between it and the duct of Wirsung (Fig. 63). A segment of rubber catheter of appropriate size is inserted and anchored with a fine silk suture to the posterior wall of the divided duct of Wirsung. With the four sutures previously placed in the duct of

Wirsung, the duct is precisely anastomosed to the opening made in the jejunum. The segment of catheter previously placed in the pancreatic duct is inserted into the lumen of the jejunum before the anterior ductal suture is tied. The anastomosis is completed by inserting a series of transverse silk mattress sutures, which approximates the anterior wall of the jejunum to the anterior surface of the neck of the pancreas.

Hepaticojejunostomy. After apposing the posterior wall of the hepatic duct to the jejunum with interrupted silk sutures approximately 9 cm distal to the pancreatojejunostomy, an opening is made in the anterior wall of the hepatic duct about 2 cm proximal to the anastomotic line. A T tube, threaded on a Bakes' dilator or grasped with a right-angle arterial clamp to facilitate its passage, is passed through the opening into the distal segment of the hepatic duct in order to splint the hepaticojejunostomy. The

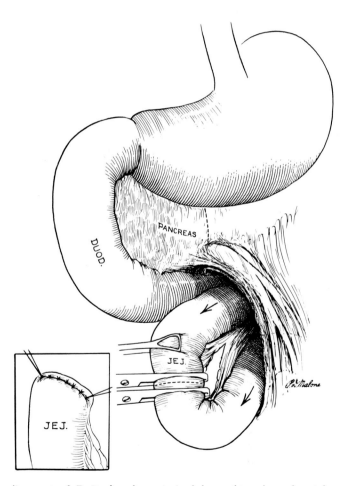

FIG. 60. The ligament of Treitz has been incised beneath and to the right of the superior mesenteric artery and vein. The ventral and dorsal leaflets of ligament of Treitz have been incised superiorly to the uncinate process. The proximal jejunum has been drawn underneath the mesenteric vessels. Two branches of mesenteric vessels supplying the proximal jejunum have been divided and ligated. The jejunum is then divided between paired clamps. *Inset:* distal stump of divided jejunum inverted. This inversion is accomplished with a continuous suture of fine catgut reinforced with interrupted sutures of fine silk.

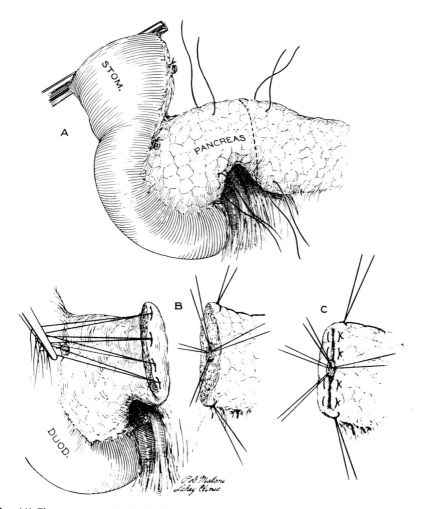

FIG. 61. (A) The superior and inferior longitudinal pancreatic arteries have been encircled with transfixion sutures of medium silk proximal and distal to the point where the pancreas will be divided. (B) The neck of the pancreas has been divided. Four fine silk sutures have been placed one in each quadrant of the duct of Wirsung. The proximal divided end of the neck of the pancreas has been secured with four interrupted sutures of medium silk held in a single clamp for future traction. (C) The cut surface of the pancreatic remnant is shown with four previously placed fine silk sutures in the duct of Wirsung. The divided end of the pancreatic remnant with the exception of the duct of Wirsung is compressed with several mattress sutures of medium silk.

two-layer mucosa-to-mucosa anastomosis is completed in the same manner as the pancreatojejunostomy.

Gastrojejunostomy. The jejunum 40 cm distal to the hepaticojejunostomy is approximated to the posterior wall of the stomach with a layer of seromuscular sutures of fine silk. A longitudinal opening is made in the jejunum and the von Petz clips are excised

from the segment of the stomach that is to be anastomosed to the jejunum. The posterior interior layers of jejunum and stomach are approximated with a continuous interlocking suture of medium chromic catgut. This suture is continued anteriorly after the manner of Connell, approximating the anterior walls of the jejunum and stomach. This is reinforced with sutures of fine silk.

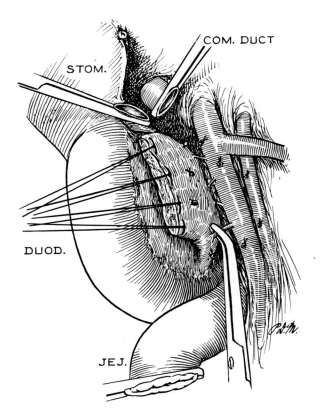

FIG. 62. Small vessels entering the superior mesenteric and portal veins from the head of the pancreas have been divided and ligated. With traction on the divided common duct above and the divided jejunum below, the uncinate process is elevated and separated from the superior mesenteric and portal veins. The uncinate process will be divided between paired right-angle clamps.

The completed reconstruction of the digestive tract is shown in Figure 64. Two sump drains and two Penrose drains are placed in Morison's pouch and the sump drains are connected to wall suction.

POSTOPERATIVE CARE

Decompression

The stomach is decompressed by gastric suction, which is not discontinued immediately after normal peristalsis returns because continued decompression eliminates the gastric phase of pancreatic secretion.

We find it expedient to continue nasogastric suction for approximately 7 days. Wound suction is maintained for 3 to 5 days, and if a biliary or pancreatic fistula occurs, wound suction is continued until the fistula has closed.

Fluid and Electrolyte Balance

During gastric drainage and until adequate oral intake is permissible, the fluid, nutritional, and electrolyte requirements are met by administration of appropriate quantities of glucose and saline solutions, supplemented by potassium chloride as required.

Because of the preceding protein deficiency, it is wise not to give too much saline solution. We prefer to keep the serum chloride on the low side of normal. A feeding jejunostomy tube (T tube) is inserted 16 inches distal to the gastrojejunostomy in the severely protein-depleted patient. The presence of this feeding tube is particularly valuable if there is delayed emptying of the stomach or if a major biliary fistula occurs. The Barron pump delivers a prepared formula of balanced food at a constant rate. The formula contains 1.5 calories in each cubic centimeter. An hourly urine output is carefully recorded, and if the urinary output falls below 25 ml per hour, 25 g of mannitol or 40 mg of furosemide (Lasix) is given intravenously. Intravenous hyperalimentation is occasionally employed, but it is not with-out danger, especially in a patient with diabetes.

Blood Transfusions

As acute pancreatitis may be precipitated by operative trauma, the serum amylase, hemoglobin, and hematocrit are measured 4 and 24 hours after operation. The rate and strength of the pulse is carefully assessed. If the amylase is elevated significantly or if the pulse is rapid and weak, there is frequently excessive fluid loss into the peritoneal cavity, and one or two units of Plasmanate is given. The value of frequent blood transfusions in maintaining the occasional patient who will have delayed opening of the gastrointestinal stoma cannot be overemphasized.

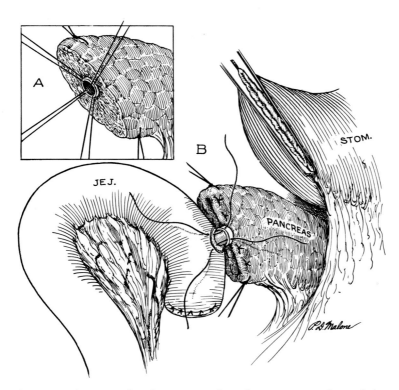

FIG. 63. The proximal jejunum has been apposed to the posterior surface of the pancreatic remnant with interrupted medium silk sutures. An opening approximately the size of the caliber of the divided duct of Wirsung has been made in the jejunum. Precise mucosa-to-mucosa anastomosis of the duct of Wirsung to the jejunum is made with previously placed interrupted fine silk sutures. A segment of rubber catheter is usually used as stent in this anastomosis.

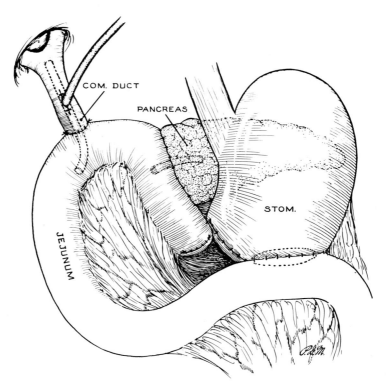

FIG. 64.   Completed reconstruction of the digestive tract. Note the end-to-side pancreatojejunostomy is proximal to other anastomoses. The anterior wall of the jejunum has been approximated to the anterior surface of the pancreas with interrupted fine silk sutures. End-to-side hepaticojejunostomy has been constructed using a T tube to splint the anastomosis. Hofmeister gastrojejunostomy has been performed 40 cm distal to hepaticojejunostomy.

Insulin

In the presence of diabetes mellitus, appropriate amounts of insulin are administered. Rarely, an apparently mild or latent preoperative diabetic state will become temporarily severe following excision of a large mass of pancreatic tissue. Diabetes may occur months or years after pancreatoduodenectomy.

Nutrition

When gastric decompression is discontinued, a liquid diet is given and selected solid foods are added gradually. Replacement of exocrine pancreatic enzymes is frequently necessary and frequently neglected. Pancreatic diarrhea is best controlled by allowing a moderate intake of fat and by the administration of pancreatin (Viokase), 15 to 20 gr (900 to 1,200 mg) with each meal. Vitamin K is administered as necessary. In severe degrees of malnutrition associated with excessive diarrhea, a typical sprue syndrome occurs and is treated with a strict gluten-free diet. Dramatic results have been observed.

Antibiotics

Chloramphenicol is administered, 4 g each day in divided doses, for 7 days.

COMPLICATIONS

Fistula.   Leakage of the pancreatojejunostomy causing a pancreatic fistula is the most common serious complication. The essential requirement in the management of such a fistula is *constant* suction until the drainage ceases. Biliary fistula occurs when there is leakage at the choledochojejunal anastomosis. Continued suction drainage will allow this to heal.

Hemorrhage. Severe hemorrhage may occur at any time in the postoperative period, either through the drainage tracts or into the intestinal tract, causing hematemesis or melena. The hemorrhage is caused by pancreatic leakage and tryptic digestion of the blood vessels near the anastomosis. If the bleeding continues after initial blood replacement, local surgical control of hemorrhage is required. Removal of the pancreatic remnant for the control of hemorrhage is rarely indicated.

Other problems. Jejunal ulceration or gastrojejunal obstruction has necessitated reoperation in a few of our patients. Peritonitis contributed to death in the only 4 patients, who died during the postoperative period.

RESULTS

We have performed pancreatoduodenectomy in 148 patients, including 20 patients who had total pancreatectomy done in one or two stages. There were four deaths in the postoperative period (2.7 percent). There were no operative deaths among the patients who had total pancreatectomy.

148 Patients

Results	Number of Patients	Percent
Excellent	52	35.4
Good	49	32.9
Poor	40	26.8
Hospital deaths	4	2.7
Unable to evaluate	3	2.4

Of these 148 patients, 90 were operated on before June 1965; 82 had pancreatoduodenectomy and 8 had total pancreatectomy. Good or excellent results were obtained in approximately two-thirds of patients treated with pancreatoduodenectomy, as shown below:

These figures show a low mortality rate and an improved rate of success in comparison with other operations advocated for the treatment of this devastating disease. Eighty-one percent of our patients had had previous unsuccessful operations for chronic relapsing pancreatitis; one-third had had sphincterotomy. Many of the patients who had unsatisfactory results after pancreatoduodenectomy were narcotic or alcoholic addicts. Therefore, we emphasize total care of the patient after pancreatic resection, including intensive and prolonged therapy for these addiction problems, either of which may be the determining factor in success or failure of surgery. In addition, we prescribe the proper diet, vitamins, and exocrine pancreatic enzymes and insulin, if necessary.

REFERENCES

1. Cattell, R. B., and Warren, K. W., Surgery of the Pancreas, Philadelphia, Saunders, 1953, p. 374.
2. Geevarghese, P. J., Pancreatic Diabetes: A Clinico-Pathologic Study of Growth Onset Diabetes with Pancreatic Calculi, Bombay, Popular Prakashan, 1968, p. 29.
3. Warren, K. W., Gastroenterology 36:224, 1959.
4. Warren, K. W., Surgery of Pancreatic Disease: Modern Trends in Gastro-enterology, London, Butterworths, 1961, pp. 264-299.
5. Warren, K. W., Henry Ford Hosp. Med. Bull. 14:143, 1966.
6. Warren, K. W., Am. J. Surg. 117:24, 1969.
7. Warren, K. W., and Cattell, R. B., New Engl. J. Med. 261:280; 333; 387; 1959.
8. Warren, K. W., and Veidenheimer, M. C., New Engl. J. Med. 266:323, 1962.

D. Pancreatolithiasis

RODNEY SMITH

The mere presence of pancreatic calculi is no indication that an operation should be performed; some patients have considerable collections of calculi with relatively minor symptoms whilst others have symptoms of pancreatic insufficiency calling for medical care (such as diabetes mellitus or steatorrhoea). *Pain* is the main indication for operation and occurs because there is not only pancreatolithiasis but chronic pancreatitis; this must always be taken into account in planning an operation. In the writer's view, the only indications for surgery are: (1) pain; (2) recurrent severe exacerbations of subacute pancreatitis; (3) major surgical complications, such as pancreatic cyst, pancreatic fistula, portal vein obstruction; and (4) suspicions of a superimposed malignant condition (e.g., a short history of increasing pancreatic pain with marked weight loss).

PREOPERATIVE CARE

When pancreatic calculi are visible in the x-ray films, diagnosis is seldom difficult; but the presence of complicating factors, such as gallstones or a pancreatic cyst, may be brought to light by routine x-ray of the stomach, duodenum, biliary tract, and colon. In some cases, further direct evidence of the state of the pancreas is obtainable via pancreatic scanning with selenomethionine, transsplenic portal venography, selective coeliac and superior mesenteric angiography, and retroperitoneal insufflation. Before operation, there should certainly be correction of anaemia, hypoproteinaemia, and electrolyte imbalance, as well as preparations for blood transfusion during operation. Arrangements for on-table cholangiograms or pancreatograms should be made.

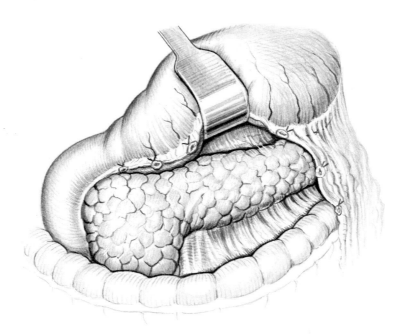

FIG. 65. An approach to the body of the pancreas through the lesser sac.

THE OPERATION

The incision should be one giving good access to the whole of the upper abdomen. Usually some modification of a left or right paramedian incision is employed, but in a thick-set muscular patient a bilateral subcostal incision may be necessary for adequate exposure of the whole pancreas. The operation should naturally begin with a general exploration, concentrating finally upon an assessment of the degree of pancreatitis and peripancreatitis and the relative involvement of its head, body, and tail, as well as consideration of such complications as pancreatic pseudocysts, coincidental biliary tract disease, and portal or splenic vein compression, the presence of which may be indicated by dilated mesenteric veins or by splenomegaly.

Selection of Technique

No single procedure is adequate to deal with all cases of pancreatolithiasis requiring surgical intervention. In the writer's view, about seven procedures should be considered, these being:

1. Transgastric or transjejunal T tube drainage of the duct of Wirsung.
2. Distal pancreatectomy and pancreatogastrostomy.
3. Subtotal (95 percent) pancreatectomy.
4. Longitudinal pancreatojejunostomy (see Puestow's contribution on this in Part B of this chapter).
5. Pancreatoduodectomy (see Warren's contribution on this in Part C of this chapter).
6. Total pancreatectomy.
7. Splanchnicectomy.

In selecting the most appropriate procedure, the surgical objectives should be clearly borne in mind. These are not merely the removal of calculi from the pancreatic duct system, but they include also (1) the eradication of disease and (2) the provision of free drainage of the duct of Wirsung.

At an early stage, therefore, examination of the duct of Wirsung is essential; this is best carried out by approaching the body of the pancreas through the lesser sac, dividing the gastrocolic omentum, and opening the

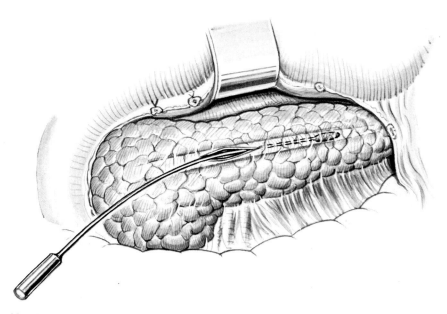

FIG. 66.   Transgastric T tube drainage of the duct of Wirsung. Examination of the duct with a dilator.

duct at the most accessible point. Calculi are removed and the state of the duct determined by: (1) the passage of probes or, if the duct is dilated, Bakes' dilator and (2) operative pancreatography. It will be found that the duct conforms to one of three descriptions:

1. It is generally dilated, without strictures, a 3-mm or larger dilator passing easily throughout the length of the duct.
2. The duct is divided into a number of dilated segments by multiple strictures (Puestow's "chain of lakes").
3. The main duct is scarcely bigger than normal. Small calculi and calcareous debris block not only the main duct but fill the main and smaller tributaries even right out to the periphery of the gland.

SIDE-TO-SIDE
PANCREATOJEJUNOSTOMY:
MUCOSAL GRAFT TECHNIQUE

Indications for use. This procedure is to be preferred to any other if there is a generalised wide dilatation of the duct of Wirsung without strictures and if the main pancreatic duct can be cleared of calculi from its head to tail. A minimal degree of peripheral calcification (nearly always being, in fact, tiny stones in the peripheral ducts rather than parenchymatous calcification) can be ignored, and, provided that there is free drainage of the main pancreatic duct, it may not result in continuing symptoms.

Anastomosis of the pancreatic duct to a Roux loop of jejunum is effected by using the "mucosal graft" method described and illustrated in *Operative Surgery*.[1] This technique is shown in Figures 67–72.

This preference arises from the following reasons: (1) it is a simple procedure and technically very easy to perform; (2) it is practically without hazard during the operation and free from postoperative complications; (3) it has a high success rate; and (4) even if, after a period of relief, symptoms recur, a further operation, e.g., distal pancreatectomy, is not made more difficult.

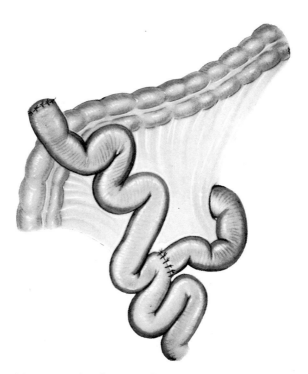

FIG. 67. Pancreatojejunostomy (employing a long Roux loop) for pancreatolithiasis. A long Roux loop of jejunum is constructed as shown. (R. Smith's technique.) (From Rob, Smith, and Morgan. *Operative Surgery*, 2d ed., 1969. Courtesy of the editors and Butterworths, London.)

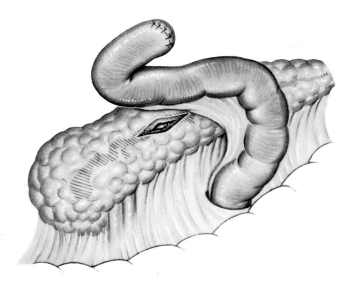

FIG. 68.   Pancreatojejunostomy for pancreatolithiasis. The incision has been made through the body of the pancreas and the duct of Wirsung. After clearing the duct of calculi, the apex of the jejunal loop will be anastomosed to the pancreatic duct. (From Rob, Smith, and Morgan. *Operative Surgery*, 2d ed., 1969. Courtesy of the editors and Butterworths, London.)

Technique. The dilated duct is already opened in the most accessible part of the body. All calculi are extracted with scoops of various sizes and a dilator passed in both directions to be sure that there is now a big empty duct from head to tail (Figs. 65 and 66).

A latex T tube is then placed in the duct and an operative pancreatogram is used to confirm filling of the whole of the duct without strictures or residual stones (Figs. 67–72).

A corrugated rubber drain is placed in the lesser sac through a separate stab incision

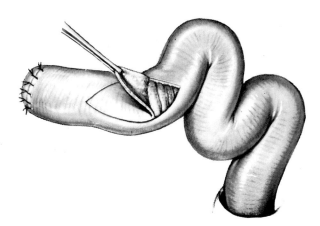

FIG. 69.   The plan is to line the track through the pancreatic substance into the duct with jejunal mucosa. An oval segment is excised exposing the mucosa. (From Rob, Smith, and Morgan. *Operative Surgery*, 2d ed., 1969. Courtesy of the editors and Butterworths, London.)

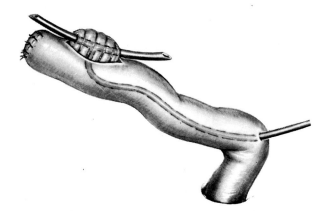

FIG. 70. Placing the latex rubber T tube in position. (From Rob, Smith, and Morgan. *Operative Surgery*, 2d ed., 1969. Courtesy of the editors and Butterworths, London.)

and the abdomen is closed.

Postoperatively, the corrugated drain is removed after 48 hours if, as is usually the case, there is no drainage. The T tube is allowed to drain freely into a plastic bag for 7 to 10 days, until the pancreatic juice is seen to be clear and free of debris. The tube is then spigotted and washed out once daily with sterile water. The patient is taught to do this and is discharged from hospital with the tube in situ. T tube drainage into the jejunum is continued for 3 months and the tube then removed.

DISTAL PANCREATECTOMY AND PANCREATOGASTROSTOMY

Indications for use. This procedure is selected when the duct of Wirsung is dilated or choked with calculi and the site of multiple strictures make simple T tube drainage inappropriate. (Puestow's technique is also logical in these circumstances but is, in the view of the writer, more complicated and subject to a wider range of possible postoperative complications.) Distal pancreatec-

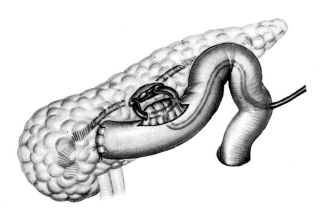

FIG. 71. The two limbs of the T tube are now inserted into the duct so that when pressed home the T tube will carry the jejunal mucosal graft with it into the duct. (From Rob, Smith, and Morgan. *Operative Surgery*, 2d ed., 1969. Courtesy of the editors and Butterworths, London.)

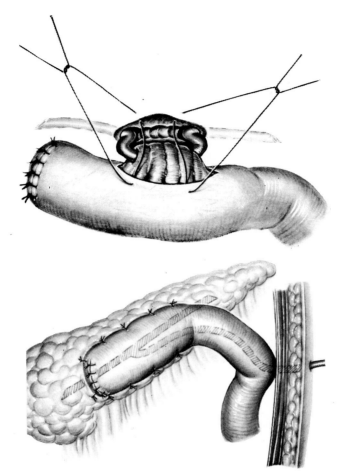

FIG. 72.   Fixing the jejunum to the pancreas. The jejunal loop is now sewn to the front of the pancreatic substance and the long limb of the T tube is brought through the abdominal wall to the exterior. (R. Smith's technique.) (From Rob, Smith, and Morgan. *Operative Surgery*, 2d ed., 1969. Courtesy of the editors and Butterworths, London.)

tomy is also indicated when the main pathological condition is in the distal pancreas with the head of the gland being relatively normal, e.g., pancreatic rupture has been followed by pancreatitis confined to the distal gland. In such a case, pancreatogastrostomy can be omitted.

Technique.   Good access is essential, and occasionally the incision should be extended across the left costal margin into the eighth intercostal space to give a thoracoabdominal approach. The lienorenal ligament is divided so that the spleen, the tail

of the pancreas. and the fundus of the stomach are mobilised. The stomach is mobilised from the spleen and pancreas by dividing between ligatures the gastrocolic omentum and all the short gastric vessels.

The peritoneum above and below the pancreatic body is then incised and a finger is passed behind the gland. Mobilisation of the distal pancreas and spleen is usually easily effected, the splenic vessels being lifted forward with the pancreas (Figs. 73 and 74).

The splenic vein is easily identified adherent to the back of the pancreas, and

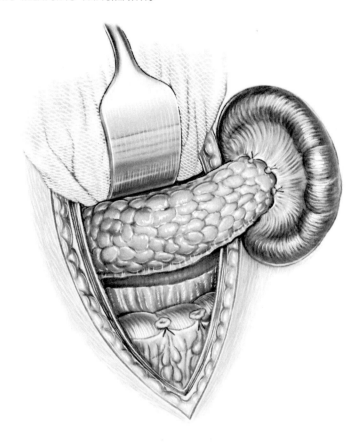

FIG. 73. Distal pancreatectomy. Mobilisation of the distal pancreas and spleen. (From Rob, Smith, and Morgan. *Operative Surgery*, 2d ed., 1969. Courtesy of the editors and Butterworths, London.)

dissection proceeds from left to right until the junction of this vein with the superior mesenteric vein is seen. The splenic vein is then divided between ligatures and the neck of the pancreas freed from the front of the portal vein (Fig. 74). The splenic artery is divided between ligatures, leaving the distal pancreas completely mobilised (Fig. 75). Two stay sutures of silk are placed in the neck of the gland, which is transected; the distal pancreas and spleen are removed. The duct of Wirsung in the head of the pancreas is then cleared of calculi and debris with scoops as a preliminary to pancreatogastrostomy (Fig. 76).

A continuous silk suture mounted on an atraumatic (eyeless) needle is used to suture the pancreatic substance to the seromuscular coat of the posterior wall of the antrum. Half of this is completed (Fig. 77), after which the junction of pancreatic duct to the stomach is effected as follows: A long polyethylene tube of a size to fit loosely in the duct is employed. One end is fitted tightly onto a Kirschner wire.

The free end of the tube is inserted into the pancreatic duct, reaching nearly as far as the duodenal papilla. A single catgut stitch tied around the tube anchors it to the pancreatic duct and prevents it from slipping out. The Kirschner wire, used as a bodkin, carries the tube across the lumen of the stomach, entering the antrum at the centre of the pancreatogastric anastomosis and leav-

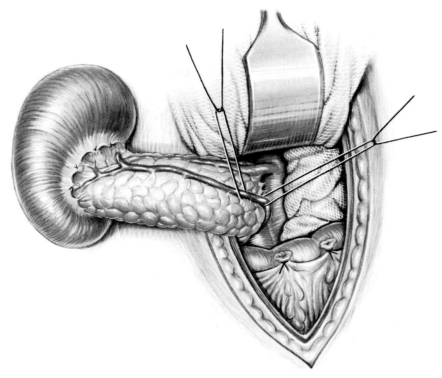

FIG. 74.   Distal pancreatectomy. Ligation of the splenic vein. (From Rob, Smith, and Morgan. *Operative Surgery*, 2d ed., 1969. Courtesy of the editors and Butterworths, London.)

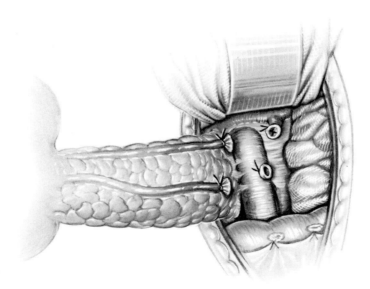

FIG. 75.   Distal pancreatectomy. Ligation of the splenic artery. (From Rob, Smith, and Morgan. *Operative Surgery*, 2d ed., 1969. Courtesy of the editors and Butterworths, London.)

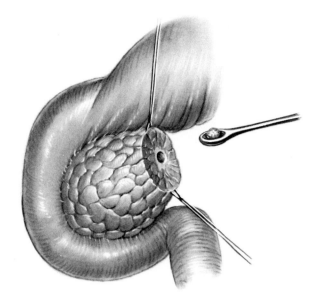

FIG. 76.   Distal pancreatectomy. Clearing the head end of the pancreatic duct of stones and debris. (From Rob, Smith, and Morgan. *Operative Surgery*, 2d ed., 1969. Courtesy of the editors and Butterworths, London.)

ing the anterior gastric wall rather to the left of this point. With the tube in situ, the continuous silk suture completes the anterior half of the pancreatogastric anastomosis. The

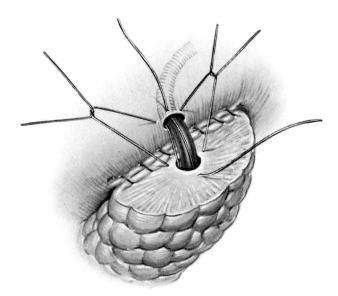

FIG. 77.   Distal pancreatectomy. The posterior half of the anastomosis between the pancreas and the back of the stomach has been completed. (From Rob, Smith, and Morgan. *Operative Surgery*, 2d ed., 1969. Courtesy of the editors and Butterworths, London.)

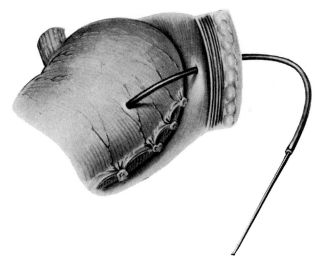

FIG. 78. Distal pancreatectomy. Method of bringing the tube through the stomach and the abdominal wall. (From Rob, Smith, and Morgan. *Operative Surgery*, 2d ed., 1969. Courtesy of the editors and Butterworths, London.)

Kirschner wire is used to carry the tube through the anterior abdominal wall to the left of the incision, and at this point the anterior wall of the stomach is sutured to the parietal peritoneum to leave no gap (Fig. 78).

A corrugated rubber drain is placed in the lesser sac through a separate stab incision and the abdomen is closed.

Postoperatively the corrugated drain is removed in from 2 to 5 days, depending upon whether there is any oozing from the pancreatic bed. The polyethylene tube drains into a plastic bag and is usually removed after a postoperative pancreatogram on the eighth to tenth day.

Subtotal (95 Percent) Pancreatectomy

If the whole of the pancreatic duct system, including the finer tributaries right out to the periphery of the gland, is choked with calculi, subtotal distal pancreatectomy is the procedure of choice.

The operation is carried out exactly as described for distal pancreatectomy (*above*) up to the point at which the splenic artery has been divided and the neck of the pancreas

isolated. The procedure then continues with a further dissection to the right, the head of the pancreas in the concavity of the duodenal loop being carefully defined. During this stage, the gastroduodenal artery is encountered and is better divided between ligatures than preserved. The head of the pancreas is then itself divided close to the duodenal wall, leaving a thin crescentic fragment protecting the common bile duct and securing, as they are encountered, the branches of the pancreatoduodenal arterial loop. The uncinate process, tucked behind the superior mesenteric vein, need not be totally removed. It is safer to leave a thin fragment of this process attached to the vein.

No ductal anastomosis is necessary after this radical removal. A corrugated drain is placed down to the divided pancreatic substance and the abdomen is closed.

Postoperatively, little leakage of pancreatic juice occurs. Diabetes mellitus is likely to develop, and plans to deal with this must be made accordingly.

Other Operations

1. *Puestow's method* of performing longitudinal pancreatojejunostomy is an al-

ternative to distal pancreatectomy and pancreatogastroscopy and is described in this chapter.

2. *Pancreatoduodenectomy,* as described by Dr. Kenneth Warren, is appropriate when the head of the gland is disorganised and some of the body and tail are nevertheless worth preserving.

Total pancreatectomy, an extension of pancreatoduodenectomy, is only occasionally indicated for pancreatolithiasis in those cases in which the disorganisation of the gland is so complete that it is not worth attempting to retain any of it. Patients in this group are always already diabetic and receiving pancreatic extracts to control steatorrhoea.

3. *Splanchnicectomy* is an operation for the relief of pancreatic pain in those patients in whom operation directed at the actual pathology present is considered *impracticable.* It is usually of temporary benefit only.

REFERENCES

1. Rob, C., and Smith, R., eds., Operative Surgery, 2d ed., London, Butterworths, 1969.
2. Smith, R., Acta Gastroenterol. Belg. 23:1031, 1960.
3. Smith, R., Basic Science and Pancreatic Surgery, Lettsonian Lecture Transactions Med. Soc. London, Vol. LXXXIV, 1968.
4. Smith, R., Proc. R. Soc. Med. 62:131, 1969.
5. Smith, R., Strictures of the Bile Duct, in J. Badenoch Bryan Brooke, ed., Recent Advances in Gastroenterology, Philadelphia, W. B. Saunders, 1972.
6. Smith, R., Am. J. Surg. (In press.)
7. Warren, K. W., Surg. Clin. North Am. 35:785, 1955.
8. Warren, K. W., and Veidenheimer, M. C., New Engl. J. Med. 266:323, 1962.

E. Total Pancreatectomy

MILTON R. PORTER

INDICATIONS

About forty years ago we were all being taught that the complete removal of the pancreas, apart from being technically virtually impossible, produced a physiological state which was in essence incompatible with continued life. It has turned out over the years that the operation is quite possible and even safe to do, but that it has acquired a very bad reputation largely because of the usually hopeless disease for which it was (at least originally) done. In this respect it has had much in common with total gastrectomy.

As time has passed and operative technique has been perfected, the indications for the performance of total pancreatectomy have broadened and the operation can be appraised "on its own merits" so to speak.

Most surgeons continue to do total pancreatectomy for what they believe to be operable tumors. Our criteria for operability have been clearly defined elsewhere.[1] As with most, the cure rate has been discouraging. In addition, one would now have to add a few other indications for total pancreatectomy. These would include:

1. Certain candidates for a Puestow-like procedure whose glands are found to be so damaged as to preclude doing that operation because of the operator's inability to find any significant ducts to open.
2. Certain cases of trauma involving large or important areas of the gland such as are seen after stabbings, gunshot wounds, and auto accidents.

Adapted from Porter, Total Pancreatectomy. In Cooper, Operative Technique, 1964. Courtesy of Little, Brown & Company.

The pancreas is in many ways a more difficult organ to manage surgically than other viscera. It is situated at a complex anatomical crossroad where its central position provides lymphatic drainage radially along several major routes (the splenic, hepatic, and superior mesenteric vessels). This makes it harder to design an operation which, in an orderly manner, removes primary, secondary, and tertiary nodal groups. Moreover, the intimate association of the pancreas with the major vessels of the epigastrium at once limits the extent of the procedure and dictates what must be removed. Thus, when a tumor spreads a short distance to involve the portal vein or the superior mesenteric artery, it becomes incurable. Similarly, if the gland is removed, the need to excise the vessels that go with it makes removal of the spleen and duodenum necessary.

If only part of the gland is removed, or if the gland is incised, safe management of any draining pancreatic juice becomes a matter of primary importance, since the enzymes, if allowed to remain in the abdomen, may wreak havoc. A first principle of pancreatic surgery is, therefore, the provision of adequate drainage. Secondly, since catgut is a protein substance that is rapidly digested by trypsin, it cannot be trusted as a ligature on major vessels or as a suture material for closing the abdomen. Silk, cotton, wire, or nylon is safer.

TECHNIQUE OF TOTAL PANCREATECTOMY

Apart from the usual preparatory measures, it is well to be certain that candidates for pancreatic resection are not deficient in vitamin K if they are jaundiced; that there is a reasonable quantity of blood on call (the average pancreatectomy requires 1,000 to 1,500 ml in the operating room); and that the patient understands in advance that he may be rendered diabetic.

The Incision

The operation is usually done through a bilateral subcostal incision with the incision longer on the right than on the left. In persons with unusually narrow costal angles, a vertical incision is made. The reasons for preferring transverse incisions in most patients are that they provide easier access to the lateral aspect of the duodenum without sacrificing good exposure of the spleen and the tail of the pancreas; they tend to run more nearly in the axis of the pancreas itself; they are relatively simple to make; and they are less apt to be complicated by weakness or intestinal obstruction postoperatively. In making the transverse incision, it is well to keep it two fingerbreadths from the costal margin, since this provides greater postoperative comfort and consequently better ventilation of the lung than would obtain otherwise.

Diagnosis in the Operating Room

One of the most difficult problems in pancreatic surgery is the differentiation between carcinoma of the head of the pancreas and chronic pancreatitis. This problem rarely occurs when the patient is jaundiced, but is more apt to come up because of a chance finding when the patient is being operated upon for other reasons. There is a small percentage of cases of carcinoma of the pancreas in which the tumor is very small and hidden in the midst of a virtually ligneous gland which is totally involved in fibrotic pancreatitis. In these instances, the diagnosis may elude discovery until the gland reaches the surgical pathology laboratory or autopsy table—no matter how great an effort is made to obtain a specimen of the growth for biopsy. Moreover, certain tumors in this area present the pathologist with a very difficult problem in identification on frozen section. It is well to remember that in the absence of *acute* inflammation and/or gallstones, solid, hard, noncystic masses in the head of the pancreas associated with obstructive jaundice and dilatation of the common bile duct are rarely due to pancreatitis and are *usually* carcinoma. Conversely, hard, noncystic masses involving a major part of the retroampullary part of the gland and unassociated with jaundice and dilatation of the biliary tree are *usually* pancreatitis. Small areas of induration in the head of the pancreas are *usually* benign, and because they are small they are more amenable to precisely placed biopsies (needle or knife) than larger masses.

Obviously, these generalizations, although helpful, will not serve to differentiate certain carcinomas from chronic pancreatitis. The surgeon must then decide whether to try to establish a diagnosis by doing frozen section biopsies. Each operator will quite properly be influenced by his own and his pathologist's experience in this field as well as by the clinical situation.

The policy in our clinic relative to biopsy can be briefly stated as follows:

1. All ampullary and small duodenal lesions are subject to biopsy through a duodenotomy. This must be done because benign growths occur in the area and gallstones impacted at the ampulla can exactly simulate tumors.
2. All inoperable tumors are diagnosed before the surgeon leaves the operating room, even if the job is time-consuming. This takes the matter out of the realm of doubt—an especially important point when a palliative procedure restores the patient to relatively good health for a long period and doubt is raised as to the diagnosis. A biopsy positive for carcinoma, on file, may then prevent a fruitless second laparotomy.
3. Frozen sections are made of lymph nodes peripheral to the proposed specimen to help establish operability.
4. Primary intrapancreatic growths are rarely subjected to biopsy when operable. (This does not necessarily apply when cystic tumors are present. They are managed differently.)

The arguments supporting these policies have been published previously. They include the following:

1. Representative sections from the pancreas are often hard to obtain because of confusion between tumor and surrounding pancreatitis.
2. Interpretation of frozen section biopsy specimens of the pancreas may be difficult because some desmoplastic carcinomas closely resemble chronic pancreatitis.
3. The establishment of diagnosis by means of frozen section biopsy specimens is often time-consuming and traumatic.

When a pancreatic biopsy is done, the operator should make great efforts to avoid the major pancreatic ducts and vessels, the typical anatomy of which must be well fixed in mind. Hemorrhage, when encountered, is often profuse and difficult to control. Silk mattress sutures are more effective than clamping and tying. Chromic catgut should not be used, since it may digest rapidly in the presence of trypsin spilled by the gland. As previously explained, pancreatic wounds should be drained.

Assessment of Operability and Choice of Procedure

Briefly stated, the lesion is considered inoperable if there are distant metastases, invasion of the major blood vessels (especially the portal vein), or extension beyond the area of the usual pancreatectomy specimen. Experience with extended resections has proved the futility of developing a more radical block than that of a total pancreatectomy.

Apart from the usual exploration of the abdomen, special care should be used in searching for involved lymph nodes in the area of the root of the small bowel mesentery, the celiac axis, and the middle colic vessels. A surprisingly large number of patients are found to have metastases below the transverse mesocolon in the root of the small intestinal mesentery and no metastases above the pancreas. Suspicious nodes in these areas should be examined by frozen section; if they are involved, there is no point in resecting. Positive nodes in the areas to be included in the specimen are no contraindication to resection. There are usually large, rubbery, greenish nodes behind the common duct in these patients; they are much less apt to reveal metastases than are smaller, harder nodes from the area under discussion.

In assessing operability, the lesser sac is entered through the gastrocolic omentum, and a thoroughgoing mobilization of the duodenum and pancreatic head is done

(Kocher's maneuver). This not only reveals invasion of the lumbar gutter structures such as the vena cava, if such invasion exists, but also facilitates examination of the portal vein and superior mesenteric artery and their relationship to the tumor. The artery can be felt with the fingers behind the gland. If the tumor invades it or completely surrounds it posteriorly, the case is considered inoperable. The portal vein cannot be felt, but it lies anterior and to the right of the artery (i.e. closer to the operator); hence, if that area is involved in tumor it is best to check the vein more carefully. This is done from the anterior aspect of the gland. First, the superior mesenteric vein is found just above the mesocolon where it ducks beneath the pancreatic neck. It can be rapidly located by following the middle colic vein to the point where it enters the superior mesenteric. As soon as it goes beneath the pancreas, the superior mesenteric is joined by the splenic to form the portal, which emerges from beneath the superior border of the pancreas. There are almost never any tributaries to the anterior surfaces of these veins behind the pancreas, and instruments and fingers can be gently inserted anterior to the portal vein to assess tumor invasion. Some prefer to enter this passage from above; if this is done, division of the gastroduodenal artery may facilitate the approach.

If the portal vein is invaded, the case is inoperable. Operable tumors located in the pancreas, whatever their cell type, are treated by total pancreatectomy. Operable tumors confined to the duodenum or ampulla are treated by resection of the head of the pancreas.

As has been previously reported, a review of our clinic's experience has shown that duodenal and ampullary lesions are often cured by resection of the head of the pancreas. On the other hand, a study of the cases of carcinoma of the pancreas has brought to light three facts, all of which are interpreted as reasons for doing total pancreatectomy. (1) Microscopic, intraglandular strands of tumor have often been cut through at the time of partial resection. (2) Scattered microscopic foci of carcinoma have been found in the tail of the gland after total resection for carcinoma of the head of the pancreas. (3)

Postoperative management of the totally pancreatectomized patient is not nearly as difficult as had been thought. To these reasons can be added our admitted prejudice against partially resecting any gland harboring a carcinoma.

One is rarely called upon to resect a carcinoma which has arisen in the tail of the gland, since such growths are virtually always inoperable by the time they come to attention. Benign lesions and cystic lesions often require resection of the tail only.

The Resection

The gastrocolic omentum is opened and the short gastric vessels are divided and ligated.

The spleen is then mobilized from its posterolateral attachments. Its pedicle is divided and ligated and it is removed, thus reducing the bulk of the specimen and getting rid of an organ which often oozes blood from its posterior bare areas. Figures 79 to 84 show the spleen attached in order to make the relations clear.

The tail of the pancreas and the splenic vessels are mobilized as one unit. One should never try to take the tail of the pancreas out and spare the splenic vessels. Too many tiny tributaries and branches would have to be managed, and saving the spleen is not worth the time or effort.

At this stage, it is usually best to divide the stomach to provide better exposure for subsequent pancreatic mobilization. Resection of the stomach and part of all of the pancreas (which contributes the major share of alkali to the intestinal tract) predisposes to marginal ulceration in long-term survivors. For this reason, it is preferable to remove all the antrum by dividing the stomach just above the incisura, rather than by dividing through the distal antrum as recommended by some. We have also recently added a complete subdiaphragmatic vagotomy to the operation. The dissection of the pancreatic tail then moves rapidly from left to right, and the point of origin of the splenic artery from the celiac axis is found and divided, care being taken to protect the axis itself and the hepatic artery.

The point of entry of the inferior mesen-

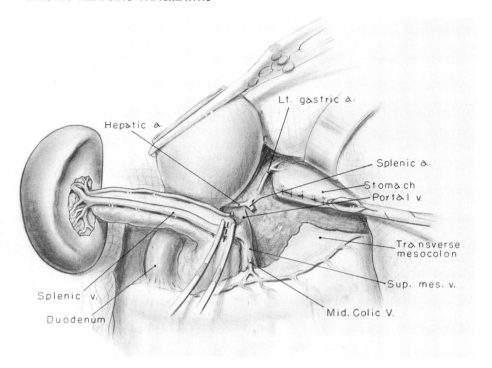

FIG. 79. The splenic vein is clamped, cut, and ligated near its junction with the portal vein. (From Porter. In Cooper, *Operative Technique,* 1964. Courtesy of Little, Brown.)

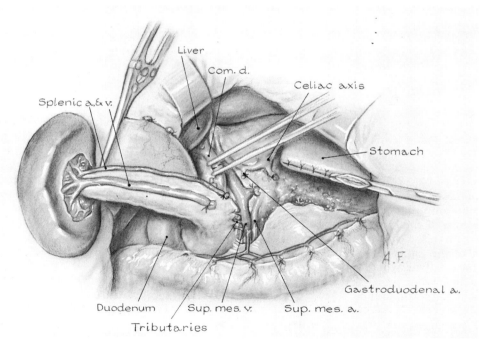

FIG. 80. The common bile duct is clamped and cut. (From Porter. In Cooper, *Operative Technique,* 1964. Courtesy of Little, Brown.)

teric vein into the splenic varies rather widely. It is divided at the point where it enters the splenic. It sometimes enters the superior mesenteric; when it does, it is not disturbed. The splenic vein is divided just proximal to its junction with the portal (Fig. 79).

The gastroduodenal artery is then divided at its origin from the hepatic. The weight of the specimen and traction often tent the hepatic artery at this moment and invite damage to it. The anatomy should be clearly defined to prevent such damage. Lymph nodes, which obscure the view, may have to be cleaned away from the front surface of this vascular junction.

The common bile duct is then divided at a convenient level between clamps. Care must be taken not to divide it too close to the junction of the right and left hepatic ducts (Fig. 80). The gallbladder is removed. In the absence of an ampulla of Vater, the previously normal gallbladder is predisposed to develop cholecystitis and may subsequently need to be removed. Moreover, the cystic

duct often implants at a low level, forcing cholecystectomy upon the operator.

The specimen now remains attached only by the bowel and vascular attachments. At this point, it is best to free the bowel completely as it passes through the transverse mesocolon, by cutting the peritoneum around the circumference of the duodenum as it emerges from beneath the superior mesenteric vessels in the area of the duodenojejunal junction.

The left hand is then placed beneath the head of the pancreas and the specimen is folded to the patient's right and held by the operator's left thumb in front. The major tributaries from the uncinate process to the portal vein are gently "wiped into view" with "peanut" sponges, divided, and ligated. There are usually about four such tributaries, and they can be easily isolated and managed.

Occasionally at this point, with all bridges burned, the portal vein is found to be invaded. In this circumstance, we elect to cut through tumor to remove the specimen, leaving the vein undisturbed—such cases in our

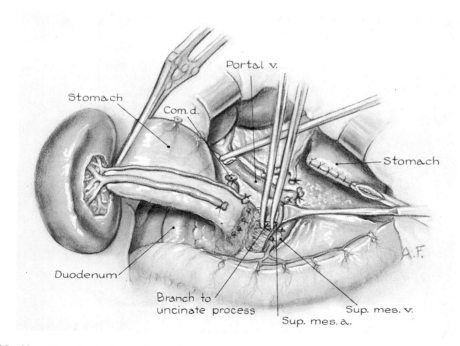

FIG. 81.   Dissection between the uncinate process and the superior mesenteric artery. The portal vein is retracted. (From Porter. In Cooper, Operative Technique, 1964. Courtesy of Little, Brown.)

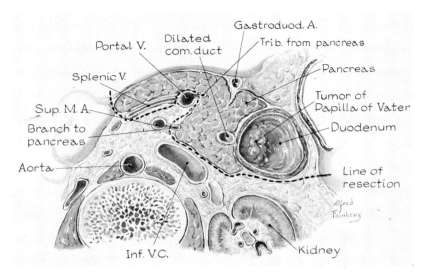

FIG. 82.   Cross section of the region of the head of the pancreas. (From Porter. In Cooper, *Operative Technique*, 1964. Courtesy of Little, Brown.)

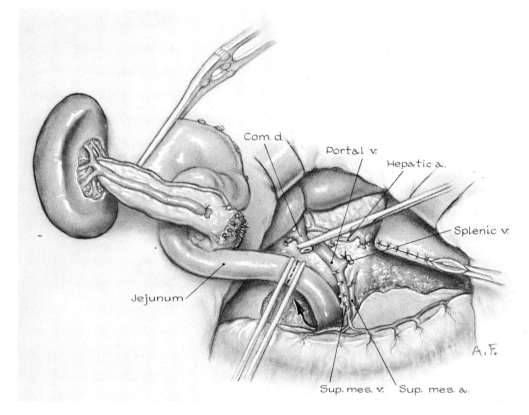

FIG. 83.   The jejunum is delivered through a rent in the mesocolon and divided. (From Porter. In Cooper, *Operative Technique*, 1964. Courtesy of Little, Brown.)

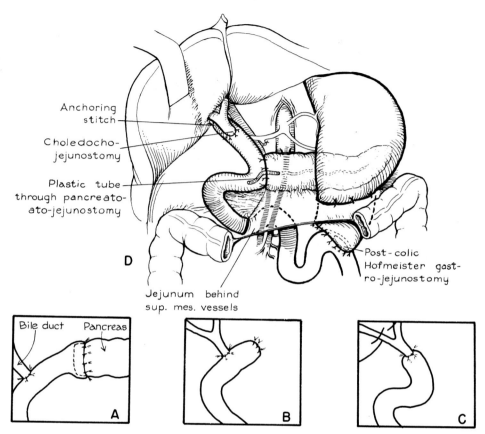

Anchoring stitch

Choledocho-jejunostomy

Plastic tube through pancreato-ato-jejunostomy

D

Jejunum behind sup. mes. vessels

Post-colic Hofmeister gastro-jejunostomy

Bile duct   Pancreas

A

B

C

FIG. 84. Biliary and pancreatic anastomoses. Unless the common bile duct is very large, it is better to put it into the side of the jejunal limb, as in (A), (B), or (D). (From Porter. In Cooper, *Operative Technique*, 1964. Courtesy of Little, Brown.)

opinion being incurable. In the past, it was decided to resect the portal vein in five patients. The vein ends were simply ligated and no anastomosis or shunt was done. All had uncomplicated postoperative courses but one, and he was found at autopsy to have a thrombosed hepatic artery. The other four died later of metastases. Since the retroperitoneal collateral circulation is adequate to manage the portal flow, we feel strongly that it is poor judgment to embark upon a portacaval shunt at this point.

The portal vein is retracted to the left with a vein retractor, and the dissection drops down one level to the bridge of tissue between the uncinate process and the superior mesenteric artery, which is defined by the left thumb anteriorly and the left forefinger behind the pancreas. Unlike the venous connections of the area, the arteries are not all easily demonstrated, and it has seemed easier and faster to divide the entire fibrofatty isthmus which contains them between serially placed clamps. Adson clamps are best for this purpose, since they have fine curved points but are long enough to reach the area. Kelly clamps are too gross for this work. About nine pairs of clamps are needed. During this step, the location of the superior mesenteric artery is constantly checked, using the left thumb and forefinger. This prevents damage to that vessel which, although palpable, is not usually clearly visible at this stage (Fig. 81). Figure 82 shows the anatomy of this area in cross section.

It is always best to tie all clamps and tidy up the field before starting this step. Otherwise, the wound will fill up with clamps and it is awkward to stop short of completion of the step. When the inferior pancreatoduodenal artery is tied, often a bridge of tissue remains which binds the bowel to the vascular structures. This can best be defined by herniating some of the upper jejunum into the right upper quadrant beneath the mesenteric vessels. When the uppermost few vessels of the jejunal mesentery are divided, the bowel slides easily into the subhepatic space where it can be divided to free the specimen (Fig. 83). It is then anastomosed to the common hepatic duct.

In many patients, the diameter of the common hepatic duct may be as great as that of the jejunum, or even greater. In such cases, an end-to-end anastomosis is done (Fig. 84C). Occasionally, however, the duct will not be very dilated, and in these patients it may be easier to close the end of the bowel and put the duct into the side of the jejunum as shown in Figure 84B and D. The arrangement in Figure 84B often proves less difficult technically.

In doing the choledochojejunostomy, 4–0 arterial silk mattress sutures are used as the outer layer, and the posterior row is placed while the common hepatic duct is still held in its clamp. The clamp is then cut off, ensuring removal of all crushed tissue. The inner layer of 5–0 atraumatic chromic catgut is then put in as a continuous locked stitch through all layers. This ensures an accurate mucosa-to-mucosa approximation and makes leakage less likely.

In the uncommon situations in which the duct is small or the tissues unusually friable, a T tube splint is used, but in the majority of instances it is not. It is interesting that in contrast to the patients with injured bile ducts upon whom plastic procedures are done (and in whom T tube splints are always used) late stenoses are rare. Recurrent tumor, however, has occluded the duct on occasion.

Some surgeons do not pull the small intestine up beneath the mesenteric vessels, but prefer to close the duodenojejunal junction as they close a duodenal stump and bring the jejunum in front of the colon to reach the duct. However, the more direct route recommended here seems to provide a more radical excision and requires one less suture line in the bowel. The mesocolon is reconstructed around the jejunum, and at a point about 14 inches below the choledochojejunostomy an antecolic or postcolic gastrojejunostomy is done according to any of the accepted techniques. The 14-inch distance ensures against reflux of gastric content into the biliary tree, which sometimes predisposes to cholangitis.

The area of the biliary anastomosis is drained and the abdominal wound closed. The deeper layers may be closed with chromic catgut, but the external oblique and anterior rectus sheath are closed with figure-of-eight mattress sutures of 30-gauge stainless steel wire. When only part of the pancreas is removed and there is the possibility of leakage of pancreatic juice, it is especially important that all layers of the wound be closed with nonabsorbable suture material, since catgut may be rapidly digested by the enzyme. For the same reason, all intra-abdominal ties and sutures are of silk.

A nasogastric tube is left in the stomach until there is evidence of return of peristaltic activity.

TECHNIQUE OF PARTIAL PANCREATECTOMY (HEAD OF THE PANCREAS)

When malignant tumors are confined to the duodenum and/or ampulla, the operation of choice (after obtaining a positive report on a biopsy specimen) is resection of the head of the pancreas. This operation is done in the same manner as the total pancreatectomy except that the neck of the gland is divided and its tail and the spleen are left in. This requires an additional anastomosis between the tail of the pancreas and the jejunum.

There are two ways of doing this: end-to-end or end of pancreas to side of jejunum. Each method has to date resulted in a few late stenoses with resultant sprue, but ordinarily either method gives satisfactory results, and it seems hard to defend simply ligating and draining the cut end of the pancreas and not doing any anastomosis.

The end-to-end anastomosis is done by plugging the pancreatic stump into the jejunal lumen and holding it with silk sutures. No attempt is made to do a mucosa-to-mucosa anastomosis. When the end-to-side method is used, fine atraumatic catgut is used at the mucosal level, and silk sutures for the outer layer of the anastomosis. A short plastic catheter is left as a splint until the fine transfixion suture of chromic catgut which holds it dissolves and it is passed down the intestinal tract (Fig. 84D).

When a partial pancreatectomy is done and the tail of the gland remains in the abdomen, a rubber tube drain is placed to the area of the pancreatojejunostomy. It is held in exactly the correct position by a suture of 3–0 plain catgut. If profuse drainage occurs, a smaller tube can be suspended in it to provide sump drainage. There is rarely much drainage, and if it does occur it rapidly dries up.

PALLIATION

It is our opinion that pancreatic resection is too formidable a procedure to be employed for palliative purposes. If cure is impossible, cholecystojejunostomy is the preferred operation for biliary decompression, since it is less apt to be obstructed by the expanding primary tumor. The likelihood of duodenal obstruction must always be considered and if it exists, or is impending, a gastrojejunostomy should be done. It is an unhappy situation to find that several months after having decompressed the biliary tree it is necessary to reoperate for duodenal obstruction. It is much wiser to anticipate the need and provide the solution at the first operation.

Pain, especially the characteristic backache, is not effectively managed by sympathectomy and is, we believe, best handled by narcotics. Unexpectedly, codeine and aspirin often seem to be more effective than meperidine (Demerol) or morphine.

Since most of these patients have complete obstruction of the alkaline pancreatic juice, they are prone to develop benign peptic ulcers of the duodenum and even hemorrhage from them. For this reason, and especially because epigastric distress is difficult to interpret in such patients, the use of an antacid is recommended.

POSTOPERATIVE PROBLEMS

Deepening Jaundice

When a biliary tree which has been completely obstructed for many weeks is suddenly decompressed it is usually found to contain light-yellow, watery bile. Within a few minutes it may become somewhat sanguineous in appearance or even grossly bloody. Occasionally the fluid which runs from the common duct or gallbladder may seem to contain more blood than bile, and the hemorrhage on a few occasions may reach alarming proportions. It has, in our experience, always stopped. The discharge seems to be analogous to the bleeding from the kidneys which occurs when long-standing urinary obstruction is suddenly relieved. The release of the dammed-up bile produces oozing from the walls of the bile passages. When this occurs, jaundice may not improve or may even deepen for a few days, but within 4 or 5 days steady improvement is noted. Fortunately, this complication is not frequent, but it has been seen after both palliative cholecystojejunostomies and pancreatic resections. We have not felt it necessary to try to arrange for a slow release of the pressure.

Diabetes Following Total Pancreatectomy

Total pancreatectomy leaves the patient with a relatively mild type of diabetes which in the average case requires only about 30 units of insulin a day to control it. In only one instance in our clinic's experience has the diabetes been difficult to control. In general the management of total pancreatectomy patients is like the management of a mild diabetic who has had a gastrectomy.

The urine must be examined every 6 hours

and standard insulin given as indicated. It is dangerous to try to switch to the long-acting type of insulin preparations until the patient's appetite and food intake have stabilized at reasonably normal levels. Chlor-propamide and talbutamide are useless, since their action depends upon the presence of pancreatic tissue.

Enzyme Replacement

The absence of pancreatic juice is compensated for by giving three pancreatin tablets (N.F.) with each meal. More may be used if evidence of greater need exists. Pancreatin powder (N.F.) is, if anything, more effective than the tablets but it is malodorous and unpleasant. Three teaspoonfuls are taken in any liquid (fruit juice is often preferred).

Sprue and/or Diabetes Following Partial Pancreatectomy

A few patients who have had the head of the pancreas resected with a pancreato-jejunostomy will develop sprue and/or diabetes after having been asymptomatic for 18 or more months. They lose weight and strength and give the impression of being patients whose tumors are metastasizing. Actually they may have developed stenosis of the pancreatojejunostomies with the late development of sprue. The diabetes seems to be due to the loss of islets because of fibrosis in the remaining tail of the gland. Care must be taken to rule out sprue and diabetes in such patients, since these disorders might otherwise go unrecognized and the patients be thought to be dying of metastases. Proper treatment rapidly restores them to normal health.

REFERENCE

1. Porter, M. R., Carcinoma of the pancreato-duodenal area, operability and choice of procedure. Ann. Surg. 148:711, 1958.

39

PANCREATIC TUMORS AND PERIAMPULLARY CARCINOMAS

A. Palliative Operations: Whipple's Pancreatoduodenectomy

RODNEY MAINGOT

CLASSIFICATION

Pancreatic and periampullary tumours may be classified as follows:

A. Primary malignant tumours.
   1. Adenocarcinoma of the head of the pancreas and periampullary carcinomas.
   2. Carcinoma of the body and tail of the gland.
   3. Sarcoma.
      a. Leiomyosarcoma.
      b. Fibrosarcoma.
      c. Lymphoma.
      d. Reticulum-cell sarcoma.
      e. Hodgkin's.
      f. Neuroblastoma.
      g. Plasmacytoma.
      h. Malignant neurilemoma.
   4. Islet-call carcinoma (insulin-secreting).
   5. Noninsulin-secreting carcinoma.
   6. Cystadenocarcinoma.
   7. Malignant carcinoid.
   8. Adenoacanthoma.
   9. Malignant melanoma.
   10. Malignant periampullary ulcer.
B. Secondary malignant tumours.
   These may be caused by the spread of cancerous growth from the stomach or transverse colon, or by metastatic carcinomas, e.g., of the lung, malignant melanomas, etc.
C. Benign tumours.
   1. Tumours of the periampullary region.
      a. Adenoma.
      b. Papilloma.
      c. Leiomyoma.
      d. Neurofibroma.
      e. Lymphangioma.
      f. Carcinoid.
      g. Heterotopic pancreatic tissue.
   2. Solid benign growths of the pancreas.
      a. Islet-cell tumours (noninsulin-secreting and insulin-secreting adenomas).
      b. Lipoma.
      c. Fibroma.
      d. Myxoma.
      e. Chondroma.
      f. Fibroadenoma.
      g. Perithelioma.
      h. Haemangioma.
      i. Lymphangioma.
      j. Haemangioendothelioma.
      k. Neuroma.
      l. Schwannoma.
   3. Cystadenoma.

CARCINOMA OF THE PANCREAS AND PERIAMPULLARY CARCINOMA

These growths are the most important and the most common malignant lesions of the pancreas, and they constitute 2 percent of all carcinomas. Cancer of the pancreas accounts for 0.5 percent of all *hospital admissions.*

Primary malignant growths are of the

spheroidal-cell pattern when they arise from the acini; they are columnar-cell carcinomas when they originate from the ducts. When malignant changes affect the islets of Langerhans, the cells are peculiarly large and possess outsize nuclei. About 80 percent of tumours are adenocarcinomas which arise from the ductular epithelium. Cancers arising from the acini account for 13 percent of growths.

Secondary growths of the gland are comman because cancer of the stomach is common and because the pancreas forms the greater portion of the bed of the stomach. It is sometimes difficult with advanced growths of the pancreas or stomach to determine whether the primary growth originated in the stomach or in the pancreas.

The most common source of cancer metastasising to the pancreas is that of malignant lesions of the lung. Other metastatic cancers found in the pancreas are, in order of frequency, malignant melanoma, and carcinoma of the breast, kidney, thyroid, uterus, colon, and prostate.

The clinical features, physical manifestations, associated laboratory findings and the operative treatment of carcinoma of the head of the pancreas and of periampullary cancers (ampulla of Vater, and distal common bile duct, and the duodenal mucosa adjacent to the major pancreatic papilla) have so much in common that these two lesions are best discussed together.

Frequency

Many cases labelled carcinoma of the head of the pancreas at operation are, in fact, cases of cancer of the lower end of the bile duct. Willis [75] found that his necropsy series included 42 proved cases of carcinoma of the pancreas and 58 of the lower end of the common bile duct and periampullary region.

About 65 percent of carcinomas of the pancreas originate in the head and ampullary area, while only 25 percent involve the body or tail of the gland.

Bell (1957) found 609 cases among 73,187 necropsies, an incidence of about 7 percent.

In England and Wales there has been a progressive increase in the mortality rate (Table 1).

Age

The majority of cases occur between the ages of 40 and 75. Wallau [60] reported on 330 autopsy cases; of these subjects, 54 percent were between 50 and 70 years old; and 73 percent between 40 and 70. Moore and Younghusband,[41] in reviewing 49 of their cases, found that four-fifths of the patients were more than 60 years of age, and one-third were over 70. The disease is rare under the age of 30. The average age of patients with malignant lesions of the head of the pancreas and ampulla of Vater is 57. Mielcarek [37] reported an adenocarcinoma with malignant deposits in the liver and regional lymph nodes in a boy of 15. He reviewed reports in the literature of cases under 20 years of age and accepted 5 of them as proved.

Cancer of the pancreas is an uncommon tumour in children. The clinical features are similar to those in adults, the main differences being the equal sex distribution and the more frequent occurrence of gastrointestinal haemorrhage.

Sex

Carcinoma of the pancreas is slightly more common in the male than in the female. (See Table 1.)

Table 1.   MORTALITY RATE OF CANCER OF THE PANCREAS AND
PERIAMPULLARY REGION (ENGLAND AND WALES)[a]

Sex	1954	1956	1958	1960	1962	1964	1969
Males	1766	1839	1980	2077	2103	2357	2666
Females	1522	1546	1747	1882	2017	2010	2318
	3288	3385	3727	3959	4120	4367	4984

[a]*Registrar-General's Statistical Reviews for the years 1954, 1956, 1958, 1960, 1962, 1964 and 1969.*

Site

Rives et al.[50] give the following ratio of distribution of carcinomas of the pancreas from a collective review of 415 cases: head, 66 percent; body and head, 18 percent; body, 6 percent; and tail, 10 percent. Duff [16] stated that from 70 to 75 percent of malignant tumours of the pancreas arise in the head of the gland. Bouchier [2] estimated that between 50 and 70 percent of cancers of the pancreas arise in the head of the gland. *The proportion of carcinoma of the head of the pancreas to periampullary carcinoma* is approximately 3:1; d'Offray's assessment [15] being 8:5.

Periampullary carcinoma may take one of three forms: (1) a small, hard, pea-like or marble-like growth distending the papilla and in intimate relation to the ampulla; (2) an ulcer of typically malignant appearance situated in the wall of the duodenum near the papilla of Vater; or (3) a growth which involves the distal 2 cm of the common bile duct. Lesions in the narrow confines of the pancreatoduodenal region offer "rich soil" for the development of carcinoma. It is generally agreed that, less eager in their growth, they spread, and that, owing to their situation, they tend to block the end of the common duct at an early stage and accordingly may be diagnosed relatively early.

Owing to these factors, and others not fully understood, the *prognosis* of periampullary carcinoma is distinctly more favourable, on pathological and surgical grounds, than the prognosis of invasive lethal lesions of the head of the pancreas proper. In the ulcerative variety, which on duodenotomy resembles *any* localised ulcer of the gastrointestinal canal, bleeding and obstructive jaundice may be notable features.

Warren et al.[62] state that the mortality rate of pancreatoduodenectomy was 13.5 percent in 253 patients with periampullary cancer treated during 1942–65. Only 1 of 35 patients died during 1966–67. The survival rate after pancreatoduodenectomy was 12.5 percent in patients with carcinoma of the pancreatic head and 30 to 41 percent in those with carcinoma of the ampulla, distal bile duct, and duodenum. Survival times after biliary bypass surgery in 332 patients and after laparotomy in 231 patients averaged 6.5 and 5 months, respectively. Ten patients with primary ductal carcinomas of the pancreatic body and tail had resection without long-term survival. The average survival of 6 patients having total pancreatectomy for ductal carcinoma of the pancreas during 1942–65 was 8 months. (Tables 2 and 3.)

Forty-one consecutive Whipple resections without operative mortality were performed by John Howard [24] in the past 13 years. The indication for operation was carcinoma of the pancreatic head or lower end of bile duct in 31 cases, chronic pancreatitis in 8, and pancreatic cystadenoma in 2. Howard's success is attributed to a careful study of patients preoperatively, decompression of the biliary tree and proximal jejunal limb, and the administration of serum albumin and, possibly, infusions of calcium postoperatively. A clinical team continuously interested in the problem is also important.

Table 2. MORTALITY RATES AFTER PANCREATODUODENECTOMY FOR PERIAMPULLARY CANCER (LAHEY CLINIC)

Site	Number of Cases	Mortality Rates (percent)
Cancer of head of pancreas	97	11.4
Ampullary cancer	93	10.8
Cancer of distal bile duct	26	19.2
Duodenal cancer	37	21.6
Total	253	13.5

Source: From Warren, Surg. Clin. No. Amer. *46:639, 1967. Courtesy of Dr. K. W. Warren and W. B. Saunders, Philadelphia.*

Table 3. SURVIVAL RATES AFTER PANCREATODUODENECTOMY FOR PERIAMPULLARY CANCER (LAHEY CLINIC)[a]

	5-Year Survivors	
	Number	Percent
Head of pancreas	9	12.5
Ampulla	20	29.8
Distal bile duct	5	35.7
Duodenum	7	41.2

Source: From Warren, Surg. Clin. No Amer. *46:639, 1967. Courtesy of Dr. K. W. Warren and W. B. Saunders, Philadelphia.*
[a]*Additional statistical data are submitted by Rodney Smith in Chapter 39, Part B.*

Diagnosis

SYMPTOMS AND SIGNS

The operability of cancer of the peri-ampullary region and of cancer of the head of the pancreas depends upon early diagnosis. In the inaugural stage of these diseases, it is almost impossible to make a correct preoperative diagnosis. Nevertheless, there are certain premonitory symptoms that are commonly present before jaundice becomes manifest. These should be carefully weighed before subjecting the patient to a few pertinent investigations.

Doubt, suspicion, and the probability of cancer arising somewhere in the upper abdomen sometimes form the basis of a precocious and life-saving diagnosis. To be able to make a certain diagnosis at the time of the bedside examination of the patient often means that the case has already reached the inoperable stage. When the so-called classic manifestations of the disease are present, the time for radical surgery has already passed for a large percentage of the patients.

The clinical features include epigastric pain, pyrexia, steatorrhoea, weakness, anorexia, indigestion, loss of weight, and jaundice. The initial symptoms simulate closely those of early cancer of the body of the stomach but, on the whole, they are less clamant and insistent. The symptom triad most frequently described by patients with cancer of the head of the gland and periampullary area is pain, weight loss, and jaundice. According to Klintrup,[32] loss of weight is one of the most characteristic symptoms, occurring in almost all patients.

The symptoms and signs of pancreatic carcinoma vary according to the situation of the growth. When the *body or tail* is involved, the clinical picture is in many ways similar to that of carcinoma of the stomach, there being, for instance, backache, anorexia, and progressive loss of weight and of strength. The fatigue syndrome, too, is marked, and the patient feels weary, disinterested, and melancholic. He sometimes senses that his is a misdiagnosed case and that all that remains is to submit with courage and patience to what Fate has in store for him.

It is rare for the tumour to be palpated in the epigastrium, even in very thin patients.

Pain is the main symptom and is felt in the epigastrium and in the back. It is constant, boring, worse at night, and unrelenting in the later stages of the disease in spite of large doses of morphine. It is one of the chief factors leading to a final decision in favour of exploratory laparotomy. Loss of weight is very marked; vomiting is present in many cases of cancer of the body of the pancreas; and anorexia and nausea are almost invariably present.

Following radiological and chemical investigations, which often throw little light on the diagnosis, an exploratory laparotomy is advisable in order to determine the true nature of the condition.

In cases of cancer of the head of the pancreas, epigastric pain, backache, weakness, nausea, anorexia, loss of weight, and cachexia nearly always precede the onset of jaundice. Pain, which is described as dull or aching in character and which is felt in the epigastrium and beneath the scapulae, is present in more than 60 percent of the patients and may arise either before or after the jaundice appears. At times it is intense and persistent, while at other times it may be intermittent and cramp-like, as in gallstone colic. The pain is frequently epigastric in cases of carcinoma of the pancreas, but is more apt to be localised to the right upper quadrant of the abdomen in cases of cancer of the ampullary zone. Extension of pain to the back is noted in 50 percent of those with pancreatic malignant disease, but is observed less frequently in patients with carcinoma of the ampulla of Vater and in those with cancer of the lower reaches of the choledochus. It is common (65 to 70 percent) in patients suffering from carcinoma of the duodenum. *Jaundice* arises insidiously; at first it is only slight, but as the disease progresses it becomes very severe and remains so until the end. The skin may be coloured a light canary yellow, olive green, light brown, or even a dark mahogany hue. Very marked and intractable jaundice, associated with a maddening torture of *itching* which is unresponsive to local applications, are often signs of malignant biliary-pancreatic disease. Jaundice occurs in 75 percent of *all* cases of carcinoma of the pancreas and in approximately 90 percent of the cases of carcinoma of the head of the gland. It is usually a late manifestation when the growth involves the body or tail of the gland. *Marked loss of weight* is observed in over 90 percent of the resected cases. A history of *vomiting* is obtained in about 40 percent of patients having carcinoma of the periampullary area, while only 15 percent of those with cancer of the head of the pancreas complain of this symptom. *Steatorrhoea* is a common symptom and occurs in approximately 30 percent of patients with resectable periampullary lesions. Brown et al.[4] state that the *stools* are often bulky and may contain *visible fat,* especially when the fat content of the diet is high. The presence of visible fat is of much greater diagnostic significance than an excess of microscopic fat, which may also occur in other forms of obstructive jaundice and in sprue (leading article, *Lancet* 2:1197, 1952).

In my opinion, a distended and *tense gallbladder* is noted before operation in about 40 percent of malignant cases. Miller and coworkers,[38] however, place the incidence higher than this and state that palpation revealed that more than 50 percent of the icteric patients in their series had enlarged gallbladders or, specifically, 68.2 percent of those with pancreatic malignant disease and 51.8 percent with papillary carcinoma. A nontender *enlarged liver* was palpated in 77.8 percent of the icteric patients having carcinoma of the pancreas and 66.6 percent of those having periampullary carcinoma. The enlarged liver is the consequence of either biliary stasis or hepatic metatases. A palpable epigastric mass is present in about 10 percent of these cases.

Cattell et al.[10] have stressed the fact that the classic hallmark of the disease, namely, a palpable gallbladder in the presence of painless jaundice, has been observed in only 30 percent of their resectable series. Inability to palpate the gallbladder does not mean that the biliary tree is not distended, for at operation the gallbladder (when present) is dilated in almost all instances (98 percent). The possibility of carcinoma of the head or of the periampullary area should not be excluded merely because the gallbladder is not palpable. It should be remembered that as the liver enlarges with pent-up bile and the gallbladder becomes increasingly distended, the fundus of the gallbladder is diverted downwards and towards the right flank.

Courvoisier's law states that if, in a jaundiced patient, the gallbladder is enlarged, the condition is not one of stone impaction of the common bile duct, as previous cholecystitis will have rendered the gallbladder fibrotic and incapable of dilatation. Moynihan[42] pointed out that Courvoisier's law, like all other laws, is capable of infraction. He showed that the law may be violated in the following circumstances:

1. When there is a stone in or stricture of the cystic duct causing mucocele or empyema together with impaction of a calculus in the common bile duct.
2. When there is a calculus in the cystic duct or in Hartmann's pouch compressing the common bile duct.
3. When there is distention of the gallbladder by an acute inflammatory process with blockage of the common bile duct by stone.
4. When there is chronic induration of the head of the pancreas with a stone in the common bile duct.

Methods of Investigation

The chronic course of the disease, which is usually apyrexial (except in patients with cholangitis due to carcinoma of the common bile duct), the previous history of epigastric pain, backache, fatigue, nausea, anorexia and loss of weight, the swollen gallbladder, the enlarged liver, the presence of jaundice of a severe character, the incessant itching, the presence of bile in the urine and its absence in the putty-like faeces are factors which proclaim or suggest a diagnosis of cancer of the head of the pancreas or of the lower end of the common bile duct.

The disease may, on occasion, be confused with hepatogenous jaundice (toxic, infective, or cirrhotic), chronic sclerosing pancreatitis, calculous obstruction of the bile passages, a postoperative stricture of the common bile duct, fibrosis of the sphincter of Oddi, or choledochal cyst. Every effort should be made to arrive at a diagnosis as soon as possible, as the longer the obstruction persists the greater the risks of operative interference.

Pain is the most common initial symptom of carcinoma of the head of the pancreas or duodenum, but chills and fever, dark urine, pruritis, and jaundice may also be initial symptoms in patients with carcinoma of the papilla and ampullary zone. *Painless jaundice is most commonly observed in patients with carcinoma of the papilla and common bile duct. The investigation and management of the jaundiced patient* receives the expert consideration of Dr. Frances H. Smith in Chapter 45.

Radiological investigations. These include: (1) plain x-ray films of the epigastric regions; (2) barium-meal x-ray examination; (3) duodenography (see Chap. 4, Part C by Louis Kreel); (4) percutaneous transhepatic cholangiography (see Chap. 46 by Geoffrey Walker); (5) operative cholangiography (see Chap. 43); (6) isotope scanning (see Chap. 38A); (7) portal venography (at operation); and (8) selective angiography (see Chap. 108). The following contributions are worthy of careful study: Sodee [56]; Brown et al.[5]; and Bouchier.[2]

Plain x-ray pictures may display the presence of pancreatic cysts, calcinosis of the gland, pancreatolithiasis, the presence of opaque gallstones, etc. Cancer of the pancreas has been reported in 25 percent of patients with calcific pancreatitis.

The barium-meal x-ray signs of duodenal involvement with carcinoma are fixation, distortion from external pressure, dilatation, narrowing, localized filling defects. and marked widening or exaggeration of the C of the duodenal loop.

A combination of invasion and oedema of the papilla of Vater may produce a typical filling defect resembling a reversed 3. The inverted 3 sign of Frostberg may be present, but this is an indication of a pancreatic mass and not necessarily a cancer. Some of the x-ray manifestations include slight alterations on the medial aspect of the duodenal loop and minor pressure defects on neighbouring viscera before any widening of the C-loop has occurred.

Wise and Johnston[76] are of the opinion that widening of the duodenal loop without distortion of the mucosa on the internal aspect of the duodenum should be regarded lightly in the interpretation of disorders of the gland. *In healthy, muscular, broad-chested men, considerable widening of the C-loop of duodenum may be commonly observed.*

Duodenography has proved to be a most helpful method of investigating the duode-num, the head of the pancreas, and the peri ampullary area. (See Chap. 4, Part C.)

It should be noted that *cholecystography* and *cholangiography* are useless, and possibly dangerous, when the serum bilirubin values exceed 3 to 4 mg per 100 ml. The illumination of the pelves and calyces of the kidneys following intravenous cholangiography is indicative of liver damage.

Percutaneous intrahepatic cholangiography supplies the surgeon with a valuable aid to preoperative diagnosis, and in special cases may be employed for therapeutic purposes (see Chap. 46). Thus, the main uses of this method of cholangiography are:

1. To diagnose the presence of obstructive extrahepatic jaundice as opposed to the intrahepatic "medical" lesions.
2. To diagnose the presence and the site of a carcinoma of the bile ducts, the ampulla of Vater, or the head of the pancreas.
3. To demonstrate the site of biliary tract calculous disease and the number and size of stones, especially in patients in whom the serum bilirubin concentration exceeds 3 mg per 100 ml.
4. To localise the presence and site of postoperative strictures of the bile ducts, especially intrahepatic and hilar strictures which prove so difficult to detect at operation, or to tap for the performance of *operative* cholangiography.
5. To elucidate the condition of the biliary tree in cases of congenital atresia of the bile ducts. In only some 20 per cent of such cases is reconstructive biliary-intestinal anastomosis possible.[36]

FIBRESCOPIC DUODENOSCOPY WITH CANNULATION OF THE SPHINCTER OF ODDI (ENDOSCOPIC PANCREATOCHOLANGIOGRAPHY)

This method is described by Louis Kreel in Chapter 34B.

SCANNING OF THE PANCREAS

See Chapter 38A.

Laboratory findings. Chapter 45 deals with the investigation and management of the jaundiced patient.

Selective arteriography. This procedure, when used on the coeliac and superior mesenteric arteries, has provided useful information. Nebesar and Pollard [44] caution against overoptimism concerning the accuracy of arteriography, however, and they find that 10 percent of patients *without* carcinoma of the pancreas will show false positive arteriographic changes.

Leucocytosis. Arkin and Weisberg [1] found leucocytosis in more than 50 percent of a series of patients suffering from carcinoma of the pancreas; they noted that it was usually associated with metastases in the liver. Increased leucocyte counts are found predominantly with carcinoma of the ampulla and lower end of the common bile duct, as lesions in this situation are usually associated with cholangitis.

Significant secondary anaemia is sometimes observed in patients with resectable carcinoma of the head of the pancreas, but with malignant lesions of the periampullary area, which are prone to bleed, this finding is quite common. Brown et al. (*Am. J. Med. Sci.* 233:349, 1952) found *occult blood* to be present in 67 of the 1,700 consecutive cases of cancer of the ampulla of Vater investigated by them. Warren (1967) found occult blood to be present in *over* 80 percent of all his cases of periampullary cancer. In carcinoma of the duodenum, occult blood was discovered in 100 percent of the cases.

Blood urea estimations. The blood urea is raised in cases of obstructive jaundice, and the higher the reading the graver the prognosis.

Serum amylase and lipase studies. In cases of cancer of the pancreas and of periampullary carcinoma, it is unusual to find any notable rise in the serum amylase or lipase estimations.

Steatorrhoea and creatorrhoea. These sequelae of grave pancreatic disease are more common with carcinoma of the head than with cancer of the periampullary area (including the lower reaches of the common bile duct).

It is possible that an examination of the stools (which are so commonly grey, frothy, greasy, and malodorous) to determine the fat content may prove of some value in indicating the site and the nature of the pancreatic lesion. In cases of carcinoma of the head of the gland, for instance, both the neutral fat content and the fatty acids of the stools are increased, while in chronic relapsing pancreatitis the increase is mainly in the fatty acids. The duct of Wirsung is not so frequently occluded in cancer of the ampulla of Vater as it is in cases of carcinoma of the body of the pancreas. In cancer of the papilla, the blockage is, as a rule, intermittent until a late stage in the disease is reached (Bockus, 1966).

Liver function tests. Elevation of the alkaline phosphatase and cholesterol values frequently supports a diagnosis of obstructive jaundice—of that and of nothing else. In most patients, the levels of serum alkaline phosphatase seldom exceed 35 K-A units. Cephalin-cholesterol floccula-

tion and thymol turbidity tests usually confirm the absence of hepatic parenchymal disease.

Mongé et al. (*Surg. Gynec. Obstet.* 118:275, 1964) found the median value of total serum bilirubin in 43 patients was 9 mg per 100 ml for those with cancer of the pancreatic head; 11.5 mg per 100 ml for those with carcinoma of the ampulla or papilla of Vater; and 16.9 mg per 100 ml for those with carcinoma of the lower end of the common bile duct. The highest individual values for the respective groups ranged from 21.2 to 28.4 mg.

Duodenal drainage. The absence of bile in the aspirated fluid is, of course, a significant finding. Laboratory methods for the analysis of pancreatic enzymes and sodium bicarbonate in the pancreatic juice which has been withdrawn from the second or third portion of the duodenum may, on occasion, be helpful in diagnosis, but such tests are not frequently employed today.

Raskin et al. (*Gastroenterology* 34:996, 1958) describe in some detail a method of intubation of the duodenum for exfoliative cytological inquiries. They investigated 203 patients by this method, and malignant cells were recovered in 28 of 43 cases of pancreatic, biliary, or duodenal carcinoma, the diagnosis being verified by subsequent operation or at postmortem examination.

Cytology. Duodenal samples obtained during the secretin test may be examined for malignant cells. Positive results have been recorded in 86 percent of proved cancers in the head and body and tail of the gland.

Plasma prothrombin response to intravenous injections of vitamin K. Ivy and Roth [27] considered this to be a good practical test for estimating hepatic insufficiency. Today this method is still occasionally performed, more particularly in the early stages of jaundice. Bouchier [3] states that vitamin K absorption will be reduced when there is steatorrhoea. There will be a raised prothrombin time.

Palliative Operations

If the surgeon decides to perform pancreatoduodenectomy in *two stages*, the first-stage operation should be simple *T tube choledochostomy or cholecystostomy* combined with drainage of the right subhepatic space. All manipulations should be reduced to a minimum, and Kocher's manoeuvre, duodenotomy, pancreatic biopsy, and such drainage operations as choledochoenterostomy or cholecystoenterostomy should not be carried out. All such bypass procedures, especially when accompanied by manipulation and mobilisation of the head of the pancreas, double the surgeon's difficulties at the second-stage operation, or they may be a cause of disseminating malignant cells.

If the malignant tumour proves to be

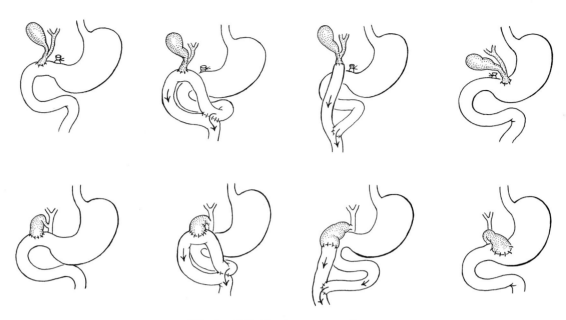

FIG. 1.   Palliative bypass operations.

irremovable, the majority of surgeons perform one of the many short-circuiting or decompressive operations as illustrated in Figures 1 to 4. These include choledochojejunostomy, choledochoduodenostomy, choledochogastrostomy, cholecystojejunostomy, cholecystoduodenostomy, and cholecystogastrostomy. Today, the choice of these palliative procedures is cholecystojejunostomy using the Roux-en-Y loop or the simple jejunal loop technique combined with side-to-side jejunojeunostomy or end-to-side choledochojejunostomy carried out on the Roux-en-Y plan [13] (Fig. 4). As a rule, supplementary gastrojejunostomy is carried out to circumvent the possibility of subsequent duodenal obstruction. The operative mortality rate of these palliative procedures varies from 5 to 10 percent.

Operations such as cholecystojejunostomy are generally inappropriate for palliative biliary bypass because, all too often, the primary malignant neoplasm relentlessly creeps upward, by direct extension, along and around the common bile duct to obstruct and strangle the cystic duct and even the choledochus itself. As this is so, the anastomosis between the intestinal tract and the gall-bladder or the common bile duct fails to provide even a reasonable period of relief from jaundice. During convalescence, many patients develop cholangitis, melaena, bouts of vomiting, or further episodes of jaundice caused by stenosis of the biliary-intestinal stoma. In most cases, relief from jaundice is obtained for from 4 to 7 months, but few of these unfortunate patients survive for 1 year.

I believe that a greater measure of relief can be obtained by displaying the biliary passages, ligating and dividing the cystic artery, transecting the enlarged common hepatic duct, excising the gallbladder together with its cystic duct and upper portion of the common bile duct, and by anastomosing the open mouth of the common hepatic duct to the apex of an antecolic loop of proximal jejunum, after which an entero-anastomosis is fashioned to deflect intestinal contents away from the biliary-jejunal anastomosis (Fig. 4). Antecolic gastrojejunostomy completes the operation.

A few of these palliative biliary bypass procedures will be described (see Figs. 1 to 4).

In cases of irremovable cancer of the head of the pancreas or of the ampulla-papillary region, there are still a number of surgeons who consider that *cholecystogastrostomy* is the operation of choice and elect this method for anatomical reasons, as the distended gallbladder lies over the pyloric region of the stomach and therefore lends itself readily to anastomosis (Figs. 1 and 3).

Cholecystogastrostomy, however, has the following disadvantages:

1. Leakage from the anastomotic line may occur, owing to the tension produced by the powerful contractions of the stomach.

2. The thick musculature and the loose redundant mucosa of the stomach lend themselves to accurate suture with the thin gallbladder wall less readily than does the wall of the jejunum.

3. Following the anastomosis, the pylorus may be kinked or partially obstructed.

4. The stoma permits the free ingress of gastric contents into the bile radicles with the result that ascending suppurative cholangitis is a common sequel.

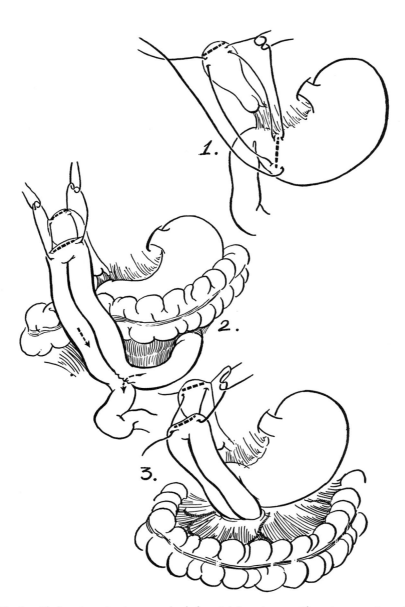

FIG. 2.   Cholecystogastrostomy and cholecystojejunostomy with entero-anastomosis.

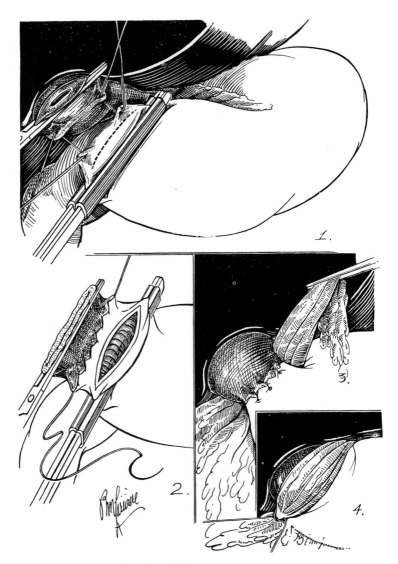

FIG. 3.   Cholecystogastrostomy.

Cholecystoduodenostomy is not advised owing to the propinquity of the stoma and the growth.

In cases of irremovable cancer of the head of the pancreas, *cholecystojejunostomy* remains a popular palliative procedure. A loop of jejunum some 20 inches (50.8 cm) from the duodenojejunal flexure is selected, brought over the transverse colon, and anastomosed to the fundus of the gallbladder. The operation is completed by performing an entero-anastomosis between the proximal and distal jejunal limbs, about 16 to 18 inches (40.6 to 45.7 cm) beyond the ligament of Treitz (i.e., just inferior to the cholecystojejunal union;

see Fig. 2), after which, for added security, the omentum is wrapped around the area where the gallbladder has been joined to the small intestine.

The anastomosis can be accomplished without any tension, the suturing is simple, the junction can be made watertight, and the entero-anastomosis deflects the intestinal contents away from the gallbladder so that cholangitis seldom occurs.

When the duodenum appears to be partially constricted by growth, I often add anterior gastrojejunostomy to the above procedures, in order to forestall the onset of acute obstruction.

The *results of these palliative operations* for

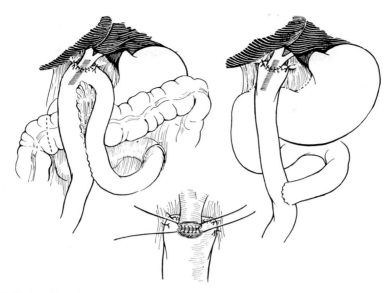

FIG. 4. Palliative hepaticojejunostomy for periampullary carcinomas and cancers of the head of the pancreas. The Roux-en-Y method is depicted on the right side of the figure. A method of anastomosing the hepatic duct to the jejunum by the end-to-side mucosa-to-mucosa method is depicted in inset.

cancer of the head of the pancreas are disappointing, as the average mortality rate is about 5 to 10 percent, and within 6 months or so of the operation all—or nearly all—such patients are dead. Few patients are alive 1 year after such operations for irremovable tumours of the periampullary region. When survival exceeds one year, the question always arises as to whether the primary lesion in the pancreas was in fact cancerous or not. The mortality rate is higher in patients who are extremely jaundiced, and when there is *white bile* the immediate death rate is as high as 15 percent. Postoperative deaths are caused by peritonitis, haemorrhage, chest complications, external biliary fistula, shock, and liver failure; more than 30 percent of the patients succumb to the "hepatorenal syndrome."

Cattell (*Surg. Clin. N. Amer.* June: 649, 1948), who was the first to suggest *anastomosis of the duct of Wirsung to the proximal jejunum* as an additional procedure to cholecystojejunostomy and entero-anastomosis for irremovable growths of the head of the pancreas and of the periampullary region, writes:

"We have accomplished this anastomosis by two technical procedures:

"1. If only *moderate* distension of the duct is present, the seromuscular coat of the jejunum is divided, exposing the mucosa. The anterior surface of the pancreas is incised over the duct but it is not entered. A braided silk suture is then passed through the anterior wall of the duct and through 1 cm of the exposed jejunal mucosa and is tied tightly. The opposite side of the jejunum

is then sutured to the upper side of the pancreatic body above the duct.

"2. If the duct of Wirsung is *large,* it is opened for a distance of 2 cm, a T-tube inserted into it and an open anastomosis performed to the jejunum, suturing the mucosa of the duct to the mucosa of the jejunum with a non-absorbable suture line outside.

"When this anastomosis has been completed, either by the necrosing suture technic or by open anastomosis, the efferent loop of the jejunum is then brought over to the gallbladder and a cholecystojejunostomy done 3 or 4 inches (7.5 to 10 cm) distal to the pancreatic anastomosis. The operation is completed by doing an enteroenterostomy 4 inches (10 cm) proximal to each of the two previous anastomoses, thus short-circuiting them to avoid regurgitation into the two duct systems."

TECHNIQUE OF CHOLECYSTOGASTROSTOMY

The gallbladder is isolated, a trocar and cannula of the Mayo pattern is introduced through the fundus, and the bile is aspirated. The fundus of the collapsed gallbladder is next seized with Ochsner forceps and drawn across to the pyloric region of the stomach to ascertain whether it can be made to lie there without undue tension. Two pairs of Allis forceps are placed, one near the lesser curvature and the other near the greater curvature, about 3 cm from the pyloric ring, and these draw the stomach to the undersurface of the gallbladder, about 2.5 cm proximal to the Ochsner clamp. The incision in the stomach will therefore be vertical or oblique (Fig. 3).

Four of five interrupted sutures of fine silk approximate the contiguous surfaces of the pylorus and the gallbladder and also act as tractor sutures. A continuous seromuscular suture of 000 chromic catgut is then introduced as a posterior layer, after which the stomach is opened and its contents are aspirated, the Ochsner clamp steadying the gallbladder being removed after that portion of the fundus which projects beyond the Ochsner clamp has been excised. After the clamp is removed, the posterior margin of the gallbladder is united to the contiguous margin of the stomach wall by a running suture, commencing at the greater curvature. When this reaches the lesser curvature, it is continued anteriorly as a Connell or loop-on-the-mucosa suture which unites the anterior margins of the gallbladder and stomach. When this suture reaches the greater curvature, it is knotted to the end that is left long. The first posterior seromuscular suture is then picked up and continued anteriorly, invaginating the anterior suture line. When this is completed, a few interrupted sutures of fine silk are placed here and there along the suture line to reinforce it even further. The stoma should admit the tip of one finger, as it invariably contracts when the gallbladder returns to its normal size.

The omentum is then drawn around the anastomotic line as an added measure of safety.

TECHNIQUE OF CHOLECYSTODUODENOSTOMY

This operation is performed without the aid of clamps. Two stay sutures are first introduced into the duodenum, fully 5 cm away from the pyloric outlet. The first suture is placed on the anterior surface of the duodenum near its outer margin, the second at a point on the inner margin of the gut but a little below the first suture. The fundus of the gallbladder is clamped with Ochsner forceps and the two stay sutures are inserted at the inner and outer margins of the gallbladder about 2 cm below the clamp. The anastomosis is then conducted in a manner similar to cholecystogastrostomy, i.e., by inserting two layers of continuous sutures with a reinforcement of interrupted seromuscular sutures.

TECHNIQUE OF CHOLECYSTOJEJUNOSTOMY

The selected loop of jejunum, which should be approximately 20 inches (50.8 cm) from the duodenojejunal flexure, is brought across the transverse colon and the selected loop is sutured about 5 mm below the clamped fundus of the gallbladder. A posterior continuous seromuscular suture unites the jejunum to the undersurface of the gallbladder, and after the redundant fundus has been trimmed away and

the Ochsner clamp removed, an opening is made into the jejunum—corresponding in length to the open end of the gallbladder. A second continuous suture draws together the posterior margins of the gallbladder and jejunum, and this is continued anteriorly as a Connell suture. The anterior suture line is invaginated by a continuous Cushing stitch and further strengthened with interrupted sutures of fine silk, after which the omentum is wrapped around the anastomosis and anchored into position with a few sutures. The extremities of the anastomosis should be sutured to the edge of the liver with a few interrupted stitches to take away the strain from the suture line.

The operation is completed by performing an entero-anastomosis between the proximal and distal limbs of the jejunum a few inches below the biliary enteric stoma.

TECHNIQUE OF CHOLEDOCHODUODENOSTOMY

As the common bile duct is usually grossly dilated, it is easy to anastomose it to the contiguous duodenum by the side-to-side method. I usually make an oblique stoma and construct the anastomosis with two layers of sutures: an outer one of interrupted sutures of fine silk and an inner one of continuous 00 chromic catgut. At the completion of this simple procedure, the surgeon should perform gastrojejunostomy.

TECHNIQUE OF HEPATICOJEJUNOSTOMY

After a Roux-en-Y loop has been fashioned, the cystic artery is isolated, tied, and divided; after which the gallbladder, cystic duct, and the upper portion of the common bile duct are excised, leaving behind the open gaping mouth of the common hepatic duct, which is anastomosed end-to-side to the ascending limb of jejunum. The closed end of this ascending limb is sutured to Glisson's capsule to prevent downward traction and to relieve any strain of the anastomosis. T tube hepaticostomy and drainage of the subhepatic space with a Penrose tube completes the operation (Fig. 4).

In conclusion, it may be said that operation is the best course to adopt, as those who survive the ordeal are rendered more comfortable, since there is often considerable relief of jaundice and of itching—life also being prolonged for a few valuable months. Again, the difficulties in diagnosis must be stressed: a simple case may be mistaken for a malignant one. This alone would justify a bypass operation.

Transduodenal Excision of Tumour of the Ampulla of Vater

Local excision of the tumour may rarely be indicated for lesions that are locally malignant and have not invaded the adjacent duodenal wall or the pancreas. This procedure is particularly suitable in elderly poor-risk patients in whom the more extensive operations, such as pancreatoduodenectomy, might be undesirable. Figure 5 illustrates the more important steps of the operation. The second portion of the duodenum is opened through a longitudinal incision to expose a tumour of the ampulla of Vater (A). The tumour with a margin of normal duodenal wall is excised by a cautery (B). The edges of the common bile duct and the pancreatic duct are seen (C), after which the common bile duct and the pancreatic duct are sutured to the duodenal wall and to each other with interrupted sutures of 0000 silk (D). The operation is completed by performing T tube choledochostomy and by closing the incision in the anterior wall of the duodenum. Recently, Kenefick [30] reported 5 cases treated by this procedure. Two patients are alive and well 3 or more years years after operation and three have died 8, 9, and 12 months after operation, respectively.

Radical Procedures

Carcinoma of the Tail and Body of the Pancreas

As the disease is insidious and is seldom recognised in its early stages, radical excision of the tail and body of the organ together with the spleen has rarely been successfully performed. Serafini [53] was the first to report a successful case of excision of the body of the pancreas for cancer. His patient, a woman, died from muscle and bone metastases 2½ years after operation. Grekoff [20] removed about nine-tenths of a pancreas, which was the seat of a large carcinoma occupying the tail and body of the gland.

About 25 percent of carcinomas of the pancreas arise in the body and tail. The disease is most frequently encountered between the ages of 50 and 70, the peak incidence being about 57. The ratio of males to females is 2.5:1.

The pathological features are in many respects similar to those of cancer of the head of the gland. The growth is eager in its spread and soon involves adjacent organs and structures, such as the aorta, the mesenteric blood vessels, the coeliac axis, inferior vena cava, the posterior wall of the stomach, and the duodenojejunal flexure. The liver and lungs soon become studded with metastatic implants.

The *clinical picture* is, at first, obscure. But, later on, pain situated in the midepigastrium or left subcostal region is usually constant and severe, and often stabs through to the back or to the left scapula. Anorexia and rapid loss of weight are early symptoms. Jaundice, when present, is always a late and ominous complication. Jaundice is often produced by metastases in the liver. Vomiting and retching are not infrequent, and diarrhoea and steatorrhoea may be troublesome features in some patients.

Physical examination may reveal nothing abnormal except, perhaps, a hard mass in the epigastrium. Laboratory data are not helpful in diagnosis, but a barium-meal x-ray investigation may show displacement of the stomach, duodenum, colon, or biliary tract. Few cases are correctly diagnosed before exploratory laparotomy.

Rodney Smith (1961) was able to resect 3 carcinomas of the tail or body of the pancreas in his series of 43 patients. None of his patients who underwent radical resection was alive 6 months after operation.

Only a few of these cancers lend themselves to "resection for cure," and only a select few patients survive the ordeal of operation for more than 6 months. For example, resection was possible in only 8 of 158 patients having adenocarcinoma of the body and tail of the pancreas operated upon at the Mayo Clinic.

We have been unable to find any mention in the literature of a patient alive and well without recurrence for more than 5 years after resection of an *unquestioned* carcinoma of the body or tail of the pancreas (Kibler and Bernatz, *Proc. Mayo Clin. 33*:247, 1958).

Sir Gordon Gordon-Taylor,[18] however, gave a detailed and vivid account of the

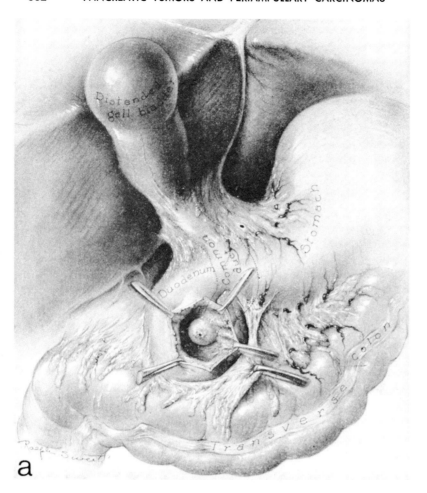

a

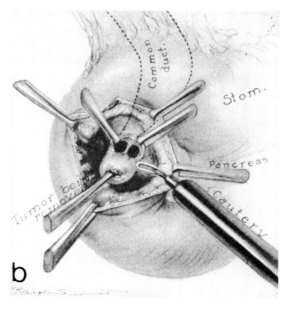

b

FIG. 5. Transduodenal resection of the ampulla of Vater for carcinoma of the distal end of the common bile duct. (From Hunt and Budd, *Surg. Gynecol., Obstet.* 61:652. Courtesy of the authors and *Surgery, Gynecology and Obstetrics*.)

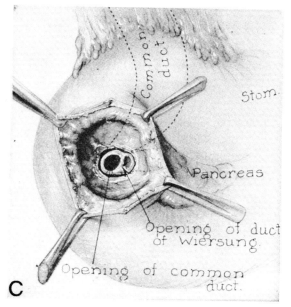

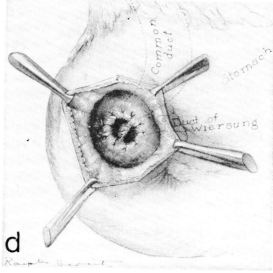

FIG. 5C. (See legend page 882.)

FIG. 5D.

heroic and highly successful operation he performed upon a man with *carcinoma of the body of the pancreas.* He wrote:

Almost seven years have now elapsed since the removal of a massive carcinoma of the body of the pancreas was performed in the case under consideration; and a recent visit of the patient in an excellent state of health, and in possession of boundless mental and physical energy, prompts the presentation of this note. The following account does not purport to be a narrative of some stupendous or venturesome operation, but merely embodies a hope that others may be encouraged to radical measures should it be their fortune to encounter a similar set of conditions. Moreover, the possibility of an enduring cure as a recompense for surgical fortitude would seem to justify a bolder attitude than has been customary in this disease. . . .

Every one of the 14 cases of cancer of the tail or body that I have encountered at operation has proved to be unresectable. The average length of life following exploratory operation was no more than 5 months.

The tumour is best approached through a long vertical or transverse epigastric incision, and the pancreas freely exposed by unpicking the greater omentum from the transverse colon and by completely severing the gastro-splenic omentum, after which the omentum and stomach are drawn firmly upward over the chest and held there in the grasp of an assistant's hand. When resection appears to be a feasible undertaking, the spleen and the tail and body of the pancreas are mobilised and drawn through the abdominal incision after the splenic artery and vein have been ligated close to the upper border of the gland and the distal portion of the pancreas has been freed from its posterior attachments; the gland is cut across at its neck, beyond the visible and palpably growing margin of the tumour. Bleeding points in the cut surface of the pancreas are picked up with mosquito forceps and tied with fine silk or underrun and ligated. The duct of Wirsung is identified and ligated with silk. The cut surface of the gland is now oversewn with mattress sutures and wrapped around with omentum. Drainage should always be provided.

Less than 5 percent of cases encountered at exploratory operation are resectable. Even when distal pancreatectomy appears to be a feasible undertaking, this operation should not be attempted *where the disease has spread beyond the confines of the gland.* To do so, in such circumstances, achieves nothing of consequence, as the life of the patient will not be prolonged by splenectomy combined with distal pancreatectomy.

PANCREATODUODENECTOMY FOR CANCER OF THE HEAD OF THE PANCREAS AND THE PERIAMPULLARY REGION

The radical procedures for resectable cancerous growths of the ampulla-papillary region and of the head of the pancreas are based upon the original and brilliant work of a distinguished American surgeon, Allen Whipple. The following historical account is based primarily on his paper,[72] from which I have drawn much valuable material.

HISTORICAL NOTE

Hopes of a radical treatment for carcinoma of the pancreas were first raised when Halsted (*Boston Med. Sci. J.* 141:645, 1899) resected a segment of the second part of the duodenum and a portion of the pancreas for an ampullary carcinoma. He implanted the pancreatic duct and the bile duct in line with the suture of the repair of the duodenal defect. His patient died six months later from recurrence of the growth.

W. J. Mayo (1900), Mayo-Robson (1900), and Koerte (1904) reported limited excisions which were unsuccessful, while Desjardins (1907), Sauve (1908), Coffey (1909), and Kehr (1914) proposed operations for cancer of the pancreas which they carried out in human cadavers. Between 1912 and 1935 there were only three successful cases of *limited* resection of a portion of the duodenum and of the head of the pancreas for cancer, and these were reported by Kausch (*Beitr. Klin. Chir.* 78:439, 1912), Hirschel (*Münch Med. Wochenschr.* 61:1728, 1914), and Tenani (*Policlinico* [*Chir*] 29:291, 1922). Hirschel's operation was an example of a one-stage *limited* duodenal resection with wedge excision of a relatively small portion of the head of the pancreas for an ampullary carcinoma, whilst Kausch and Tenani's cases were subjected to the two-stage procedure. In 1935, Whipple, Parsons, and Mullins (*Ann. Surg. 102:* 763, 1935, following a systematic study of the subject and considerable experimental work, published the first report of their successful two-stage procedure for radical en bloc resection of the duodenum and head of the pancreas for a growth of the ampulla of Vater (Fig. 6).

During the period, 1935 to 1946, a number of surgeons recorded their modifications of the two-stage procedure, notably Cooper (*Ann. Surg. 106:*1009, 1937), Orr (*Surg. Gynecol. Obstet.* 73:240, 1941), Hunt (*Ann. Surg. 114:*570, 1941), Illingworth (*Edinburgh Med. J. 46:*331, 1939), Maingot (*Lancet 2:*798, 1941), Whipple (*Ann.*

*Surg. 114:*612, 1941; *Surg. Gynecol. Obstet. 82:* 623, 1946), Cattell (*Surg. Clin. North Am. 23:*753, 1943), Child (*Ann. Surg. 119:*845, 1944), and Waugh and Clagett (*Surgery 20:*224, 1946) (Fig. 7).

Brunschwig (*Surg. Gynecol. Obstet. 65:*681, 1937; *The Surgery of Pancreatic Tumours,* 1942) was the first surgeon to perform successfully an *extensive* radical pancreatoduodenectomy for carcinoma of the head of the pancreas, including the head and neck of the gland together with 90 percent of the duodenum. In March 1940 Whipple performed the first recorded *one-stage removal* of the entire head of the pancreas and all of the duodenum with occlusion of the pancreatic stump, while a few weeks later Trimble, Parsons, and Sherman (*Surg. Gynecol. Obstet. 72:*711, 1941) reported a similar procedure.

RADICAL PANCREATODUODENECTOMY

Radical pancreatoduodenectomy is the standard operation for resectable growths of the head of the pancreas and of the periampullary region. In ampullary cancer, the operative mortality rate is low and the cure rate is relatively high.

In cases of cancer of the head of the pancreas, the radical operation is attempted only when a careful preliminary mobilisation fails to reveal any local (i.e., to the portal vein) or distant extension, in other words, when the tumour is well circumscribed and without demonstrable metastases.

One reason why the surgical results in cancer of the head of the pancreas are disappointing is because the tumour is frequently of the anaplastic invasive variety, rarely produces any significant symptoms in its *early* stages, and the radiological and biochemical investigations afford but little help in diagnosis. When jaundice is well established, the growth is often in the exuberant stage. Unfortunately, the majority of patients are referred to the surgeon when jaundice, which is a late sign, has been present for a number of weeks. Much valuable time is often wasted on numerous laboratory tests. Any case of extrahepatic obstructive jaundice demands early surgical intervention following a brief but intensive course of preoperative therapy.

Exploration of the abdomen. Many incisions have been employed, including the following: right or left epigastric paramedian, right rectus muscle-splitting, and trans-

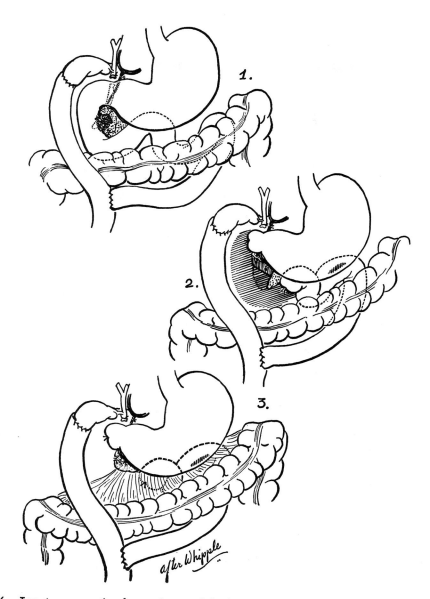

FIG. 6. Two-stage operation for carcinoma of the head of the pancreas—Whipple, Parsons, and
Mullins' original technique.

verse. In most instances, a right paramedian or rectus muscle-splitting incision suffices.

The exploration of the abdominal viscera should be thorough and methodical. The case is obviously *inoperable* when the liver is studded with secondary deposits, enlarged malignant nodes are crowded into the portal fissure, implants are scattered on the peritoneal surfaces of the omenta or mesenteries, the pelvic shelf is implicated with nodular malignant seedlings, ascites is present, or the mass in the pancreatic head is fused to the inferior vena cava. The case is also beyond the reach of radical surgery when there is local spread (with direct invasion) beyond a possible limit of resection; the superior mesenteric vessels are adherent to cancerous tissue, or the portal vein is involved by ex-

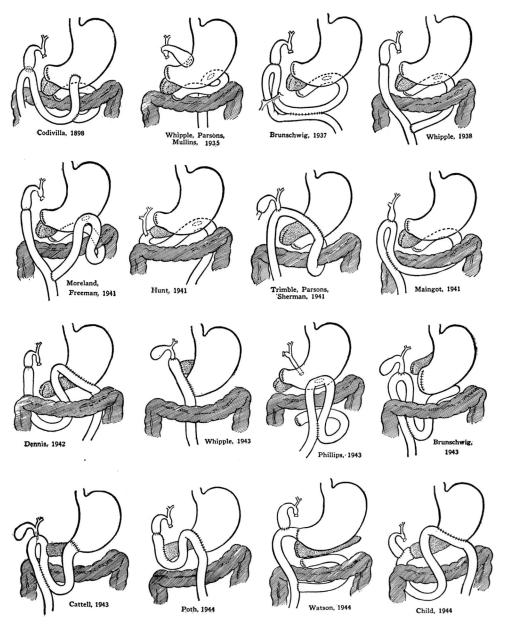

FIG. 7. Various *early* techniques of pancreatoduodenectomy.

tension of the growth.

About 40 percent of malignant lesions involving the periampullary region can be resected. These, as already described, are the most favourable growths (about 31 to 40 percent of 5-year cures). About 20 percent of cancers of the head of the pancreas lend themselves to radical surgery. The operative mortality rate is high (10 to 20 percent) and the 5-year survival rate following the extensive procedure of pancreatoduodenectomy is depressingly low: about 10 to 15 percent in expert hands. *Therefore, only the early and most favourable carcinomas of the head of the pancreas should be selected for resection.* When a hard craggy mass is found to occupy

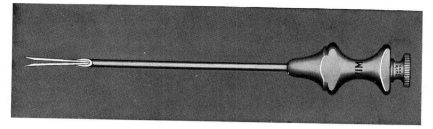

FIG. 8. Vim-Silverman needle.

the head of the pancreas, the diagnosis is rarely in doubt. In such cases, a search should be made for spread beyond the confines of the gland, for secondary deposits, and for any involvement of the *vital large vessels* which are intimately associated with the gland.

The position is different when a solitary indurated nodule is felt in the head of the pancreas or at the lower end of the chole-dochus. In such cases, the whole of the gland should be carefully examined and if it is found to be normal in consistency, the common bile duct should be opened and probed. The bile that pours through the incision in the duct should be aspirated; the gallbladder should be emptied to exclude the presence of stone; a Bakes' dilator should be passed through the choledochotomy incision downward toward the ampulla; and the anterior wall of the second part of the duodenum should be incised so that a clear view of the papilla of Vater can be obtained. The "nodule" can now be investigated by inspection, palpation, or by excision or needle biopsy (Fig. 8). Its position in relation to the papilla and to the bulbous end of the dilator can be ascertained.

Should biopsy of the duodenal wall, the papilla, the ampulla, or of the head of the pancreas (by means of a Vim-Silverman needle) confirm a diagnosis of cancer and there are no contraindications to the performance of the radical operation, the surgeon would be well advised to carry out a *one-stage procedure* without much ado, as previously emphasised. In all cases where there are *no distant metastases* and the growth appears to be limited to the head of the gland, the operator should satisfy himself that the in-

ferior vena cava, the portal vein, the superior mesenteric vessels, and the base of the meso-colon are not involved in malignant tissue before proceeding with this extensive operation. The entire gastrocolic omentum should be divided and freed from the greater curvature of the stomach in order to gain access to the lesser peritoneal sac and to the anterior surface of the pancreas and the superior mesenteric vessels. When this is completed, the lateral ligamentous and peritoneal attachments of the hepatic flexure of the colon are divided and the right colon is "dropped" together with the right half of the transverse colon and then "tucked away" into the left side of the abdominal cavity. This manoeuvre provides an excellent view of the first three parts of the duodenum; division of the ligament of Treitz and cautious dissection in this area will reveal the anterior surface of the fourth portion of the duodenum. The superior mesenteric vessels should next be lifted upward as they cross the third part of the duodenum and the uncinate process. The inferior margin of the head of the gland is displayed, and a finger is passed into the groove where the vessels disappear beneath the neck of the pancreas. (Fig. 9A.) Some pancreatic cancers have a predilection for streaming downward along the superior mesenteric vein to invade the root of the transverse mesocolon. This area should be visually and palpably explored. Should this structure be infiltrated with tumour, the lesion is considered nonresectable (Child and Frey [13]). The peritoneum at the outer convex border of the duodenum is incised, the right gastric vessels are isolated and divided, and the duodenum is freely mobilised by Kocher's method, turned over medially and to the left in order to display the posterior portion of the common bile duct and the head of the pancreas. The pylorus and the first part of the duodenum are retracted firmly downwards to bring the portal vein, the supraduodenal portion of the dilated common duct, and the curving hepatic artery into view. The gastrohepatic omentum should be divided as close to the inferior margin of the liver as is possible, and the dissection should proceed outward into the hepatoduodenal ligament. Any enlarged lymph nodes that are encountered above or below the pylorus, in the hepatic pedicle or elsewhere should be removed and handed to the pathologist for a prompt report on the frozen sections. *I do not believe that strictly local and minimal adjacent lymphatic extension is necessarily a contraindication to resection.*

Mongé et al.[39] state that metastasis to lymph nodes occurs in 53.6 percent of the carcinomas of the head, in 62.5 percent of duodenal carcinomas, in 23.1 percent of those of the papilla, and in 33.3 percent of those of the common duct.

When biopsy of the head of the gland is considered necessary, I invariably use a Vim-Silverman needle to obtain the specimen. By one method, the duodenum is opened near the papilla and the needle is plunged into the hard craggy mass and rotated. The cylindrical specimen is immediately subjected to microscopical investigation. Usually the Vim-Silverman needle is inserted into the hardest portion of the mass and one or more specimens obtained.

In order to obtain a suitable portion of tissue for microscopical examination, the head of the pancreas should not be incised by a knife.

The pancreatic incision is difficult to close, as the sutures often tear out; fistula formation, peritonitis, and subphrenic abscess are frequent complications; and, above all, the interpretation of the true nature of the sections is frequently open to doubt. A wrong diagnosis, such as chronic pancreatitis. is recorded in more than 40 percent of the cases. Positive results as to the presence of cancer in the tissue are frequently obtained in the advanced or *inoperable* cases.

Operative cholangiography is a useful aid in localising the position of the obstructing agent.

Portal venography may, on occasion, provide valuable information. Prior to commencing pancreatoduodenectomy in a patient with a tumour of questionable resectability, x-ray visualisation of the portal and superior mesenteric veins should be secured. Satisfactory films of this kind can usually be obtained by introducing 70 percent Hypaque into a small branch of the superior mesenteric vein. If these vessels are seriously distorted or occluded, any thought of pancreatoduodenectomy should be abandoned (Child and Frey [13]).

These and other methods of exploring the vital vessels will demonstrate the presence or the absence of involvement of adjacent tissues (Fig. 9A). If, as I have emphasised, any of the large and important vessels are involved in the growth, the case should be deemed inoperable.

At the present time, the majority of surgeons favour a one-stage operation, namely, pancreatoduodenal resection. Most authorities consider that the advantages of the single-stage procedure far outweigh its disadvantages. Whipple,[72] more than 25 years ago, was the first to emphasise that with careful preoperative treatment, blood replacement, and the use of synthetic vitamin K, a two stage operation was not necessary in the majority of cases.

Rodney Smith (1970) writes:

The view held today is that radical pancreatoduodenectomy should be performed in one stage unless there is some very good reason for preferring a two-stage procedure. It is doubtful if a one-stage operation should be rejected on the score of the age or infirmity of the patient, for no conclusive evidence exists to show that a one-stage operation, performed with all the modern aid to procedures of this kind, carries any higher risk to life than a two-stage operation, with its inevitable chance that the actual resection at the second stage may be made more difficult by complications arising as a result of the first stage.

The Technique of Single-Stage Radical Pancreatoduodenectomy

Whipple's operation. Any operation as extensive as radical pancreatoduodenectomy may, of course, be carried out in different ways.

The following is an account of radical

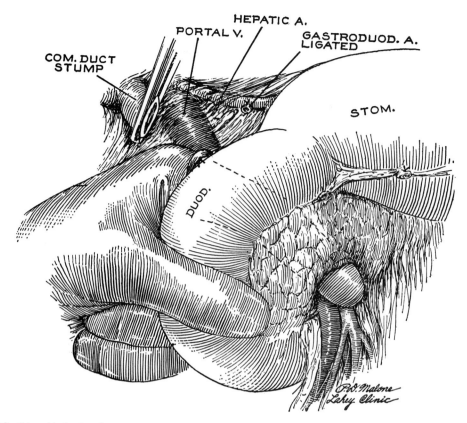

FIG. 9A. Methods of investigating whether the superior mesenteric blood vessels are adherent to a malignant lesion of the head of the pancreas. (Courtesy of Dr. R. B. Cattell, Dr. K. W. Warren, and W. B. Saunders Company, Philadelphia.)

pancreatoduodenectomy based on Whipple's technique.[68]

There is a choice of three incisions: (1) right paramedian, which starts at the right costal margin lateral to the xyphoid process and extends downwards to a point some 3 inches (7.6 cm) to the right of the umbilicus: (2) the right vertical rectus muscle-splitting incision; and (3) a curved subcostal (inverted U) incision (see Chap. 1).

An abdominal exploration is conducted on the lines previously described, a few regional nodes are removed, and biopsy specimens obtained. Biopsy will not be advisable in the majority of the patients who have carcinoma of the head of the pancreas unless the surgeon chooses to use a Vim-Silverman needle. I agree with Lemuel Bowden[33] that this method of biopsy is of absolute

value only when a frozen-section analysis for cancer is obtained. When the diagnosis is established, the next step is to determine the feasibility of radical excision. It should be noted that in almost all cases of carcinoma of the head of the pancreas, the duct of Wirsung and the biliary passages are dilated. The right half or more of the gastrocolic omentum is divided and the adhesions which exist between the posterior aspect of the mesocolon and the inferior surface of the pyloric portion of the stomach are freed, thus exposing the middle colic vessels. The peritoneal incision is continued laterally, liberating the hepatic flexure and the right half of the transverse colon, and displacing the large bowel downwards and medially.

A good view is thus obtained of the anterior surface of the pancreas. The perito-

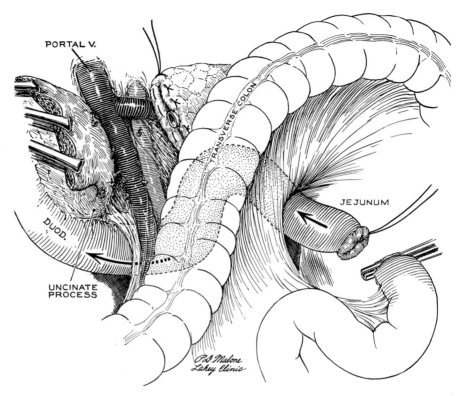

FIG. 9B. The ligament of Treitz is severed and the body of the pancreas and the proximal jejunum are divided. (From Cattell and Warren, *Surgery of the Pancreas*, 1953. By kind permission of W. B. Saunders Company, Philadelphia and London.)

neum is incised at the inferior border of the gland in order to display the superior mesenteric vessels. The inferior pancreatoduodenal artery is next isolated, ligated, and divided. The inferior cervical pancreatic vein, which drains into the superior mesenteric vein, and a number of small vessels that are exposed are all ligated with silk or cotton before they are divided. The peritoneum lateral to the duodenum is incised and the head of the pancreas and the duodenum are liberally mobilised and turned over toward the middle line. The spermatic or ovarian vessels and the upper portion of the ureter are visualised and a long segment of the inferior vena cava is bared. The gastrohepatic omentum is incised and the right gastric artery is ligated and divided, after which the course of the hepatic artery is determined.

The gastroduodenal artery is identified where it springs from the hepatic artery. This artery is tied with strong silk mounted on an aneurysm needle and divided.

The common bile duct is then dissected free and the point of entry of the cystic duct noted. A piece of tape is passed around the common bile duct and the ends of the tape clamped with a haemostat. By applying outward traction on the tape sling, the portal vein will be brought into view. The index finger of the left hand can then be passed under the neck of the pancreas on top of the portal vein so as to emerge below the body of the gland anterior to the superior mesenteric vein (see Fig. 9A). This is an excellent method of ascertaining if the portal or superior mesenteric veins are adherent to the growth. If the cancerous lesion is not adherent to these large vessels, the common bile duct should be doubly clamped, transected, and the distal end of the duct ligated with stout silk. The portal vein is then freed from the posterior aspect of the common hepatic duct, after which the cystic artery is isolated, doubly ligated, and cut across.

The gallbladder is pierced by a Mayo-Ochsner trocar and cannula and its contents are aspirated by an electric suction machine. When the gallbladder and common hepatic duct appear to be empty, *the common hepatic duct is transected;* the gallbladder is mobilised and then removed together with the clamped upper portion of choledochus. The raw surface in the liver bed is reperitonealised, and a warm pack of gauze is "crammed" into the porta hepatis to prevent blood or bile contaminating and spilling over the operative field.

The left gastric artery is isolated and ligated and divided between ligatures, some 3 or 4 cm from the cardia. The left gastro-epiploic vessels are secured and divided close to the lower pole of the spleen and the stomach is prepared for transection. A von Petz machine is crushed home at the junction of the upper and middle third of the body of the stomach, and the organ is transected with a knife or cautery between the rows of the neatly applied metal clips. The distal end of the stomach is caught in a large Payr's clamp which acts as a useful tractor during the subsequent stages of the operation. The upper one-half of the crushed portion of the gastric remnant (together with its contained von Petz clips) is inverted with a running suture of 00 chromic catgut, after which it is further in-turned with a series of closely applied sutures of fine silk. The gastric remnant is then snugly placed below the left lobe of the liver and kept out of sight by means of a large gauze swab. The distal portion of the stomach embraced by the Payr's clamp is drawn firmly over to the right in order to obtain an unhindered view of the pancreas. A finger is next inserted under the neck or (preferably) the body of the pancreas and haemostatic silk suture-ligatures are inserted on the superior and inferior aspects of the pancreas to control the corresponding longitudinal pancreatic arteries. These suture-ligatures are placed in the distal part of the pancreas near the line of transection.

The pancreas is then divided and haemorrhage is controlled from the proximal side with three or four Allis or Babcock forceps.

The duct of Wirsung is identified and dissected out before division, and left to project from the cut surface of the body of the pancreas. The portal vein, the superior mesenteric vein, the splenic vein, and the superior mesenteric artery are exposed by the division of the gland. The distal raw surface of the pancreas is next closed with a series of interrupted mattress sutures of silk or cotton, leaving the duct of Wirsung projecting for one-third of an inch (8.5 mm) from it. (Fig. 9B.)

The proximal portion of the pancreas is drawn across to the right to display the posterior aspect of the head and neck of the gland. Numerous thin-walled vessels that emerge from the neck and head of the pancreas enter and drain into *the right margin of the superior mesenteric vein.* These should be isolated individually, underrun with an aneurysm needle, and ligated with fine silk or cotton. They are carefully divided between ligatures, and care is taken not to injure the superior mesenteric vein.

The transverse colon is drawn vertically upwards and a point selected for division of the proximal jejunum about 6 inches (15.24 cm) distal to the ligament of Treitz. This ligament is divided, opening up a way through into the retroperitoneal tissues and exposing the third and fourth parts of the duodenum.

The mesentery of the proximal jejunum is cut through with scissors and the blood vessels are secured. The jejunum is clamped with two Kocher's forceps and the bowel is transected with a cautery, after which the proximal end of the jejunum is ligated with tape or floss silk and the clamp is removed. The ends of the ligature are kept long to act as a tractor. The clamp on the distal jejunum is not removed at this stage, since it also serves as a useful tractor. (Fig. 9B.)

The distal portion of the duodenum and the short segment of proximal jejunum are freed by blunt dissection beneath the superior mesenteric vessels, and the liberated intestine is drawn through to the right and away from the overhanging vascular mesenteric root. The portal vein, the splenic vein, the superior mesenteric vein, and the superior mesenteric artery can then be clearly seen as they lie slightly to the right of the pulsating aorta and in the centre of the operative field, between the ends of the pancreatic stumps.

By elevation of the duodenum and the head of the pancreas, the uncinate process can be freed up posteriorly. By elevation of the distal end of the stomach, head of the pancreas and duodenum, *the short branches of the superior mesenteric vein and the arteries* which go to the head of the pancreas, the uncinate process and the fourth and third portions of the duodenum are then divided between clamps, permitting delivery of the specimen. This is the most difficult part of the operative procedure (Cattell and Warren, 1953). (See Fig. 9B.)

After removing the specimen [which consists of the duodenum, 70 percent of distal stomach, the gallbladder, the cystic duct, the choledochus, the head and neck (and possibly a portion of the body) of the pancreas, and 6 inches (15.24 cm) of the proximal jejunum], and confirming that haemostasis is satisfactory and complete, the reconstruction of the pancreatic, biliary, and gastrointestinal tracts is carried out. The opening in the mesocolon is closed with a running silk stitch, and a generous loop of proximal jejunum is drawn upwards and over the transverse colon for anastomosis to the common hepatic duct, the duct of Wirsung, and the stomach.

Antecolic anastomoses are preferred to the retrocolic unions because the recurrence rate following this radical resection is high and invasion of the stomas by growth do not appear to occur as rapidly if they are performed in front of, rather than behind, the colon.

The steps of the *reconstruction* are described as follows:

Anastomosis of the common hepatic duct to the end of the ascending (antecolic) limb of the proximal jejunum. The clamp that was applied to the distal end of the jejunum is now drawn upward towards the porta hepatis to determine if there might be any tension after completing this anastomosis. If the limb of mobilized jejunum is ample in length, the end of the bowel is closed with a sewing-machine stitch and then inverted with a series of closely applied Lembert sutures of 0000 silk. The closed end of the bowel is passed *beneath* the common hepatic duct and sutured to Glisson's capsule in order to prevent any subsequent downward retraction and possible traction of the biliary-

intestinal stoma. The open end of the common hepatic duct is then anastomosed—end-to-side—to the apex of the jejunal loop, using two rows of interrupted sutures of 000 catgut. A T tube is inserted into the common hepatic duct and then downwards through the stoma into the jejunal limb. (Fig. 11.)

Anastomosis of the duct of Wirsung to the jejunum. Careful anastomosis of the duct of Wirsung to the jejunum can be carried out in most cases and in all cases in which the duct is dilated. *Mucosa-to-mucosa suture is accomplished.* A point is selected on the loop of jejunum for the anastomosis of the pancreatic duct, which is a few inches *below* the biliary-jejunal anastomosis. A small seromuscular incision is made on the antimesenteric surface of the bowel. The jejunum is sutured to the edge of the posterior margin of the pancreas with interrupted silk stitches passed through the area of pancreas previously closed by mattress sutures; this prevents these latter sutures from pulling out. When the posterior suture line has been completed, the pouting jejunal mucosa is opened and 4 interrupted sutures of fine chromic catgut are taken between the mucosa of the duct and the mucosa of the jejunum. A latex tube of appropriate size is inserted into the pancreatic duct and then led into the jejunum for a distance of 5 cm. This tube is anchored with a fine catgut suture to the *posterior portion of the suture line.* The pancreato-jejunostomy is completed by inserting a few interrupted sutures through the anterior wall of the jejunum and pancreas. This will buttress the closed end of pancreatic tissue against the intact mucosa of the jejunum. A further "buttressing" of the cut end of the pancreas to the jejunal wall is often practised in order to reduce the incidence of fistula formation (Fig. 10). The four sutures which unite the open end of the duct of Wirsung to the adjacent jejunal mucosa are depicted in Figure 11 inset. Where possible, a good mucosa-to-mucosa approximation should be achieved in order to circumvent the possibility of subsequent fibrotic contraction of this important stoma.

Anastomosis of the gastric pouch to the jejunum. The stomach is withdrawn from the hidden recess below the left lobe of the liver and led through the incision on to the abdominal wall. An antecolic Billroth II operation is now carried out, the stoma being

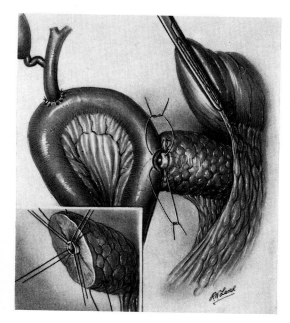

FIG. 10.   Radical   pancreatoduodenectomy.   (After Cattell.)

placed a few inches below the previous pancreatojejunostomy. This completes the operation, but drainage of the right subhepatic space is provided (Fig. 11). The abdominal incision is closed with interrupted sutures of 0 silk or Deknatel for the peritoneum and the posterior rectus sheath, and with a series of interrupted nylon sutures for the anterior rectus sheath. The skin margins are approximated with 00 Mersilk or Deknatel.

In those cases in which the caliber of the pancreatic duct is on the small size, use of the technique advocated by Child and Waugh may become obligatory (Fig. 12).

COMPLICATIONS

Pancreatic fistula. This is the most common complication and the most common cause of death following pancreatoduodenectomy. It occurs in approximately 10 to 20 percent of patients following resection for cancer of the periampullary region and in about 5 percent of patients following resection for carcinoma of the head of the pancreas. Fistula is more rare after operation for the latter disease because the duct is quite dilated and it can usually be anastomosed to the jejunum by precise mucosato-mucosa sutures.

Warren et al.[66] stated that the overall in-cidence of pancreatic fistula for patients having pancreatoduodenectomy for cancer of the periampullary region is 16 percent. The incidence during the last 5 years was 12 percent. In the Mongé et al.[39] series, fistula occurred in 18.5 percent—most frequently in patients with carcinoma of the papilla and duodenum. The discharge from the fistula usually ceases by the end of the seventh postoperative day.

In the management of such cases, the best results are obtained by constant suction applied to a Foley catheter which has been inserted into the fistulous tract. The catheter is fixed to the skin wtih Steristrips, and one of the many adhesive liquid plastic agents is applied to the skin in the region of the fistula. Constant suction must continue during the day and night, without interruption, and for a period of at least two days after the fistula has ceased to discharge its eroding contents. It is doubtful whether fasting, special diets, and certain anticholinergic drugs (such as Pro-Banthine and the like) have any appreciable effect on slowing down the rate of pancreatic secretion. Where drainage is excessive and prolonged, the pancreatic juice may advantageously be returned to the intestinal tract through an indwelling intestinal tube.

Haemorrhage. Severe haemorrhage after pancreatoduodenectomy may occur early or late. There are four varieties: (1) intraperitoneal; (2) extraperitoneal, i.e., through the Penrose drainage tube as the result of generalised oozing or a slipped ligature; (3) gastrointestinal bleeding—haematemesis or melaena; and (4) in association with a pancreatic fistula. The incidence varies from 3 to 6 percent.

Intraperitoneal haemorrhage may be caused by a slipped ligature or by erosion or digestion by pancreatic juice of a vessel in the operative field which was ligated with catgut.

Early bleeding into the retroperitoneum is frequently a harbinger of a pancreatic fistula. Postoperative haemorrhage and pancreatic fistula or biliary fistulas have frequently co-existed.

Bleeding into the gastrointestinal canal may result from hypoprothrombinaemia, avitaminosis, excessive oral ingestion of antibiotic agents, or acute gastric erosions. It is therefore necessary to administer vitamins B, C, and K in liberal amounts for several

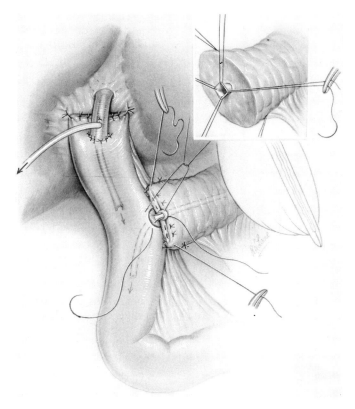

FIG. 11.   Whipple's radical pancreatoduodenectomy. The operation is completed by anastomosing the gastric pouch to the jejunum a short distance below the stoma of the pancreatojejunostomy by the antecolic Schoemaker-Billroth II procedure.

days following operation.

Blood studies and liver function tests should be carried out as routine procedures in the early postoperative period, and anaemia and hepatic impairment should be corrected by blood transfusions, serum albumin, infusions of calcium, and dietary measures.

OTHER PROBLEMS

These include wound infection, peritonitis, subphrenic abscess, partial obstruction of the hepaticojejunostomy stoma, anastomotic ulcer, hypoproteinaemia, hepatic failure, atelectasis, and diabetes mellitus. Wound infection and peritonitis are occasionally seen in combination with pancreatic fistulas. The incidence of wound infection is about 6 to 12 percent. In a number of series presented in 1963–66, the incidence of jejunal ulcer was about 14 percent.

I believe that some 70 percent of the distal stomach should be resected when pancreatoduodenectomy is being performed for cancer of the head of the pancreas or periampullary region, or if hemigastrectomy is the selected procedure, it should be combined with vagotomy.

Today the incidence of stomal ulceration following pancreatoduodenectomy for cancer of the head of the pancreas and periampullary region does not exceed 2 percent.

A few patients will experience a transient disturbance of carbohydrate metabolism. It is, however, uncommon for diabetes mellitus to develop after the operation if there has been no previous evidence of the disease.

An additional reason for implantation of the pancreas or for anastomosis of the duct of Wirsung to the jejunum is the fact that

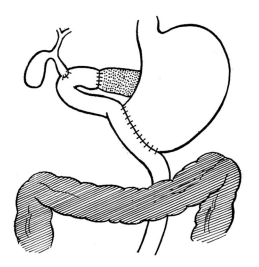

FIG. 12. One-stage pancreatoduodenectomy, with triple anastomosis, as practised by Child, Waugh, and many surgeons. In most cases, it is advisable to excise the gallbladder and to anastomose the hepatic duct to the jejunal limb.

such measures do, in fact, reduce the incidence of *anastomotic ulceration* following this radical operation.

In the reconstruction that follows the resection of the pancreas and duodenum, the bile and pancreatic secretion should be directed past the gastroenteric orifice. The occurrence of anastomotic ulcer is a valid reason for the removal of *at least 70 percent of the stomach* rather than performing a pylorectomy or antrectomy.

It would appear that stomal ulceration is more frequently observed in those cases in which the main pancreatic duct has been ligated or buried in the sutured cut end of the pancreatic remnant.

In a few cases *benign obstruction of the biliary-jejunal anastomosis* has been observed as a late complication. The obstruction is usually caused by fibrotic constriction of the stoma, an impacted gallstone, or a retained rubber prosthesis.

These cases are best treated by reoperation, removal of the gallbladder (when present), and repair of the stricture. This reconstruction procedure includes excision of the stenosed stoma, exploration of the biliary tree, removal of any residual stones, irriga-

tion of the ducts, refreshening the end of the duct, mucosa-to-mucosa anastomosis between the duct and jejunum, followed by prolonged T tube hepaticostomy.

MORTALITY AND 5-YEAR SURVIVAL RATES

The literature relative to mortality and 5-year survival rates following pancreatoduodenectomy for cancer of the head of the pancreas and for periampullary carcinoma is immense and *conflicting*. I have therefore thought it best to present to our readers the well-documented data from selected papers and personal communications submitted by certain surgeons who have specialised in this field.

I have drawn freely from the contributions of such well-known surgeons as the following:

Rodney Smith (*Br. J. Surg. 44*:294, 1956; *London Clin. Med. J. 2*:32, 1961; *Progress in Clinical Surgery*, Series III, 1966; *personal communications*, 1970–71); Warren et al. (*Surg. Clin. North Am. 39*:799, 1958; *44*:743, 1964; *47*:639, 1967); Mongé et al. (*Surg. Gynec. Obstet. 118*:275, 1964); Mongé, Judd, and Gage (*Ann. Surg. 160*:711, 1964); Child and Frey (*Surg. Clin. North Am. 46*:1201, 1966); Cleveland (*Ann. Surg. 159*:469, 1964) and ReMine and Kelly (*Mayo Clinic*) 1973.

Mongé, Judd, and Gage [40] have shown that in a review of 239 cases involving radical pancreatoduodenectomy for cancers of the periampullary area and covering a 22-year experience at the Mayo Clinic, the overall hospital mortality rate was 19.2 percent and, except for the favourable results of resection for islet-cell carcinoma of the pancreas, prognosis could not be related to histological type. The approximate 5-year survival rates were 18 percent for patients with carcinoma of the head of the gland, 39 percent for the 77 cases with carcinoma of the papilla of Vater and for the 25 cases with cancer of the duodenum, and 11 percent for the 18 with carcinoma of the lower end of the bile duct. High histological grade or lymph node involvement or perineural metastasis did not preclude 5-year survival.

Mongé et al.[39] state that the overall operative mortality rate was 12.3 percent. The 5-year survival rate based on patients surviving operation was 25 percent for carcinoma of the pancreatic head; 34.8 percent for carcinoma of the papilla; 14.3 percent for duodenal carcinoma; and *zero* for carcinoma of the common duct.

SARCOMA OF THE PANCREAS

Sarcoma of the pancreas is a clinical rarity. The first tumour of the pancreas to be removed successfully was a fibrosarcoma, and this was performed by Trendelenburg in 1882. Walters and Cleveland (*Arch. Surg. 42*:819, 1941) found only 1 case of sarcoma of the pancreas in 185 malignant growths of this gland seen at the Mayo Clinic between 1935 and 1939. The majority of the authentic cases are of the spindle-cell type of sarcoma. Bockus (1966) points out that sarcomas described in the past as round-cell and giant-cell varieties may represent lymphoid infiltrations or inflammatory lesions rather than new growths of connective tissue originating primarily in the pancreas.

Angiosarcomas have been reported and have been classified as an entity. It is doubtful if malignant lymphomas arise in the organ, and the diagnosis of some of the earlier reported cases of lymphosarcoma of the pancreas are open to question. Ross (*Br. J. Surg. 39*:53, 1951) recorded a case of leiomyosarcoma of the pancreas and states that this is the first case to be reported in the literature. He is of the opinion that many cases reported as primary lymphosarcoma or round-cell sarcoma do not bear close criticism, and several authors have suggested that only malignant connective-tissue tumours can be accepted with any degree of confidence as being truly of pancreatic origin.

The disease is most frequently observed in infancy and childhood.

TREATMENT

Operation is usually advised for an epigastric tumour of undetermined pathology. The mass is commonly large, dome-like, hard and nodular, as well as fixed and tender. The main symptoms, such as backache, epigastric uneasiness, indigestion, flatulence, icterus, loss of weight, the heavy ache associated with hepatic engorgement and bouts of vomiting, are caused by pressure of the slowly expanding malignant tumour on neighbouring structures.

At exploratory laparotomy, the physical characteristics of the lump will at once proclaim its ominous malignant features: it is firm, nodular, and inseparable from the pancreas, and it commonly invades adjacent structures, such as the stomach and transverse colon. As the disease is rare, the surgeon may believe that he is dealing with a rapidly growing carcinoma or cystadeno-carcinoma of the pancreas, or a luxuriating retro-peritoneal sarcoma. A biopsy specimen examined immediately may clinch or cloud the diagnosis.

Excision, if this is technically feasible, should be carried out in the manner already described for a carcinoma of the organ. Deep x-ray treatment affords no palliation. I have been unable to find in the literature a single case of prolonged survival.

OBSERVATIONS ON TOTAL AND SUBTOTAL PANCREATECTOMY

Waugh [68] gives the following indications for total pancreatectomy:

Islet-cell tumour of the head of the pancreas. Before subjecting a patient to total pancreatectomy for islet-cell tumour of the head of the pancreas, it is imperative to determine that: (a) the patient's symptoms are a result of spontaneous hypoglycaemia; (b) the tumour is not in the tail or body where about 45 percent are found or in an accessory pancreas; (c) a local excision preserving the pancreas is not possible, e.g., if it is in the head and is large; and (d) the symptoms and disability produced by the tumour outweigh the magnitude of the operation and the disturbance in metabolism that follows it. (See Part E of this chapter.)

Carcinoma of the pancreas. Growth of the pancreas confined to the gland (without metastases), yet involving so much of its substance that removal of the head and body would be insufficient for their proper excision is an exceptional condition.

Certain cases of calcification of the gland. Carcinoma develops in 25 percent of patients suffering from *calcification of the pancreas*. In some cases, the malignant process in the gland tends to "absorb" or dissipate the calcific areas. Total or subtotal pancreatectomy is indicated in selected cases of widespread calcification of the gland.

Large cystadenoma of the pancreas. Rockey [51] reported a case of almost total pancreatectomy. The patient survived 15 days and only 1 g of pancreatic tissue was found on postmortem examination.

Priestley [46] was the first surgeon to report a successful case of total pancreatectomy. He performed total pancreatectomy for the relief of hyperinsulinism in a patient in whom no *adenoma of the pancreas* could be seen or palpated. When the organ was sectioned, an adenoma, 1.5 mm in diameter, was discovered. The patient was relieved of hyperinsulinism and was alive and fit 6 years later.

Fallis (quoted by McClure)[34] was the first surgeon to perform total pancreatectomy successfully for a carcinomatous lesion. The patient lived for 14 months after this operation. According to Waugh, the first total pancreatectomy for *chronic relapsing pancreatitis associated with calcification of the pancreas*

was carried out by Clagett in 1944. This patient died in her home some 3 months later from an overdose of insulin. Nardi[43] collected 27 instances of total pancreatectomy, but this report did *not* include cases previously reported by Greenfield and Sanders,[19] Rhoads et al.,[49] Jarrin (1950); and Warren et al.[66] Cattell and Warren[11] collected from the literature 33 cases of total pancreatectomy. In 23 instances, the lesion was malignant—including 20 carcinomas and 3 sarcomas—and in 10 cases the lesion was benign —including 8 patients with chronic pancreatitis and 2 with hyperinsulinism. There were

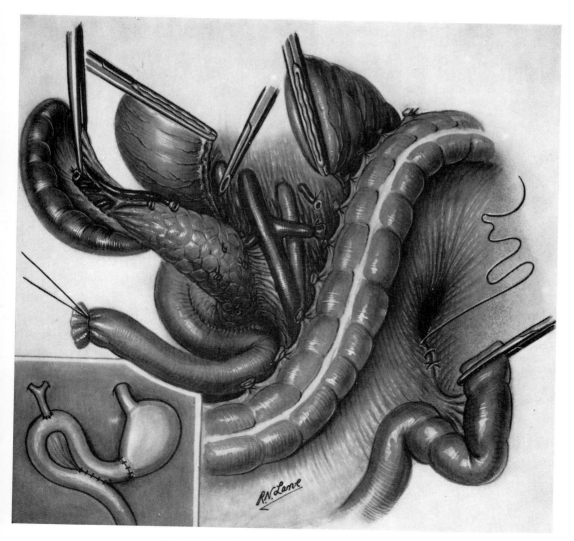

FIG. 13. Total pancreatectomy. (After Cattell.)

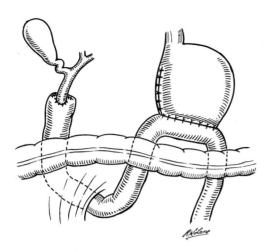

FIG. 14. Total pancreatectomy. In most instances, it is advisable to excise the gallbladder and choledochus. The end of the common hepatic duct is anastomosed to the top end of the jejunum. Partial gastrectomy followed by *posterior* gastrojejunostomy and T-tube hepaticojejunostomy complete the operation. (After Waugh.)

12 deaths in the 33 cases, a mortality rate of 36.4 percent. Brooks (1970), who has successfully performed total pancreatectomy on 12 cases cogently advises this operation for malignant lesions of the pancreas. ReMine et al.[48] reported 35 total pancreatectomies in a 25-year period; 21 of these were for malignant disease of the gland.

Hicks and Brooks,[22] in an excellent article presented their series of 116 patients with cancer of the pancreas. They performed Whipple's operation in 36 and total pancreatectomy in 11. Their hospital mortality rate was 9.1 percent. *In their opinion, total pancreatectomy offers the best chance of cure for cases of carcinoma of the pancreas.* At the completion of total pancreatectomy, they perform hepaticojejunostomy, three-quarter gastrectomy plus vagotomy and gastrostomy. The common hepatic duct is drained with a T tube for about 2 weeks.

In the *operation of total pancreatectomy,* the whole pancreas, the spleen, the duodenum, 70 percent of the stomach, the common bile duct, and the gallbladder are removed en masse, after which a loop of proximal jejunum is brought *anterior* to the transverse colon for anastomosis with the cut end of the common hepatic duct and the cut end of the stomach, or a *retrocolic gastrojejunostomy* may be conducted on the plan suggested by Waugh (Fig. 14).

The subject of total pancreatectomy is fully discussed by Milton Porter in Chapter 38, Part E.

Cystadenoma and cystadenocarcinoma of the pancreas. *Cystadenoma of the pancreas* is a rare tumour which, in some respects, resembles the papillary cystadenoma of the ovary. *Nine out of 10 cystadenomas of the pancreas are found in women.*

This innocent tumour may arise in any portion of the gland, but it shows a predilection for the tail and body. It grows slowly and may reach a considerable size; it has a translucent capsule. As it expands, it compresses the pancreas, adjacent large blood vessels, the duodenum, and (when arising from the head) it may block the lower end of the bile duct and give rise to obstructive jaundice. It is frequently diagnosed as pseudopancreatic cyst or a retroperitoneal sarcoma. The cut surface presents a honeycombed appearance, with cysts of various sizes separated by interlacing masses of fibrous strands and neoplastic tissue. In some specimens, one or more large cysts are present, or a solitary cyst may fill the interior and cause pressure necrosis of the peripheral growth. The fluid may be clear, opalescent, or turbid, yellowish-green, or brown, and may contain altered blood or debris. The fluid in the cysts does not contain pancreatic ferments. (See Chap. 39C, Figs. 29 and 30.)

Cystadenocarcinoma of the pancreas. This is a nodular, low-grade malignant tumour, which often contains cysts of various proportions. It has no capsule; it is invasive; and nodal involvement and liver metastasis occur at an early stage of the disease.

Diagnosis is often not made until a palpable epigastric tumour is discovered. Barium-meal x-ray examination may show displacement of the stomach and colon by the pancreatic mass. Selective angiography and scanning of the pancreas have afforded considerable help in diagnosis (See Chap. 108).

The *Prognosis* is extremely grave, as few patients survive radical resection for more than 2 years.

Treatment. If a cystadenoma is definitely encapsulated, it is best removed by simple enucleation, but usually a distal pancreatectomy will be necessary to obtain adequate excision. The resectable cystadenocarcinomas of the tail or body of the pancreas are treated by distal subtotal pancreatectomy, that is, by excision of the spleen, and the tail, body, and neck of the pancreas. The large malignant cystadenocarcinomas that fill the left upper quadrant of the abdomen should be exposed through a lengthy left abdominothoracic incision. Local invasion of the stomach, colon, or small bowel does not preclude resection (see R. Smith, Part B of this chapter.)

When these malignant growths occupy the head of the gland, pancreatoduodenectomy should be carried out—provided there is no local or distant cancerous spread and the portal vein and superior mesenteric vessels are not implicated in the cancerous mass.

BENIGN PANCREATIC NEOPLASMS

TYPES

Benign pancreatic neoplasms may be classified as follows:

Benign ampullary tumours: adenoma, papilloma, melanoma, neurofibroma, lymphangioma, carcinoid (Vaughan Hudson, 1952; Mrazek, 1953).

Benign pancreatic tumours: lipoma, fibroma, myxoma, chondroma, adenoma (insulin-secreting and noninsulin-secreting), fibroadenoma, leiomyofibroma, perithelioma (Polya, 1921), haemangioma, lymphangioma, haemangio-endothelioma (Dixon and Whitlock, 1938).

Treatment

Abdominal exploration is, in most cases, performed to ascertain the nature of the lesion, which is often diagnosed as a pancreatic tumour or cyst of unknown pathology.

Benign ampullary growths often declare their presence by obstructing the bile duct. At operation, the exact nature of these benign tumours is often impossible to determine without the aid of a pathologist.

One of the following operations will be indicated: (1) enucleation of the tumour;

(2) wedge resection; (3) excision of the tail or of the tail and body of the pancreas, together with the spleen; (4) duodenotomy with local excision of a benign papillary or ampullary tumour; (5) transduodenal resection of the ampullary area, followed by implantation of the bile duct and the duct of Wirsung into the posterior wall of the duodenum; or (6) pancreatoduodenectomy.

REFERENCES

1. Arkin and Weisberg, Gastroenterology 13:118, 1949.
2. Bouchier, Br. Med. J. 2:169, 1968.
3. Bouchier, Br. Med. J. 173, 1969.
4. Brown et al., Am. J. Med. Sci. 223:349, 1952.
5. Brown et al., Lancet 1:160, 1968.
6. Brunschwig, Surg. Gynecol. Obstet. 65:681, 1937.
7. Brunschwig, The Surgery of Pancreatic Tumours, 1942.
8. Cattell, Surg. Clin. North Am. 23:753, 1943.
9. Cattell, Surg. Clin. North Am. 6:649, 1948.
10. Cattell et al., Surg. Clin. North Am. 39:781, 1959.
11. Cattell and Warren, Surgery of the Pancreas, Philadelphia, Saunders, 1953.
12. Child, Ann. Surg. 119:845, 1944.
13. Child and Frey, Surg. Clin. North Am. 46:1201, 1966.
14. Cooper, Ann. Surg. 106:1009, 1937.
15. d'Offray, Br. J. Surg. 34:116, 1946.
16. Duff, Bull. Johns Hopkins Hospital 65:69, 1939.
17. Fish and Cleveland, Ann. Surg. 159:469, 1964.
18. Gordon-Taylor, Ann. Surg. 100:206, 1934.
19. Greenfield and Saunders, Surgery 25:828, 1949.
20. Grekoff, Surg. Gynecol. Obstet. 36:327, 1923.
21. Halsted, Boston Med. Sci. J. 141:645, 1899.
22. Hicks and Brooks, Surg. Gynecol. Obstet. 133:16, 1971.
23. Hirschel, Munch Med. Wochenschr. 61:1728, 1914.
24. Howard, J., Ann. Surg. 168:629, 1968.
25. Hunt, Ann. Surg. 114:570, 1941.
26. Illingworth, Edinburgh Med. J. 46:331, 1939.
27. Ivy and Roth, Gastroenterology 1:655, 1943.
28. Jordan, Am. J. Surg. 107:313, 1964.
29. Kausch, Beitr. Klin. Chir. 78:439, 1912.
30. Kenefick, Br. J. Surg. 59:50, 1972.
31. Kibler and Bernatz, Proc. Mayo Clin. 33:247, 1958.
32. Klintrup, Acta Chir. Scand. Suppl. 362, 1966.
33. Lemuel Bowden, Ann. Surg. 139:403, 1954.
34. McClure, Ann. Surg. 120:416, 1944.
35. Maingot, Lancet 2:798, 1941.
36. Maingot, Proc. R. Soc. Med. 55:587, 1962.
37. Mielcarek, Am. J. Path. 11:527, 1935.
38. Miller et al., Cancer 4:233, 1951.
39. Mongé et al., Surg. Gynecol. Obstet. 118:275, 1964.
40. Mongé, Judd, and Gage, Ann. Surg. 160:711, 1964.
41. Moore and Younghusband, Br. J. Surg. 41:562, 1954.
42. Moynihan, Edinburgh Med. J. 19:410, 1906.

43. Nardi, New Engl. J. Med. 247:548, 1952.
44. Nebesar and Pollard, Radiology 89:1017, 1967.
45. Orr, Surg. Gynecol. Obstet. 73:240, 1941.
46. Priestley, Ann. Surg. 119:211, 1944.
47. Raskin et al., Gastroenterology 34:996, 1958.
48. ReMine et al., Ann. Surg. 172:604, 1970.
49. Rhoads et al., Surg. Clin. North Am. Dec. 1801, 1949.
50. Rives et al., Surg. Gynecol. Obstet. 65:164, 1937.
51. Rockey, Ann. Surg. 118:603, 1943.
52. Ross, Br. J. Surg. 39:53, 1951.
53. Serafini, Gior. Accad. Med. Torino 20:204, 1914.
54. Smith, R., Br. J. Surg. 44:294, 1956.
55. Smith, R., London Clin. Med. J. 2:32, 1961.
56. Smith, R., Progress in Clinical Surgery, Series III, 1966.
57. Sodee, Geriatrics 22:133, 1967.
58. Tenani, Policlinico [Chir.] 29:291, 1922.
59. Trimble, Parsons, and Sherman, Surg. Gynecol. Obstet. 72:711, 1941.
60. Wallau, Arch. Path. Anat. 283:321, 1932.
61. Walters and Cleveland, Arch. Surg. 42:819, 1941.

62. Warren, K., Lahey Clin. Bull. 7:86, 1951.
63. Warren, K., Surg. Clin. North Am. 46:639, 1967.
64. Warren et al., Surg. Clin. North Am. 39:799, 1958.
65. Warren et al., Surg. Clin. North Am. 44:743, 1964.
66. Warren et al., Surg. Clin. North Am. 47:639, 1967.
67. Warren et al., Surg. Clin. North Am. 48:601, 1968.
68. Waugh, Proc. Mayo Clin. 21:25, 1946.
69. Waugh and Clagett, Surgery 20:224, 1946.
70. Whipple, Ann. Surg. 114:612, 1941.
71. Whipple, Ann. Surg. 115:1066, 1942.
72. Whipple, Ann. Surg. 121:847, 1945.
73. Whipple, Surg. Gynecol. Obstet. 82:623, 1946.
74. Whipple, Parsons, and Mullins, Ann. Surg. 102:763, 1935.
75. Willis, Pathology of Tumours, 4th ed., 1967.
76. Wise and Johnston, Surg. Clin. North Am. 36:699, 1956.

B. Radical Pancreatoduodenectomy for Carcinoma of the Pancreas and Periampullary Growths

RODNEY SMITH

Radical resection of a malignant tumour obstructing the terminal common bile duct is a logical procedure in rather less than one case in three. The favourable cases are usually carcinomas arising in the "periampullary" region, including primary carcinoma of the bile duct itself. Carcinoma of the head of the pancreas may be resectable, but all too frequently by the time exploration is undertaken the growth has already involved the superior mesenteric or portal vein. If this is the case, most surgeons are satisfied with a biliary short-circuiting operation to relieve jaundice. Carcinoma of the head of the pancreas not involving the superior mesenteric or portal vein should, in the opinion of the writer, be resected; although the long-term survival rate is poor, resection is a better palliative operation than short-circuit alone, particularly in that intractable pancreatic pain may be avoided.

The operative hazard and long-term outlook in a series of cases (the author's patients) between the years 1946 and 1972 are summarised in Tables 4 and 5.

PREOPERATIVE ASSESSMENT: SPECIAL INVESTIGATIONS

Diagnosis will not be discussed in detail. Some preoperative forecast of the type of tumour present may be made on clinical grounds. For instance, marked anaemia and occult blood persistently present in the stools usually mean an ampullary tumour. Backache as the first symptom usually means a pancreatic tumour.

Both pancreatic scanning with seleno-methionine and selective pancreatic arterio-angiography may yield evidence of value, but in the main both investigations have proved disappointing. Percutaneous trans-hepatic cholangiography may be useful, but it is not indicated in every case. In the ab-

Table 4.   PANCREATODUODENECTOMY 1946-72: THE OPERATIVE RISK

Location of Tumour	Number	Deaths	Mortality Rate (percent)
Duodenum; ampulla	120	3	2.5
Distal common bile duct	60	5	8.3
Head of pancreas	44	9	20.5
Total	224	17	7.6

Table 5.   PANCREATODUODENECTOMY: LONG-TERM SURVIVAL AFTER RESECTION BETWEEN 1946 and 1966

Location of Tumour	3-year Survival Rate (percent)	5-year Survival Rate (percent)
Duodenum; ampulla	50	35
Distal common bile duct	36	19
Head of pancreas	10	6

sence of a palpable "Courvoisier" gallbladder, however, transhepatic cholangiography should immediately precede surgery and may well show, for instance, that the tumour is sited high up in the common hepatic duct and is not pancreatic at all.

THE OPERATION

Various upper abdominal incisions have been employed. A long right paramedian or, better, Mayo Robson incision usually gives ample access. Epidural anaesthesia is particularly suitable.

Exploration

It is not uncommon for evidence to present itself at once confirming not only the malignant nature of the obstruction but also its inoperability, such as the escape of ascitic fluid and palpation of nodules of carcinoma involving the peritoneum. Examination of the liver may reveal metastases. In the absence of either, confirmation of the presence of a mass in the region of the head of the pancreas and of dilatation of the common bile duct and gallbladder is sought. More detailed evidence is looked for to indicate the degree of pathology and operability. The coeliac and para-aortic lymph nodes are

palpated and a hand is placed in the pelvis, seeking a possible Krukenberg tumour. In particular, the transverse colon should be elevated and the inferior surface of the transverse mesocolon examined. It is not uncommon to find that a pancreatic carcinoma has already penetrated through the root of the mesocolon alongside the superior mesenteric vessels. If so, resection should not be attempted.

Mobilisation of the Right Colon

Assuming that at this point no contraindication to resection has been found, the next step is to clear the colon completely from the right upper quadrant of the abdomen. The hepatic flexure and ascending colon are mobilised and drawn down and to the left, and the transverse colon is cleared from the front of the head of the pancreas and second part of the duodenum. The exposure of the duodenum is continued to display the third part and the superior mesenteric vein where it lies on the uncinate process of the pancreas (Fig. 15).

Mobilisation of the Duodenum

The duodenum is mobilised by dividing the peritoneum lateral to the second part (Fig. 16). It is then lifted forward with

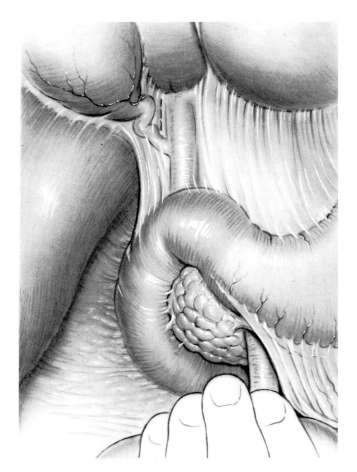

FIG. 15.   Exposure of the front of the head of the pancreas and the second part of the duodenum.

the head of the pancreas—exposing, behind it, the inferior vena cava and right ovarian or spermatic vein. With the fingers of the left hand behind the head of the pancreas and the thumb in front, the area of the tumour can then be palpated (Fig. 17).

The findings conform to one of three patterns:

(1)   A large carcinoma of the head of the pancreas is present, clearly involving the portal vein and superior mesenteric vessels. Resection is abandoned and a short-circuit is performed.

(2)   The tumour is clearly confined to the pariampullary region and resection can proceed.

(3)   The tumour appears to be pancreatic

but is not large. Involvement of the portal vein is in doubt. In this case resection may proceed, but the early stages should be so managed that no irrevocable step is taken until resectability is established beyond doubt; otherwise the surgeon may find himself in a position from which it appears impossible either to advance or retreat.

Recent experiences with the use of cytotoxic agents (mainly 5FU) delivered by a Seldinger catheter in the coeliac artery have shown that this can be very effective, particularly in the treatment of pancreatic pain. The view that it is necessary to resect all resectable tumours on account of pain clearly

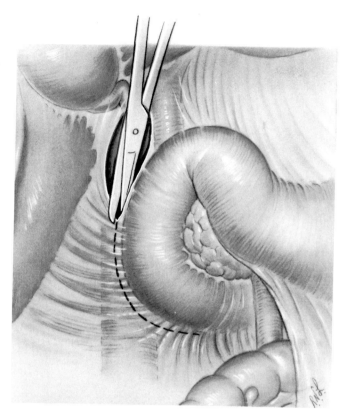

FIG. 16. Division of the posterior peritoneum and mobilisation of the second part of the duodenum.

needs reassessment. In the "doubtfully re-sectable" group, a reasonable compromise is to perform, as a first stage, a biliary short-circuit operation, allow the jaundice to disappear, subject the patient to a full course of intra-arterial chemotherapy, and then proceed to a "second look" in the hope of re-secting the tumour.

Mobilisation of the Distal Stomach and Bile Duct

The lower half or more of the stomach is mobilised (Fig. 18), the right gastric and right gastroepiploic arteries being divided between ligatures. The plan is to remove this part of the stomach, for if the stomach is divided just proximal to the pylorus and later anastomosed to the jejunum, there is a considerable risk of a jejunal ulcer developing.

If the tumour is ampullary, the stomach is divided between clamps at this point; if it is pancreatic, a gauze sling or sling of rubber tubing is placed around the antrum to use as retractor. The supraduodenal portion of the common bile duct is then isolated and, if the tumour is ampullary, it is divided. A sucker is used to evacuate the bile gushing from the dilated proximal bile passage and gallbladder, after which a bulldog clip is placed on the divided duct to prevent further bile from escaping. If the tumour is pancreatic, a piece of capillary rubber tubing is placed temporarily around the duct as a retractor.

Exposure of the Portal Vein

The gastroduodenal artery is next sought, a short distance to the left of the common bile duct, just above the head of

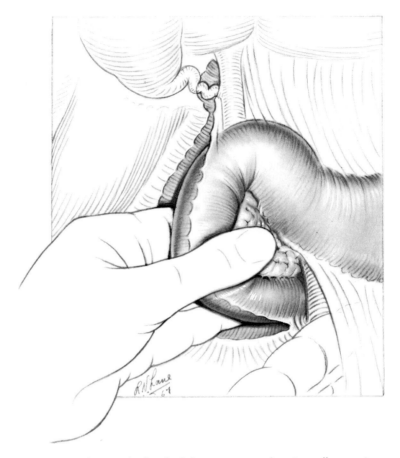

FIG. 17.   Palpating the head of the pancreas and periampullary region.

the pancreas, and its origin from the hepatic artery is demonstrated. It is divided between ligatures—exposing, rather more deeply placed, the front of the portal vein (Fig. 19).

The plane behind the pancreas and in front of the portal vein is now opened up, using very gentle dissection with Lahey swabs and the left forefinger (Fig. 20). If this stage is carried out incorrectly or roughly, the portal vein may be torn and severe haemorrhage result. Two points are important. First, it is much easier to enter the correct plane and stay in it if a finger is passed from above than if the superior mesenteric vein is identified first and a finger passed upwards from below. Secondly, pancreatic venous tributaries entering the superior mesenteric

vein are all located to the right of the vein. None enters the front of the vein. The finger opening up the space between pancreas and vein should thus keep in front of the vein. If it strays into the groove to the right of the vein, a venous tributary may be torn from the side of the vein with resultant severe haemorrhage.

This last step establishes resectability. If the space between vein and pancreas cannot be opened up because it is invaded by carcinoma, resection is abandoned. If it is clear of tumour, resection proceeds.

Recently Eiseman has described his experiences with resection of carcinoma of the head of the pancreas infiltrating the portal vein, the excision including a length of vein which is then replaced with a synthetic graft

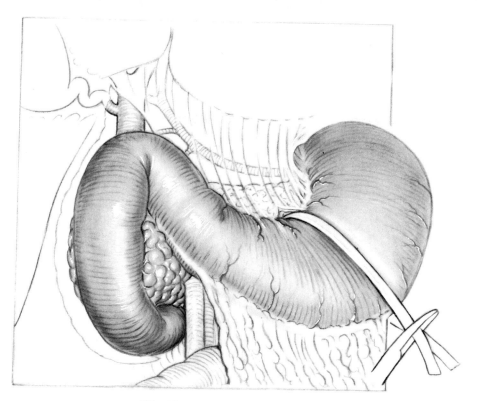

FIG. 18.   Mobilisation of the stomach.

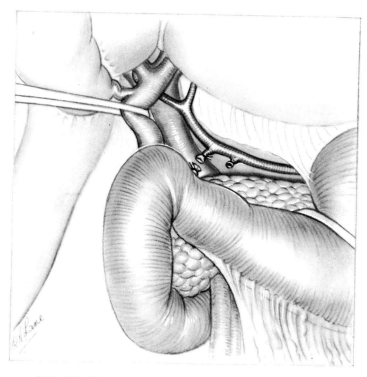

FIG. 19.   Exposure and division of gastroduodenal artery.

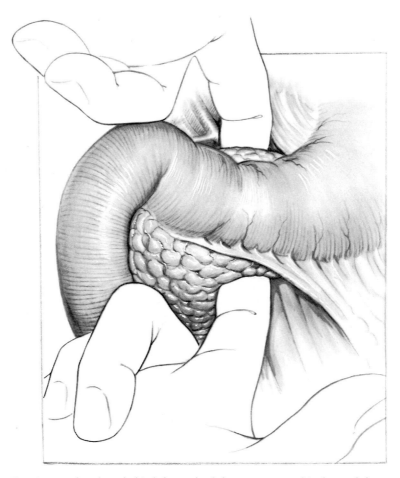

FIG. 20.   Opening up the plane behind the neck of the pancreas and in front of the portal vein.

(Eiseman, 1972). This would not appear to be a surgical advance. Early, disseminated, metastatic cancer is so common in patients with lesions of this kind that resection is illogical. Palliative surgery plus chemotherapy would appear to have a better chance of helping the patient.

Division of the Stomach, Bile Duct, and Pancreas

Unless this procedure has already been carried out, the stomach and the common bile duct are divided (Figs. 21 and 22). If the cystic duct joins the common hepatic duct very low down, it is probably better to mobilise and remove the gallbladder, dividing the common hepatic duct. If the ducts join higher up, it is safe to leave the gallbladder.

The body of the pancreas, already freed from the front of the portal vein, is further elevated; four stay sutures are placed to control bleeding from the cut surface and the gland is divided (Figs. 23 and 24). Gentle dissection with Lahey swabs allows the head to be drawn over to the right and the portal vein and the superior mesenteric vein lying on the uncinate process of the pancreas to be fully exposed. The venous tributaries entering this vein are subject to wide variation, but they always require care and gentleness in isolating and dividing them between ligatures.

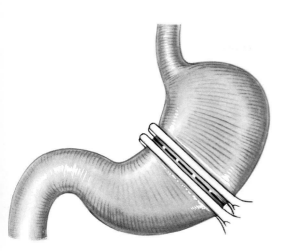

FIG. 21. Division of the stomach.

Division of Jejunum and Mobilisation of Distal Duodenum

The plan being to remove the whole of the duodenum and a few inches of the upper jejunum, attention is then turned to the jejunum. With the transverse colon and mesocolon elevated, the ligament of Treitz is divided and the duodenojejunal flexure fully exposed.

The jejunum is divided between clamps some 4 to 6 inches (10 to 15 cm) distal to the flexure, and the lower end inverted and closed. Vessels in the mesentery supplying the proximal jejunum are divided between ligatures. The divided jejunum and freed duodenal flexure are then passed beneath the superior mesenteric vessels from left to right, into the original operative field; the trans-

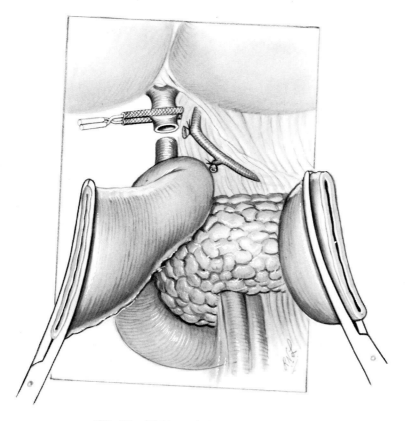

FIG. 22. Division of the common bile duct.

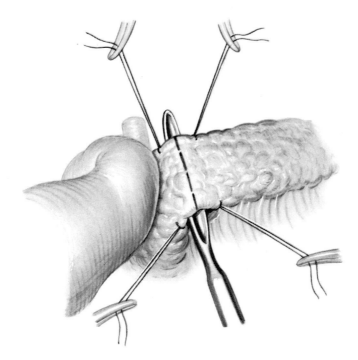

FIG. 23. The body of the pancreas is about to be divided. Four stay sutures have been inserted as shown.

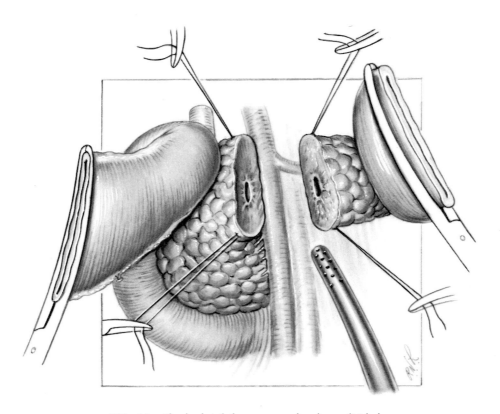

FIG. 24. The body of the pancreas has been divided.

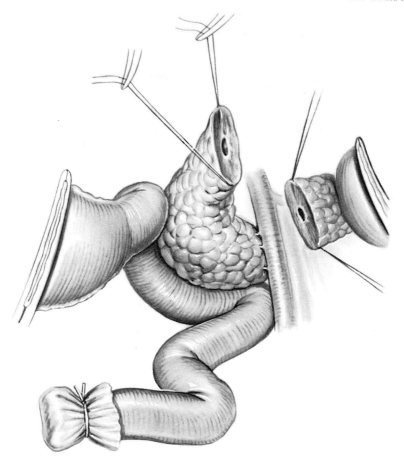

FIG. 25. The jejunum has been divided and drawn through beneath the superior mesenteric vessels and to the right.

verse colon and mesocolon are allowed to drop down again into their former position (Fig. 25).

Gentle traction on the duodenum identifies the inferior pancreatoduodenal artery running from the superior mesenteric artery into the groove between the duodenum and the pancreas. This and other smaller inconstant vessels supplying the duodenum are divided between ligatures.

Division of the Uncinate Process

It remains to deal with the uncinate process, tucked in behind the superior mesenteric vessels. Total removal of the uncinate makes it difficult to secure the several fragile veins running directly into the back of the

superior mesenteric vein. It is safer to place a row of haemostats directly on the substance of the uncinate, ligating these individually with fine silk—thus leaving a very thin margin of the uncinate itself protecting the vein (Fig. 26).

Reconstruction: Bile Duct Anastomosis

The operative field is inspected and haemostasis confirmed. Reconstruction can then begin. The end of the jejunum, already closed, is brought up into the porta hepatis and end-to-side choledochojejunostomy performed, employing a single layer of inverting fine catgut sutures (Fig. 27). To cover the anastomosis and to support the jejunal loop,

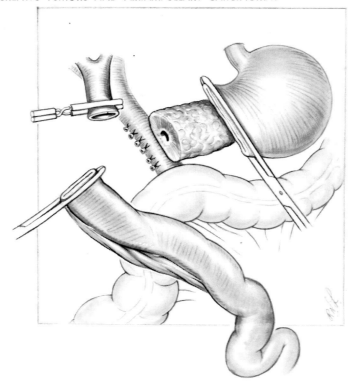

FIG. 26. Division of the uncinate process of the pancreas completes the removal of the specimen.

several further catgut stitches are inserted between the seromuscular coat of the jejunum and the peritoneum covering the common bile duct.

Pancreatic Anastomosis

The divided pancreas is anastomosed to the side of the jejunal loop 2 to 3 inches (5 to 7.5 cm) distal to the biliary anastomosis. Before this anastomosis is begun, a piece of capillary rubber tubing 4 inches (10 cm) long is selected which fits loosely in the duct, leaving 2 inches (5 cm) projecting. A continuous silk suture mounted on an atraumatic (eyeless) needle is then used to suture the cut surface of the pancreas to the seromuscular coat of the jejunum. When the posterior half of this suture line has been completed, a tiny stab incision is made into the jejunal lumen at a point opposite to the pancreatic duct, and the projecting 2 inches (5 cm) of capillary rubber tubing is inserted. The anterior half of the suture line of continuous silk is then completed. This 4-inch (10-cm) length

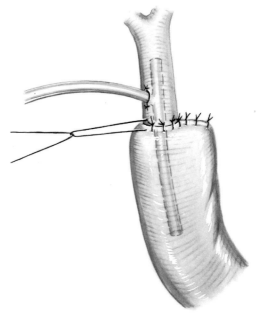

FIG. 27. Anastomosis of the common bile duct to the jejunum.

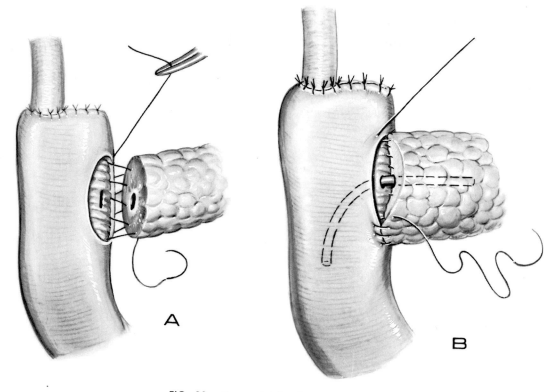

FIG. 28.   Pancreatojejunal anastomosis.

of fine capillary tubing is usually passed some weeks later, after the patient has left hospital (Fig. 28).

Alternatively, and perhaps better, a plastic "Redivac" tube with many lateral holes is placed in the pancreatic duct running from there through the stab incision, into the jejunal loop, down this loop for 10 to 12 cm and then out via a small puncture in the jejunal wall and parietes to the exterior. Suction is applied to this tube for several days to divert pancreatic juice; it is removed about 2 weeks postoperatively after a pancreatogram has shown that there is no extravasation.

Gastrojejunostomy

Reconstruction is completed by a standard anastomosis (in two layers) of the divided stomach to the jejunal loop (Fig. 29). Although it has been suggested that this should be a considerable distance from the biliary anastomosis in order to avoid the late complication of ascending cholangitis, the writer believes that this complication is more often related to stenosis of a biliary-intestinal anastomosis than to reflux. Stenosis of the biliary-intestinal anastomosis after pancreato-duodenectomy is quite rare because the bile duct is nearly always a very big one, dilated by obstruction. It is safe to site the gastrojejunostomy 6 to 8 inches (15 to 20 cm) from the biliary anastomosis, 3 to 5 inches (7.5 to 12.7 cm) below the pancreatojejunal anastomosis; this will avoid the kinking and stasis that may occur in an overlong loop of jejunum proximal to the gastrojejunostomy.

Closure of the Abdomen

A corrugated rubber drain is placed down to the area of the biliary and pancre-

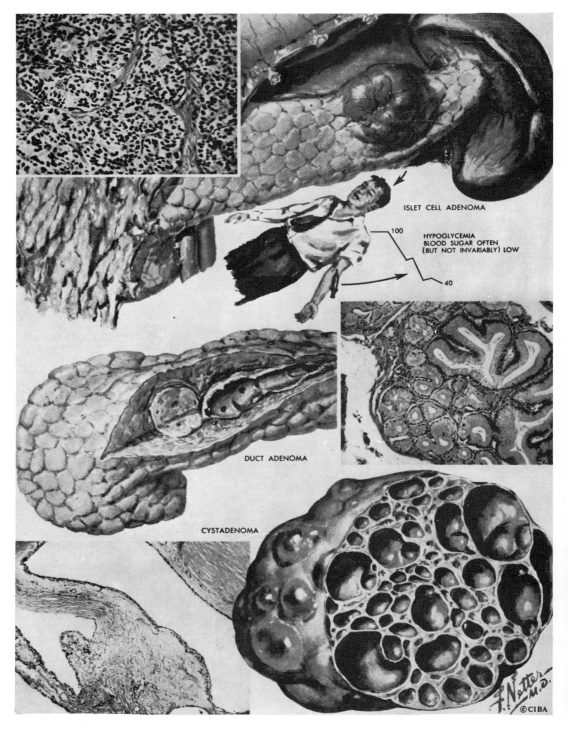

ISLET CELL ADENOMA

HYPOGLYCEMIA
BLOOD SUGAR OFTEN
(BUT NOT INVARIABLY) LOW

DUCT ADENOMA

CYSTADENOMA

FIG. 29.   Islet-cell adenoma of the tail of the pancreas. (Upper portion of Figure.) (Courtesy of
the CIBA Collection of Medical Illustrations by Frank H. Netter, M.D.)

atic anastomoses through a separate stab incision and the abdomen is closed.

POSTOPERATIVE CONSIDERATIONS

Leakage of bile and pancreatic juice is not uncommon, but the risk is much reduced by the use of indwelling biliary and pancreatic tubes, as described above. If, nevertheless, the patient recovers but with a persistent fistula, the treatment is patience, and even if several weeks pass, the fistula eventually closes.

Gastric delay is a common postoperative nuisance and is maximal if insufficient stomach has been removed. Reoperation is never called for, but gastric suction is occasionally necessary for 10 to 14 days postoperatively.

The most common fatal complication in patients surviving the actual resection in good shape is secondary haemorrhage occurring 7 to 10 days later. This is probably due to retroperitoneal digestion and sepsis associated with leakage of pancreatic juice into a retroperitoneal haematoma. Prevention is probably the only treatment for this compli-

cation. Once established, the mortality rate is very high.

Stomal ulceration is a major, late complication if the stomach is divided just above the pylorus. A high division of the stomach will usually avoid an initial troublesome delay and later stomal ulceration.

Stricture and obstruction of the biliary-jejunal anastomosis are rare. Obstruction of the pancreatojejunal anastomosis is probably relatively common, for without pancreatic exocrine replacement therapy, steatorrhoea occurs in some 10 to 20 percent of patients.

REFERENCES

1. Cattell, R. B., and Warren, K. W., Surg. Pract. Lahey Clin. Philadelphia, Saunders, 1962.
2. Smith, R., Br. J. Surg. 44:294, 1956.
3. Smith, R., Basic Science and Pancreatic Surgery. Lettsomian Lecture, Trans. Med. Soc. Lond., Vol. LXXXIV, 1968.
4. Smith, R., Pancreatic Surgery, 2d ed., in C. G. Rob and R. Smith, eds., Operative Surgery, London, Butterworths, 1969.
5. Smith, R., Progress in Clinical Surgery. London, Churchill, 1969.
6. Smith, R., Am. J. Surg. (in press) 1973.
7. Warren, K. W., Cattell, R. B., Blackbury, J. P., and Nova, P. F., Ann. Surg. 155:653, 1962.

C. Insulin-Producing Islet-Cell Tumors of the Pancreas: Insulinomas

RODNEY MAINGOT

Deficiency of the internal secretion from the islands of Langerhans (diabetes) does not primarily concern the surgeon except insofar as some of its remote complications require treatment. But hypersecretion of the β-cells of the islet tissue—as the result of overactivity, adenoma, or carcinoma—is of great surgical interest and produces a definite syndrome which, if recognised in good time, will prove amenable to surgical measures. One is reminded of the similarity between the rapid increase in knowledge of hyperparathyroidism and that of hyperinsulinism—small active tumours of endocrine tissue dominating from their special angles the whole picture of

metabolism. The effect of this internal overdosage of insulin is to reduce the blood sugar level to such an extent that hypoglycaemic symptoms appear.

It should be remembered that the control of the blood sugar is not solely dependent upon the islands of Langerhans' secreting insulin, but it is affected also by the pituitary, the suprarenals, the liver, and the thyroid. Hypoglycaemia also occurs in the terminal stages of diabetes after the withdrawal of insulin, in exhaustion of the glycogen reserve (such as is found in many diseases of the liver), and in the muscular dystrophies. *The non-beta-celled, noninsulin-secreting ulcerogenic tumours of the pancreas* are discussed in Chapter 13 by Dr. Robert Zollinger and his colleagues.

When islet-cell tumours do not generate hormones, that is, when they are *nonfunctioning,* their presence in the pancreas may or may not be of clinical significance. Adenocarcinoma is an important exception, as are the rare types of nonfunctioning malignant tumours that arise in the head of the pancreas and cause biliary obstruction. The latter type of islet-cell tumours have been reported by Kalish and Shapiro [19] and Wastell and Ellis.[35] It is often difficult to distinguish the nonfunctioning islet-cell tumours that cause obstructive jaundice from other malignant tumours of the head of the pancreas.

No study of this subject would be complete without reference to the recent authoritative reviews by Buckle et al. (*Proc. R. Soc. Med. 57*:675, 1964); Ernesti et al. (*Lancet 1*:628, 1965); Ford and Bailey (*Br. Med. J. 2*:343, 1965); Roth et al. (*New Eng. J. Med. 274*:493, 1966); Mengoli and Le Quesne (*Br. J. Surg. 54*:749, 1967); Gutman et al. (*New Eng. J. Med. 284,* 1003, 1971); Wolfe et al. (*Arch. Surg. 104*:56, 1972); and Ruskin et al. (*Surg. Gynecol. Obstet. 133*:1, 1971).

CLASSIFICATION OF SPONTANEOUS HYPOGLYCAEMIA

Spontaneous hypoglycaemia can be classified by aetiology as follows:

A. *Organic*—recognisable anatomical lesion:
    1. Hyperinsulinism:
        a. pancreatic islet-cell carcinoma;
        b. pancreatic islet-cell adenoma;
        c. generalised hypertrophy and hyperplasia of the islands of Langerhans.
    2. Hepatic disease:
        a. ascending infections—cholangitis;
        b. toxic hepatitis;
        c. diffuse carcinomatosis;
        d. fatty degeneration or metamorphosis;
        e. glycogenosis (von Gierke's disease).
    3. Pituitary hypofunction (anterior lobe):
        a. destructive lesions (chromophilic tumours, cysts, etc.);
        b. atrophy and degeneration (Simmonds' disease);
        c. thyroid hypofunction—secondary to pituitary hypofunction.
    4. Adrenal hypofunction (cortex); atrophy or destruction of cortex.
    5. Lesions of the central nervous system (some interfere with nervous control of the blood sugar).
B. The result of *excessive insulin administration.*
C. Sensitivity to certain amino acids such as *leucine.*
D. *Functional*—no recognisable lesion:
    1. Hyperinsulinism (imbalance of the autonomic nervous system).
    2. Renal glycosuria.
    3. Pregnancy and lactation.

HISTORICAL NOTE

The pancreatic islets were first described by Langerhans in 1869. Banting and Best (*J. Lab. Clin. Med. 7*:251, 1922) reported the momentous discovery of insulin in 1922. Neve (*Lancet 2*:659, 1891) was the first to describe an adenoma of the pancreas, which he discovered at autopsy. Nicholls (*J. Med. Res. 8*:385, 1902) in reporting on another adenoma of the pancreas, drew attention to its resemblance to normal islet tissue, while Lang (*Arch. Path. Anat. 257*:235, 1925) published the first account of a case of multiple adenomas—adenomatosis. Seale Harris (*J.A.M.A. 83*:729, 1924), in his stimulating article, suggested that there was a clinical possibility of spontaneous hyperinsulinism as opposed to the hypoinsulinism of diabetes, and Wilder and his colleagues (*J.A.M.A. 89*:348, 1927), benefiting by Harris's research (1924), were the first to operate upon a case of tumour of the pancreas associated with hyperinsulinism. At operation, W. J. Mayo found a primary malignant insulinoma which had produced metastatic implants in the liver, in the regional lymphatic nodes, and in the mesentery. Two years later Roscoe Graham (quoted by Howland et al. (*J.A.M.A. 93*:674, 1929) excised an islet-cell tumour with complete remission of symptoms owing to hypoglycaemia. In the previous year Finney (*Ann. Surg. 88*:584, 1928) had explored a patient and, finding no adenomatous tumour, had resected 22.5 g of the pancreas without alleviation of the symptoms.

Following the report of these early cases, which stimulated interest in the subject, Allan, Carr, Whipple, Walton, Conn, Rayner, and Lups described their experiences and results in patients who were successfully operated upon for growths of the islet cells associated with hypersecretion of insulin. Whipple and Frantz (*Ann. Surg. 101*:

1299, 1935) were able to report 35 cases in which operation had been performed up to 1935.

These authors gave a detailed description of 6 cases of their own. Meyer et al. (*J.A.M.A. 117*: 16, 1941) recorded 53 cases successfully treated surgically, and Holmes et al. (*Br. J. Surg. 33*:330, 1946) reported 9 more cases and added one of their own.

In Whipple's review (*Ann. Surg. 121*:847, 1945) of 149 cases of islet-cell tumour showing hypoglycemia, there were 106 that were considered benign, 28 questionably malignant, and 15 definitely malignant with metastases in the liver.

Howard, Moss, and Rhoads (*Int. Abst. Surg. 90*:417, 1950) collected 398 cases of islet-cell tumour from the literature. In a more recent report, Moss and Rhoads (*Surgical Diseases of the Pancreas*, Howard and Jordan, eds., London, Pitman, 1960) surveyed the world literature on hyperinsulinism prior to 1958 and found 766 islet-cell tumours. Today, move than 1,000 cases have been reported in the literature.

AETIOLOGICAL FACTORS AND PATHOLOGY

Islet-cell tumours *may occur at any age,* but are rare in infancy and after the age of 60. Most cases are found between the ages of 15 and 55; the peak age incident being 45. A case of a 24-hour-old infant has been reported by Sherman,[30] and Roxburgh[25] reported a case in a child aged 7 years.

According to reports submitted in the literature, these tumours are slightly more common in the *female,* the ratio being 1.5:1.

Lopez-Kruger and Dockerty[20] discovered 44 islet-cell tumours in 10,314 consecutive necropsies, 8 of which were judged to be functioning and 80 percent of which had produced no symptoms. This frequency conforms to the generally held view that some 20 percent of islet-cell tumours are hormonally active. About 14 percent of patients with islet-cell tumours have multiple lesions. Lopez-Kruger and Dockerty offer the following *classification of islet-cell tumours;* this is based on the pathological and the clinical features of these growths:

1. Adenomas of islet cells without hypoglycaemia.
2. Adenomas of islet cells with hyperinsulinism.
3. Metastasising carcinoma of islet cells without hypoglycaemia.
4. Metastasising carcinoma of islet cells with hyperinsulinsm.
5. Borderline malignant islet-cell tumours with or without hyperinsulinism.

Frantz,[10] on the basis of microscopical study, divided these tumours into: (1) benign, (2) questionably malignant, and (3) malignant growths. Then, again, there is a fourth type—diffuse hyperplasia of the islet cells without localized tumour.

Duff,[5] in an authoritative contribution concerning the pathology of islet-cell tumours, stated that some of them show no histological manifestations of malignant change; others grow eagerly, invade, and metastasise, and are obviously cancerous; still another group displays microscopical evidence of capsular and blood-vessel invasion but shows no metastases.

These tumours of *doubtful malignant nature* do not, as a rule, recur after excision and must therefore be regarded as benign. Hanno and Banks[14] stated that the histological appearance of malignancy in cases of islet-cell tumour is not a valid index of malignancy. According to them, the only safe index is the presence of extraglandular metastases. They were able to collect 21 cases that showed involvement of other organs.

Campbell et al.[3] estimated that the incidence of islet-cell adenomas was one in 1,000 autopsies and that the clinical manifestations were evident in approximately 20 percent of these subjects.

The adenoma may be found in any part of the pancreas, with a remarkably even distribution throughout the organ (Fig. 29).

Thus in Marshall's series[21] of 19 cases the locations were as follows: 7 in the body of the pancreas, 5 in the tail, 6 in the head, and 1 extrapancreatic tumour in the gastrosplenic omentum.

Whipple,[36] on the other hand, believed that *multiple adenomas* are more often found in the *tail of the pancreas,* almost as frequently in the head, and somewhat less frequently in the body of the gland. He reported an interesting case in which 7 adenomas of the pancreas were removed. Thus, as Marshall reminds us, even though a single adenoma of the pancreas is discovered at exploratory operation, other pancreatic tumours should be searched for as a routine measure.

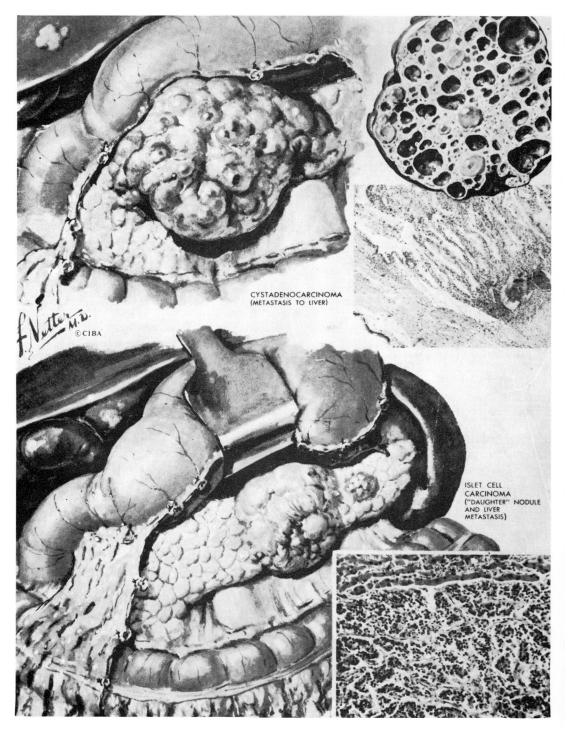

CYSTADENOCARCINOMA
(METASTASIS TO LIVER)

ISLET CELL
CARCINOMA
("DAUGHTER" NODULE
AND LIVER
METASTASIS)

FIG. 30.   Islet-cell carcinoma of the tail of the pancreas with daughter tumour and secondary deposits in the liver. (Lower portion of figure.) (Courtesy of the CIBA Collection of Medical Illustrations by Frank H. Netter, M.D.)

Adenomas are sometimes found in *ectopic pancreatic tissue;* when a meticulous exploration fails to reveal a tumour in the pancreas itself, a methodical search should be conducted for a localised mass in or at the common sites of aberrant pancreatic tissue, e.g., in or about the duodenum, stomach, proximal jejunum, gastrosplenic ligaments, gastrocolic and gastrohepatic ligaments, the mesocolon, the greater omentum, and the retroperitoneal area immediately adjacent to the pancreas and kidneys. According to Fonkalsrud, Dilley, and Longmire,[9] only 15 cases of ectopic functioning islet-cell tumours have been reported.

Of the 398 adenomas collected by Howard and co-workers,[17] 78 percent were benign, 12 percent were borderline carcinomas, and 9.3 percent were frankly malignant lesions.

Mervyn Smith (1959) stated that the types of pancreatic lesion that may be associated with spontaneous hypoglycaemia include benign adenoma (84 percent), adenocarcinoma (9.3 percent), and a diffuse hyperplasia of islet tissue (6.7 percent).

The majority of the adenomas are reddish or mauve in colour and are not large, averaging 1 to 3 cm in diameter. Tumours smaller than 4 mm do not usually produce hyperinsulinism. The smallest tumour in the series reported by Marshall was 1 cm in diameter and the largest measured 9.5 by 6.5 cm.

Graham and Womack,[12] Brunschwig[2] and Gorden et al.[11] have reported unusually large islet-cell tumours.

These tumours have a firmer consistency than the surrounding normal gland, and because of their extensive capillary network they have a brownish red, pinkish-violet, or mauve colour as compared with the amber-

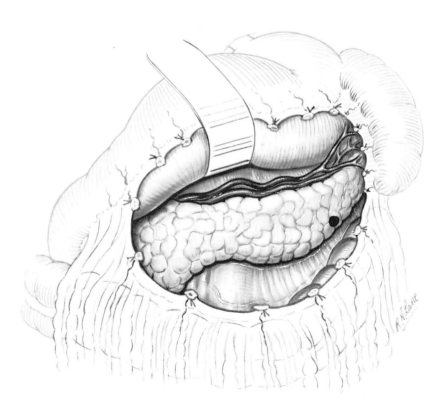

FIG. 31. Exposure of the pancreas by liberal division of the gastrocolic and gastrosplenic omenta. The insulinoma was discovered in the inferior margin of the pancreas. (Drawing done during operation. Author's patient.)

coloured pancreas. In certain instances, when the blood supply is meagre, they may be dark yellow or greyish-white in colour.

They are extremely difficult to find if situated in the central part of the head or uncinate process. Palpation is the surest way of locating them, but in order *to examine all parts of the organ. the pancreas has to be freely mobilised.* Fortunately, the majority of adenomas present on the surface of the gland and project above it.

The *malignant insulinoma* with hypoglycaemia is much more rare than the benign tumour and is *likely to grow to a greater size.* It is invasive, devoid of a capsule, and spreads to neighbouring structures as soon as it becomes sizeable. Metastases to the liver and the regional lymph nodes occur, and later spread to more distant sites (Fig. 30).

The *microscopical appearances* have been described by Lopez-Kruger and Dockerty,[20] Marshall,[21] Willis,[37] and Bockus.[1]

Lopez-Kruger and Dockerty analysed 17 cases of metastasising and hyperfunctioning, islet-cell carcinoma; Howard[17] in 1950, collected a total of 22 functioning islet-cell carcinomas, while Cunliffe Shaw[4] gave a detailed account of 2 metastasising insulinomas with hypoglycaemia. Fonkalsrud et al.[9] stated that during the previous 8 years, 10 patients had been explored for hypoglycaemia. A single adenoma was found in 7 patients, and from another patient 2 separate adenomas were removed. In 4 of these 8 patients, the tumours were found in the head of the gland. Kenneth Warren[34] and his colleagues at the Lahey Clinic reviewed 24 patients in whom a diagnosis of hyperinsulinism had been made. Four of the patients had previously had blind distal pancreatectomy before admission to the clinic. Solitary adenomas were excised in 10 cases, blind pancreatic resection was performed in 13, and total pancreatectomy was carried out in one patient.

The *"suspiciously malignant tumours"* appear to be cancerous in histological appearance only, and at exploratory operation they do not show any evidence of extraglandular spread. Those cases that show *doubtful* malignant change constitute but 10 percent of approximately 1,000 insulinomas recorded up to 1972.

Cases of *metastasising insulinomas* with hypoglycaemia have a bleak prognosis, and only 1 patient of the 37 reviewed by Howard[17] was alive and well 4 years after operation.

Diffuse hypertrophy of islet-cell tissue is much more rare than the adenoma group, which is fortunate, as the prognosis after blind partial or subtotal pancreatectomy is poor when compared with the good or excellent results following excision of an adenoma (or adenomas).

CLINICAL FEATURES AND DIAGNOSIS

The clinical picture of hyperinsulinism and hypoglycaemia is that of chronic disease characterised by periodical attacks of nervous disorders coming on at irregular intervals. As a rule, the attacks occur during the fasting period or after severe exertion. The attacks are relieved promptly on the administration of sugar. The symptoms of this syndrome are as various and variable as those caused by an overdosage of insulin.

Whipple has shown that the severity of the symptoms does not necessarily correspond to the degree of hypoglycaemia in different individuals or at different times in the same individual; nor does the size of the tumour determine the severity of the symptoms. Wilder grouped the symptoms as follows: (1) those relating to disturbance of the sympathetic nervous system, (2) those involving the central nervous system, and (3) those of psychic origin.

According to Rogers[24] a huge swirl of insulin into the blood stream not only generates initial hypoglycaemia, but also evokes a prompt epinephrine response wherein the adrenal medulla endeavours to restore homeostasis by stimulating glycogenolysis. The consequences of concurrently increased circulating levels of insulin and epinephrine are frequently clinically indistinct. The following symptoms have been summarised by Rogers:

1. Central nervous system activity
    a. Restlessness
    b. Diplopia
    c. Muscle spasm
    d. Maniacal seizures
    e. Convulsions
    f. Coma

2. Sympathetic nervous system activity
   a. Sweating
   b. Flushing
   c. Nausea
   d. Chilliness
   e. Trembling
   f. Weakness
   g. Rapid pulse
   h. Epigastric pain
   i. Hunger
3. Psychiatric disturbances
   a. Unconsciousness
   b. Emotional lability
   c. Disorientation
   d. Amnesia

The hypoglycaemic state has often been confused with psychosis, epilepsy, and alcoholism, and it is not surprising that some of these patients are found in mental institutions. During the attacks, the blood sugar level is low, the recorded figures varying from 4 to 58 mg per 100 ml.

Whipple [36] has presented an essential *triad* that must be satisfied before surgical search for a hyperfunctioning islet-cell tumour is justifiable: (1) The attacks of insulin shock must come during periods of fasting or after exertion. These attacks are often accompanied by central nervous, psychiatric, or vasomotor symptoms. (2) The blood sugar value during an attack or after 24 hours of fasting must be below 50 mg per 100 ml. (3) The symptoms must be relieved promptly by the oral or intravenous administration of glucose. When this triad is present, the possibility of islet-cell tumour owing to spontaneous overdosage of insulin must be seriously considered. Whipple found a functioning tumour of the pancreas in 34 of the 39 patients upon whom he operated for the relief of hypoglycaemia.

After the diagnosis of chronic hypoglycaemia has been established, and adrenal, hepatic, thyroid, pituitary, and other extrapancreatic causes have been eliminated, the patient should be given a course of medical treatment for 2 or 3 weeks to determine his response to conservative measures.

Laboratory Investigations

Serial blood specimens must be taken during the height of the attack. Howard et al.,[17] in reviewing 398 cases, found that the mean minimal fasting blood sugar level was 32 mg per 100 ml, and rarely did this value exceed 50 mg. Bockus [1] emphasised that the ordinary glucose tolerance test, whether oral or intravenous, and even when extended to 5 hours, is seldom worthwhile in the diagnosis of functioning islet-cell tumour.

The simplest and the surest *provocative test* is total deprivation of food. Starvation (with or without strenuous exercise) will induce a typical attack of symptoms and provide an opportunity to verify the characteristic hypoglycaemia within 24 to 36 hours in most patients. Such were the findings of 59 of 79 patients studied by Scholz et al.[28]

Another provocative test is the tolbutamide test.[7, 29] The usual response to sodium tolbutamide, injected intravenously, is a steep and spontaneous fall in the blood sugar level for a period of 30 to 50 minutes, followed by spontaneous recovery. In a patient harbouring a functioning islet-cell adenoma, the fall is very deep, rapid, and lasting, and it may fail to return to 75 to 80 percent of control levels in three hours. Tompkins et al.[32] stated that the 72-hour fast with exercise and the test with intravenously administered tolbutamide are the most reliable means of establishing a diagnosis of insulinoma. Hunt [18] maintained that an intravenous tolbutamide test should be made only when facilities for insulin assay are available. This test will increase diagnostic accuracy though not all insulinomas will give positive results. Plasma insulin assay will reveal normal levels in the presence of extrapancreatic neoplasm with hypoglycaemia.

If it is found that the blood sugar values are continuing to remain low, e.g., 50 mg per 100 ml or lower, and that the fits and attacks can be controlled with a high carbohydrate intake, exploratory laparotomy is indicated.

Other Investigations

These include: (1) *duodenography* (see Chap. 4, Part C); (2) *retrograde pancreatography by fibre-duodenoscopy* (see Chap. 34, Part B); (3) *coeliac angiography* (see Chap. 108, also Thomas et al.[31] give an excellent account of angiography and radioisotopic scanning in the diagnosis of pancreatic tumours); and (4) *selenium scan* (see Chap. 38A) and *laparoscopy* (see Chap. 4, Part D) to exclude secondary deposits in the liver or omenta.

OPERATIVE TREATMENT

The treatment of hyperinsulinism caused by an islet-cell adenoma is enucleation of the tumour. As soon as the diagnosis of organic hyperinsulinism has been made and other causes of hypoglycaemia have been excluded, the pancreas should be explored because of the possibility of a malignant lesion and the risk of permanent damage to the central nervous system.

A few hours before the operation is undertaken, the patient is given 500 ml of a 5 percent solution of glucose intravenously and the stomach is emptied of fluid and gas by aspiration. An intravenous infusion of 10 per-

cent glucose solution is continued throughout the operation and for a few hours afterwards.

Most surgeons prefer the sequence pentothal-gas-oxygen-muscle relaxant, as complete relaxation is essential; however, McCaughan preferred ether anaesthesia because of its reputed effect in sustaining and even elevating the normal level of the blood sugar.

Whipple recommended a transverse epigastric incision, but here again there are a number of surgeons who maintain that a long right or left paramedian incision gives adequate access to the pancreas.

In the average case, the best access is obtained by a liberal division of the gastrocolic omentum. It is essential that the whole organ —the head, the tail, and the body of the pancreas—should be visualised (Figs. 32 to 36).

A search should be made for accessory pancreatic tissue in and about the stomach,

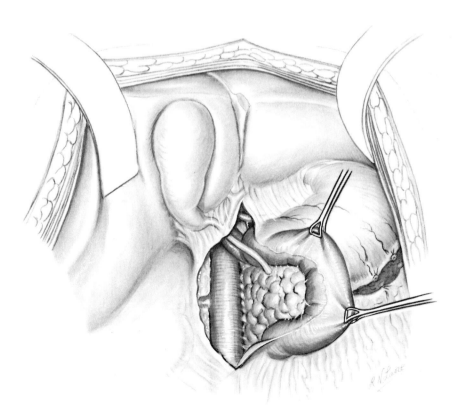

FIG. 32.   Mobilisation of the duodenum and head of the pancreas by Kocher's method.

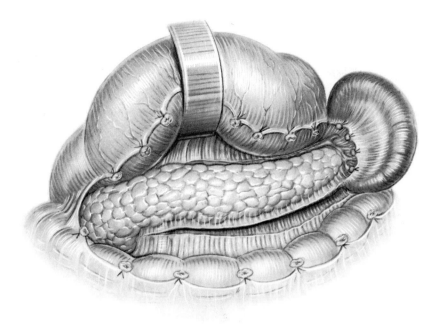

FIG. 33.   Exposure of the pancreas and hilus of the spleen. The peritoneum on the posterior wall just inferior and superior to the pancreas is incised to allow manipulation of the organ. (From Rob, Smith, and Morgan. *Operative Surgery*, 2d ed., 1969. Courtesy of Rodney Smith and Butterworths, London.)

duodenum, gastrosplenic omentum, and so forth. The reader is referred to Rudd and Walton's classic article [26] and a paper by Holman et al.,[16] both of which deal with *extrapancreatic islet-cell adenomas.* More than 35 islet-cell tumours have been reported in ectopic pancreatic tissue.

When the gastrohepatic omentum is fully divided, the hepatic flexure of the colon is mobilised by division of the phrenocolic ligament and by incising the peritoneum lateral to the ascending colon, after which the liberated bowel is "dropped" and retracted downward and inward. The duodenum and entire head of the pancreas are mobilised by Kocher's method (Figs. 32 to 34), and the gastrocolic ligament is completely divided in order to facilitate inspection along the course of the superior mesenteric vein up to the point where the vessel disappears from sight under the neck of the gland. In some instances, it may be advisable to detach the greater omentum from the transverse colon in order to obtain the best possible view of the lesser sac. One of the most inaccessible areas of the pancreas is the inferior aspect

of the uncinate process as it sweeps behind the superior mesenteric vein and extends to within a few millimetres of the superior mesenteric artery.

Unless the adenoma lies upon or is close to the anterior face of the pancreas, it cannot be felt except by bidigital palpation. As I have said, it is advisable in all cases to divide the peritoneum along the inferior border of the pancreas in order to facilitate the methodical bidigital palpation of the neck, body, and tail of the pancreas. The head of the gland should be carefully felt between the fingers of both hands, and the posterior surface should be visualised and palpated after turning it over, as on a hinge, toward the midline (Fig. 34).

Sometimes it may be helpful to incise the gastrohepatic omentum and to pass two slings of gauze around the antrum and body of the stomach in order to elevate and retract it upwards and away from the entire operative field.

At this stage, the abdominal incision should be widely retracted with Deaver retractors and the bridge of the operating table should be elevated to arch the patient's back and to bring the pancreas closer to the surface. As previously emphasised, *the whole gland must then be carefully inspected and palpated*. Care should be taken in searching for an adenoma in the hilus of the spleen as the tail of the pancreas normally insinuates itself among the tributaries of the splenic vein (Fig. 36). In some cases, when a prolonged search for a tumour has been unrewarding, it is necessary to incise the filmy sheet of peritoneum *above and below the body and tail of the pancreas* and to elevate the gland from the posterior abdominal wall with encircling fingers. The posterior aspect of the pancreas can, in such circumstances, be cautiously and methodically explored for the presence of the peccant lesion. The superior mesenteric vein and portal vein, in their hidden tunnel of pancreatic tissue, should

be daintily palpated with the index finger in the hope of detecting a "wary" tumour. When all fails, an assiduous search should be conducted to locate a cryptic *ectopic* tumour.

An islet-cell tumour is usually seen as a small rounded body, 1 to 3 cm in diameter, brownish pink or purplish pink in colour, and readily recognisable in the amber substance of the pancreas. It is covered with numerous small blood vessels which bleed freely while the adenoma is being removed from the pancreas. The malignant tumours are, however, invasive. If one adenoma is found, a search should be made for others by exploring and carefully palpating the anterior and posterior surfaces of the gland.

In the majority of cases, the adenoma can easily be enucleated from the substance of the pancreas. (Fig. 35.)

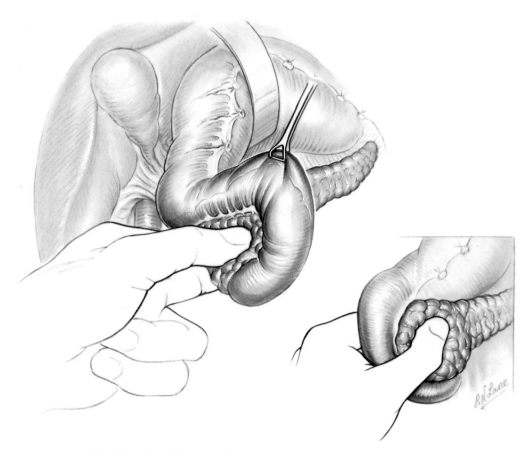

FIG. 34.   Search for an islet-cell tumour in the head of the pancreas.

Enucleation of a Benign Insulinoma

When the tumour is single and appears to be a well-encapsulated adenoma, the peritoneum over it is incised and a plane of cleavage between the capsule of the tumour and the surrounding pancreas is developed by dissection with a pair of curved dissecting scissors.

The capsule is seized by an Allis forceps and the tumour lifted from its bed as dissection proceeds on its deeper aspect; finally, removal is completed by enucleation (Fig. 35). The cavity from which the tumour has been enucleated should be carefully inspected, but if the indications for enucleation are correct, there is no danger of damaging a pancreatic duct. Rodney Smith states: "Similarly, there is no need to insert sutures in order to obliterate the little hollow space from which the tumour has been removed." *If a major duct is transected during the performance of enucleation, distal resection is preferable to attempted repair.*

Again, if the tumour appears to be *infiltrating the pancreas* without a proper capsule, partial pancreatectomy rather than enucleation should be performed.

I believe that *palliative partial pancreatectomy* is advisable even in the presence of obvious metastases. In about one case in ten, the tumours are malignant.

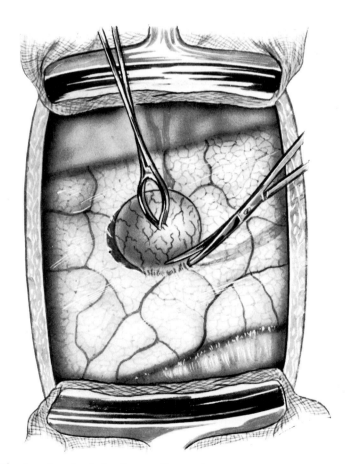

FIG. 35.   Enucleation of a simple insulinoma. (From Rob, Smith, and Morgan. *Operative Surgery,* 2d ed., 1969. Courtesy of Rodney Smith and Butterworths, London.)

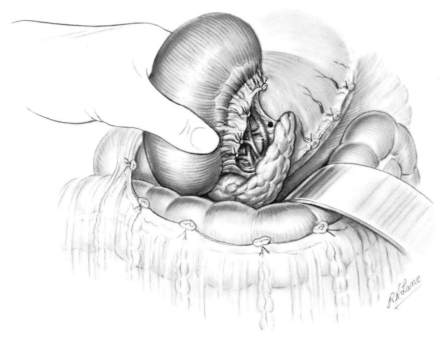

FIG. 36.   The search for an insulinoma in the hilus of the spleen and near the tail of the pancreas.

Distal pancreatectomy is in order when the malignant adenoma is situated in the body or tail of the gland (Fig. 37). A radical operation should not be enjoined in the presence of a *questionably malignant adenoma* when it is situated in the head of the gland.

If no adenoma is found and if no firm nodule can be palpated in the mobilised pancreas, the surgeon is then justified in resecting the tail and body of the pancreas and the spleen up to the superior mesenteric vein in the hope that a small adenoma will thus be removed.

If there is no relief following blind distal pancreatectomy or subtotal pancreatectomy at the primary operation, at the next or final exploratory operation the head of the pancreas should once again be completely mobilised and a scrupulous search be carried out for a tumour in the substance of the head of the pancreas. It is surprising how frequently a second or even a third look will reveal the presence of a hidden tumour, not only in the head (or proximal remnant) of the pancreas itself, but in ectopic pancreatic tissue situated in the hilus of the spleen. A possible explanation may be that the period of delay occasioned by fruitless surgical efforts to locate the adenoma will have afforded the growth ample time in which to blossom into a tumour of some proportions.

If, in these circumstances, no tumour can be detected in the head of the pancreas or in ectopic pancreatic remains, *total pancreatectomy* should be performed as a final solution to the problem.

It is necessary to add the following. (1) With blind distal or subtotal pancreatectomy and total pancreatectomy, the spleen is removed en bloc with the specimen. (2) Following blind subtotal pancreatectomy, the duct of Wirsung should be clearly identified and ligated with silk or with a transfixion suture. (3) The transected neck or body of the pancreatic remnant should be closed with a series of interrupted mattress sutures of silk (Fig. 37). (4) The lesser sac should be drained with one or two rubber tubes in the event that suction may prove to be necessary in the early postoperative days. In cases of *hyperplasia* (or adenomatosis), total pancreatectomy may be necessary, while for large

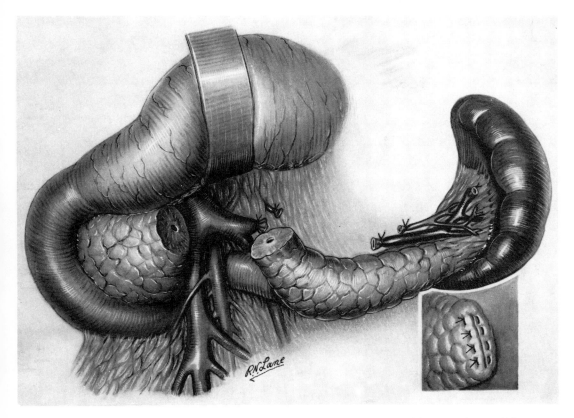

FIG. 37.   Blind resection of the body and tail of the pancreas; a case of hyperinsulinism. (After Cattell.)

tumours in the head of the gland, a Whipple operation is advisable.

A diuretic, Diazoxide, has recently been found effective in controlling hypoglycaemia from insulinoma as well as leucine.sensitivity. The drug is administered in doses of 400 to 600 mg orally, per day. The only noticeable side-effect has been elevated blood uric acid. "To date, the drug shows great promise and may solve what has traditionally been a perplexing clinical problem." (Edwin Ellison and Larry Carey, 1969.)

PROGNOSIS

The immediate and late operative results are excellent or good. Howard et al.[17] found that simple *enucleation* of the adenoma relieved the symptoms in 86.4 percent of cases. (They reported an operative mortality rate of 9.3 percent. Today, the opera-

tive mortality rate for simple enucleation is about 1 to 3 percent, and for blind subtotal pancreatectomy, 4 to 5 percent.) *Blind subtotal pancreatectomy* was performed in 77 of Howard's patients because of failure of the surgeon to find an adenoma. Only 43 percent of this group obtained relief from this operation, but an additional 9 percent were "improved."

The death rate following blind subtotal pancreatectomy was 14.3 percent. Of 46 patients in whom the excised portion of the gland was microscopically normal, 11 were found later to have an islet-cell tumour. Two patients were cured by *total pancreatectomy*, with no operative mortality.

Lopez-Kruger and Dockerty[20] reported excellent results in a collected series of 99 cases of islet-cell adenoma associated with hyperinsulinism. In their series, one adenoma was found in ectopic pancreatic tissue near the duodenum. Howard, in a collected review of

398 cases, recorded only 9 instances of such ectopic islet-cell tumours. In Marshall's series of 19 patients, symptoms of hyperinsulinism were cured in 17, and most of the patients had a follow-up of 1 to 13 years. (The operative mortality rate was 4.2 percent.)

The surgeon can expect to find and excise the adenoma in some 75 to 80 percent of cases in which the diagnosis has been supported by sound clinical and chemical tests. Whereas total relief of symptoms is assured in 80 to 90 percent of patients in whom an adenoma is identified and resected, *"blind"* pancreatic resection will uncover 22 to 25 percent of tumours in the specimen. Total pancreatectomy should not be carried out as a primary procedure when a discrete adenoma is not found. If distal (two-thirds) pancreatectomy does not relieve symptoms, it is always possible to resect the remaining portion of the pancreas.

Mengoli and Le Quesne [22] supply further details on Prognosis. They wrote:

Moss and Rhoads (1960) surveyed the world literature on hyperinsulinism prior to 1958 and found 766 islet cell tumours. Surgery was the definitive therapy in 453 of these patients. In 165 patients with suspected insulinoma no tumour could be palpated at laporotomy and a blind distal resection of the pancreas was carried out. In only 36 instances was an occult tumour found in the resected specimen. In a further 30 patients an adenoma of the pancreas was found at a later

procedure. No tumour was ever found in the remaining 99 patients (60 per cent), although half were said to be cured or improved [Fig. 38]. This finding is in contrast to that of Breidahl, Priestley, and Rynearson (*Ann. Surg. 142*:698, 1955 and *J. Am. Med. Ass. 160*:198, 1956), who reported that the chances of cure were slight when no tumour was found in the resected specimen. However, on the basis of their survey, Moss and Rhoads advised distal pancreatic resection if no tumour could be palpated at laparotomy.

Many of the patients reported prior to 1958 would not satisfy present criteria for the diagnosis of insulinoma, and the high incidence of cure in patients without tumour makes the diagnosis of organic hypoglycaemia suspect in many instances. The introduction, by Fajans and Conn in 1959, of the *intravenous tolbutamide test* has done much to make the diagnosis of insulinoma more accurate, and in recent years it has been further refined by the development of *plasma insulin assay* (Yalow and Berson, *J. Clin. Invest.* 39:1157, 1960 and Samols and Marks, *Brit. Med. J. 1*:507, 1963). As a result many patients with hypoglycaemia of nonpancreatic origin, who might previously have been treated by laparotomy and blind distal pancreatectomy, can now be accurately assessed and spared a fruitless operation.

. . . The problem of blind distal pancreatectomy for suspected insulinoma is reviewed, based on an analysis of the 47 examples reported in the English literature, since 1958, together with 3 hitherto unreported cases.

A tumour was found in the resected specimen in 11 patients (22 per cent), and in 24 (48 per cent) a tumour was found at a later procedure. In 1 patient an insulinoma was found in the remaining pancreas at the time of blind resection. No tumour was ever found in 12 patients and in the remaining 2 patients the presence or absence

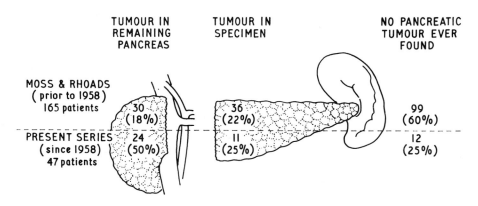

	TUMOUR IN REMAINING PANCREAS	TUMOUR IN SPECIMEN	NO PANCREATIC TUMOUR EVER FOUND
MOSS & RHOADS (prior to 1958) 165 patients	30 (18%)	36 (22%)	99 (60%)
PRESENT SERIES (since 1958) 47 patients	24 (50%)	11 (25%)	12 (25%)

FIG. 38. Diagram summarising main findings in present study of patients subjected to blind distal pancreatectomy for suspected insulin tumour, compared with those of Moss and Rhoads (1960). Only 47 of the 50 cases in present study are included in this diagram, as final diagnosis in remaining 3 remains uncertain. (Courtesy of Mr. Mengoli and Mr. LeQuesne and the *British Journal of Surgery*.)

of an insulinoma is not certain. Eighty-one operations were performed on these 50 patients, and 26 (52 per cent) required second, third, and fourth operations for recurrence of symptoms. There were 6 deaths in the entire series, 4 being related to surgery; 2 died following the initial blind resection and 2 following a subsequent procedure.

On the subject of *diabetes after removal of insulin tumours of the pancreas:* A long-term follow-up survey of 11 patients is presented by D. C. Dunn,[6] who writes:

Eleven patients who had islet-cell tumours of the pancreas removed over a 20-year period were reviewed. Two have died, one in the postoperative period and one 10 years postoperatively. The remaining 9 were traced and 8 of them were personally interviewed and tested. All 9 patients were well and free from recurrent symptoms.

Five of the 8 patients had evidence of subnormal insulin production in response to oral glucose. The glucose-tolerance test was impaired in 3. Minor abnormalities were found in the electrocardiograms of all these patients and major abnormalities in two. The results of this survey suggest that other patients who have had islet-cell tumours removed may now have unsuspected diabetes.

Postoperative Treatment

The glucose drip should be continued until the patient is able to take nourishment by mouth. A fasting blood sugar estimation should be carried out 3 hours and 6 hours after the cessation of the drip.

In my opinion, if the operation has been successful, the blood sugar level should rise to normal or higher, with some temporary glycosuria. Routine blood sugar estimations should be performed every 6 hours for the next few days and thereafter at regular intervals. The patient should be kept under supervision for some years. In my experience, permanent diabetes rarely occurs even after subtotal pancreatic resections.

REFERENCES

1. Bockus, Gastro-Enterology, Vol. III, 2d ed., Philadelphia, Saunders, 1966.
2. Brunschwig, The Surgery of the Pancreas, Philadelphia, Saunders, 1942.
3. Campbell et al., Am. J. Med. Sci. 198:445, 1939.
4. Cunliffe Shaw, Br. J. Surg. 43:579, 1956.
5. Duff, Am. J. Med. Sci. 203:437, 1942.
6. Dunn, Br. Med. J. 2:84, 1971.
7. Fajans et al., J. Clin. Endocrinol. Metab. 21:371, 1961.
8. Fajans et al., J. Clin. Endocrinol. Metab. 85:166, 1962.
9. Fonkalstrud, Dilley, and Longmire, Ann. Surg. 159:730, 1964.
10. Frantz, Ann. Surg. 112:161, 1940.
11. Gorden et al., J. Clin. Endocrinol. Metab. 33:983, 1971.
12. Graham and Womack, Surg. Gynecol. Obstet. 56:728, 1933.
13. Gutman et al., New Engl. J. Med. 284:1003, 1971.
14. Hanno and Banks, Ann. Surg. 117:437, 1943.
15. Hartsuck and Brooks, Am. J. Surg. 117:541, 1969.
16. Holman et al., Arch. Surg. 47:165, 1943.
17. Howard et al., Surg. Gynecol. Obstet. 90:417, 1950.
18. Hunt, Surg. Gynecol. Obstet. 125:371, 1967.
19. Kalish and Shapiro. Ann. Surg. 158:222, 1963.
20. Lopez-Kruger and Dockerty, Surg. Gynecol. Obstet. 85:495, 1947.
21. Marshall, Surg. Clin. North Am. 39:775, 1947.
22. Mengoli and Le Quesne, Br. J. Surg. 54:749, 1967.
23. Randall, Mayo Clin. Proc. 41:390, 1966.
24. Rogers, Am. J. Surg. 99:268, 1960.
25. Roxburgh, Lancet 1:1057, 1954.
26. Rudd and Walton, Br. J. Surg. 29:266, 1941.
27. Ruskin et al., Surg. Gynecol. Obstet. 133:1, 1971.
28. Scholz et al., Proc. Mayo Clin. 35:545, 1960.
29. Schwartz et al., Arch. Surg. 86:166, 1962.
30. Sherman, Am. J. Dis. Child. 74:58, 1947.
31. Thomas et al., Am. J. Roentgenol. 104:646, 1968.
32. Tompkins et al., Surg. Gynecol. Obstet. 125:1069, 1967.
33. Tompkins et al., Surg. Gynecol. Obstet. 85:166, 1960.
34. Warren et al., Surg. Clin. North Am. 44:757, 1964.
35. Wastell and Ellis, Proc. R. Soc. Med. 58:432, 1964.
36. Whipple, Can. Med. Assoc. J. 66:334, 1952.
37. Willis, Pathology of Tumours, 5th ed., London, Butterworths, 1972.
38. Wolfe et al. Arch. Surg. 104:56, 1972.

Gallbladder and Bile Ducts

40

CONGENITAL ANOMALIES OF THE GALLBLADDER, THE BILE DUCTS, AND THE HEPATIC AND CYSTIC ARTERIES

RODNEY MAINGOT

The surgeon should be familiar not only with the anatomy of the gallbladder, the biliary passages, and the associated blood vessels, but also with the various abnormalities which may from time to time be encountered during operation in these areas (Figs. 1 and 2).

Inadequate knowledge of the course and relations of the structures of the hepatic pedicle, combined with poor visualisation of the operative field during cholecystectomy, are responsible for most of the major postoperative complications such as ductal stricture, bile peritonitis, subphrenic abscess, haemorrhage, and profuse and persistent discharge of bile through the wound.

I would estimate that about 85 percent of all postoperative bile duct strictures are caused by errors in surgical technique at the time of the original cholecystectomy.

Gerald Dowdy, Jr.,[23] in his excellent book *The Biliary Tract,* writes:

Practically every article on biliary tract surgery acknowledges the frequent variations found in biliary tract anatomy. But even though the importance of these differences has been emphasized, recent studies show that a significant number of technical errors still occur in surgery . . . Although "normal anatomy" is non-existent in reference to the pancreatobiliary system, dissections have established a common pattern which serves as a base line. One should recognize, however, that numerous deviations from this pattern are normal anatomical variations.

The anomalies will be discussed in the following order: (1) anomalies of the gallbladder, (2) anomalies of the bile ducts, and (3) anomalies of the hepatic and cystic arteries.

ANOMALIES OF THE GALLBLADDER

Congenital anomalies of the gallbladder may be classified as follows: (1) *anomalies of number:* absent (agenesis), double, triple, or replaced by a fibrous nodule; (2) *anomalies of size:* very large or "giant" gallbladder, rudimentary gallbladder; (3) *anomalies of shape:* partitioned, bilobed, folded fundus or Phrygian cap, Hartmann's pouch, septate, hourglass, with diverticulum; kinking; and (4) *anomalies of position:* intrahepatic, transverse, left-sided, one gallbladder on the right side (in normal position) with another gallbladder on the *left* side, retrodisplacement, lumbar, iliac, pelvic, retroperitoneal, and ptosis of the gallbladder. See Figures 3, 4, and 5.

Anomalies of Number

ABSENCE OF THE GALLBLADDER

Congenital absence, or agenesis, of the gallbladder is a rare anomaly in the human subject. There are less than 200 recorded cases up to 1972. According to Danzis,[21] Courvoisier collected and reported 25 cases in 1890. Gross [33] collected 38 cases in which the patients' gallbladder and cystic duct were absent, the hepatic and other ducts being present and functioning normally.

Bower [10] reported 60 cases; Finney and Owen,[26] 10 cases; Stolkin,[95] 31 cases; and Latimer and co-workers,[50] 74 cases. Gerwig

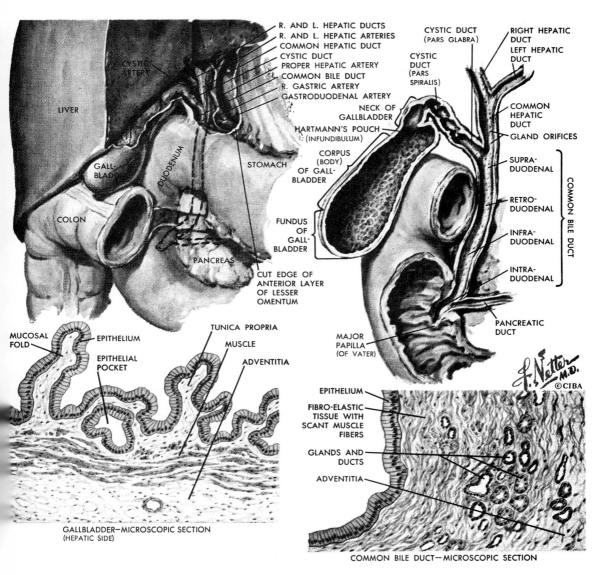

FIG. 1. Anatomy of the gallbladder and bile ducts. (Copyright The CIBA Collection of Medical Illustrations (III) and Frank H. Netter, M.D.)

et al.[30] reviewed the literature from 1947 to 1960 and found 139 authentic cases.

Rabinovitch and his colleagues[76] reported a series of 5 cases of complete absence of the gallbladder.

McIlrath et al.,[56] in an important contribution, state that the total number of cases of agenesis reported in the literature is 143 (they reported 10 cases of their own). Sei-

fert[86] collected, from the literature of that time, 148 cases of congenital absence of the gallbladder without other biliary tract abnormalities. Sterson[93] reported one case of agenesis of the gallbladder and found 139 publications pertaining to this abnormality.

During the last 10 years, cases have been recorded by Seifert,[86] Hammond et al.,[35] Satpathy,[83] Richards,[80] Yamashita,[102] Sterson,[93] and other authors.

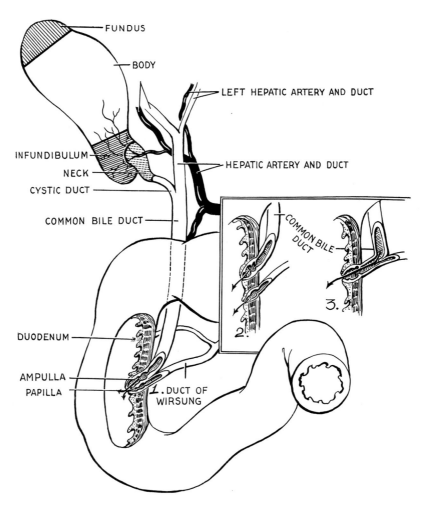

FIG. 2.   Anatomical subdivision of the gallbladder and biliary passages. "Normal" arrangements of the arteries and some of the modes in which the common bile duct and the pancreatic duct enter the second part of the duodenum are illustrated.

Necropsy incidence is computed to be between 0.03 and 0.09 percent. In 185 recorded cases, Stolkind[95] found 70 with complete absence of the gallbladder, 55 replaced by a fibrous cord, and 60 rudimentary gallbladders.

The ratio of male to female is 1:1.2.

The anomaly may be observed at any age, the average age being 35. In 96 cases, Danzis[21] found 31 were infants less than 1 year old. Gross found the condition to occur twice as frequently in females. At autopsy, however, agenesis of the gallbladder is found equally in both sexes. Smyth[91] has reminded us that most cases are associated with stones in the ducts, malformation or agenesis of the extrahepatic ducts, and that many of the patients die in the first 6 months of life. When only the gallbladder and cystic duct are absent, survival to adult life is, of course, possible.

In the majority of patients with absence of the gallbladder who have come to operation, the signs and symptoms were those of choledocholithiasis, cholangitis, jaundice, and icterus.

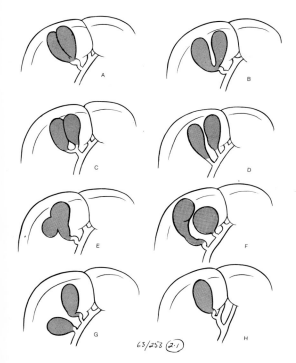

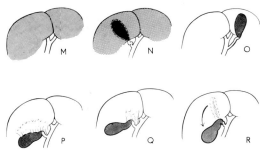

FIG. 5. Anomalies of the gallbladder. (M) Absence, or agenesis. (N) Intrahepatic gallbladder. (O) Gallbladder on the left side. (P), (Q), and (R) Gallbladder with and without a mesentery. Ptosis. (After Gross.)

FIG. 3. Anomalies of the gallbladder. (A), (B), and (C) The three types of bilobed gallbladder—septal, T-, and Y-shaped. (D), (F), and (G) Double gallbladders—H-type. (E) Diverticulum of the gallbladder. (H) High position of the gallbladder with its cystic duct draining into the right hepatic duct. (Adapted from Dr. Robert E. Gross, Archives of Surgery, Courtesy of Butterworths, London.)

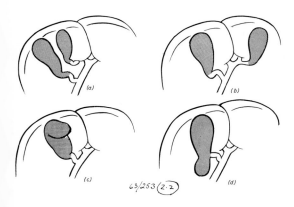

FIG. 4. Anomalies of the gallbladder. (A) Double gallbladder. (B) One gallbladder in its normal position and another on the left side. (C) Phrygian cap. (D) Hartmann's pouch. (After Gross.)

Preoperative and operative cholangiography reveal complete lack of filling of the gallbladder. If at exploration no gallbladder is found in the normal position, search should be made in the recognised abnormal positions and especially for a prominence on the anterior surface of the right lobe of the liver (caused by an intrahepatic gallbladder).

Malmstrom[62] described a case of agenesis of the gallbladder diagnosed at operative cholangiography. If no gallbladder is found, congenital absence may be diagnosed; in this case there will probably be calculi in the choledochus, which should be opened, probed, and drained with a T tube after removal of all the stones and sediment, and after an adequate dilatation of the sphincter of Oddi and papilla of Vater with graduated Bakes' dilators. In many cases, it may be necessary to perform sphincterotomy or sphincteroplasty followed by T tube drainage. Drainage of the biliary tract should, in most cases, be carried out for a period of at least 3 months.

There appears to be a definite association between congenital biliary tract abnormalities and cholelithiasis. This subject is reviewed and many cases are recorded in papers by Harding Rains[77] and Mouzas and Wilson.[70] Dixon and Lichtman,[22] who analysed 60 cases of gallbladder agenesis, found symptoms suggestive of gallbladder disease in 58 percent; jaundice was present in 48 percent, stones in the choledochus in 27 percent, and dilatation of the common bile duct in 32 percent.

DOUBLE GALLBLADDER

In the condition termed *double gallbladder*, there are two separate organs and two separate cystic ducts (Figs. 6, 7, and 8). Clyde Wilson [101] stated that duplication of the gallbladder is rare, occurring only about once in every 3,000 to 4,000 human beings. According to Boyden,[11] it is common in cats (12 percent), pigs, calves, and lambs, but extremely rare in humans. Boyden found 2 cases in 9,221 anatomical dissections and 3 cases in 9,970 cholecystograms.

Dunkerley described a specimen removed from a patient at operation. In this patient there was one normal gallbladder and another that was the seat of calculous cholecystitis. Dunkerley [24] remarks that rather more than 100 cases were reported up to 1964. Up to the present time, I have been able to trace 124 cases of double gallbladder in the literature. In most cases of double gallbladder, there are two well-formed vesicles (one may be larger than the other), each with its own cystic duct that drains into the main extrahepatic bile duct. On occasion, one gallbladder is situated on the right side of the other on the *left side* (beneath the left lobe of the liver); or, again, one organ may lie in its rightful fossa with its cystic duct emptying into the common hepatic duct while its companion is perched higher up and has a cystic duct which pierces the hepatic substance to drain into the intrahepatic portion of the *right* hepatic duct. The *size* of the accessory gallbladder usually approximates that of the normal gallbladder, but occasionally it is considerably smaller and may be globular instead of pyriform.

Accessory, anomalous or rudimentary gallbladders which arise from the common duct

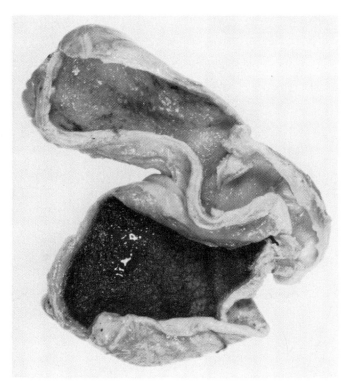

FIG. 6.   Double gallbladder, one cavity showing cholecystitis, the other normal. Rodney Smith's patient. (Courtesy of Butterworths, London.)

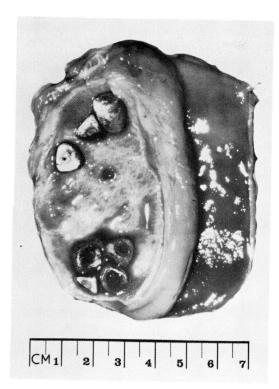

FIG. 7. Double gallbladder, one normal and the other containing many stones. The patient was operated on successfully by Martin Birnstingl of St. Bartholomew's Hospital, London. (From Dunkerley, and Birnstingl. *Proc. R. Soc. Med.* 57:331, 1964.)

by a narrow neck, lie along the free margin of the hepatoduodenal ligament and are commonly partially intrahepatic. Gross [33] refers to the finding in infants and children of a small rudimentary gallbladder, which is lit-tle more than a nuggin. He believes that this is due to congenital hypoplasia. Rudimentary gallbladders are invariably small and have no remaining function. They measure from ½ to ¾ inch (12.7 to 19 mm) in length. In the H type, in which each gallbladder has its own cystic duct emptying separately into the extrahepatic biliary system, *two cystic arteries are usually present.*

Sherren [88] of the London Hospital, was the first surgeon to record a case in which a double gallbladder was successfully removed, while Climan [20] was the first to demonstrate the condition on cholecystography.

Schachner's case [84] was one of great interest. He operated upon a patient, aged 52, for acute cholecystitis, and on finding a double gallbladder he drained each viscus.

Hicken and his associates [38] reported four cases of true double gallbladders, each with its own cystic duct. In two cases, the diagnosis was confirmed at operation, and two were diagnosed radiographically without operative confirmation.

Gross,[33] in his excellent review of 148 cases of congenital anomalies of the gallbladder, reported only 1 case of a double gallbladder.

Further cases of double gallbladder have been reported by Kennon.[45] Boyden [13] reported 20 cases and Rabinovitch et al.[76] reviewed 12 cases of anomalies of the gallbladder which were observed at operation or at autopsy. Further reports have been made by Hurwitz,[42] Mackie,[58] and Guyer et al.[34] *It is estimated that 10 percent of human subjects have some anomaly of the biliary tract.*

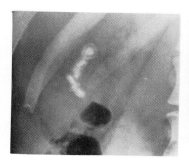
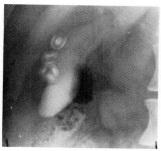
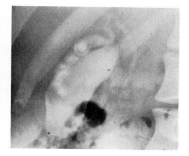

FIG. 8. Double gallbladder, radiological appearances. The patient was operated on successfully by Martin Birnstingl of St. Bartholomew's Hospital, London. (From Dunkerley, and Birnstingl. *Proc. R. Soc. Med.* 57:331, 1964.)

Recht [79] gives an excellent and interesting account of *torsion of a double gallbladder*.

Lumsden and Truelove, in their work *Radiology of the Digestive Tract* (1970), confirm that the x-ray incidence of double gallbladder is low. In the cases reported by Sherren (1911), Braun,[14] and Nichols,[73] the plain x-ray films showed two distinct rows of stones.

According to Gross, the presence of the congenital anomaly is often not diagnosed before operation because there are no characteristic symptoms or signs. When the accessory organ is the seat of inflammatory change or stone formation, the symptoms and signs closely resemble those occurring with cholecystitis or cholelithiasis in a normally formed gallbladder. It is difficult to state whether an accessory organ is more prone to be involved in disease processes, but the fact that most of these anomalies have been discovered during operations and only a few at postmortem examination certainly indicates that the accessory structure is probably more likely to undergo pathological changes than is a normally formed organ.

Dunkerley [24] has stressed the fact that double gallbladders are subject to the same pathological processes as are single ones. Acute and chronic cholecystitis, gallstone formation, volvulus, and carcinoma have all been described:

The presence of a double gallbladder may pose special problems. The cholecystogram in a patient who clinically has cholecystitis may be absolutely normal, masking a second inflamed gallbladder with function too poor for visualization. At operation, if a preoperative diagnosis has not been made, an inflamed gallbladder may be left behind after cholecystectomy. Ryrberg reports that in one such case the surgeon was sued.

TRIPLE GALLBLADDER
(VESICA FELLEA TRIPLEX)

In 1958, Skielboe [89] reported the only case on record of triple gallbladder in man. The anomaly is not uncommon in certain animals. Skielboe's patient was a woman, aged 53, who gave a history suggestive of chronic cholecystitis. Cholecystograms suggested the presence of gallstones in a double gallbladder of the H Type.

Cholecystectomies were performed, and the pathological examination revealed three distinct separate gallbladders, each with its own cystic duct, emptying into the common bile duct. Two of the gallbladders were of normal size, the other was somewhat smaller. Each gallbladder contained bile and stones.

The second case of *triplication of the gallbladder* was recorded by Roeder, Mersheimer, and Kazarian [81] in 1971. At operation, two gallbladders with their own cystic ducts were excised. One gallbladder was inflamed and contained stones, while the other harboured a papillary adenocarcinoma. The third gallbladder was shown, on operative cholangiography, to be intrahepatic.

Anderson and Ross [3] reported a case of the *septal type* which was diagnosed by cholecystography. They reviewed the literature up to 1958 and could find only five V- or Y-shaped and three septal types.

They believe that this malformation may be the result of failure of refusion of the paired buds of the gallbladder primordium or of the incomplete recavitation of the embryonic structure early in foetal life.

The most common symptoms are colic and icterus. Gallstones are found in one or both cavities in some 70 percent of the cases. Radiography will frequently confirm the diagnosis, and the treatment recommended is cholecystectomy, with or without exploration of the biliary system.

Anomalies of Shape

BILOBED GALLBLADDER

In this anomaly, the gallbladder has two cavities that drain by a single duct into the common bile duct.

So far, 14 cases have been reported including a recent one by Hobby [39] and the one described by Cecil Wakeley.[98] In Wakeley's case, a gallbladder of the Y variety was successfully excised, and, on examination, one sac was found to contain many stones while the other contained only bile and mucus. There are three varieties of bilobed gallbladder:

1. The cavities may be divided by a septum (septal type).
2. There may be two cavities which coalesce at their "necks" to join a cystic duct which empties into the common bile duct.

3. There are two vesicles (of about equal size) which have their own cystic ducts which unite to form a single duct before this drains into the main bile duct. Bilobed gallbladders (V-, Y-, or T-shaped types) must be clearly distinguished from double gallbladders, in which there is two cavities, *each* drained by its *own* cystic duct. Double gallbladder is more common than bilobed gallbladder, which was first described by Cruveilhier in 1860.

DIVERTICULUM OF THE GALLBLADDER

This may be found in any position along the surface of the organ from the fundus to the neck. The most common site for such a diverticulum is in Hartmann's pouch. Beluffi (1939) described a case of congenital diverticulum of the fundus of the gallbladder. These diverticula vary in size from 0.6 to 9 cm in diameter. Only a few of them have been observed at operation, but they are occasionally seen when the gallbladder is examined at cholecystography. True congenital diverticulum (containing all three layers of a normal gallbladder) is a very rare anomaly of the gallbladder.

I have performed cholecystectomy upon one patient in whom diverticulum was diagnosed preoperatively by means of an oral cholecystogram. The diverticulum arose from the body of the gallbladder and measured 2 cm in diameter; it contained all three coats of the normal organ and the connecting channel was narrow—3 mm in diameter.

Clinically, a diverticulum may be symptomless. It may be the seat of diverticulitis or contain calculi and, rarely, it may perforate and give rise to a subhepatic abscess or spreading peritonitis. The first description of the diverticular type of gallbladder was made by von Jeister in 1717, and, as early as 1890, Courvoisier found 28 cases in the literature, of which 18 had stones.

Acromond and Barnett [1] reported three cases and gave a review of the literature.

Blalock found diverticula to be present in 0.2 percent of 727 surgical gallbladder cases. Weisel and Waltman Walters,[99] of the Mayo Clinic, state that in a series of 29,701 sur-gically removed gallbladders, 25 specimens had a diverticulum.

Cholecystectomy is the treatment indicated when this abnormality of the gallbladder produces symptoms or harbors calculi.

Multiple diverticula do occur, but they are exceedingly rare.

STRICTURES, DUMBBELL, OR HOURGLASS GALLBLADDER

Various malformations in the contour of the gallbladder—such as strictures, dumbbell, and hourglass—are observed. They may be congenital or acquired in origin, but it is probable that most of them are acquired. Thompson and Dormandy [97] give an account of *torsion of an hourglass gallbladder* with focal arteritis. They believe that secondary constriction of the gallbladder proximal to an impacted calculus in the fundus is not uncommon, but that as a primary condition, hourglass deformity of the organ is rare. Flannery and Caster [27] were able to confirm their x-ray diagnosis by operation, and found gallstones confined to the distal loculus.

Michels [67] states that hourglass gallbladder may be congenital or acquired in origin. The condition is likely to be congenital when there is no evidence of cholecystitis, whereas if the constriction is near the neck and the vesicle is inflamed or contains calculi, the abnormality will, in all probability, prove to be of the acquired type.

Figure 9 is an x-ray reproduction of a case of the author's, in which the hourglass constriction involving the middle portion of the body of the viscus can be clearly seen. The proximal compartment appears to be normal on the cholecystogram, while the distal pouch is filled with numerous small tightly packed calculi. Cholecystectomy confirmed the preoperative findings.

KINKING OF THE GALLBLADDER

Boyden,[11] in 165 anatomical studies, found that 18 percent showed a marked kinking of the gallbladder between the body and infundibulum or between the body and the fundus. Feldman (1957) states that cholecystography offers the best means of disclosing changes in the shape of the gallbladder. Con-

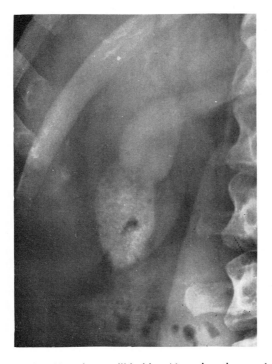

FIG. 9. Hourglass gallbladder. Note that the proximal pouch appears normal on the cholecystogram, but the distal pouch of the hourglass gallbladder contains many closely packed gallstones. (R. Maingot's patient.)

strictions are often observed in routine studies, many of which have no important clinical significance.

Phrygian Cap Gallbladder ("phrygische mutze, spitzendivertikel")

The Phrygian cap gallbladder has been described as a congenital malformation, and the significance of this finding on radiology or at operation is discussed by Lichtenstein.[53] Lichtenstein placed the incidence at 3 to 8 percent, and Boyden[13] at 18 percent.

It is more common in women than in men, the ratio being 3:2, and may be found at any age. I believe that while such a vesicle may be involved by disease, folded fundus or *phrygische Mutze* has no pathological significance.

Bartel,[6] who was the first to describe this peculiar anomaly, collected 43 autopsy speci-

mens. It is also known as liberty cap, a pointed form of headgear commonly worn by the people of Phrygia and by the sansculottes in the time of Robespierre. Bronner[16] believed that the condition was pathological, but Boyden considered that it was of no clinical significance. Boyden, in his series of 200 collected cases, found that in 18 percent there was kinking of the gallbladder either between the body and the infundibulum (24 cases) or between the body and the fundus (6 cases).

The septum may vary from one-quarter to the entire diameter separating the fundus from the body. The gallbladder functions normally and, in itself, has no clinical implication, as Meyer et al.[65] and other clinicians have emphasized.

Hartmann's Pouch

Hartmann's pouch is simply an asymmetrical bulging or ballooning of the infundibulum and neck of the gallbladder near the point of exit of the cystic duct. It is a congenital condition, but may be of surgical importance during cholecystectomy when it is unduly large and firmly adherent to the cystic or common bile duct, or both. The choledochus may be injured during liberation of this pouch.

Multiseptate Gallbladder

This anomaly of the gallbladder is an extremely rare congenital one of *form*. I can find only eight cases recorded in the literature. Knetsch,[47] in 1952, reported the radiological findings in three cases of multiseptate gallbladders showing a few septa in each instance. Dr. F. Netter[71] illustrated a case in the CIBA collection in 1957. Simon and Tandom,[90] Haslam et al.,[36] Bigg,[8] and Bhagavan[7] each reported a case with many septa. Cholecystography (sometimes combined with intravenous cholangiography) showed normal-sized gallbladders with excellent concentration of the dye and satisfactory contraction after a fatty meal. "There was however, a striking subdivision of the contrast material by multiple, thin, crisscrossing septa, producing an irregular mosaic pattern. The cystic duct also showed some septation, but none was found in the common duct."[82] Simon and Tandom[90] state that the gallbladder they excised was normal in size and without any evidence of acute or chronic inflammation. In most cases, a striking feature was the peritoneal surface, which presented a number of bulging or pouting elevations that appeared and felt cystic.

The multiseptate gallbladder is of rubbery consistency, and when it is compressed, it feels as though it might contain a minute sponge.

Since the honeycombed septa are formed by fibromuscular shelves lined by epithelia, it is postulated that the wall is either pushed or drawn into the gallbladder during embryogenesis. Perhaps the appearances of these gallbladders are best explained as resulting from incomplete cavitation of the developing gallbladder.

The majority of the patients are young; and surgery is indicated only where *recurrent* colicky pains cannot be controlled by medical measures.

Anomalies of Position

A normally formed gallbladder has been found: (1) within the hepatic substance; (2) under the left lobe of the liver (left-sided gallbladder); (3) posteriorly under the inferior aspect of the right lobe of the liver; and (4) horizontally in the transverse fissure of the liver. In the latter instance, the gallbladder lies in the transverse position and the right and left hepatic ducts (or the common hepatic duct) drain separately into the vesicle while the common bile duct "arises" from the inferior margin, proceeding downward to empty its contents into the duodenum. Further positional anomalies are: (5) retrodisplacement; (6) lumbar, iliac (Fig. 10), pelvic; (7) ptosis or floating gallbladder.

LEFT-SIDED GALLBLADDERS

Kehr gave a description of a left-sided gallbladder found accidentally at laparotomy in 1902. According to Newcombe and Henley,[72] Hochstetter[40] described the condition in three cases in 1886. C. W. Mayo and Kendrick[64] reported a case found at operation in 1950. There are two types of left-sided gallbladder: (1) when the liver and gallbladder are in the left hypogastrium in *sinus inversus viscerum* and when there is (2)

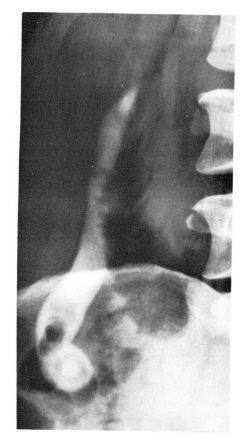

FIG. 10. Iliac gallbladder. Note the large gallstone lying in the right iliac fossa. In such cases, the gallbladder usually has a complete mesentery. (From May. *Br. J. Clin. Pract.* 21:191, 1967.)

transposition of the gallbladder to the left in the absence of *sinus inversus viscerum*. In the latter condition, the gallbladder is situated under the left lobe of the liver and to the left of the falciform ligament. This is a medical curiosity: Complete *sinus inversus viscerum* (thoracic and abdominal) has been reported in 0.002 to 0.005 percent of hospital and clinic admissions.

Bleich and co-workers[9] describe a case of *left-sided gallbladder* which was the twelfth case to be recorded in the literature and the fourth case to be diagnosed preoperatively by means of cholecystography. Transposition of the gallbladder to the left in the absence of *sinus inversus viscerum* is very rare.[37, 49] In 1948, Gowan, reporting a left-sided gallbladder, found only seven previous cases in the literature. In such cases the cystic duct may drain into the left hepatic duct or the common hepatic duct. *An exceptional finding is a left-sided gallbladder associated with a normal vesicle on the right side.*

RETRODISPLACEMENT OF THE GALLBLADDER

Here the gallbladder does not rest in its own fossa and the fundus extends backward in the free margin of the hepatoduodenal ligament and may point in any direction. Excision of this type of gallbladder may present unusual technical difficulties.

INTRAHEPATIC GALLBLADDER

McNamee,[57] in his much quoted article, states that over 56 percent of the collected cases of intrahepatic gallbladder were found in infants.

Many animals normally have intrahepatic gallbladders. When occurring in man, the gallbladder is found partially or completely embedded in liver substance. Bockus (1966) pointed out that 60 percent of adult patients with intrahepatic gallbladders had gallstones.

Preoperative and operative cholangiography supplies the most accurate means of diagnosis. At operation, cholecysostomy should be carried out, as attempts to remove intrahepatic gallbladders may be associated with *severe haemorrhage.*

PTOSIS AND VOLVULUS OR TORSION

There are three types of floating gallbladder: (1) the organ is completely invested by peritoneum and possesses no mesentery—in such cases the only attachment between the gallbladder and the liver is the cystic duct and cystic artery; (2) the vesicle is suspended from the liver by a complete mesentery (Fig. 11); and (3) the cystic duct and the neck of the gallbladder have a mesentery in which the cystic artery lies, but the fundus and body are free and ptosed.

This condition is by no means rare, and is seen in some 5 percent of all gallbladders—84 percent of such cases occurring in women and 16 percent in men.[89] Its main interest lies in the fact that only when the gallbladder has a long mesentery or is quite free is it capable of undergoing torsion.

It is said that the majority of the cases of *torsion of the gallbladder* occur in late life, the maximum incidence being between the ages of 60 and 80. It is difficult to understand why this should be so, but it may possibly be due to the fact that with advancing age

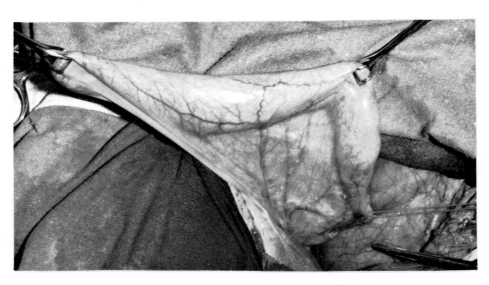

FIG. 11. Gallbladder with complete mesentery. The cystic artery and the cystic duct have been ligated prior to excision of the gallbladder. (From May. *Br. J. Clin. Prac.* 21:191, 1967.)

the supporting fat tends to disappear from the surrounding structures, and when atrophy of the tissues permits increased ptosis of the viscera (including the gallbladder), there is an increase also in the mobility of the vesicle—which predisposes to twisting. Rais and Thuzen[78] reported a case in a boy 12 years of age, and traced the original reports of four other cases in children under the age of 15.

Rawson described torsion of the gallbladder in a child of 12, and also reviewed the literature. He considered that torsion in children was by no means rare.

Recht,[79] in describing his case of *torsion of a double gallbladder,* remarks that all the published cases of torsion occurred in the floating type of gallbladder. On the other hand, in the 40 cases of double gallbladder reported up to that time, only 1 case of torsion had occurred. Recht's patient was a man aged 48. Wendel[100] reported the first case of torsion of the gallbladder in 1898.

Leger et al.[51] and Anschutz[4] collected 91 cases of torsion up to 1945, to which they added one of their own. Twenty-three further cases had been reported in the literature by the end of 1951, bringing the total to 115 (Rawson). Arnold Levene,[52] in reporting two cases, states that the number of recorded cases amounted to about 200 in 1958. Carter et al.,[18] writing nearly 6 years later, give the same figure! The number of reported cases in English medical literature is, at the present time (1973), 250.

The writer has successfully operated upon two patients with gangrene of the gallbladder caused by acute torsion. The first patient was a woman of 72 years of age, and the second a man of 81. Neither case was diagnosed preoperatively.

Short and Paul[89] believed that "acute pain and vomiting, without jaundice, in an elderly female, and the appearance within a few hours of onset of the greatly enlarged and palpable gallbladder are highly suggestive of the diagnosis of acute torsion of the gallbladder." If, they say, the tumour comes and goes, it can scarcely be anything else."

McCrea[55] described a unique case of *herniation of the gallbladder through the foramen of Winslow.* The gallbladder, which was devoid of mesentery—the floating type—was disimpacted and excised. The patient made a good recovery from this operation.

Nearly all patients who suffer from torsion of the gallbladder are thin, asthenic, and visceroptotic. When torsion occurs, the patient experiences abrupt and acute pain below the right costal margin, which continues unabated and with extreme severity. Immediately after the onset, collapse is marked, vomiting is frequent, the temperature rapidly rises, and the pulse rate is quickened. The pain, although mainly localised to the right of the epigastrium, is often keenly felt below the right shoulder blade. Over the gallbladder, which may be palpable, the signs of tenderness and rigidity may also be observed.

A diagnosis of acute obstructive cholecystitis or empyema of the gallbladder is usually made, and operation is frequently advised during the first 48 hours. It is well that this is so, as after this time peritonitis rapidly ensues owing to gangrene and perforation of the organ. At operation, the gallbladder is tensely swollen, oedematous, haemorrhagic, or necrotic; it may be red, dark brown, or black in colour. The true state of affairs is immediately recognised, as the twisted pedicle and infarcted gallbladder present a characteristic picture.

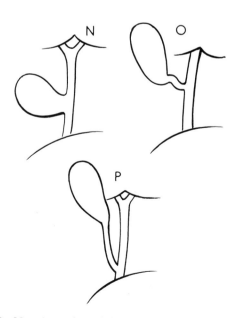

FIG. 12.   Anomalies of the ducts. (N) No cystic duct. (O) No extrahepatic right and left hepatic ducts. (P) Low insertion of the cystic duct.

The subject of volvulus or torsion of the gallbladder has been ably discussed by Sullivan and Appleby,[96] Cartorel et al.,[18] Shah,[87] May,[63] and by Clarence Schein, in his book *Acute Cholecystitis.*[85]

The *treatment* is simple and consists in detorsion of the organ, isolating the cystic duct and artery, and ligaturing and dividing them, after which the loose attachment of the gallbladder to the liver is clamped and severed and the organ removed. In a collected series of 70 patients subjected to a cholecystectomy, Arthur[5] found the mortality rate to be about 16 percent. Today, however, *the operative mortality rate is less than 3 percent.* All authors comment on the ease of removing the gallbladder and the smoothness of the patient's convalescence.

For further description of various anomalies of the gallbladder the reader is referred to Grosberg,[32a] Hoslam,[36] Richards,[80] and Dowdy.[23]

ANOMALIES OF THE BILE DUCTS

The right and left hepatic ducts unite in the portal fissure or just below it to form the common hepatic duct, which is usually 1 to 1½ inches (2.5 to 3.8 cm) in length. The cystic duct, which is normally about the same length, unites with the common hepatic duct to form the common bile duct which, in most individuals, is about 3 inches (7.6 cm) long. The length of the supraduodenal portion of the common bile duct, however, varies with the level of the duodenum and also with the point at which the cystic and common hepatic ducts join. (See Figs. 1 and 2.)

In some cases the *cystic duct is absent,* and when this is so the neck of the gallbladder—or rather the infundibulum—enters the main bile passages by a wide mouth (Fig. 12). According to Sperling,[93] congenital absence of the cystic duct has been reported only 16 times. Langer and Pearson[48] reported three cases in 1963. There are numerous cases of congenital absence of the cystic duct that have not been recorded in the world literature. In my last 500 consecutive cholecystectomies, the cystic duct was absent in seven cases.

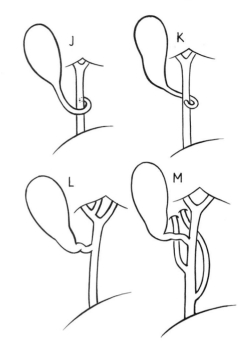

FIG. 13. Anomalies of the ducts. (J) and (K) Spiral types of cystic duct (present in 8 percent of cases). (L) Double right hepatic duct. (M) Showing a right and left accessory hepatic duct.

Perelman[75] has described a case of *cystic duct reduplication.*

I believe that there are instances in which the cystic duct and the neck of the gallbladder become obliterated by a large impacted calculus which slowly ulcerates through into the common duct. Niemeier[74] described a case in which the gallbladder was interposed in the course of the common bile duct so that no cystic duct was present. The common hepatic duct emptied directly into the anomalous "gallbladder," while the lower end of the bile duct issued from its inferior surface—thus carrying the bile into the duodenum beyond. (See Fig. 14(1).)

I have had one case, at the Royal Free Hospital, London, in which the two hepatic ducts drained into a transverse thin-walled sac—the remnant of the gallbladder—and the choledochus was attached to its inferior wall. An operative cholangiogram (through the common bile duct) showed that the choledochus adequately drained the transversely interposed "vesicle." No surgical procedure was carried out in this instance.

The medial aspect of the lower quarter or half, or sometimes even more, of the cystic duct is often firmly adherent to the lateral margin of the common bile duct, being fixed to the duct by inflammatory adhesions or swathed by an enveloping sheet of fibrous tissue. The cystic duct may join the common duct at any point between the usual anatomical position (i.e., within ½ inch [1.27 cm] of the upper border of the duodenum) and the ampulla of Vater, and in exceptional circumstances it may even open into the second portion of the duodenum separately. (Fig. 12.)

The cystic duct normally opens on the right side of the main bile duct, but in 8 to 10 percent of cases it enters on the anterior surface, the posterior surface, or even on the medial side, *twisting spirally* around the main duct (Fig. 13). In 15 percent of cases, the cystic duct enters the *left* side of the com-

mon duct. In rare instances, two cystic ducts may be present, each draining separately into the common bile duct.

The cystic duct may drain into the right hepatic duct and may prove a source of "confusion" and danger during cholecystectomy.

An *accessory bile duct,* which is in fact an anomalous right hepatic duct, emerges from the portal fissure, lies in Calot's triangle and at a somewhat posterior plane to the cystic duct, and *usually* unites with the extrahepatic ducts at some point between the union of the right and left hepatic ducts and the opening of the cystic duct into the main bile duct.

An accessory hepatic bile duct may open: (1) into the neck of the gallbladder, (2) into the right hepatic duct, (3) into the right side of the common hepatic duct, (4) at a point at or very close to the site where the cystic and common hepatic ducts join, (5) into the common bile duct below the insertion of the cystic duct or (6) into the gallbladder (Fig. 14).

I have never seen a sizeable accessory hepatic duct open into the body or fundus of the gallbladder.

Accessory ducts are present in about 10 percent of human subjects. Flint [28] found 29 cases of accessory (or anomalous) bile ducts among his 200 dissections. Eisendrath [25] reported that anomalous bile ducts were found in 8 percent of a series of necropsies. Michels [67] found accessory hepatic ducts in 18 percent of 200 specimens.

An accessory duct is usually about the same size as a normal cystic duct, but in some cases it may be minute. An undetected injury to one of these accessory ducts during cholecystectomy may subsequently produce a troublesome external biliary fistula or bile peritonitis, with attendant complications.[29]

As has been emphasized, injuries to the extrahepatic ducts and their associated blood vessels occur most frequently during the excision of the gallbladder. Such injuries should not arise if the surgeon ensures good exposure of the parts at operation, if he constantly bears in mind during every gallbladder operation that such variations as I have described are by no means uncommon, and if he makes it a rule never to clamp or divide any structure in this region until he has identified it beyond all cavil and demonstrated it to an

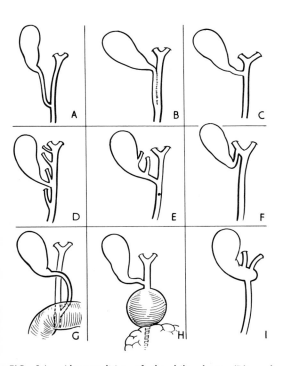

FIG. 14. Abnormalities of the bile ducts. (D) and (E) Accessory hepatic ducts. (G) Low insertion of the cystic duct. (H) Choledochus cyst. (I) No cystic duct. "Interposition" of the gallbladder. (After Gross and Hollinshead, Courtesy of Butterworths, London.)

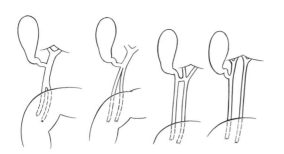

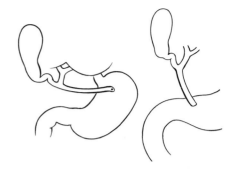

FIG. 15. Malpositions and reduplications of the choledochus. (Adapted from Swartley and Weeder. *Am. Surg.* 101:912, 1935. From Smith and Sherlock, *Surgery of the Gallbladder and Bile Ducts,* 1964. Courtesy of Butterworths, London.)

FIG. 16. Ectopia of the common bile duct. (Adapted from Swartley and Weeder. *Am. Surg.* 101:912, 1935. From Smith and Sherlock, *Surgery of the Gallbladder and Bile Ducts,* 1964. Courtesy of Butterworths, London.)

assistant. Mossman [69] pointed out that a dissection of Calot's triangle in 147 cadavers revealed that within this area lay part of the courses of the cystic artery in 90 percent, the right hepatic artery in 82 percent, and 91 percent of the 23 accessory hepatic bile ducts found in the specimens investigated.

The surgical significance of anomalies of the right and left hepatic ducts, of the common hepatic duct, of the cystic duct, of the common bile duct and of aberrant accessory hepatic ducts is ably discussed by Alden and Sterner,[2] Braasch,[13a] Linder and Green,[54] and Dowdy.[23]

MALPOSITIONS AND REDUPLICATIONS OF THE CHOLEDOCHUS

If, at operation, an anomaly of the main extrahepatic bile ducts is found, an anomaly of the blood supply should be looked for and vice versa.

Malpositions and reduplications of the bile ducts are rare, and chiefly found at postmortem examination. When encountered during operations on the biliary system, they are a source of "apprehension" and misgivings owing to their peculiar anatomical relations.

Seven different variations have been reported:

(1) A single common bile duct entering the pylorus or antrum.
(2) A duct joining the duodenum independent of the pancreatic duct.

(3) Bifurcation of the common bile duct with separate openings into the duodenum.
(4) Duplications of the main bile ducts.
(5) A bifurcating duct, with one branch entering the duodenum and the other entering the stomach.
(6) A separate common bile duct, with two openings of the single duct into the duodenum.
(7) A single common bile duct opening into the fundus of the stomach (Figs. 15 and 16).

ANOMALIES OF THE HEPATIC AND CYSTIC ARTERIES

Weiss, Eisendrath, Harberland, Holmes, Kehr, Ladd, Friend, Flint, Michels, and others have ably drawn attention to the normal and the abnormal arrangements of the arteries in relation to the gallbladder and biliary passages, and have emphasized the surgical importance of these structures.

The following is a brief summary based chiefly upon the anatomical studies of Flint [28], Michels [67] and Hollinshead (see below) (Fig. 17).

A detailed description of examples of *replacing* accessory and aberrant hepatic arteries is given by Hollinshead in Anatomy for Surgeons.[41a]

The *common hepatic artery* is normally a branch of the coeliac axis, and gives off the gastroduodenal artery and right gastric artery before ascending in the outer border of the

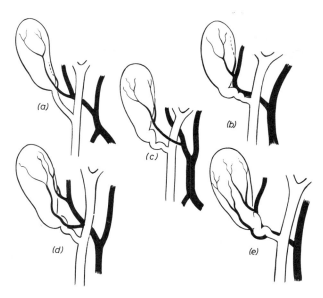

FIG. 17.   Hepatic and cystic arteries. (A) Normal anatomy. (B) to (E) A variety of abnormalities. (After Hollinshead.)

hepatoduodenal ligament toward the liver. It runs parallel and medial to the common bile duct and divides into the right and left hepatic branches just below the junction of the three hepatic ducts.

In 80 percent of instances, both branches lie on a plane behind the corresponding hepatic ducts.

The important variations in the hepatic arteries are those of (1) origin, (2) number, and (3) position.

The *right hepatic artery* arises from the main hepatic trunk in 79 percent of cases; it reaches the liver by passing behind the common hepatic duct in 68 percent of cases and in front in 12.5 percent. In 21 percent of cases, the right hepatic artery originates from the superior mesenteric artery, and when this is so it almost invariably runs upward toward the portal fissure behind the common duct. In 3.5 percent of cases, there are two right hepatic arteries, one arising from the main hepatic artery and the other—usually a smaller branch—from the superior mesenteric artery. In 1 percent of cases, there are two right hepatic arteries, both arising from the common hepatic trunk. When this is so, one blood vessel passes in front and the other

behind the main bile duct. In 2 percent of cases, in addition to passing behind the ducts, the main hepatic or the right hepatic artery also passes behind the portal vein. The main or (more commonly) the left hepatic artery arises from the left gastric artery in 3 percent of cases, and may be in danger during the performance of a subtotal or total gastrectomy. One of the most common causes of postopeative stricture of the common hepatic duct is injury to the right hepatic artery or from injudicious attempts to control bleeding from it during cholecystectomy.

The right hepatic artery is likely to be injured during cholecystectomy: (1) when it lies parallel with and close to the cystic duct; (2) when it forms a loop in front of the common hepatic duct; (3) when it projects markedly forward, forming as it were a knuckle close to the upper margin of the neck of the gallbladder before sweeping backward to the portal fissure; (4) *when the gallbladder has a mesentery (as in such instances the artery often lies within this on its way to the right lobe of the liver);* and (5) when it is dragged out of position by a sclerosing, contracted gallbladder.

When this artery lies across or ascends on

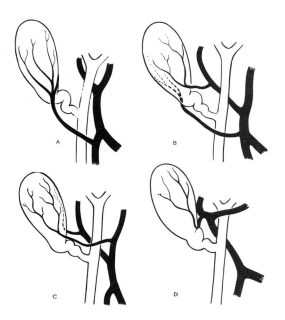

FIG. 18.   Some anomalies of the origin of the cystic artery. (A) The cystic artery arises from the gastro-duodenal artery. (B) Presence of two cystic arteries, one from the common hepatic artery and the other from the right hepatic artery. (C) Presence of two cystic arteries. (D) Abnormal left hepatic artery; and short cystic artery stemming from the right hepatic artery. (After Hollinshead.)

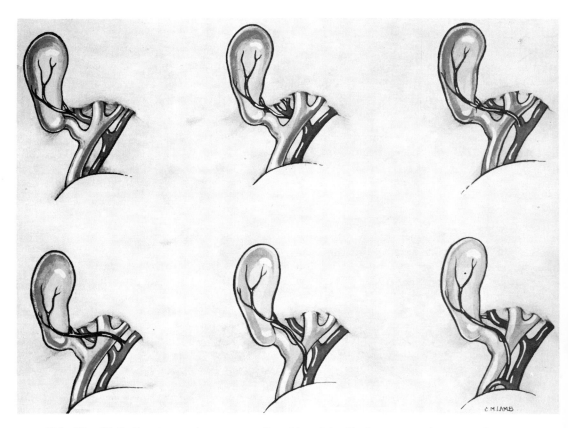

FIG. 18.   (E) Cystic artery and some anomalies of its origin. The bottom row shows a cystic artery arising from the left gastric artery; one from the common hepatic artery; and one arising from the gastroduodenal artery. (Adapted from Gray and Whitesell.)

top of the common hepatic duct, it may also be inadvertently clamped or divided during a difficult cholecystectomy or during a secondary operation upon the bile passages. When there is a wide communication between the gallbladder and bile duct, and no cystic duct is visible, the right hepatic artery, which may be lying behind the gallbladder, may be traumatised when the broad isthmus is being clamped or divided. It should be remembered that the following arteries may pass anterior to the bile ducts: the cystic, the common hepatic, the gastroduodenal, and the superior pancreaticoduodenal.

The *cystic artery* springs from the right hepatic artery in 95 percent of cases. In the remaining 5 percent, it arises from the left hepatic artery, from the main parent trunk, from the junction of the right and left hepatic arteries, or even from the gastroduodenal or inferior mesenteric artery (Fig. 18). In 16 percent of cases, it passes in front of the common hepatic duct, while in 84 percent, it arises medial to or immediately posterior to this duct. Michels [67] pointed out that a crossing of the common hepatic duct by the cystic artery was found in 50 out of 200 cases (25 percent).

Gray and Whitesell [32] have reviewed the variation in the morphological arrangement of the right hepatic and cystic arteries encountered in a series of 100 consecutive cases of cholecystectomies. In 54 of these cases, the right hepatic artery paralleled the cystic duct for a considerable distance before giving off its cystic branch (Figs. 19, 20).

An *accessory cystic artery* is found in 12 percent of cases. In 8 percent, two cystic arteries arise from the right hepatic artery. In but 1 percent of cases: (1) one artery arises from the right hepatic artery and the other from the gastroduodenal artery; (2) the accessory artery arises from the main hepatic trunk; (3) both vessels arise from the left hepatic artery; or (4) the accessory artery arises from the gastroduodenal, the superior pancreaticoduodenal, or superior mesenteric artery.

When an accessory cystic artery is present, it frequently passes in front of the bile duct. Ignorance of the presence of accessory cystic arteries may be responsible for a severe haemorrhage during the preliminary dissection in Calot's triangle, which is necessary prior to cholecystectomy or exploration of the common duct.

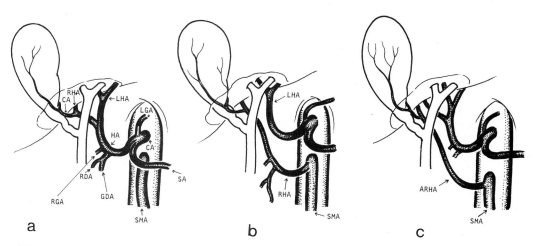

FIG. 19. Some anomalies of the hepatic arteries. CA, coeliac axis. SA, splenic artery. LGA, left gastric artery. HA, hepatic artery. CHA, common hepatic artery. RHA, right hepatic artery. LHA, left hepatic artery. CA, cystic artery. GDA, gastroduodenal artery. RGA, right gastric artery. SMA, superior mesenteric artery. ARHA, anomalous right hepatic artery. First picture on the left shows so-called normal arrangements of the feeding vessels of the liver and gallbladder. RDA, retroduodenal artery. Note the replacing and aberrant right hepatic arteries. (After Hollinshead.)

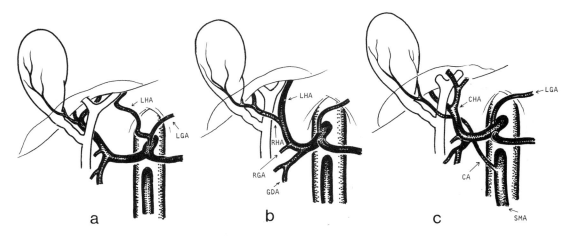

FIG. 20. Some anomalies of the hepatic arteries. (A) An aberrant left hepatic artery arising from the left gastric artery. (C) An aberrant cystic artery arising from the superior mesenteric artery. (Adapted from Gross, Hollinshead, and Netter, copyright The CIBA Collection of Medical Illustrations (III).)

The *gastroduodenal artery* is of importance in operations involving the common bile duct, as in 20 percent of cases it crosses in front of the supraduodenal position of the common duct, while in a further 36 percent it reaches across the left border of the duct. In 76 percent of cases, the superior pancreaticoduodenal artery, which is a branch of the gastroduodenal artery, crosses the lower end of the common bile duct.

Grant, Fitts, and Ravdin,[31] in reporting two cases of *aneurysm of the hepatic artery,* offer the following conclusions:

1. Aneurysm of the hepatic artery, although a rare cause of biliary symptoms, must be considered in the differential diagnosis of jaundice. Hepatic aneurysm produces pain, jaundice, and bleeding into the gastrointestinal tract. Heretofore, the diagnosis has rarely been made before death and only 14 patients with aneurysm had been operated upon up to 1950.

2. Two additional hepatic aneurysms, both diagnosed at operation, are reported. Both patients died—one from massive hepatic necrosis, the other from recurrent haemorrhage.

3. The only reported cures of hepatic aneurysm have been achieved by ligation of the artery.

Several recent developments may improve the results of treatment, although to our knowledge they are still untested in humans: (a) the use of antibiotics in the prevention of liver necrosis following ligation; (b) reconstruction of the artery by grafts of artery or veins; and (c) anastomosis of the ligated hepatic artery to the portal system.

Browning, Clauss, and MacFee[17] state that aneurysm of the hepatic artery is infrequently diagnosed during life, and rarely treated successfully. To date, 124 cases have been reported in the literature. Kirklin[46] reviewed 105 published cases and added one of his own, this being the first aneurysm to be successfully excised. Since Kirklin's paper, 18 other cases have been reported by Inui (1956), Mainette (1956), Sheridan (1956), Hejnal (1957), Merle (1957), and others. Jewett,[43] in reporting a case of aneurysm of the hepatic artery in a girl of 13, states that in childhood lesions such as choledochal cyst and malignant tumours enter into the differential diagnosis. The presenting clinical picture is often that of abdominal pain, fever, jaundice, epigastric mass, anaemia, and gastrointestinal haemorrhage. It is important to establish a correct preoperative diagnosis.

This, according to Jewett, can be effectively done by angiogram with catheterisation of the aorta, either through the femoral or brachial artery. At the conclusion of the aortogram, intravenous pyelograms can be done with the same injection of dye, which will define the position and contour of the right kidney. (See Chapter 108 on selective angiography.)

Jewett[109] says that ligation, surgical excision, or aneurysmorrhaphy, under hypothermia, is the treatment of choice. Recently, Bristol et al.[15] reported the second case of aneurysm of the hepatic artery which was successfully treated by *resection followed by end-to-end anastomosis*. The presenting symptoms were severe and persistent pain in the gallbladder area and in the back, and indigestion. Cholecystography showed negative results and the aneurysm was diagnosed by means of coeliac arteriograms.

Hepatic artery injury. Karasewich and Bowden[44] have submitted a valuable report on seven patients with hepatic artery injury who had been admitted to the Memorial Hospital, New York. Their reviews of some of the established facts about such injuries in experimental animals and in human beings and their discussion of worthwhile approaches to treatment constitute a valuable document which calls for careful study. Karasewich and Bowden submit the following summary:

Six instances of accidental, obligatory, or deliberate injury to the hepatic artery occurred during operations at the Memorial Center for Cancer between 1950 and 1966. Two patients in whom the artery was immediately repaired survived, but 4 patients died with massive ischemic necrosis of the liver possibly aggravated by superimposed infection. One other patient survived gradual occlusion of the hepatic artery during the infusion of 5-fluorouracil for metastatic carcinoma of the liver, but died later from staphylococcal pneumonia and septicemia.

If injury to the hepatic artery is recognized during an operation, reconstitution of the vessel should be carried out promptly. If such reconstitution is impossible, and if part of the hepatic arterial supply is intact, resection of the infarcted portion of the liver is recommended.

If hepatic artery occlusion is suspected postoperatively, surgical re-exploration is probably indicated. If this is not feasible, the patient should be vigorously treated with broad spectrum antibiotics, adequate blood replacement, and hyperbaric oxygen.

REFERENCES

1. Acromond and Barnett, Am. J. Dig. Dis. 4:556, 1959.
2. Alden and Sterner, Ann. Surg. 145:269, 1957.
3. Anderson and Ross, Arch. Surg. 76:7, 1958.
4. Anschutz, Bol. Acad. Cir. 31:806, 1947.
5. Arthur, Br. Med. J. 2:265, 1937.
6. Bartel, Wien Klin. Wochenschr. 31:605, 1916.
7. Bhagavan, Arch. Path. 89:382, 1970.
8. Bigg, Arch. Surg. 88:501, 1964.
9. Bleich et al., J.A.M.A. 147:849, 1951.
10. Bower, Ann. Surg. 88:80, 1928.
11. Boyden, Am. J. Anat. 38:177, 1926.
12. Boyden, Surg. Gynecol. Obstet. 104:641, 1957.
13. Boyden, Am. J. Roentgenol. 33:589, 1935.
13a. Braasch, Surg. Clin. North Am. 38:627, 1958.
14. Braun, Chirurg. 53:1055, 1926.
15. Bristol et al., Am. J. Surg. 120:97, 1970.
16. Bronner, Botr. Klin. Chir. 145:132, 1928.
17. Browning, Clauss, and MacFee, Ann. Surg. 150:320, 1959.
18. Carter et al., Surg. Gynecol. Obstet. 116:105, 1963.
19. Caster, Int. Abstr. Surg. 103:439, 1956.
20. Climan, Med. J. Rec. 130:73, 1929.
21. Danzis, Am. J. Surg. 29:202, 1935.
22. Dixon and Lichtman, Surgery 17:11, 1945.
23. Dowdy, G., Jr., The Biliary Tract, Philadelphia, Lea & Febiger, 1969.
24. Dunkerley, Proc. R. Soc. Med. 57:331, 1964.
25. Eisendrath, J.A.M.A. 71:864, 1918.
26. Finney and Owen, Ann. Surg. 115:736, 1942.
27. Flannery and Caster, Am. J. Gastroenterol. 46:402, 1966.
28. Flint, Br. J. Surg. 10:509, 1923.
29. Foster and Mayson, Am. J. Surg. 104:14, 1962.
30. Gerwig et al., Ann. Surg. 153:113, 1961.
31. Grant, Fitts, and Ravdin, Surg. Gynecol. Obstet. 91:525, 1950.
32. Gray and Whitesell, Surg. Clin. North Am. 30:1001, 1950.
32a. Grosberg, Am. J. Dig. Dis. 7:1039, 1962.
33. Gross, Arch. Surg. 32:131, 1936.
34. Guyer et al., Br. J. Radiol. 40:214, 1967.
35. Hammond et al., J. Med. Soc. N. J. 62:514, 1965.
36. Haslam et al., Am. J. Dis. Child. 112:600, 1966.
37. Herrington, L., Jr., Am. J. Surg. 112:106, 1966.
38. Hicken et al., Surgery 25:431, 1949.
39. Hobby, Br. J. Surg. 57:870, 1970.
40. Hochstetter, Arch. Anat. Entwick., pp. 369-384, 1886.
41. Hollinshead, Textbook of Anatomy, 2d ed., Cassell, 1968.
41a. Hollinshead, Anatomy for Surgeons, New York, Hoeber, 1968, Vol. 2.
42. Hurwitz, J. Maine Med. Assoc. 55:79, 1964.
43. Jewett, Ann. Surg. 150:951, 1959.
44. Karasewich and Bowden, Surg. Gynecol. Obstet. 124:1057, 1967.
45. Kennon, Br. J. Surg. 20:522, 1933.
46. Kirklin, Ann. Surg. 142:110, 1955.
47. Knetsch, Fortschr. Geb. Roentgenstr. Nuklearmed. 77:587, 1952.
48. Langer and Pearson, Canad. J. Surg. 6:29, 1963.
49. Large, Arch. Surg. 87:982, 1963.
50. Latimer et al., Ann. Surg. 127:810, 1947.
51. Leger et al., J. Chir. 61:21, 1945.
52. Levene, A., Br. J. Surg. 45:338, 1958.
53. Lichtenstein, Surg. Gynecol. Obstet. 64:684, 1937.
54. Linder and Green, Surg. Clin. North Am. 46:1273, 1964.
55. McCrea, Br. J. Surg. 38:386, 1951.
56. McIlrath et al., J.A.M.A. 180:782, 1962.
57. McNamee, Am. J. Roentgenol. 33:603, 1935.
58. Mackie, Postgrad. Med. J. 42:213, 1966.

59. Maingot, Br. J. Clin. Pract. 26, 1972.
60. Maingot, in Smith and Sherlock, eds., Surgery of the Gallbladder and Bile Ducts, London, Butterworths, Chaps. 2 and 4, 1964.
61. Maingot, in Rob and Smith, eds., Operative Surgery, Vol. 4, London, Butterworths, 1969.
62. Malmstrom, Acta Chir. Scand. 105:440, 1953.
63. May, Br. J. Clin. Pract. 21:191, 1967.
64. Mayo, C. W., and Kendrick, Arch. Surg. 60: 668, 1950.
65. Meyer et al., Am. J. Roentgenol. 37:788, 1937.
66. Michaels, J.A.M.A. 172:125, 1960.
67. Michels, Ann. Surg. 133:503, 1951.
68. Monroe and Ragan, Calif. Med. 85:422, 1956.
69. Mossman, Anat. Rec. 100:289, 1948.
70. Mouzas and Wilson, Lancet 1:628, 1953.
71. Netter, F., The CIBA Collection of Medical Illustrations, Vol. III, Part III, 1957, p. 123.
72. Newcombe and Henley, Arch. Surg. 88:494, 1964.
73. Nichols, Radiology 6:255, 1926.
74. Niemeier, Surgery 12:584, 1942.
75. Perelman, J.A.M.A. 175:710, 1961.
76. Rabinovitch et al., Ann. Surg. 148:161, 1958.
77. Rains, Harding, Br. J. Surg. 39:37, 1951.
78. Rais and Thuzen, Acta Chir. Scand. 113:289, 1957.
79. Recht, Br. J. Surg. 39:342, 1952.
80. Richards, Can. Med. Assoc. J. 94:859, 1966.
81. Roeder, Mersheimer, and Kazarian, Am. J. Surg. 121:746, 1971.
82. Rothman, in H. Bockus, ed., Gastroenterology, 2nd ed., Vol. III, Philadelphia, Saunders, 1966, Chap. 108, p. 595.
83. Satpathy, J. Indian Med. Assoc. 47:130, 1966.
84. Schachner, Ann. Surg. 64:419, 1916.
85. Schein, Acute Cholecystitis, New York, Harper & Row, 1972.
86. Seifert, Wis. Med. J. 62:259, 1963.
87. Shah, Br. J. Clin. Pract. 20:535, 1966.
88. Sherren, Ann. Surg. 54:206, 1911.
89. Short and Paul, Br. J. Surg. 22:301, 1934.
90. Simon and Tandon, Radiology 80:84, 1963.
91. Skielboe, Am. J. Clin. Path. 30:252, 1958.
92. Smyth, Lancet 1:301, 1949.
93. Sperling, Arch. Surg. 88:1077, 1964.
94. Stearson, Aust. N.Z. J. Surg. 39:255, 1970.
95. Stolkind, Br. J. Child. Dis. 36:115, 1939.
96. Sullivan and Appleby, Wis. Med. 62:149, 1963.
97. Thompson and Dormandy, Br. J. Surg. 47:203, 1959.
98. Wakeley, C., Br. J. Surg. 15:334, 1927.
99. Weisel and Walters, W., Am. J. Surg. 16:753, 1941.
100. Wendel, Ann. Surg. 27:199, 1898.
101. Wilson, C. Ann. Surg. 110:60, 1939.
102. Yamashita et al., Am. J. Surg. 46:402, 1966.

41

A. GALLSTONES: NATURE AND AETIOLOGY

A. J. HARDING RAINS

Gallstones are common. *Surveys have shown that in the "developed" countries gallstones are present in at least 20 percent of women over the age of forty.*[1] In men, the incidence is less, but it increases with age, and by the seventh or eighth decade reaches 20 percent. Even in children, infants, and in the newborn, the disease is no longer a curiosity and several series have been published.[2] Overweight people are a little more prone than are those who are thin or underweight, and, in general, repeated pregnancies favour stone formation (see below). The old axiom that a typical gallstone sufferer is a woman who is fat, forty, and fertile is only partly true, and in recent years there has been an increase in the number of relatively young women admitted for cholecystectomy soon after their first pregnancy.

Operations on the biliary tract, of which the majority are for gallstones (cholecystectomy and choledocholithotomy) are amongst the operations most commonly performed in large communities today. Surgeons and physicians have often remarked on "epidemics" of gallstones in various countries, the most notable being manifest in Scandinavia by the dramatic fourfold rise, in some city hospitals, in operations for stones, which reached 1,000 per year between 1945 and 1955.

This marked incidence of gallstones is not characteristic of some parts of the world, however. For example, in Egypt the incidence is curiously low and the fat and fertile women of forty seem to be relatively immune.[3] In Japan and in Korea, the incidence of the type of gallstone seems to be related to class, occupation, and the degree of affluence.[4, 5] In India, gallstones are found in some districts but not in others. In Bogota, Columbia, the poorer classes are most commonly afflicted. Such findings suggest that diet must play a significant role in the aetiology of stones (see below).

NATURE OF GALLSTONES

Gallstones are crystalline bodies formed from the constituents of bile; the character of the stone depends mainly upon the predominance of one or more constituents (Fig. 1). Amongst the constituents of bile are found types of cholesterol, bile acids, bile pigments, protein, carbonate, phosphate, calcium, sodium, potassium, and enzymes (such as glucuronidase and phosphatase). Crystallisation takes place most commonly in the gallbladder. Primary stones in the hepatic and common bile ducts are less crystalline than primary gallbladder stones and are more like a concretion of sludge (Fig. 1).

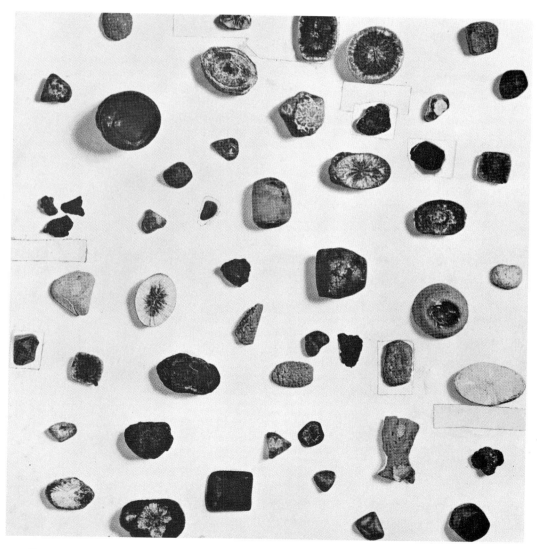

FIG. 1. Gallstones. (Courtesy of the editor, Spectrum International, Pfizer International Subsidiaries.)

Classification

In general, gallstones are divided into three groups by the naked eye appearance of the constituent in major proportion: (1) cholesterol, (2) pigment, and (3) mixed cholesterol/pigment stones. With such a classification, up to 10 percent are solitary or multiple cholesterol stones; 75 to 80 percent are mixed; and the rest (about 15 percent) are pigment stones. This is an inaccurate classification if more than a working knowledge is required. The old established chemical methods of analysis have now given way to the separation and identification of the constituents by the methods of column chromatography, thin-layer chromatography, infrared spectrophotometry (Fig. 2), and x-ray diffraction.[6] These methods may, for example, reveal the presence of bile acids, protein, carbonate, and phosphate in a stone regarded as pure pigment or pure cholesterol by the naked eye—a matter of some moment if any special consideration is to be given to the cause of the stone in a particular patient.

The centre of a gallstone varies in appearance and constituents. In some stones, there is a clear crystalline pattern radiating from the centre; in others the centre may be homogeneous and irregular, and crystallisation may begin at a little distance therefrom. Occasionally the centre is hollow and creviced in a triradiate (Mercedes Benz) or biradiate (Seagull) pattern. Gas has been reported in these crevices, and it may be discernible on plain x-ray (Mercedes Benz sign, Seagull sign).[7]

Analysis of the centre of the stone may give an indication of the origin of the gallstone. Unfortunately, no one single constituent predominates, be it bilirubin, cholesterol, protein, unconjugated bile acids,[8] cells, ova, etc. It is a mistake to think that all gallstones come from one cause—even observations by the naked eye and the analytical evidence of the centre suggest otherwise.

Size and Shape

Gallstones may be single or multiple, small or large, round, mulberry, coral-like, and facetted. These characteristics are an expression of the environment in which the

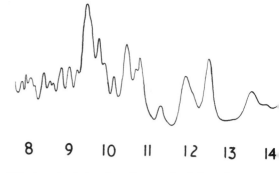

FIG. 2. Analysis of gallstones by infrared spectrophotometer. Cholesterol was detected in peaks at 9.5, 10.5, 11.95, and 12.59 wavelength microns.

stone or stones began and continued to grow. For example, a single cholesterol "solitaire" is classically supposed to form in an aseptic environment of bile stasis in a gallbladder, while multiple mixed stones denote infection. Sometimes a single cholesterol stone is found together with a number of mixed stones, the former being called primary and the latter secondary. Mulberry stones bespeak crystallisation in a proteinous (or colloid) medium, while coral-like (largely pigment) and sharply edged stones (cholesterol) are formed in a more aqueous phase. The appearance of facets between stones owes to irregular crystallisation caused by the juxtaposition of other stones. Very rarely, with large stones, a facet may be caused by fracture of the stone.

Aetiology

Cholesterol and bile pigment are insoluble in water and would be insoluble in bile if it were not for the formation of soluble complexes and compounds. Disturbance of these complexes will result in the emergence of these substances in crystalline or paracrystalline forms.

BASIC METABOLIC CONSIDERATIONS (SOLUBILITIES)

Cholesterol/bile acid relationship. It is in the liver that the structure of a quantity of cholesterol is altered to form bile acids.

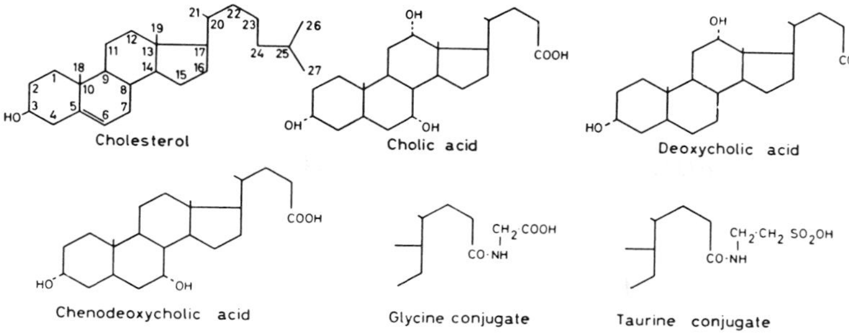

FIG. 3.   The main human bile acids.

In the human, these acids are either the unconjugated cholic, deoxycholic, or chenodeoxycholic types, or the conjugated glycocholic and taurocholic acids (Fig. 3). The old chemical axiom that "like dissolves like" applies in this instance; the bile acids dissolve cholesterol—or, more exactly, they render cholesterol soluble. The mystery surrounding this phenomenon was clarified when it was discovered that the bile acids form molecular aggregates (micelles) in solutions at physiological concentrations and at body temperature.[9] These molecular aggregates behave like modern detergents and, having water-attracting and water-repellent parts, are able to absorb and carry an insoluble substance in an aqueous medium (Fig. 4).

Cholesterol/bile acid ratio. The cholesterol-dissolving power of the bile acids increases with their concentration. Providing the ratio of cholesterol to bile acid is no more than 1:12 at 37.5° C, the cholesterol will remain in solution (critical ratio) (Fig. 5). Should the cholesterol content of bile be increased or the bile acid concentration be reduced, cholesterol will come out of solution. A significant increase in cholesterol excretion by the liver is unlikely. Curiously enough, a relative increase occurs in starvation, and cholesterol-rich diets [10] or hypercholesteraemic states [11] may not cause cholesterol-rich bile or, in any case, upset the ratio. Only in some types of cholecystitis (empyema) does the cholesterol exceed the ratio, probably as a result of an increased exfoliation of cells.

Bile acid production by the liver may be reduced by feeding sucrose,[12] and by liver poisons. Currently it is believed that a lithogenic bile, low in bile acid content, is the consequence of a reduction of the constituents of the bile acid pool in the liver, especially chenodeoxycholic acid [13, 14] (see below). The association between gallstone formation and disease or removal of the ileum [15] is considered to be due to reduced reabsorption of bile acids in the lower small intestine (i.e., a break in the enterohepatic circulation of bile acids). Also, the bile acid content of gallbladder bile may be reduced by absorption through an inflamed gallbladder wall. One other important way in which the critical cholesterol/bile acid ratio may be upset is by the presence of an interface (discussed below).

Bile pigment solubility. This depends upon the catalytic action of glucuroni-

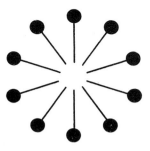

FIG. 4.   A spherical micelle formed by the aggregation of bile acid molecules. The rounded end of each molecule is water-loving (hydrophilic), whilst the stick end is the hydrophobic part to which the water-insoluble cholesterol is absorbed. (From Bailey and Love. *Short Practice of Surgery*, 15th ed., Courtesy of Professor A. H. Rains, H. K. Lewis and Co., Ltd., London.)

dase for the formation of bilirubin diglu-curonide. Bile pigment overload on the liver —such as occurs periodically with the haemo-lytic crisis of various haemolytic diseases, in-cluding malaria—may result in the extrusion into the biliary canaliculi of unconjugated and insoluble bilirubin particles which may fuse to form larger pigment stones or act as the centre of a larger and mixed gallstone. Liver poisons [16] and infection also result in a similar state of pigment insolubility. That bile pigment particles are the basis of the formation of all gallstones was the thesis of Rovsing (Fig. 6); it is true that pigment may be found in the centre of most but not all stones.

DIET AND GALLSTONES

Reference has already been made to the variations in the incidence of gallstones according to geography. Probably the geo-graphic location and the climate play little part, but rather the incidence varies accord-ing to dietary intake. For example, in Bogota, Columbia, situated at a high altitude, the incidence of mixed stones in those who are well off is said to be very low, while that in the poorer classes is high. A possible explana-tion is that the poor exist on a diet which is low in protein and vitamins; they sustain themselves almost entirely upon cane sugar. In Japan and Korea, pigment stones in the bile ducts have been the most common type of gallstone in the agricultural and poorer classes.[17, 18] In Japanese urban communities, however, the mixed cholesterol/bile pigment stone predominates, the professional classes and housewives being affected as in the West. Certainly whenever diets are generous and high in caloric value (e.g., in the United States, Scandinavia, Belgium, Holland, France, and Germany), the incidence of stones is at its greatest. Probably the sucrose and general carbohydrate intake is more to blame than is the intake of cholesterol. In-deed most of the cholesterol absorbed from the intestine is believed to be endogenous (from exfoliated gastrointestinal cells).

Experimental diets. Bile duct stones have been produced in rats fed on a diet which is deficient in vitamin A.[19] Cattle fed in stall during the winter produce bile duct

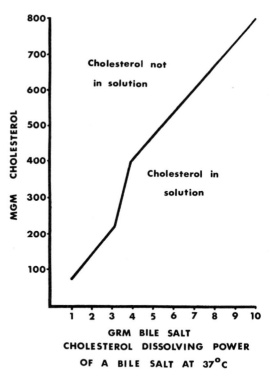

FIG. 5. Solubility of cholesterol in bile acid—the critical cholesterol/bile acid ratio at 37° C.

concretions, while they are free from them when grazing in open pastures during spring and summer. Hamsters are specially prone to gallstone formation and have been used extensively in experiments.[20, 21] It has been found that a diet lacking in fats and oils rather than in calories is lithogenic and that stone formation may be prevented by adding yeast and soya bean to the animals' daily intake.

The body of knowledge concerning diet and the incidence of gallstones begins to point to a high caloric intake (mainly in the form of confectioneries and the cereal foods with a high extraction rate).

OTHER FACTORS

Infection. The oldest theory about gallstone formation is that the nucleus or starting point of a stone arises from an in-flammatory exudate, a cellular exfoliation,

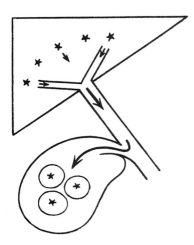

FIG. 6.   Rovsing's theory. Stones are formed around pigment particles from the liver.

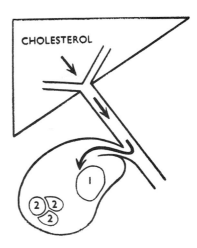

FIG. 8.   Aschoff and Bacmeister theory. (1) Cholesterol from the liver forms a primary aseptic cholesterol stone. (2) Later, secondary mixed stones form as a result of cholangitis.

or the presence of bacteria in the bile. Naunyn's thesis "no infection—no stones" (Fig. 7) was challenged by Rovsing ("all stones commence as pigment stones") and by Aschoff and Bacmeister (Fig. 8), who claimed that primary stones form in an aseptic environment purely as a result of biliary stasis. This last theory is often refuted on the grounds that all gallbladders containing stones show histological evidence of disease (though this

could be post hoc rather than propter hoc).

Firm support for the infective theory came many years ago from examples of typhoidal cholecystitis resulting in gallstones containing typhoid bacilli, and streptococcal inflammation with stones containing streptococci. Similarly, coliform organisms, staphylococci, and actinomyces have been implicated. (The last named is a common finding in salivary calculi and dental tartar.)

Parasites and parasite ova may also be found in the centre of stones (usually common duct stones), the best known examples being ova of the nematode *Ascaris lumbri-*

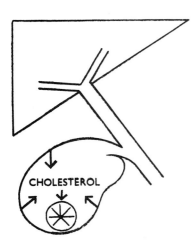

FIG. 7.   Naunyn's theory. Cholesterol comes from an inflamed gallbladder wall.

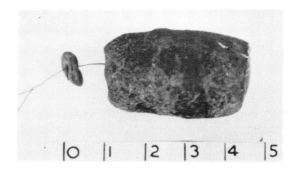

FIG. 9.   Large barrel-shaped and smaller ring-doughnut gallstone formed on a nylon suture; it was found in a dilated common bile duct.

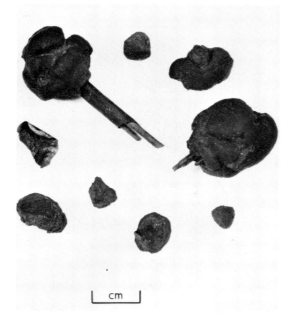

FIG. 10. Common bile duct gallstone; it had formed around a rolled-up plum skin.

coides or the fluke *Clonorchis sinensis* [22] (which causes Asiatic cholangiohepatitis [see Chap. 49]). In this context, comparison is frequently made between the pearl of the oyster, which Du Bois called "the brilliant sarcophagus of a worm," and the gallstone, which Moynihan said is "a tombstone erected to the memory of the organism within it."

Foreign bodies. These, like bacteria and parasites, act as centres (see *interfaces,* below) for stone formation. Unabsorbable sutures used in a previous biliary operation have been found on occasion (e.g., see Fig. 9), while a rolled-up tomato skin and a plum skin (Fig. 10) have worked their way into the common bile duct and caused a stone to form.

Stasis. Stasis is another factor in the formation of gallstones. In a gallbladder without some degree of stasis, any gallstones would be voided while very small. Stasis occurs most commonly during the last 3 months of pregnancy,[23] and that may be the cause of the increased incidence of gallstones in the woman who is blessed with fecundity rather than the existence of any hypercholesteraemia associated with pregnancy. Three

months is long enough for stones to crystallise into an appreciable size (see also *layering,* below).

Linked diseases. The stasis of gallbladder bile incurred by pregnancy suggests an overall and temporary variation of the balance of the autonomic nervous system—possibly emanating from the hypothalamus. Other conditions of what may be a similar aetiology are pyloric dysfunction with oesophageal regurgitation and (hiatal hernia) and diverticulosis. Cardiac irregularities may also be linked to the function and disease of the gallbladder (the cardiac link). Many of the patients with gallstones suffer from migraine.

pH. Hepatic bile is slightly alkaline and gallbladder bile is acid. In the presence of stasis or infection, the acidity increases. Precipitation from the cholesterol/bile acid complex occurs if the natural buffering power of bile acids is overcome. This favours stone formation and, perhaps, the type of crystal formation (see below). On occasion, as in the condition misguidedly called "empyema" of an inflamed gallbladder, the "pus" is a cream of cholesterol, lecithin, and, sometimes, calcium carbonate; it is usually sterile. With stasis and the precipitation of calcium salts, the cream may be radiopaque and is called "limey" bile.

Residual bile. Any cholecystogram demonstrates that it is unlikely that the gallbladder ever empties itself completely. There is always some residual bile, and in pregnancy the residuum is greater.[24] It has been shown that fresh incoming bile from the liver does not mix easily with this residuum, and it may well be that some of the residuum remains stagnant in the gallbladder.

Layering and interfacial tension. If the incoming bile does not mix freely with the residuum, *layering* occurs between these biles—biles which are of differing specific gravity, concentration of constituents, and pH. Layering is sometimes clinically evident on a cholecystogram (Figs. 11 and 12). When this occurs, an interface (with interfacial tension) exists between the layers. It has been shown that there is a migration of cholesterol and bile acids at different rates across the interface, with resultant local disturbance of the critical cholesterol/bile acid ratio.[25] Here, too, pH difference favours cholesterol

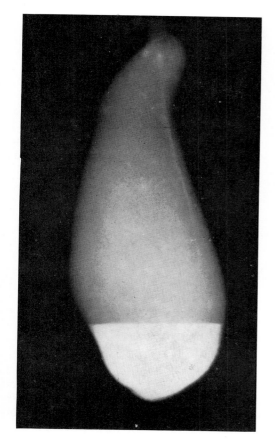

FIG. 11.   Limey (limewater) bile. X-ray taken after cholecystectomy.

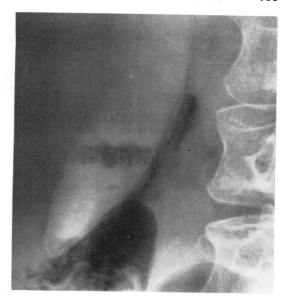

FIG. 12.   Layering of bile. Stones are floating at the interface between biles of different specific gravity.

precipitation if the buffering power of the bile is overcome.

Crystallisation. When any interface is present in a solution in which the solubility of a constituent is critical, crystal formation may begin. When the solution is colloidal, owing to the presence of protein, the crystallisation begins in what is called a paracrystalline form—as minute amorphous spheroliths.[26] These spheroliths coalesce to form larger spheres and change within from an amorphous to a radiating crystalline structure (Fig. 13). The phenomenon can be demonstrated experimentally with cholesterol and also calcium carbonate, and it is often manifest to the surgeon in practice when he finds mulberry stones in a gallbladder (Fig. 14). In an aqueous phase, however, cholesterol crystallises in wavy criss-crossing bundles (rather like a ball of wool), and this (the myelin form of cholesterol) also may be encountered in practice.[27, 28] The pH of the bile at the time of stone growth is also believed to affect the form that the crystals take, but the detail of this influence has yet to be worked out.

DISSOLVING GALLSTONES

Once crystallisation of stones of visible size takes place, the problem of dissolving them will only be resolved by the application of further knowledge of the chemistry of gallstone formation and the physical chemistry of crystallisation. The curious phenomenon of stone formation in cattle fed in stall during the winter (with immunity when fed on fresh grass during the summer) first requires a biochemical explanation rather than the empirical adoption of bizarre fresh-vegetable and grass diets. So far, low cholesterol diets and the exhibition of cholesterol-inhibiting substances have no effect in reducing the size of a stone.[29] Theoretically, the aim should be to produce secretion of a bile with a low cholesterol and a high bile acid content in order that sufficient bile acid

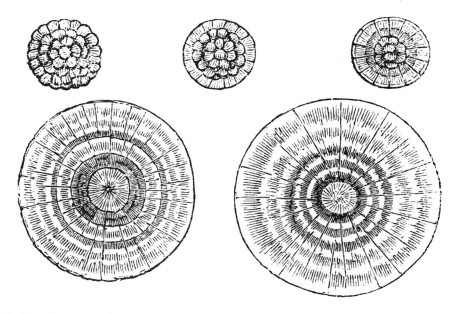

FIG. 13.   Formation of concretions and stones. The top left shows coalescence of spheroliths which gradually merge to form a concretion with concentric laminae and radiating lines of crystallisation. (After Rainey.)

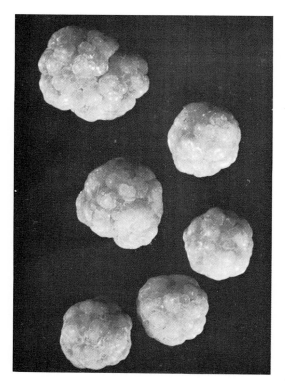

FIG. 14.   Mulberry cholesterol gallstones formed by coalescence of smaller stones measuring less than 1 mm.

micelles are available for bringing the cholesterol in a stone into solution. Recently,[30] cholesterol stones were dissolved in one patient and partially dissolved in three patients (no effect on another three) following prolonged administration of chenodeoxycholic acid) (see above and Fig. 3). The rationale for this treatment was based on the finding of reduced chenodeoxycholic acid in total bile acid pools of gallstone sufferers. Treatment has to be prolonged (about 2 years) and the bile acid may have side effects and toxicity.

Using a T Tube

Stone-dissolving substances have been injected down a T tube for the purpose of dissolving a stone left in the common bile duct after choledochotomy. Certainly, in vitro, a human gallstone can be dissolved in dog's bile, which has a high concentration of bile acids. Unfortunately, this method appears to be of doubtful practical value, as it means prolonged hospitalisation; further, it is uncertain if all the constituents and any organic matrix of a stone will be dispersed. A similar application has been made for many years of the cholesterol-dissolving power of ether, but, in practice, it is also of doubtful value and certainly the introduction of more than 2 ml ether down a T tube may be dangerous (1 ml ether at body temperature can evaporate to 200 ml vapour).[31]

Spontaneous Disappearance

That gallstones can disappear spontaneously is undoubtedly true.[32] Patients in whom stones were known to be present on x-ray examination have been found to be free from them on subsequent laparotomy, while on other occasions a gallbladder has emptied itself after a series of attacks of gallstone colic. In order to pass down the ducts, these stones are rarely larger than 3 to 5 mm in diameter and may be of recent origin; the patient most likely to have this condition is a woman just after a pregnancy.

CONCLUSION

It is probable that there is no single cause of gallstones. Chemical analysis and bacteriological examination do not pinpoint a common factor. In general, a gallstone is primarily a crystallisation of those constituents of the bile which would be insoluble if it were not for the formation of special soluble complexes or compounds (cholesterol/bile acid micelle complex, bilirubin glucuronide). Any disturbance in the formation or maintenance of these complexes or compounds—occasioned by diet (carbohydrate) and infection in the case of the pigment—make stone formation likely. The act of crystallisation probably depends upon the appearance of an interface (and interfacial tension) in a more or less colloid (proteinous) environment in varying hydrogen ion concentrations. Epithelial cells, organisms, foreign bodies, parasites, and small particles of pigment are likely causes of an interface. Layering of bile, particularly when stasis occurs, produces another kind of interface which may explain the so-called aseptic primary stone formation of Aschoff and Bacmeister.

References

Most of the material used for this chapter is derived from the monograph *Gallstones—Causes and Treatment* by A. J. Harding Rains, published by William Heinemann Medical Books Ltd., London, 1964. A selection of references cited therein is included here together with other publications.

1. Horn, G., Br. Med. J. 2:732, 1956.
2. Soderlund, S., and Zetterstrom, B., Arch. Dis. Child. 37:174, 1928.
3. Zaki, O. A., and Kamel, R., Br. J. Surg. 54:8, 713, 1967.
4. Maki, T., Arch. Surg. 82:599, 1961.
5. Yagi, T., Tohoku J. Exp. Med. 72:117, 1960.
6. Juniper, K., Am. J. Med. 20:383, 1956.
7. Hay, H. R. C., Gut 7:387, 1966.
8. Schoenfield, J., Sjovall, J., and Sjovall, K., J. Lab. Clin. Med. 68:186, 1966.
9. Rains, A. J. H., and Crawford, N., Nature 171: 829, 1953.
10. Patey, D. H., Br. J. Surg. 22:378, 1934.
11. Piper, J., and Orrild, L., Am. J. Med. 21:34, 1956.
12. Wright, A., and Whipple, G. H., J. Exp. Med. 59:411, 1934.
13. Vlahcevic, Z. R., Bell, C. C., Jr., and Swell, L., Gastroenterology 59:62, 1970.
14. Vlahcevic, Z. R., Bell, C. C., Jr., Buhac, I., et al., Gastroenterology 59:165, 1970.
15. Heaton, K. W., Read, A. E., Br. Med. J. 3:494, 1969.
16. Naunyn and Minkowski. Cited by O. Hammarsten, in A Textbook of Physiological Chemistry. 7th ed., trans.: J. A. Mandel, New York, Wiley, 1914.
17. Jessen, C., Acta Chir. Scand. (Suppl.) 283:242, 1961.
18. Hur, K. B., Rice, R. G., and Sa Suk Hong, Yonsei Med. J. 4:103, 1963.
19. Fujimake, Y., Jap. Med. World 6:29, 1926.
20. Dam, H., and Christensen, F., Acta Path. Microbiol. Scand. 30:236, 1952.
21. Christensen, F., Dam, H., and Kristensen, G., Acta Physiol. 36:329, 1956.
22. Stock, F. E., in C. Wells and J. Kyle, eds., Scientific Foundation of Surgery. London, Heinemann, 1967.
23. Gerdes, M. M., and Boyden, E. A., Surg. Gynecol. Obstet. 66:145, 1938.
24. Tera, H., Acta Chir. Scand. (Suppl.) 256, 1960.
25. Fitz-James, P., and Burton, A. C., Canad. J. Res. (Sect. E.) 27:309, 1949.
26. Rainey, G., On the Mode of Formation of Shells of Animals, of Bone, and of several Other Structures by a Process of Molecular Coalescence Demonstrable in Certain Artificially Formed Products. London, Churchill, 1858.
27. Montgomery, E., Proc. R. Soc. 15:314, 1866.
28. Ord, W. M., On the Influence of Colloids upon Crystalline Form and Cohesion (with Observations on the Structure and Mode of Formation of Urinary and other Calculi). London, Stanford, 1879.
29. Johnston, C. G., and Nakayama, F., Arch. Surg. 75:436, 1957.
30. Danzinger, R. G., Hofmann, A. F., Schoenfield,

L. J., Thistle, J. L., Dissolution of cholesterol gallstones by chenodeoxycholic acid. New Engl. J. Med. 286:1, 1972.

31. Rains, A. J. H., Br. J. Surg. 39:37, 1951.
32. Oschner, S. F., and Giesen, A. F., Am. J. Roentgenol. 83:831, 1960.

B. TYPES OF CHOLECYSTITIS: THE MANAGEMENT OF ACUTE AND CHRONIC CALCULOUS CHOLECYSTITIS

RODNEY MAINGOT

CHOLECYSTITIS GLANDULARIS PROLIFERANS

In a small percentage of patients with gallbladder disease, the gallbladder, either on radiological examination or pathological examination or on both, will show one or more of the following changes: (a) a transverse stricture, (b) a fundal nodule—the so-called fundal adenoma, or (c) extramural sinuses, which together make up the condition most commonly known as cholecystitis glandularis proliferans. In describing the radiological and pathological features of this disease, Le Quesne and Ranger [29] point out that the essential features of the condition are the presence, in localised areas, of epithelial sinuses (Rokitansky-Aschoff sinuses) which penetrate through the muscle coat of the gallbladder to expand in the subserous layer, together with localised hypertrophy of the muscularis of the gallbladder. These changes may or may not be accompanied by a varying degree of chronic inflammation, and often the gallbladder also contains stones or biliary gravel.

As opposed to chronic cholecystitis, which affects the whole gallbladder, the changes of cholecystitis glandularis proliferans occur in localised areas, forming either a stricture at a varying site in the gallbladder (Fig. 15), or a fundal adenoma (Fig. 16)—although in some

instances the two lesions may coexist and extend to surround the distal portion of the gallbladder (Figs. 15, 16, 17, 18). The typical distribution of the lesions is shown in Fig. 18. In a recent study of transverse strictures of the gallbladder, Beilby [30] has produced strong evidence that these defects are congenital in origin, that the changes of epithelial sinus formation and muscular hypertrophy are secondary to the narrowing produced by the stricture, and that, similarly, a fundal "adenoma" develops only in the presence of such a stricture or of a narrowing at the junction of the gallbladder and cystic duct.[3] Cholecystitis glandularis proliferans is not a premalignant condition, but it is commonly associated with gallstones which probably form on small concretions originating in the epithelial sinuses.

The condition is usually recognised on cholecystography performed in the investigation of a patient with symptoms suggesting gallbladder disease. The radiological appearances of the condition are well described by Colqhoun.[9] When gallstones are also present, cholecystectomy is indicated; however, it is not certain that a stricture or fundal adenoma are by themselves capable of producing symptoms of sufficient severity to warrant this operation. When there is well-marked sinus formation, clearly visible on cholecystography, and when the stricture is broad, it is probable that the condition gives rise to significant symptoms warranting cholecystec-

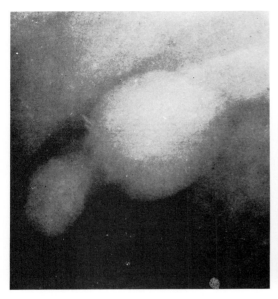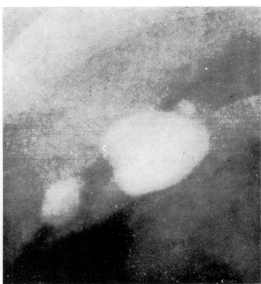

FIG. 15. Cholecystitis glandularis proliferans. (A) Cholecystogram showing a broad stricture dividing gallbladder into two unequal portions, the distal loculus having irregular walls. (B) When the gallbladder contracts after a fatty meal, a contraction of hypertrophied muscle in the stricture divides the lumen of gallbladder into two separate cavities. Examination of the excised gallbladder showed a narrow stricture; proximal to this area the gallbladder was normal but the wall of the distal loculus was thickened, with multiple cystic spaces containing calculi; microscopy also showed muscular hypertrophy with chronic inflammatory changes. (From LeQuesne and Ranger. *Br. J. Surg.* 44:447, 1957.)

tomy, but care should be taken before symptoms are ascribed to a small fundal adenoma or narrow stricture.

CHOLESTEROSIS OF THE GALLBLADDER

This condition, sometimes known as the *strawberry gallbladder,* in which the epithelial lining and stroma of the mucous membrane of the gallbladder are infiltrated with lipid and especially with cholesterol esters, is of comparatively frequent occurrence. It affects middle-aged patients, and the incidence bears no relation to sex or social status. There are two types: in the first, there is a diffuse infiltration of the entire mucous membrane of the gallbladder, while in the second, small lipoid-laden papillomas are seen. The detachment of these may furnish the nuclei for mulberry-like cholesterol stones. Virchow (1857) was one of the first to describe the presence of lipoid material in the epithelium of a gallbladder obtained at postmortem examination. Naunyn (1896) reported that there was a marked concentration of cholesterol esters in the bile of many patients with calculous cholecystitis.

McCarty[32] was the first to use the term *strawberry gallbladder.* Moynihan[39] gave a vivid description of the macroscopic appearance of the disease (for which he advocated cholecystectomy) while Mentzel[35] was the first to make use of the term *cholesterosis.*

Much of our present knowledge of strawberry gallbladder we owe to Boyd,[6] who accurately described the nature of the lipid material involved in the infiltration. The aetiology of the condition is as yet obscure.

Cholesterosis usually occurs in association with a mild catarrhal cholecystitis, and cholesterol stones are found in the gallbladder in nearly half of the cases. The *necropsy incidence* of cholesterosis varies from 12 to 38 percent, while the incidence in cases of excised gallbladders ranges from 9 to 20 percent. To the naked eye, the exterior of the

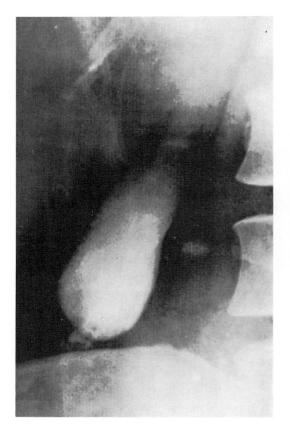

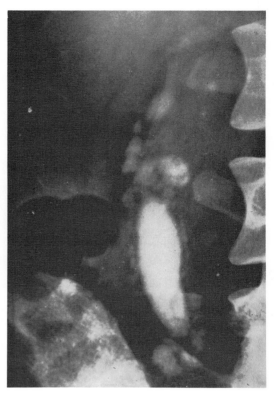

FIG. 16. Cholecystitis glandularis proliferans. Cholecystogram showing fundal filling defect with irregular, dye-filled spaces projecting into the centre—typical appearances of so-called fundal adenoma. (From LeQuesne and Ranger. *Br. J. Surg.* 44:447, 1957).

FIG. 17. Cholecystitis glandularis proliferans. Cholecystogram showing the main portion of the gallbladder surrounded by multiple, extraluminal dye-filled spaces. The stricture was close to the neck of the gallbladder, and the whole distal loculus was surrounded by large epithelial sinuses, with gross thickening of the wall of the gallbladder. (From LeQuesne and Ranger. *Br. J. Surg.* 44:447, 1957).

gallbladder may appear healthy or slightly thickened, and when the organ is slit open the characteristic brick-red congested mucous membrane will be seen to be speckled with bright yellow nodules (Fig. 19). In some specimens, the villi are markedly rugose and appear to be overburdened with lipoid, while in others only a few scattered white "warts" or "papillomas" can be discerned.

The condition is of clinical importance because it is the forerunner of single or multiple mulberry-like cholesterol stones in fully 40 percent of cases of cholesterol stones. Even when stones are absent, abdominal pain, biliary colic, and transient attacks of jaundice may occur (Fig. 20).

Some patients, and especially those suffering from recurrent attacks of biliary colic, are operated upon as cases of cholecystitis, with or without calculi. At *operation* the gallbladder may appear healthy, may show evidence of a mild degree of chronic inflammatory change, or may contain a few rounded bead-like gallstones.

The correct treatment is cholecystectomy, but the immediate and late results are only moderately good, as MacKey[33] has shown.

Mitty and Rousselot,[38] however, reported that following cholecystectomy the majority of their patients were relieved of symptoms. In one of my series, in 35 patients suffering from cholesterosis (with or without stones), cholecystectomy proved unrewarding in 8. The best results were obtained in those pa-

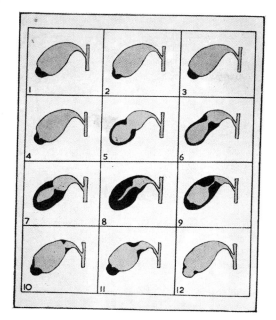

FIG. 18. Cholecystitis glandularis proliferans. Characteristic distribution of lesions. (From LeQuesne and Ranger. *Br. J. Surg.* 44:447, 1957.)

tients in whom cholesterosis was associated with multiple calculi. The operative mortal-

ity rate of cholecystectomy for this condition is less than 0.5 percent.

MUCOCELE OF THE GALLBLADDER

A solitary stone may form and lie in the gallbladder for many months or years without giving rise to any symptoms at all. The stone may, perchance, become impacted in the neck of the gallbladder or in the cystic duct; when it does so, a sharp attack of biliary colic results. The colic is severe but usually afebrile, and after a few hours the pain disappears and the patient is left with a sore aching area below the right costal margin. A few days after such an attack, the patient feels well again and does not suffer any dyspeptic symptoms, but sooner or later it is common for these attacks of colic to recur and become more frequent until eventually the stone becomes entrapped in the cystic duct and cannot escape. A mucocele of the gallbladder then develops (Fig. 21). With this

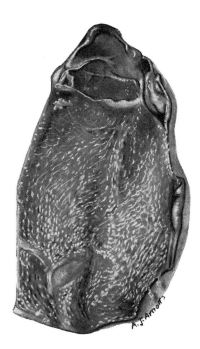

FIG. 19. Cholesterosis of the gallbladder. (Museum, London Hospital.)

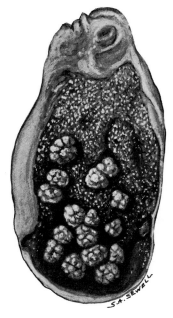

FIG. 20. Strawberry gallbladder, showing multiple pure cholesterol stones situated in gallbladder, which is the seat of cholesterosis. (Hunterian Museum, Royal College of Surgeons.)

is associated a chronic dull pain in the right upper quadrant of the abdomen, and flatulence and epigastric distress—especially after fatty meals.

On examination, the painless, tense, distended gallbladder can often be felt as a pyriform tumour beneath the right costal margin. Cholecystography will show that the organ has failed to fill with bile-laden dye. At operation, the pale, distended, freely mobile, pear- or sausage-shaped gallbladder should be emptied of its mucoid contents to facilitate the performance of cholecystectomy. In cases such as these, there is usually no obligation to explore the common bile duct. The operative mortality rate of cholecystectomy with or without exploration of the bile passages is about 0.5 percent.

A *pyocoele* or *empyema* of the gallbladder caused by infection of the wall of the vesicle or of its entrapped contents demands an expeditious cholecystectomy to forestall perforation, peritonitis, and other grave complications.

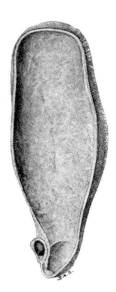

FIG. 21.   Mucocele of the gallbladder caused by impaction of small calculus in cystic duct. (Museum Royal College of Surgeons.)

EMPHYSEMATOUS CHOLECYSTITIS

Historical Note

Cases of acute emphysematous cholecystitis (acute gaseous cholecystitis, acute pneumocholecystitis, pyopneumocholecystitis, or gas phlegm of the gallbladder) have been reported by Stolz (*Virchow Arch. Pathol. Anat. 165*:90, 1901); Lobinger (*Ann. Surg. 48*:72, 1908); Cottam (*Surg. Gynecol. Obstet. 25*:192, 1917); Kirchmayr (*Chirurg. 52*: 1522, 1925); Hegner (*Arch. Surg. 22*:992, 1931); McCorkle and Fong (*Surgery 11*:851, 1942); Heifetz and Senturia (*Surg. Gynecol. Obstet. 86*:424, 1948); Jemerin (*Surgery 25*:237, 1949); Zaccone (*Radiol. Med. 37*:622, 1951); Hutchinson (*Br. Med. J. 1*:915, 1956); and Wilson (*Br. J. Surg. 45*:333, 1958), who reviewed 56 cases. Heifetz and Rifkin (*J. Abdom. Surg. 3*:75, 1961), in a review of the literature to 1961, found reports of only 87 cases. Up to September 1967, this figure has increased by the reports of 30 new cases, making a grand total of 117. Rosoff and Meyers (*Am. J. Surg. 111*:410, 1966) reported from the University of California School of Medicine 10 patients with acute emphysematous cholecystitis.

Acute emphysematous cholecystitis is a severe infection of the gallbladder characterised by the production of gas within the lumen, with or without concomitant pericholecystitic infiltration of gas.

In most instances, the main aetiological factors are obstruction of the neck of the gallbladder or the cystic duct caused by a stone, kinks, acute angulation, enlarged lymph nodes, tumours, or anomalous blood vessels. The blood supply to the vesicle eventually becomes impaired or occluded, and when this occurs the stage is set for acute obstructive gangrenous or emphysematous cholecystitis.

Clostridium perfringens was found in the majority of patients with recorded bacteriological findings. The infection may reach the gallbladder (and sometimes the bile ducts) through the arterial, venous, or lymphatic vessels, or through the bile. Many of the patients with this grave disorder were diabetic. Males are more frequently affected than females, the ratio being 3:1. The average age incidence is about 67.

The onset is acute, as in biliary colic, and it is ushered in by hyperpyrexia and intense right subcostal pain. Jaundice is rare, but a palpable mass is found in most cases. The clinical picture is that of acute cholecystitis. Diabetes mellitus is present in some 20 percent of the cases.

The condition takes longer to settle than does the more usual type of acute cholecystitis, and the physical signs take longer to subside. There is frequently a leucocytosis of 15,000 to 20,000 per cu mm of blood.

According to Green (1958), Hegner [21] was the first to describe the radiological findings in this disease. The typical appearances on x-ray films are an area of gas in the gallbladder outlining the organ and, on occasion, gas in the surrounding tissues. There is usually a fluid level in the gas-filled gallbladder. In clinching the diagnosis, one must, of course, exclude other sources of gas in the biliary system, such as spontaneous biliary-enteric fistula, previous cholecystoenterostomy, and reflux of gas through an incompetent or unduly relaxed sphincter of Oddi.

At *operation,* gas and evil-smelling brownish exudate are found in and around the gallbladder. Crepitus can be elicited in the wall of the gallbladder. Stones are frequently present.

The operation advised is cholecystectomy with drainage of the operative field. *Antibiotic and replacement therapy are called for before and after operation.*

G. Smith et al.[48] and others have shown that *oxygen administered in a hyperbaric chamber* is an effective means of treating infections with anaerobic organisms. There is no doubt that oxygen therapy constitutes one of the most important methods of treating acute emphysematous cholecystitis, both before and after operation. Some patients have been successfully treated by conservative medical or expectant treatment. But, in my opinion, such nonoperative measures constitute the best form of *preoperative treatment.* Sarmiento [45] reviewed 105 cases in 1966. All the patients had gallstones; and the mortality rate was 12 percent in both conservatively and surgically treated groups. Most of the deaths in the surgically treated group occurred in patients subjected to operation because conservative treatment had failed. The death rate rises to 50 percent with free perforation. Most surgeons advise *early* operation, more especially in those cases in which a mass is palpable.

ACUTE CHOLECYSTITIS

By far the most common single cause of acute cholecystitis is obstruction of the neck of the gallbladder or of the cystic duct by a stone (Fig. 22). This is confirmed by postmortem examination and by operative findings.

Acute noncalculous cholecystitis is on rare occasions encountered in the course of acute infective diseases such as typhoid, pneumonia, streptococcal and *Escherichia coli* septicaemia, or even in the more virulent forms of influenza. The infection in such cases is blood-borne or "lymphatic"-borne or bile-borne (rarely). Some cases of acute noncalculous cholecystitis are undoubtedly produced by chemical agents in the bile, pancreatic juice, or regurgitated duodenal contents.[52]

It is true that gallstones may lie dormant in a chronically inflamed gallbladder for an indefinite period and give rise to little more than occasional bouts of flatulence, epigastric

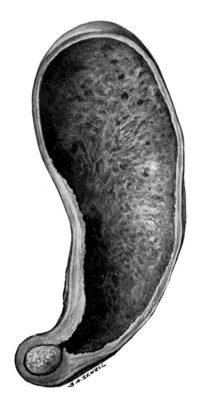

FIG. 22. Acute obstructive cholecystitis. (Hunterian Museum, Royal College of Surgeons.)

uneasiness, or a feeling of localised discomfort. When impaction occurs—and this is by no means an infrequent event, even in cases of so-called symptomless or silent stones—acute obstructive cholecystitis results.

Clinical Picture

The onset may be gradual, but more often it is sudden. In the former case, a persistent ache under the right costal margin is by degrees replaced by a sharp pain which increases in intensity and reaches a maximum in about 48 hours, while in the latter an unusually severe attack of biliary colic denotes that impaction has occurred. The patient is doubled up at the height of each seizure and writhes in agony as each gripping pain attains a crescendo-like ferocity. A measure of relief is afforded when the stone loosens and allows the putrid bile to drain into the common duct, or when liberal doses of propantheline, dihydrocodeine, pentazocine, or atropine are given. Morphine and pethidine (meperidine) have the great disadvantage of causing increased tone of the smooth muscle "sphincters" of the cystic and common bile ducts. The pain of biliary colic is chiefly localised to the right upper quadrant of the abdomen, but at times it may be diffused over the entire epigastrium or be referred mainly to the right flank or back or between the scapulae.

After a variable period, usually some hours, the pain changes in character. Its colicky nature is replaced by a dull throbbing ache which is felt most acutely near the tip of the ninth right costal cartilage or lower down on a level with the umbilicus. Nausea, retching, vomiting, and the belching up of large quantities of gas, as well as mild rigors, a rise in temperature and pulse rate, a sensation of tightness or girdle pain, and a catch in the breathing are all characteristic features of the early stages of acute cholecystitis.

At the end of 48 hours after the onset of the acute attack—and this is the critical period—either resolution will follow with disimpaction of the stone, or complications (e.g., empyema, gangrene, perforation, or peritonitis) will ensue.

The clinical manifestations *after* the first 48 hours are most variable and at times even misleading. *It is not uncommon to find that serious complications are present in the absence of significant signs or symptoms which would point to a grave pathological condition of the gallbladder.*

I also observe that the gallbladder in acute cholecystitis may proceed in its pathological course to gangrene and perforation in the presence of subsiding and minimal signs and symptoms.[21a]

When the patient is examined during the acute phase, he will be apprehensive and distressed, his face flushed, his tongue coated white or yellow and the upper half of the right rectus muscle on guard, fixed and tender; and the caecum and ascending colon will be distended and tympanitic. Jaundice may or may not be in evidence, and there may be traces of bile in the urine—which is often scanty, highly coloured, and concentrated.

In some cases the tensely swollen gallbladder may be felt through the stiffened abdominal muscles, or an indefinite tender mass may be made out below the inflamed liver margin, while in others the ballooned caecum may suggest a diagnosis of acute retrocaecal appendicitis or obstruction of the large intestine.

An examination of the chest will commonly show a slight degree of congestion of the lower lobe of the right lung, this being due to fixation of the right cupola of the diaphragm.

Aetiology

According to Glenn and Thorjarnarson,[18] about 95 percent of patients with acute cholecystitis have gallstones. As has been said, acute cholecystitis is initiated by obstruction of the cystic duct by a stone. The failure to find microorganisms in the bile or in the walls of the gallbladder in some 50 percent of the cases suggests that it is not primarily caused by bacterial infection. It is generally believed that acute cholecystitis is a chemical inflammation frequently augmented by bacterial invasion.

Pathology

In the early stages of the disease, the gallbladder will be distended, congested, and angry with inflammation. Its walls are thickened, oedematous, and fleshy; the mucous membrane is swollen, haemorrhagic or ulcerated. The mucous surface is red or maroon in colour, and may show areas of necrosis. The contents consist of thin white bile, yellowish mucopus, or dark brown decomposing blood laden with bacteria and leucocytes. The most common organisms cultivated from the contents of the gallbladder are *E. coli* and streptococci. In some of the fulminating cases *C. perfringens* or other anaerobic organisms may be discovered. The liver is often enlarged, pale yellow-brown in colour, with rounded edges, and friable to a marked degree. The omentum and the adjacent portions of the colon, stomach, and duodenum may be attached by fibrinous or fibrous adhesions to the inflamed surface of the gallbladder. When disimpaction occurs, the bile is free to be discharged through the cystic duct into the common duct. The gallbladder then shrinks, and the oedema slowly disappears. The gallbladder is now a chronically inflamed organ, crippled in the extreme, surrounded by fibrous adhesions, tethered to the hepatic flexure of the colon or anterior surface of the duodenum, and prone to future attacks of acute or subacute inflammation.

In those cases in which the acute inflammatory process continues unabated, serious complications such as gangrene, perforation, subphrenic abscess or suppurative pyelophlebitis may arise.

Gangrene may lead to perforation of the gallbladder with a localised abscess or spreading peritonitis. A localised abscess, however, is a more common occurrence. Gangrene is more prone to occur in elderly patients, owing to vascular rigidity. It is difficult to determine the incidence of gangrenous cholecystitis, as reports from different sources show wide variations. Barndale and Johnston,[2] in analysing a large series of cases of acute cholecystitis, found that 95 percent of the cases were caused by an impacted stone in the cystic duct, in the neck of the gallbladder, or in the region of the infundibulum. After a searching study of the recent literature on this subject, I would estimate that gangrene supervenes in 10 to 15 percent of cases of acute calculous cholecystitis.

What is the total incidence of *perforation* of the gallbladder?

I believe that the incidence of *free per-* *foration into the peritoneal cavity* with spreading or general peritonitis is about 3 percent. Diffenbaugh et al.[11] collected from the literature 630 cases of perforation of the gallbladder. The average incidence was 11.9 percent, but it varied in different hospitals from 2.5 percent to 25 percent. In the 328 cases of acute cholecystitis reported by Massie et al.,[34] there were 1.44 percent of acute perforations with spreading peritonitis. These authors recorded one case of perforation of an acute condition within the gallbladder with *massive intraperitoneal haemorrhage* which was the thirteenth such case to be found in the literature. The findings of Massie and his colleagues were confirmed by Ellis and Cronin [13] in their review of 795 patients who were admitted to the Radcliffe Hospital, Oxford, with acute cholecystitis. Only 11 (1.4 percent) of these patients suffered acute perforation, with bile peritonitis.

There are three types of perforation of the gallbladder:

1. *Acute perforation.* Here rupture has occurred with leakage into the general peritoneal cavity (3 percent). The peritonitis which has resulted owes to a lack of protective adhesions. The prognosis in such cases is always grave, especially in aged subjects (i.e., in patients more than 60 years of age).

2. *Subacute perforation.* Here the perforated gallbladder is surrounded by an abscess which is sealed off by adhesions from the peritoneal cavity (10 to 15 percent).

3. *Chronic perforation.* Here there is fistulous communication between the gallbladder and some other viscus— generally the duodenum or hepatic flexure of the colon (about 1 percent of all cases of calculous cholecystitis). It is in such cases as these that *gallstone ileus* may occur (see Chap. 86).

Differential Diagnosis

1. Perforated peptic ulcer
2. Appendicitis
3. Acute pancreatitis; pancreatic abscess or infected pseudocyst.
4. Strangulation—obstruction
5. Mesenteric occlusion
6. Pyelonephritis

7. Salpingitis; ruptured pyosalpinx
8. Acute hepatitis
9. Myocardial infarction
10. Acute congestive heart failure
11. Right lower lobe pneumonia

In the average case, the *history and the physical signs* leave little room for doubt. Plain x-ray pictures of the abdomen rarely show a calculus or calculi. There is, as a rule, no visualization of the gallbladder on cholecystography or intravenous cholangiography. The leucocyte count is elevated.

Treatment: Early or Late Operation

One of the most difficult problems concerning the subject of acute cholecystitis is that of fully comprehending the various terms used by surgeons to indicate when operation should in fact be performed for this acute abdominal condition. What is the difference between *immediate* and *early* operation? Can we distinguish between *delayed* and *late* operation with any degree of accuracy? The term *immediate operation* to my mind implies that the patient is hurried into hospital and is forthwith rushed into the operating room!

Immediate diagnosis of acute cholecystitis with immediate hospitalisation for such cases is the essence of good management, but immediate operation for the acutely inflamed gallbladder implies a rushed laparotomy.

I use the term *early* when operation is carried out some 12 to 48 hours after the patient's admission to hospital—when the surgeon has had sufficient time to establish the diagnosis, to evaluate the risk of surgical interference, to restore fluid balance, and to correct alterations in the blood chemistry. It is generally agreed that early cholecystectomy is the treatment of choice for acute cholecystitis in most patients.

By *late* operation I mean that surgical interference is postponed for some days after the patient's admission to hospital. It is "delayed" because the patient has shown a steady and progressive improvement under medical care, operation being performed when the symptoms and signs suggest that the acute inflammatory stage has subsided or is smouldering.

In most cases of acute cholecystitis, operation should be performed as soon as adequate preoperative treatment has been carried out. Cholecystectomy for *chronic* calculous cholecystitis was first advised and carried out by Carl Angenbuch [26] in 1882, but it was James Walton,[51] of the London Hospital, about 58 years ago, who performed the first excision of the gallbladder for *acute* cholecystitis.[51] There should be no undue haste, and no item in the investigation or in the preoperative treatment should be omitted. Some hours may be required to prepare these patients, and in a few instances it may be well to wait a day or two until they are deemed fit for operation. This preparation does not constitute the irksomeness of "conservative treatment," however. *Early surgery is not emergency surgery.* Once the patient is prepared, the operation should be performed—the nature and the extent of the procedure being determined by the findings and the general condition of the patient.

With the exception of certain cases, I am opposed to the so-called conservative or expectant treatment of acute cholecystitis, and to those who would regard this treacherous disease (which displays such great discrepancies between clinical signs and pathological changes) as a medical problem.

The proponents of *early operation* believe as follows:

1. In cases of acute cholecystitis, it is extremely difficult to decide whether the condition will subside under conservative treatment or become progressively worse. The exact nature and the extent of the inflammatory lesion are often a matter of speculation until the abdomen has been opened, as advanced grades of inflammation of the gallbladder *may* exist in the complete absence of signs and symptoms, whereas in patients presenting the same condition clinically, wide variations in the pathological changes may be observed at operation. For instance, it is not an uncommon experience after a period of watchful waiting (during which time the patient may have been afebrile and symptomless) to find at operation that the gallbladder is a bag of pus and

that a localised abscess or gangrene is present.

2. Some 20 percent of the patients fail to respond to conservative treatment or they show such rapid progression of their symptoms that they must be operated upon as soon as fluid balance is established.

3. Early operation is technically easier because *fibrinous* adhesions are encountered without the strong *fibrous* adhesions which are the rule later.

4. Both the mortality rate and the morbidity rate are lower with early operation. At the present time, the surgical treatment of acute cholecystitis can be accomplished by an experienced surgeon with an operative mortality rate comparable with that of nonacute biliary tract disease. Eliason and Stevens (1944) reported a series of 135 cases of acute cholecystitis in which early operation was performed with a mortality rate of 1.5 percent. In a consecutive series of 101 patients of mine, who were operated upon for acute cholecystitis within 48 hours of admission to hospital, there was but one fatality. Marshall reported a consecutive series of 64 cases of acute cholecystitis, in which the patients were subjected to operation during the early stage, with one hospital death. Hinchey and Hampson [22] write:

During the 7-year period from 1955 to 1962, 441 patients with acute cholecystitis were treated surgically at the Montreal General Hospital. The overall death rate was 0.45 percent. . . . Operation was carried out on 80 percent of the patients after the third day of admission to hospital. Definitive surgery was possible in 95 percent of the group, cholecystostomy being required for general or local reasons in only 5 percent of the patients.

This subject is also ably discussed by Essenhigh [15] and by Rosi and Midell,[42] who presented data derived from the records of 514 consecutive private patients who had clinical diagnosis of acute cholecystitis, and who were operated upon by board-certified surgeons in a 14-year period, with a mortality rate of about 2 percent.

The concept of conservative or nonoperative management ignores the fact that individual responses vary considerably. Thus, it is my practice to advise early operation after essential laboratory tests and other investigations have been carried out and when the patient has obtained the anticipated beneficial effects of well-applied supportive treatment.

But there are *exceptions* to this rule, and these include:

1. Obese patients who show unmistakable evidence of hypostatic congestion of the base of the lungs or cardiac embarrassment.

2. Debilitated *patients* including many poor-risk cases.

3. Those suffering from associated disorders such as marked hypertension, severe diabetes, phthisis, nephritis, and the like.

4. Those in whom the attack has been *very mild* and appears to be subsiding as previous attacks have done, or those in whom serum amylase values are very high suggesting that *acute pancreatitis* may be a primary or a complicating factor.

The ideal treatment is cholecystectomy (combined with exploration of the common bile duct and T tube choledochostomy (when indicated) for these reasons:

1. The useless, damaged, and infected organ is removed.

2. The operation in *experienced hands* presents no special difficulties as a rule.

3. An otherwise-necessary secondary operation is avoided.

4. Convalescence is shorter, smoother, and attended by fewer complications. There is, in addition, less pain, and fewer dressings are required. Too, the economic factor must be borne in mind.

Prognosis

This depends upon the following factors:

The age of the patient. All writers on the subject are in accord in stating that *the older the patient the higher the mortality rate and morbidity rate.*

Glenn and Thorbjarnarson [18] wrote:

For almost 30 years we have adhered to the policy of early operation for acute cholecystitis. Our definition of early surgical treatment provides that the operation be performed when the patient has been adequately prepared, unless some co-existing condition, not immediately reparable contraindicates surgery. During the period September 1, 1932 to September 1, 1961, 1130 patients with acute cholecystitis have been operated upon with a total mortality of 2.9 percent. The mortality rate for patients under the age of 50 was 1.1 percent.

Sex. The operative mortality rate is slightly higher in men than in women.

Duration of the acute attack. The time that elapses between the onset of the symptoms and surgical interference has a definite bearing on the mortality rate. Heyd showed in 3,986 cases that the safest time for operation was between 12 and 48 hours. This may be so, but each case must be judged on its own merits. Ellison,[14] who made a special study of biliary-tract diseases wrote:

During the period from 1948 through 1954, 152 patients with acute cholecystitis were treated by early operation on the surgical service of University Hospital, Ohio, with one death, or a *mortality of 0.6 percent.* Sixty-five, or 43 percent, came to operation within 48 hours following admission. Of these, 37 either had failed to improve with supportive measures or had had such rapid progression of signs and symptoms that operation was performed soon after fluid balance had been established. Cholecystostomy was considered the procedure of choice in 11 instances. The one death in this series occurred in one of the 6 patients with gallstone ileus. Of the total patients, 22, or 14 percent, were operated upon electively within 48 hours of the onset of their disease. The remaining 87, or 57 percent, were hospitalised for 48 hours or more before operation. *The gallbladder was removed in 135 patients, with no deaths.* These figures compare favorably with the mortality rate and complications in 887 instances of cholecystectomy for chronic cholecystitis in the same period, i.e., 1.4 percent. Choledochostomy was added to the procedure in 51, or 37.7 percent, of the 135 patients, and common duct stones were removed in 20, or 39.1 percent, of the ducts explored.

The presence of jaundice. The operative mortality rate is more than trebled when jaundice is present.

The type of operation. The choice of operation in acute cholecystitis is cholecystectomy, with or without choledochostomy. The excision of the gallbladder interrupts the pathological process and averts the danger of gangrene and perforation of the viscus.

Cholecystectomy is, however, contraindicated under the following circumstances:

1. When it is impossible to identify the biliary passages and the all-important blood vessels (*cholecystostomy* is obviously indicated in these cases).
2. When the patient's general condition is so serious that use of a general anaesthetic and performance of a prolonged operation are not justified.

To recapitulate, the indications for *cholecystostomy* may be summarised as follows:

1. Poor general condition of the patient.
2. Anatomy obscuration.
3. Acute cholecystitis associated with acute pancreatitis.
4. Jaundice associated with cholaemia and grave condition of the patient.
5. Technical reasons, e.g., extreme obesity.

In actual practice, I perform cholecystectomy in about 96 percent of my cases. The bile ducts are explored at the time of the cholecystectomy if the clinical, operative, and radiological findings support a diagnosis of choledocholithiasis. It has been my experience that the mortality rate in acute cholecystitis is increased by at least 2 percent when exploration of the bile ducts and T tube choledochostomy is carried out at the same time as the cholecystectomy.

CHRONIC CHOLECYSTITIS AND CHRONIC CALCULOUS CHOLECYSTITIS

Chronic cholecystitis is caused by chemical inflammation plus bacterial infection. With bacterial infection, the common organisms are: coliform bacilli and/or non-haemolytic streptococci; less commonly Clostridium welchii, other anaerobic bacilli, staphylococci, and bacilli of the typhoid-paratyphoid group.

The possible routes of infection include: (1) the ascending or chologenous route; (2) descending biliary infection *via* the hepatic ducts into the gallbladder; (3) lymphogenous infection; (4) haematogenous group; and (5) extension from adjacent viscera. Stagnation of bile, disturbances of lipoid or cholesterol metabolism, and haemolytic diseases are well-known predisposing factors. As previously stated, chronic cholecystitis may precede gallstones or may follow them as a result of their obstructive effects. Warren Cole believes that cholecystitis starts primarily as a chemical lesion. He has found that cultures of the bile and wall of the gallbladder in early cases of acute cholecystitis are frequently sterile. He states that all the infectious phase of cholecystitis is usually superimposed on an initial chemical inflammation.

The average *age* of males and females suffering from calculous cholecystitis is 53 years. The ratio of females to males is 2:1.

Gallstones are exceedingly common, being present in at least 20 percent of women over the age of 50 and in 20 percent of men over 70. Children, infants, and even premature babies may be afflicted. The number of gallstone sufferers is increasing yearly. (See Part A of this chapter.) Clarence Schein [46] states that gallstones and their complications constitute the fourth most frequent cause for hospitalization and the most common indication for abdominal surgery in the adult in America. About 500,000 operations are performed annually for gallstones and the complications of gallstones. The disease is on the increase and, at present, affects about 20 percent of the mature population.

The normal gallbladder is sea-green or blue-green in colour. This is because the walls of the organ are translucent and transmit the colour of the bile within. When the gallbladder is gently compressed with the fingers and thoroughly emptied of its contents, it will be seen that its walls are thin and flexible and that it takes on a pale salmon-pink hue.

When cholecystitis is well established, the

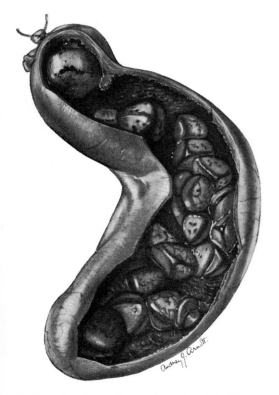

FIG. 23. Specimen of an enlarged gallbladder containing multiple faceted stones with one stone impacted in the neck of the gallbladder. (Museum, London Hospital.)

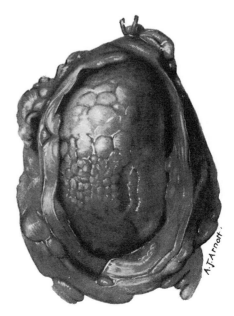

FIG. 24. Gallbladder showing marked chronic cholecystitis. Gallbladder has contracted down on single stone within its lumen. (Museum, London Hospital.)

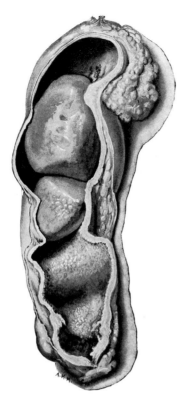

FIG. 25. Chronic calculous cholecystitis. Gallbladder contains two large faceted stones.

walls of the gallbladder become thickened and inelastic and present a pearly white appearance (Figs. 23, 24, and 25). The gallbladder may be normal in size or it may be enlarged and tense with bile and with contained stones when impaction has occurred; again, it may be small and shrunken, fibrotic, calcific, and deformed. In an extreme case, it may be represented as a thickened fibrous cord containing a few faceted stones. The mucous membrane may show early inflammatory changes—catarrhal cholecystitis—or it may be markedly congested, ulcerated from the pressure of calculi, pitted, or scarred. In a few late cases, *the walls may become calcified* (Fig. 26).

About 100 cases of *calcified cholecystitis* (porcelain gallbladder, enamelled gallbladder, or petrified gallbladder) have been reported. According to Biocca,[5] the condition is rare; he states that Kirklin recorded only

4 cases in 6,000 cholecystograms. Of the 10 cases reported by Phemister, 4 were found at autopsy.

The *diagnosis* of porcelain gallbladder is made by x-ray examination, which reveals a radiopaque shadow in the right upper quadrant. Cholecystectomy is advised for this disease. Scirrhus carcinoma has been observed in a few cases of porcelain gallbladder.

In chronic cholecystitis, the bile may be a healthy green or yellowish hue; it may be odourless and free from organisms, while on the other hand it may be pale and opalescent (white bile), turbid or muddy (mucopus), dark brown, or thick and tarry and laden with biliary mud.

The gallbladder may be adherent to the surrounding structures: the pylorus, the first portion of the duodenum, the hepatic flexure of the colon, or the greater omentum.

Clinical Features

Clinical features depend upon dysfunction of the gallbladder caused by inflammation or the presence of stones, or upon *reflex pylorospasm*. In more advanced cases,

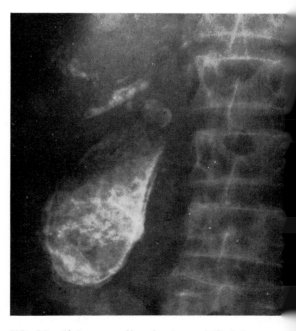

FIG. 26. Plain x-ray film showing calcified (porcelain) gallbladder.

some of the clinical manifestations are due to toxic absorption from the diseased gall-bladder. The patient complains of flatulent dyspepsia after meals—particularly after fatty food has been taken. A large meal often aggravates the epigastric distress and never brings relief as might be the case in uncomplicated chronic duodenal ulcer. In some instances, the bloating of the epigastrium may be extreme and be associated with a marked degree of belching. Heartburn is present in 30 percent of such patients. The patient frequently complains of a pain below the angle of the right scapula, beneath the right costal margin and sometimes in the right flank—particularly on stooping, during exercises, or occasionally after a cold bath and, owing to this pain, exercise is avoided and weight is consequently increased. When impaction occurs, there may be a dull constant ache in the right upper quadrant of the abdomen, or there may be intermittent attacks of biliary colic associated with the so-called bilious vomiting and marked nausea. Jaundice occurs in some 10 percent of patients with gallstones that are limited purely to the gall-bladder; when migration of the stones into the main ducts takes place, the incidence rises to 50 percent. In some patients with gallstones, the symptoms may be vague and signs entirely absent. In such anomalous cases, nausea, frequent headache, and "rheumatic pains" (chiefly felt in the neck, in the back, and in the joints) are complained of. This is a manifestation of a chronic toxaemia and it is extremely difficult to trace the trouble to the gallbladder. Nevertheless, when the presence of chronic cholecystitis is proved conclusively and cholecystectomy is undertaken, in many cases the rheumatic manifestations disappear.

In some patients, too, *cardiac symptoms*—precordial pain, palpitation, breathlessness—are much in evidence. It would appear that in some instances the myocardium becomes secondarily affected by prolonged biliary disease, and severe cardiac pain may occur, simulating angina pectoris. This condition has been termed the *cholecystitic heart,* and is no bar to operation.

Not infrequently, as Miller,[37] Rutledge,[43] and Colcock[7] have pointed out, the cardiac condition may improve considerably after cholecystectomy. Laird[25] considered that

chronic cholecystitis was associated with cardiac lesions in more than 70 percent of cases and that in some of these patients excision of the gallbladder would effect a cure or at least afford considerable amelioration of symptoms. Walters and Master[50] stated that following cholecystectomy for an inflamed gallbladder or for gallstones in such cases, the electrocardiograms may demonstrate considerable improvement. *The underlying disease of the coronary arteries, however, is seldom affected by such surgical procedures.*

In the quiescent period, physical examination of the abdomen will often be negative, although Murphy's sign may be positive. Following an attack of biliary colic, there may be some rigidity and tenderness in the right upper quadrant of the abdomen, but apart from this, little else can be discovered.

Silent or Symptomless Gallstones

A few words are pertinent on *so-called silent or symptomless gallstones.* Admittedly, silent stones do exist, but it is impossible to concede that gallstones are harmless because they are symptomless. Gallstones are often discovered accidentally during x-ray examination carried out for some other reason, or at autopsy in a patient who has died from some other cause. Sir Henage Ogilvie maintained that these silent stones are not really symptomless. He wrote:

A careful enquiry will nearly always elicit many of the prodromal symptoms of gallstones—a dislike of certain articles of diet, a tendency to upper-abdominal distension after meals, attacks of vomiting associated with blinding headaches that have been put down to migraine, long periods of lassitude, fatigue, and inability to carry out duties that were formerly a pleasure. Most striking is the fact that after cholecystectomy (and cholecystectomy must always be advised when gallstones have been demonstrated), the patient immediately experiences a joy in life and a feeling of fitness that makes him realise he was unfit before.

I say with all seriousness that when gallstones have been found, operation should be advised, even if they are not giving rise to symptoms, or even if the symptoms of which the patient complains are thought to be due to something else.

Lund[31] reported a study of 526 calculous-cholecystitis patients, most of whom were not operated upon and who were followed for 5 to 20 years. He found that irrespective of previous symptoms, severe symptoms or complications (or both) subsequently developed in about 50 percent of the patients. Approximately 30 percent of patients harbouring gallstones have no symptoms (the "symptomless gallbladder"). Most of the grave complications of calculous cholecystitis —fistula, choledocholithiasis, pancreatitis, etc. —are seen in elderly patients, and especially in those who have had "silent gallstones" for many years but who have obstinately and steadfastly refused the benefit of a well-performed cholecystectomy.

Method et al.[36] are convinced that the only way to reduce the mortality rate in chronic and acute cholecystitis and their complications is to make a more diligent search for the "silent" gallstone, especially in those over 50 years of age, and to remove the gallbladder as an elective operation. Colcock et al.[8] believe that early surgical treatment of cholelithiasis, when the patients are still asymptomatic, will reduce the incidence of common duct disease and will also reduce the mortality and morbidity rates associated with disease of the biliary tract. I agree with the views expressed by the authorities quoted above. Nevertheless, I am of the opinion that patients who have silent gallstones and do NOT want an operation should not be "intimidated" into surgery.

Disappearing Gallstones

This subject has been studied by Gardiner et al.[17] and Sing and Howard.[47] The latter authors state that the presence of multiple gallstones was clearly demonstrated radiologically in the gallbladder of one of their patients. After the patient suffered multiple attacks of biliary colic, exploration of the biliary tract demonstrated that each of the stones had been passed into the duodenum via the bile ducts. Gardiner and his colleagues (1966) discussed the clinical history in 9 patients in whom gallstones had disappeared. Fifteen similar cases from the literature were reviewed. Because of this disappearance, these authors conclude that in patients in whom small residual stones are found in the choledochus on postoperative cholangiography, a conservative attitude can safely be adopted.

This subject—spontaneous disappearance of gallstones—is also discussed by Linsman and Corday,[10] Dworken,[12] and Appleman.[1] Patients frequently inquire whether gallstones can be dispersed without operation. The answer must be in the negative at the moment. Certain diets low in cholesterol and the administration of cholestyramine and chenodeoxycholic acid have been given a trial without any promising effects.[28] In some cases, however, where the cystic duct is dilated by the passage of the first calculus, the rest follow and negotiate the common bile duct and the sphincter of Oddi if their diameter is no more than 5 to 7 mm. According to Harding Rains,[41] there is nothing in this phenomenon on which to base any regular and satisfactory treatment policy. (See Chap. 41A.)

Diagnosis

On many occasions chronic calculous cholecystitis can be diagnosed on the presenting symptoms alone, as they may be strikingly characteristic. But at times the disease may be confused with chronic appendicitis, chronic peptic ulcer, chronic gastritis and duodenitis, carcinoma of the colon, gastric tumours, chronic relapsing pancreatitis, renal disease, hiatal hernia, or angina pectoris.

An accurate preoperative diagnosis is often achieved by employing the following tests:

1. Plain radiographs of the gallbladder region.
2. Cholecystography (oral), intravenous cholangiography, and percutaneous transhepatic cholangiography.
3. Barium-meal x-ray examination of the oesophagus, stomach, duodenum, and intestines.
4. Duodenal drainage.
5. Complete examination of the blood, urine, and faeces, including liver function tests; differential diagnosis of jaundice; determinations of serum amylase and lipase and of urinary diastase.
6. Fibre-duodenoscopy.

RADIOLOGY OF THE BILIARY TRACT

Plain x-ray films of the gallbladder area will demonstrate the presence of stones

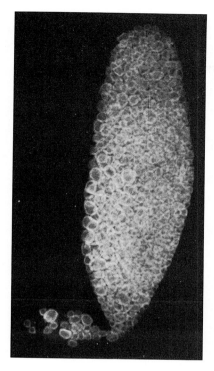

FIG. 27. Plain x-ray film of gallbladder immediately after removal shows gallbladder and cystic duct tightly packed with small multiple faceted stones.

in more than 15 percent of the patients studied. Stones in the common bile duct rarely throw a shadow, but the barrel-shaped and mixed stones in the gallbladder, which often have an outer shell of calcium, the so-called signet-ring stone (with its cholesterol core and coating of calcium bilirubinate), and calcium carbonate stones are easily recognised in plain radiographs (Figs. 27 to 30).

CHOLECYSTOGRAPHY AND CHOLANGIOGRAPHY

This technique is now universally used, and the profession owes a great debt to Graham and Cole [19] for the introduction of this valuable test. The dye is excreted in the bile and is carried to the gallbladder and there concentrated. The concentrated dye, being radiopaque, clearly outlines the gallbladder. The test is a gauge of gallbladder function. In most instances, it determines the presence or absence of stones, and also determines the character, number, and position of the stones. It is also valuable in differentiating gallstones from other opacities in the right upper abdomen which might otherwise be misinterpreted.

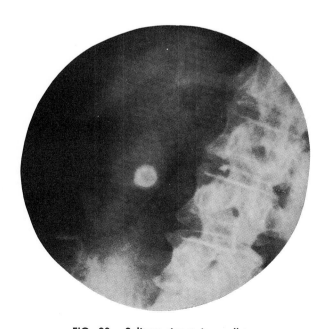

FIG. 28. Solitary signet-ring gallstone.

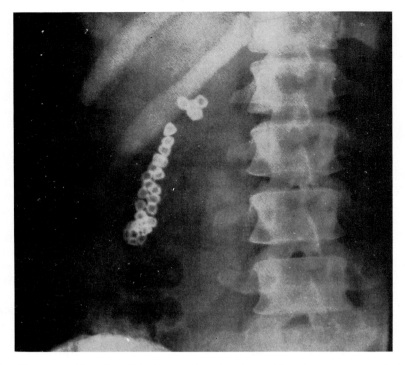

FIG. 29.   Plain x-ray film of gallbladder region, showing multiple faceted stones of signet-ring type. (Courtesy of Dr. Laurie.)

I have said that this test determines the number of gallstones in the gallbladder, but this statement requires qualification; at times, many more gallstones may be present than is suggested by the x-ray pictures. The dye should not be given to patients who are jaundiced or to those in whom the serum bilirubin level is higher than 3 to 4 mg per 100 ml, as it is then not free from danger and a pyelogram rather than a cholecystogram is frequently obtained.

The compounds or contrast media now employed are Priodax, iopanoic acid (Telepaque), Biloptin, Osbil, and Bilopaque. In recent years, iodipamide (Biligrafin), an *intravenous excretion medium,* first introduced by Frommhold,[16] has been employed with gratifying results. In fact, during the last 10 years, radiological examination of the biliary tract by simple intravenous injection of iodipamide has become a routine procedure and *operative* and *postoperative cholangiography* by direct injection of the biliary ducts has been increasingly practised. Duff Gray[20] says that coincident with the development of new contrast media there has been a striking development of radiological methods generally, so that today the advantages of many accessory techniques are available that serve to improve the value of the radiological investigation of the biliary system.

As examples of these newer methods, the following may be mentioned: multiple localised films under screen observation, permitting minor variations in applied pressure over the gallbladder; postural alterations of the patient to displace intestinal gas and to show "levels;" tomography, especially to demonstrate the common bile duct; and, most recently, the use of the image amplifier with ciné recording.

Various combined techniques have also been carried out by Alridge (1955), Mitchell (1956), Johnstone and Sumerling (1957), and Macfeat (1973). In a leading article in Lancet,[27] the value of intravenous cholangiography is cogently stressed. It is generally accepted that the biliary passages are displayed in a higher proportion of cases by this method than by oral techniques. This is

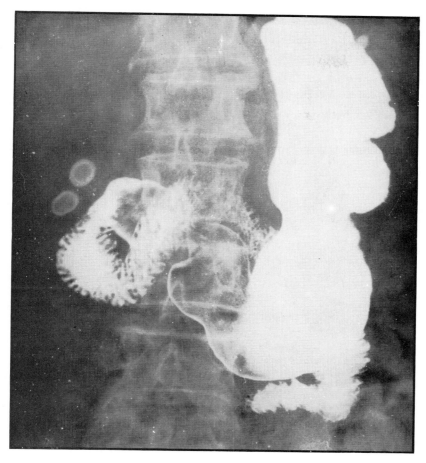

FIG. 30.   Barium-meal x-ray examination of stomach and duodenum shows no organic lesion in stomach or duodenum. Two gallstones, however, are clearly demonstrated situated to outer aspect of duodenal cap. (Courtesy of the late Dr. Leo Rau.)

so because the dose of contrast medium entering the blood stream is fixed and controlled, whereas with oral methods the proportion of medium absorbed from the intestine cannot be predicted and may be negligible. It is often advisable to combine oral cholecystography with intravenous cholangiography. Failure to display the gallbladder by the intravenous technique is a far more certain index of disease than is failure by the oral method, as Stenhouse [49] has stressed. When the bile ducts are demonstrated by iodipamide cholangiography but the gallbladder is not shown, a diagnosis of calculous cholecystitis with obstruction of the cystic duct may be made with a degree of confidence.[24, 40, 44]

Don and Campbell (1956) believe that physiological dilatation of the ducts after cholecystectomy is not the rule in man, and that dilatation of the ducts is a permanent result of back pressure owing to obstruction of the duct at some stage by stones. This subject is discussed by Le Quesne, Whiteside, and Hand.[30] Their summary and conclusions follow:

In a series of 73 patients undergoing cholecystectomy measurements were made of the diameter of the common bile duct as revealed on operative cholangiography, and on intravenous cholangiography performed 12 months or more after operation. At the time of this latter examination the patients were interviewed and placed in one of four categories according to their clinical symptoms.

There is a wide variation in the calibre of the normal common bile duct. It is suggested that, as seen on radiology, an image of 10 mm. diameter represents the usual upper limit of normal, and that an image of 12 mm. or greater is evidence of dilatation of the duct.

There is no evidence that the common bile duct becomes dilated after cholecystectomy.

There is no evidence that a dilated common bile duct diminishes significantly in calibre after cholecystectomy and removal of stones from the duct.

There is no correlation between the continuance of symptoms after cholecystectomy and the calibre of the common bile duct.

The finding of a dilated bile duct on intravenous cholangiography performed after cholecystectomy is of no significance in itself in the absence of information about the size of the duct at the time of operation.

Operative and postoperative cholangiography is described by Leslie Le Quesne in Chapter 43A.

INTERPRETATION OF CHOLECYSTOGRAMS

Normal gallbladder. Here there is a good uniform shadow of the gallbladder, which contracts rapidly and satisfactorily after a fatty meal. It indicates definitely that the liver is capable of excreting the dye, that the bile ducts are patent, and that there is no impairment of the walls of the gallbladder.

The gallbladder outlines well, but contains negative shadow or shadows. This implies that the dye-laden bile has freely entered the gallbladder, the walls of which may or may not be chronically inflamed, and that the negative shadows are caused by nonopaque gallstones which have displaced the dye. In a fair proportion of cases, the gallbladder concentrates the dye normally and the stones are clearly visible in it. In some 2 percent of cases, a gallbladder containing small cholesterol stones concentrates the dye in a normal manner and the contrast medium conceals the stones.

No gallbladder shadow. When the gallbladder is not visualized, the finding indicates that the neck of the gallbladder or cystic duct is blocked by a stone or by some disease process.

Nonvisualisation of the gallbladder, following one or more oral or intravenous dye tests in a patient giving a history of gallbladder disease, indicates the presence of cholelithiasis in 97 percent of cases.

No shadow should be reported as being *faint* unless it is persistently so thin that it is scarcely discernible, and every gallbladder should be judged by its best shadow, not by its worst.

The terms *faint shadow, poor concentration,* and *poor emptying* are not significant if gallstones are not irrefutably demonstrated. These findings often suggest the presence of some derangement of function at the time of the investigation, and such radiological signs are an indication for further x-ray studies following a course of medical treatment. It is necessary to emphasize the fact that the combination of faint shadow and poor emptying does not necessarily denote that the gallbladder is organically diseased, although diagnosis of chronic cholecystitis is frequently made in these circumstances. *The radiological diagnosis of chronic cholecystitis, in the absence of calculi, can rarely be upheld with conviction.*

Gallbladder irregular in outline. These may be filling defects suggestive of papillomatous or malignant growths. (See Chap. 50.)

Percutaneous intrahepatic cholangiography is discussed in Chapter 46.

BARIUM MEAL

A barium-meal x-ray examination of the stomach and duodenum and possibly the colon is desirable to exclude the presence of concomitant disease such as hiatal hernia, duodenal ulcer, or chronic appendicitis. An article by John and Raymond Beeler [23] on barium-meal studies of the gastrointestinal tract in determining the cause of jaundice contains many helpful points.

Duodenography is discussed in Chapter 4; and *fibre-duodenoscopy* in Chapter 34, Part B by Louis Kreel.

DUODENAL DRAINAGE

This step consists of passing a duodenal tube and, after ensuring that the point of the tube is lying in the duodenum, running in a concentrated solution of magnesium sulphate through the tube. After a short while, the bile is recovered from the duodenum and examined. In marked disease of the gallbladder and bile passages, biliary sand, bile salts, cholesterol crystals, pus cells, and organisms may be recovered. A negative finding is of no value, as normal bile may be obtained even in the presence of calculus cholecystitis. The Meltzer-Lyon test is of some value in diagnosis and in assessing the effects of medical treatment in those cases in which the common bile duct is infected.

LABORATORY INVESTIGATIONS

Pertinent laboratory tests are discussed in Chapter 45 by Frances H. Smith.

The subjects of *choledocholithiasis* and *exploration* of the *bile ducts* are discussed by Le Quesne in Chapter 43A. The techniques of *cholecystostomy* and of *cholecystectomy* are described by Maingot in Chapter 42.

REFERENCES

1. Appleman, Am. J. Gastroenterol. 37:656, 1962.
2. Barnsdale and Johnston, Ann. Surg. 127:816, 1948.
2a. Beeler, J., and Beeler, R., J.A.M.A. 151:268, 1953.
3. Beilby, Br. J. Exp. Pathol. 48:455, 1967.
3a. Beilby, J. Path. Bact. 93:175, 1967.
4. Bell et al., Ann. Surg. 138:268, 1963.
5. Biocca, Policlinico [Chir.] 54:173, 1947.
6. Boyd, Br. J. Surg. 10:337, 1927.
7. Colcock, Surg. Gynecol. Obstet. 117:529, 1963.
8. Colcock et al., Am. J. Surg. 113:44, 1967.
9. Colqhoun, Br. J. Radiol. 34:101, 1961.
10. Corday, J.A.M.A. 171:1098, 1959.
11. Diffenbaugh et al., Arch. Surg. 59:742, 1949.
12. Dworken, Gastroenterology 38:76, 1960.
13. Ellis and Cronin, Br. J. Surg. 48:166, 1960.
14. Ellison, Current Surgical Management, Philadelphia, Saunders, 1957.
15. Essenhigh, Br. J. Surg. 53:1032, 1966.
16. Frommhold, Fortschr. Geb. Röntgen. 79:283, 1953.
17. Gardiner et al., Br. J. Surg. 53:114, 1966.
18. Glenn and Thorbjarnarson, Surg. Gynecol. Obstet. 116:61, 1963.
19. Graham and Cole, J.A.M.A. 82:613, 1924.
20. Gray, Duff, Proc. R. Soc. Med. 51:793, 1958.
21. Hegner, Arch. Surg. 22:993, 1931.
21a. Heuer, Surg. Gynecol. Obstet. 83:50, 1946.
22. Hinchey and Hampson, Surg. Gynecol. Obstet. 120:475, 1965.
23. Beeler, J. and Beeler, R., J.A.M.A. 151:268, 1953.
24. Kreel, L., Personal communication, 1972.
25. Laird, Lancet 1:884, 1938.
26. Langenbuch, Carl, Berl. Klin. Wochenschr. 19: 725, 1882.
27. Leading article, Intravenous Cholangiography, Lancet 2:49, 1959.
28. Leading article, Dissolving Gallstones, Lancet 2:525, 1972.
29. LeQuesne and Ranger, Br. J. Surg. 44:447, 1957.
30. LeQuesne, Whiteside, and Hand, Br. Med. J. 1:329, 1959.
31. Lund, Ann. Surg. 151:153, 1960.
32. McCarty, Am. Surg. 51:651, 1910.
33. MacKey, Br. J. Surg. 28:462, 1941.
34. Massie et al., Ann. Surg. 145:825, 1957.
35. Mentzer, Am. J. Path. 1:383, 1925.
36. Method et al., Arch. Surg. 85:338, 1962.
37. Miller, Lancet 1:767, 1932.
38. Mitty and Rousselot, Gastroenterology 32:910, 1957.
39. Moynihan, Ann. Surg. 50:1265, 1909.
40. Norman, Acta Radiol. Suppl. 84, 1959.
41. Rains, H., on Gallstone Disease, in Diseases of the Digestive System, British Medical Journal, 1969.
42. Rosi and Midell, Surg. Clin. North Am. 47:147, 1967.
43. Rutledge, Surg. Clin. North Am. June:660, 1943.
44. Samuel, Lancet 1:454, 1959.
45. Sarmiento, Arch. Surg. 93:1009, 1966.
46. Schein, Acute Cholecystitis, New York, Harper & Row, 1972.
47. Sing and Howard, Ann. Surg. 160:119, 1964.
48. Smith, G., et al., Lancet 2:756, 1962.
49. Stenhouse, J. Fac. Radiol. 9:223, 1959.
50. Walters and Master, Surg. Gynecol. Obstet. 94: 152, 1952.
51. Walton, J. A., Textbook of the Surgical Dyspepsias, London, Arnold, 1925.
52. Womack and Bricker, Arch. Surg. 44:658, 1952.

42

THE TECHNIQUES OF CHOLECYSTOSTOMY AND CHOLECYSTECTOMY

RODNEY MAINGOT

CHOLECYSTOSTOMY

Colecystostomy may be, and often is, as Glenn [3] remarks, a procedure of compromise, but it is frequently a life-saving one. It is a measure that meets the immediate demands to save the patient's life, and it also paves the way for safety at a later time for performing a definitive operative procedure.

Indications

The indications for the performance of cholecystostomy may be summarised as follows:

1. Acute cholecystitis with gallstones—

When the patient is aged and infirm.
When cholecystectomy presents unusual technical difficulties (for example, anatomical obscuration or extreme obesity) or involves great risk (such as the possibility of injury to the bile ducts).
When the condition of the patient is grave (toxaemia being pronounced) or other serious renal, cardiovascular, or pulmonary complications being present.
As a preliminary measure in certain selected cases of acute cholecystitis and suppurative cholangitis associated with obstruction of the distal end of the common bile duct.
When there is cardiac or respiratory distress during the early stages of the exploratory laparotomy.

2. Chronic calculous cholecystitis

When the surgeon is lacking in experience of operating on the biliary tract, and when the risks involved in excising the gallbladder appear to be unusually great in the particular case.

3. Acute pancreatitis with obstructive jaundice

When committed to operation for such a grave event, the surgeon would be well advised to adopt the simplest procedure—cholecystostomy or, possibly, T tube choledochostomy.

4. In some instances of cancer

In *certain* cases of cancer of the head of the pancreas or of the periampullary region, as a first stage operation to relieve jaundice. In such instances, cholecystostomy should only be employed with full control of dehydration and electrolyte depletion and with the intent of carrying out pancreatoduodenectomy within 7 to 10 days.

Positioning the Patient

The patient lies in the dorsal recumbent position with the head and chest slightly raised and with the knees supported by means of a soft pillow to afford some relaxation of the abdominal muscles. The operating table is adjusted to a *slight* reversed Trendelenburg position to aid in a minor degree in the downward displacement of the viscera. The bridge in the operating table is not raised and no pillow or other support is employed to throw the epigastric region forward, as this position causes a great deal of backache in the postoperative phase and does not facilitate the exposure of the gallbladder and bile ducts. The hyperextended position of the body for gallbladder surgery was abandoned by the writer many years ago.

Instruments

Some of the more important instruments that are used in gallbladder surgery are as follows: Harrington or Deaver retractors (four sizes—small, medium, large, and extra large); long dissecting (nontoothed) forceps (15 in. [38 cm]); Lahey cholecystectomy forceps; Mayo-Ochsner trocar and cannula; T tubes such as the modified (latex or red rubber barium-impregnated) Kehr's T tubes in different sizes, as made by the Davol Rubber Company, and Maingot's gutter T tubes (as supplied by Down Brothers, London); gum-elastic bougies and Bakes' dilators (in sizes from 3 to 11 mm); various scoops; suction tubes; Desjardins forceps; Priestley's malleable tube for irrigation of the ducts, and modified Denis Browne forceps. These instruments need no special description (Fig. 1).

Incisions

A large number of incisions have been employed in operative procedures on the gallbladder and bile passages. These include the median vertical epigastric, right paramedian, rectus muscle-splitting, the Bevan S-shaped, Mayo-Robson, Kehr, transverse, and Kocher subcostal. In actual practice, I employ only three incisions: the paramedian, in which the upper half of the right rectus muscle is retracted outward; the rectus muscle-splitting incision; and Kocher's right oblique subcostal incision. The incision of choice is a lengthy right paramedian incision starting at the costal margin and finishing 2 inches (5 cm) or so to the right and below the umbilicus. Kocher's incision is employed for obese patients and broad-chested muscular patients (Fig. 2). (Also see Chap. 1). For secondary operations, or when there has been a previous paramedian incision, the vertical epigastric rectus muscle-splitting incision is undoubtedly the best.

At the completion of the operation, the edges of the peritoneum, and the posterior sheath of the rectus muscle are drawn together with a continuous suture of 0 chromic catgut, at times using a double strand of this material. The margins of the anterior sheath of the rectus muscle are approximated with interrupted sutures of 0 chromic catgut, medium silk, cotton, monofilament nylon or

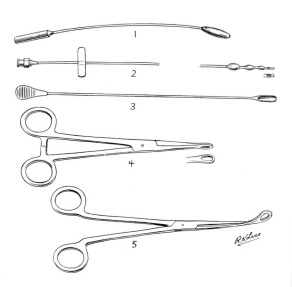

FIG. 1. A few popular sounds, scoops, and other instruments used in biliary tract surgery. 1. Bakes' dilators in sizes of from 3 to 11 mm. 2. A useful combined bile duct dilator and irrigator. 3. A malleable scoop. 4. Maingot's modification of Denis Browne forceps. 5. Modified Desjardins forceps.

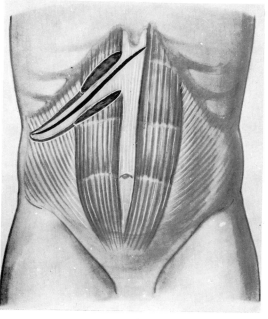

FIG. 2. Kocher's incision. This right subcostal muscle-dividing incision is sometimes employed in obese broad-chested patients.

Dexon. The skin is closed with vertical mattress sutures of fine Deknatel or black serumproof silk. Occasionally, however, in very obese patients and in cases in which speed is imperative owing to the grave condition of the patient, all the layers of the abdominal wall, with the exception of the skin and subcutaneous tissues, may be approximated with a series of vertical through-and-through sutures or figure-of-eight sutures of stainless steel wire or stout monofilament nylon. The skin is closed with vertical mattress sutures of Deknatel or with Mersilk. When the patient is obese, in order to facilitate exposure of the ducts and to make all intra-abdominal manipulations easier, the incision through the skin and subcutaneous tissues is made very much longer than that through the muscles. In many cases, it is wise to drain the subcutaneous space with fine corrugated sheets of latex.

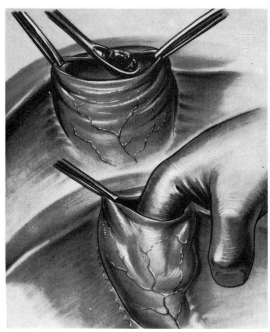

FIG. 4. Cholecystostomy. Removal of gallstones by scoops, and exploration of the interior of the gallbladder with the index finger.

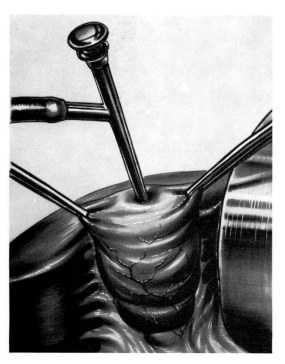

FIG. 3. Cholecystostomy. The contents of the gallbladder are withdrawn by suction through a Mayo-Ochsner trocar and cannula. (From Maingot, Cholecystostomy, in Rob, Smith, and Morgan. *Operative Surgery*, 2d ed., 1969. Courtesy of Butterworths, London.)

Technique

The edges of the wound and the region around the gallbladder should be well protected with abdominal pads, cellophane-gauze squares, or acrylic sheets, as the bile may be highly infective in cases in which cholecystostomy is performed. Inflammatory adhesions, and in particular inflamed oedematous omentum that is walling off the gallbladder should be disturbed as little as possible.

The contents of the gallbladder are next aspirated with a wide-bore aspirating needle, or if the gallbladder is unduly distended, the isolated fundus may be pierced by a Mayo-Ochsner trocar and cannula and the infected bile be withdrawn into a receptacle by suction (Fig. 3).

The fundus is now seized with Allis or Babcock forceps on either side of the puncture spot to prevent the gallbladder from retracting when it is empty and also to prevent any leakage when the needle or cannula

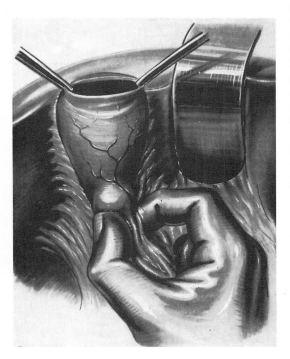

FIG. 5. Cholecystostomy. Dislodging a stone impacted in the neck of the gallbladder. (Courtesy of Butterworths, London.)

is withdrawn. An incision of sufficient length to admit the finger is then made through the fundus, a suction tube is introduced into the gallbladder, and the septic bile and inflammatory debris and gravel are withdrawn (Fig. 4). The gallbladder should then be collapsed unless its walls are thickened and rigid with inflammatory exudate, or stones occupy its interior. The index finger of the right hand is passed under the cystic duct and the neck of the gallbladder, and the stones are worked upward with the fingers toward the opening in the fundus. The calculi may be expressed through this opening or be extracted from the gallbladder with special scoops or forceps (see Fig. 4). When no further stones can be palpated either in the cystic duct or in the gallbladder, the forefinger of the right hand is once again introduced into the gallbladder to feel if any fragments or grit remain; if so, these may be removed by passing strips of gauze into the gallbladder with dissecting forceps and by packing the gauze strips firmly in and then withdrawing them. Small particles will be-

come entangled in the gauze meshes and can then be extracted. If there is much inflammatory debris or pigment putty-like substance, the gallbladder should be gently irrigated with warm weak antiseptic or normal saline solution by means of a rubber catheter attached to a syringe. The returning fluid should be aspirated at once with a suction tube.

When calculi are felt to be firmly impacted in the neck of the gallbladder or in the cystic duct, it is usually possible to milk them back into the gallbladder (Fig. 5). This is done by passing the finger and thumb down and along the outer side of the neck of the gallbladder until the fingertip enters the foramen of Winslow. In this way, the lowest part of the cystic duct is reached. From this point the fingers are worked gently upward, pushing any stones that may be encountered back into the gallbladder. If a stone is firmly lodged in the cystic duct, firm pressure is applied with the finger and thumb to the duct's lower end, thus coaxing the stone back into the gallbladder. If the stone cannot be dislodged or if the cystic duct or neck of the gallbladder is inadvertently torn during this manoeuvre, cholecystectomy should be carried out.

Eliason and Ferguson devised a *cholecystoscope* which is in the nature of a short sigmoidoscope and carries a light and suction channel. This, they consider, is of great assistance in visualising the inaccessible portions of the gallbladder. *"This instrument has enabled us to recover stones in 15 percent of cases in which our fingers and scoops have missed."*

When the surgeon has made quite sure that no more stones remain in the gallbladder and that the cystic duct is patent, a rubber tube or a Malecot catheter with an outside diameter of about $\frac{1}{3}$ to $\frac{1}{2}$ inch (8.4 to 12.7 mm) is passed for 2 to 3 inches (5 to 7.6 cm) into the gallbladder and secured by a stitch at the opening (Figs. 6 and 7). When tied, this stitch anchors the rubber tube to the gallbladder and further tends to invaginate a portion of the edge of the opening.

The incision in the gallbladder is now closed by a series of interrupted sutures or by means of one or two purse-string sutures (see Figs. 6, 7, and 8). When the walls of the gallbladder are very thick or friable, interrupted sutures will have to be used, but

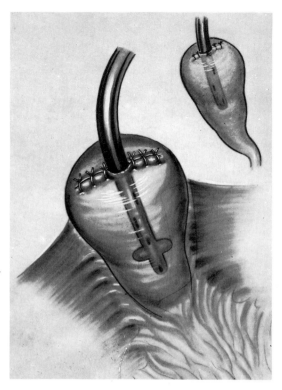

FIG. 6. Cholecystostomy. A Malecot catheter is used to drain the gallbladder.

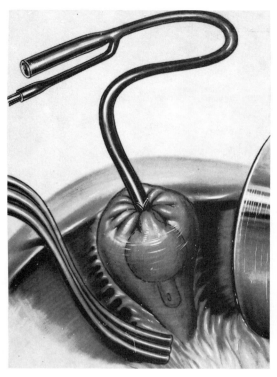

FIG. 8. Cholecystostomy. The Foley catheter method. (Courtesy of Butterworths, London.)

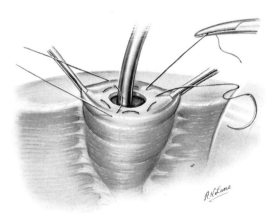

FIG. 7. Cholecystostomy. The purse-string method of closure of the opening in the fundus of the gall-bladder. Note how the tube is stitched to the adjacent walls of the gallbladder.

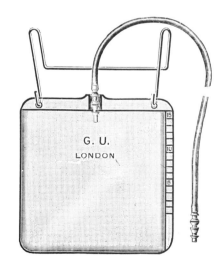

FIG. 9. URI-BAG. (Courtesy of the Genitourinary Mfg. Co., Ltd., London.)

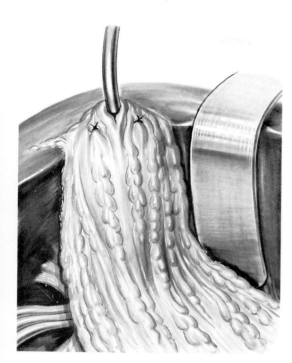

FIG. 10. Cholecystostomy. Completion of the operation. Note the position of the tubes and also the method of cloaking the gallbladder with the greater omentum. (Courtesy of Butterworths, London.)

when, on the other hand, the walls are flexible and firm, purse-string sutures are to be preferred.

A Malecot catheter or, better still, a *Foley catheter is often used in draining the gallbladder.* The latter, when attached to a URI-BAG (Figs. 8 and 9) which is affixed to the side of the patient's bed, affords good drainage, permits intermittent irrigations with antibiotic solutions, and assures a degree of safety in that it is unlikely to be inadvertently withdrawn before its terminal balloon is deliberately deflated (Fig. 8).

Adjacent omentum is next brought up and wrapped around the tube or stitched to the fundus of the gallbladder to afford assurance against leakage (Fig. 10). Some surgeons advocate suturing the fundus of the gallbladder to the parietal peritoneum, but in my opinion this step is unnecessary. Another rubber tube,

a piece of corrugated rubber or a Penrose drain, is then placed below the gallbladder in case there is any leakage, and the abdominal wound is closed. If an oblique subcostal incision has been used, at the end of the operation the tubes are drawn through the wound at its most dependent point and they are tied to the margins of the incision. The tube that has been inserted into, or adjacent to, the foramen of Winslow to drain the right subhepatic region is withdrawn on the second, third, or fourth postoperative day. The cholecystostomy tube is left in situ until it works loose on or about the twelfth to fifteenth postoperative day.

In some instances in which the *fundus* of the gallbladder is or appears to be gangrenous and cholecystectomy is contraindicated owing to the poor condition of the patient, it may be advisable to excise the major portion of the distal end of the gallbladder (subtotal cholecystectomy), and then drain the remnant of gallbladder with an indwelling Foley catheter (Fig. 11).

MANAGEMENT OF THE CHOLECYSTOSTOMY TUBE

This tube should be secured to the abdominal wall with strips of adhesive tape, Micropore, Steristrips (Fig. 11B), and then connected to a URI-BAG. The amount of bile passed into the URI-BAG should be measured daily. The cholecystostomy tube should not be removed until it works loose. This usually takes place between the twelfth and fifteenth postoperative days. It should on no account be removed before the fourteenth postoperative day.

In some instances, it may be advisable to irrigate the gallbladder with warm saline solution, or with an antibiotic solution.

The rubber drainage sheet that was inserted toward the foramen of Winslow should be removed on the third or fourth postoperative day. If there is an excessive amount of discharge of blood, purulent material, or bile from this tube, it is advisable to leave it in for a longer period.

The skin stitches are removed between the seventh and ninth postoperative day.

POSTOPERATIVE COMPLICATIONS

These include the complications common to all abdominal operations, such as atelectasis, infection of the wound, stitch abscess, disruption of the abdominal wound, and venous thrombosis; the hazards peculiar to this operation are: sub-

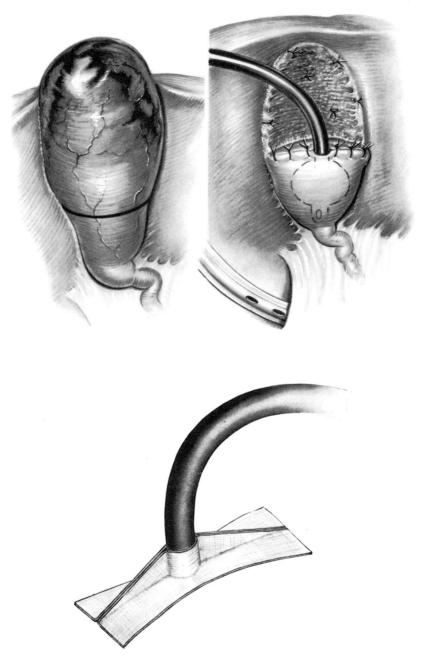

FIG. 11.   (A) Subtotal cholecystectomy for gangrene of the fundus of the gallbladder. The remaining portion of the gallbladder is drained with a Foley catheter and the subhepatic space is likewise drained with the Maingot latex tube. (B) The drainage tube is securely held in position with Steristrips.

phrenic abscess, cellulitis of the abdominal incision, and intractable external biliary fistula.

It is therefore important to provide free drainage of the operative field and to persevere with antibiotic treatment until the temperature remains normal for a few days.

CHOLECYSTECTOMY

Carl Langenbuch,[5] in 1882, performed the first cholecystectomy and it was successful. According to Madden et al.,[6] it is estimated that 400,000 cholecystectomies are performed yearly in the United States—or more than 1,000 daily. In America, cholecystectomy is now the most commonly performed abdominal operation, exceeding in frequency that of appendectomy.

Today, in the British Isles, cholecystectomy is the second most commonly performed intra-abdominal operation, being *marginally* exceeded by appendectomy for acute or chronic recurrent appendicitis. The numerous complications of gallstones are due to delay in diagnosis and surgical treatment, and are thus, in large measure, avoidable.

In most cases, cholecystectomy, when carefully performed, is one of the simplest and safest of all abdominal operations and is associated with a low operative mortality rate (about 0.5 percent) and gratifying immediate and late results.

On the other hand, it may be a most difficult and hazardous procedure demanding the greatest technical skill, experience, and endurance. Inadequate knowledge of the anatomy of the gallbladder, cystic duct, the hepatic ducts and their vascular supply, the various anomalies, as well as the course and relations of the structures in the hepatic pedicle and in Calot's triangle, combined with inadequate visualisation of the operative field during excision of the viscus, are responsible for most of the major postoperative complications, such as ductal stricture, bile peritonitis, subphrenic abscess, and profuse and persistent discharge of bile through the wound.

Indications

1. Most cases of traumatic rupture of the gallbladder or cystic duct.

    One of the possible exceptions would be rupture of the fundus of the gallbladder, when cholecystostomy may be indicated.

2. Carcinoma of the gallbladder.

    Here the operation involves: cholecystectomy alone; or wedge excision of a portion of the liver to include the gallbladder, cystic duct, and adjacent lymph nodes; or total right hepatic lobectomy (see Chap. 50). The choice of operation would depend upon the extent of the disease and upon the skill of the surgeon.

3. Resectable cancers of the bile duct which involve the cystic duct, and benign tumours of the gallbladder.
4. Cases of internal biliary fistula associated with calculous cholecystitis and/or choledocholithiasis.
5. Cases of persistent biliary or mucous fistula following cholecystostomy for acute or chronic calculous cholecystitis.
6. During a *second-stage resection* for cancer of the head of the pancreas, or the periampullary region.

    This would obtain when the first operation has been cholecystostomy, cholecystogastrostomy, cholecystoduodenostomy, or cholecystojejunostomy.

7. During pancreatoduodenectomy for carcinoma of the head of the pancreas, periampullary cancers, and some cases of chronic relapsing pancreatitis. (See Chap. 39A and B.)
8. Cases of biliary peritonitis, with or without demonstrable perforation.
9. Cholecystitis, with or without gallstones.

This would include strawberry gallbladder; calcinosis or porcelain gallbladder; calcium bile, usually associated with stone in the cystic duct; mucocele of the gallbladder; chronic calculous cholecystitis; most cases of acute cholecystitis in the absence of gross complications or anatomy obscuration; volvulus or empyema of the gallbladder; gangrene of the gallbladder, with or without perforation; cases of noncalculous cholecystitis associated with intermittent attacks of right subcostal pain, colic or jaundice; cases of *cholecystitis glandularis proliferans;* and patients with acute emphysematous cholecystitis who show immediate satisfactory response to supportive measures and antibiotic therapy.

SPECIAL CONTRAINDICATIONS

Poor-risk, aged, and feeble patients suffering from calculous cholecystitis should not be subjected to cholecystectomy—including patients with another *grave* complicating medical disorder. Another contraindication is the presence of acute cholecystitis when the general and local conditions do not permit cholecystectomy.

When, however, pain is intractable or recurrent attacks of colic are associated with bouts of pyrexia, rigors, and/or jaundice, the gratifying results of judicious, expeditious, and skillful surgical intervention should be carefully weighed against the calculated risks that are entailed.

The operative mortality rate is greatly increased in old age and in the presence of jaundice, and in cases of liver damage caused by recurrent attacks of cholangitis or of obstruction of the bile duct.

Cholecystectomy Technique

STARTING FROM THE FUNDUS END

The gallbladder may be removed by starting the dissection from the fundus or from the cystic duct end.

When the dissection commences from the *fundus* end, the blood oozes from the raw surface of the liver and tends to obscure the field of operation, thus rendering the isolation of the cystic artery and duct difficult. Nevertheless, when the gallbladder is encompassed by dense adhesions, when an extra large ovoid or barrel-shaped stone occupies Hartmann's pouch and by its bulk distorts and obscures the ducts, or when in some cases of acute cholecystitis these vital structures are hidden by oedematous peritoneal bands and membranes, rendering dissection precarious, the plan of excising the gallbladder by starting the dissection at the fundus end may be recommended. For many years I have employed this method in selected cases of *acute* obstructive cholecystitis, especially when the right border of the gastrohepatic omentum was dense and felted with adhesions. Kenneth Warren [13] disagrees with this view. He writes:

Many surgeons prefer to remove the gallbladder from above downward, waiting to identify the precise anatomical structures, including the cystic artery, the cystic duct and the common bile duct, until the gallbladder has been mobilized to the general level of these structures. This procedure has been employed for a sufficient number of years by so many surgeons that it can be performed with relative safety. Our concern with the protection of the common bile duct is so acute, however, that we never mobilize the gallbladder until the vital structures around the common duct have been identified. Once these structures have been identified, clamped and divided and the stump of the cystic artery and cystic duct secured, it makes very little difference whether the gallbladder is removed from below upward or from above downward. We are reluctant to accept the premise that it is safe to remove the gallbladder from above downward, leaving the identification of the vital structures until the region of the common duct has been approached.

CHOLECYSTECTOMY— FIRST METHOD. STARTING AT THE FUNDUS

There are two methods of performing retrograde cholecystectomy:

A trocar and cannula are plunged into the cavity of the gallbladder (Fig. 12). The cannula is attached to a suction apparatus and the gallbladder is speedily emptied of its contents. When this instrument is withdrawn, the puncture hole in the fundus is immediately grasped in the jaws of Denis Browne forceps to prevent any leakage of bile during subsequent manipulations. The adhesions between the gallbladder and adjacent viscera are cautiously separated as shown in Figure 13 and the organ is gradually detached from its vascular bed by dissection with the point of a knife. *When the neck of the gallbladder is reached, great care must be taken to isolate the cystic artery and to tie it in continuity close to the gallbladder, using an aneurysm needle.* It is advisable to tie the cystic artery proximally *twice* with 0 chromic catgut.

After dividing the artery, the fatty envelope around the cystic duct is dissected clear and the duct is traced to its junction with the common hepatic duct and the common bile duct. When these three ducts have been freed and displayed, an aneurysm needle threaded with a strand of 0 or 00 chromic catgut is passed underneath the cystic duct and this duct is ligatured *almost* flush with the main

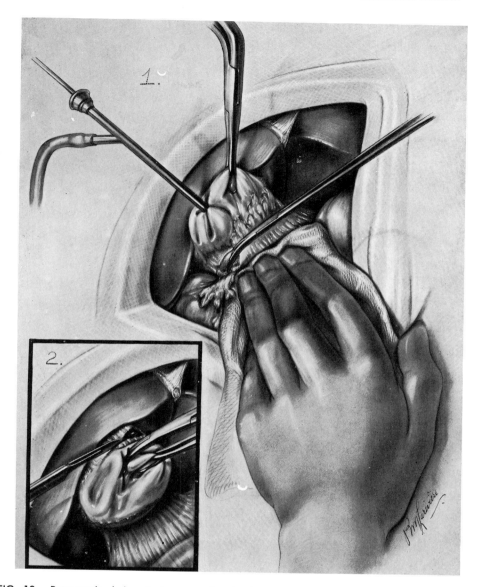

FIG. 12.   Retrograde cholecystectomy, starting the dissection from the fundus end. The gallbladder
contents should be emptied with a trocar and cannula before proceeding with the dissection.

ducts. The portion of the cystic duct close to the neck of the gallbladder is clamped with slender cholecystectomy forceps and the duct is divided between the haemostat and the catgut ligatures. Here, again, the cystic duct stump should be ligated close to the common duct *twice* with 0 or 00 chromic catgut. Broadman and Ghazi,[1] the writer, and many other surgeons have emphasised the point that no sizeable cystic duct stump should be left in situ following a well-performed cholecystectomy. The cystic stump may or may not be symptomatic.

Symptomatic causes include:

1.   Acute or chronic inflammation.
2.   "Residual" or newly formed calculus.
3.   Neuroma of the parasympathetic nerve filaments.

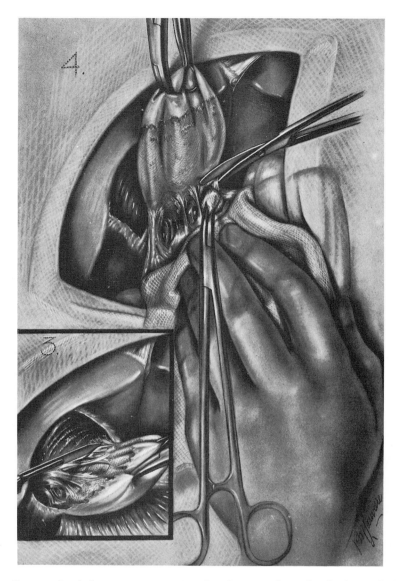

FIG. 13.　Retrograde cholecystectomy, starting the dissection from the fundus end. Adhesions are being cautiously separated.

4. Pressure from dilated stump on adjacent common bile duct.
5. "Tumour" formation.
6. Empyema.

A swab soaked in a hot saline solution is applied to the bleeding gallbladder fossa for a few moments to control the oozing from this region, after which the raw area is re-peritonealised with a series of interrupted mattress sutures of 00000 chromic catgut.

Sometimes the margins of the gallbladder fossa are so widely separated and the liver is so fatty and friable that it is impossible to close the defect by means of sutures. In such cases, after transfixing and ligating any bleeding points and coagulating (with a diathermy needle) oozing areas, a portion of the greater omentum should be drawn into the gaping gallbladder fossa and then plugged into this area and carefully sutured into position (Fig. 14). The operative field is always drained through the top end of a vertical incision or through a literally placed stab incision, as there may be oozing of blood or bile or both during the first few days following operation.

Second method. By this method, which was advocated by Lahey,[4] no clamp or haemostat is applied to the friable wall of the gallbladder. The gallbladder and its contents are removed intact.

The operation is performed by incising the medial peritoneal reflection of the gallbladder close to the liver and well above the neck of the viscus, so as to avoid the cystic artery, and *by passing a finger behind the gallbladder into the loose layer of tissue which lies between the gallbladder wall and the layer of fascia over the liver.* The finger is swept upward and readily detaches the body and fundus of the gallbladder from its fossa, after which the cystic duct is cleared and the cystic artery is displayed (Figs. 15, 16, 17, and 18).

The cystic artery and the three ducts are clearly brought into view by drawing the gallbladder downward and cautiously clearing the fibro-fatty tissues which obscure these vital structures. The cystic artery is ligated twice and divided to enable the cystic duct to be straightened out by traction and gauze dissection. This duct is tied $\frac{1}{8}$ inch (3.15 mm) away from its junction with the common ducts and then divided, leaving a little cuff of tissue projecting distal to the ligature. The stump of the cystic duct is next transfixed and ligated with 00 or 0 chromic catgut. The gallbladder bed is, when possible, obliterated with interrupted mattress sutures of 00000 chromic catgut. Drainage of the operative field is provided.

Before the abdominal incision is closed, an *operative cholangiogram* is frequently performed to exclude the possibility of stones being lodged in the bile ducts. Experience has shown that the incidence of choledocholithiasis is higher in cases of *acute* cholecystitis than in cases of *chronic* calculous cholecystitis. The approximate ratio is estimated as being 14 to 10. Incidentally, it is now the practice of most surgeons to perform operative cholangiography in the majority of cases in which cholecystectomy is indicated for calculous cholecystitis.

Preexploratory cholangiography as performed by Leslie LeQuesne is described and illustrated in Chapter 43. The writer's techniques are illustrated in Figures 19 and 20.

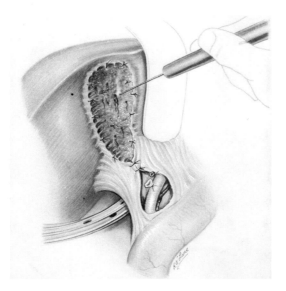

FIG. 14.   A method of dealing with the raw surface of the gallbladder fossa where reperitonealisation is not possible. (From Maingot, Cholecystectomy, in Rob, Smith, and Morgan. *Operative Surgery*, 2d ed., 1969. Courtesy of Butterworths, London.)

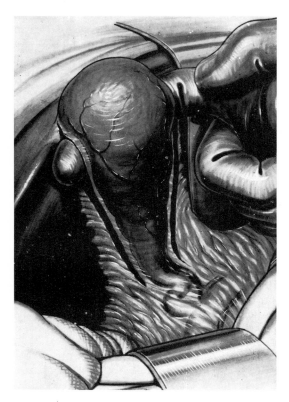

FIG. 15. Cholecystectomy, by the so-called retrograde method. Mobilisation of the gallbladder. (After Lahey.)

CHOLECYSTECTOMY— SECOND METHOD. STARTING AT THE CYSTIC DUCT END

In this operation, *which is the procedure of choice,* the cystic artery and cystic duct are displayed early in the operation, and after these have been ligatured and divided the gallbladder is freed from its bed in the liver and removed. The operation is greatly simplified by ensuring the maximum degree of exposure of the gallbladder and bile passages. This is obtained by:

1. Making an adequate right paramedian or Kocher's incision (in obese patients).
2. Illuminating the area well.
3. Administering perfect anaesthesia with complete muscular relaxation.
4. Passing the right hand between the liver and diaphragm and retracting the liver downwards to facilitate the introduction of air into the subphrenic spaces. Two packs of gauze are then inserted between the liver and diaphragm, superiorly and laterally, to assist the downward displacement of the liver.[12]
5. Carefully freeing any adhesions that may exist between the gallbladder and adjacent viscera.
6. Aspirating the contents of the gallbladder (some cases).
7. Grasping the fundus of the gallbladder with Denis Browne forceps and drawing the viscus firmly downward and outward.
8. Inserting a long roll of gauze to act as a barrier between the pyloric end of the stomach, the first part of the duodenum, and the hepatic flexure of the colon on the one hand and the gallbladder on the other. Morison's pouch is also filled with gauze. Three Deaver retractors are then inserted: one keeps the stomach away from the operative field; one, when slipped in between the neck of the gallbladder and the duo-

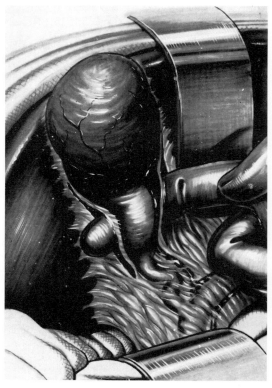

FIG. 16. Cholecystectomy, by the retrograde method. (From Maingot, Cholecystectomy, in Rob, Smith, and Morgan. *Operative Surgery,* 2d ed., 1969. Courtesy of Butterworths, London.)

denum and drawn downward, effectually keeps the duodenum out of sight and puts the *common bile duct on the stretch;* the other is applied to the right lobe of the liver medial to the gallbladder to draw the undersurface of the liver upward and outward. The placing of the rolls into Morison's pouch between the gallbladder and the duodenum and over the stomach and the correct placing of the Deaver retractors are all essential to good exposure (Fig. 21). If the retractors have been correctly placed, the stomach, duodenum, colon, and omentum are not seen throughout the essential steps of the operation (Figs. 22 and 23).

Before the dissection commences, another long strip of gauze is passed into the foramen of Winslow to prevent blood or bile from reaching the lesser sac; this is removed just before the operation is completed. A curved

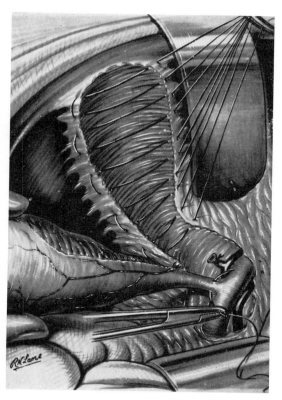

FIG. 18. Retrograde cholecystectomy. The cystic duct is transfixed and tied with chromic catgut before being divided. Note the method of suturing the margins of the gallbladder fossa with fine chromic catgut. (Courtesy of Butterworths, London.)

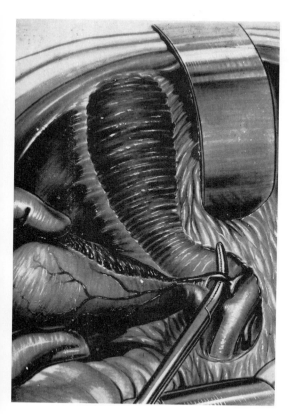

FIG. 17. Retrograde cholecystectomy. The gallbladder is liberated from its bed before the cystic artery and duct are dealt with. Isolation of the cystic artery.

haemostat or another pair of Denis Browne forceps is fixed to Hartmann's pouch (infundibulum). This is drawn downward and outward, while the forceps on the fundus are pulled upward, thereby putting the cystic duct on the stretch so that this structure and Calot's triangular space above it in which the cystic artery lurks may be readily recognised.

A small incision is now made in the peritoneum over the neck of the gallbladder or over the common bile duct, and the serofatty tissues in this region are cautiously dissected away until the supraduodenal portion of the common bile duct and the cystic duct can be clearly defined (Fig. 23). The dissection now proceeds a little further inward and upward in Calot's space in order to display the cystic artery and also the common bile duct, the

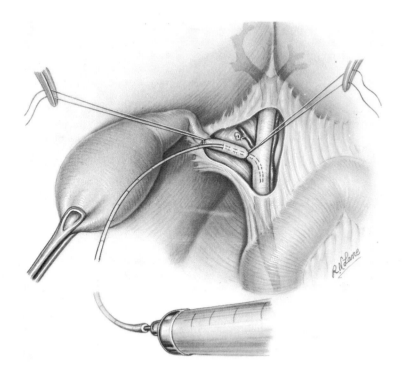

FIG. 19.   Preexploratory cholangiography. (Courtesy of Butterworths, London.)

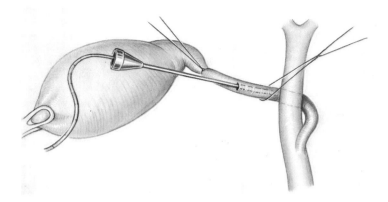

FIG. 20.   Preexploratory cholangiography.

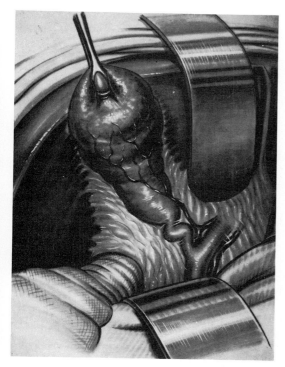

FIG. 21. Cholecystectomy. Note the positioning of the Deaver retractors.

right margin of the hepatic duct, and the point where the cystic duct joins the common ducts (Figs. 24 and 25).

I have already discussed the various anatomical points in connection with the cystic artery and how the right hepatic artery may be mistaken for it and be inadvertently ligatured. I feel sure that some of the so-called "liver deaths" or unexplained fatalities following "straightforward" cholecytstectomy operations are due to ligature of the main hepatic artery, or its right branch in mistake for the cystic artery. As a rule, the cystic artery lies in a more posterior plane than the cystic duct, slightly above it and in close proximity to the liver. A little dissection in this obscure area will reveal the artery travelling toward the gallbladder. It should, when possible, be traced to the point where it arises from its parent vessel to the exact site where it bifurcates into anterior and posterior branches—in fact, the point where it enters the wall of the gallbladder, usually near the

neck. When it has been isolated, an aneurysm needle threaded with 0 or 00 chromic catgut is passed behind it and tied three times—twice proximally and once laterally, well away from the right hepatic artery or its parent trunk, and close to the gallbladder itself. The artery is then divided close to the lateral ligature. Sometimes the artery is fan-shaped, i.e., there are several little radiating branches arising from the main short parent stem. In such instances, it is safer to underrun and ligate each branch separately rather than to dissect, strip, and isolate the main cystic artery.

The cystic artery is usually a small vessel and should be handled gently and with the greatest care. Haemostats are often clumsy instruments and they should certainly not be used to catch this delicate structure. The aneurysm needle method ensures the neatness and tidiness that accompany precise work.

The surgeon must always be on his guard when he sees an unduly large cystic artery. Here again the dissection cannot be too meticulous and the vessel must be cautiously freed to demonstrate its true anatomical relations. *Too often what the surgeon considers to be a large cystic artery is, in fact, the right hepatic artery.* He should also proceed with circumspection when the right hepatic artery has a caterpillar-like hump or when it jostles the cystic duct on its way to the right lobe of the liver, as the cystic artery in these cases is often stumpy and cunningly hidden behind the neck of the gallbladder. The surgeon should constantly bear in mind that the right hepatic artery frequently runs parallel to and in close company with the cystic duct and the neck of the gallbladder. He should proceed cautiously with the dissection of the cystic artery when the gallbladder possesses a mesentery, as in such instances the right hepatic artery (or the common hepatic artery itself) may course through this structure on its way to the porta hepatis. Again, a meticulous search should always be made for two or more cystic arteries and for the slender trunk of an accessory hepatic bile duct. The cystic duct lymph gland nearly always lies on top of the cystic artery and is a good guide to this vessel. This lymph node should invariably be removed during cholecystectomy.

It is, as a rule, better and safer to isolate

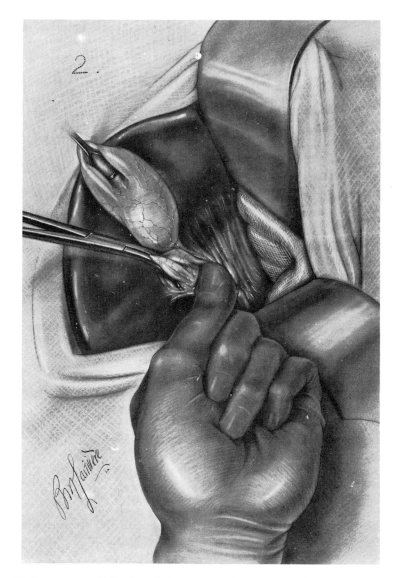

FIG. 22.   Cholecystectomy. Palpation of the common ducts between the index finger and thumb.

and tie the cystic artery before ligaturing the cystic duct. Bentley Colcock[2] writes:

By securing the cystic artery first, three things are accomplished:

1.   The subsequent dissection is carried out in a relatively dry field;
2.   When the cystic artery is divided and released from the gallbladder, the convolutions of the cystic duct can be straightened out and the junction of this duct with the common duct more clearly and accurately defined; and,
3.   It eliminates the danger of serious bleeding from tearing the cystic artery through traction upon the gallbladder. (See **Figs.** 25 and 26.)

It should be remembered that an accessory cystic artery is found in about 12 percent of cases, and that in 8 percent two cystic arteries

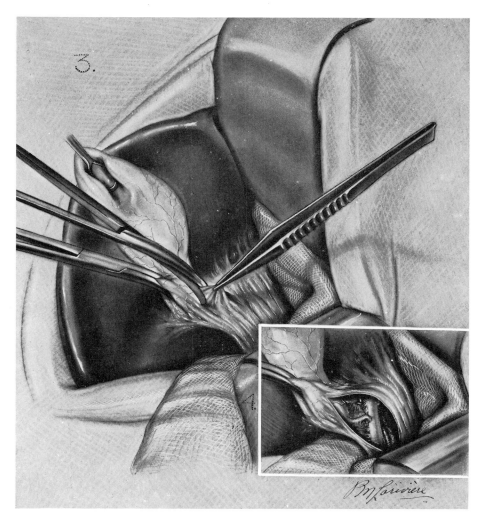

FIG. 23. Cholecystectomy. The three ducts are exposed.

arise from the right hepatic artery. (See Chap. 40.)

The cystic duct is never ligatured until it has been followed upward into the neck of the gallbladder and inward to the point where it unmistakably joins the common ducts, and it is a good rule at this stage to demonstrate to an assistant the three ducts as they are clearly displayed (Fig. 27).

Before ligating the cystic duct, it is important to remove all fatty and areolar tissue that may surround it, and also to identify, isolate, sever, and sweep away the fine fila-

mentous strands of parasympathetic nerves which so frequently lie on its surface. This step eliminates any possibility of the subsequent formation of *neuroma of the stump of the cystic duct.*

The cystic duct is then rendered as straight and taut as possible and an aneurysm needle threaded with a strand of 0 or 00 chromic catgut is passed underneath the duct, which is tied securely in two places. The duct is divided between ligatures, after which the neck of the gallbladder close to the stump of the cystic duct is seized with curved artery

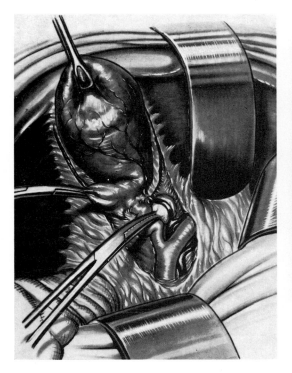

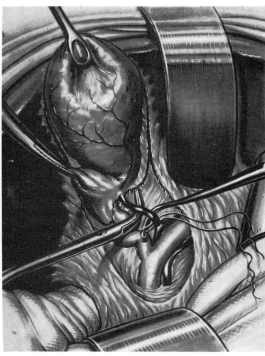

FIG. 24. Cholecystectomy. Isolation of the cystic artery. This artery must be dissected free and displayed where it gives off its anterior and posterior branches to the gallbladder. Its site of origin should, in most instances, be identified. Here the cystic artery is arising from the right hepatic artery.

FIG. 25. Cholecystectomy. Isolation of the cystic artery. Note that the *origin* and *distribution* of this artery should be identified before ligating it with 0 chromic catgut. (Courtesy of Butterworths, London.)

forceps and rotated outward to display a small area of the posterior wall of the viscus so that any vascular adhesions that may have developed here may be ligated and divided by sight.

In those cases in which the cystic duct is unusually large or fibrotic, it is better to apply a transfixion ligature of 00 or 0 chromic catgut to ensure that there will be no subsequent slipping off of this all-important ligature. This step in the operation is clearly depicted in Figure 27 (inset). It is always wise to ligate the stump of the cystic duct *twice*.

A few large veins—which run from the gallbladder to the liver substance and which are usually situated at about the middle and on either side of the body of the gallbladder—are divided during the peritoneal separation, the bleeding points being picked up

with mosquito forceps and ligatured. The gallbladder is freed from its bed, with knife dissection, in an upward direction towards the fundus and, when it is removed, the edges of the peritoneum on each side of its fossa are approximated with a continuous catgut suture or a series of interrupted sutures (Fig. 28). A small "window" in the free margin of the lesser omentum is, however, left open where the ligated stumps of the cystic duct and artery can be seen (Fig. 29). I believe that it is unwise to suture the margins of the peritoneum over the common ducts and the stumps of the cystic duct and cystic artery, as these structures would thereby be placed in the retroperitoneum and, should bleeding or leakage of bile occur in the early postoperative period, extravasation would take place in a confined area and the pent-up fluids, being denied free drainage

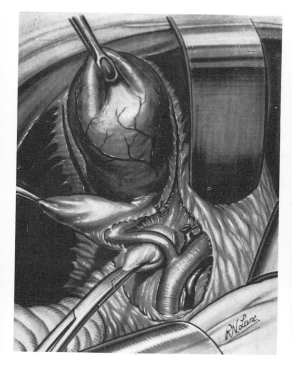

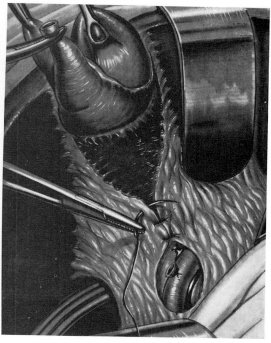

FIG. 26. Cholecystectomy. Ligation and division of the cystic artery. Note how the cystic duct straightens out after division of the cystic artery.

FIG. 28. Cholecystectomy. Liberation of the gallbladder and suture of the peritoneal margins of the gallbladder fossa.

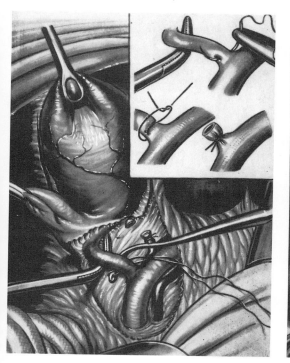

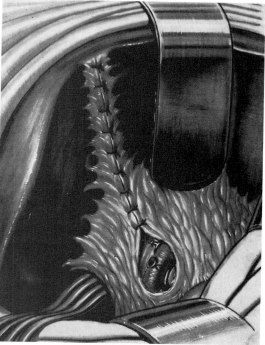

FIG. 27. Cholecystectomy. Isolation and ligation of the cystic duct. If the cystic duct is large, it is better to use a transfixion suture rather than an ordinary one. (Courtesy of Butterworths, London.)

FIG. 29. Cholecystectomy. Note the closure of the margins of the gallbladder fossa, and the drain to the foramen of Winslow. Note also the little "window."

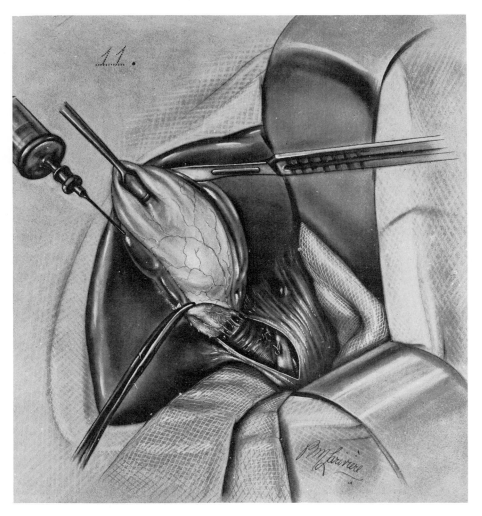

FIG. 30.   Cholecystectomy. In order to facilitate the division of the peritoneal reflections of the gallbladder, saline solution may be injected underneath the peritoneum, where it is reflected from the gallbladder onto the liver.

to the surface, might become infected and lead to serious complications.

Drainage of the sutured or unsutured gallbladder fossa is never omitted in this operation, for if bile escapes into the general peritoneal cavity, it is prone to become infected and to give rise to peritonitis or subphrenic abscess. The tube is left in situ for 2 or 3 days, as there may be leakage of bile from an unrecognised severed accessory hepatic duct or from the raw surface of the liver itself and, however carefully the operation is per-

formed, such leakage is apt to occur from time to time.

Arthur Allen repeatedly emphasised the importance of draining the right subhepatic space by tubes which drain dependently through a stab wound in the flank rather than through the original vertical exploratory incision. Some surgeons, however, prefer to lead these drainage tubes (and T tubes) through the top end of vertical epigastric incisions and through the most dependent point of subcostal incisions, while others con-

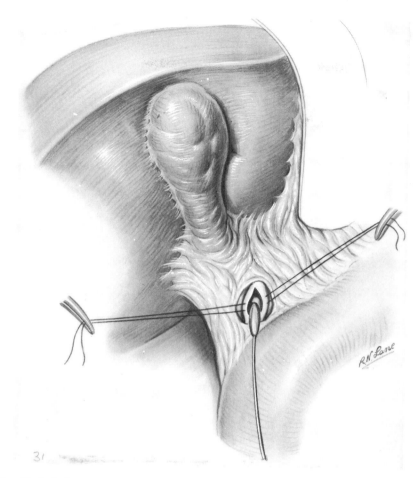

FIG. 31. Choledochotomy, and guiding a Bakes' dilator into the right hepatic duct. A wise precaution before performing a difficult cholecystectomy. (After Warren and Braasch. Courtesy of Butterworths, London.)

tinue to use separate laterally placed stab incisions for drainage purposes.

If the essential precepts of a safe cholecystectomy are carefully pursued in every case, injury to the choledochus would almost never occur. Most of the injuries to the bile ducts, occurring because of haemorrhage (and haemorrhage is the most common complication), result from the panic generated by the magnitude of the bleeding and from the blind application of clamps indiscriminately applied to the area of bleeding. This is an invitation to disaster!

A final word: in some cases of cholecystectomy, in order to facilitate the division of the peritoneal reflections of the gallbladder,

saline solution may be injected underneath the peritoneum where it is reflected from the gallbladder on to the liver (Fig. 30).

In certain cases, when the surgeon anticipates that cholecystectomy will prove a difficult undertaking owing to the portal fissure and right border of the gastrohepatic omentum being shrouded in dense fibrous adhesions, it may be advisable to display the accessible supraduodenal portion of the common bile duct, to open it, and then to insert a Bakes' dilator upward into the right hepatic duct.

When in position, this sound or dilator acts as a useful guide to the vital structures lying on its lateral border (Fig. 31).

POSTOPERATIVE COMPLICATIONS

Atelectasis and other pulmonary complications are fairly commonly seen in a severe or lesser degree in about 10 percent of patients who have undergone cholecystectomy.

The immediate hazards are internal or external haemorrhage, bleeding from the cystic artery or an unrecognised accessory artery, or from the gallbladder fossa. Discharge of bile from the wound is unusual, but if it is copious and persistent, it may give rise to alarm and suggest that some injury has been inflicted on the common bile duct, the ligature on the cystic duct has slipped, or an accessory hepatic duct has been divided. External duodenal fistula is a rare complication and may be caused by pressure necrosis from a drainage tube or to (inadvertently) incising the lumen of the bowel during the freeing of dense adhesions between the gallbladder and the first part of the duodenum.[10]

Jaundice in the early postoperative stage is always a danger signal, as it may be due to improper blood grouping and matching, injury to the common bile duct, an overlooked stone in the choledochus, or the obstruction of the bile duct by large extraductal collections of bile and blood.

REFERENCES

1. Broadman and Ghazi, Am. J. Surg. 37:427, 1971.
2. Colcock, Surg. Clin. North Am. June, 641, 1949.
3. Glenn, Surg. Clin. North Am. 39:1128, 1966.
4. Lahey, Surg. Gynecol. Obstet. 91:25, 1950.
5. Langenbuch, Berl. Klin. Wehirschr. 19:725, 1882.
6. Madden et al., Current Problems in Surgery, Surgery of the Common Duct, May, 1968.
7. Maingot, Ann. R. Coll. Surg. Engl. 24:186, 1959.
8. Maingot, London Clin. Med. J. 2:11, 1961.
9. Maingot, Proc. R. Soc. Med. 55:587, 1962.
10. Maingot, Ann. R. Coll. Surg. Engl. 32:42, 1963.
11. Maingot, Cholecystostomy and Cholecystectomy, in Rob, Smith, and Morgan, eds. Operative Surgery, 2d ed., London, Butterworths, 1969.
12. Sanders, Surgery 69:115, 1971.
13. Warren, Surg. Clin. North Am. 40:681, 1960.

43

A. CHOLEDOCHOLITHIASIS: INCIDENCE, DIAGNOSIS, AND OPERATIVE PROCEDURES

LESLIE P. LE QUESNE

Stone in the common bile duct is one of the most common and most serious of the complications of gallstones. The great majority of stones present in the common duct originally formed in the gallbladder, later passing down the cystic duct into the common duct. Usually patients with a stone, or stones, in the common duct also have calculi in the gallbladder; however, such is not always the case, although in these latter patients the gallbladder almost invariably shows chronic inflammatory changes—suggesting that it previously harboured stones.

Stones or soft concretions of biliary mud may form in the bile duct in the presence of stasis and infection. Madden (1968) has suggested that the incidence of such primary duct stones is possibly higher than has been previously thought, and the mechanism by which such concretions develop has been reviewed by Scott (1971). Stones can also form in the bile ducts in the type of suppurative cholangitis seen in certain Asian countries. In this latter condition, the stone formation has been attributed to infestation of the bile ducts with the parasite *Clonorchis sinensis* (Fung, 1961), although Ong (1961) has shown that this parasite is not always present and suggested that infection of the ducts with *Escherichia coli* or enterococci may be the critical cause of the ductal stone formation. In a more recent study, King (1971) was only able to isolate *C. sinensis* in one of 44 patients with oriental cholangitis, and he also emphasises that the clinical and pathological features of this condition differ from those of the usual Western type of gallstone disease.

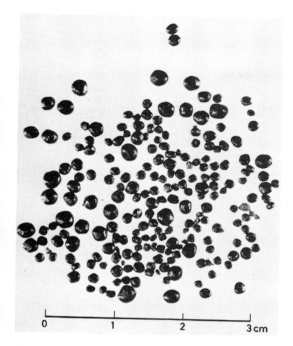

FIG. 1. Multiple small stones removed from the common bile duct.

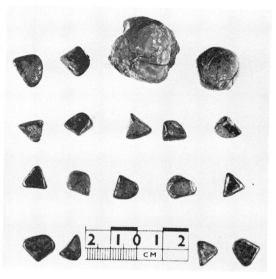

FIG. 2. Multiple stones removed from a dilated common bile duct. Many of the stones are facetted, revealing their origin in the gallbladder. The two large, barrel-shaped stones were impacted in the intrapancreatic portion of the duct: they are covered with a layer of soft pigment and debris laid down in the duct, and are mutually congruent where they have been in contact.

Stones in the common duct may be single or multiple, 100 or more sometimes being present in a dilated duct (Fig. 1). Very commonly the origin of the stones in the gallbladder is shown by their facetted shape (Fig. 2). From the narrow calibre of the cystic duct, it is evident that, in the absence of fistula formation, only relatively small stones can pass into the common duct but, once in this duct, they may enlarge as the result of the deposition of soft pigment and debris on their surface. When this occurs, the stones may become barrel-shaped and mutually congruent (Fig. 2). On section, such stones will usually be found to contain in their centre a small, hard, and often facetted calculus, betraying their origin from the gallbladder.

STONES IN THE COMMON DUCT

Incidence

The incidence of stone in the common duct is difficult to determine with accuracy, partly because many such stones do not give rise to symptoms; at operation, stones in the common duct may be overlooked; and comparison of reported series of patients may be misleading owing to the differing composition of the various series. This latter point is particularly important in relation to the age of the patients in any series, for there is evidence that the incidence of stones in the common duct increases with age (Appleman, Priestley, and Gage, 1964). Despite such difficulties, there is reasonable uniformity in the published data on this point, and from Table 1 it can be seen that stones are present in the common duct in from 10 to 15 percent of all patients subjected to cholecystectomy for gallstones. This figure may be taken as representing reasonably accurately the true incidence of choledocholithiasis as a complication of gallstones, for in view of the wide range of the figures for these purposes, the small incidence of residual stones can be overlooked.

Table 1.   CHOLECYSTECTOMY: INCIDENCE OF EXPLORATION
OF COMMON DUCT AND OF DISCOVERY OF STONES

| Author | No. of Cases | Exploration of Common Bile Duct | | Stones Found in Common Bile Duct | | |
		No.	Percent	No.	Ducts Explored (percent)	Total (percent)
Adams and Stranahan (1947)	1,051	451	43	161	36	15
Walters, Gray, and Priestley (1948)	1,259	301	24	–	–	12[a]
McLaughlin and Kleager (1951)	230	71	31	24	34	10
Glenn (1952)	3,367	359	10.6	234	65	6.9
Zollinger, Boles, and Crawford (1955)	676	333	49	117	46	18
Thomson (1956)	745	106	14	45	41	6
Bartlett and Waddell (1958)	2,243	–	–	–	–	16
Harvard (1960)	702	148	21	84	57	12
Appleman, Priestley, and Gage (1964)	4,948	1,127	22.8	480	42.6	9.7
Glenn (1967)	4,677[b]	694	14	416	59	9

[a]Approximate figure given in text.

[b]Stones not present in gallbladder in a small but unspecified number.

Fate

ANATOMY OF THE CHOLEDOCHODUODENAL JUNCTION

There is no doubt that some stones that enter the common duct pass on into the duodenum. Evidence in support of this outcome is provided by patients who pass gallstones per rectum and at a subsequent operation are shown to have no fistula between the gallbladder and intestines. Occasionally radiographic examination may provide similar evidence (Fig. 3). How often this occurs is not known, and it may well be that small stones pass on more often than is realised. It is believed that the majority of stones that pass from the gallbladder into the common duct remain there until removed surgically, but there is no real evidence in support of this belief.

The intrinsic anatomy of the common duct makes it unlikely that any but small stones pass with much frequency into the duodenum. The anatomy of the choledochoduodenal junction is admirably described by Hand (1963), and the following brief account is based on his paper. The detailed anatomy of this area is also described by Hughes and Kernutt (1954) and by Kune (1964).

The main portion of the common bile duct, lying in the free edge of the lesser omentum and in relation to the posterior surface of the head of the pancreas, is a tube of relatively wide bore, with thin walls which contain little or no muscle. Shortly before it passes obliquely through the posteromedial wall of the second part of the duodenum, the lumen of the common duct narrows abruptly as a result of a thickening of its walls (Fig. 4). This thickening is due almost entirely to the appearance of a copious amount of circular smooth muscle in the wall of the duct; the major portion of this muscle is the intrinsic sphincter of the duct, with a relatively small contribution from the musculature of the duodenum. Having pierced the muscle wall of the duodenum, the duct runs obliquely through the submucosa to open into the duodenum on the summit of the papilla. The terminal segment of the duct, alternatively referred to as the thickened or narrow segment, depending upon whether it is the wall or lumen that is being described, varies in length from 11 to 27 mm and it is important to appreciate that it commences some 2 mm before the duct enters the muscle coat of the duodenum. Hand (1963) found that in the majority of instances (80 percent) the terminal segment was joined in its passage through the submucosa by the main pancreatic duct, giving a common channel varying in length from 2 to 17 mm, but usually measuring some 5 mm in length. The common bile duct is at its narrowest just before this junction, but there is no true ampulla in that the diameter of the common channel does not exceed the sum of the diameters of the two ducts; further, the common channel itself narrows throughout its length (Fig. 5).

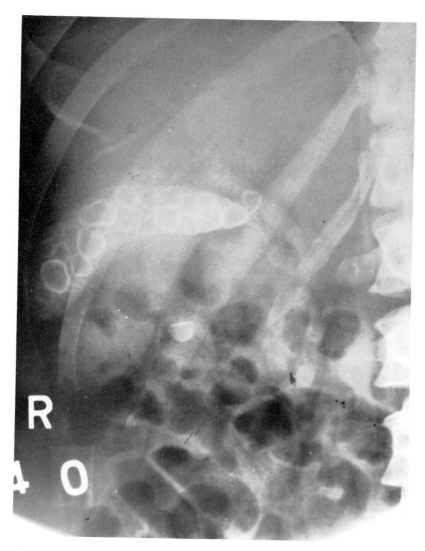

FIG. 3. Intravenous cholangiogram showing multiple stones in the gallbladder, with a single facetted calculus lying separate from the gallbladder, probably in the colon. Subsequent radiographs showed this separate stone to have disappeared, and operation showed no fistula between the gallbladder and intestines.

This division of the common duct into two portions, viz., the main portion (with a wide lumen and thin walls) and the terminal segment (with a relatively narrow lumen and thick walls), has an important bearing on many aspects of the problem of stone in the duct. Furthermore, appreciation of this anatomy is essential for the correct interpretation of many types of cholangiogram. The junction between the main portion of the duct and the terminal segment is clearly seen on operative cholangiograms (Fig. 6), and there is often a distinct notch in the image of the duct lumen at this junction. In the past this abrupt narrowing of the terminal portion of the duct has often been interpreted as representing a pathological stricture.

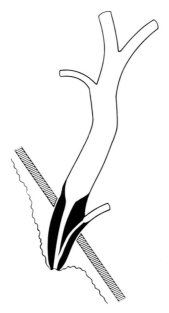

FIG. 4. The intrinsic anatomy of the termination of the bile duct. The main portion of the duct is a relatively wide-bore tube with thin walls. Shortly before piercing the muscle coat of the duodenum, the lumen of the duct narrows abruptly, owing to thickening of its wall due to the presence of circular muscle forming the sphincteric mechanism of the duct. Note (1) the abrupt junction between the main portion of the duct and its narrow, terminal segment; (2) the length of the terminal segment, which begins outside the duodenal wall and runs obliquely through the submucosa; and (3) the formation of a common channel with the pancreatic duct in the submucosa of the duodenum.

Effects

In rare instances, a stone impacts in the terminal narrow segment of the common duct, giving rise to a complete obstruction to flow of bile into the duodenum and resulting in an obstructive jaundice closely resembling that seen in patients with carcinoma of the head of the pancreas. Much more commonly, the stone remains in the wider portion of the duct, where it may move up and down—causing chronic, intermittent, and partial obstruction to the flow of bile; when the stones are large, they may become impacted in the intrapancreatic portion of the duct, just above the narrow segment, giving rise to acute obstruction with jaundice.

ACUTE OBSTRUCTION

Acute obstructive jaundice caused by a stone in the common duct is not unusual; it is usually due to a stone impacting in the intrapancreatic portion of the duct, at the junction of the main portion of the duct with the terminal segment. The obstruction is caused partly by the actual presence of the stone, partly by oedema of the wall of duct, and partly by spasm of the sphincteric musculature of the terminal segment. The obstruction to the flow of bile is rarely com-

LEVEL	Av Diam mms.	
At entry into Pancreas	6·5	A········
Above Notch.	5·7	B·······
Below Notch	3·9	C········
In Submucosa	3·3	D········
At Junction with Pancreatic Duct.	1·9	
Common Channel	2·9	E········ F········ G········
Orifice of Papilla	2·1	

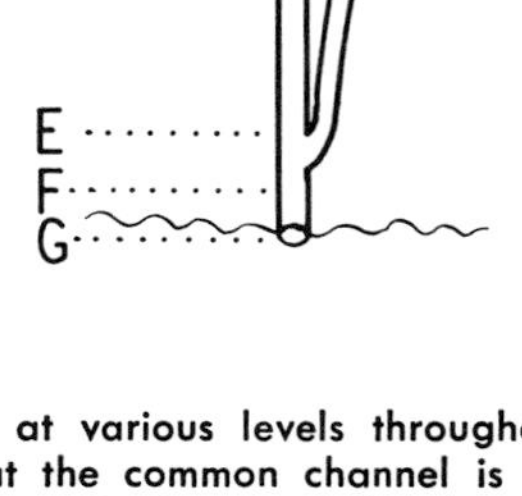

FIG. 5. The average diameter of the common duct at various levels throughout its passage through the pancreas and duodenal wall. Note that the common channel is not wider than the combined width of the terminal bile duct and pancreatic duct, and that the common channel narrows throughout its length.

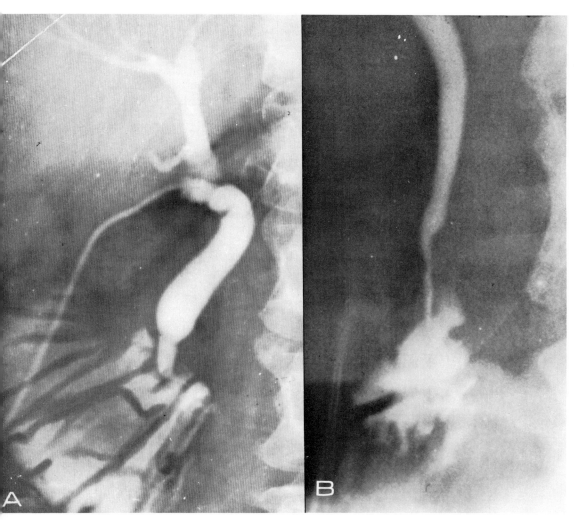

FIG. 6A and B. Two normal operative cholangiograms, showing the well-marked notch at the junction of the main portion of the duct with the narrow, terminal segment. A also illustrates an abnormal tributary of the right hepatic duct opening into the common hepatic duct.

plete, so that although the stools are pale they contain some bile pigments and, accordingly, some urobilinogen is usually present in the urine. Further, the degree of obstruction tends to vary from day to day, with the result that the jaundice is characteristically fluctuant. In view of the fact that the obstruction is rarely complete, "white bile" is rarely seen in the ducts of patients with calculous obstruction. In the majority of instances, the stone either passes on into the duodenum or, with subsidence of the oedema and spasm, free flow of bile is reestablished, resulting (in either case) in a clearing of the jaundice.

CHRONIC OBSTRUCTION

Stones may be present in the common duct for many months or years—causing chronic, intermittent obstruction but in an insufficient amount to cause jaundice, although at times the obstruction may temporarily become sufficiently severe to cause transient icterus. During the time they are in the common duct, the stones may markedly increase in size owing to the laying down of pigment and debris on their surface. As with acute obstruction, the impedence to the flow of bile is partly caused by the mechanical presence of the stone, and partly by intermittent spasm of the sphincteric mechanism; in addition, in some patients there may be actual fibrosis of the sphincteric musculature as a result of prolonged irritation from a stone in the duct.

Chronic obstruction results in dilatation of the ducts, which may become twice their normal calibre. This dilatation affects not only the main portion of the common duct but extends also up into the intrahepatic ducts—although these latter are rarely so greatly dilated as they may be in patients with malignant obstruction to the terminal common duct. The dilatation does not affect the terminal segment of the common duct, with the result that the sudden narrowing of the duct at its junction with the terminal segment becomes even more prominent than in the normal. In addition to becoming dilated, the walls of the common duct also become thicker because of an increase of fibrous tissue in their walls. In rare instances, an impacted stone causes ulceration of the wall of the duct, and on healing this ulceration can uncommonly cause a fibrous stricture of the duct.

Chronic obstruction also gives rise to changes in the liver, eventually resulting in biliary cirrhosis; however, this is usually marked only in patients with long-standing obstruction of severity sufficient to cause jaundice, as in patients with a stricture of the duct. The essential change in the liver is the deposition of fibrous tissue in the portal tracts, spreading out to surround the liver lobules; together with this, there is proliferation of the bile canaliculi and the formation of bile thrombi in the smaller ducts (Fig. 7). These changes, when mild, are reversible following relief of the obstruction.

A serious complication of stone in the common duct is infection, which may not be apparent either clinically or at operation. The studies of Scott and Khan (1967) and Flemma et al. (1967) show that in the majority of patients with stone in the common duct the bile is infected, the most common organism being *E. Coli*. When infection is

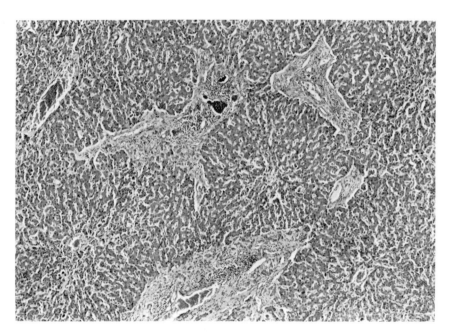

FIG. 7. Section cut from a liver biopsy obtained at operation from a patient with multiple stones in a dilated common duct, showing the changes of biliary cirrhosis. Note the periportal fibrosis, with bile-duct proliferation and bile thrombi (×50).

severe, in addition to the changes already mentioned, the walls of the ducts are infiltrated by an inflammatory exudate, and these acute inflammatory changes extend up into the portal tracts. The bile itself contains pus cells and inflammatory exudate, and in severe instances the bile ducts are full of purulent bile; rarely, multiple liver abscesses may develop.

Clinical Features

Stones may be present in the common duct for months or years without causing symptoms, but sooner or later they almost invariably give rise to the typical picture of severe upper abdominal pain, accompanied or followed by jaundice, with pale stools and dark urine. Often these attacks come on after ingestion of a rich or fatty meal; they characteristically occur in women previously subject to a flatulent dyspepsia suggestive of gallstones.

The pain is usually sudden in its onset, reaching its maximum intensity in 20 to 60 minutes, and the attack may last many hours before subsiding—usually relatively slowly, but sometimes suddenly. The pain is commonly described as "biliary colic." Correctly used, the word "colic" describes an intermittent pain, coming in waves; in relation to the pain caused by impaction of a stone in the common duct, the word is most often either incorrectly used or is misleading. In a most valuable analysis of the pain in "biliary colic," French and Robb (1963) found that once it reaches its intensity, the pain is almost invariably constant and that true colic is very rare. Our own clinical experience would strongly support this conclusion. The pain is commonly epigastric in onset, and characteristically radiates to the right hypochondrium or through to the region of the right scapula. It may, however, originate to the right or left of the midline or in the umbilical region, and may radiate retrosternally, to the left, or to the umbilicus. During an attack, the patient is usually restless (French and Robb, 1963), often sweats, and commonly feels sick (although vomiting is rarely prominent). There is usually some tenderness in the upper right quadrant of the abdomen during the attack, and as the attack subsides the patient often feels sore and "bruised" in this area.

In a typical attack, the pain usually subsides within 12 to 24 hours, toward the end of which time (or shortly afterwards) the patient may become jaundiced, and excrete pale stools and dark urine. The jaundice is rarely deep, so that pruritus is uncommon and is usually short-lived—though often within a few days or weeks there may be a recurrence of the pain with reappearance of the icterus. In obstructive jaundice caused by a stone in the bile duct, a palpably distended gallbladder is very rarely found, in contrast to the jaundice in association with carcinoma of the head of the pancreas when such a finding *is* common (Courvoisier's law). The reason for this difference between the two common causes of obstructive jaundice is twofold: (1) In patients with calculous obstruction, the gallbladder is almost invariably affected by chronic cholecystitis with fibrosis, and so cannot readily dilate; in patients with carcinoma of the pancreas, the gallbladder is usually normal. (2) In patients with stone in the duct, the obstruction is usually incomplete, so that the pressure in the ductal system does not rise as high as in malignant obstruction when the obstruction, once established, is usually complete and continuous.

By no means all patients with stones in the common duct present with a typical picture. As already mentioned, *patients can harbour stones in their common duct for years with no symptoms or only insignificant ones.* They may present with jaundice that is not accompanied by real pain; alternatively, they may complain of pain typically biliary in origin without jaundice, or any change in the colour of their stools or urine. Further, it is important to stress that subsidence of a typical attack of painful jaundice does not necessarily imply that the obstructing stone has passed into the duodenum, and following such an attack a patient may go for months or years without symptoms but with a stone still in the common duct.

In addition, whilst an attack of severe biliary pain with jaundice most commonly indicates the presence of a stone in the common bile duct (Watkin and Thomas, 1971), this is not always the case. On occasions the oedema around a stone impacted in the cystic duct may cause transient jaundice. It has been suggested that an acutely enlarged cystic lymph node may also cause obstructive jaundice; however, there is little, if any, concrete evidence to support this view.

If stones in the common duct are accompanied by overt cholangitis, in general the illness is altogether more severe. In addition to the pain and jaundice, there is a high fever, often with severe sweating and prostration, and there may be rigors. The fever tends to be intermittent (Charcot's intermittent hepatic fever), and it is thought that the periods of high fever coincide with obstruction of the duct and that when this relents the fever falls—only to rise once more when the obstruction again becomes more complete. In general, the jaundice tends to be deeper than in patients with simple obstruction, and often there is a hepatocellular element in the jaundice in addition to the obstruction.

Many patients with stones in the common duct and infected bile have no clinical evidence of infection, however, and in all patients with stone in the duct, the presence of infection should always be suspected (see below).

Diagnosis

In most instances, the diagnosis of stone in the common bile duct is fairly clear on clinical grounds, and biochemical and radiological information is required mainly to confirm the diagnosis. The diagnosis may sometimes be difficult, however, even with the help of all possible aids.

Commonly, the urine is dark and contains both bile salts and bile pigments; as the obstruction to bile flow into the duodenum is rarely complete, in most instances urobilinogen is present in the urine (although in reduced amounts). For the same reason, if the pale stools are tested, they will be found to contain stercobilin. The jaundice is rarely severe, and the moderately raised serum bilirubin concentration is accompanied by the typical biochemical changes of an obstructive jaundice, namely, a positive direct Van den Bergh reaction and a raised alkaline phosphatase level; the transaminases may show a slight rise, especially if there is concomitant cholangitis, but this is rarely great. Characteristically, the jaundice wanes within a few days, a change accompanied by a return to normal of the various other indices. If the jaundice is prolonged, vitamin K absorption may be sufficiently impaired to cause a fall in the plasma prothrombin concentration, but this is unusual. If, as a result of quite prolonged obstruction or severe cholangitis, there is significant liver-cell damage, not only will the concentration of serum transaminases rise but there may also be a fall in the plasma albumen concentration and further impairment of prothrombin synthesis; these changes are uncommon with jaundice due to calculous obstruction.

A plain x-ray film of the upper abdomen may show radiopaque calculi; such stones are usually in the gallbladder and it is uncommon to demonstrate a stone in the duct on plain radiography (Fig. 8). Failure to demonstrate the presence of gallstones on plain radiography in no way invalidates the diagnosis, as only some 30 percent of gallstones are radiopaque. At the same time, the demonstration of gallstones does not of necessity clinch the diagnosis; they may be an incidental finding in a patient jaundiced for some other reason. Neither cholecystography nor oral intravenous cholangiography are of any assistance in the diagnosis in the presence of jaundice, as no opacification of the biliary apparatus will be seen. Following clearing of the jaundice, cholangiographic findings may give conclusive information (Fig. 9) but it is wise to wait at least 2 weeks after the serum bilirubin has returned to normal before performing the investigation. In an indirect way, intravenous cholangiography is a very sensitive test of liver function; thus satisfactory films will not be obtained until several days after all the usual biochemical parameters of liver function have returned to normal. In a patient who has recently been jaundiced, the demonstration of a stone in the common duct is clearly of diagnostic significance, but failure to demonstrate such a stone does not mean that the duct is free of stone: on intravenous cholangiography it may be impossible to demonstrate small stones and the duct may appear in all respects normal.

Reflecting the variable way in which it

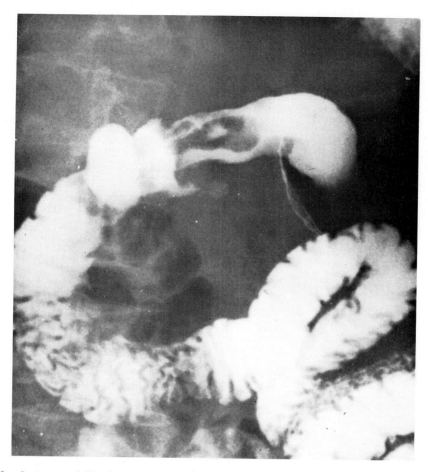

FIG. 8. Barium-meal film from a patient with obstructive jaundice. A rounded shadow is seen below the pylorus, and operation confirmed this to be a stone in the common duct. The pyloric mucosa is deformed by oedema in the pylorus and pancreas resulting from impaction of the stone.

can present clinically, stone in the common duct may have to be differentiated from a wide range of conditions, and the differential diagnosis is greatly influenced by whether pain or jaundice is the predominant symptom. *The differential diagnosis and investigation of jaundice is considered in detail elsewhere (Chap. 45), and here only the outline of the problem is discussed.* If jaundice is prominent and pain unobtrusive or absent, the condition must be distinguished not only from other causes of obstructive jaundice (notably carcinoma involving the lower end of the common duct) but also from virus hepatitis, drug-induced jaundice, and a number of other conditions of which

secondary deposits in the liver is a common cause of jaundice that is easily overlooked initially. Classically, the jaundice caused by malignant obstruction to the common duct is painless and is accompanied by a palpably distended gallbladder (Courvoisier's law), although neither feature is constant. In all patients with jaundice, careful palpation for a distended gallbladder is essential; it may be quite low in the abdomen if the liver is greatly enlarged. The various liver function tests may be of diagnostic aid, but they are not always so and too much should not be expected of them. At best, the tests can only distinguish between jaundice predominantly due to obstruction or to hepatocellular dam-

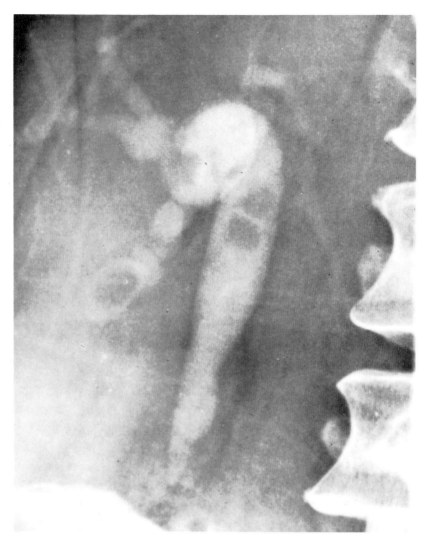

FIG. 9. Intravenous cholangiogram showing several stones in a moderately dilated common duct: there are also stones present in a contracted gallbladder.

age; they cannot distinguish between jaundice caused by obstruction at multiple sites within the liver or at one site in the extrahepatic biliary passages. In general, jaundice due to a stone in the common duct has the features of a fluctuant, incomplete obstruction; however, in difficult cases, the correct diagnosis may only be revealed by liver biopsy or even laparotomy.

Depending upon its exact location and accompanying features, the pain of so-called "biliary colic" may have to be distinguished from a wide range of conditions, including not only other abdominal conditions but also various intrathoracic diseases. Thus the pain of a myocardial infarction may closely resemble that of a stone in the common duct, and an electrocardiogram may be a most valuable investigation in distinguishing between the two. Of the various abdominal conditions that may give rise to pain similar to that of a stone in the common duct, the most common are peptic ulcer, chronic pancreatitis, and, on occasions, carcinoma of the pancreas.

The diagnosis of stone in the common duct involves not only the problem of the differential diagnosis of a patient presenting with pain and/or jaundice, but also the problem of determining whether any individual patient with gallstones has a stone in the common duct; this latter problem is discussed fully in the section on indications for exploration of the duct.

MANAGEMENT

There is no reliable method available either for causing dissolution of stones in the common duct or for causing them to pass on into the duodenum. The only certain method of treatment is surgical removal of the stones, and for practical purposes this should be advised in all instances. Even though at the time of making the diagnosis the stones may be giving rise to no symptoms, it is almost certain that sooner or later they will do so, and by the time they do so they may well have resulted in dilatation of the ducts and some liver damage. For these reasons, it is only on rare occasions that, because of advanced age or concurrent disease, surgical removal of stones in the common duct is not advisable. If the alleviation of an acute attack (see below) is excluded, the only common preoperative treatment that may be indicated —save for routine measures, such as required in patients with chronic bronchitis—is weight reduction. As in all patients with gallstones, many patients with stones in the common duct are overweight, and the operation is greatly facilitated if these patients are helped by the usual dietary measures to lose weight before the operation is performed (assuming that circumstances allow time for this).

It is usually unwise and unnecessary to operate on a patient during an acute attack of pain and jaundice caused by a stone in the common duct; as explained previously, in the majority of instances, the acute attack will subside and the operation can then be undertaken at leisure at a later date when there has been time to assess the patient's condition fully. The first essential in an acute attack is the relief of pain. It is widely taught that morphia should not be given for this purpose, as it causes spasm of the musculature surrounding the termination of the common duct, and that pethidine is the drug of choice. In fact Boulter (1961 *a*) showed that the action of these two drugs on the sphincteric mechanism of the common duct is essentially similar, though that of morphia may be more prolonged. He also showed that the effect of both drugs on the sphincteric mechanism was largely abolished by the simultaneous administration of propantheline bromide (Pro-Banthine), and suggested that combination of this drug with either morphia or pethidine is probably advisable in the treatment of so-called "biliary colic."

Aside from bed rest and the relief of pain, little active treatment is required. Fluids can be administered by mouth and only rarely is the vomiting sufficiently severe to require use of the intravenous route. With the subsidence of the pain and vomiting, solid food can be taken again, but fats should be avoided. When the jaundice has cleared, any necessary radiological examinations can be carried out, and with confirmation of the diagnosis, the operation can be performed at a suitable time. Often the radiological examinations only demonstrate the presence of stones in the gallbladder, but this does not exclude the presence of a stone in the common duct and is in itself an indication for operation following an acute attack of biliary pain and/or jaundice. Occasionally the jaundice does not relent and may even increase as the days pass; if an hepatic cause for the jaundice can be excluded, it is wise in these circumstances not to delay operation for too long in the hope that the jaundice will eventually clear. Before operating on such patients, the prothrombin time should be estimated, and if there is any doubt, it is wise to give a dose of vitamin K. In those patients in which the condition is complicated by cholangitis, an antibiotic should be administered; ampicillin is probably the drug of choice, as it is concentrated in the bile (Ayliffe and Davies, 1965), though the excretion of the penicillins in the bile may be impaired if there is liver damage (Zaslow et al., 1947), and also in the presence of obstruction to the flow of bile in the common duct (Mortimer, Mackie, and Haynes, 1969). For this reason, if, despite antibiotic treatment, the patient remains febrile and jaundiced, it becomes urgent to relieve the obstruction to prevent severe liver damage; usually definitive exploration of the bile duct should be performed, but rarely, if the patient is very ill, simple drainage of the duct via a T tube may be advisable, with removal of the stones at a later date.

EXPLORATION OF THE COMMON BILE DUCT

Except in the case of patients with a residual stone in the common duct, exploration of the common bile duct and removal of stones (choledocholithotomy) are carried out at the same time as removal of the gallbladder. A second operation to remove stones from the common duct of necessity implies that the patient has experienced additional discomfort and distress; further, such an operation is in general more difficult and hazardous than exploration of the common duct at the time of the first operation on the biliary tract. For these reasons, it is of the utmost importance that at the time of cholecystectomy stones in the common duct are not overlooked; this may occur from either (a) failure to explore a duct containing stones or (b) failure to remove all the stones from a duct, despite exploration.

Indications. Exploration of the common duct is classically indicated in patients (a) who are or recently have been jaundiced, (b) who are found to have a palpable stone in the common duct, and (c) whose common duct is found to be dilated. The importance of these three criteria was brought out in a study by Bartlett and Waddell (1958), based on an analysis of 900 patients undergoing primary operation on the biliary tract for gallstones; exploration of the common duct revealed a stone or stones in 56.5 percent of 382 patients with a clear history of jaundice, in 55 percent of 354 patients with a dilated duct (defined as measuring more than 10 mm at operation), and 95.8 percent of the 96 patients with a "palpable stone" in the duct.

Despite the value of these indications, there is now abundant evidence that if the common duct is explored only when one of these factors is present, stones in the duct will be overlooked in an unacceptable number of patients. This is not surprising in view of the fact, previously stressed, that stones may well be present in the common duct without causing pain or jaundice, or indeed any symptoms at all. Further, in patients with multiple small stones in the gallbladder, it may well be possible to dislodge a stone into the common duct in the course of cholecystectomy (see below). In addition, it is well established that even quite large stones in the duct can be overlooked on palpation, even by an experienced operator (Fig. 10). It is certain that the common duct does not require exploration in every patient undergoing cholecystectomy for gallstones, but at the same time it is clear that if the decision to explore is based on the obvious indications set out above, ductal stones will be missed and wider indications are clearly required.

To meet this situation, a set of indications (based on all features of the case, both clinical and operative) has been worked out by men experienced in this branch of surgery. Thus Adams and Stranahan (1947) gave the following indications for exploration of the duct:

(1) Frequent, acute attacks of biliary colic, chills or fever ; (2) past or present history of obstructive jaundice, or biochemical evidence thereof; (3) dilated or thickened common bile duct; (4) multiple, small stones in the gallbladder; (5) unsatisfactory or suspicious findings on palpation of the common duct; (6) sediment in bile aspirated from the common duct; (7) a gallbladder empty of stones (but presumably showing some chronic inflammatory changes) in a patient with biliary tract symptoms; (8) small, contracted gallbladder; and (9) acute or subacute pancreatitis. Very similar indications are set out by Glenn (1952 and 1967), Maingot (1961), and Colcock and Perey (1964), and they are widely accepted in many centres.

The use of these wide indications undoubtedly gives fairly satisfactory results, and there is evidence (Havard, 1960) that the higher the incidence of exploration of the common duct the lower is the incidence of residual stones. The use of wide indications for exploration of the common duct may, however, be criticised on two grounds. First, it still results in an appreciable incidence of residual stones. This problem is discussed in full in a later section and it must suffice here to note that the incidence of this complication is in

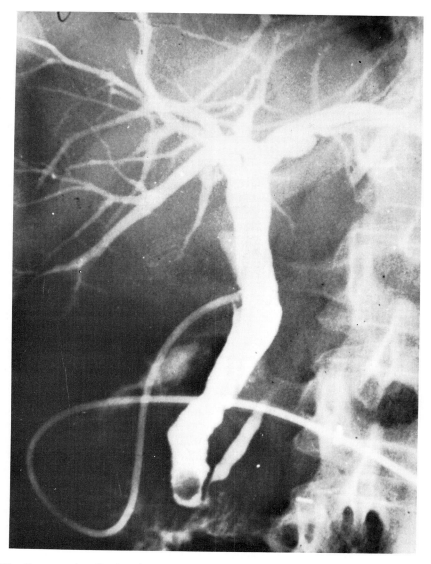

FIG. 10.   Postoperative, T tube cholangiogram showing a large residual stone in the lower portion of the common duct.

the region of 4 percent, and many figures in excess of this have been reported. Secondly, it undoubtedly results in a large number of negative, and thus unnecessary, explorations of the duct. Table 1 shows that in many of the reported series of cases, exploration of the duct failed to reveal a stone in more than half the patients submitted to this procedure. It is clearly of importance to determine whether this high incidence of negative exploration has any deleterious consequences. Colcock (1958) reported a mortality rate of 0.9 percent following cholecystectomy, and one of 1.1 percent following cholecystectomy with exploration of the common duct. Bartlett and Waddell (1958), in their large series from the Massachusetts General Hospital, reported a mortality rate of 0.6 percent following cholecystectomy and that addition of choledochostomy to the operation increased the mortality rate to 1.8 percent. Havard (1961) gave similar evidence that the addition of choledochostomy to the operation doubles the mortality rate, whilst Glenn (1967) reported a mortality rate of 0.7 percent in 3,983 patients undergoing cholecystectomy or cholecystostomy and that in 687 patients who underwent exploration of the common duct in addition to cholesystectomy the figure was 4.3 percent. These figures, however, can easily be misinterpreted; there is no doubt but that *most of the deaths following exploration of the duct occur in elderly patients who are jaundiced at the time of operation, and often have the additional complication of cholangitis.* The critical point in question is whether a simple, negative exploration of the duct increases the mortality rate of cholecystectomy. The evidence from Colcock (1958) suggested that it does not, and Adams and Stranahan (1947) are also of this opinion. This view is supported by the figures of Larson et al. (1966), who reported a mortality rate of 0.5 percent in 207 patients undergoing negative exploration of the common duct, whilst that in 208 patients in whom stones were removed from the duct the figure was 4.3 percent. Aside from mortality, there is evidence that the addition of choledochostomy to the operation of cholecystectomy increases the postoperative morbidity, largely due to infective complications (Keighley and Graham, 1971), and further that it increases the length of the patient's stay in hospital (Hight, Lingley, and Hurtubise, 1959; Nienhuis, 1961). Thus it would appear that the addition of a negative exploration of the common duct does not, at least appreciably, increase the mortaliyt rate of cholecystectomy but that it does increase the morbidity and the period of stay in hospital. Clearly it would be advantageous to reduce the incidence of such explorations if this can be done without increasing the incidence of residual stone in the duct.

In recent years much attention has been given to increasing the accuracy of the diagnosis of stone in the common duct, particularly by the use of the various types of cholangiography. *Intravenous cholangiography* is undoubtedly capable of demonstrating the presence of stones in the duct in many instances, but an apparently normal intravenous cholangiogram cannot be depended upon as evidence that the duct is stone-free. In general, this is due to the fact that by this technique the finer details of the duct are not delineated with sufficient clarity. The method suffers the additional disadvantage that there is, if not of necessity then certainly in usual practice, a significant passage of time between the radiological examination and the operation on the biliary tract. The surgeon wants to know not whether the duct does or does not contain stones at some time, even one day, before the operation, but the state of the duct after the cystic duct has been ligated. *Percutaneous transhepatic cholangiography* has little part to play in the problem for, as already mentioned, stones can well be present in the common duct without causing dilatation of the ductal system, and this type of cholangiogram is usually impossible when the ducts are of normal calibre. Similarly the 4-day Telepaque test, though occasionally useful, cannot be relied upon in the diagnosis of stone in the common duct (Grundy, King, and Lloyd, 1972).

In contrast to these techniques, *operative cholangiography* can make a major contribution to the diagnosis and management of stone in the common duct. Introduced by Mirizzi in 1932, the technique was at first unsatisfactory owing to the use of oil contrast material, but with the development of water-soluble media, its value was soon appreciated. Two types of operative cholangiogram can be performed (a) before the duct is explored, *preexploratory cholangiography,* or (b) after the duct has been explored, *postexploratory cholangiography.* The purpose of the preexploratory examination is to determine whether the common duct contains a stone or stones and hence whether it requires exploration. The purpose of the postexploratory examination is to determine whether exploration has succeeded in removing all the stones from the duct. This latter examination is discussed later.

Preexploratory cholangiography
TECHNIQUE. To produce reliable films capable of critical interpretation, preexploratory cholangiography demands scrupulous attention to details in technique; many of the disappointing results that have been reported with this examination can be ascribed

to faults in technique. The examination can be carried out either by inserting a catheter into the common duct via the cystic duct, or by direct injection via a needle inserted into the common duct. In the writer's opinion the former technique is the more satisfactory and reliable.

For operative cholangiography, the patient is placed on the operating table on a shallow box into which the x-ray cassettes can be placed (Fig. 11). This can conveniently be done from the side or, alternatively, from the head of the table (Samuel, 1959). In order to avoid obscuring the films, towels should be fixed to the patient with sutures or adhesives, not clips. The usual steps in the performance of a cholecystectomy are carried out, up to the exposure of the cystic duct. A catheter is then inserted into the cystic duct, in a fashion similar to the insertion of a cut-down intravenous drip (Fig. 12). An ureteric catheter, provided it has no proximal holes, is most suitable for this purpose, but a length of polythene tubing can be used if preferred. To avoid introducing bubbles into the ductal system, it is essential, before insertion of the catheter, to attach it to a syringe filled with isotonic saline and to fill the catheter with this fluid. The catheter is then inserted through an incision in the cystic duct and passed some 2 cm down the common bile duct. Occasionally the spiral valve in the cystic duct will make insertion difficult, and the cystic duct will require gentle dilatation before this can be achieved. When the catheter has been manipulated into the common bile duct, the distal ligature is tightened; gentle suction is then applied with the syringe to remove any bubbles accidentally introduced into the system, after which a few millimetres of saline are injected to test that flow is free.

Before taking the films, all instruments are removed from the operation site, as are swabs marked with a radiopaque filament, and the table is tilted some 15 degrees to the right (Fig. 13) to throw the image of the common duct clear of the vertebral column. A towel is placed over the operation area and the x-ray machine wheeled into position. The syringe containing isotonic saline is then replaced with one filled with 20 ml of sodium

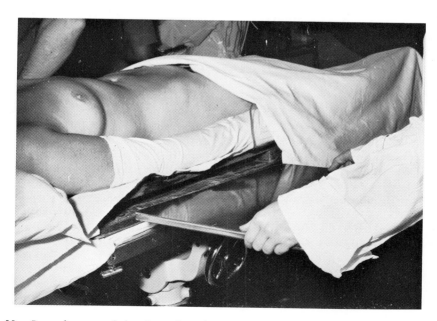

FIG. 11. Preexploratory cholangiography. The patient is shown in position on the operating table, lying on a box into which the x-ray cassettes can be inserted. For clarity, the towels are not in position but the cassettes can easily be inserted beneath the towels without contaminating the operative field.

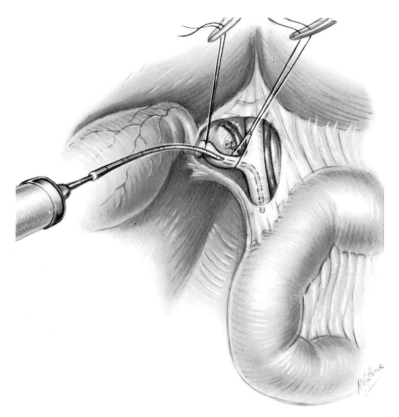

FIG. 12. Preexploratory cholangiography. The catheter, filled with saline from the attached syringe, is inserted into the common duct via the cystic duct. After tightening the ligature, gentle suction is applied to remove any bubbles before a few milliliters of saline are injected to test the system.

diatrizoate (Hypaque) and (again, before any injection is made) suction is applied via the syringe to remove any bubbles that may have entered the system during the exchange of syringes. The use of a relatively dilute contrast material is essential, as strong solutions may obscure small filling defects (Ashmore et al., 1956).

Films are exposed after the slow injection of 2 to 3 ml, 5 to 7 ml, and 9 to 10 ml of contrast material, the anaesthetist being asked to arrest all respiratory movement at the time of each exposure. If the common duct is dilated, the amount of contrast medium injected before each exposure is increased, but in all instances it is essential that the first film is taken after only a small volume of medium has been injected. If this

is not done, the image of the lower part of the common duct may easily be obscured by contrast medium in the duodenum, with the result that small stones and other abnormalities can be missed (Fig. 14). Failure to appreciate this point was the cause of misleading results in some of the earlier reported series of operative cholangiograms.

After the films have been exposed, the table is returned to its horizontal position, and retractors and the like are replaced. The catheter is removed from the cystic duct, which is then ligated and divided in the usual way, followed by removal of the gallbladder. Whenever possible, the films should be processed by a rapid development technique so that they are available for study at the conclusion of the cholecystectomy. If

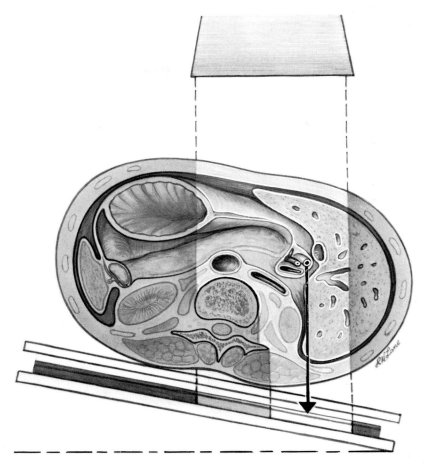

FIG. 13.   Preexploratory cholangiography. Before injection of the contrast medium and exposure of the films, the table is tilted 15 degrees to the right, to throw the image of the common duct clear of the spine.

for any reason it is thought that the films may be unsatisfactory and require to be repeated, it is usually possible to leave the catheter in situ, divide the cystic duct close to the gallbladder, and then (if indicated) repeat the cholangiogram after removal of the gallbladder. On completion of this examination, the catheter is removed, the cystic duct ligated, and the redundant portion excised.

INTERPRETATION OF FILMS. Interpretation of the films demands attention to a number of points beyond looking for filling defects. A normal preexploratory cholangiogram shows the following features [Le Quesne, 1960 (Fig. 15)]: (1) there is a free flow of contrast medium into the duodenum in all three films; (2) the narrow, terminal portion of the duct is clearly seen; (3) the main portion of the duct is of normal calibre; as measured on an x-ray film the diameter of the duct is usually 10 mm or less, and a diameter in excess of 12 mm should be considered abnormal (Le Quesne, Whiteside, and Hand, 1959); (4) there are no filling defects in the ducts; and (5) there is no excess retrograde filling of the intrahepatic radicles. If all these criteria are strictly fulfilled, the cholangiogram can be relied upon as evidence of a normal duct, not requiring exploration for removal of stones. If, however, the films show any abnormality, this should

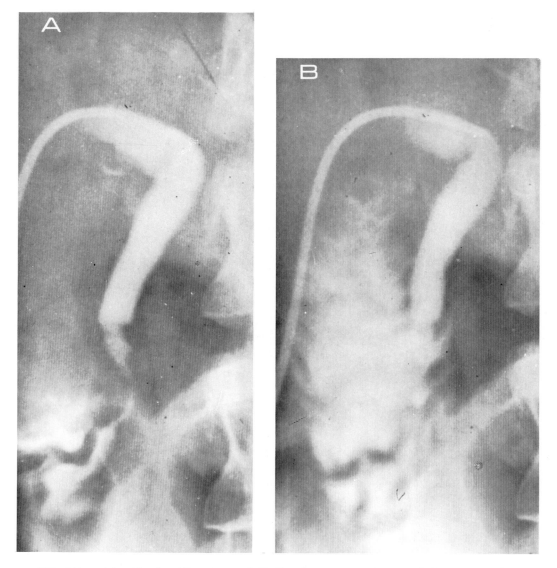

FIG. 14A and B. The first (A) and second (B) films from a preexploratory cholangiogram, illustrating how the flow of contrast material into the duodenum can easily obscure the detail of the terminal segment, thus emphasising the importance of the first film taken after the injecion of only 2-3 ml. of contrast medium.

be taken as evidence of an abnormal duct probably requiring exploration. The sole exception to this rule is failure to demonstrate flow in the first film; if the examination is in all other respects normal, particularly if the narrow segment is seen in the first film, it can be taken as indicating a normal duct.

The most obvious indication of a stone in the common duct is a filling defect, which may be single or multiple (Figs. 16 and 17). Often the defect is accompanied by dilatation of the duct, failure of flow of contrast medium into the duodenum, failure to demonstrate the terminal narrow segment, and by excess retrograde filling of the intrahepatic ducts (Fig. 18). In some cases a filling defect is not seen, and the only evidence of a stone is failure of flow of contrast medium into the duodenum with failure to visualise the narrow segment; especially if associated with dilatation of the duct and excess retrograde filling, these findings strongly suggest the presence of a stone or sludge at the lower end of the duct (Fig. 19). It must be emphasised that the examination should be accepted as indicating a normal duct only if it fulfills all the criteria set out above.

The presence of bubbles in the duct can occasionally give rise to difficulties in interpretation, although these should be avoided by attention to details in technique. The fact that a filling defect is caused by an air bubble is usually suggested by the circular outline and a cholangiogram that is in all other respects normal. If the presence of a bubble or bubbles is suspected, the difficulty can usually be resolved by repetition of the examination after thoroughly flushing the duct (via the catheter) with normal saline, which will remove bubbles (Fig. 20).

In rare instances, difficulties can also arise as the result of spasm of the sphincteric mechanism surrounding the terminal portion of the duct for reasons other than the presence of stones in the duct. Spasm of this sphincteric mechanism will prevent flow of the contrast medium into the duodenum and also prevent visualisation of the terminal segment of the duct. Usually these abnormalities are caused by the presence of a stone in the duct or by pancreatitis, but occasionally they may be due to extraneous causes, such as the preanaesthetic drugs, etc. If this is thought to be the case, the examination should be

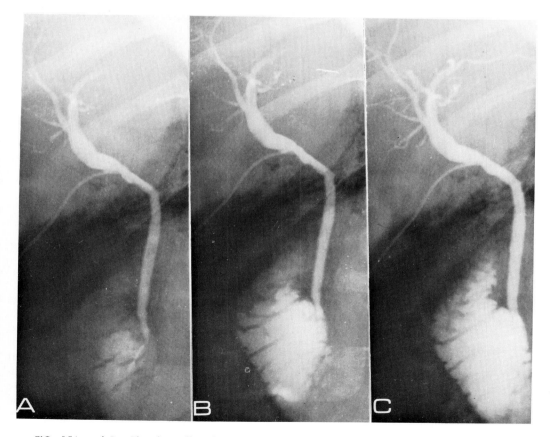

FIG. 15A and B. The three films from a normal, preexploratory cholangiogram. Note (1) the free flow of contrast material into the duodenum, (2) the clear delineation of the narrow, terminal segment in (A), (3) the normal calibre of the duct, (4) the absence of filling-defects.

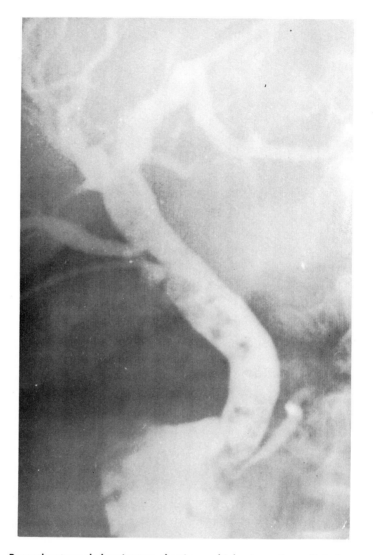

FIG. 16.   Preexploratory cholangiogram showing multiple stones in a dilated common duct.

repeated after asking the anaesthetist to give the patient amyl nitrite by inhalation; in the absence of a stone in the duct, this will usually relax the spasm, resulting in a normal cholangiogram (Fig. 21); if the appearances are still abnormal, exploration is indicated.

EVALUATION OF THE EXAMINATION. In assessing the value of preexploratory cholangiography, the critical question to be faced is not whether this form of examination can demonstrate stones in the common duct (for this is manifestly the case), but whether the information it gives is more accurate in the diagnosis of stone in the duct than that provided by a combination of the clinical and operative findings, including exploration of the duct. To pose the problem in a different way: Does the use of preexploratory cholangiography reveal stones that might otherwise have been overlooked? Does it cut down the incidence of negative, and hence unnecessary, explorations of the duct? It is difficult to give a final, definitive answer to these questions, but there is now considerable weight of evidence suggesting that this examination gives the most accurate information available as to whether there are stones in the duct, and that its use does greatly cut down the number of negative explorations of the duct.

A wealth of literature on the value of pre-exploratory cholangiography is now in existence. In 1956, Ferris and Weber recorded their experiences with this technique in 185 patients undergoing cholecystectomy and reported that in 7 instances it revealed stones in the duct that would otherwise have been overlooked. Hutchinson and Blake (1957) reported that prior to using operative cholangi-ography they explored the common duct in 63 percent of patients undergoing cholecystectomy, but found stones only in 23 percent; following the introduction of operative cholangiography, and after they had gained experience with the technique, in a series of 143 cholecystectomies the common duct was explored in 27 patients (18.8 percent), with removal of stones from 23 of these subjects. Commenting on their experience with the examination, they noted that apart from revealing a number of unsuspected stones, "our most striking triumph has been the marked reduction in the number of ducts explored."

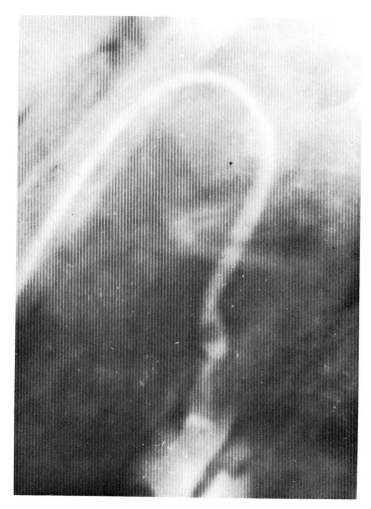

FIG. 17. Preexploratory cholangiogram showing a single stone in a duct of normal calibre.

Nienhuis (1961), Schulenburg (1969) and Grundy, King, and Lloyd (1972) all give useful reports of their experience with this technique and confirm its value both in detecting unsuspected stones and demonstrating a normal duct. Nienhuis (1961) reports that in a series of 171 patients in whom preexploratory cholangiography was carried out, unsuspected stones were revealed in 7 patients —although in 2 patients a palpable stone was not demonstrated and in two other patients the cholangiogram was interpreted as being abnormal even though no stone could be found on exploration of the duct.

Our own experience in our first 109 patients in whom preexploratory cholangiography was used was reported previously (Le Quesne, 1960). In 4 patients, unsuspected stones that would otherwise have been overlooked were demonstrated and successfully removed. In 18 patients the duct, which would otherwise have been explored, was

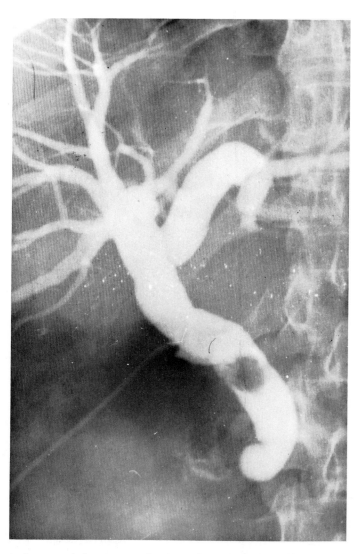

FIG. 18.   Preexploratory cholangiogram showing a large stone in a dilated duct. Note also the absence of flow of contrast material into the duodenum, and failure to delineate the terminal segment.

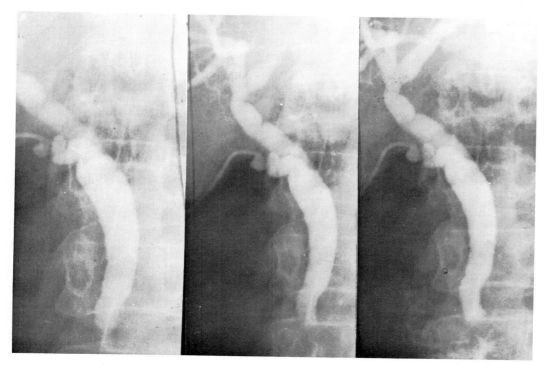

FIG. 19.   The three films from a preexploratory cholangiogram showing a duct of normal calibre with no filling defect, but with no flow of contrast material into the duodenum and failure to demonstrate the terminal segment. Repetition of the examination after the inhalation of amyl nitrite showed no change in these appearances, and on exploration a stone was found in the lower portion of the duct. Note the superimposition of the duct image on that of the spine, owing to failure to tilt the table sufficiently.

not opened because of normal cholangiographic findings. Filling defects caused by bubbles were seen in 3 patients; after repetition of the examination (see above), exploration of the duct was required in only one of the patients. Spasm of the sphincteric musculature of the terminal duct was seen in 5 patients; after repetition of the examination with inhalation with amyl nitrite, exploration was required in none of them. Further experience with more than 400 cases has amply confirmed the value of the examination; in our practice it is now unusual to explore a duct not containing stones. The reliance that can be placed on this examination in demonstrating a normal, stone-free duct was shown by a follow-up study of 90 patients whose common duct was not explored at the time of cholecystectomy because of a normal preexploratory cholangiogram

(Chapman, Curry, and Le Quesne, 1964). All these patients were reviewed one year or more after operation, and in all an intravenous cholangiogram was performed at the time of this review; in no patient was there any evidence, clinical or radiographic, of a residual stone in the duct.

The examination has been criticised as being time-consuming, and it certainly adds a few minutes to simple cholecystectomy. With efficient radiographic technique, however, the films should be available for study by the time the gallbladder has been removed, and it is very doubtful whether routine cholangiography takes up more time than a large number of unnecessary explorations of the common duct. Further, by preventing unnecessary exploration of the duct, the examination reduces the average postoperative stay in hospital. The examination

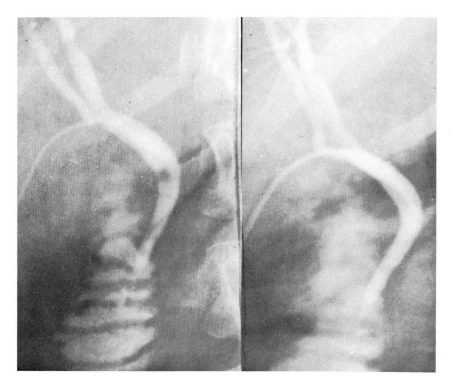

FIG. 20.   Preexploratory cholangiogram showing, in the left-hand film. (A) A defect due to an air-bubble in the duct. Note that the defect is circular and that the cholangiogram is normal in all other respects. After flushing the duct with saline, a repeat cholangiogram showed a normal duct with no defect (B). *Note that in this patient the cystic duct joins the right hepatic duct.*

has also been said to carry the risk of causing an attack of pancreatitis; Schulenburg (1961), from an experience of 353 patients, states that he has never seen this complication, nor have we in our series of more than 400 such examinations.

The examination has an additional advantage that it may demonstrate abnormalities in the bile duct system. Schulenburg (1961) reported that the examination showed ductal anomalies in 9.8 percent of his series. The most important abnormalities that the examination may reveal are drainage of the cystic duct into the right hepatic duct (Fig. 20), and a low insertion of the cystic duct into the common duct.

SUMMARY OF INDICATIONS FOR EXPLORATION OF THE COMMON DUCT.   Preexploratory cholangiography is not a foolproof method of investigation. To give good results, it requires careful attention to the details of technique and scrupulous regard for the criteria of normality in interpreting the films. Furthermore, it is not a technique that can be relied upon to give good results if only used occasionally in difficult cases: the best results are obtained by those who use it routinely. In addition, the information it provides, though of paramount importance, must be interpreted in the light of all available information. Provided due regard is paid to these considerations, the evidence strongly suggests that preexploratory cholangiography is the best available technique for determining whether the common duct requires exploration. If this method of examination is not used, the decision should be based on the wide criteria set out previously.

TECHNIQUE OF EXPLORATION OF THE COMMON DUCT.   The operation area is exposed through whichever incision is preferred for cholecystectomy, and before removal of the gallbladder is begun the common duct is carefully palpated. Exploration of the common duct is usually performed after removal of the gallbladder, though some surgeons recommend that it should be performed after division of the cystic duct so that the gallbladder itself can be used to retract the liver. It is doubtful whether such retraction is of real benefit, but whichever course is chosen it is essential that the cystic duct is ligated before the duct is explored; if this is not done, there is a risk that manipulation of the gallbladder will force small stones down the cystic duct into the common duct after the latter has been explored. *Exploration of the common duct through the stump of the cystic duct does not give adequate access and is a procedure to be condemned.*

The decision to explore the common duct having been taken, the area of the free edge of the lesser omentum is exposed by the suitable positioning of retractors and packs, the essential steps being the retraction of the right lobe of the liver upwards, the displacement of the duodenum downwards, and the retraction of the stomach to the left. The peritoneum over the anterolateral surface of the common duct is divided, and the duct exposed by clearing away any fatty tissue overlying it.

In view of the high incidence of infected bile in patients with stone in the common duct, a sample of bile should be taken by needle aspiration before the duct is opened; the sample is sent for bacteriological examination, so that appropriate antibiotic treatment can be given at an early stage if there are postoperative infective complications.

Two stay sutures of fine chromic catgut on an (eyeless) atraumatic needle are then inserted some ⅛ to ¼ inch (about 0.4 to 0.7 cm) apart on the anterior surface of the duct (Fig. 22), and the duct opened longitudinally between them with a scalpel (Fig. 23). This opening is usually made below the point where the cystic duct enters the common duct, but if this is unduly low, the common duct is opened above the junction. The initial incision is enlarged to a length of ½ to ¾ inch (1.25 to 1.89 cm) either by stretching or with scissors; any escaping bile is removed by a sucker. If this initial incision exposes calculi in the duct, they should immediately be removed with forceps.

With the margins of the incision in the common duct held open by the stay sutures, common-duct (Desjardins) forceps are passed up into the common hepatic and right and left hepatic ducts, any calculi encountered being extracted with the forceps. It is essential to make certain that the forceps enter both the main hepatic ducts, and in doing so care should be taken not to push stones far up into these ducts. Removal of stones from the region of the junction of the two ducts is often difficult, and sometimes they are most easily removed by the insertion of a fine sucker up the duct. On occasions, patients are encountered who have many small stones lying in widely dilated intrahepatic ducts, and the removal of all of them is impossible: in such circumstances, it is probably wise to perform a choledochoduodenostomy. On completion of exploration of the proximal ducts, if it is thought that the lower reaches of the common duct contain many stones, it is wise to insert into the common hepatic duct a dental roll or suitable small swab, to prevent stones passing up toward the liver during subsequent manipulations; a marker length of suitable ligature material must be attached to this swab, and care taken to see that it is removed at the end of the operation (Fig. 24).

Any stones in the lower portion of the duct are now removed by passing the forceps down towards the duodenum. Often if there is a large stone in the intrapancreatic portion of the duct it can be removed only by mobilising the duodenum and head of the pancreas and manipulating the stone with fingers inserted behind the head of the pancreas at the same time as attempts are made to grasp it with forceps passed down the duct through the choledochotomy incision. In order to achieve a thorough clearance if the duct contains many small stones, sludge, or grit, it is usually necessary to irrigate the duct with isotonic saline via a catheter inserted into the duct; it is in just these circumstances, especially if the duct is dilated, that it is often advisable to perform either a sphincterotomy or a choledochoduodenostomy. To complete exploration of the duct, an instrument, either a gum-elastic bougie or a Bakes' dilator, must be passed down the duct into the duodenum (Fig. 25).[2] In doing this, it is very easy to push the duodenal

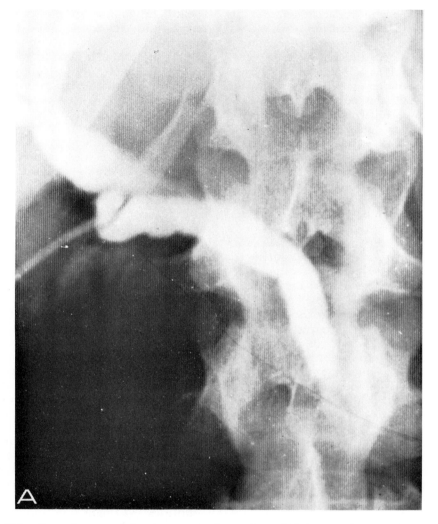

FIG. 21A. Preexploratory cholangiogram showing a duct which is normal except that no flow into the duodenum is demonstrated.

papilla forward against the anteromedial wall of the duodenum, and on palpation it may appear that the instrument has entered the duodenal lumen when it is still within the duct. To be sure that the instrument has entered the duodenum, it is essential either (a) to feel the cuff of the papilla around the bougie where it is entering the duodenum (Fig. 26) or (b) to feel the instrument several inches down the duodenum, well beyond the opening of the duct. It is a common practice to complete the explora-

tion by dilating the terminal portion of the duct by the passage of increasingly large bougies; this may be beneficial, but there is no concrete evidence that such is the case, and it may be harmful.

Finally, a T tube is inserted in the common duct (Fig. 27), which is closed around the tube with a 00 chromic catgut suture. To avoid pulling on the suture line when the T tube is removed, the tube projects from the lower end of the incision in the duct (Fig. 28). After performance of a postexplora-

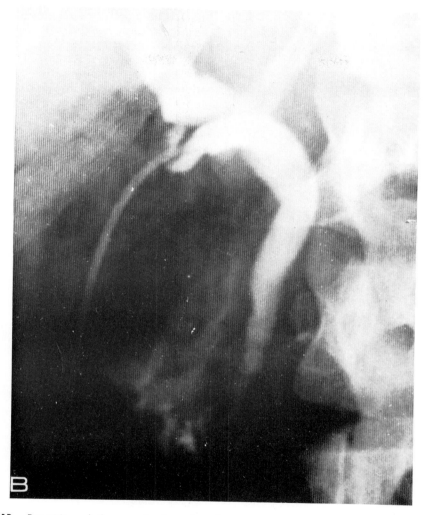

FIB. 21B. Repetition of the examination after the inhalation of amyl nitrite shows free flow into the duodenum, with a normal terminal segment. In this patient, the spasm of the sphincteric mechanism was presumably due to some extraneous cause, such as the preanaesthetic drugs.

tory cholangiogram, the T tube, together with a corrugated drain, is brought out through a stab in the right flank; after exploration of the common duct, this corrugated drain should not be omitted. The T tube is fastened to the skin by an encircling stitch, and on the patient's return to bed the tube drains into a bottle or plastic bag suspended from the side of the bed. *It is important that the T tube is made of latex rubber and not of polyvinylchloride or other plastic materials, as such materials are so inert in the tissues that they cause no adhesive reaction around themselves with the result that on removal of the tube biliary peritonitis may develop* (Winstone et al., 1965).

A number of surgeons claim that T tube drainage of the common duct after choledochotomy is unnecessary and that simple closure of the incision in the duct, with a corrugated drain to the operation site, is perfectly safe. They maintain that the inser-

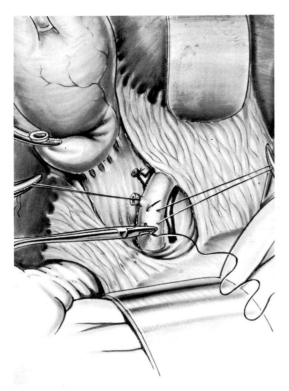

FIG. 22. Exploration of the common duct: insertion of the stay sutures.

tion of a T tube increases the patient's discomfort and length of stay in hospital, as well as resulting in an avoidable loss of water and electrolytes. Collins, Redwood, and Wynne-Jones (1960), in an admirable review of this problem, report that in a series of 198 patients undergoing exploration of the duct with immediate suture there was an intraperitoneal collection of bile in only 2 patients, in one of whom the operation site was inadvertently not drained; they show that, on the average, the postoperative stay in hospital of these patients was several days shorter than in a comparable series of patients in whom the duct was drained with a T tube. Sawyers, Hemington, and Edwards (1965) reported the results in 250 patients undergoing exploration of the common duct with T tube drainage compared with 250 patients undergoing the same operation with primary closure of the duct; they encountered no untoward results from primary closure of

the duct, and on grounds of postoperative morbidity, mortality rate, and shorter stay in hospital found that the procedure compared favourably with the conventional technique of T tube drainage. Recently Collins (1967) has reported no complications with the use of immediate closure in 69 patients undergoing exploration of the duct. It is to be noted, however, that in discussing the paper by Sawyers and his colleagues (1965), Glenn reports that he has seen "a group of complications that are extremely difficult to manage," and is clearly reluctant to adopt the procedure.

From the evidence available, it appears that the technique of immediate closure of the duct does not carry the risks hitherto ascribed to it—provided the duct is carefully

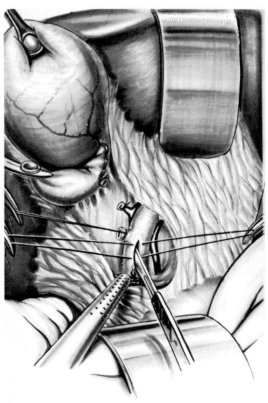

FIG. 23. Exploration of the common duct: the duct is incised between the stay sutures. Note the sucker, to remove escaping bile. (After Maingot.)

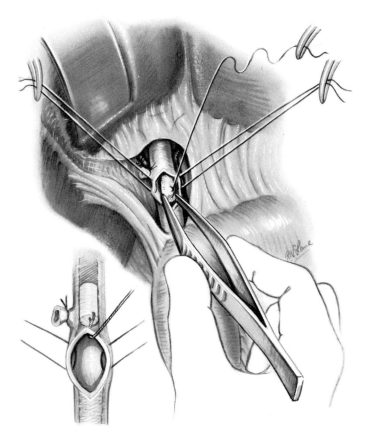

FIG. 24. Exploration of the common duct: insertion of a small swab into the common hepatic duct. When the lower duct is thought to contain small stones and debris this manoeuvre is useful in preventing the passage of small stones up into the proximal duct. Note the stay suture attached to the swab.

closed with fine catgut sutures (preferably not piercing the whole thickness of the duct wall) and that the operation site is properly drained. Adoption of the technique does mean that postoperative cholangiography is impossible, with the result that an overlooked stone in the common duct may not be recognised until it gives rise to trouble months or years later. With properly performed postexploratory operative cholangiography (which can be performed before final closure of the duct), the risk of overlooking a stone is slight so that this advantage of T tube drainage can be overemphasised. There is no question but that at the present time the majority of surgeons experienced in biliary tract surgery recommend and practise T tube drainage of the duct after exploration. It may be that it is wrong to consider the two techniques of T tube drainage and immediate closure as being mutually exclusive and that there is a place for both. Sawyers, Herrington, and Edwards (1965) recommend T tube drainage if the exploration has been difficult, or if there is pancreatitis or cholangitis. It may well be that immediate closure is the procedure of choice following simple, uncomplicated choledocholithotomy, with the addition of T tube drainage in complicated cases. Further experience and investigation are needed to clarify this problem in surgical technique.

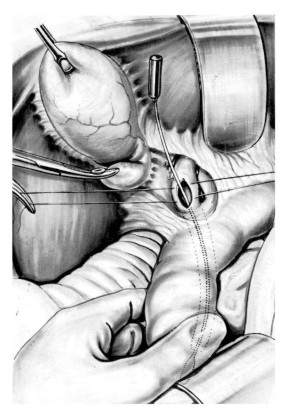

FIG. 25.   Exploration of the common duct: passage of a sound down the duct into the duodenum.

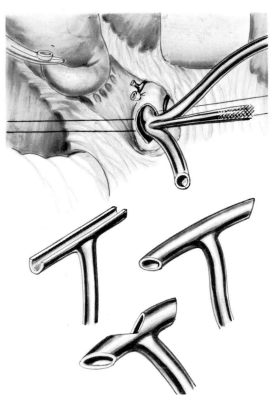

FIG. 27.   Exploration of the common duct: insertion of the T tube. Insert shows the various types of T tube available: Maingot's split tube (top left) is that most commonly used, and is the easiest to insert. Before inserting the tube its patency should be tested by flushing it with saline.

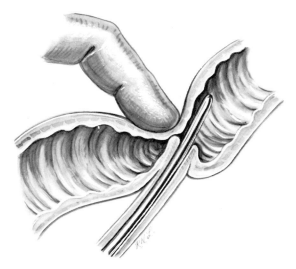

FIG. 26.   Exploration of the common duct: palpation of the papilla as a cuff surrounding the bougie, to make certain that the bougie has entered the duodenum.

Postexploratory cholangiography. The purpose is to determine whether exploration of the duct has succeeded in removing all stones from it, or whether some still remain. The examination is performed by the injection of a water-soluble radiopaque solution into the common duct via the T tube, 25 percent Hypaque being a suitable medium for the purpose. As with the preexploratory examination, all instruments, etc., must be removed from the operation site and the table tilted some 15 degrees to the right before the films are exposed. It is, of course, necessary that the patient should be lying on the table on a suitable box into which the cassettes can be placed. Owing to the dead space in the T tube, larger quantities of the contrast medium have to be injected than in the preexploratory examination; it

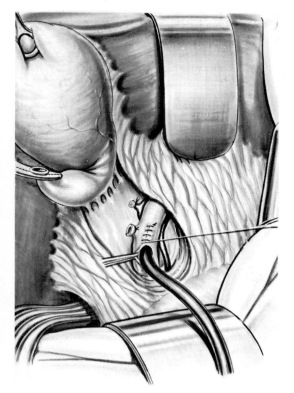

FIG. 28. Exploration of the common duct: closure of the duct, with fine catgut on an atraumatic needle, around the emergent T tube. Note that the tube protrudes from the lower end of the incision. The corrugated drain to the subhepatic space is shown in position.

common, presumably as a result of spasm of the sphincteric mechanism following either instrumental exploration of the duct or sphincterotomy. Accordingly, the only reliable indication of a residual stone in the duct is a filling defect (Fig. 30) and to this extent postexploratory cholangiography is not so sensitive a method of investigation as is the preexploratory examination.

Despite these problems, postexploratory cholangiography is a procedure of great value. In a series of 146 patients undergoing exploration of the common duct followed by postexploratory cholangiography, Mixter, Hermanson, and Segal (1951) reported the discovery of residual stones in 19 (13 percent), in all of whom they were successfully removed at the initial operation. Hight, Lingley, and Hurtubise (1959) recorded the demonstration and successful removal of residual stones in 7 of 134 patients having exploration of the common duct, and Nienhuis (1961) reported the demonstration of residual calculi in 3 out of 36 patients similarly treated. In our own experience (Le Quesne, 1960), postexploratory cholangiography re-

is our practice to expose two films after the injection of 6 to 8 ml and 10 to 12 ml of the medium—if the duct is markedly dilated, even larger quantities may be required.

A difficulty in this examination is to rid the common duct of air bubbles. To achieve this, the T tube should be flushed with isotonic saline on a number of occasions whilst the incision in the duct is being closed (Fig. 29); after a watertight closure has been achieved, the duct should be freely irrigated with 20 to 40 ml of isotonic saline down the T tube. This technique usually succeeds in washing all the bubbles from the duct, but if this is to be done with certainty, the irrigation must be generous. The interpretation of the films of a postexploratory cholangiogram is further complicated by the fact that failure to demonstrate flow of contrast medium into the duodenum and to visualise the terminal (narrow) segment of the duct is

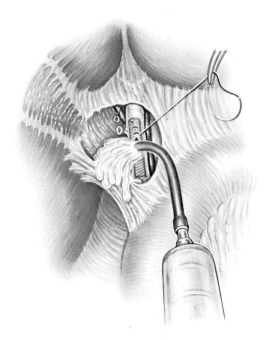

FIG. 29. Postexploratory cholangiography: to remove bubbles from the duct, the T tube is flushed with saline at intervals during closure of the duct.

the frequency of their demonstration by post-operative cholangiography. The great majority of stones demonstrated by postoperative cholangiography can be revealed by post-exploratory cholangiography immediately subsequent to exploration of the duct and then removed at the time of this first operation, thus saving most of these patients the necessity of a second operation. As with pre-exploratory cholangiography, the examination is not foolproof, but it is a safe and simple investigation which takes little time and adds distinctly to the certainty of operative exploration of the duct; for these reasons, it is difficult to avoid the conclusion that it should always be performed after removal of stones from the common duct.

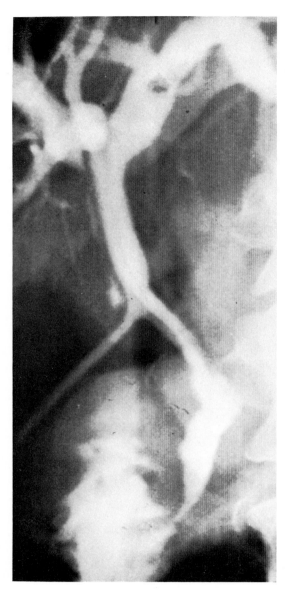

FIG. 30. Postexploratory cholangiogram showing an overlooked stone in the left hepatic duct; this stone was successfully removed, thus probably saving the patient from a second operation.

SPHINCTEROTOMY, CHOLEDOCHODUO-DENOSTOMY, AND SPHINCTEROPLASTY

Indications

The removal of multiple stones from the lower end of the bile duct through a supraduodenal choledochotomy incision may be a difficult procedure, and particularly if there are small stones and debris in a dilated duct it can be impossible to be certain that the duct has been completely cleared. Under these circumstances, there is a risk that the patient may have further symptoms from residual or recurrent stones. For this reason, an additional operative procedure is often thought wise, though the exact indications for any such procedure are not clear. The procedures available are those of transduodenal sphincterotomy, choledochoduodenostomy, and transduodenal sphincteroplasty. In the operation of sphincterotomy the distal part (approximately 1 cm) of the sphincteric musculature surrounding the terminal segment of the common duct is divided to allow thorough exploration of the duct, with the object of complete removal of grit and debris. In contrast, the other two operations are based on the belief that even if the duct is completely cleared, there is a real risk of recurrent stone formation in a dilated, infected duct: accordingly, they are designed to

vealed stones in 2 of 34 patients following exploration of the duct, and in both the stone was removed at the first operation. It is surprising what large stones can be overlooked on exploration of the duct (Fig. 31), even by experienced surgeons, and the risk of overlooking stones is emphasised by

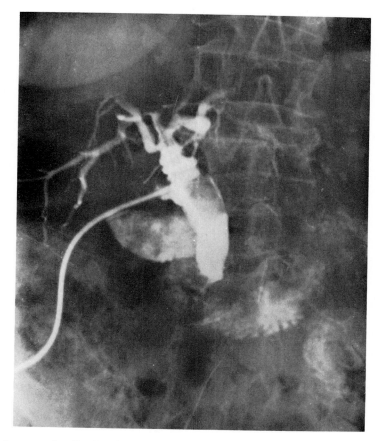

FIG. 31. Postoperative T tube cholangiogram demonstrating a large stone overlooked on exploration of the duct: a second operation was required to remove this stone, which almost certainly would have been revealed by a postexploratory cholangiogram.

create a wide, patulous opening between the duct and the duodenum, so that infected bile can drain freely into the duodenum. In the operation of choledochoduodenostomy, this is achieved by an anastomosis between the supraduodenal common duct and the duodenum, whereas in sphincteroplasty, it is achieved by complete division of the musculature surrounding the terminal segment of the common duct. (In effect, a sphincteroplasty is an internal choledochoduodenostomy.)

At the present time, there is no clear evidence as to which of these procedures is preferable, or the circumstances in which one rather than the other is indicated. In a valuable study of 110 patients undergoing either choledochoduodenostomy or sphinc-terotomy, Thomas, Nicholson, and Owen (1971) report that both operations were effective in overcoming obstruction at the lower end of the duct and in preventing recurrent disease, and Jones and Smith (1972) report equally satisfactory results from sphincteroplasty. There is no doubt that sphincterotomy is an effective operation for removing stones and debris from the lower end of the duct; in that it leaves a more normal state of affairs with the opening of the common duct still controlled by a functioning sphincteric mechanism capable of preventing reflux, it would seem to be the more logical operation for this procedure. If the duct is considerably dilated, however, the operation may be followed in a small percentage of patients by recurrent stone

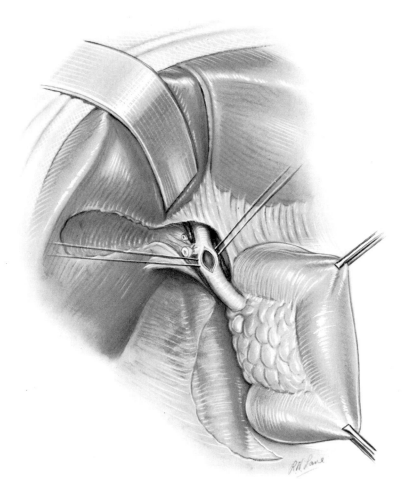

FIG. 32.   Sphincterotomy: mobilisation of the duodenum and head of the pancreas. Note the exposure of the inferior vena cava.

formation, probably resulting from continuing infection in a duct which does not drain properly. Choledochoduodenostomy is a quicker, simpler operation, but may be followed by complications arising from the collection of debris in the terminal portion of the duct (Wilson, 1970), and Jones and Smith (1972) point out that sphincteroplasty is free from these complications.

It is becoming clear that these operations should not be looked upon as simple alternatives, but rather that we should seek to determine the particular circumstances under which one or the other is appropriate. Thomas, Nicholson, and Owen (1971) suggest that sphincterotomy is the operation of choice if the common duct is not significantly dilated and if the main problem is the removal of stones impacted in the lower end of the duct, whereas choledochoduodenostomy is indicated if the common duct is widely dilated, if for any reason it is difficult to identify or expose the opening of the common duct, and in the presence of suppurative cholangitis. It must, however, be repeated that at the present time the advantages of one procedure over the other are not clear, and the choice of operation will often be dictated by the surgeon's experience and preference. It must additionally be emphasised that there is a small but definite morbidity related to both operations: they are not indicated whenever a stone is removed from the duct, but only when the presence of multiple or impacted stones and debris, and/or a dilated, infected duct suggests that recurrent (or residual) stone formation is likely.

SPHINCTEROTOMY

The main indication for performance of a sphincterotomy is the presence in the lower portion of the common duct of a stone or stones which cannot be removed by exploration from above. It is also indicated when there is much debris and sludge in the duct, particularly if the duct is dilated. Often in these circumstances a bougie cannot be passed into the duodenum, and if this cannot be done in a duct containing stones or debris, a sphincterotomy should be performed to elucidate the cause of the obstruction; usually it is due either to biliary grit in the lower duct or to fibrosis of the papilla. In addition, the operation is often recommended in a more ill-defined group of patients when it is thought desirable to increase

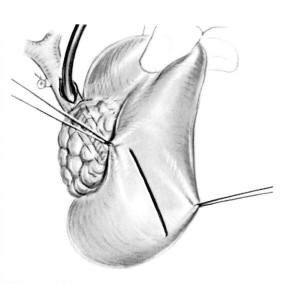

FIG. 33. Sphincterotomy: opening of the duodenum by an oblique incision at the level of the papilla, which is demonstrated by the passage of a bougie down the common duct.

the flow of bile into the duodenum, especially in patients with a dilated and infected duct that has contained stones. It is believed that in some of these patients, either as a result of a disturbance of muscle function or of fibrosis, there is a functional obstruction in the terminal segment of the duct, which may lead to bile stagnation (possibly with the formation of further stones) unless improved drainage of the duct is provided. This concept of a partial, functional obstruction at the lower end of the duct—despite the absence of a demonstrable organic obstruction—has been postulated by a number of surgeons, notably by Mallet-Guy and his colleagues at Lyons (Mallet-Guy, Jeanjean, and Marion, 1947), but it has yet to win general acceptance. Often in patients with multiple stones in a dilated duct a sphincterotomy is necessary to make certain that all the stones have been removed, and this additional procedure is probably wise in all such patients—especially if the duct is dilated. There does not appear to be any certain evidence, however, that the postoperative course of such patients is improved as a result of any functional effect of the operation on the sphincteric mechanism.

The use of the operation of sphincterotomy in the treatment of chronic pancreatitis and fibrosis of the sphincter of Oddi is discussed in Chapter 43, Part A and 47.

TECHNIQUE. When carried out for the removal of stones from the lower end of the common duct, the procedure is performed after exploration of the common duct. The first step is to mobilise the second part of the duodenum and head of the pancreas. To perform this, the posterior peritoneum is divided just lateral to the duodenum along the whole length of its second portion and around its upper curve to the region of the common duct. The plane of cleavage behind the duodenum and pancreas is entered and the pancreas mobilised forward by dissecting medially in this plane, by a mixture of sharp and blunt dissection, to expose the anterior surface of the inferior vena cava (Fig. 32). To complete the mobilisation of the duodenum and head of the pancreas, it is often necessary to free the hepatic flexure of the colon and push it downward, exposing and freeing the third part of the duodenum.

With the duodenum and pancreas turned

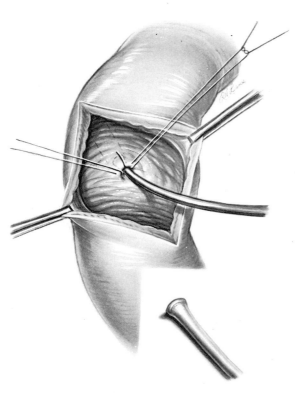

FIG. 34. Sphincterotomy: the papilla is incised in its right, upper quadrant between stay sutures. A bougie with an expanded base has been passed down the duct, enabling the papilla to be drawn forwards so that it can be manipulated with ease.

forward, a bougie is passed down the common duct from above to locate the level at which the duct enters the duodenum. Two stay sutures are inserted into the duodenum, and the duodenum opened at the appropriate level with an incision 1 to 1½ inches (1.3 to 3.8 cm) long; this incision may be placed longitudinally and later closed transversely, but it is neater to make an oblique incision which is closed in its long axis (Fig. 33). With a bougie passed from above, the opening of the common duct is identified; almost invariably the tip of a gum-elastic bougie can be coaxed into the duodenum, where it can be grasped and pulled down, but sometimes it may be necessary first to dilate the opening from above with Bakes' dilators.

To perform the actual sphincterotomy, the author prefers a technique using gum-elastic bougies with a slightly expanded base. When such a bougie of suitable size is passed down the duct from above, its expanded base impacts in the terminal duct and gentle traction on the bougie lifts the papilla up into the wound where it can be inspected and manipulated freely. Two 000 chromic catgut sutures on an atraumatic needle are then passed through the tip of the papilla in its right upper quadrant, opposite to the opening of the pancreatic duct, and the opening of the common duct incised for 5 mm between these sutures (Fig. 34). The bougie can now be withdrawn easily and a pair of forceps is inserted into the enlarged opening of the duct, following which the incision can be enlarged for a further 3 to 5 mm. Usually when this has been done the end of the duct gapes open. Care must be taken not to extend the incision too far upward or the duodenal wall itself is encroached upon. Two or three fine chromic catgut sutures are inserted to oppose the adjacent cut edges of the duodenal and bile duct mucosae; it is often advised that these sutures should be omitted, but there seems no reason to neglect the general principle of mucosal apposition; in addition, these stitches control oozing from the cut mucosal edges.

It is now possible to explore the duct by passing forceps up from below, and stones in the lower reaches of the duct can usually be removed with ease (Fig. 35). To make certain that the duct is free of small calculi and debris a catheter should be inserted into the duct both from above and below and the duct freely irrigated with saline.

To complete the operation, it is wise to identify the opening of the pancreatic duct (Fig. 35) on the medial wall of the papilla and insert a fine bougie; this manoeuvre is not essential, but it is reassuring to know that the duct is patent at the conclusion of a sphincterotomy.

The incision in the duodenal wall is closed in two layers, with an inner continuous inverting Connell suture of fine chromic catgut and an outer layer of interrupted silk stitches. If the incision has been a longitudinal one, it should be closed transversely to prevent narrowing of the duodenal lumen; however, if an oblique incision has been made, this

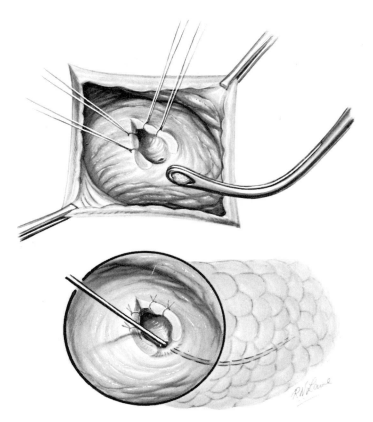

FIG. 35. Sphincterotomy: exploration of the common duct from below, with removal of a calculus. Note the sutures coating the mucosae of the duodenum and bile duct. Insert shows the passage of a bougie to demonstrate the patency of the pancreatic duct.

can be closed in its own longitudinal axis. This latter technique gives the neater result (Fig. 36). The incision in the common duct is then closed around a T tube as described previously and a postexploratory cholangiogram performed.

Some surgeons recommend that after this operation a *long-limb T tube* should be inserted, its long distal limb passing down into the duodenum, as recommended by Cattell (1948). It is claimed that this long limb prevents the enlarged opening of the common duct from narrowing down, but there is no evidence in support of this claim; it seems just as likely that the irritation of the tube may actually increase the fibrosis as the incision in the papilla heals. In addition, the use of a long-limb tube has been held responsible for causing acute pancreatitis in

the immediate postoperative period by obstruction of the opening of the pancreatic duct (Diffenbaugh and Strohl, 1956; Thompson, Howard, and Vowles, 1957). *There seems to be no good reason for the use of a long-limb tube; the usual, short tube is to be preferred.*

Various other techniques are described for performance of sphincterotomy. Rodney Smith (1958) uses a modification of Bakes' dilator with a groove cut into the bulbous end (Fig. 37); after mobilisation and opening of the duodenum, this instrument is passed down the duct from above and the sphincterotomy performed by inserting a scalpel blade into the groove and slitting the opening of the duct in its right upper quadrant. Maingot (1961) prefers to dilate the papilla from below and then cut the duct orifice with

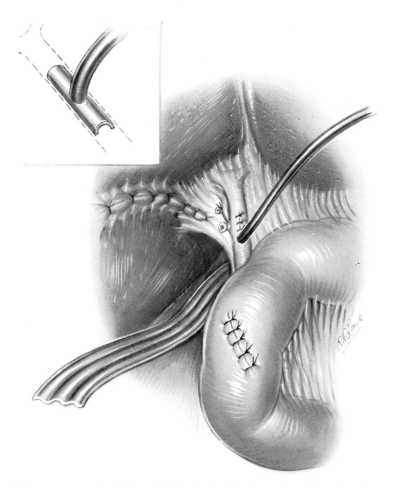

FIG. 36.   Sphincterotomy: the oblique incision in the duodenum has been closed in two layers, and the common duct closed around a short T tube. Note the corrugated drain to the subhepatic and retroduodenal areas.

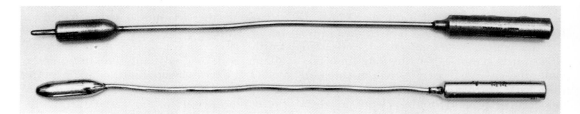

FIG. 37.   Rodney Smith's modification (top) of Bakes' dilator (bottom). Note the narrow termination, with a groove cut into the head. To perform sphincterotomy, this instrument is passed down the duct, until the narrow termination protrudes into the duodenum: a knife is then inserted into the groove and the lower portion of the sphincter slit open.

scissors. Both these techniques give excellent results, and Maingot's technique is particularly applicable in the unusual patient in whom it is not possible to insert a bougie into the duodenum from above.

There is no doubt that sphincterotomy greatly facilitates the removal of stones from the lower end of the common duct and adds to the certainty with which the duct can be cleared of small stones and sludge. The complications of acute pancreatitis and duodenal fistula have been described as occurring after the operation (Blatherwick and Pattison, 1954), but in an extensive experience with the operation, we have found it to be safe and have never seen these complications. Maingot (1961) writes that he has never seen a duodenal fistula following the transduodenal approach to the termination of the common duct. Nevertheless, the opening of the common duct should be handled with gentleness, and the utmost care must be taken not to damage the opening of the pancreatic duct. Despite its name, the operation of sphincterotomy does not divide the whole length of the sphincteric musculature surrounding the termination of the common duct. As described previously, the terminal segment of the duct is some 15 mm long, and begins some 2 mm outside the duodenal wall. The operation of sphincterotomy only divides the muscles surrounding that portion of the common duct lying obliquely in the submucosal plane of the duodenum. The sphincteric mechanism left intact represents about one-half of the entire sphincter musculature, and is more than adequate to prevent reflux of duodenal contents into the bile duct. Following the operation, a postoperative cholangiogram clearly shows the notch at the junction of the main portion of the duct with the terminal segment, and on this examination it is usually impossible to detect that the operation has been performed. The operation does, however, slit open the narrowest portion of the duct, and this may explain why flow studies 10 to 14 days after operation (Boulter, 1961b) show that the flow characteristics are altered and that bile drains more easily into the duodenum, though this effect may not be permanent (Eisman et al., 1959).

CHOLEDOCHODUODENOSTOMY

In patients with multiple stones in a dilated common bile duct, some surgeons recommend side-to-side choledochoduodenostomy in preference to sphincterotomy. The purpose of the operation is to create a wide opening into the duodenum, so that if any small stones remain in the duct, they will pass on into the duodenum, and so that there is permanently free drainage of bile into the duodenum.

The operation is performed by enlarging the choledochotomy incision downward to the point where the common duct enters the pancreas, giving an incision some 3 cm long (Capper, 1961). A transverse incision of the same length is then made at the junction of the first and second portions of the duodenum, so positioned that it lies comfortably against the incision in the common duct. The opening in the duodenum is stitched to that in the common duct with a continuous fine chromic catgut suture, reinforced with a few interrupted fine silk sutures. The site of the anastomosis is drained through a stab in the right flank.

It is claimed that this operation is safer and simpler than a sphincterotomy, and gives freer drainage to the biliary tract. Capper (1961), in a most valuable review of the operation, reported on its use in 125 patients, in 79 of whom it was performed for stones in the common duct. Based on a careful follow-up with repeated barium-meal studies, he showed conclusively that the stoma remains patent, and that though free reflux of duodenal contents into the bile duct occurs, this does not appear to give rise to pain or significant cholangitis provided the opening is large. At varying times after the operation, 5 patients developed signs of recurrent obstruction of the common duct, but in each case there was evidence either that the stoma was too small or that the common duct was of normal calibre; Capper recommended that the operation should be performed only when the common duct is dilated. Apart from these cases, the rest of the 79 patients remained well and symptom-free after the operation. Barner (1966) and Burgess and

Kidd (1967) also reported favourably on the use of this operation in patients with multiple stones in a dilated duct, the latter authors recommending it as the operation of choice in this situation.

There seems no doubt that, provided an *adequate stoma* is fashioned, the operation of choledochoduodenostomy in general gives satisfactory results in patients with multiple stones in a dilated duct, and that in years past the risk of ascending cholangitis with recurrent jaundice has been overemphasised. Rodney Smith (1964), however, drew attention to the fact that patients may develop symptoms from the impaction of vegetable material in the lower cul-de-sac of the bile duct.

In those rare patients with multiple stones in dilated intrahepatic ducts, when complete clearance of the stones is impossible, choledochoduodenostomy is the operation of choice and probably the only method of preventing recurrent jaundice. It may also be the operation of choice for patients with multiple choledochal stones associated with chronic pancreatitis.

Choledochoduodenostomy may also be used in the treatment of stricture of the lower end of the common duct and in patients with chronic pancreatitis; its use in these conditions is discussed in Chapters 38A, 47, and 48B.

SPHINCTEROPLASTY

The technique of sphincteroplasy is essentially the same as that of sphincterotomy, except that the incision in the terminal duct is carried sufficiently far proximally to divide all the musculature surrounding the lower end of the common bile duct. Of necessity, this means that the incision traverses the full thickness of the duodenal wall, so that the cut edges of the incision must be carefully sutured, particularly at the apex of the incision. The technique and results of this operation are fully described by Jones and Smith (1972), who claim that it has advantages over both sphincterotomy and choledochoduodenostomy. At the present time, its exact place in the treatment of choledochal stones remains to be defined.

Postoperative Care

Management of T tubes. Following straightforward exploration of the common duct with removal of calculi, the patient usually makes an uneventful recovery, especially if jaundice is absent or only slight. In such patients, intravenous fluids are not required; on recovery from the anaesthetic, they can be given fluids by mouth, with the addition of a light diet from the second or third postoperative day, as indicated by the wishes of the patient. By the seventh to tenth day, the patient is usually taking a normal diet. Many of the patients requiring this operation are overweight and with a tendency to bronchitis, so that vigorous attention to postoperative breathing exercises, etc., is needed to prevent sputum retention; if such retention does occur, it may be wise to prescribe a suitable antibiotic. The patient should be encouraged to move as freely as possible; if they so desire they can sit out of bed on the first postoperative day, and should certainly be encouraged to be out of bed for increasing periods from the second day onward. The patient will return to the ward with a T tube and corrugated drain protruding from a stab incision in the right flank. The management of the T tube is discussed below. For the first 48 to 72 hours after operation, there is usually a moderate discharge of serosanguineous fluid alongside the corrugated drain, sometimes accompanied by a transient bile leak. It may be necessary to change the dressings over the tube once or twice a day, but by the third day the discharge is usually diminishing rapidly. At this stage, the drain can be shortened, and removed completely 24 to 48 hours later. The skin sutures are usually removed on the tenth day, as after a cholecystectomy.

Complications. Although the postoperative course is usually uneventful, the operation of choledocholithotomy may be a serious undertaking—especially in elderly patients with marked jaundice, and particularly if in addition there is cholangitis. Glenn (1967) reports a mortality rate of 6.1 percent in 428 patients aged 50 years or more undergoing cholecystectomy and exploration of the common duct, whilst the mortality rate in a group of 259 patients less than 50 years old undergoing the same operation was only 1.5 percent. The common causes of death in elderly patients are cardiac complications, and complications such as liver failure, pancreatitis, bacteriaemic shock, etc., arising as a result of the severity of their primary condition. Many of these patients have a degree of liver damage before operation, because of biliary cirrhosis, and despite the most careful anaesthesia and skillful surgical technique, liver function may be further impaired in the postoperative period. The peculiar combination of hepatic and renal failure, the so-called hepatorenal syndrome, is particularly likely to occur in patients with some degree of preexisting renal and hepatic damage. Bacteriaemic shock is a well-recognised complication of operations on patients with heavily infected gallbladders and/or bile ducts, and is particularly dangerous in the elderly.

In view of these considerations, after choledocholithotomy in the elderly the postoperative course must be watched particularly carefully, especially if at operation the duct was found to be dilated, infected, or full of multiple stones. The urine output and concentration must be recorded regularly and the blood urea concentration measured at intervals to detect signs of renal failure; if this is found to be developing, either restriction of fluids or (if the failure is of the polyuric type) an increased intake may be indicated. In the latter situation, intravenous fluids may be required. Similarly, liver function should be checked by estimation of the serum bilirubin; the prothrombin content of the plasma should also be measured to make certain that the patient is not developing a bleeding tendency. To protect the liver in the postoperative period, whenever possible an intake of not less than 200 gm of carbohydrate a day should be given; if there is an acute, temporary impairment of function, not only may vitamin K be required intravenously but the plasma albumen concentration should also be watched—if it falls below 2 gm percent, an intravenous infusion of albumen may be required.

Following sphincterotomy, many surgeons give fluids by mouth as after simple exploration of the duct. After this operation, however, there is almost certainly some oedema surrounding the orifice of the pancreatic duct, causing some obstruction to the exit of pancreatic juice. It seems wise to avoid any stimulation of pancreatic secretion during this period. For this reason, it is our practice (1) to keep the stomach empty by suction via a Ryle tube or preferably a small gastrostomy tube inserted through a stab in the epigastrium at the time of operation, (2) to give only minimal fluids by mouth, and (3) to give fluids intravenously for 48 to 72 hours after operation. If at this stage the recovery is uneventful, fluids by mouth can be increased rapidly and intravenous fluids—stopped—although if there is any sign of gastric stasis, it may be necessary to continue them for a short while longer. It must be emphasised that this line of treatment is based on theoretical considerations and that there is no concrete evidence that it is required.

On the patient's return to the ward from the theatre the T tube is allowed to drain freely into a bottle or plastic bag (Uri-bag) suspended from the patient's bed, and free drainage should continue for 4 to 5 days. Preparatory to its removal, the tube is clamped or spigotted for an increasing time each day, starting with a period of 2 to 4 hours and ending with continuous occlusion on the eighth or ninth day after operation. Alternatively, the height of the receptacle for the bile may be raised each day or the tube itself (en route to the receptable) raised to an increasing height daily—both these methods depending upon increasing the hydrostatic pressure in the drainage system—until it reaches such a height that all the bile flows down the duct into the duodenum. Until such a time as all, or nearly all, the bile is passing into the intestine the patient's motions will be pale, but it is essential to see that he passes a normal coloured motion before the tube is removed. If for any reason, such as a retained stone, there is an obstruction to the flow of bile, not only may the stools remain pale but in addition there is likely to be pain on clamping the tube, together with a leak of bile alongside the T tube. It is, however, perfectly possible a residual stone to be in the duct with none of these manifestations, and for this reason the tube should not be removed until a postoperative cholangiogram has been performed.

Postoperative cholangiography. This is performed by the injection of a water-soluble contrast medium, such as Hypaque 25 percent, down the T tube. The flow of contrast medium into the duodenum is watched on the x-ray screen and films taken both to show the details of the termination of the duct and to provide a permanent record of the postoperative state of the duct. The interpretation of the films is essentially similar to that of a preexploratory cholangiogram, except that the calibre of the duct is only of significance if it exceeds that of the previous examination. By far the most common indication of a residual stone is the finding of a filling defect in the duct. Postoperative cholangiography is a very accurate method of investigation; it is free of risk, causes the patient little or no discomfort, and is an examination which should never be omitted—both for its immediate information and because, if the patient later develops symptoms possibly related to the biliary tract, its evidence is of great value.

Provided the cholangiogram findings are normal, the patient's stools have returned to normal, and the tube has been occluded for 48 hours without untoward symptoms, the T tube is removed. This is done by gentle but firm traction on the tube; it causes little pain. Usually there is only a slight discharge from the track for a few hours, after which time it dries up completely; persistence of a bile leak is strong evidence of obstruction in the duct.

Residual stones. *The demonstration on cholangiography of a residual stone poses a difficult problem.* The incidence of this finding is variable, and depends not only upon the skill with which the common duct has been explored but also upon whether postexploratory cholangiography has been performed. Bartlett and Dreyfuss (1960), reviewing a series of 355 postoperative cholangiograms performed at the Massachusetts General Hospital (postexploratory cholangi-ography apparently had not been used in these patients), reported an incidence of definite residual calculi in 2.8 percent, with a probable incidence of 4.2 percent. On occasions, postoperative cholangiography reveals the presence of surprisingly large residual calculi, emphasising the inaccuracy of trying to detect the presence of such stones at operation by palpation and exploration of the duct, especially when the stones are soft and even when the surgeon is experienced.

The treatment of a residual stone diagnosed in the immediate postoperative period poses difficult problems, and the correct procedure is by no means well defined. In some instances, if the stone is small and for other reasons a further procedure is considered undesirable, it may be justifiable to remove the T tube in the hope that the stone will pass. There is no doubt that this can occur, though how often is not known, but there is also the risk that if the stone does not pass it will enlarge, giving rise to further symptoms at a later date. For this reason, this course of action is seldom wise. If it is carried out, the patient must be watched for the development of symptoms due to the stone in the duct, and it is also wise to perform intravenous cholangiography together with estimation of the serum bilirubin and alkaline phosphatase concentrations at regular intervals until such time as it is clear that the stone has either passed or that a further operation is required.

Until recently the only certain method of removing a residual stone was by a further operation. In the last few years, however, attention has been directed to two additional methods of treatment. Coincident with the development of drugs that may be able to dissolve stones in the gallbladder, there has been a reawakening of interest in the idea that it may be possible to dissolve stones in the common duct by the irrigation of the duct with appropriate solutions, but to date this method remains experimental. In addition, there have been a number of reports of the successful removal of stones by the passage into the duct, down the track formed by the T tube, of Desjardins forceps, a wire ureteric basket (Dormia catheter) or other similar instruments (Magarey, 1971; Mahorner and Bean, 1971). These manipulations must be carried out under careful radiographic control, preferably using an image intensifier. The exact place of this form of treatment cannot be assessed until further experience has been obtained, but initial reports are promising, and given adequate facilities, a careful attempt to remove a residual stone (provided it is not too large) by these means would seem to be the preferred first line of treatment. It must be emphasised that this procedure should not be attempted without adequate x-ray facilities, and it is probably wise to desist if initial attempts to remove the stone are unsuccessful.

If instrumental attempts to remove the stone are either inadvisable or unsuccessful, and the stone is too large to leave in the hope that it will pass, the only alternative is to perform a further operation. The timing of this operation is difficult, but in general it should be undertaken as soon as the patient has recovered adequately from the first operation, due regard being paid to the patient's age and general condition. If, for any reason, the operation must be delayed for a number of weeks, the problem arises as to whether or not the T tube should be removed. If the tube is removed, it is probable that the fistulous track will heal and the patient have no symptoms in the relatively short time before the second operation is performed. There is always the risk, however, that a fistula may develop through the T tube track, and that symptoms may arise from the residual stone. For this reason, most surgeons advise leaving the tube in situ, with a spigot in place. The actual operation itself differs in no significant detail from primary exploration of the duct, save that exposure of the duct may be difficult owing to adhesions.

REFERENCES

Adams, R., and Stranahan, A., Surg. Gynecol. Obstet. 85:776, 1947.

Appleman, R. M., Priestley, J. T., and Gage, R. P., Proc. Mayo Clin. 39:473, 1964.

Ashmore, J. D., Kane, J. J., Pettit, H. S., and Mayo, H. W., Surgery 40:191, 1956.

Ayliffe, G. A. J., and Davies, A., Br. J. Pharmacol. 24:189, 1965.

Barner, H. B., Ann. Surg. 163:74, 1966.

Bartlett, M. K., and Dreyfuss, J. R., Surgery 47:202, 1960.

Bartlett, M. K., and Waddell, W. R., New Engl. J. Med. 258:164, 1958.

Blatherwick, N. H., and Pattison, A. C., Am. J. Surg. 88:129, 1954.

Boulter, P. S., Guy Hosp. Rep. 110:246, 1961 (a).

Boulter, P. S., Br. J. Surg. 49:17, 1961 (b).

Burgess, J. N., and Kidd, H. A., Br. Med. J. 1:607, 1967.

Capper, W. M., Br. J. Surg. 49:292, 1961.

Cattell, R. B., Surg. Clin. North Am. 28:659, 1948.

Chapman, M., Curry, R. C., and Le Quesne, L. P., Br. J. Surg. 51:600, 1964.

Colcock, B. P., Surg. Clin. North Am. 38:663, 1958.

Colcock, B. P., and Perey, B., Surg. Gynecol. Obstet. 118:20, 1964.

Collins, P. G., Br. J. Surg. 54:854, 1967.

Collins, P. G., Redwood, C. R. M., and Wynne-Jones, G., Br. J. Surg. 47:661, 1960.

Diffenbaugh, W. G., and Strohl, E. L., Arch. Surg. 72:931, 1956.

Eisman, B., Brown, W. H., Virabuts, S., and Gottesfeld, S., Arch. Surg. 79:24, 1959.

Ferris, D. O., and Weber, H. M., Arch. Surg. 73:197, 1956.

Flemma, R. J., Flint, L. M., Osterhout, S., and Shingleton, W. W., Ann. Surg. 166:563, 1967.

French, E. B., and Robb, W. A. T., Br. Med. J. 2:135, 1963.

Fung, J., Br. J. Surg. 48:404, 1961.

Glenn, F., Surg. Gynecol. Obstet. 95:431, 1952.

Glenn, F., Surg. Gynecol. 124:974, 1967.

Grundy, D. J., King, P. A., and Lloyd, G., Br. J. Surg. 59:205, 1972.

Hand, B. H., Br. J. Surg. 50:486, 1963.

Havard, C., Ann. R. Coll. Surg. Eng. 26:88, 1960.

Hight, D., Lingley, J. R., and Hurtubise, F., Ann. Surg. 150:1086, 1959.

Hughes, E. S. R., and Kernutt, R. H., Aust. New Zeal. J. Surg. 23:223, 1954.

Hutchinson, W. B., and Blake, T., Surgery 41:605, 1957.

Jones, S. A., and Smith, L. L., Surg. 71:565, 1972.

Keighley and Graham, 1971, p. 16.

King, M. S., Br. J. Surg. 58:829, 1971.

Kune, G. A., Arch. Surg. 89:995, 1964.

Larson, R. E., Hodgson, J. R., and Priestley, J. T., Surg. Gynecol. Obstet. 122:744, 1966.

Le Quesne, L. P., Proc. R. Soc. Med. 53:852, 1960.

Le Quesne, L. P., Whiteside, C. G., and Hand, B. H., Br. Med. J. 1:329, 1959.

Madden, J. L., Current Problems in Surgery, Chicago, Year Book, 1968.

Magarey, C. J., Lancet 1:104, 1971.

Mahorner, H., and Bean, W. J., Ann. Surg. 173:857, 1971.

Maingot, R., Abdominal Operations, 4th ed., New York, Appleton-Century-Crofts, 1961.

Mallet-Guy, P., Jeanjean, R., and Marion, P., La Chirurgie Biliaire Sous Controle Manométrique et Radiologique Peroperatoire. Paris, Masson, 1947.

McLaughlin, C. W., and Kleager, C. L., Nebraska Med. J. 36:17, 1951.

Mirizzi, P. L., Bol. Soc. Cir. B. Air. 16:1133, 1932.

Mixter, C. G., Hermanson, L., and Segal, A. L., Ann. Surg. 134:346, 1951.

Mortimer, P. R., Mackie, D. B., and Haynes, S., Br. Med. J. 3:88, 1969.

Nienhuis, J. I., Ann. Surg. 154:192, 1961.

Ong, G. B., Arch. Surg. 84:199, 1962.

Samuel, E., Br. J. Radiol. 32:669, 1959.

Sawyers, J. L., Herrington, J. L., and Edwards, W. H., Am. J. Surg. 109:107, 1965.

Schulenburg, C. A. R., S. Afr. Med. J. 35:202, 1961.

Schulenburg, C., Surgery 65:723, 1969.

Scott, A. J., Gut 12:487, 1971.

Scott, A. J., and Khan, G. A., Lancet 2:790, 1967.

Smith, R., in Rob, Smith, Morgan, eds., Operative Surgery, Progress Volume, London, Butterworths, 1958.

Smith, R., in Smith and Sherlock, eds., Surgery of the Gall-Bladder and Bile Ducts, London, Butterworths, 1964.

Thomas, C. G., Nicholson, C. P., and Owen, J. D., Ann. Surg. 173:845, 1971.

Thompson, J. A., Howard, J. M., and Vowles, K. D. J., Surg. Gynecol. Obstet. 105:706, 1957.

Thomson, F. B., Surg. Gynecol. Obstet. 103:78, 1956.

Walters, W., Gray, H. K., and Priestley, J. T., Proc. Mayo Clin. 23:40, 1948.

Watkin, D. F. L., and Thomas, G. G., Br. J. Surg. 58:570, 1971.

Wilson, H., Am. J. Surg. 119:52, 1970.

Winstone, N. E., Golby, M. G. S., Lawson, L. J., and Windsor, C. W. O., Lancet 1:843, 1965.

Zaslow, J., Counseller, V. S., and Heilman, F. R., Surg. Gynecol. Obstet. 84:140, 1947.

Zollinger, R. M., Boles, E. T., and Crawford, G. B., New Engl. J. Med. 252:203, 1955.

B. *SPHINCTEROPLASTY (NOT SPHINCTEROTOMY) IN THE PROPHYLAXIS AND TREATMENT OF RESIDUAL COMMON DUCT STONES*

S. AUSTIN JONES

The bête noire of the biliary tract surgeon is the occasional residual stone or stones which usually require further surgery. The overall incidence of calculi following initial choledocholithotomy is 10 percent. Even more significant, this figure rises to 25 percent following an operation for residual stones.[17] Calculi may be overlooked at the initial duct exploration and discovered later by postoperative cholangiography. Stones, especially in the hepatic ducts, may be irremovable at the first operation and eventually lodge in the common duct. Any narrowing at the distal end of the common duct, if unrecognized and untreated at the primary procedure, may produce intermittent obstruction and sufficient stasis to cause reformation of calculi within the ductal system.[6]

Many ingenious and helpful operative methods have been designed to reduce the number of residual calculi, but none of these

Adapted from Austin Jones and Smith. A reappraisal of sphincteroplasty (not sphincterotomy). Surgery 71:565–575, 1972.

has been uniformly successful. Our philosophy has been in agreement with that of Best, who stated that no matter how carefully a duct is explored, some calculi will be left behind.[3] This is substantiated by the results of different prophylactic approaches used at surgery and outlined in Table 2. It must be stressed that these figures are among the best reported, and are not representative of the general surgical population.

With these considerations in mind, our approach to the prophylaxis and treatment of residual common duct stones has been to create a permanent, noncontractile opening between the distal end of the common duct and the side of the duodenum, with a stoma equal in diameter to that of the widest portion of the common duct. Such a widely patent noncontractile opening should permit any overlooked stones to pass easily into the bowel, and bile stasis, which has been known to contribute to stone reformation, will be eliminated. Hepatic duct stones, which move later into the common duct, should pass harmlessly into the duodenum.

Table 2.   METHODS USED TO PREVENT RESIDUAL STONES

Technique	Author	Residual Stones (percent)		
		Proven	Probable	Total
Operative cholangiography	Jolley et al.[12]	3.5	3.5	7.0
Sphincterotomy	Backer[2]	3.9	2.6	6.5
Ampullary dilatation	Chodoff[7]	7.0	—	7.0
Fogarty balloon	Fogarty et al.[10]	7.6	—	7.6
Choledochoscope	Shore and Shore[21]	3.3	—	3.3
Sphincteroplasty	Present series	0	0	0

Source: From Austin Jones and Smith. Surgery 71: 565-575, 1972.

In order to produce this type of opening, it is necessary to perform a transduodenal sphincteroplasty using the technique discussed in detail below. A *sphincterotomy* fails to destroy all the muscular sphincters that surround the distal common and pancreatic ducts, and leaves behind a constricting mechanism that may retain residual calculi.

HISTORICAL NOTE

Anatomical

The presence of a sphincter mechanism at the distal end of the common duct has been known since 1681, when it was described by Glisson.[11] The common and pancreatic ducts parallel each other as they pass obliquely through the duodenal wall. In this intramural course, the common duct is reduced in caliber, producing the distal narrowing seen in a normal cholangiogram. As the ducts pass through the bowel wall, their lumens are affected not only by contraction of the duodenal muscle per se, but also by a thin sheath of specialized musculature lying in a submucosal position as described by Boyden.[4, 5] The fibers of this submucosal sheath mingle with those of the duodenal wall where the common duct enters the bowel, forming the superior sphincter of Boyden. At the termination of the duct, it forms the papillary or inferior choledochal sphincter, a series of stout circular muscular trabeculae some 6 mm in length (Fig. 38). It is clear that to eliminate the entire complex of sphincteric muscular mechanisms, the full length of the intramural course musculature must

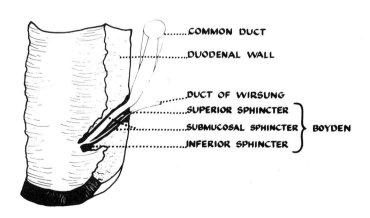

FIG. 38.   The lumens of the distal ducts are affected by both the duodenal wall muscle and the sphincter of Boyden. (From Austin Jones and Smith. *Surgery* 71:565–575, 1972. Courtesy of The C. V. Mosby Company.)

be destroyed, and the incision must therefore extend through the entire thickness of the duodenal wall.

Clinical

The first sphincterotomy was performed by McBurney in 1891, enabling him to extract a common duct calculus.[20] Four years later, Kocher performed a lateral choledochoduodenostomy 1 cm above the papilla and removed a stone.[19] Sphincterotomy was first used to treat recurrent pancreatitis by Archibald,[1] and this approach was subsequently employed extensively by Doubilet and Mulholland.[8, 9]

Sphincteroplasty was developed in 1951 in an effort to improve upon the poor results that had been obtained with sphincterotomy in the treatment of recurrent pancreatitis.[14] It was recognized early that any procedure on the distal end of the common duct and pancreatic duct would be of value only in the absence of parenchymal destruction and fibrosis or intrapancreatic ductal obstruction, and that an operative ductogram would be mandatory in choosing the optimum surgical approach.[16]

As very few patients with recurrent pancreatitis meet these criteria, the operation has an extremely limited value in this disease, and the indications for its use are not applicable to this discussion. *It soon became apparent, however, that this ablation of the distal sphincter mechanism affecting both the common and pancreatic ducts was of real value in the prophylaxis and treatment of residual common duct stones. At present we consider this to be by far the most important indication for transduodenal sphincteroplasty.*[15]

TECHNIQUE OF SPHINCTEROPLASTY

Sphincteroplasty is performed by approaching the papilla of Vater transduodenally and, by serial clamping, division, and suture approximation of the duodenal and common duct walls, creating a wide anastomosis between the end of the common duct and the side of the duodenum.

Figure 39 shows the anatomical relationship of the ducts and sphincter mechanism in the normal, postsphincterotomy and postsphincteroplasty states. It is clear that if one wishes to eliminate the sphincters completely and to produce a stoma as large as the widest part of the common duct, sphincterotomy will be inadequate. To achieve these objectives, a sphincteroplasty must be performed.

This operation can be performed by anyone familiar with biliary tract surgery, but we urge that the points outlined below be followed carefully:

1. The duodenum must be thoroughly mobilized by Kocher's maneuver. This includes the division of the peritoneal reflection which forms the in-

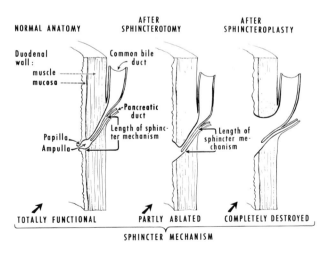

FIG. 39. Comparison of the normal anatomy with that following sphincterotomy and sphincteroplasty. Note that after sphincteroplasty the diameter of the stoma created equals that of the common duct. The ampulla shown and frequently described is usually not present. (From Austin and Smith. *Surgery* 71:565–575, 1972. Courtesy of The C. V. Mosby Company.)

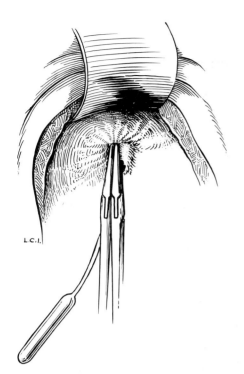

FIG. 40. Technique of sphincteroplasty. Placing the first pair of clamps at ten o'clock avoids pancreatic duct injury. (From Austin Jones and Smith. *Surgery* 71:565–575, 1972. Courtesy of The C. V. Mosby Company.)

ferior border of the foramen of Winslow.

2. We open the duodenum longitudinally, as we are never absolutely certain of the level of the papilla. Regardless of the axis of the duodenotomy, in order to avoid tension on the suture line the incision must always be closed in the same direction in which it is made.

3. The papilla may be located by: (1) palpation; (2) by using a small glass circle to depress the mucosa; [13] or (3) passage of a No. 10 Robinson catheter downward through a choledochotomy incision. If metal instruments such as Bakes' dilators are employed, there is a definite risk of producing a false passage.

4. In patients who have had previous

surgery in the right upper quadrant, the initial approach should be made transduodenally to avoid the problems of choledochotomy in such a situation.

5. In opening the papilla from below, care must be taken not to mistake the pancreatic duct for the common bile duct. If the anatomical relationships are in doubt, the common duct must be opened from above and the papilla located by gentle downward passage of a catheter.

6. The first pair of clamps must be placed in an anterolateral position at ten o'clock (Fig. 40). This avoids damage to the pancreatic duct which, in our dissections, always entered the medial side of the common bile duct.

7. After the initial opening of the papilla and visualization of the pancreatic duct, clamps are placed anteriorly (Fig. 41). Otherwise, the operator may find himself outside of the common duct on its lateral aspect.

8. Each successive pair of clamps is placed parallel, one to the other, and not over 3 mm of common duct and duodenal wall are included at a time. The tissue between the clamps is divided, and the clamps oversewn. The sutures are tied as each clamp is removed. We do not excise a wedge of tissue unless biopsy is indicated.

9. The diameter of the stoma produced must equal the largest diameter of the common bile duct. After we believe we have completed the operation, we check the opening under direct vision from below using Bakes' dilators, and if there is any question of constriction further division is done. *The length of the incision is not a criterion of the adequacy of the sphincteroplasty, as the length of the intramural course varies with different patients (Fig. 42). Only when the diameter of the stoma has been made equal to that of the common duct are we assured that the constricting mechanism in that particular patient has been eliminated. The apical stitch is of utmost importance, as at this point*

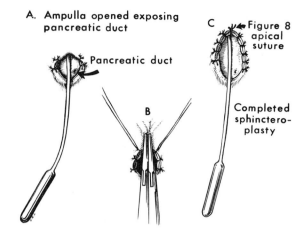

FIG. 41. Technique of sphincteroplasty, continued. After the pancreatic duct is visualized (A), clamps are placed anteriorly (B). The important apical stitch is shown in (C). (From Austin Jones and Smith. *Surgery* 71:565–575, 1972. Courtesy of The C. V. Mosby Company.)

the incision made is actually through the duodenal wall, and suture approximation is mandatory to avoid a leak (Figs. 41C and 43).

10. As we consider this operation an end-to-side choledochoduodenostomy per-

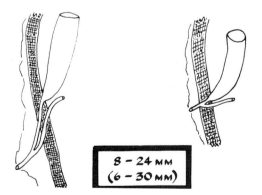

FIG. 42. The length of the intramural course varied from 8 to 24 mm in our dissections and from 6 to 30 mm in other series reported. Hence, the length of the incision varies with different patients, and must be continued until the diameter of the stoma created equals that of the widest part of the common duct. (From Austin Jones and Smith. *Surgery* 71:565–575, 1972. Courtesy of The C. V. Mosby Company.)

formed transduodenally, we have used 00000 silk interrupted mattress sutures. With a one-layer anastomosis, we feel more secure with nonabsorbable material, and to date have seen no contraindications to its use.

11. We remove the gallbladder following sphincteroplasty, as it will no longer function.

12. If choledochotomy has been done, a short-limbed T tube is used. If the patient has been operated upon for residual or multiple common duct stones, a completion cholangiogram can be obtained by placing the patient in a deep Trendelenburg position, or by occluding the distal common duct with an inflated balloon catheter prior to injection.

13. Routine cholangiograms are made on the eighth postoperative day, using a deep Trendelenburg position. If the ducts are clear, the T tube is withdrawn and the patient is discharged the following morning.

14. If the sphincteroplasty is done from below without a choledochotomy, neither T tube nor stent is employed.

15. Although not pertinent to this dis-

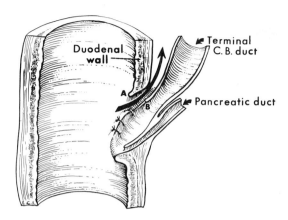

FIG. 43. The location of a retroperitoneal leak if the apex suture is not properly placed. (From Austin Jones and Smith. *Surgery* 71:565–575, 1972. Courtesy of The C. V. Mosby Company.)

cussion on residual stones, comments on technique should include two points which we feel are important in the rare case where this surgery is performed for recurrent pancreatitis. As previously stated, a pancreatic ductogram is mandatory in selecting the proper surgical approach. This always requires that the first part of a sphincteroplasty be done to visualize the pancreatic duct opening. The sphincteroplasty should always be completed, or the remaining sphincteric mechanism may contribute to postoperative pancreatitis. Also, the avascular septum between the pancreatic and common duct terminations should be divided.

PHYSIOLOGICAL DIFFERENCES BETWEEN SPHINCTEROTOMY AND SPHINCTEROPLASTY

The physiological differences between the two procedures has been presented in detail in previous reports.[17, 18] An outline of the methods used is given below:

Postoperative T Tube Pressure Studies

Intravenous morphine will constrict any remaining sphincteric mechanism at the lower end of the common duct. Following the administration of this drug, the postsphincterotomy patients show an abrupt rise and sustained pressure elevation, while the postsphincteroplasty group demonstrate only a transient immediate pressure elevation due to reflux of contents from the contracting duodenum followed by a rapid fall to base line pressure (Fig. 44).

Postoperative T Tube Cholangiography

ROUTINE CHOLANGIOGRAPHY

When the sphincterotomized patient is given intravenous morphine sulfate and dye is injected into the T tube, complete occlusion of the distal common duct is demonstrable, proving that the sphincteric complex has not been eliminated (Fig. 45). In marked contradistinction, the postsphincteroplasty patients demonstrate a wide opening with free flow both before and after morphine,

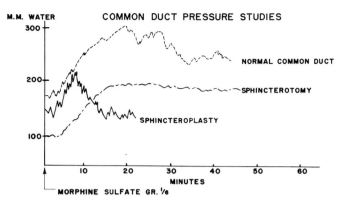

FIG. 44. Common duct pressure studies. The initial transient rise in the postsphincteroplasty group is due to reflux of duodenal contents from the contracting duodenum. (From Austin Jones and Smith. *Surgery* 71:565–575, 1972. Courtesy of The C. V. Mosby Company.)

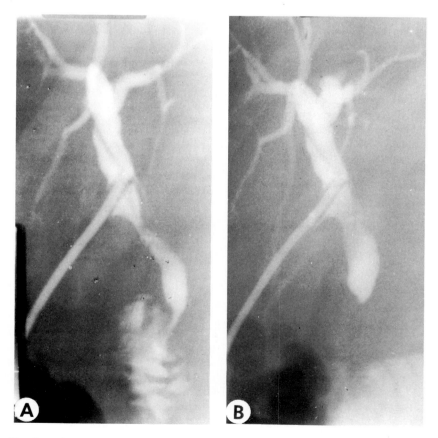

FIG. 45. Postsphincterotomy cholangiograms before (A) and after (B) administration of intravenous morphine. (From Austin Jones and Smith. *Surgery* 71:565–575, 1972. Courtesy of The C. V. Mosby Company.)

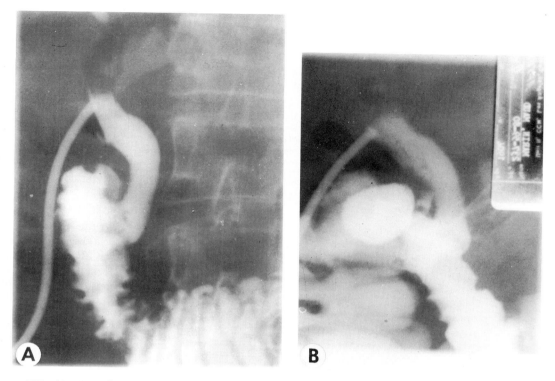

FIG. 46.   Postsphincteroplasty cholangiograms before (A) and after (B) morphine. (From Austin Jones and Smith. *Surgery* 71:565–575, 1972. Courtesy of The C. V. Mosby Company.)

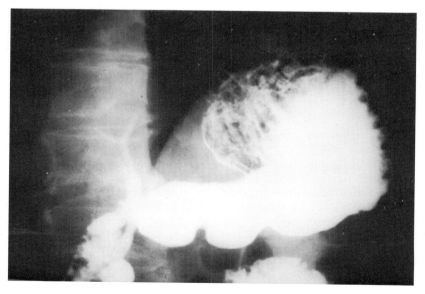

FIG. 47.   Desired reflux of barium on postoperative upper gastrointestinal series following an adequate sphincteroplasty. This case also demonstrates permanence of the stoma, as the film was made 12½ years after sphincteroplasty. (From Austin Jones and Smith. *Surgery* 71:565–575, 1972. Courtesy of The C. V. Mosby Company.)

Table 3.   POSTOPERATIVE T TUBE CINERADIOGRAPHY

Factors To Be Considered	After Sphincterotomy	After Sphincteroplasty
Position of patient	Supine	45-degree Trendelenburg
Rate of Hypaque infusion	15 to 30 drops per minute	150 drops per minute
Amount of Hypaque needed for study	30 to 60 cc	180 to 240 cc
Following intravenous morphine		
Distal duct	Occluded	Wide open
Proximal ducts	Dilated	Normal size
Pain	Marked	None
Nausea	Marked	None
Reflux from duodenum	None	In all cases

Source: From Austin Jones and Smith. Surgery 71: 565-575, 1972.

proving the complete ablation of the distal sphincters (Fig. 46).

CINERADIOGRAPHIC T TUBE STUDIES

Postoperative cinecholangiography in the two groups verified the points that were demonstrated by standard postoperative cholangiography. In addition, discomfort occurred routinely in the postsphincterotomy patients when dye was injected following morphine, and this group also demonstrated proximal dilatation of the common duct. Neither pain nor ductal distension developed after morphine was given to patients upon whom sphincteroplasty had been performed (Table 3).

Postoperative Barium Reflux with Upper Gastrointestinal Studies

Reflux of barium on postoperative upper gastrointestinal films was not seen after sphincterotomy. In contrast, all patients who had had a complete sphincteroplasty demonstrated free reflux of barium into the biliary tree (Fig. 47).We consider the absence of such reflux to be evidence of an incomplete operation.

Permanence of the Stoma Following Sphincteroplasty

While the opening produced by sphincterotomy has been shown to constrict with the passage of time, this does not occur with sphincteroplasty. Very late autopsy studies have demonstrated wide open stomas. Barium reflux has been noted following sphincteroplasty many years after the operation (Fig. 47).

We believe that the opening created by sphincteroplasty remains patent because only the anterior portion of the stoma is sutured. In contradistinction, a standard end-to-side choledochoduodenostomy requires suture closure of the entire circumference of the anastomosis, and late constriction is not unusual.

INDICATIONS AND CONTRAINDICATIONS FOR SPHINCTEROPLASTY

It is clear that sphincteroplasty and sphincterotomy are separate and distinct operations, and that a properly constructed sphincteroplasty should be of practical value in the prophylaxis and treatment of residual common duct stones. It should be stressed, however, that any surgery in this area carries a certain risk, and that the operation must not be used indiscriminately.

It has been our policy to perform a sphincteroplasty whenever we operate for residual stones or when irremovable hepatic duct stones are present. The operation is recommended at primary duct exploration whenever the surgeon encounters thick mud or sludge, ampullary stenosis, or multiple common duct stones. Admittedly the term *multiple stones* presents a gray area of decision. We believe sphincteroplasty is indicated when there is a sufficient number of calculi present to make complete clearing of the ducts questionable.

Sphincteroplasty is contraindicated at primary choledocholithotomy where only a few large stones are present, the bile is clear, the papilla is at least 3 mm in diameter, and a negative completion cholangiogram is obtained. It is not advised in the presence of a peri-Vaterian diverticulum or any inflammatory process involving the distal duct, or when there is gross enlargement of the common duct. Under these circumstances, a Roux-en-Y choledochojejunostomy or a lateral choledochoduodenostomy should be considered. In general, we do not favor the latter operation for the prophylaxis and treatment of residual calculi, as the distal segment may collect stones or food. We reserve this procedure for certain patients with a malignant obstruction of the distal duct where a bypass operation is indicated.

RESULTS

Our conclusions are based upon 280 sphincteroplasties performed over the past 20 years. In 170 cases, the primary indication was the presence of multiple common duct stones. Five had irremovable hepatic duct stones, and 20 were sent to us with residual stones. To date, there have been no patients with residual stones following sphincteroplasty. In four cases, postoperative cholangiograms demonstrated overlooked calculi, which were immediately washed into the duodenum by saline irrigation through the T tube.

There were four deaths in the 280 cases. Three of these were due to postoperative pancreatitis. In two of this group the cause was iatrogenic, and in the third no explanation was found. The fourth patient developed a duodenal fistula at the site of the duodenotomy. This was repaired twenty-three months later and a distal pancreatectomy performed. At autopsy the duodenal closure was intact, and the cause of death was reported as peritonitis and sepsis.

To emphasize the importance of making the stoma co-equal with that of the common duct, there were three other deaths not reported in this series where small plastic sphincterotomies were performed to extract stones from below in patients with grossly di-

lated common ducts. One patient died of postoperative pancreatitis, the second of generalized sepsis and cholangitis, and the third of septicaemia, cholangitis and a lung abscess.

The overall morbidity of 4.7 percent included five wound infections and three cases of transient postoperative pancreatitis. It is important to point out that none of the 280 patients developed cholangitis following sphincteroplasty, as no bile stasis is present following this operation. We believe that the low incidence of leakage at the duodenal suture line is associated with our insistence upon closing the duodenal incision in the same direction in which it was opened, thus avoiding suture line tension.

CONCLUSION

It is our conviction that no matter what operative techniques are used to clear the biliary tree of multiple calculi, occasionally stones will be left behind. The principle of permanent wide open distal drainage of the duct, when the indications given are present, appears to be a rational one. To obtain this result, a sphincterotomy is inadequate, and a transduodenal sphincteroplasty must be performed.

REFERENCES

1. Archibald, E., Surg. Gynecol. Obstet. 28:529, 1919.
2. Backer, O. G., Personal communication.
3. Best, R. R., Surg. Gynecol. Obstet. 78:425, 1944.
4. Boyden, E. A., Anat. Rec. 66:217, 1936.
5. Boyden, E. A., Surg. Gynecol. Obstet. 104:641, 1957.
6. Cattell, E. G., Colcock, G. P., and Pollack, J. L., New Engl. J. Med. 256:429, 1957.
7. Chodoff, R. J., J. Einstein M. Cent. 8:215, 1960.
8. Doubilet, H., and Mulholland, J. H., Ann. Surg. 128:609, 1948.
9. Doubilet, H., and Mulholland, J. H., J.A.M.A. 160:521, 1956.
10. Fogarty, T. J., Krippaehne, W. W., Dennis, D. L., and Fletcher, W. S., Am. J. Surg. 116:177, 1968.
11. Hendrickson, W. F., Johns Hopkins Hosp. Bull. 9:223, 1898.
12. Jolley, P. C., Baker, J. W., Schmidt, H. M., Walker, J. H., and Holm, J. C., Am. Surg. 168:551, 1968.
13. Jones, S. A., Surgery 54:480, 1963.
14. Jones, S. A., and Smith, L. L., Ann. Surg. 136:937, 1952.
15. Jones, S. A., and Smith, L. L., Surgery 71:565, 1972.
16. Jones, S. A., Smith, L. L., and Gregory, G., Ann. Surg. 147:180, 1958.
17. Jones, S. A., Smith, L. L., Keller, T. B., and

Joergenson, E. J., Arch. Surg. 86:1014, 1963.
18. Jones, S. A., Steedman, R. A., Keller, T. B., and Smith, L. L., Am. J. Surg. 118:292, 1969.
19. Kocher, T., Korrespondenz-blatt fur Aerzte
7:193, 1895.
20. McBurney, C. L., 53:520, 1891.
21. Shore, J. M., and Shore, E., Ann. Surg. 171:269, 1970.

44

POSTCHOLECYSTECTOMY SYMPTOMS

LESLIE P. LE QUESNE

Viewed overall, the removal of a gallbladder containing stones is one of the most satisfactory operations in abdominal surgery, and the great majority of patients with definite symptoms arising from stones in the gallbladder or bile ducts are permanently relieved by operative treatment. Reviewing a series of 141 patients undergoing cholecystectomy, Burnett and Shields (1958) found that 75 percent had been completely relieved of all preoperative symptoms, and that in a further 6 percent the symptoms were so mild that in fact they could be considered to be "within the bounds of normal." Le Quesne, Whiteside, and Hand (1959) similarly found that 75 percent of 73 patients reviewed after cholecystectomy for other purposes were symptom-free, and Schofield and MacLeod (1966) reported that 88 percent of 407 patients followed up for several years after surgical treatment for gallstones had experienced no abdominal pain following the operation. These figures in fact underestimate the success of the operation, for of the remaining patients in these three series, only a minority had severe symptoms and only a small percentage had significant symptoms arising from continuing or recurrent disease in the biliary tract.

As is to be expected, despite the excellent results from the operative treatment for gallstones, much attention has been directed to the small group of patients who continue to get symptoms after removal of their gallbladder. It has been suggested that after cholecystectomy some patients may develop a postcholecystectomy syndrome, in the same way that patients may develop one of the specific postgastrectomy syndromes. This concept of a specific postcholecystectomy syndrome was particularly prevalent before modern, accurate cholecystography and chol-

angiography were freely available—at a time when it was not uncommon to remove gallbladders which did not contain calculi. With increasing accuracy in the diagnosis of gallstones, and with the recognition of the fact that a number of conditions, such as hiatal hernia, can give rise to symptoms closely simulating those of gallstones, the existence of such a specific syndrome has been increasingly questioned; there is now no good evidence that such a condition exists. Glenn and Johnson (1955), Burnett and Shields (1958), and Schofield and MacLeod (1966)—from their studies of patients after cholecystectomy—all concluded that there is no such entity as a specific postcholecystectomy syndrome. Cholecystectomy must affect the mechanisms normally controlling the discharge of bile into the duodenum; nevertheless, there is no evidence that the operation gives rise to any detectable alteration in the absorption of foodstuffs, or to any specific, recognizeable clinical syndrome.

It is obvious that following removal of the gallbladder patients may develop abdominal symptoms due to some totally unrelated abdominal condition. The problem of postcholecystectomy symptoms really centres around that small group of patients who after operation continue to experience the same symptoms as they had before operation, or who develop symptoms suggestive of disease of the biliary apparatus. In these patients, the symptoms may be caused by (a) extrabiliary disorders or (b) disorders of the extrahepatic biliary tract.

EXTRABILIARY DISORDERS

The most common cause of postcholecystectomy symptoms, as defined above, is some extrabiliary disorder. Burnett and Shields (1958) found that 20 patients in their series complained of significant abdominal symptoms after cholecystectomy, and in 18 of the patients these symptoms could be accounted for by some condition unrelated to the biliary tract. These findings emphasise the well-established fact that in many patients stones in the gallbladder may cause no symptoms, and that the demonstration of stones in the gallbladder does not per se imply that the stones are responsible for a patient's symptoms.

Many conditions can give rise to symptoms mistakenly thought to be caused by gallstones, and then continue to cause symptoms after removal of the gallbladder. *The most common of these conditions are hiatal hernia, peptic ulceration, and chronic pancreatitis.* All three of these conditions often occur in patients who also have gallstones, thus adding to the preoperative difficulty of determining the main cause of the patient's symptoms; this is particularly the case in patients presenting with chronic indigestion as opposed to isolated attacks of pain, and it is this group of patients who make up the bulk of those presenting after cholecystectomy with symptoms due to some extrabiliary disorder. Hiatal hernia, a common condition in overweight women, is often present in patients with gallstones, and although the symptoms of reflux oesophagitis do not resemble those of gallstones, the flatulent dyspepsia that accompanies both conditions is very similar. In view of this difficulty, it is wise always to perform a barium-meal examination in a patient with gallstones before proceeding to cholecystectomy and, similarly, to perform a cholecystogram before undertaking repair of an hiatal hernia. If necessary, both conditions can be dealt with at the same operation, either through a midline upper abdominal incision or through a Kocher's, right subcostal incision with a midline extension upward with excision of the xiphisternum.

The diagnosis of extrabiliary disorders giving rise to symptoms after cholecystectomy is based on the careful taking of the history and an examination, followed by such investigations as are indicated—barium-meal x-ray examination usually being the most important of these. In general, once a diagnosis has been made, the condition should

be treated on its merits; only rarely does the previous cholecystectomy influence the treatment.

DISORDERS OF THE EXTRAHEPATIC BILIARY TRACT

The common disorders of the biliary tract giving rise to symptoms after cholecystectomy are: (1) stricture of the bile duct, (2) residual stone in the common duct, (3) cystic duct syndrome (see below), and (4) fibrosis of the sphincter of Oddi. Stricture of the bile duct and fibrosis of the sphincter of Oddi are discussed in Chapters 34 and 48B.

Residual Stone in the Common Duct

As emphasised previously, the great majority of stones present in the common duct were originally formed in the gallbladder, later migrating into the common duct—although on occasions soft stones may form in a dilated duct, especially if there is also cholangitis and/or some obstruction to the flow of bile into the duodenum. From this it follows that in the great majority of instances the demonstration of a stone in the common duct of a patient who has previously had a cholecystectomy implies that this stone was present in the duct at the time of removal of the gallbladder. Usually such residual stones are single, but on occasions they may be multiple and then only one of the ductal stones may be truly residual, the remainder having formed in the partially obstructed duct.

Residual stones are the most important and most common cause of symptoms arising in the biliary tract in patients who have had a cholecystectomy. Such stones may occur either after simple cholecystectomy (as a result of failure to explore the duct) or after cholecystectomy and exploration of the duct (as a result of failure either to detect a stone in the duct or to remove all those present therein). The true incidence of residual stone is difficult to determine and varies considerably in reported series, as shown in Table 1, but there is general agreement that the incidence is higher in those patients in whom the common duct was explored at the time

Table 1.   INCIDENCE OF RESIDUAL STONE ON THE COMMON BILE DUCT

Author	No. of Cases	Total Incidence of Residual Stone (percent)	Incidence Following Simple Cholecystectomy (percent)	Incidence Following Cholecystectomy plus Exploration of Common Bile Duct (percent)
Glenn (1952)	200	5.5	4	7
Hicken et al. (1954)	400	—	—	20
Thomson (1956)	106	—	—	11
Colcock and Liddle (1958)	100	—	—	2
Bartlett and Dreyfuss (1960)	355	—	—	4.2
Havard (1960)	702	4.2	2.3	13.5
Smith et al. (1963)	316	7[a]	—	—
Larson et al. (1966)	415	—	—	3.1[b]

[a]Proved and suspected stones.

[b]The incidence in 207 patients with negative exploration of the duct was 1 percent and 5.3 percent in 208 patients in whom stones were removed from the duct.

of cholecystectomy. The figures of Larson et al. (1966) also emphasise the difficulty of making certain that all the stones have been removed from a duct containing several. The varying incidence of residual stone is an expression both of the varying length of the follow-up period in the different series and also of differences in the original patient material, for there is clear evidence that the incidence of stone in the duct as a complication of gallstones rises with age (Appleman, Priestley, and Gage, 1964). From these figures, it can be concluded that the average, overall incidence of residual stones is in the region of 4 percent—though with the increasing use of operative cholangiography, both before and after exploration of the duct, this figure is likely to fall.

CLINICAL PRESENTATION AND DIAGNOSIS

A residual stone may give rise to symptoms at any time after cholecystectomy, from a few days following the operation to many years later. In an analysis of 102 patients with residual stones in the common duct, Glenn and McSherry (1965) found that 25 percent caused symptoms within one month of operation but that more than 25 percent did not cause trouble for 5 years or more after removal of the gallbladder.

In the immediate postoperative period, the presenting manifestations of a stone in the common duct will largely depend upon whether there is a T tube in the common duct. If the duct has been drained, the presence of a residual stone may be suggested by the development of pain and a leak of bile around the T tube when it is spigotted; alternatively, the patient may develop a biliary fistula following removal of the T tube. It is perfectly possible, however, for a residual stone to be present without any of these manifestations and for the patient to make an uneventful recovery from operation. By far the most accurate method of diagnosing a residual stone in the early postoperative period in a patient with a T tube in the common duct is by the performance of a postoperative cholangiogram (Fig. 1). It is for this reason that such a cholangiogram should always be performed before the T tube is removed. If the common duct has not been explored and drained, a residual stone may cause pain and jaundice in the immediate postoperative period, the picture in no way differing from the presentation of such a stone later in the postoperative period except that in rare instances the obstruction to the duct may cause the cystic duct to blow open, leading either to biliary peritonitis or a biliary fistula.

The majority of patients with a residual stone in the duct make an uneventful recovery from operation, and it is not until

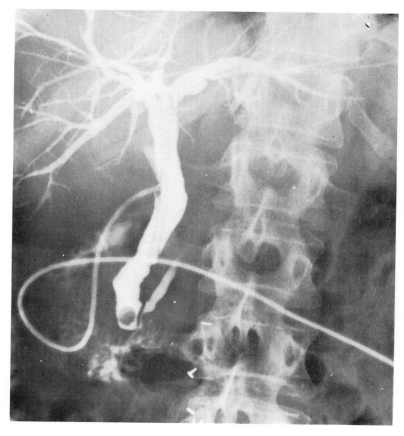

FIG. 1. Postoperative T tube cholangiogram showing a residual stone in the common bile duct. (Courtesy of Butterworths, London.)

weeks, months, or years thereafter that the stone gives rise to trouble. The symptoms and signs of a stone in the common duct after a cholecystectomy are essentially the same as in a patient who has not had her gallbladder removed. The outstanding manifestations are pain (so-called biliary colic) and jaundice; the characteristics of this pain and jaundice have been described previously. The biochemical features of the obstruction of the duct as well as its consequences and complications are also similar to those in a patient who has an intact gallbladder, as is the differential diagnosis—except that after cholecystectomy, stone in the common duct has to be differentiated from a traumatic stricture of the duct. The majority of patients with a traumatic stricture of the duct develop symptoms shortly after the operation;

however, some make an uneventful recovery to present later with pain and jaundice, and in these patients the differential diagnosis (between stricture and residual calculus) may be difficult. Usually jaundice owing to a residual calculus is fluctuant and not very deep whilst that caused by a stricture is constant and often deep; however, these features are not reliable, and if a stricture is associated with cholangitis and the presence of mud in the duct, the jaundice may be episodic.

The most important investigation in the diagnosis of residual stone in the common duct is an intravenous cholangiogram, and this may give conclusive information by the demonstration of a filling defect (Fig. 2). Tomograms are often of value in revealing filling defects not visible on routine radiographs. Attention must also be paid to other

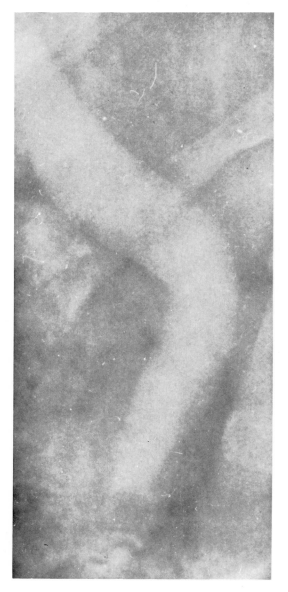

FIG. 2.   Intravenous cholangiogram showing a residual calculus at the lower end of a dilated common duct. (Courtesy of Butterworths, London.)

the 2-hour film shows as dense an image of the duct as that at 1 hour after the injection, and the chronic obstruction caused by a stone may result in dilatation of the duct. The finding of a dilated common duct on intravenous cholangiographic examination of a patient who has previously had his gallbladder removed, however, must be interpreted with caution. In a study of a series of patients who had undergone cholecystectomy a year or more previously, Le Quesne, Whiteside, and Hand (1959) showed that a normal common duct does not increase in size after removal of the gallbladder, and that a common duct dilated at the time of cholecystectomy does not significantly diminish in calibre following removal of the gallbladder and any stones in the duct. From these facts, it follows that the demonstration of a dilated duct in a patient who has undergone cholecystectomy is not, per se, significant of continuing obstruction of the duct unless there is clear evidence that the duct has increased in calibre since the removal of the gallbladder. Per contra, definite evidence that the duct has increased in calibre following cholecystectomy signifies that there is some obstruction to the flow of the bile in the duct. These considerations are an important argument in favour of the routine performance of operative cholangiography, for this examination not only gives important immediate information but is also of the utmost value in the interpretation of intravenous cholangiograms at a later date, should they be required.

If the patient is jaundiced, intravenous cholangiography is not possible to perform, and in these circumstances either the diagnosis must be made on clinical and biochemical evidence or time must be allowed for the jaundice to subside so that intravenous cholangiography becomes feasible; on occasions, percutaneous transhepatic cholangiography may give valuable information. This examination, which is discussed in full elsewhere (see Chap. 46) is possible only when the intrahepatic ducts are dilated, but it may be particularly useful in a deeply jaundiced patient in whom the differentiation between a residual stone and a traumatic stricture must be made.

features of the examination beside the presence or absence of a filling defect. Small stones, mud, and grit may not give rise to a filling defect, but they may cause delayed emptying of the duct (Wise, 1962) so that

MANAGEMENT

In the great majority of instances, a residual stone in the common duct should be removed surgically; it is only rarely that concurrent disease or other factors make conservative management advisable. The longer a stone remains in the duct, the more likely is it to cause liver damage or cholangitis; thus in general the sooner it is removed the better.

The detection of a stone in the common duct in the immediate postoperative period raises particular problems (see below). The discovery of a residual stone in the common duct of a patient who has been free of symptoms for several months or more after removal of the gallbladder almost of necessity implies the development of unpleasant symptoms demanding relief, and for this reason (in addition to those mentioned above) it is usually wise to proceed to remove the stone as soon as feasible. Before operation, the same investigations and precautions should be taken as before a primary operation on the duct, particular attention being paid to the prothrombin and albumen concentrations in the plasma. The essential step in the operation itself is the exposure of the common bile duct, which may be difficult owing to adhesions from the previous operation. To avoid adhesions to the original incision, it may be prudent to open the abdomen by a different incision, but this does not confer a major advantage and it is probably wise for the surgeon to use the incision and route with which he is most familiar.

On opening the abdomen, the duodenum will usually be found adherent to the gallbladder bed and must be separated with care to expose the common duct, which is often dilated and thus more readily identified. If the adhesions surrounding the supraduodenal portion of the common duct are particularly dense, it may be hazardous to persist in a direct exposure; under these circumstances, it is helpful to mobilise the duodenum and head of the pancreas (Chap. 42) and approach the duct from below and behind. By this approach it is often possible to expose the duct with safety and comparative ease despite the presence of dense adhesions. Once the duct has been exposed, it should be carefully palpated, and before it is opened it is wise to perform a cholangiogram to obtain further information about the number of stones in the duct and any additional changes in the duct. Save for the fact that the contrast material is introduced into the duct by direct needle puncture, the technique and interpretation of this examination are in all respects similar to ordinary preexploratory cholangiography. Following this examination, the duct is opened and explored as described previously, with removal of all stones and debris. In patients requiring reexploration, the duct is often dilated and contains much debris, and to ensure free drainage of bile an additional procedure (either a sphincterotomy or a choledochoduodenal anastomosis) may well be required. The purposes of these two operations are different and their relative merits as yet incompletely established; the technique of these two operations and their respective advantages and disadvantages are discussed in full elsewhere. On rare occasions the adhesions surrounding the duct may be so dense as to render the exposure of its supraduodenal portion impossible or unacceptably dangerous, and it will then be necessary to mobilise the pancreas, open the second part of the duodenum, identify the papilla, perform a sphincterotomy by Maingot's technique (see Chap. 48) and explore the duct from below.

At the conclusion of the exploration, the common duct is closed around a T tube and a postexploratory cholangiogram performed. This examination is not foolproof, but on occasions it may prevent a third operation on the duct for removal of twice-overlooked calculi. The operation site is drained with a corrugated drain which, together with the T tube, is brought out through a separate stab incision. The postoperative management of the drain and T tube is similar to that following primary exploration of the duct—as is the general management of the patient.

When a residual stone is detected in the immediate postoperative period, it may well be wise to defer operation, save in the rare patient when this stone is causing biliary peritonitis. Attempts may be made to flush the stone down into the duodenum by irrigating the duct with saline via the T tube, but such attempts are rarely successful. Similarly, attempts to dissolve the stone by injecting ether or other substances into the duct (Pribram, 1935) are usually fruitless and often painful, so that these procedures should not be performed. If the residual stone is small and thought likely to pass spontaneously, the T tube should be removed and events awaited. It is not known how often such stones will pass, but they undoubtedly may. The patient should be watched carefully, with repeated estimations of the serum bilirubin and alkaline phosphatase concentrations, and with performance of intravenous cholangiography at suitable intervals. If the patient develops any symptoms of biliary obstruction, or if there is biochemical or radiographic evidence of such obstruction, operation should be advised; but in the absence of such evidence there is no immediate urgency to remove the stone. If the residual stone is large and thought unlikely to pass, little is to be gained by delaying the second operation, which should be performed as soon as the patient has recovered from the initial operation. In all instances the general condition, age, and circumstances of the patient must be taken into account; in *any* given patient, the decision as to when to advise a further operation must be based on all the relevant considerations. This problem is discussed in Chapter 43A.

Cystic Duct Stump

It is widely taught that if, in performing cholecystectomy, a portion of the cystic duct is left in situ, this may give rise to symptoms which can only be relieved by the stump's excision at a second operation. Beye (1936) put on record one of the earliest of such cases, and with the introduction of intravenous cholangiography the number of such cases recorded has increased. Garlock and Hurwitt (1951) reported 30 patients with "the cystic duct syndrome"; 24 of these patients had the cystic duct stump removed, with relief of their symptoms. Larmi and Fock (1958) recorded 13 similar cases, and

Glenn and Whitsell (1961) described their experience with 60 patients operated upon for removal of the cystic duct stump. From the descriptions of these and other writers, it appears that the majority of these patients

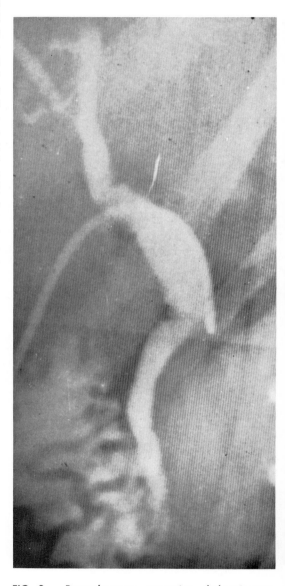

FIG. 3.   Preexploratory, operative cholangiogram; the catheter appears to be lying outside the common duct, and is in the lumen of an anatomically abnormal cystic duct which passes behind the common duct, runs down closely applied to its left side, and enters it at a lower level than normal.

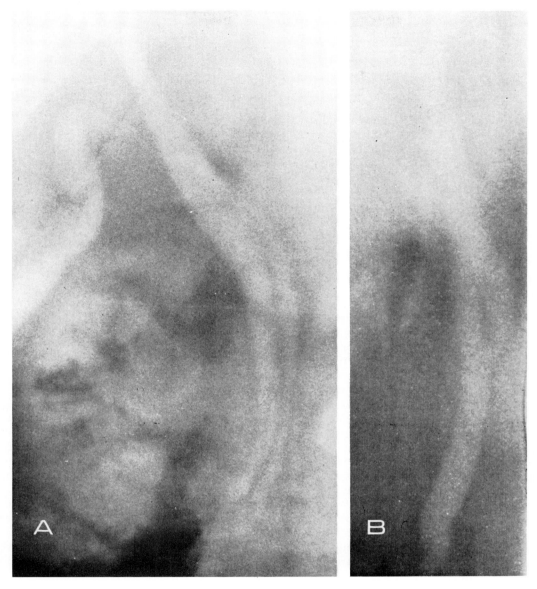

FIG. 4. (A) Preoperative intravenous cholangiogram showing an anatomically abnormal cystic duct which runs down along the left side of the common duct, to join it just proximal to its termination. (B) Postoperative, intravenous cholangiogram showing an abnormal cystic duct entering the left side of the common duct at an abnormally low level.

complained of symptoms suggestive of calculous cholecystitis, often accompanied by transient jaundice and sometimes with quite severe pain similar to that of a stone in the common duct. In most cases the cystic duct stump was demonstrated by intravenous chol-angiography; in some the duct stump was dilated, resembling a miniature gallbladder, but in others it was apparently normal in calibre.

As a result of these reports, the doctrine has developed that in performing a cholecystectomy it is unwise to leave behind a portion of the cystic duct, as it may at a later date give rise to undesirable complications and symptoms. This view was clearly stated by Garlock and Hurwitt (1951), who wrote that the cystic duct stump "becomes, in effect, a diseased gallbladder of small size, undergoing inflammatory changes of varying degree, and . . . capable of forming calculi which pass into the common duct. . . ." It is clearly an obvious extension of such a doctrine to recommend that removal of the entire cystic duct is an essential part of the operation of cholecystectomy, as recommended by Hicken, White, and Coray (1947), who stated: "It is essential that the entire gallbladder and its cystic duct be removed whenever a cholecystectomy is being performed . . . operators incapable of performing complete anatomic dissections of the cystic duct should not elect to remove the gallbladder."

For many years it has been known that the cystic duct does not always open into the right lateral border of the common duct in the free edge of the lesser omentum; however, the introduction of the various forms of cholangiography has shown that such congenital abnormalities are more common than was previously realised. A common abnormality is for the cystic duct to pass behind the common duct and then to run down within the sheath of the common duct, closely applied to the left lateral wall of the duct, and to open into the common duct a variable distance from its termination. At operation, such a cystic duct appears to join the common duct in the usual position, but if an operative cholangiogram is performed, the true anatomical arrangement becomes evident (Fig. 3), and it may be thought necessary to remove this terminal portion of the cystic duct to prevent the development of postcholecystectomy symptoms. Similarly, cystic ducts with a low insertion into the common duct may be demonstrated on intravenous cholangiography (Fig. 4), and the demonstration of a residual portion of cystic duct in a patient with symptoms following cholecystectomy may lead to a second operation for the removal of the part. The removal of a length of cystic duct lying within the sheath of the common duct

is a difficult and potentially dangerous procedure, and now that such ducts can be demonstrated easily the doctrine that they are harmful demands critical reconsideration.

When the literature concerning the *cystic duct stump syndrome* is reviewed, it is to be noted that many of the patients considered to be suffering from symptoms due to this condition also had an additional abnormality in the biliary tract. Thus, Hicken, White, and Coray (1947) reported 7 patients with this condition of whom 6 had a residual calculus in either the cystic duct or common duct or both, and in the seventh the stump of the cystic duct was adherent to the gallbladder bed, kinking the common duct. Twenty-one of the 30 patients reported by Garlock and Hurwitt (1951) had stones in either the cystic duct remnant or common duct or both, and the same is true of 26 of the 60 cases reported by Glenn and Whitsell (1961). Furthermore, of the remaining 9 patients reported by Garlock and Hurwitt (1951), 6 were at some time jaundiced; the authors wrote: "In every instance (that is, in all 30 cases) the common bile duct was thickened and dilated, at times up to 3 cm in diameter, irrespective of an antecedent history of jaundice or the presence or absence of calculi." Similarly, Beargie and his colleagues (1962), reporting the experience of this condition at the Mayo Clinic, record that of 27 patients with cystic duct remnants, 18 had residual stones in some part of the biliary tract.

Considering the problem from another angle, from the cholangiography evidence now obtainable it is clear that cystic duct remnants of significant size are much more common than was previously thought, and that if such remnants were commonly a cause of symptoms, the cystic duct syndrome should be more common than in fact it is. Millbourn (1951) studied 294 patients who had undergone cholecystectomy and found that the average length of the cystic duct stump was 2.7 cm, and that in 17 percent of these patients it was 4 cm or more long—although none of these patients with long stumps had symptoms. Millbourn, in the same paper, records 21 patients with a cystic duct stump who underwent a second operation; in each patient the symptoms could be accounted

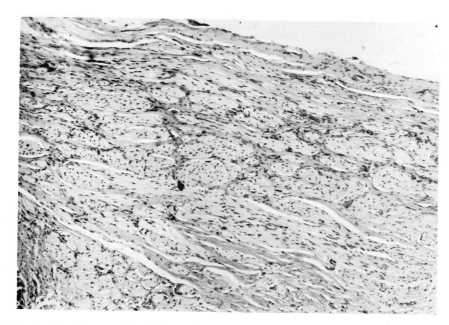

FIG. 5.   Section of a small nodule at the tip of a cystic duct stump excised from a patient with upper abdominal symptoms following cholecystectomy. The section shows nerve elements in dense fibrous tissue, a so-called "stump neuroma." The patient's symptoms were unaffected by this operation (×90.) (Courtesy of Butterworths, London.)

for by some other lesion, usually a stone in the common duct. Seven patients were relieved of their symptoms by removal of a stone from the common duct, despite leaving in situ a cystic duct stump 5 cm or more in length.

It has been suggested (Womack and Crider, 1947) that symptoms can arise as the result of the formation of a neuroma on the cystic duct stump from the ends of the severed autonomic nerves which run alongside the duct (Fig. 5). There is no critical evidence in support of this hypothesis and no evidence that such neuromas are present more frequently in patients with symptoms following cholecystectomy than in those without symptoms.

In the light of these considerations, it seems that it is only possible to conclude there is no convincing evidence that the leaving behind of a portion of normal, healthy cystic duct gives rise to symptoms following cholecystectomy, or that such a remnant can result in the formation of new stones. If a portion of diseased gallbladder

is overlooked, or if a portion of cystic duct containing calculi is left in situ, or if the cystic duct stump is associated with some condition causing interference with the flow of bile into the duodenum, the patient may develop symptoms; but these symptoms should be ascribed to the factor additional to the presence of a cystic duct stump, and they will be relieved only by dealing with this additional factor.

From this analysis of the problem, two conclusions emerge. First, if during the performance of a cholecystectomy an abnormally low insertion of the cystic duct is demonstrated (usually by preexploratory cholangiography), there is no need to dissect the duct down to its termination, and it is both immediately safer and in the long term free from the risk of causing postcholecystectomy symptoms to ligate and divide the duct in the usual site 2 to 3 mm from the right lateral border of the common duct—assuming that there is clear evidence that the portion of cystic duct left in situ does not contain calculi. Second, in a patient with symptoms following removal of the gallbladder, the demonstration by intravenous cholangiography of a cystic duct stump should not be interpreted as evidence that the cause of the symptoms has been demonstrated, for in the great majority of instances the symptoms will be caused by some other factor. The author has experience of 4 patients in whom the cystic duct stump was removed in an attempt to relieve symptoms following cholecystectomy, in one of whom a neuroma was demonstrated in the cystic duct remnant (Fig. 5); none of these 4 patients benefitted from the operation. Wise (1962), basing his opinion on the experience of the Lahey Clinic, wrote: "Cystic duct remnants per se, not being regarded as a cause of symptoms, are not regarded in our institution as an indication for surgical exploration." Beargie and his colleagues (1962), writing from the Mayo Clinic, urged that surgeons should be very cautious in advising the removal of cystic duct stumps.

REFERENCES

Appleman, R. M., Priestley, J. T., and Gage, R. P., Proc. Mayo Clin. 39:473, 1964.
Bartlett, M. K., and Dreyfuss, J. R., Surgery 47:202, 1960.
Beargie, J. R., Hodgson, J. R., Huizenga, K. A., and Priestley, J. T., Surg. Gynecol. Obstet. 115:143, 1962.
Beye, H. L., Surg. Gynecol. Obstet. 62:191, 1936.
Burnett, W., and Shields, R., Lancet 1:923, 1958.
Colcock, B. P., and Liddle, H. V., New Engl. J. Med. 258:264, 1958.
Garlock, J. H., and Hurwitt, E. S., Surgery 29:833, 1951.
Glenn, F., Surg. Gynecol. Obstet. 95:431, 1952.
Glenn, F., and Johnson, G., Surg. Gynecol. Obstet. 101:331, 1955.
Glenn, F., and McSherry, C. K., Surg. Gynecol. Obstet. 121:979, 1965.
Glenn, F., and Whitsell, J. C., Surg. Gynecol. Obstet. 113:711, 1961.
Havard, C., Ann. R. Coll. Surg. Eng. 26:88, 1960.
Hicken, N. F., McAllister, A. J., and Call, D. W., Arch. Surg. 68:643, 1954.
Hicken, N. F., White, L. B., and Coray, Q. B., Surgery 21:309, 1947.
Larmi, T. K. I., and Fock, G., Acta Chir. Scand. 114:361, 1957–8.
Larson, R. E., Hodgson, J. R., and Priestley, J. T., Surg. Gynecol. Obstet. 122:744, 1966.
Le Quesne, L. P., Whiteside, C. G., and Hand, B. H., Br. Med. J. 1:329, 1959.
Maingot, R., Personal communication, 1972 and 1973.
Millbourn, E., Acta Chir. Scand. 100:448, 1951.
Pribram, B. O., Surg. Gynecol. Obstet. 60:55, 1935.
Schofield, G. E., and MacLeod, R. G., Br. J. Surg. 53:1042, 1966.
Smith, R. B., Conklin, E. F., and Porter, M. R., Surg. Gynecol. Obstet. 116:731, 1963.
Thomson, F. B., Surg. Gynecol. Obstet. 103:78, 1956.
Wise, R. E., Intravenous Cholangiography. Springfield, Ill., Thomas, 1962.
Womack, N. A., and Crider, R. L., Ann. Surg. 126:31, 1947.

45

THE INVESTIGATION AND MANAGEMENT OF THE JAUNDICED PATIENT

FRANCES HAYWARD SMITH

Recent research in liver disease has discovered new means of investigating and managing the jaundiced patient. Chief among them are: the identification of the Australia antigen and the role of immunology in liver disease; the increased knowledge of the relationship of drug and bile pigment metabolism; the discovery of hepatic cytoplasmic organic anion-binding proteins; the intensive work in viral and drug-induced hepatitis; and the development of sophisticated endoscopes that permit visualization of the biliary tree and the cannulation of the ampulla of Vater.

"Surgical" jaundice may be distinguished from its medical counterpart by relatively simple means in approximately 80 percent of cases. A thorough history, an observant physical examination, a few hematological studies (including hemoglobin, hematocrit, erythrocyte, and leukocyte counts, and direct and indirect bilirubin determinations), and an examination of the urine with respect to color and the presence of bile and urobilinogen will give sufficient information for appropriate management.

The remaining 20 percent demand not only a working knowledge of bilirubin production, transport, storage, conjugation, and excretion, but a knowledge of the means to detect the abnormalities in these mechanisms.

A representative but by no means complete classification of jaundice is given below:

Unconjugated Hyperbilirubinemia

Increased production (hemolytic states)
  Hereditary or congenital
    Spherocytosis
    Nonspherocytic hemolytic anemia
    Thalassemia
    Sickle cell disease
  Acquired (Coombs' positive anemia)
  Paroxysmal nocturnal hemoglobinuria
  "Shunt" hyperbilirubinemia
  Infectious agents
  Chemical agents
  Physical agents (severe burns)
  Poisons
Transport and storage
  Congenital (Gilbert's disease)
  Acquired
    Postviral hepatitis
    Postportacaval shunt—clears after splenectomy
  Drugs
    Novobiocin
    Rifamycin
    Flavaspidic acid
    Others
  Metabolic defects
    Crigler-Najjar syndrome
    Jaundice of premature infants
    Jaundice of neonates
      Deficiency of glucuronyl transferase and uridine diphosphate, glucuronic acid dehydrogenase
      Decreased cytoplasmic-binding protein (Y and Z)
      Abnormal steroids in breast milk or maternal plasma (Lucey-Driscoll type)

Conjugated Hyperbilirubinemia

Excretion
  Congenital secretory failure
    Dubin-Johnson syndrome
    Rotor syndrome
  Intrahepatic obstruction
    Cirrhosis
    Hepatitis
      Infectious
      Alcoholic
      Amyloidosis of the liver *
      Carcinoma
      Granulomatous disease
Drugs
  Promazine
  C-substituted compounds of testosterone
  Halothane
  Others
Extrahepatic obstruction
  Cholelithiasis
  Choledocholithiasis
  Bile duct strictures
  Pancreatitis
  Carcinoma of the head of the pancreas
  Carcinoma of the bile ducts
  Carcinoma of the ampulla of Vater
  Sclerosing cholangitis

BILIRUBIN METABOLISM

Bilirubin is a yellowish organic anion that is transported, conjugated, stored, and excreted by the liver cells in processes similar to but less important than other organic anions, such as steroids, drugs, and dyes. It is a catabolic waste product derived from several sources. In the normal human subject, about 85 percent of the bilirubin production of 250 to 300 mg a day comes from the breakdown of erythrocytes 100 to 120 days old. Ten to 20 percent arises from other sources. One source is nonerythropoietic, i.e., principally enzymes in the liver, such as catalase, peroxidase, tryptophan, pyrrolase, and cytochromes; heme or porphyrin not

---

* From *Levy, Fryd, and Eliakim, Gastroenterology 61:234, 1971.*

used in hemoglobin synthesis; and turnover of nonhemoglobin heme-containing proteins. The other source is erythropoietic, i.e., intracorpuscular degradation of hemoglobin during erythrocyte maturation in the bone marrow and intramedullary destruction of newly formed erythrocytes.

This 10 to 20 percent is called the "early labeled fraction" since, when ^{15}N glycine is given, the isotope occurs in stercobilin in 5 to 10 days rather than 100 to 120 days later when the larger fraction appears from the breakdown of senescent erythrocytes. The early labeled fraction is greatly increased in pernicious anemia, porphyria, thalassemia, and after hemorrhage.

Much of the information as to how hemoglobin is converted first to biliverdin and then to bilirubin is based on inconclusive evidence from artificial model systems, most of which are lacking in enzymes. A condensed summary of current opinion is given in Figure 1. The globin is hydrolyzed to amino acids; the iron fraction of the heme

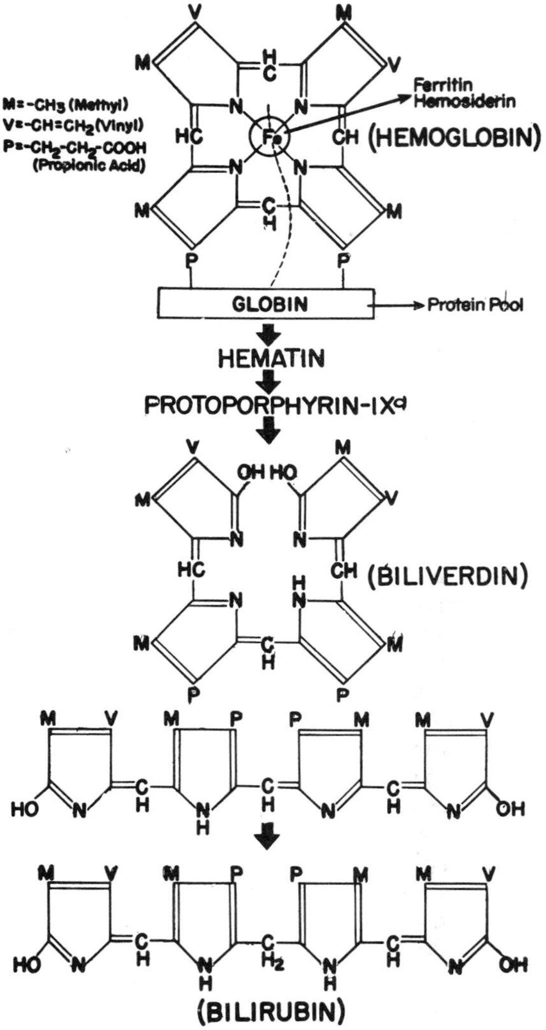

FIG. 1. Bile pigment metabolism.

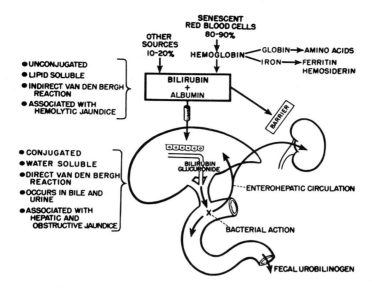

FIG. 2. Direct and indirect van den Bergh reaction.

molecule is oxidized to the ferric form and stored as ferritin or hemosiderin; and the heme ring opens at the α-methane bridge with the loss of a carbon atom as carbon monoxide to form a linear tetraypyrrole. The reaction requires iron to be present and is catalyzed by a microsomal membrane-bound heme oxygenase found in liver, brain, spleen, and lung.

Biliverdin reductase is present in liver and kidney in excess; the presence of heme oxygenase and biliverdin reductase in phagocytic cells accounts for the demonstrable conversion of heme to bilirubin after trauma.[1]

Unconjugated bilirubin is a lipoid-soluble nonpolar pigment that gives an indirect van den Bergh reaction (Fig. 2). It is released from the reticuloendothelial system primarily in the liver, spleen, and bone marrow, but also in other sites throughout the body and is transported in the plasma attached to albumin, for which it has an extremely high affinity. A negligible amount of unbound bilirubin is also carried by the blood. Other factors, such as plasma pH, organic anions which compete for albumin, and physiochemical factors, may influence bilirubin transport. The bilirubin-albumin complex enters the sinusoidal circulation of the liver from either the portal vein or the hepatic artery, where the intricate process of changing nonwater-soluble nonpolar unconjugated bilirubin into water-soluble polar conjugated bilirubin begins at the plasma membrane of the liver cell. Carrier mechanisms at this site have been postulated but have not been demonstrated.

Within the cell, bilirubin is bound and stored by two basic acceptor proteins, Y and Z. The concentration of Y and Z in the cytoplasm may determine the rate of transfer across the hepatic cell membrane as well as the amount and rate of reflux.[2]

It is now recognized that the conjugation of bilirubin is a complex process involving a variety of monosaccharides and disaccharides. Many investigators consider conjugation with glucuronide the most important of these, although the recent work of Kuenzle and others suggests that the major bilirubin conjugates are not excreted as glucuronides but as ester glycosides of uronic acid-containing disaccharides: 3-aldobiouronic acids, 1-hexuronosylhexuronic acid, and 1-pseudo-aldobiuronic acid.[3]

When liver function is impaired, conjugation may take place in the kidney, small intestine, and other tissues. Other hydro-

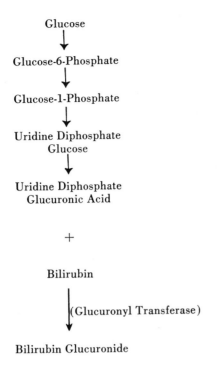

FIG. 3.   Derivation of bilirubin glucuronide.

philic groups, such as sulfates, methyl, acetyl, and glycine, may also be used as conjugates but are of limited functional use, if any, since in glucuronyl transferase deficiency no increase in nonglucuronide conjugates has been found.[1]

Bilirubin glucuronide is excreted either as a monoglucuronide with a 1:1 ratio or a diglucuronide in which 2 moles of glucuronic acid are attached to 1 mole of bilirubin by an ester linkage. The steps by which glucuronide is derived from glucose or glycogen are summarized in Figure 3.

The steps in the intracellular transport system, which are partly established and partly conjectured, are shown in Figure 4.

After bilirubin leaves the cell, it enters biliary channels of increasing caliber until it reaches the intestine, where bacteria, primarily in the distal half of the ileum, reduce it to urobilinogen. Urobilinogen is the name given to an entire group of colorless chromogens some of which are further converted to stercobilin, which gives a characteristic brown color to the feces, and urobilin. It is absent after external biliary drainage, after

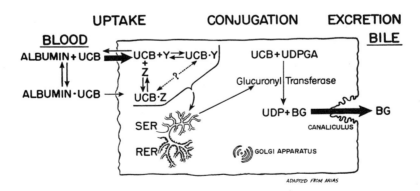

UCB = Unconjugated bilirubin
SER = Smooth endoplasmic reticulum
RER = Rough endoplasmic reticulum

UDP = Uridine diphosphate
UDPGA = Uridine diphosphate glucuronic acid
BG = Bilirubin glucuronide

FIG. 4.   Unconjugated bilirubin is separated from albumin at the plasma membrane and enters the cell where it is bound to acceptor proteins, Y and Z, and stored. There is some bidirectional flux across the membrane. Within the cell, it is subsequently conjugated with glucuronic acid in a reaction involving glucuronyl transferase from the smooth membrane portion of the endoplasmic reticulum and then transferred against a concentration gradient into the bile canaliculus by a presumed energy-dependent system in which the endoplasmic reticulum and Golgi apparatus may function.

therapy with broad-spectrum antibiotics, and in germ-free animals. About 10 to 20 percent is absorbed from the terminal ileum and colon and then reexcreted by the liver and kidney. The major portion is lost directly in feces.

In the liver, urobilinogen is excreted in bile directly without the need for reconjugation.[4]

Urine urobilinogen concentration is a function of multiple variables:

1. Bilirubin formation and output
2. Intestinal absorption
   Decreased with diarrhea
   Decreased to absent after broad-spectrum antibiotics
3. Hydration of the patient
   Renal function
   Urine pH
   Increased in alkaline urine

Urine urobilinogen should be measured under standard conditions of hydration and controlled pH. If collected between 12 noon and 4:00 P.M., blood levels may be high and the urine alkaline.[5] The range of daily excretion by the kidney in the normal adult is 0 to 4 mg; for fecal urobilinogen, the range is 40 to 280 mg. The absence of urobilinogen from the urine and feces indicates complete obstruction. Some of the bilirubin glucuronide is hydrolyzed in the intestine to bilirubin and returned to the liver by way of the portal circulation. Here, after reconjugation, it may be excreted in the bile or may pass into the general circulation to be excreted in the urine.

JAUNDICE

Several conditions may simulate mild jaundice.

Hypercarotenemia. This is the most common. The body areas for which this pigment shows an affinity are the palms of the hands, soles of the feet, and the pilosebaceous areas of the face, in contrast to the affinity for elastic tissue, primarily the mucous membranes and bulbar conjunctiva seen in patients with hyperbilirubinemia. The nor-

mal serum carotene, 40 to 300 μg per milliliter, is increased. Usually the patient has a history of eating large amounts of heavily pigmented vegetables, such as carrots, beets, squash, spinach, and the like. The condition also occurs in some patients with myxedema and panhypopituitarism when the ability to metabolize carotene is impaired.

Lycopenemia. This produces a skin discoloration more deeply orange than that seen in "pure" carotenemia and may be found in patients who consume large quantities of tomatoes.

Other rare forms of yellowish pigmentation may come from drugs, such as atabrine and quinacrine, dyes, such as fluorescein sodium used diagnostically, and some industrial chemicals. Patients with xanthochromia and uremia may also exhibit pigmentation which is usually easily distinguished from jaundice. Discoloration from picric acid, which produces a pigmentation most like jaundice and is found in the same areas of distribution, that is, the elastic tissues, occurs in patients who are malingerers or who are using picric acid ointment. The presence of picrates in the urine distinguishes it from jaundice.

Addison's disease. This may be mistaken either for jaundice or for normal tanning of the skin, which in these patients is unusually persistent. The pigmentation occurs on both exposed and unexposed skin, in the palmar creases, and occasionally as black patches on the buccal mucosa. It may present with such gastrointestinal manifestations as nausea, vomiting, diarrhea, anorexia, and weight loss. The diagnosis is made by noting lack of response to infusions in saline of ACTH, which fail to show a rise in either the 17-hydroxycorticoids or the 17-ketosteroids.

Diagnosis

In attacking the problem of diagnosis, the importance of the history and physical examination should not be minimized in deference to widely publicized liver function tests which continue to grow in number and complexity. The duration of symptoms, age, and enlargement of the liver and spleen were found to be the most useful of 60 indicants in the history and physical examination of 200 jaundiced patients in respect to histological, operative, and autopsy findings. Of surprising lack of significance were a history of contact, nausea, vomiting, pale stools, myalgia, or location of abdominal pain.

The best 5 of 20 laboratory tests were, in order, γ-globulins, prothrombin time, serum aspartate transaminase, α-2 globulins, and bilirubin. Of the three immunoglobulins measured, only IgG was an effective discriminator. In the liver scan, the best differentiators were spleen length and uptake. Liver size was of little value. Diagnoses from scan measurements were correct in 42 percent of these patients; 52 percent of the laboratory tests yielded correct information; and from the clinical features, 60 percent were correct. Using the best features from each group further improved accuracy.[6]

HISTORY

It may be helpful to note that congenital and inflammatory liver diseases are more common in children and young adults. Cirrhosis and neoplastic disease, while more frequent in the older age group, cannot be excluded from consideration in the young. Alcoholic cirrhosis is more frequent in men and is an occupational hazard of bartenders, while cholelithiasis and intrahepatic cholestasis caused by taking steroids are more common in women. Reports of jaundice in patients using steroids for the control of ovulation as well as most of the large series of patients with cholestatic jaundice of pregnancy have come from the Scandinavian countries and Chile. Geographical factors may also suggest the possibility of parasitic infestation or fungal disease. In the Mississippi Valley, histoplasmosis is common.

A history of jaundice occurring in more than one member of a family suggests an hereditary or infectious origin. A history of both jaundice and neurological disease may be the clue to Wilson's disease, while farmers and sewer workers may have leptospirosis (Weil's disease). Brucellosis is more common in farmers and packing house workers. A history of travel or environmental catastro-

phe may give the clue to the diagnosis of hepatitis.

Particular attention should be given to eliciting a history of (1) drug ingestion; (2) parenteral injections, a potential source of infectious hepatitis; (3) transfusions, a source of serum hepatitis; (4) abdominal or thoracic surgical procedures, as well as the type of anesthesia, for example, halothane; (5) exposure to toxic volatile solvents used in various manufacturing processes, such as synthetic textiles and plastics, and exposure to cleaning fluids, paints, and explosives; (6) the amount, frequency, and nature of the alcoholic intake; and (7) the nature of the patient's hobbies, which may involve exposure to hepatotoxins, for example, airplane glue.

The symptoms of liver dysfunction—anorexia, asthenia, malaise, and depression as well as weight loss, pain, and jaundice—may occur in the prodromal, acute, or chronic stage of the disease. Patients with viral hepatitis frequently feel better after the appearance of jaundice and experience relief from anorexia and malaise. Nausea and vomiting, if severe, are usually associated with extrahepatic obstruction; in milder forms they may occur with parenchymal damage to the liver. Right upper quadrant abdominal pain, which is dull or dragging in nature, is associated with hepatitis and cirrhosis. When it is colicky, with radiation to the right scapula, tip of the shoulder, or right periauricular area, it suggests extrahepatic biliary obstruction. Epigastric pain radiating through to the back occurs with posterior penetrating ulcer, pancreatitis, and carcinoma of the pancreas.

Weight loss may be obscured by the accumulation of ascitic fluid. A history of an increase in abdominal circumference may help to clarify this.

Pruritus occurs more often in obstructive jaundice and almost never in hemolytic jaundice.

Fever suggests hepatitis, cirrhosis, or neoplastic disease. When fever is accompanied by chills, cholangitis or liver abscess should be suspected. A history of dyspnea—either on exertion or at rest—distended neck veins, and edema of the extremities suggest congestive heart failure as a factor in the diagnosis.

HEREDITARY HYPERBILIRUBINEMIA

Several syndromes of hereditary or familial nonhemolytic jaundice are of considerable interest. In Gilbert's disease and the Crigler-Najjar syndrome, the bilirubin is unconjugated. In the Dubin-Johnson and Rotor syndromes, the bilirubin is conjugated.

Gilbert's disease. This was first described early in the twentieth century, and is the most common form of chronic unconjugated hyperbilirubinemia not associated with overt signs of hemolysis, although it may represent compensated hemolytic processes.

In some patients it may be associated with a wide variety of acquired diseases; in others, none. Serum bilirubin values are usually less than 5 mg per 100 ml. Frequently, jaundice is present from infancy or early childhood, but occasionally it is not recognized until the third or fourth decade.

In the differential diagnosis of this condition, cholecystitis, pancreatitis, hemolytic anemia, and the recovery phase of viral and other forms of hepatitis should be considered.

The consensus of opinion is that this disorder results from genetically determined factors in the production, transport, and excretion of bilirubin. The recognition of this common benign entity is of prime importance so that treatment other than reassurance may strictly be avoided.[1]

Crigler-Najjar syndrome. There are two types which are phenotypically homogeneous but genotypically heterogeneous. In type 1, the bilirubin concentration may rise to 20 to 30 mg per 100 ml, and the occurrence of kernicterus is frequent, with residual spasticity and mental deficiency. The bile is colorless and contains only traces of unconjugated bilirubin. The conjugation defect is transmitted as an autosomal recessive. Phenobarbital is ineffective as treatment.

In type 2, the bilirubin values are less than in type 1 (9.1 to 17 mg per 100 ml). Kernicterus does not occur. In the bile, pigments and bilirubin glucuronide are present in small amounts. The conjugation defect is an autosomal dominant.

Striking improvement in the jaundice within 2 to 3 weeks follows treatment with phenobarbital in doses of 30 to 120 mg a day. It is thought that all patients with long-standing unconjugated hyperbilirubinemia who respond well to phenobarbital probably have type 2 of this disease.

It might be mentioned here that phenobarbital given in doses of 150 to 200 mg a day for 2 weeks had no effect on lowering the bilirubin levels in extrahepatic obstruction. Since there is a significant decrease in patients with Dubin-Johnson syndrome, primary biliary cirrhosis, and drug jaundice, this finding may be of help in differentiating extrahepatic from the intrahepatic diseases previously mentioned.[7]

Phenobarbital is known to increase hepatic glucuronyl transferase activity, increase thyroxine-binding by liver protein, and increase the synthesis of Y (the predominant acceptor protein in the liver cell) but not Z. It may also increase formation of achromatic biliary metabolites.

Lucey-Driscoll syndrome. This syndrome is characterized by transient familial unconjugated neonatal hyperbilirubinemia with a severe risk of kernicterus. In this disorder, an unidentified factor, presumably a steroid, which inhibits glucuronyl transferase activity in vitro, is found in the mother's serum in the last trimester of pregnancy. It increases as term approaches and disappears rapidly after delivery from both maternal and infant serum.[1]

Familial benign unconjugated hyperbilirubinemia may occur in infants whose mothers excrete pregnane-3α, 20β-diol in their milk and urine during lactation. Severe jaundice usually appears from the seventh to the tenth day and may reach levels of 15 to 25 mg per 100 ml. No signs or symptoms of kernicterus have been reported. The clinical course of the jaundice may be ameliorated by substituting cow's milk for breast milk on alternate days.[8]

Dubin-Johnson syndrome. In this, the "black liver disease," increased amounts of lipofuscin-like pigment are found in the centrilobular parenchymal cells. The jaundice is characterized by elevation of direct, water-soluble bilirubin so that bile may appear in the urine. Although the disease apparently represents an inborn error of metabolism, it may not appear until adult life, with exacerbations and remissions. The defect is a failure in the secretory apparatus for organic anions. In this syndrome, urinary coproporphyrin I, an excretory product without known function, is greatly increased. Urinary coproporphyrin III, an intermediate in the formation of heme, is decreased by 83 percent with no difference in the total urinary coproporphyrins. An amount greater than 80 percent of urinary coproporphyrin I indicates Dubin-Johnson syndrome.[9]

Rotor syndrome.   This is a variant of the Dubin-Johnson syndrome. It differs chiefly in the fact that no pigment is found in the liver.

It has been suggested that the physiological jaundice of the premature and the newborn infant is due to immaturity of the glucuronyl transferase activity. This enzyme system is not completely developed even in the term infant until about the tenth postnatal day. Fluctuation in the serum bilirubin in individual cases may reflect variations either in enzymatic activity or in the load presented to a defective enzyme system. Furthermore, the enzyme system may be damaged by various toxins, viruses, or bacteria so that impairment of bilirubin conjugation may be the result of multiple factors rather than solely a congenital defect. Recent work has raised the question of the importance of the acceptor mechanisms Y and Z, among others.[10]

PHYSICAL EXAMINATION

The physical examination for jaundice should be carried out in daylight (but not in direct sunlight) whenever possible. Artificial light, yellow walls, drapes, and bedclothes may obscure the early manifestations of jaundice. By careful observation, jaundice may be detected in the bulbar conjunctivae when the bilirubin level is 2 mg per 100 ml. When the level reaches 6 mg per 100 ml or more, jaundice becomes readily noticeable in the skin and mucous membranes. The color of the icterus may suggest its etiology: the obstructive type is charac-

teristically dark green while the hepatocellular type is orange or yellow.

A large, hard, nodular liver is almost certainly indicative of carcinoma; conversely, if the liver is not palpable, the possibility that carcinoma obstructs the biliary outflow is remote. A palpable gallbladder associated with long-standing jaundice also suggests carcinoma (Courvoisier's law), although this sign is considerably less helpful in practice than in theory.

Nodes in the supraclavicular or infraclavicular area are indicative of carcinoma until proved otherwise. Nodes elsewhere in the body may indicate metastatic nodules, Hodgkin's disease, or inflammatory lesions such as infectious mononucleosis.

Spider angiomas occur in many patients with cirrhosis, in some pregnant patients, and in others without known cause. They are most frequently observed above the diaphragm, especially on the anterosuperior aspect of the thorax, and on the neck, face, and upper arms. An obvious venous pattern on the abdominal or chest wall and an enlarged spleen are most common in patients with cirrhosis of the liver but are also found in obstruction to the portal circulation. The same is true of the presence of ascites. In the male, feminizing characteristics such as soft skin, loss of male hair distribution, and gynecomastia are common in advanced liver disease because of the inability of the liver to catabolize estrogens. It is important to determine the size, consistency, and degree of tenderness of the liver. Long-standing biliary obstruction, acute inflammation, and fatty infiltration give rise to hepatomegaly. In fibrotic liver disease, the liver may be small or only slightly enlarged but it is usually hard, as it is in neoplastic disease. An acutely tender liver indicates either inflammation or stretching of the capsule. The spleen is usually palpable in patients with hemolytic anemia and portal hypertension but rarely in those with obstructive jaundice unless the condition is of long duration.

Dupuytren's contracture is found occasionally in patients with alcoholic cirrhosis. Palmar erythema may also be found in this condition but, like Dupuytren's contracture, it is seen in many other diseases and is of little help in diagnosis.

One of the simplest and most useful examinations of the jaundiced patient is the daily visual examination of the stool. The acholic stool, characteristic of obstructive jaundice, may be recognized easily by its gray appearance, which is due to an increased fat content and a decreased or absent bile pigment. It is readily differentiated from the light stool seen in children and ulcer patients who ingest large amounts of milk, but it is somewhat more difficult to differentiate from the barium stool if barium studies have been carried out within a day or two before the stools are collected. If stools are difficult to obtain, a gloved finger specimen will usually reveal the desired information.

The dark urine of obstructive jaundice must occasionally be differentiated from hemoglobinuria and porphyrinuria as well as from normally concentrated urine. Bile pigments in the urine in significant amounts are most easily demonstrated by the foam test. This is positive when there is a yellow tint to the foam that appears after urine is vigorously shaken. The test is positive in patients with hepatic and obstructive jaundice but negative in patients with hemolytic jaundice.

ROUTINE LABORATORY EXAMINATIONS

Much helpful information may be gathered from simple laboratory studies of the blood and urine. Although anemia may be present in any one of the three categories of jaundice under discussion, the absence of bile pigments in the urine will suggest a prehepatic jaundice just as the absence of urobilinogen will denote obstructive jaundice. If glucose is present in the urine, a pancreatic lesion must be considered. Leucine and tyrosine crystals in the urine suggest hepatic necrosis. A smear of the peripheral blood and the blood indices will identify 20 to 25 percent of the forms of macrocytic anemia as well as other forms of anemia associated with increased fragility, such as hereditary spherocytosis, sickling, and so forth.

OSMOTIC FRAGILITY TEST. In most cases of hereditary spherocytosis, the erythrocytes hemolyze in concentrations of saline solution in which normal erythrocytes do not. Although increased osmotic fragility may be found in the acute phase of acquired spherocytosis, this is not a common finding.

MECHANICAL FRAGILITY TEST. Increased mechanical fragility occurs with congenital hemolytic anemia, sickle cell anemia, and in some cases of atypical hemolytic anemia in which normal or decreased osmotic fragility is present.

COOMBS' TEST. Neither the direct nor the indirect Coombs' test is positive in hereditary spherocytosis unless it is associated with transient episodes of acquired hemolytic anemia. In the acquired type, both the direct and indirect tests are positive when circulating antibodies are present. When they are not, only the direct Coombs' test is positive.

Liver Function Tests

The general purpose of liver function tests is to establish the presence, type, and severity of liver disease as an aid to prognosis and management. Most of these fall into three categories which evaluate the excretory, metabolic, and enzymatic functions of the liver. The excretory function may be estimated by measuring the bile pigments or substances such as bromsulphalein (BSP), rose bengal, and indocyanine green. The BSP test, one of the most useful in nonicteric patients, is of little value when the serum bilirubin is 2 mg per 100 ml or more, except in patients with the Dubin-Johnson syndrome. In this abnormality, there is characteristic regurgitation of the BSP back into the circulation beginning 60 minutes after the dye is given. The 45-minute value is usually normal or only slightly elevated, but at 60, 90, and 120 minutes the values may be markedly increased.

When the standard dose of 5 mg per kilogram of body weight is infused slowly into the venous circulation, less than 6 percent should be retained in 45 minutes. Such factors as increased age, cachexia, fever, pregnancy, and obesity may account for higher values in patients without liver disease. The failure to get the entire dose into the vein may give a false normal value or a low value, as well as a severe local reaction. Rose bengal is now used primarily as the isotope ^{131}I rose bengal. It is removed, unlike BSP, exclusively by the liver cells and excreted into the bile without reabsorption. The maximum hepatic uptake occurs in 20 minutes and gastrointestinal tract activity begins at 25 minutes. Its ^{131}I energy of 364 kev (kilo electron volts) is readily detected by scintiscanning and somewhat less efficiently detected by the standard gamma camera.

The disadvantages include biliary excretion into the small intestine, which may add confusing background activity, but which is of paramount importance in excluding the diagnosis of obstructive biliary disease. When prolonged intrahepatic retention is present, renal excretion may be mistaken for gastrointestinal activity, and the diagnosis of biliary obstruction may be missed.[11]

The use of indocyanine green has recently enjoyed a renaissance utilizing the dichromatic ear densitometer. Like rose bengal, this dye has no extrahepatic excretion, and there have been no serious side-effects when the usual dose of 5.0 mg per kilogram of body weight is used. From 22 to 25 percent per minute is the maximum removal capacity of the dye which permits detection of minimal alterations in liver function and, as a follow-up procedure, gives accurate information of repair of liver damage.[12] Although this test has had extensive use in following the progress of alcoholic cirrhosis, it would seem to be of value in other diagnostic problems because of its ease of administration and lack of serious side-effects.

BILIRUBIN.   Frequent bilirubin determinations should include estimates of the total bilirubin and the one-minute direct (conjugated water-soluble) fraction. The upper limit of normal for total bilirubin is 1.5 mg per 100 ml; for the one-minute direct fraction, 0.3 mg per 100 ml.

If the total bilirubin is elevated and the one-minute fraction is 0.3 mg or less, the diagnosis lies between hemolytic jaundice and decreased liver function as seen in cardiac decompensation and in the convalescent stage of infectious hepatitis. If the direct fraction is increased and the total bilirubin is normal or only slightly elevated, common duct stone, cirrhosis, and carcinoma should be considered.

METABOLIC FACTORS.   Of the several tests that provide some information about the metabolic activities of the liver, the oldest and perhaps most useful is the determination of the *total protein* and the *albumin-globulin ratio*. In uncomplicated prehepatic and posthepatic jaundice, these values show little, if any, abnormality. In hepatocellular jaundice, the most common finding is reversal of the albumin-globulin ratio. A serum albumin below 3 mg per 100 ml should be considered a contraindication to surgical intervention until corrected. Elevation of total serum globulin levels occurs in most forms of intrahepatic disease. The significance of the changes in the various fractions will be discussed separately.

The *serum mucoprotein* is uniformly elevated in posthepatic jaundice and depressed in acute liver cell damage.

The *serum monamine oxidase* [13] (MAO) level is elevated in liver disease only when hepatic fibrosis is present. and is not related to abnormalities of other liver enzymes. MAO may be a valuable early clue to the development of cirrhosis.

Although *flocculation tests* have largely been replaced by fractionation of the globulin moiety, at the present time it seems to provide little more diagnostic precision.

The flocculation tests were based on the observation that sera from patients with hepatic disease react with various substances to produce turbidity or precipitation. The most commonly used test, the *cephalin flocculation,* was not always reliable because of the instability of commercial antigens and the fact that it was positive in other diseases, for example, collagen disease and subacute bacterial endocarditis.

The test depended upon a colloidal balance between stabilizing factors in the albumin and α-globulin fractions, and precipitants in the γ-globulin fraction. A positive test associated with a prompt direct-reacting bilirubinemia indicated but was not specific for parenchymal necrosis. The test was of less diagnostic value than the transaminase determinations, but was occasionally useful in differentiating acute from chronic hepatitis, and in selecting patients for whom anti-inflammatory rather than surgical therapy was indicated.

In acute viral hepatitis, the flocculation tests were positive in 80 to 90 percent of cases; in obstructive jaundice in the absence of cholangitis, these tests were positive in only 25 percent. If the serum glutamic oxaloacetic transaminase (SGOT) is less than 400 units, flocculation tests can help to provide a diagnosis of hepatitis. Flocculation tests are usually negative in recurrent cholestatic jaundice of pregnancy, hyperemesis gravidarum, and congenital hyperbilirubinemia.

The *zinc sulfate turbidity* is a highly accurate measurement of γ-globulin and has the added advantage of being inexpensive. The *thymol turbidity* measures the lipoprotein fraction chiefly associated with β-globulin. This fraction is increased in infectious hepatitis and in subacute and chronic liver atrophy, but not in nutritional cirrhosis.

Fibrinogen and prothrombin are generally conceded to be formed solely in the liver so that abnormal values in these substances indicate hepatic dysfunction. An increase in the prothrombin time may arise from several causes: (1) liver damage which decreases the synthesis of various activation factors; (2) diminished absorption of vitamin K because of decreased bile salts in the intestinal lumen; (3) the prolonged use of parenteral feeding; (4) sterilization of the gut; and (5) use of anticoagulants. Except in patients with severe parenchymal disease, parenteral administration of vitamin K quickly returns the prothrombin time to normal.

The prothrombin time is also of considerable value in prognosis. If it is less than 40 percent of the normal control, and persists in spite of adequate parenteral doses of vitamin K, the prothrombin time is one of the most accurate indices of fulminating necrosis in patients with viral, toxic, or drug-induced hepatitis.

Although *cholesterol* is synthesized by organs other than the liver, the liver appears to be the site of much of its synthesis, esterification, degradation, and excretion. With obstruction, the cholesterol level rises; with hepatocellular disease, it falls; and in severe liver damage, the esters may almost disappear. Normal plasma cholesterol varies from 130 to 250 mg per 100 ml; the normal cholesterol esters vary from 66 to 78 percent of the cholesterol value.

SERUM ENZYMES. Although *alkaline phosphatase* is not elaborated in the liver in ap-

preciable quantities, it is excreted in the bile and is a sensitive indication of biliary obstruction. High serum levels are observed in complete obstruction either from extrahepatic causes or in patients suffering from cholangitic or chlorpromazine hepatitis. Elevation of the serum alkaline phosphatase in the presence of normal serum bilirubin is a common finding in infiltrative diseases such as sarcoid, tuberculosis, Hodgkin's disease, metastatic carcinoma, as well as metabolic bone disease. When the serum alkaline phosphatase is combined with measurement of serum leucine aminopeptidase (LAP) or 5'-nucleotidase, a more accurate evaluation of the liver alkaline phosphatase is possible, since neither LAP nor 5'-nucleotidase derives from bone. It should be pointed out that the sensitivity of each of these three tests is not always uniform, so that a lack of increase in LAP or nucleotidase combined with a slight elevation of alkaline phosphatase may not exclude hepatic disease. In pregnancy, the alkaline phosphatase, which is derived from the placenta, is heat-resistant, while that derived from bone shows marked heat sensitivity. The phosphatase derived from liver lies somewhere between the two.

After a review of 271 papers or titles dealing with the *transaminases* as liver function tests, Clermont and Chalmers [14] found that transaminase determinations were the most valuable of any of the 36 enzymes studied. When SGOT was related to serum alkaline phosphatase, the distinction between hepatocellular and obstructive jaundice could be determined with considerable accuracy. The lower values were found in obstructive jaundice, and the higher, especially those in the 400 to 500 range or above, were found in hepatocellular involvement.

Although an inverse ratio between increased SGOT and serum bilirubin has been suggested as a criterion for hepatitis, the finding is not sufficiently constant to be of diagnostic value.

Comparing the SGOT and alkaline phosphatase within a certain range of values is more helpful; for example, when the SGOT is 250 units or lower and the alkaline phosphatase less than 25 King-Armstrong units, no differentiation between hepatocellular and obstructive jaundice is possible. In a series of 28 patients, however, when the alkaline phosphatase was below 25 and the SGOT above 250 units, 26 had hepatitis and 2 were obstructed. When the SGOT was below 250 units and the alkaline phosphatase above 25 units, 29 of 32 patients had biliary obstruction.

In infectious hepatitis, the transaminases are usually elevated before the appearance of jaundice, an important finding in the early diagnosis of anicteric or preicteric viral hepatitis, when the patient may not show signs of illness, but the danger of infection is present nonetheless. It is also useful in assessing a relapse during convalescence and in the early diagnosis of parenchymal drug toxicity.

It is useful to remember that the very high transaminase values found in early viral hepatitis often fall to less than 300 units in $1\frac{1}{2}$ to 3 weeks after the onset of jaundice.

In alcoholic hepatitis the SGOT is low in contrast to the high values found in acute cellular injury following viral or toxic invasion. This finding may result from one or both of two factors: First, because alcoholic hepatitis is accompanied by malnutrition, pyridoxine deficiencies may be present. The serum amino transferase is dependent on the coenzyme, pyridoxal phosphate. Second, the necrosis and malnutrition are chronic processes so that the steep rise seen in acute conditions is absent.[15]

LIVER BIOPSY. Results of needle biopsies are enthusiastically reported by numerous investigators, especially when preceded by liver scans which greatly increase the percentage of meaningful biopsy specimens. There are, however, two objections to the procedure. First, it is not without the danger of bile peritonitis and hemorrhage, which is occasionally fatal. Second, if the biopsy specimen is normal, it does not necessarily exclude disease nor do positive biopsy specimens always give a complete picture.

Liver biopsies should be avoided in patients in whom any abnormality of the clotting mechanism exists, in those with ascites, infections of the right lung or pleura (when the intercostal approach is used), when compatible blood in emergency amounts is not immediately available, or in patients who are unable to cooperate intelligently with the examining physician.

Roentgenological and Other Tests

A flat plate of the abdomen may reveal biliary or pancreatic calculi, calcified nodes, or soft tissue masses. The cholecystogram tests the ability of the liver cells to excrete dye, shows the patency of the biliary tree, and may demonstrate disease in the gallbladder, cystic duct, or both. If biliary structures cannot be visualized after oral cholecystography, either or both of two additional procedures may be useful before resorting to intravenous cholangiography. In the first, a double dose of the dye is given; in the second, iopanoic acid (Telepaque), 1 gm is given 3 times a day for 4 days before films of the gallbladder are made. In the latter procedure, stones have been visualized in more than 75 percent of the patients with cholelithiasis.

If these examinations fail to permit visualization of the gallbladder, intravenous cholangiography should be carried out. In patients with a history of allergy, administration of an antihistamine, such as promethazine hydrochloride (Phenergan), 25 mg intramuscularly or intravenously before the cautious administration of the dye, will permit the use of the test. No fatalities have occurred in approximately 10,000 patients studied at the Lahey Clinic Foundation, and reactions have been held to approximately 4 percent by strict adherence to a slow injection rate, the use of antihistamines, and hydration.[16]

A barium-meal examination may show evidence of displacement or compression of the upper gastrointestinal tract from extrinsic masses. A widened duodenal loop occurs routinely with obesity. If *any* of the borders is irregular, not only the medial one, carcinoma of the head of the pancreas should strongly be suspected. In patients with obstruction to the common duct from stones, from fibrosis with narrowing from previous surgery, carcinoma of the head of the pancreas, or from enlarged periampullary nodes, the dilatation proximal to the area of obstruction may be visualized occasionally as a cordlike structure. It may appear on the lateral border of the duodenal bulb or lie between the bulb and the descending limb of the duodenum. Enlargement and irregularity of the ampulla of Vater may be noted when carcinoma invades this structure. When this is present, stiffening and irregularity of the duodenal borders may result as well. Cineradiography may increase the accuracy of diagnosis of lesions in the ampullary area by as much as 82 percent.[17]

A barium-enema examination may reveal displacement of the colon from above downward when the liver, spleen, or pancreas is enlarged. There may also be displacement, irregularities, or filling defects in other areas from by retroperitoneal or pelvic tumors.

RADIOISOTOPES. All radioisotope techniques used in the diagnosis of liver disease fall into one of two categories: (1) those which depend upon the excretion of the radioactive substance by the hepatocytes, and (2) those in which the radioactive substances are phagocytosed by the reticuloendothelial cells of the liver. These modalities have their greatest usefulness in detection of tumors, both solid and cystic, cirrhosis, and bile duct obstruction. ^{131}I scintiscanning, in conjunction with the percent of the isotope found in the stool, can differentiate obstructive from nonobstructive jaundice. In obstructive jaundice, less than 5 percent of the dose appears in the stool in 72 hours, and with no evidence of biliary excretion on scanning, the diagnosis of obstruction is usually confirmed. Rare cases of ascending cholangitis or diffuse hepatocellular disease have shown similar findings, however. Severe constipation with poor evacuation may also give misleading values.

Biliary cirrhosis or atresia may give intrahepatic retention of the isotope long enough to cause dissociation of ^{131}I with release of free iodine. This results in high urinary activity and a false diagnostically low fecal activity. Extrahepatic causes of jaundice may show low fecal activity without high urinary activity.

Accuracy of 80 to 90 percent has been reported in the detection of metastatic disease of the liver.

^{198}Au and ^{99m}Tc are both taken up by the Kupffer's cells and may provide more information than ^{131}I, which is taken up solely by the hepatocyte. ^{99m}Tc is taken up by the spleen in larger amounts than ^{198}Au and often provides a satisfactory scan of that organ.

Angiography

This modality has been of especial value in studying patients with portal hypertension in whom portacaval shunts were being considered. With the development of selective catheterization of the celiac axis and hepatic artery, reliable information in the diagnosis of primary hepatomas and metastatic lesions in the liver is obtained by demonstrating increased vascularity as a "tumor stain" or vascular displacement by intrahepatic masses. Selective arteriography and arterial study of the liver before chemotherapy have been useful in evaluating the results of treatment.

In acute alcoholic hepatitis, not only do the common hepatic and intrahepatic arteries show marked dilatation, but the major divisions of the entire celiac axis may be dilated, with marked hypervascularity in the parenchymatous structures of the upper abdomen. Increased filling of the hepatic artery within the liver and of its terminal ramifications may result in "smudging" suggestive of neoplastic disease.[18]

Angiography in the diagnosis of gallbladder disease may be useful in the early diagnosis of malignant tumor, in differentiating between inflammation and tumor, in demonstrating the extent of advanced tumor, and in evaluating operability.[19]

A further use of angiography is in the control of bleeding in the gastrointestinal tract by the infusion of vasopressin. In a series of 48 patients, Baum and Nusbaum found 28 who were actively bleeding from varices; 14 were infused electively at the time of portal systemic shunt surgery; and 6 were infused because of hemorrhage from a previously demonstrated arterial or capillary source. A superior mesenteric artery catheter was placed, and continuous infusion with vasopressin with a signal motor pump begun at the rate of 0.2 pressor units per milliliter per minute. After 10 minutes, the angiogram was repeated and if a satisfactory response had been obtained, the catheter was secured and vasopressin continued for 3 to 14 days. Bleeding was controlled by this method in all but 1 of 28 patients with active variceal hemorrhage.

For portal hypertension, the arterial infusion of vasopressin for 1 hour prior to elective surgery and continuing through the shunt procedure was found to provide significant collapse of the collateral pathways with improved surgical exposure. Dissection was facilitated, blood loss was diminished, and operative time was decreased.[20]

To overlook an unusual site of gastrointestinal bleeding may be to lose a patient. Angiography can be of definitive help in such instances as in the patient reported by Ranninger et al., in whom a ruptured intrahepatic aneurysm was found.[21]

Of the 176 patients with hepatic artery aneurysm reported up to 1970, only one third who reached surgery survived. The aneurysm usually ruptured into the peritoneal cavity or common duct, and occasionally into the gallbladder, stomach, or duodenum. The diagnosis is suggested by the symptoms of pain, hemorrhage, and jaundice, and is confirmed by angiography if time allows. Aggressive surgery is the only method of treatment.[22]

Ultrasonography

This modality has been helpful in differentiating between solid and cystic masses in the liver and has been able to detect approximately 95 percent of liver abscesses greater than 2 cm in diameter. In experienced hands, it is capable of detecting as little as 300 ml of ascitic fluid.[23]

As duodenography and cannulation come into wider use, it is reasonable to assume that attempts will be made to dissolve stones within reach of these instruments, following the lead of successful procedures already performed with ureteral stones.

No controlled studies on the injury to the tissues involved are as yet available, however, and the long-term effects of such procedures must await further study.

Duodenal Intubation

The use of duodenal intubation as a diagnostic tool has largely been abandoned because of the frequently equivocal results. It has the advantage, however, of employing inexpensive and readily available equipment which does not require unusual skill or experience to use. A Rehfuss tube is passed into the stomach through the pylorus and into the second portion of the duodenum. Accurate placement of the tip of the tube is important and should be verified by fluoroscopy. With the tube in place, the duodenal contents are recovered by aspiration. Cholesterol crystals or aggregates of calcium bilirubinate crystals are pathognomonic of gallstones. The flow of bile is stimulated by magnesium sulfate or olive oil introduced through the tube. This may dislodge mucus or small stones and result in clinical improvement, in addition to providing information. Complete absence of bile is most often found in malignant lesions of the extrahepatic biliary tract, although this may also occur with a stone in the common duct, and rarely when there is obstruction from a mucus plug. Bourke and coworkers found in a series of 75 patients that laparotomy was indicated by the tests in 40 and, in fact, would have been justified in 39. The other patient had associated intrahepatic disease. In the remaining 35 patients, laparotomy was considered not to be indicated despite the fact that 13 had gallstones in the common bile duct and 5 had high bile duct carcinomas which were not revealed.[24] Abnormalities in the pancreas, the duodenum, or at the ampulla were more readily detected.

Even with successful cannulation of the pancreatic ducts, tumors in the body and tail of the pancreas are often impossible to detect.[25]

Perineoscopy, which enjoyed a considerable vogue in the 1930s and 1940s as a diagnostic procedure, is again being used to determine the presence and cause of ascites, to observe the abdominal viscera for evidence of bleeding or masses, and most especially to inspect the liver for the presence of metastases or other abnormalities.

Recent studies have shown the abnormal lipoprotein, *LP-X,* to be a sensitive indicator of cholestasis, although it does not distinguish between the extrahepatic and intrahepatic forms. It has been suggested, however, that if LP-X is combined with lecithin-cholesterol acyl transferase (LCAT), such differentiation will be possible. Further confirmation of these hypotheses is eagerly awaited.[26]

Percutaneous transhepatic cholangiography is being used with increasing frequency. Its method and importance will be discussed in Chapter 46.

Immunological Studies

Within recent years, interest in the role of immune processes in liver disease has been increasing. Fractionation of total serum globulin has revealed a number of immune globulins. IgG, IgA, and IgM have been studied extensively, and IgD, IgE, and others less extensively. Although there was hope that certain fractions might be associated with specific liver diseases, for example, IgA with alcoholic hepatitis and IgM with primary biliary cirrhosis, further experience demonstrated that the presence of immune globulins merely indicates liver disease, since the normal liver does not elaborate these substances.

The mesenchymal cell is the presumed site of origin, although a high level of serum immune globulin is not necessarily associated with high levels of immune globulin-containing cells in the liver.

Antinuclear factor, of both the speckled and diffuse varieties, occurs in 30 to 50 percent of patients with active chronic hepatitis as well as primary biliary cirrhosis. In active chronic hepatitis, the antinuclear antibody correlates with the serum γ-globulin.

Despite the logical inference that after viral or nutritional damage, components of the liver cell might become antigenic and evoke an auto-immune reaction, no evidence of an organ-specific antigen has been demonstrated.

Another factor of great promise involved the use of *antimitochondrial (M) antibody (AMA).* The antigen involved, a lipoprotein, is part of the inner membrane of mitochondria, possibly a membrane transport protein. Early studies showed it to be present in approximately 85 percent of patients with primary biliary cirrhosis as compared to less than 1 percent of those with extrahepatic obstruction. Here, at last, it seemed was a pre-cise measurement to distinguish medical from surgical disease. Further experience, however, revealed that if the obstruction had been present for 60 days or longer, the percentage of positive tests increased greatly. When the obstruction was relieved, the test became negative.

Lam and his associates suggested two factors that might be responsible for the difference between the previously published reports (which considered a positive AMA test presumptive evidence that laparotomy was unnecessary) and their own findings. Both had to do with information *not* included in most of the previous reports. First was the length of time the obstruction existed. In acute obstruction, the percent of AMA positive tests was indeed low. The second factor was the age of the antigen. Serum may be stored at minus 20°C for approximately 10 months. When older, activity is diminshed or lost. In one report in which the age of the serum was specified, it was more than 4 years old.[27]

AMA is present in low titer in virus hepatitis and drug-induced jaundice and is absent in pericholangitis and sclerosing cholangitis secondary to chronic ulcerative colitis, and alcoholic hepatitis. The AMA test correlates fairly well with IgM.[28]

The smooth-muscle antibody test (SMA) is neither species-specific nor organ-specific, nor is it an antibody against any known component of the liver cell. It is not an antibody to the Australia antigen and is usually absent, but it may occur in low titer in some patients with Australia-antigen-associated liver disease. It has been reported in approximately 70 percent of patients with active chronic hepatitis and in 50 percent of those with primary biliary cirrhosis.

Serum alpha-feto proteins (AFP) have been detected in patients with primary carcinoma of the liver. This protein is a normal component of the plasma in the fetus from the age of 6 weeks until a few weeks after birth, when it disappears from the circulation. It reappears in high titer in some patients with hepatoma as well as in a small number of embryonal tumors of the ovary and testis in childhood.

Alpert and co-workers have demonstrated AFP in serum by a sensitive detection method in 50 percent of whites, and 75 to 95 percent of nonwhite patients with hepatoma. The positive reactions correlated with larger and more undifferentiated tumors. The production of AFP was more frequent in younger patients and in men, but neither age nor sex difference was statistically significant.[29]

Stillman points out that while positive tests for AFP are rare if hepatoma or hepatoblastoma is absent, false negative tests are common. It is proposed that this is due to the inability of present techniques to detect extremely small concentrations of AFP.[30]

VIRAL HEPATITIS

The discovery of Australia antigen quite by accident in 1968 has resulted in an explosion of research not only in liver disease and virology but in many other fields where important contributions have increased the understanding of viral hepatitis and provided stimuli to still further investigation.

The Australia antigen is a virus (or a virus-like particle) detectable by its reaction with antibody. Until the recent development of increasingly sensitive and sophisticated methods of detection, it was found in high titer only in the serum of patients who had already received large numbers of transfusions.

Viral hepatitis may be divided into two groups. The first, virus A (IH—infectious hepatitis), has a short incubation period and a low fatality rate, but occurs more frequently than virus B (SH—serum hepatitis). The Australia antigen is found only in the latter group and has not been prevalent in common source epidemics.

About 25 percent of patients with posttransfusion hepatitis are HAA-positive. In chronic active hepatitis, the presence of HAA antigen is extremely variable.

The ability to detect antibody (anti-HAA) in patients who have been exposed to HAA-positive hepatitis has been greatly improved by the use of radioimmuno-assay (RIA), radioimmunoprecipitation (RIP), and passive hemagglutination, which calls for reinterpretation of early statistics.

Lander et al. found anti-HAA in 20 percent of 324 serum samples of a human population in Washington, D.C. There was no sex difference, but the HAA-positive samples were greater as the age of the patients increased. It was only 6 percent in those under 20 years of age and 31 percent in those over 20 with the highest percent (39) in patients between the ages of 40 and 49. The differences noted between the age groups may reflect differences in the immunological response of children and adults. Anti-HAA may be either IgG or IgM, but the antibody response to HAA was unlike the typical response to soluble proteins (transient IgM and persistent IgG) and also unlike the response to the bacterial polysaccharides or lipoproteins (predominantly IgM response either transient or persistent).[31]

DISSEMINATION

The means of dissemination of hepatitis are varied. Originally it was believed that the most important, if not the only, means of spread was by transfusion of Australia antigen-positive blood or by contaminated needles.

More recently Prince et al. has postulated that oral transmission may account for the majority of instances of adult hepatitis.[32]

Garibaldi et al. reported an outbreak of hepatitis in nine members of a group caring for a renal hemodialysis patient. The patient had received 58 units of blood and was found to be HAA-positive before he hemorrhaged at home. Five of the nine attendants involved in the emergency became ill 60 to 95 days later. Three of these were HAA-positive. All were presumed in good health before the incident, with no history of exposure to patients with liver disease. None had cuts or abrasions of the skin, although all came in some contact with the patient's blood directly or on clothing, walls, or furniture.[33]

The possibility that HAA may pass the placental barrier has been the subject of intensive study. Schweitzer et al., in a series of 56 mothers who had acute viral hepatitis during pregnancy or within 6 months of delivery, found 26 who were HAA-positive in the acute illness; ten of their babies were HAA-positive. In 19 babies whose cord blood was tested, 2 were positive. It was postulated that with more sensitive techniques this percentage might have been considerably higher.

None of the 20 HAA-negative mothers had HAA-positive babies. Ten other mothers were not HAA-tested during the period of acute illness; none of their babies was HAA-positive.

Three possible means of transmission are suggested: The antigen may cross the placental barrier in some, but not in all cases; there may be contamination of the baby with maternal blood and feces during the second and third stages of labor; or there may be a transmission from mother to child during the normal care of the newborn.

In none of these patients were the babies breast-fed so that the antigen was not transmitted in the mother's milk.[34]

INCIDENCE

It has been estimated that of the approximately 100,000 cases of hepatitis that occur each year in the United States in which 1,500 to 3,000 succumb, a substantial number is due to HAA-positive blood transfusions. It is further estimated that if all HAA-positive donors could be excluded, 500 to 1,000 lives might be saved each year, and morbidity from liver disease drastically decreased.[35]

This would seem somewhat at variance with Reinicke et al., who screened 13,300 consecutively registered Danish voluntary blood donors, of which only 24 had persistent HAA antigen. In this study, none of the HAA-positive donors had any clinical signs of disease and, although liver biopsy specimens were taken from all 24, in only 1 was cirrhosis demonstrated. None of the remaining 23 showed the changes seen in viral hepatitis, but only 6 had completely normal liver findings. A retrospective study of the recipients of the HAA-positive blood showed no evidence of past or present acute hepatitis. Nor were HAA antigens or antibodies found in any of the surviving recipients. In the retrospective study, which may have dated back at least 3 years from detection of the antigen, it was not known with certainty whether or not the donor had been HAA-positive at the time his recipients received their blood transfusions.[36]

Some work suggests that multiple donations of blood may in some way alter the blood constituents. More work will be re-

quired before the importance of this finding can be evaluated.

There were no marked changes in immunoglobulins or SGOT values in any case.

Chalmers and his group postulate that patients with demonstrable HAA antigen can be divided by the transaminase values into two groups: those with acute or chronic hepatitis, and those with no significant liver disease. Asymptomatic carriers of HAA have normal transaminase levels. When the transaminase is elevated in a small number, the abnormality will be transient (acute hepatitis); in the rest it will be persistent (chronic hepatitis). In the latter group, 10 to 25 percent of the patients with chronic active hepatitis with positive HAA and persistent elevation of the transaminase value should have liver biopsy. If the aggressive form of the disease is present, steroids can be life-saving. In other forms of the disease, they are not only of no use, but may be seriously harmful.[35]

Nielsen et al. made a prospective study of 253 consecutively admitted patients with biopsy-verified acute viral hepatitis and showed Australia antigen in 44 percent (112). In 88 of these, the antigen was transiently detectable from 1 to 13 weeks. It was persistent (greater than 13 weeks) in 4.3 percent. In the latter group, all developed clinical and chemical signs of chronic hepatitis verified by repeated liver biopsies. Chronic aggressive hepatitis developed in eight and chronic persistent hepatitis in two. In this group, it was felt that drug addiction played no major role in the progression from acute to chronic hepatitis.[37]

A chronic carrier state of Australia antigen is found in three types of patients: healthy persons, patients with various chronic disorders (for example, those with Down's syndrome and in patients maintained on hemodialysis), and patients with an initial acute viral hepatitis associated with Australia antigen. Persistent Australia antigen in the general population is estimated to be 3 to 4 percent, in whom a gene-dependent susceptibility or an immune deficiency state may be present.

TREATMENT

Although the value of γ-globulin in preventing infectious hepatitis if given early enough after exposure is well known, it is thought to be totally ineffective in preventing posttransfusion hepatitis. However, since the possibility that the hepatitis may have been incurred by other than parenteral means, even though parenteral sources are strongly suspected, γ-globulin should be given prophylactically if intimate exposure to patients with HAA-positive hepatitis or accidental inoculation with trace amounts of HAA-positive blood has occurred.[35]

Further justification for this opinion comes from the Armed Forces. Of United States soldiers in Korea, 107,803 were given injections ranging from 2 to 10 ml of γ-globulin or a placebo; 65 percent of personnel were given a second injection in 5 to 7 months. It was found that the 5-ml dose gave the best results. The incidence of hepatitis was significantly decreased and passive protection was provided for 6 months in both HAA-positive and HAA-negative hepatitis. There was no significant alteration in the incidence of other commonplace infectious diseases.[38]

In another study of 1,133 military personnel, only 3 were found to be HAA-positive by complement-fixation. Seven more were discovered when RIA was used.

In serum collected from 211 patients with hepatitis during the first week of jaundice, 25 percent were HAA-positive by RIA.

Of 52 patients with HAA-positive hepatitis, five received 5 ml of γ-globulin and six patients received 10 ml. The γ-globulin had a high anti-HAA titer and gave significant protection against the development of symptomatic icteric hepatitis. Lower doses were ineffective.

The conclusion from this study is that the important determinants of the effectiveness of γ-globulin are: (1) the size of the infective dose of virus, (2) the amount of γ-globulin given, and (3) a high titer of antibody. A fourth factor may be the means by which the antigen was transmitted, parenterally or nonparenterally.[39]

The recent findings reported from the National Transfusion Hepatitis study strongly emphasize that intramuscular injections of normal immune serum globulin with only a small amount of hepatitis B antibody are worthless. The use of immune serum globulin with a high titer is being reported, however, with increasing frequency as a possible effective agent in prevention and treatment of Australia antigen-positive hepatitis.[40]

These encouraging reports and the fact that in the fulminant form of the disease treatment with transfusions, steroid therapy, and intensive supportive care resulted in almost 100 percent fatality have tempted clinicians to use high-titer antibody indiscriminately. In the best interest of the patient, this should not be used until carefully controlled studies have established what types of patients are appropriate recipients, what the useful dosages are, and how fresh the antigen should be. This will help to conserve available antigen now in short supply and avoid possible harm such as injury to the liver and other organs by immune complex mechanisms.[41]

Duodenography and Cannulation of the Pancreatic and Biliary Ducts

Two of the most interesting and promising tools for the investigation of pancreatic and biliary disease are the use of duodenography and cannulation of the pancreatic and biliary ducts. In addition to the ability to visualize and biopsy both normal and abnormal tissue, their possible use in connection with ultrasound has already been mentioned. Further discussion of the use of these modalities will be found in Chapters 4C and 34B.

INDICATIONS FOR SURGICAL INTERVENTION

The indications for operation in the jaundiced patient may be summarized as follows:

1. Splenectomy is the treatment of choice for patients whose familial hemolytic anemia gives rise to hemolytic crises. A large percentage of these patients have gallstones for which cholecystectomy is required.

2. Selected cases of acquired hemolytic anemia are benefited by splenectomy,

although the percentage is decidedly smaller than that in the familial group.

3. Surgical intervention is indicated when obstruction results from extrahepatic causes. Exceptions to the rule (unless palliative measures are imperative) have always been thought to be the presence of metastases discovered in palpable nodes (including those in a rectal shelf), through x-ray study, or by finding tumor cells in ascitic fluid.

Although at the present time only 17.9 percent of untreated patients with liver metastases are alive at the end of one year, the survival time increases to 36.6 percent following hepatic artery infusion with 5-fluoro-2'-deoxyuridine (5-FUDR).[42] It is to be hoped that further progress in oncology will increase the survival time even more.

Although intrahepatic cholestasis may occasionally be confused with extrahepatic cholestasis, certain findings will help to distinguish the two (Table 1).

Surgery should not be undertaken until the diagnosis is as clearly established as circumstances permit and the vital functions of the patient are restored to normal insofar as the underlying disease will allow. In obstructive jaundice, there is rarely any necessity for emergency surgery, and usually ample time is available for optimum preoperative treatment. Arbitrarily, this may be taken as anywhere from 3 to 6 weeks, but it varies widely in individual patients. More specifically, the limit of such a period is defined by evidences of progressive parenchymatous damage. Any sharp elevation in the serum bilirubin, drop in the prothrombin level with decreased response to the administration of vitamin K_1, or a rise in the blood urea nitrogen (BUN) is an indication for immediate surgical intervention.

PREOPERATIVE PREPARATION

In the preparation of the jaundiced patient for surgery, the most important problems for consideration are those of deficits in

Table 1. CHOLESTASIS

Findings	Extrahepatic	Intrahepatic
Jaundice as an early symptom	+ +	+
Sudden onset, fever, sweats, chills	+ +	+
Liver size	+ +	±
Right upper quadrant pain	+ +	±
Palpable gallbladder	±	0
Histological findings		
Eosinophils	0	+ +
Dilated ducts	+	±
Percutaneous cholangiographic findings	Dilated ducts and demonstrable block	0
Cannulation of common duct	Dilated ducts and demonstrable block	0
History of exposure to jaundiced patients, raw shellfish, drugs	0	+
Acholic stools with absent urine urobilinogen	+	0—+
Melena	±	0
Leukocytosis	+	0
Alkaline phosphatase	+ +	+
SGOT		
<250 units	+ +	+
>250 units	0—+	0—++
Response to phenobarbital, 150 to 200 mg per day	0	+ +
M antigen		
Early	0	+ +
2 months or more	+	+ +

the various components of the blood, malnutrition, avitaminosis, and deranged fluid and electrolyte balance.

Blood Deficits

If time allows, the blood should be brought to normal values in respect to volume, number of cells, hemoglobin, platelets, and prothrombin. In addition, the amount of blood that may be lost during any surgical procedure should be estimated in advance and supplied *before* the operation in order to avoid transfusion reactions modified or obscured by anesthesia, and because the quantity needed to maintain adequate volume, osmotic pressure, and oxygenation rises steeply with each hour after the time of blood loss. Replacement ensures a smoother operative course, less danger of shock in the postoperative period, and a shorter convalescence. Blood given in the operating room should be limited to the amount imposed by unforeseen contingencies.

Transfusions of whole blood are rarely needed except in patients with acute blood loss. Replacement should be selective: if erythrocytes are needed, transfusions of washed erythrocytes which lessen the risk of reactions and of overexpanding the blood volume should be given; if platelets are low, platelet transfusions are more effective than transfusions of whole blood; if iron is needed, oral or parenteral iron should be given unless surgery cannot be delayed; vitamin B_{12} or folic acid deficiencies should be corrected with the appropriate factors.

In hemolytic anemia, if the blood volume has not been significantly improved after three or four transfusions, splenectomy should be carried out at once so that the general condition does not further deteriorate.

In patients who have lost considerable weight, normal blood findings give a false security. The normal blood volume in an adult bears a relationship to his height and normal weight. A rough method for calculating the patient's needs allows 30 ml of blood for every pound of normal weight or 65 ml for each kilogram. If the patient's actual blood volume is subtracted from his normal blood volume and the amount of blood equal

to the difference given in small daily transfusions before operation, the result in decreased morbidity and mortality rates is well worth the effort and expense involved, especially in the elderly patient in whom the vital functions are maintained in more precarious balance.

Malnutrition

In the preoperative period, the problem of malnutrition is closely linked to the restoration of normal blood constituents and electrolyte balance. It is often impossible to correct the malnutrition completely before its cause is surgically removed. The need for and success of preoperative nutritional measures may be gauged approximately by the absolute amounts of albumin and globulin present per 100 ml of blood. It should be stressed that these values are grossly inaccurate and may be gravely misleading if the patient is dehydrated, as dehydration is one of the common causes of elevation of the serum globulin.

The method of choice in correcting malnutrition is to provide the patient with high-caloric, well-balanced, attractively served meals. For patients with liver damage, experimental work has shown that while carbohydrates are necessary, an abundant supply of sulfur-bearing amino acids is even more important to protect the liver from the effects of surgical intervention and to restore it to health when diseased. In addition, the diet should be high in protein except in impending coma. Only moderate restriction of fat (80 to 85 gm a day) need be imposed. If steatorrhea is a severe problem, the usual dietary fat is decreased empirically, and medium-chain triglycerides (octanoic to decanoic acids) prepared from coconut oil are used to supplement the fat intake. These are hydrolyzed in the absence of pancreatic lipase and absorbed principally by the portal vein in the absence of bile salts. Supplementary vitamins, especially B complex and vitamin C, as well as A and D, should be given either by mouth or by parenteral injection.

Although a diet containing approximately 2,850 calories with 150 gm of protein, 388 gm of carbohydrates, and 85 gm of fat is desirable, the most important consideration is to get the patient to eat, and foods of his own choosing may be of more ultimate value than an imposed regimen. When vigorous measures are required, hyperalimentation may be used. An intracaval infusion of a high-caloric hyperosmolar solution containing approximately 25 percent glucose and 6.8 gm of nitrogen as amino acids and peptides with vitamins and minerals is given at the rate of 1 to 2 liters per day and, if tolerated, cautiously increased to 3 to 4 liters per day.

Great care and constant surveillance of the catheter must be exercised to avoid such serious and even fatal complications as septicemia and Candida fungemia. Other complications include hyperglycemia, which may precipitate diabetic coma, and hepatic decompensation. When there is fluid retention and hepatic coma threatens, the amino acid and sodium content of the infusion must be drastically curtailed.

If the blood glucose concentration becomes greater than 350 mg per 100 ml, the infusion rate should be slowed and signs of a depressed neurological state and dehydration be watched for. This is particularly true in the diabetic patient, who may require additional insulin.

Hepatic decompensation with fluid retention requires drastic curtailment of amino acid and sodium. If there is impairment of renal function, the possibility of fluid overload must be kept constantly in mind.[43]

In addition to dietary management when hyperalimentation is not used, the following measures help to correct major deficiencies: intravenous infusions of 1,000 to 2,000 ml of 10 percent glucose in distilled water with vitamins B and C; intravenous infusions of 25 to 50 gm of albumin daily for 6 to 10 days; parenteral injections of menadiol sodium diphosphate, 20 mg daily for 3 to 5 days, or in more severe prothrombin deficiencies, an emulsion of phytonadione (vitamin K_1) in intravenous doses of 50 mg a day. Broad-spectrum antibiotics such as tetracycline, 250 to 500 mg every 6 hours, are prescribed for cholangitis and infections other than liver disease.

Electrolyte Imbalance

The problem of correcting electrolyte imbalance is primarily that of restoring and maintaining the electrolytic constituents of the intracellular and extracellular components of the body. The chief of these is extracellular sodium and intracellular potassium. The average daily sodium requirement of the normal adult is 5 to 6 gm. Unless abnormal amounts are lost, as in profuse diaphoresis, vomiting, diarrhea, fistulas, or drainage from the gastrointestinal tract—in which case sodium should be replaced measure for measure—administration of sodium should be rigorously restricted to this amount.

In patients with hypochloremia, which is the usual finding in those who have lost or are losing large volumes of fluid from the gastrointestinal tract, an attempt should be made to restore electrolyte balance by increasing the salt intake. If the serum chloride fails to rise despite the administration of adequate amounts of salt solution, the probability of potassium deficiency must be considered. In its early stages, potassium deficiency may be manifested by drowsiness, apathy, weakness, abdominal distention, urinary depression, and constipation or diarrhea. The administration of potassium salts frequently brings about dramatic symptomatic relief and results in elevation of the serum chloride even if infusions of chlorides are stopped during the potassium therapy. In the absence of renal insufficiency, the amount of potassium that may be given orally with safety is limited only by the patient's gastrointestinal tolerance. If parenteral administration is necessary, plasma reaching the heart should not contain more than 7 mEq of potassium per liter. In a solution containing 40 to 80 mEq of potassium per liter (the latter amount given only in severe potassium deficiency), the rate should never exceed 12 ml (180 drops) per minute and preferably is given at about 8 ml (120 drops) per minute. If the solution is not given with careful attention, the threat of cardiac arrest, which is always present, may occur without premonitory signs.

As important as electrolyte balance and closely associated with it is the *fluid balance*. The decisive factor is a urinary output sufficient to prevent elevation of the BUN. The amount of urine required varies with the concentration. Thus, 600 ml a day with a specific gravity of 1.030 will be as efficient as

2,500 to 3,000 ml with a specific gravity of 1.008 or less; 1,000 to 1,500 ml a day with a specific gravity of 1.015 may be considered an average minimum. The injudicious use of "unphysiological saline" especially in the presence of impaired renal function and low protein intake may lead to edema, oliguria, and even anuria.

Sedatives and Analgesics

Although surgical patients are carefully screened to detect allergies, in the jaundiced patient more than ordinary attention should be given to the choice of sedatives. Morphine, the drug most frequently used in the preoperative and postoperative care of surgical patients, should be avoided in those with liver disease. About 90 percent of the detoxification of morphine occurs in the liver, so that if liver function is impaired, the effect of an overdose can result in respiratory depression. Meperidine hydrochloride (Demerol), 50 to 100 mg every 4 hours, may be as effective with less danger of unwanted side-effects. The same is true of codeine sulfate, which frequently provides adequate analgesia in doses of 30 to 60 mg every 3 to 4 hours.

Since 1954, when glutethimide (Doriden) was introduced as a substitute for barbiturates, it has become the sixth most frequently prescribed sedative (after five barbiturates). Although originally it was thought to have all of the advantages of the older drugs with fewer of the side-effects, increasing knowledge has revealed many instances of glutethimide intoxication, several of poisoning, and a few fatalities. It is now regarded as having no advantage over barbiturates.

Methyprylon (Noludar), introduced in 1955, may also be used instead of barbiturates. It has less respiratory depressive effect, but has an equally toxic effect on the cardiovascular system.

Nitrazepam (Mogadon) is useful in patients whose need for sedation is associated with emotional disorders. It has some muscle relaxant and anticonvulsant properties as do the drugs previously mentioned. These drugs should be prescribed initially in small infrequent doses and increased as indicated. A related benzodiazepine compound, flurazepam

hydrochloride (Dalmane), is also useful as a hypnotic and has few reported side-effects.[44]

A case report of cholestatic hepatitis following the use of propoxyphene (Darvon), which is widely used as an analgesic, has recently appeared. Symptoms cleared within 18 hours after discontinuing the drug and reappeared within 24 hours after three 65-mg capsules were administered as a challenge. In the initial instance, all laboratory findings were normal after 3 weeks; after the challenge, they were normal in nine days.[45]

Pruritus

The magnitude of the problem of pruritus is evident when an estimated 10 to 25 percent of all patients with hepatobiliary disease are so afflicted; of these, 60 to 70 percent have partial bile duct obstruction, and half of these (30 to 35 percent) are the result of malignant disease.

Approximately 75 percent of patients with pruritus have a serum bilirubin level of more than 5 mg per 100 ml and a greater concentration of bile acids, primarily deoxycholic, on the skin. The bile acids correlate well with the degree of pruritis; the bilirubin does not.

Anabolic agents may relieve pruritus presumably by acting on the sweat glands to prevent the accumulation of bile salts in the skin similar to their cholestatic action in the liver. It has been postulated that free bile acids may be secreted onto the skin surface by nonionic diffusion or that they may be present there because of deconjugation by skin bacteria.[46]

Although sponging the skin with acetone affords temporary relief, it is not recommended as a general measure.

Cholestyramine, a nonabsorbable anion exchange resin, is the drug of choice in the treatment of pruritus. It increases fecal bile acid excretion and decreases serum bile acid with relief from itching in most, but not all, patients with incomplete biliary obstruction. Relief of itching can occur without decrease in the serum bile acid level, and cholestyramine can sequester factors other than bile acids which may, in turn, be responsible for the pruritus. The prolonged use of cholestyramine in doses of 30 gm a day may give rise to diarrhea and acidosis. The diarrhea is controlled with diphenoxylate (Lomotil), 20 to 30 mg a day; the acidosis is controlled by decreasing the dose of cholestyramine to 6 to 12 gm a day and adding sodium bicarbonate in a like amount.[47]

Occasionally, a diet rich in polyunsaturated fatty acids promotes increased fecal excretion of bile acids with decrease in the serum bile acid level and relief of pruritis. External biliary drainage has also afforded relief from severe itching.

Other measures include intravenous injections of 10 ml of a 10 percent solution of calcium gluconate administered over a 5- to 10-minute period once or twice a day, starch and oatmeal baths, calamine lotion with 0.5 percent phenol, and the use of such antihistamines as promethazine hydrochloride (Phenergan), 25 mg 3 to 4 times a day, or diphenylhydramine hydrochloride (Benedryl), 25 to 50 mg 3 to 4 times a day. Relief of pruritus has been obtained after 4 to 7 days by giving 10 mg of phenobarbital per kilogram of body weight a day in patients with intrahepatic biliary atresia and benign recurrent cholestasis.[48]

Preparations of ergot should not be used in the presence of liver disease.

NONSURGICAL TREATMENT OF JAUNDICE

Chenodeoxycholic acid, alone of the bile acids, increases the secretion of lecithin, which forms the center of the bile acid lecithin micelle and acts as a solvent for cholesterol. Cholesterol stones account for 95 percent of cholelithiasis, which occurs in about 10 percent of the population. Since gallstones may be due to decreased bile acid secretion rather than increased cholesterol secretion, various bile acid preparations have been tried in the hope of increasing bile acid secretion, but only chenodeoxycholic acid has had the desired effect. In a small series, this has resulted in disappearance of small stones and diminution of large ones over periods ranging from 6 to 18 months.

No side-effects except for diarrhea and abdominal cramps were noted.[49] Although it

has no place in acute situations in which surgery can be life-saving, in other circumstances, either in patients with asymptomatic gallstones or in those in whom surgery is contraindicated, this therapy warrants further trial.

Phototherapy for the treatment of unconjugated hyperbilirubinemia in premature and term neonates was first reported by Cremer, Perryman, and Richards in 1958.[50] A flood of enthusiastic reports appeared in the English, French, Italian, and South American literature in the decade following. It was not until 1968, however, that the method began to be used to any extent in the United States.

Because phototherapy is a readily available and relatively simple procedure, its indiscriminate use has led to serious and even fatal results. Since jaundice may be a manifestation of infection—which is difficult to detect early in the neonate—or erythroblastosis, or liver disease, appropriate measures for management may be delayed if phototherapy is used without proper controls.

These should include the following tests: hemoglobin, hematocrit, blood type, Rh factor, Coombs' test, cultures for suspected infection, and in black males and Orientals, glucose-6-phosphate-dehydrogenase deficiency.

A serum bilirubin level of 12 to 15 mg per 100 ml, which has been shown to be rapidly rising, warrants a brief trial of phototherapy (12 to 36 hours). After 6 to 12 hours, it should be discontinued and the response evaluated before it is continued. Frequent hemoglobin, hematocrit, and bilirubin determinations, two to four a day, should be made during therapy, and at weekly or biweekly intervals for 1 to 2 months thereafter in order to detect the possible development of the delayed severe anemia of erythroblastosis fetalis or other side-effects.

Optimum methods of administration, metabolic effects, modes of excretion, and long-term physical and neurological results of this relatively new modality are unknown. Caution is urged in its use.[51]

REFERENCES

1. Fleischner, G., and Arias, I. M., Am. J. Med. 49:576, 1970.

2. Arias, I. M., New Engl. J. Med. 285:1416, 1971.

3. Kuenzle, C. C., Biochem. J. 119:411, 1970.

4. Lester, R., and Troxler, R. F., Gastroenterology 56:143, 1969.

5. Schenker, S., Liver Function Tests. Clinician—2, New York, Medcom, Inc., 1971, p. 12.

6. Knill-Jones, R. P., Maxwell, J. D., Thompson, R. P. H., et al., Digestion 4:158, 1971.

7. Manenti, F., Carulli, N., and Zeneroli, L., Digestion 4:163, 1971.

8. Washburn, T. C., letter to the Editor, J.A.M.A. 219:220, 1972.

9. Wolkoff, A., abstract, program of American Gastroenterological Association 73d Annual Meeting, Dallas, Texas, May 21–27, 1972, pp. A–127.

10. Arias, I. M., Birth Defects 6:55, 1970.

11. Potchen, E. J., and Holzer, M. E., Radionuclide Hepatography. Clinician—2, New York, Medcom, Inc., 1971, p. 88.

12. Leevy, D. M., Alcoholic Liver Diseases. Clinician—2, New York, Medcom, Inc., 1971, p. 40.

13. Kirchner, J. P., and Castell, D. O., abstract, program of American Gastroenterological Association 73d Annual Meeting, Dallas, Texas, May 21–27, 1972, pp. A–58.

14. Clermont, R. J., and Chalmers, T. C., Medicine 46:197, 1967.

15. Gregory, D. H., and Levi, D. F., Am. J. Dig. Dis. 17:479, 1972.

16. Wise, R. E., Personal communication.

17. Adler, D. C., and Meyers, H. I., J.A.M.A. 199:709, 1967.

18. Rourke, J. A., Bosniak, M. A., and Ferris, E. J., Radiology 91:290, 1968.

19. Rösch, J., Grollman, J. H., Jr., and Steckle, R. J., Radiology 92:1485, 1969.

20. Baum, S., and Nusbaum, M., Radiology 98:497, 1971.

21. Ranninger, K., Menguy, R., Kittle, L. F., et al., Radiology 90:507, 1968.

22. Ryan, R. J., letter to the Editor, J.A.M.A. 219:1762, 1972.

23. McCarthy, C. F., Wells, P. N., Ross, F. G., et al., Gut 10:904, 1969.

24. Bourke, J. B., Swann, J. C., Brown, C. L., et al., Lancet 1:605, 1972.

25. Sedgwick, C. E., Personal communication.

26. Seidel, D., letter to the Editor, New Engl. J. Med. 285:1538, 1971.

27. Lam, K. C., Mistilis, S. P., and Perrott, N., New Engl. J. Med. 286:1400, 1972.

28. Sherlock, S., Am. J. Med. 49:693, 1970.

29. Alpert, E., Hershberg, R., Schur, P. H., et al., Gastroenterology 61:137, 1971.

30. Stillman, A., and Zamchek, N., Am. J. Dig. Dis. 15:1003, 1970.

31. Lander, J. J., Holland, P. V., Alter, H. J., et al., J.A.M.A. 220:1079, 1972.

32. Prince, A. M., et al., Quoted by T. Hersh, J. L. Melnick, R. K. Goyal, et al., New Engl. J. Med. 285:1363, 1971.

33. Garibaldi, R. A., Hatch, F. E., Bisno, A. L., et al., J.A.M.A. 220:963, 1972.

34. Schweitzer, I. L., Wing, A., McPeak, C., et al., J.A.M.A. 220:1092, 1972.

35. Chalmers, T. C., and Alter, H. J., New Engl. J. Med. 285:613, 1971.

36. Reinicke, V., Dybkjaer, E., Poulsen, H., et al., New Engl. J. Med. 286:867, 1972.

37. Nielsen, J. O., Dietrichson, O., Elling, P., et al., New Engl. J. Med. 285:1157, 1971.

38. Prophylactic gamma globulin for prevention of endemic hepatitis: A cooperative study. Arch. Intern. Med. 128:723, 1971.

39. Ginsberg, A. L., Conrad, M. E., Bancroft, W. H., et al., New Engl. J. Med. 286:562, 1972.

40. Roche, J. K., and Stengle, J. M., New Engl. J. Med. 287:251, 1972.

41. Gerber, M. A., Brodin, A., Steinberg, D., et al., New Engl. J., Med. 286:14, 1972.

42. Oberfield, R. A., Med. Clin. North Am. 56:665, 1972.

43. Rosenoer, V. M., and Gokim, G., Jr., Med. Clin. North Am. 56:759, 1972.

44. Goodman, L. S., and Gilman, A., eds., The Pharmacological Basis of Therapeutics: A Textbook of Pharmacology, Toxicology, and Therapeutics for Physicians and Medical Students, New York, Macmillan, 1970.

45. Klein, N. C., and Magida, M. G., Am. J. Dig. Dis. 16:467, 1971.

46. Schoenfield, L. F., The Relationship of Bile Acids to Pruritus in Hepatobiliary Disease, in L. Schiff, J. B. Carey, Jr., and J. M. Dietschy, eds., Bile Salt Metabolism, Springfield, Ill., Thomas, 1967, pp. 257–262.

47. Stanley, M. M., Steroid-wasting Enteropathy: Clinical Picture, Bile Salt Absorption and Fecal Excretion, and Therapy, in L. Schiff, J. B. Carey, Jr., and J. M. Dietschy, eds., Bile Salt Metabolism. Springfield, Ill., Thomas, 1967, p. 266.

48. Stiehl, A., Thaler, M., and Admirand, W. H., New Engl. J. Med. 286:858, 1972.

49. Danzinger, R. G., Hofmann, A. F., Schoenfield, L. J., et al., New Engl. J. Med. 286:1, 1972.

50. Cremer, R. J., Perryman, P. W., and Richards, D. H. Lancet 1:1094, 1958.

51. Behrman, R. E., and Hsia, D. Y., Summary of a symposium on phototherapy for hyperbilirubinemia, Birth Defects 6:131, 1970.

46

PERCUTANEOUS TRANSHEPATIC CHOLANGIOGRAPHY

J. GEOFFREY WALKER

Cholangiography performed by percutaneous puncture of intrahepatic bile ducts was first described more than 30 years ago by Huard and Do-Xuan-Hop (1937). It was 15 years later, however, before further successful application of the technique was reported by Carter and Saypol (1952). Numerous larger series of cases studied by this method have subsequently been published and the investigation has become widely accepted in many centres.

The procedure is of great help to the surgeon in elucidating the difficult case of jaundice and in demonstrating the pathological anatomy when biliary obstruction is known to be present. Complications described in earlier studies, chiefly biliary peritonitis and haemorrhage, were often attributable to unwise selection of patients or failure to operate following successful demonstration of a dilated duct system. A major advance, however, was in the use of a flexible catheter introduced by means of a needle after which the latter was removed, thus minimising the chance of subsequent damage to the liver caused by movement. Leger, Zara, and Wargnier (1953) used this technique to study a small number of patients and it was later independently developed by Fernström and Seldinger (1956), Wiechel (1960), Shaldon, Barber, and Young (1962) and Arner, Hagberg, and Seldinger (1962).

TECHNIQUE

Various minor differences in the technique of introducing the cannula and locating a biliary radicle have been described. With the method of Shaldon, Barber, and Young, a polyethylene tube is threaded onto a fine needle and introduced percutaneously into the liver. The needle is at once removed, leaving the polyethylene tubing in situ. This is then attached by way of an adaptor to a syringe. Constant suction is maintained while the tube is gradually withdrawn. Once a duct is entered, bile is aspirated into the tube and syringe. Under screen control, sufficient radiographic contrast material to fill the duct system is then injected, and films are taken.

Preparation of the Patient

The prothrombin time is checked and corrected, if necessary, by administration of vitamin K. The patient is tested for sensitivity to the contrast material. Food and drink are withheld on the morning of the procedure. The patient is premedicated with meperidine (pethidine) 50 to 100 mg and scopolamine 0.4 to 0.6 mg. General anaesthesia is used only in children or unduly nervous patients.

Preparation of Equipment

The tubing used is thin-walled flexible polyethylene of internal diameter 1.5 mm and approximately 20 cm long. A flange is made at one end by rotating the tip over a small flame. Six tubes together with flexible 20-gauge steel needles 15 cm in length and ground with a short-bevel cutting point and three tap adaptors are kept presterilized.

A polyethylene tube is drawn, flange first, over one of the needles. While the tube and needle are held in one hand, the free end is pulled out and stretched so that its calibre

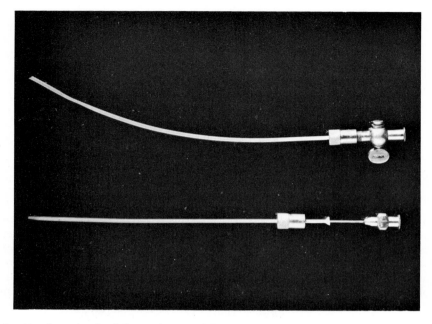

FIG. 1.   Needle and polyethylene tubing used for percutaneous cholangiography. (From Shaldon, Barber, and Young, *Gastroenterol.* 42:371, 1962.)

is reduced and it grips the end of the needle. The tube is cut off flush with the bevel and an adaptor threaded over the needle and catheter, which are then ready for use (Fig. 1).

The Procedure

The investigation is carried out in the x-ray department on a standard tilting screening table; image intensification is an advantage. It is best performed by two persons, one of whom intubates the biliary tree while the other operates the fluorescent screen and takes the films. For an anterior approach, the site chosen for insertion of the needle is 2 cm below and 2 cm to the right of the xiphisternum. This may be varied to avoid old operation scars. Local anaesthetic is injected into skin, subcutaneous tissues, and down to the liver capsule while the patient holds his breath. For a lateral approach, a point in the right mid-axillary line is chosen over one of the intercostal spaces, below the level of the costophrenic angle—on full inspiration as shown on preliminary screening. Other puncture sites have been advocated. Prioton (1960)

has supported a posterior approach. This is said to obviate the risk of blood or bile leaking into the peritoneal cavity (as it is not transperitoneal). This is a questionable advantage, as the posterior or lateral sites are not readily accessible in the event of complications.

Following a small skin incision, a track is made through subcutaneous tissues and muscle using mosquito forceps. This is particularly important if there has been a previous abdominal operation, as scar tissue causes buckling of the polyethylene tubing. In patients with extreme abdominal scarring, the lateral approach may be preferable. With the patient holding his breath, the needle and polyethylene tubing are introduced rapidly into the right lobe of the liver, in a slighly cephaled direction, to a depth of approximately 10 cm. The needle itself is swiftly withdrawn and the patient may then freely breathe. The collar adaptor is then connected to a tap connector and a 20-ml syringe containing saline. The system is flushed and the catheter slowly withdrawn as suction is applied.

When a bile duct is entered, there is an

immediate change of pressure in the syringe, and bile is aspirated. If so-called "white" bile is present, a colourless fluid, sticky to the touch, flows up the tube. A few millilitres of bile are taken for culture. If a vessel is inadvertently entered, the catheter immediately fills with blood. This is of no consequence; the tube is flushed with saline and withdrawal is continued. When bile is aspiated, the tap adaptor is strapped to the skin and the syringe removed; 5 ml of contrast medium is then injected by way of a further flexible polyethylene cistern. The radiologist operating the screen can see immediately whether the material is flowing into the duct system. If it is, the injection is continued until the biliary tree is filled sufficiently to provide maximum information. The quantity of contrast material injected varies according to the capacity of the duct system.

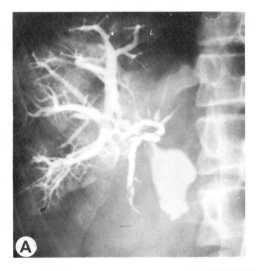

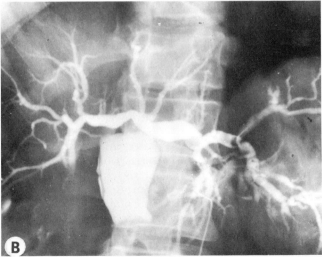

FIG. 2. Initial intubation has produced filling of only the right main hepatic duct system (A). The left main hepatic duct and its branches have been demonstrated by separate intubation with a second cannula (B). High stricture of common hepatic duct and dilatation of duct system above and below this following multiple operations; previous anastomosis to bowel almost totally occluded.

About 20 ml is usually sufficient, but 60 ml or more may be required if there is marked dilatation.

If the tube is completely withdrawn without bile being aspirated, a second puncture is made using a fresh needle and tube, the needle being directed a little to the right of the first puncture. If this fails, yet a different direction of insertion is used. If the biliary system is dilated, it is usually successfully entered in two or three attempts. When the obstruction is believed to be intermittent or partial, however, as many as 10 punctures may have to be made. To demonstrate a high lesion involving the origins of both left and right hepatic ducts, it may be necessary to cannulate separately both duct systems (Fig. 2).

A number of methods have been suggested for increasing the precision of the procedure and checking the position of the cannula during puncture. Laparoscopy has been used for this purpose, as has insertion of a radiopaque probe or suffusion of gas into the duodenum. Wiechel (1964) describes the use of previously obtained pictures of the stomach and duodenum to estimate the position of the hilum of the liver in combination with films taken in frontal and lateral projections with an indicator in the midaxillary line. Felci (1962) employed indicators placed on the skin over the lower border of the liver and duodenal bulb as located on survey films. These added measures, however, have not achieved wide popularity or usage. Probably of greater value is the use of television monitoring and image intensification along with injection of contrast medium to demonstrate puncture of a small biliary radicle in those instances when no bile has passed up the cannula. This technique has been successfully employed by Arner et al. (1962) and James (1971).

Aspiration of as much bile as possible before injection of contrast material so as to reduce dilution has been recommended by Kidd (1956), Wiechel (1964), and others. In my opinion, this practice is best avoided; the slight advantages offered are far outweighed by the real chance of the cannula's becoming dislodged from a small duct during this manipulation in patients in whom biliary dilatation is minimal and a duct has been located with some difficulty. Bile and contrast material are, moreover, readily miscible.

Films should always be obtained with the patient in various positions; the value of pictures taken during the actual injection has been stressed by Flemma, Schauble, Gardner, Anlyan, and Capp (1963). Later films, obtained up to an hour after injection, may show increased spread of the contrast material and the gallbladder may become outlined—having not been previously visualised. More important, passage of this material beyond a hitherto-appearing "complete" obstruction may occur, thus providing further invaluable anatomical information.

Percutaneous cholangiography has recently been used in conjunction with duodenography by Raia (1966). The nature and extent of pancreatic and duodenal lesions causing biliary obstruction may be defined by this method. The further addition of pancreatic scintiscanning to these procedures may lead to even more accuracy in diagnosis (Baum and Howe, 1968). Boijsen and Reuter (1967) have successfully combined the investigation with selective coeliac angiography in the demonstration and delineation of growths of the pancreas, ampulla, bile ducts, and liver. Myers, Deaver, Haupt, and Birkhead (1968) have employed cinecholangiography in the context of the percutaneous procedure, and the possibilities here merit further attention.

A novel development in recent years has been that of transjugular percutaneous cholangiography as described by Hanafee and Weiner (1967) and Hanafee, Rösch, and Weiner (1970). The latter authors have used this procedure, in addition, to carry out dilatation of biliary strictures. These reports, however, deal with very limited numbers of cases, and overall results in a representative series would be necessary for full evaluation of the advantages of the technique, and its complications. The creation of an extensive, internal, bile-blood fistula may prove to be too hazardous for the technique to be used in all save exceptional and particular cases.

INDICATIONS AND RESULTS

It is convenient to discuss results obtained with this technique along with the different indications for its use. Success rate varies widely under different circumstances, and discussion of overall results on a percentage basis irrespective of diagnosis has little meaning, as will be seen below.

The Elucidation of Jaundice

If jaundice has persisted for more than 4 weeks, and the diagnosis remains obscure despite the usual clinical, biochemical, and x-ray investigations and possibly liver-biopsy procedures, percutaneous cholangiography may offer a means of differentiating primary "hepatocellular" disorders from various forms of obstructive biliary disease. In the former group of conditions, the biliary tree is undilated and may in fact be reduced in calibre and attenuated in such diseases as primary biliary cirrhosis. Successful demonstration of such a biliary system is not usually possible with the method currently outlined. It was achieved in 15 percent of cases in the series of George, Young, Walker, and Sherlock (1965), while an overall success rate of 7.5 percent is recorded by Seldinger (1966) in a review of 131 procedures carried out by 23 groups of workers investigating primary hepatocellular conditions. Success in cannulating a biliary radicle depends, of course, upon the size of the lumen. Seldinger (1966) has studied the relationship between bile duct width and successful cannulation. Taking the upper limit for maximal intrahepatic duct calibre to be 4 mm in the presence of patent main ducts, he achieved success in 3 out of 10 patients studied without the aid of injection under television monitoring, but a 53 percent success rate was achieved with use of this refinement in a further 68 cases. In patients with jaundice due to hepatocellular disease, 3 positive results were obtained out of 9 attempted procedures using television monitoring. This technique offers no significant advantage when jaundice is caused by main duct obstruction. James (1971), also employing these refinements, reports that half the patients with normal diameter ducts can have these satisfactorily demonstrated in this way. He employs a "blind" filling of the liver under television monitoring and image intensification, if the "withdrawal" technique of cannulation has failed after four attempts.

That a biliary radicle has not been entered after five attempts at cannulation by the standard technique is good evidence that the patient has an undilated biliary system and in all probability a primary hepatocellular disease. He may thus be spared an unnecessary operation. It is perfectly safe for him to be returned to the ward and observed closely for 48 hours; there is no necessity for surgical intervention. The dangers of operation in these disorders have been stressed by Harville and Summerskill (1963). The information obtained must be weighed along with the results of all clinical and other investigations, however, before a final decision to withhold surgical intervention at any stage is reached. Negative cholangiograms are obtained in a significant proportion of patients with organic biliary obstruction—particularly that due to stricture, gallstones, and sclerosing cholangitis (see below)—and the biliary tree may be only minimally dilated (if at all) in these conditions. Atkinson, Happey, and Smiddy (1960) and Shaldon and co-workers (1962) regarded a negative cholangiogram as virtually exclusive of extrahepatic biliary obstruction. It is, however, wise to view such a result as of inferential value only. In 418 cases of failed puncture attempts reviewed by Seldinger (1966), interference with extrahepatic bile flow was subsequently found in 61 (14.5 percent). Negative cholangiograms were obtained in the presence of organic obstruction of the main bile ducts in 16 percent of 112 patients studied by George et al. (1965). In cases subsequently shown to have a biliary stricture or gallstones, the failure rate was higher (23 percent). Negative cholangiography may also result from "technical" causes, however, such as failure of the patient to tolerate the procedure, faulty technique in introduction of the cannula, and insufficient attempts at puncture.

In the uncommon event of successful cannulation of an undilated biliary tree (Fig. 3) in the presence of hepatocellular disease, the cannula may be safely removed and the patient carefully observed over the following 48 hours for signs of peritonitis. Such has not developed in a personal experience of 4 cases managed in this way. If, however, a lesion producing biliary obstruction is demonstrated and the biliary tree found to be dilated, surgical relief of the obstruction should be undertaken within a matter of a

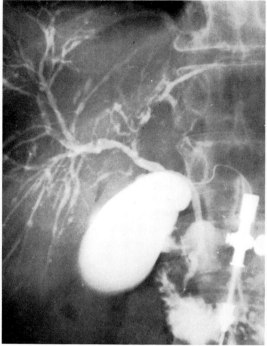

FIG. 3. Undilated biliary tree in a case of primary biliary cirrhosis demonstrated by percutaneous cholangiography. Intrahepatic radicles are irregular.

mises risk of trauma to other structures. The exact nature of the operation to be performed may also be decided upon beforehand. A simpler operation than had been expected may in some instances be possible. Reconstruction of a previous anastomosis may be deemed unnecessary and simple dilatation may suffice (Fig. 4). The procedure is perhaps of greatest value in patients with a stricture high in the biliary tree, for whom a knowledge of the line of direction of the main ducts is invaluable when dilators and tubes are to be passed (Fig. 5). In other patients, the demonstration of multiple pathological conditions such as stricture and stones or of multiple strictures is of value (Figs. 6 and 7). Occasionally, when percutaneous cholangiography reveals a slightly dilated or undilated biliary tree with little or no obstruction, operative intervention may be avoided altogether. Recurrent attacks of cholangitis may occur in patients in whom no organic obstruction to biliary flow exists. This is, however, uncommon. In these circumstances, adequate films cannot be obtained.

In a detailed study by Walker, Young,

few hours. Percutaneous cholangiography has no place in the investigation of jaundiced patients too old, too ill, or in any way unsuitable for surgical treatment. There must be no serious defect in the coagulation mechanism. Investigation of cases of obscure jaundice by this means requires previous strategic planning by physician, radiologist, and surgeon together.

Recurrent Obstructive Jaundice and Cholangitis

A second group of patients who benefit particularly from this procedure are those with recurrent cholangitis or obstructive jaundice, usually occurring after a previous biliary operation. Maingot (1962, 1964) has strongly advocated its routine use in all such instances. Preoperative definition of the site and extent of the stricture saves invaluable time used in searching for a dilated duct at the beginning of the operation and mini-

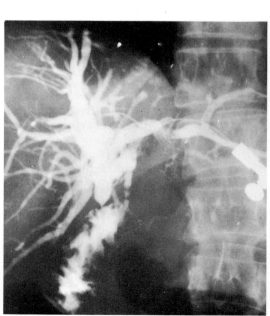

FIG. 4. Stricture of the common hepatic duct at the site of a previous anastomosis to the jejunum. Contrast medium enters the bowel.

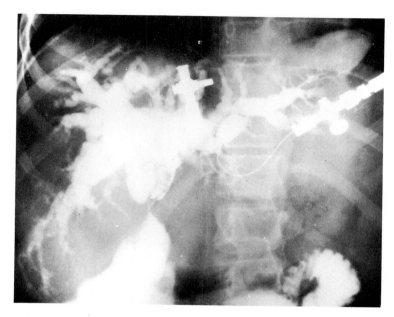

FIG. 5. Strictures of right and left main hepatic ducts at the site of a previous anastomosis to the bowel. (From Walker et al., *Gut* 7:164, 1966.)

George, and Sherlock (1966) of 35 cases of stricture of the bile ducts, successful cholangiography was achieved in 75 percent. Twenty-five of the patients had already undergone operations for biliary reconstruc-

tion. It is stressed that absence of jaundice does not preclude success under these cir-

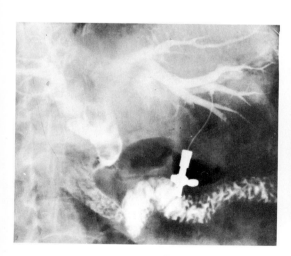

FIG. 6. Multiple stones and biliary sludge above a stricture at the site of a previous anastomosis to the jejunum.

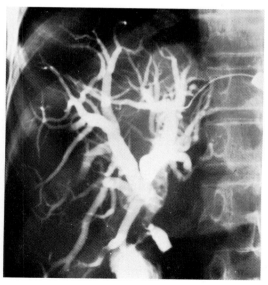

FIG. 7. Stricture of the common hepatic duct at the site of previous repair. There is a fistulous communication between the duodenum and the common bile duct which is completely obstructed at the site of a previous anastomosis to the jejunum.

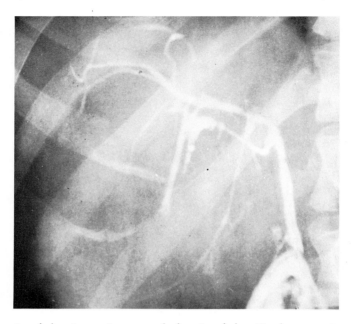

FIG. 8. Operative cholangiogram in a case of sclerosing cholangitis where percutaneous cholangiography was unsuccessful. The narrowed, attenuated intrahepatic biliary radicles are clearly seen.

cumstances, for in one-third of the successful cases the serum bilirubin level was less than 2 mg per 100 ml. In patients with biliary stricture, obstruction is often intermittent or partial, and the degree of biliary dilatation variable. As many as ten attempts at puncture may be necessary before eventual success. This is more than the number suggested as the maximum for the differential diagnosis of jaundice (see above). In nine instances in which percutaneous cholangiography was unsuccessful, subsequent laparotomy revealed no significant biliary dilatation in eight. Three of these patients were believed to be suffering from sclerosing cholangitis which in all instances was preceded by a long history of gallstones and recurrent cholangitis (Fig. 8). In a smaller number of cases (23) Seldinger (1966) reports 70 percent success in a series of his own.

When cholangiography is negative, a decision about the advisability of operation must be based on the clinical picture and biochemical investigations. In patients with a stricture, however, the history is usually fairly typical—with attacks of jaundice or pain or of cholangitis. Laparotomy is then undertaken irrespective of the cholangio-graphic result. A positive cholangiogram must always be followed shortly by surgical exploration. Broad-spectrum antibiotic cover for the procedure and routine culture of bile is of particular importance in patients with biliary stricture in whom leakage of potentially infected bile and consequent peritonitis or septicaemia are possible.

Known Obstructive Jaundice When Exact Cause and Site Are in Doubt

Even in the presence of known biliary obstruction, percutaneous cholangiography may augment the diagnosis and be of value —allowing accurate planning of the correct operation beforehand (Fig. 9). Thus, a previous diagnosis of malignancy may be changed to one of gallstones or benign stricture while the reverse is also true (Figs. 10 and 11). A diagnosis of intrahepatic bile duct carcinoma may often be established when previous laparotomies have proved negative and operative cholangiography has not been performed (Fig. 12). It may in certain instances of malignant disease demonstrate the presence

Percutaneous cholangiography has been successful in demonstrating less common biliary lesions. Kaplan, Traitz, Mitchel, and Block (1961) have demonstrated extrahepatic congenital atresia with its use while Felci (1962) and Glenn, Evans, Mujahed, and Thorbjarnarson (1962) visualised localised areas of inflammation in the common duct. Hepp and Vayre (1959) noted compression and retraction of the bile ducts at the hilum of the liver in a case of hydatid disease, but any suspicion of this condition is a positive contraindication to the procedure because of the dangers of cyst rupture. Wiechel (1964) has demonstrated bile fistulae with percutaneous cholangiography, while Isley and

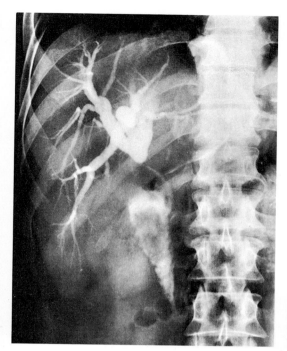

FIG. 9. Percutaneous intrahepatic cholangiography. At first operation inadvertent excision of the gallbladder (which contained stones) together with the common hepatic duct and a major portion of the common bile duct had occurred. External drainage of the hepatic duct remnant for 6 weeks; when the tube was removed, the patient developed jaundice. At the second operation, hepaticoduodenostomy was carried out successfully. (R. Maingot's patient.)

of a dilated bile duct suitable for surgical anastomosis and palliative decompression or may even help the surgeon to decide if partial hepatectomy is feasible. Advantages over preoperative cholangiography include the necessity for surgical intervention before the latter investigation can be performed. Location of a duct for the procedure is, moreover, time-consuming and not without hazard to other structures. Operative cholangiography often demonstrates only that part of the biliary tree below an obstruction when visualisation of the duct system above the lesion would be of more practical value.

In this group of patients, just as in the two already described, operative intervention is necessary if an obstructive lesion is demonstrated, while conservative management is satisfactory when no biliary radicle is cannulated.

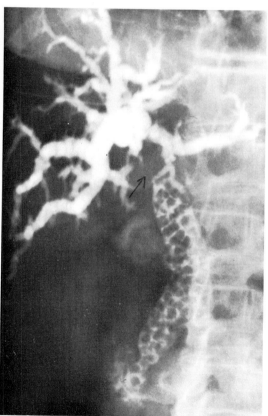

FIG. 10. Multiple stones in a dilated common bile duct. An irregular filling defect (arrow) proved to be due to concurrent carcinoma of the gallbladder. A diagnosis of pancreatic new growth had previously been made. (From George, et al. *Brit. J. Surg.* 52:779, 1965.)

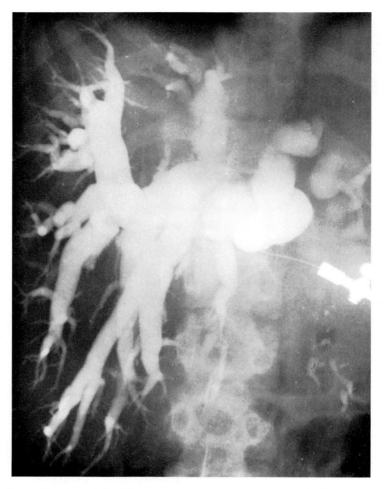

FIG. 11.   Gross dilatation of the biliary tree in a young man previously diagnosed as suffering from inoperable carcinoma of the liver. A benign stricture was located at operation at the level demonstrated by the cholangiogram. (From George, *Postgraduate Gastroenterology*, 1966. Courtesy of Baillière, Tindall, and Cassell, London.)

Schauble (1962) visualised communication between a liver abscess and the bile ducts. Intrahepatic congenital biliary atresia, on the other hand, has been invariably associated with a negative cholangiogram (Leger et al., 1953; Castiglioni and Petronio, 1964; George et al., 1965).

It is not claimed that percutaneous cholangiography offers certain diagnosis of the exact cause and extent of an obstructive lesion in 100 percent of cases. Diagnosis of calculous obstruction usually presents little difficulty, but differentiation of the processes causing narrowing of the ducts (stenosis) is less reliable on cholangiographic appearances alone. Assessment of tumour spread has been found notably difficult by Atkinson et al. (1960) and Shaldon et al. (1962).

In Seldinger's review (1966) of 44 series of cases submitted to percutaneous cholangiography, an overall success rate of 92 percent is reported in those instances in which interference to extrahepatic bile flow was adjudged to be present (763 cases). The success rate in his own series was 81 percent but only patients with a known final diagnosis were considered (90 cases). George et al. (1965) report a figure of 84 percent under

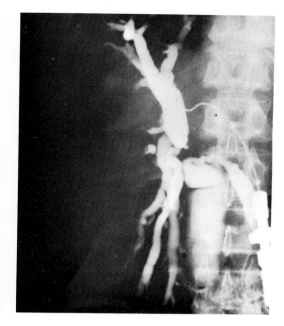

FIG. 12. Extensive carcinoma of the intrahepatic ducts. Gross dilatation of the right duct system; nonvisualisation of the left. The common bile and cystic ducts and the gallbladder are outlined and are normal. No cause for the patient's jaundice had been found at two previous operations.

count the relative proportions of the different types of cases studied.

The technique has been used for biliary decompression in inoperable carcinoma (Shaldon et al., 1962; Kaude, Weidenmier, and Agee, 1969), but this procedure is of questionable value because of the very serious risk of infection and of biliary leakage and peritonitis.

COMPLICATIONS

Significant intra-abdominal haemorrhage occurred in only 5 out of 685 percutaneous cholangiograms (0.7 percent) reviewed by Wiechel (1964). Uncorrected hypoprothrombinaemia was present in the fatal outcomes described by Nurick, Patey, and Whiteside (1953) and Barbier (1959) and could be held responsible for the train of events. A clinically insignificant amount of blood is not uncommonly found in the peritoneal cavity at laparotomy, but bleeding has by that time stopped in almost all cases. Blood clot may also be found in the bile ducts at operation, but it seldom causes real trouble.

Some degree of biliary peritonitis was present in 28 of 1,372 cases (2 percent) reviewed by Seldinger (1966). This figure could probably have been much reduced had operation followed the same day in all patients in whom a cholangiogram had demonstrated an obstructive lesion, and biliary leakage through the puncture track thereby avoided. In three reported cases in which death could be attributed to biliary peritonitis, operation had been delayed despite demonstration of an obstructed biliary tree (Leger et al., 1953; Zinberg, Berk, and Plasencia, 1965; Stiris, 1962). The recommended practice of leaving the polyethylene catheter in place to decompress the biliary tree while operation is awaited minimises the chance of biliary leakage into the peritoneum and, more rarely, nearby blood vessels during this period.

On occasion, the biliary tree is outlined by puncture of the gallbladder itself. This does not seem to increase the rate of biliary peritonitis *provided* the general principles laid out above are adhered to, and laparotomy follows promptly in obstructed cases

similar circumstances. Apart from technical reasons (insufficient puncture attempts, etc.) and minimal dilatation or actual sclerosis of ducts in patients with biliary stricture, another significant cause of failure reported in this work was extensive infiltration of the liver with neoplasm or stones. Similar overall figures are reported in two more recent series from Canada (Turner and Costopoulos, 1968; Ritchie, Jackson, and Eaglesham, 1969). *Success rate,* however, is an unfortunate term, as a negative cholangiographic result does not mean that the investigation has failed but simply that no dilated duct has been punctured. Success rate is high in cases of carcinoma of the pancreas in which the ducts themselves are uninvolved by the disease process and when infection is uncommon, cholangiograms being obtained in all such patients studied by George and her coworkers. It is at its lowest in cases of biliary stricture. Any significant appraisal of statistics in individual series must take into ac-

(De Masi, Akdamar, Sparks, and Hunter, 1967).

Haemorrhage and biliary peritonitis are by far the most serious, although uncommon, complications of the procedure. Probably the most important single factor in reducing the incidence is the use of a soft catheter with removal of the needle. This obviates the need to prevent extensive or unexpected liver movements by general anaesthesia or by "blocking" the ipsilateral phrenic nerves, as has been suggested. Other important principles which mitigate these complications include (1) nonintervention in patients with an abnormal coagulation mechanism and (2) the necessity to relieve organic obstruction after dilated bile ducts have been successfully demonstrated. The examination is contraindicated when intrahepatic sepsis is strongly suspected. Uncommonly, a bile-blood fistula may be caused by simultaneous puncture of a biliary radicle and a blood vessel (Arner et al., 1962; Koch and Gorder, 1969), but it is difficult to know with centainty if and when this occurs to a *significant* degree.

Intra-abdominal organs other than the liver have at times been punctured during attempts at cholangiography; these include stomach, duodenum, small and large bowel, and kidney. Such mistakes can be recognised at once if injection of contrast medium is performed under screen control and the tube can then be instantly withdrawn. Little serious harm occurs under such circumstances. Less serious side-effects consisting of local pain at the site of puncture and mild pyrexia after the procedure settle with conservative management in the vast majority of cases.

It may finally be concluded that the technique is safe so long as it is applied to suitable cases and it is appreciated by all concerned that it is, in essence, a "preoperative" procedure in the majority of instances.

REFERENCES

Arner, O., Hagberg, S., and Seldinger, S. I., Surgery 52:561, 1962.

Atkinson, M., Happey, M. G., and Smiddy, F. G., Gut 1:357, 1960.

Barbier, F., Belg. T. Geneesk. 15:1019, 1959.

Baum, M., and Howe, C. T., Am. J. Surg. 115:519, 1968.

Boijsen, E., and Reuter, S. R., Am. J. Roentgenol. 99:153, 1967.

Carter, R. F., and Saypol, G. M., J.A.M.A. 148:253, 1952.

Castiglioni, G. C., and Petronio, R., Surgery 56:635, 1964.

De Masi, C. J., Akdamar, K., Sparks, R. D., and Hunter, F. M., J.A.M.A. 201:225, 1967.

Felci, U., Minerva Med. 53:858, 1962.

Fernström, I., and Seldinger, S. I., Nord. Med. 55:344, 1956.

Flemma, R. J., Schauble, J. F., Gardner, C. E., Anlyan, W. G., and Capp, M. P., Surg. Gynecol. Obstet. 116:559, 1963.

George, P., Young, W. B., Walker, J. G., and Sherlock, S., Br. J. Surg. 52:779, 1965.

Glenn, F., Evans, J. A., Mujahed, Z., and Thorbjarnarson, B., Ann. Surg. 156:451, 1962.

Hanafee, W., and Weiner, M., Radiology 88:35, 1967.

Hanafee, W., Rösch, J., and Weiner, M. Radiology 94:429, 1970.

Harville, D. D., and Summerskill, W. H. J. J.A.M.A. 184:257, 1963.

Hepp, J., and Vayre, P., Rev. Int. Hépatol. 9:633, 1959.

Huard, P., and Do-Xuan-Hop, Bull. Soc. Méd. Chir. Indochine 15:1090, 1937.

Isley, J. K., and Schauble, J. F., Am. J. Roentgenol. 88:772, 1962.

James, M., Arch. Surg. 103:31, 1971.

Kaplan, A. A., Traitz, J. J., Mitchel, S. D., Block, A. L., Ann. Intern. Med. 54:856, 1961.

Kaude, J. V., Weidenmier, C. H., and Agee, O. F., Radiology 93:69, 1969.

Kidd, H. A., Arch. Surg. 72:262, 1956.

Koch, R. L., and Gorder, J. L., Radiology 93:67, 1969.

Leger, L., Zara, M., and Wargnier, M., Arch. Mal. Appar. Dig. 42:967 1953.

Maingot, R., Proc. R. Soc. Med. 55:588, 1962.

Maingot, R., in Smith and Sherlock, eds., Surgery of the Gall Bladder and Bile Ducts, London, Butterworths, 1964.

Myers, R. N., Deaver, J. M., Haupt, G. J., and Birkhead, N. C., Arch. Surg. 97:51, 1968.

Nurick, A. W., Patey, D. H., and Whiteside, C. G., Br. J. Surg. 41:27, 1953.

Prioton, J-B., Presse Méd. 68:2308, 1960.

Raia, S., Surgery 60:1125, 1966.

Ritchie, G. W., Jackson, D. C., and Eaglesham, H., Can. Med. Assoc. J. 100:110, 1969.

Seldinger, S. I., Acta Radiol. Scand. (Suppl.) 253, 1966.

Shaldon, S., Barber, K. M., and Young, W. B., Gastroenterology 42:371, 1962.

Stiris, G., T. Norske Laegeforen. 82:443, 1962.

Turner, F. W., and Costopoulos, L. B., Can. Med. Assoc. J. 99:513, 1968.

Walker, J. G., Young, W. B., George, P., and Sherlock, S., Gut 7:164, 1966.

Wiechel, K-L., Opusc. Med. 5:287, 1960.

Wiechel, K-L., Acta Chir. Scand. (Suppl.) 330, 1964.

Zinberg, S. S., Berk, J. E., and Plasencia, H., Am. J. Dig. Dis. 10:154, 1965.

47

SOME BENIGN STRICTURES
OF THE BILE DUCTS:
Operations for These Lesions

RODNEY MAINGOT

CHOLEDOCHUS CYST

Congenital cystic dilatation of the common bile duct (choledochus cyst, or idiopathic dilatation of the common bile duct) is a rare anomaly. Rogers and Priestley,[23] in a masterful and comprehensive review, state that Beverley Smith [27] collected reports of 118 cases and that Shallow, Eger and Wagner [24] recorded 175 cases 4 years later.

The number of authentic cases of this anomaly reported to date is more than 600.

Alonso-Lej et al.[1] state that the review of Tsardakas and Robnett [32] included 232 cases, and that 2 years after publication of this article they were able to find 161 more cases in the literature. These figures suggest that many more cases are now diagnosed, and the total number of cases reported is not a reliable indication of the incidence of the disease. Recently, Tsuchida and Ishida [33] who reported 16 cases, Trout and Longmire [31] 7 cases, and O'Neill and Chatworthy [22] 11 cases all agree that considerably more than 600 cases have been reported up to and including 1971.

The *crude anatomy of this congenital anomaly* was first described by Vater in 1723, but Douglas [6] was the first to give an accurate account of the symptomatology and pathological characteristics of this lesion.

The most complete reviews of this subject were submitted by Yotuyanagi,[35] Shields,[25] Farris and Yadeau,[8] Fonkalsrud and Boles,[10] Gross,[14] Warren et al.,[34] Lees et al.,[19] and Jones et al.[16]

In the majority of recorded cases, the cyst (which in some respects resembles a saccular aneurysm) has involved either the supraduodenal portion of the common bile duct or an area of the main ducts above this region, and including the intrahepatic portions of the hepatic ducts.

Gross [13] analysed 100 authentic cases which he was able to collect from the literature. Of these 100 patients, 52 had had symptoms from the ninth year of life or earlier; 45 of the 52 were under 15 years of age, and 32 of that 45 were under the age of 10 at the time of the discovery of the cyst. Eighty percent of the patients were under 30 years of age.

These anomalies have been observed in the foetus, in the still-born, and in infants a few days old.[26] They have been observed in association with other anomalies. All age groups are affected, but 75 percent of the patients presenting are under 25 years of age.

Yotuyanagi [35] considered the condition to be congenital and probably dependent upon inequalities in the rate of epithelial proliferation during the stage of occlusion of the primitive choledochus. Alonso-Lej believes that the aetiology consists of a weakness in the specific portion of the common bile duct caused by hyperproliferation and hypervacuolisation of that area during embryonic development. Such a weakness, he says, constitutes a protodilation status which develops into the clinical pathological entity when the ductal pressure increases because of an obstructive factor.

Shallow [24] considered that in these cases there was some congenital weakness of the common bile duct, possibly allied to Hirschsprung's disease or congenital idiopathic hydronephrosis.

Alonso-Lej stated: "Our most recent analysis of 91 surgically treated cases shows a mortality of 12 percent." [1] I believe that, at the present time, the mortality rate for the *short-*

circuiting operations is in the region of 2 percent, while it is approximately 4 percent for *excision* of the "sac," combined with biliary-enteric anastomosis. P. Jones and his colleagues,[17] however reported 5 patients who were successfully treated by excision of the sac followed by hepaticojejunostomy with a Roux-en-Y loop, and this is the procedure of choice for the majority of cases.

The Japanese race seems to be particularly affected. The condition is commoner in females than in males, the ratio being 4:1.

The cyst varies considerably in *size;* the largest on record—that described by Neugebauer—contained one gallon of bile. Many of the cysts have been described as being the size of an orange, a grapefruit, a clenched fist, or a child's head.

There is little if any relation between the size of the cyst and the duration of the symptoms. There is also no constant correlation between the size of the cyst and the age of the patient, although the larger sacs are more commonly found in older patients. The wall of the cyst is firm and varies from 2 to 8 mm in thickness.

Epithelium is generally absent in the lining of the cyst, the wall of which is composed of dense, fibrous, inflammatory tissue.

Although the distal portion of the common duct is generally narrowed, a great diversity of findings in this region has been seen to exist. Valve-like folds, an abnormal course of the duct through the duodenum, or one or more kinks in its course have all been reported. In some instances the caliber of the distal end of the duct has been adequate. In those cases where little or no opening was found to exist in the distal end of the common duct it is believed that inflammation produced an obliteration of a pre-existing congenital stenosis, as there were periods of months or years during which the patients in such cases were free of jaundice. The gallbladder is usually normal in size irrespective of the existence of a dilated cystic duct. The presence of stones within the gallbladder or the cyst has been reported in less than 1 per cent of cases. The bile within the cyst has varied in color and consistency depending upon the degree of obstruction and infection that exists. There may be dilatation of the extrahepatic ducts joining the upper pole of the cyst, but usually the intrahepatic ducts are of normal size. The condition of the liver apparently depends upon the duration and nature of the biliary obstruction. Cirrhosis and cholangitis are not uncommon. Ascites and splenomegaly have existed in some cases.[23]

Multiple choledochal cysts were first reported in 1964 by Arthur and Stewart[2] and also by Engle and Salmon.[7]

Separate cystic swellings of the intrahepatic biliary passages, of the choledochus, and of the cystic duct were observed. The importance of illuminating the cysts by means of operative cholangiography was emphasized by these authors. Tsuchida and Ishida,[33] in 1971, stated: "Surveys of our serial operative cholangiograms disclosed intrahepatic dilatation of apparently congenital origin in 9 of our 16 cases. This malformation is not necessarily confined to the common bile duct; it may occur in multiple areas of the whole biliary tree." This is a significant and important finding.

Diagnosis

The *symptoms and signs,* however, are sufficiently characteristic to make the disease readily recognisable if the surgeon is fully acquainted with the gross anatomy of the lesion. *Pain, jaundice, and mass are the classic diagnostic triad.* Intermittence of these symptoms increases the probability of congenital cystic dilatation.

The patient is usually a young girl who has a smooth spherical *tumour* on the right side of the abdomen, which is continuous with the liver dullness. The tumour, which feels solid when it is tense with fluid, is movable from side to side but not in an upward or downward direction. Few of these cystic tumours can be detected on palpation in infancy and childhood; the older the patient and the longer the duration of symptoms, the greater are the chances of detecting the mass —which may be fixed or mobile. There may be a band of colonic resonance over it. Right-sided epigastric *pain* is a constant symptom, and the presenting signs of biliary or duodenal obstruction—such as *intermittent jaundice, colic,* cholangitic fever and rigors, and occasional attacks of vomiting, indigestion, and flatulence—are evident.

Radiology

Radiological investigations are of the greatest value in diagnosis. For instance:

1. Excretion pyelography may show a right-sided hydronephrosis from pressure of the cyst on the ureter.
2. A barium-meal x-ray examination may show the duodenum, the hepatic flexure of the colon, and the pylorus to be displaced downward or over to the left.
3. Cholecystography may demonstrate a characteristic picture of a high gallbladder, compressed into a comma shape by the cyst but still able to receive bile and concentrate it. Intravenous cholangiography has proved valuable in diagnosis, provided the patient is not jaundiced.
4. Calcification in the cyst wall and hepatic ducts can sometimes be made out. In McLaughlin's patient,[21] a plain x-ray film of the abdomen showed a fluid level and gas in the cyst.
5. An operative cholangiogram should, as a rule, be carried out in all cases; it has proved to be the most useful of the radiological procedures. Although a choledochus cyst should be recognisable at exploratory laparotomy by an experienced surgeon, in a few instances difficulty may be encountered in differentiating a choledochus cyst from other intra-abdominal or retroperitoneal cysts. It is in such cases as these that an operative cholangiogram may prove to be a valuable aid in diagnosis. A postoperative *air cholangiogram* is sometimes carried out to determine the presence or absence of stenosis of the cysto-enteric or hepaticoenteritic stoma.
6. *Percutaneous intrahepatic cholangiography* rarely affords any help in diagnosis. (See Chap. 46.)
7. Coeliac and superior mesenteric arterial angiography and scanning of the pancreas are valuable aids in diagnosis.

Complications

Complications are mainly those due to biliary obstruction (such as suppurative cholangitis), liver abscess, biliary cirrhosis, stone formation, thrombosis of the portal vein, fibrosis of the stoma, and rupture of the cyst.

More than 20 cases of *rupture of a choledochal cyst* during pregnancy have been re-ported, including the one so ably presented by Friend,[11] and the 14 cases summarised by Chesterman.[4] Traumatic rupture of a choledochus cyst has been described by Blocker et al.[3] and others. Swartley and Weeder[30] reported a case of choledochus cyst associated with double common bile duct. *I can find only 4 cases of cystic dilatation of the common bile duct associated with malignancy.* The first was described by Irwin and Morison,[15] the second by Fischer,[9] the third by Sterry Asby,[28] and the fourth by Lorenzo et al.[20]

A choledochus cyst occurring in the presence of a primary carcinoma of the liver was described by George and Maingot,[12] and they cited two other similar examples. These patients all died and the condition was diagnosed postmortem. Dexter[5] had a patient with a choledochus cyst and multiple carcinomas of the hepatic and pancreatic ducts, also diagnosed at necropsy.

Differential Factors

A choledochus cyst may be mistaken for mucocele of the gallbladder; calculous cholecystitis; solitary nonparasitic cyst of the liver; hydatid cyst; a new growth of the liver, suprarenal gland, or pancreas; pancreatic cyst; mesenteric cyst; polycystic disease of the kidney; a right hydronephrosis; or a large epigastric retroperitoneal tumour.

Operative Treatment

There is a choice of four operations:

1. Choledochocystogastrostomy.
2. Choledochocystoduodenostomy. (See Figs. 1, 4, 5, and 6.)
3. Choledochocystojejunostomy.
   a. With entero-anastomosis in order to deflect gastric contents away from the sac.
   b. With Roux-en-Y loop. (See Figs. 2 and 3.)
4. Excision of the sac with the gallbladder followed by
   a. Hepaticojejunostomy combined with side-to-side entero-anastomosis.

b. Hepaticojejunostomy with Roux-en-Y loop. (Figs. 7 and 8.)

Choledochocystogastrostomy is rarely, if ever, performed today, as the irritating and erosive gastric and duodenal chyme is very prone to light up a persistent cholangitis which may lead to stenosis of the stoma and a recurrence of symptoms including jaundice.

A popular operation consists of short-circuiting the cyst into a loop of proximal jejunum—*choledochocystojejunostomy.* This is performed as follows: a portion of the proximal jejunum is selected and brought in front of the transverse colon to the *inferior border* of the cyst, and anastomosis is carried out as in the operation of gastrojejunostomy. At the completion of this anastomosis, a *jejunojejunostomy* is performed between the proximal and distal limbs of the jejunum, about 3 inches (7.6 cm) from the duodenojejunal flexure (Fig. 2). The entero-anastomosis deflects the intestinal chyme away from the biliary system, thus diminishing the likelihood of the subsequent onset of an ascending cholangitis.

Priestley was the first surgeon to perform the *Roux-en-Y type* of anastomosis in the treatment of choledochus cyst (Fig. 3). This method of anastomosis should appeal to the

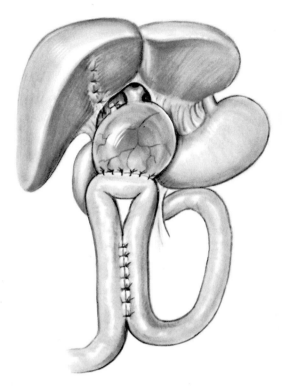

FIG. 2. Choledochocystojejunostomy: jejunal loop method. (Courtesy of Ethicon, Ltd., and Butterworths, London.)

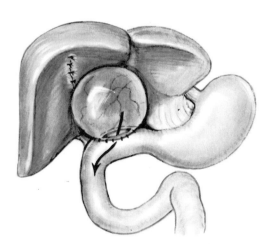

FIG. 1. Choledochocystoduodenostomy. (Courtesy of Ethicon, Ltd., and Butterworths, London.)

surgeon who encounters a choledochus cyst on exploration, as it frequently overcomes cholangitis and any tendency to stricture formation at the cystojejunal stoma.

It is most important that the choledochocystojejunostomy stoma should be sited at the *most dependent portion of the cyst,* otherwise drainage of the cystic contents will not be entirely effective. In all cases, a *large cystoenteric stoma* must be fashioned—5 cm (at least) in length. It should be noted that many cases of stricture or stenosis of the stoma have been reported in the literature following anastomosis of the cyst to the duodenum or proximal jejunum. When there is a recurrence of symptoms following stenosis of the anastomosis, at the second operation, the surgeon would be well advised to perform cystectomy and hepaticojejunostomy on the Roux-en-Y plan. (Figs. 7 and 8.)

Alonso-Lej [1] and other authorities, includ-

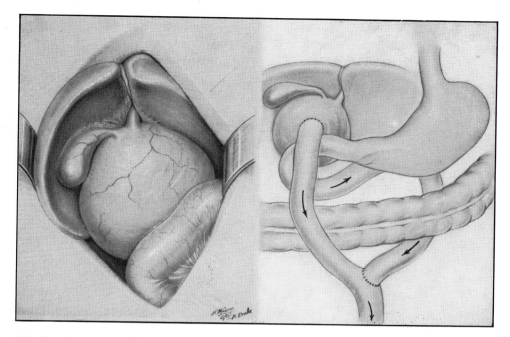

FIG. 3.   Congenital cystic dilatation of the common bile duct and drainage of a choledochus cyst by the Roux-en-Y method suggested by Priestley. The cystojejunostomy stoma should, of course, be placed at the most dependent portion of the cyst.

ing Arthur and Stewart, [2] and Tsuchida and Ishida,[33] advocate *excision of the cyst* followed by anastomosis of the remaining biliary tree (the common hepatic duct) to the jejunum employing a Roux-en-Y loop, as illustrated in Figure 8. This procedure is. however, associated with greater risks than is choledochocystojejunostomy, which has an immediate mortality rate of only 2 percent, compared with 4 percent for cystectomy. The *late results* of excision of the cyst combined with hepaticojejunostomy are excellent, however, and postoperative complications are rare.

The subject of ascending cholangitis and stricture formation at the cystoenteric stoma is discussed by Swartley,[29] McLaughlin,[21] Jones, et al.[16]; Kasi and Asakura,[18] and Trout and Longmire.[31]

The operative mortality rate some 30 years or so ago was high on account of "delayed" operation. Today it is about 4 percent in expert hands. The treatment of choledochus cyst by procedures such as cystogastrostomy,

external drainage, and marsupialization have been abandoned.

It must be emphasized that excision of the choledochus cyst followed by anastomosis of the common hepatic duct to a loop of proximal jejunum is becoming increasingly popular with surgeons who are expert in biliary-tract surgery.

The technique of excision of a choledochus cyst followed by hepaticojejunostomy, based on the Roux-en-Y plan, is illustrated in Figures 7 and 8.*

* I should like to express my thanks and appreciation to Ethicon Ltd., and to R. Smith and S. Sherlock, editors of Surgery of the Gallbladder and Bile Ducts (1964), and Butterworths & Co., London, for allowing me to reproduce the illustrations depicting operations for choledochus cyst, which appeared in my contribution (Chap. 3): Congenital Abnormalities of the Bile Ducts.

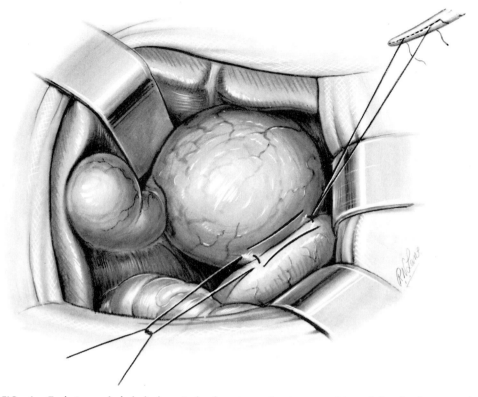

FIG. 4.   Technique of choledochocystoduodenostomy showing apposition of the duodenum to the cyst wall and sites of incisions in the gut and the cyst. (After Ethicon, Ltd. Courtesy of Butterworths, London.)

CONGENITAL ATRESIA OF THE BILE DUCTS

John Thomson [58] first aroused interest in this condition by his careful analysis of 50 cases. Holmes [47] collected 120 cases from the literature, described a large number of variations in malformations, and concluded that about 16 percent of the patients could be amenable to surgical treatment.

Ladd [50] was the first surgeon to operate successfully upon a case of congenital atresia of the bile ducts. Gray et al.,[43] in reporting on two of their own patients successfully treated by cholecystogastrostomy, stated that between 1928 and 1948 only 17 such cases were recorded in the literature.

Durell and Halliwell [39] described a case of congenital atresia of the biliary duct which

was cured by cholecystogastrostomy, and they remarked that up to 1949 surgical intervention had been successful apparently in only 21 instances. Since that time, further successes have been reported, including one of Maingot's patients.[53] Moore [54] gave his experiences with 31 proved cases and reported one case which was treated successfully. Gross [45] found that at operation nothing could be done (owing to obliteration of the ducts) in 119 cases; but in 15 patients of his who had a nubbin of common or hepatic duct available for anastomosis 12 were restored to good health. Greaney et al.[44] explored 33 cases, 9 of which were suitable for biliary-intestinal anastomosis; 3 patients were cured. Schnug [55] recorded a series of 10 proved cases, with one cure. He stated that a total of 39 patients treated successfully have been reported, which is relatively few considering the total number listed—together

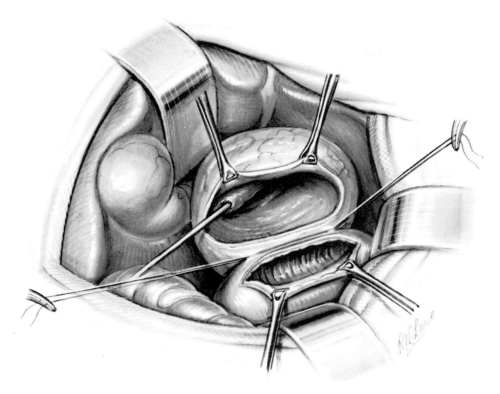

FIG. 5. Choledochocystoduodenostomy. Lateral wall of the duodenum is sutured to the cyst wall with a series of interrupted sutures of fine serumproof silk. Incisions are next made in the anterior duodenal wall and cyst. The interior of the cyst is explored for stone, biliary sand, or neoplasm. The entrance of the hepatic duct is probed and dilated with Bakes' dilators. Wide cystoenteric stoma should be assured. (After Ethicon, Ltd. Courtesy of Butterworths, London.)

with the fact that many unsuccessful cases have not been recorded. Some authorities have estimated that, up to 1973, about 100 patients with congenital biliary atresia have been cured by some type of biliary-intestinal anastomosis. Beaven and Duncan[36] reported the first successful cholecystogastrostomy case in Great Britain. Durell and Halliwell[39] reported the second such case. In 1951, Maingot recorded a case which was successfully treated by cholecystojejunostomy combined with jejunojejunostomy. Cameron and Brunton[37] reported one successful operation at University College Hospital, London. Further operative successes have been recorded by Krovetz,[49] Longmire,[52] and Foukalsrud et al.[41]

Ladd,[51] who based his instructive article on the study of 45 cases of congenital obstruction of the bile duct treated at the Children's Hospital, Boston, considered that while it was true that *almost no two cases were precisely alike,* it was nevertheless possible to *classify* the various malformations into a number of groups. The following arrangement has been suggested:

1. Cases in which there are no extrahepatic ducts.
2. Cases in which there is an atresia of the hepatic ducts.
3. Cases in which there is an atresia of the common bile duct.
4. Cases in which the gallbladder is represented as a moderate-sized cyst, not connected with the common duct, and in which there may or may not be any common or hepatic ducts.
5. Cases in which the gallbladder connects directly with the duodenum, but in which there are no other extrahepatic ducts—i.e.,

no ducts connecting the liver and gallbladder or the liver and intestine.

6. Cases in which the gallbladder and its cystic duct connect with a patent common hepatic duct.

7. Cases where there is a stenosis of the common duct, which is plugged with inspissated bile, causing complete obstruction.

8. Cases in which there is narrowing of the common duct, causing partial obstruction (Fig. 9).

Aetiology

Approximately 60 percent of the patients who have congenital atresia of the bile ducts are males.

In discussing embryological development, Chesterman [38] states:

Embryologically the liver and bile passages start in the third week of intra-uterine life as a diverticulum which grows from the ventral aspect of the foregut between the stomach and the yolk sac. This enlarges into the *septum transversum* and gives off two solid buds of cells which later form the right lobe of the liver, while the more caudally located cells of the diverticulum proliferate to form the extra-hepatic biliary passages. The hyperplasia of these caudally located cells is so rapid that it remains as a solid cord until the fourth month, when clefts appear between the cells, coalescing to re-establish a lumen shortly before the fifth month. This is roughly a month before bile pigment is found in the secretion of the liver.

Howard Gray [43] adds:

Irregular cleft formation or atypical fusion may lead to accessory ducts or reduplication. Lack of canalisation gives rise to complete atresia; partial canalisation gives rise to partial atresia.

Pathology

One or more parts of the external biliary tract are either absent or exist as fibrous cords. The extent of any such obliteration determines the operability of the case. The case will be operable if the atresia exists in the lower part of the common hepatic duct, in the common duct, or if the

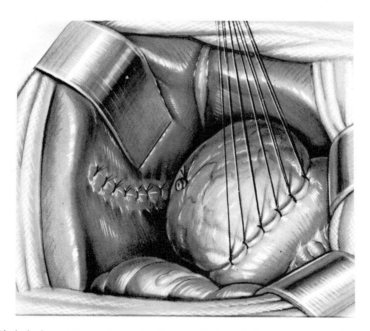

FIG. 6. Choledochocystojejunostomy. At the completion of the anastomosis, the gallbladder is dissected free, the cystic artery and cystic duct are ligated and divided, and after the removal of the gallbladder, the fossa in the liver is reperitonealised. Note that the anterior suture line consists of a number of interrupted sutures of fine silk. (After Ethicon, Ltd. Courtesy of Butterworths, London.)

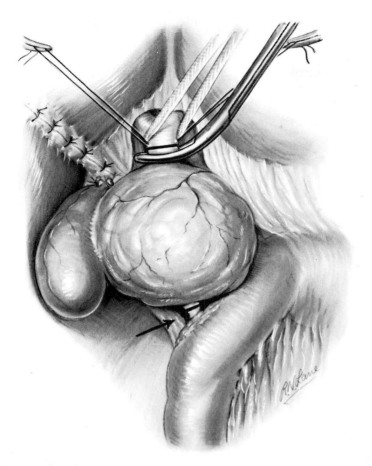

FIG. 7. Resection of a choledochal cyst. (After Ethicon, Ltd. Courtesy of Butterworths, London.)

gallbladder and cystic duct communicate with the common hepatic duct—which is distended with bile.

The *gallbladder* may be found in one of four pathological conditions: (1) it may be absent or atretic; (2) it may contain a small lumen which does not communicate with the ductal system; (3) it may be distended with white bile—mucocele; or (4) it may be normal or enlarged and contain normal bile, indicating that the obstruction is in the common bile duct. (See Fig. 9.)

The *liver* is enlarged, stained dark green in colour, and diffusely nodular, giving the picture of portal cirrhosis of the obstructive type.

The *spleen* is usually moderately enlarged, and *portal hypertension* is a common feature.

Ascites may or may not be evident. Petechiae, extravasation of blood into the subcutaneous tissues, and cerebral haemorrhage have been observed in some of these cases.

Diagnosis

The *clinical picture* is similar in most cases. The outstanding symptom is *jaundice*. The infant with biliary atresia is *not jaundiced at birth* because the bilirubin is cleared by the mother via the placenta. Holder [46] stated that the patient usually becomes icteric during the middle or later part of the first week of life.

Jaundice is at first mild, the skin being merely tinted pale yellow, but it gradually increases until at the end of a month or so

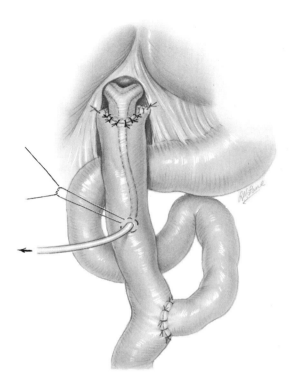

FIG. 8.   Resection of the gallbladder and choledochus cyst. Roux-en-Y anastomosis. Note the Y tube drainage of the hepatic ducts.

it is very intense and gives place to a greenish yellow hue. The cirrhotic liver at the same time slowly enlarges and feels unduly hard on palpation, its edge being rounded and firm. The spleen is usually palpable. The stools are white, putty-like, and acholic, while the urine is bile-laden and coloured dark brown. It should be noted that the stools are always white from birth, even though jaundice may not be noticed until the second week of life. The icteric index varies in different patients and from day to day in the same patient, ranging mostly between 50 and 200; the blood picture shows a secondary anaemia; the erythrocytes are not unduly fragile; there is no microspherocytosis; the clotting time is seldom increased; the prothrombin values may be somewhat lowered; and the liver function tests support a diagnosis of obstructive jaundice. The serum bilirubin estimations steadily increase, usually becoming stable in the 10- to 20-mg range. Diagnostic measures, although more

sophisticated than they were 20 years ago, are not as accurate as needed. Usually, as Holder has pointed out, the cause of the jaundice is not totally obstruction or totally disease of the liver cells, but a combination of the two, and usually the primary disease is one, with some degree of the other being present.

The serum transaminase estimations are occasionally of real value; [48] and the ^{131}I rose bengal test has proved most helpful in detecting complete obstruction.[42, 59] Percutaneous intrahepatic cholangiography has proved of little help in diagnosis. (See Chap. 46.)

The *condition may be confused with* icterus neonatorum, erythroblastosis foetalis, jaundice of haemolytic sepsis, obstruction of the bile ducts by biliary mud or sand, congenital syphilis, familial haemolytic anaemia, choledochus cyst, galactosemia, toxoplasmosis, and fibrocystic disease.

Every attempt should be made to reach a diagnosis within the first 4 weeks of life, and to correct the atresia at operation, as the majority of patients will die within 14 to 24 months if the obstruction is not relieved.

The diagnosis can be arrived at with a fair degree of certainty by the end of the first month of life by a process of elimination, and sometimes earlier than this. In other words, the diagnosis is arrived at with considerable certainty by excluding other causes of jaundice and by proving that the patient under investigation is suffering from obstructive jaundice.

About 10 to 15 percent of these babies present conditions of the extrahepatic ducts which are correctable only by operative measures. The mortality rates of the patients with total atresia is (obviously) 100 percent.

It is evident that if no patent duct exists outside the liver, the patient's condition will become progressively worse and he will die of biliary cirrhosis and its complications. Holder (1964) stated that in an effort to avoid this fate, a number of heroic attempts have been made to salvage some of these infants. Efforts to prolong life in some of these "inoperable cases" is being made by the implantation of "artificial bile ducts."

Dr. T. E. Starzl, of Denver, a pioneer in *liver transplantation,* presents a classic and

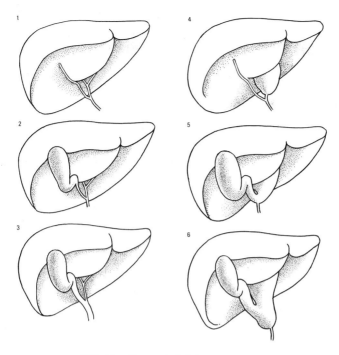

FIG. 9. Congenital biliary atresia.

illuminating account of his operation in Chapter 54.

The editorial comment in the Lancet [40] on *Congenital Atresia of the Bile Ducts* merits careful study.

Ladd and Gross, in their superb monograph: *Abdominal Surgery of Infancy and Childhood,* published by Saunders in 1941, state that they explored 45 cases of congenital atresia of the bile ducts; 9 of these patients were found to have a patent hepatic or common bile duct connecting with the intrahepatic ductal system but not with the duodenum. Of these 9, 3 died and 6 survived. Choledochoduodenostomy was performed 4 times and was followed by one death and three survivals. Cholecystoduodenostomy was carried out once—and with success. Cholecystostomy was performed once, with a fatal issue. *The six patients who have survived have been in excellent general health and have no symptoms suggesting ascending cholangitis or hepatitis.* One of their patients was alive and in splendid health more than 12 years after operation.

According to Gross,[45] *choledochoduodenostomy or hepaticoduodenostomy* is the operation of choice when the lower end of the common duct is atretic and when only a nubbin of the main bile duct is available for anastomosis to the intestine.

During recent years, a considerable amount of research work has been carried out on *human liver transplantation.* Nearly all early references on liver transplantation are concerned with experimental work in the dog or pig. Starzl et al.,[56, 57] however, have dealt with human liver transplantation: *(Extended survival in three cases of orthotopic homotransplantation of the human liver.)* Great credit is due to Starzl and his colleagues in Denver for achieving long-term survivals and for publishing results of human liver transplants. In his three successful cases, who had long-term survivals, two of these heroic operations were carried out for congenital biliary atresia and one for primary hepatoma of the liver. Starzl has brought this interesting subject up to date and has submitted his recent statistics, in his brilliant contribution in Chapter 54, to which the reader is referred.

Operative Treatment

Preoperative measures include small transfusions of blood and the administration of vitamin K. Penicillin is given before and after operation.

The *best incisions* are: (1) right upper paramedian; (2) rectus muscle-splitting incision; (3) transverse incision; or a McBurney right subtotal incision. (See Chap. 6.)

Considerable difficulty may be experienced in determining the type of malformation which is present. All the structures are small, the anomalies show wide variations, and from the duodenum and transverse colon there may be anomalous folds of membrane which tend to obscure the operative field. If the gallbladder is present and the common bile duct cannot be seen, a wise manoeuvre consists in inserting a hypodermic needle into the fundus of the gallbladder and distending the gallbladder with coloured saline solution. When the cystic duct is patent and the common bile duct is present, the fluid will distend the common bile duct and bring it rapidly into view. In some cases in which the lower reaches of the common bile duct are plugged with inspissated bile salts and biliary mud, this method may be sufficient to produce displacement of the obstructing "clump" and cause it to pass into the duodenum, thus relieving the obstruction.

Most surgeons practise operative cholangiography with the object of illuminating the existing ductal system. A hypodermic needle is introduced into the gallbladder or common hepatic duct and 5 ml of 40 percent hypaque injected slowly, carefully, and daintily. X-ray films should be taken immediately following the injection of the dye. Cholangiography takes little time and carries little risk, even to the patient with hepatic disease. If the cholangiogram reveals a segmental atresia of the choledochus, this condition is corrected. Where, however, there is a diffuse stenosis of the common bile duct, liver biopsy should be carried out as a routine measure alone. Although *cholecystogastrostomy* has been frequently practised for the relief of this condition, it is generally held that

choledochoduodenostomy, when feasible, is a superior operation in spite of its presenting greater technical difficulties.

When *choledochoduodenostomy* is being performed, the lower end of the common duct should be freed and divided, and a small, short, ureteric catheter about 1.5 cm long should be inserted upwards toward the common hepatic duct. An opening is made in the duodenum opposite the end of the duct and the small segment of catheter is led through the hole into the lumen of the bowel. With the tube in place, a row of six carefully applied interrupted through-and-through all-coats sutures of 5-0 chromic catgut or Dexon on a ½ circular 20 mm atraumatic (eyeless) intestinal needle are placed so as to anchor the wall of the duct to the duodenum. A mucosa-to-mucosa approximation must be achieved.

Hepaticoduodenostomy is likewise performed with one row of interrupted sutures of fine catgut.

When the gallbladder obviously contains bile, as demonstrated by aspiration into a Record syringe, the organ may be anastomosed to the stomach—*cholecystogastrostomy;* to the duodenum—*cholecystoduodenostomy;* or to a Roux-en-Y loop of proximal jejunum —*cholecystojejunostomy.*

In *cholecystogastrostomy,* the gallbladder is mobilised from the substance of the liver and swung over with the cystic duct and cystic artery as a pedicle. It is important to see that the cystic duct does not become kinked or twisted while the gallbladder is being anastomosed to the stomach. A side-to-side anastomosis is then made between the gallbladder and the anterior wall of the pyloric antrum. One row of fine chromic catgut sutures is used. Holden's views on the operation of choice may be summed up in his own words: *"In those patients who have lumen in an extrahepatic duct, the duct is anastomosed by a Roux-en-Y procedure to the jejunum"* [italics mine].

The operation of *cholecystojejunostomy* is described in the report of the author's case, in which the patient made a splendid recovery.

Case Report

History. Full-term breast-fed male infant (T.S.), normal at birth (Oct. 8, 1951), with weight of 7 lbs. The delivery was uneventful. During the second week of life jaundice was noticed, the urine was dark, and the stools became clay-coloured or white. No drugs or vaccines had been administered. The parents and two other children were alive and well. There was no family history of jaundice, syphilis, or congenital deformity. The patient was admitted under my care at the Southend General Hospital.

Examination. The infant was one month old, and his weight was 7 lbs., 11 oz. He was ill, apathetic, and jaundiced. No petechial haemorrhages or rashes could be seen and there was no evidence of sepsis of the skin or umbilicus. On inspection, the abdomen was slightly enlarged and there were no distended veins. There was a moderate degree of hepatomegaly as the rounded edge of the liver could be felt three fingerbreadths below the right costal margin. The spleen could not be felt. A nystagmus was present, with no other abnormal neurological signs. The urine was dark in colour and contained bile salts and pigments. No urobilinogen was present. The stools were white and obviously contained no bile pigments. The value for haemoglobin was 5.6 gm./100 ml. of blood (or 36 percent); the red cell count was 2,300,000; the colour index was 0.8; and leucocytes numbered 13,000/cu. mm. Red blood cells were of normal fragility, and 20 nucleated red cells were seen while 100 white blood cells were being counted. The Wassermann and Kahn reactions were negative. The Van den Bergh test gave a direct positive reaction and the serum bilirubin was 10.3 mg. percent. Blood grouping showed that both parents belonged to Group A and Rh-positive.

A diagnosis of congenital atresia of the bile ducts was made. The infant's general condition was improved by intravenous infusion of 120 ml. of blood, which raised the haemoglobin to 80 percent, and by the intramuscular administration of vitamins B and K.

Four days after admission to hospital the child's condition deteriorated, opisthotonus developed, and the nystagmus increased. The condition was diagnosed as an intracranial haemorrhage, and lumbar and ventricular punctures were performed. No cerebrospinal fluid was obtained on lumbar puncture and the ventricular fluid was tinted with blood.

The ventricular tap was repeated 2 days later and the fluid was blood-stained and xanthochromic. Six days later the circumference of the head had increased and bulging of the anterior fontanelle was prominent. The subdural spaces on each side were explored and 4 ml. of dark brown blood was removed from the right side. As no further haemorrhages occurred, operation was carried out, under ether anaesthesia, on Nov. 29, 1951.

Operation. The abdomen was explored through a right epigastric rectus muscle-splitting incision. Exposure revealed an enlarged cirrhotic dark green liver. The spleen was larger than normal and a small amount of yellowish ascitic fluid was removed by aspiration. The tiny gallbladder was tensely distended and the common bile duct

ended in a bulbous nubbin above the duodenum. A hypodermic needle was inserted into the fundus of the gallbladder and yellow bile was aspirated into a Record syringe, after which saline solution was forcibly injected to distend the minute ducts. The common bile duct ended abruptly about 3 mm. below the point of entrance of the cystic duct.

Cholecystojejunostomy was performed in order to bypass the obstruction. The fundus of the gallbladder was partially mobilised; a long loop of the proximal jejunum was drawn upward in front of the transverse colon; and the apex of the loop was anastomosed to the full length of the gallbladder by the side-to-side method, using one row of interrupted sutures of 4-0 chromic catgut mounted on an eyeless needle. Portions of the jejunum proximal and distal to the stoma were anchored to the capsule of the liver to relieve any tension on the suture line. The operation was completed by performing a Braun's side-to-side jejunojejunostomy with the object of diverting gastric and intestinal contents from the cholecystojejunal anastomosis. The individual layers of the abdominal wall were approximated with interrupted sutures of fine silk and a small dressing was strapped over the incision.

Postoperative progress. Bile was noticed in the vomitus the night after the operation and in the stools two days after. During the next week the jaundice began to fade and the urine became lighter in colour. The liver was not palpable 3 weeks after operation. The wound healed soundly; no further haemorrhages occurred; the appetite rapidly improved; and the infant made an uninterrupted recovery. He was discharged from hospital 6 weeks after operation, weighing 9 lbs., 2 oz. When examined at 15 months and 26 months after the operation, the infant looked the picture of health and was developing normally. At this writing, he is fat and well, and he is looking forward to celebrating his twenty-first birthday on Oct. 8, 1972.

PRIMARY SCLEROSING CHOLANGITIS

Primary sclerosing cholangitis is an uncommon condition in which a unique fibrosis of the submucosal and serosal layers of the wall of the duct is associated with marked narrowing of its lumen. The constricted area may be limited or segmental, or it may be diffuse, involving the major portion of the choledochus and even the right and left hepatic ducts. The disease was first described by Delbet[61] in 1924, and the first reference in English was submitted by an American, Dr. R. Miller, Jr., in 1927.

Classification

The *primary type,* of unknown aetiology, is very rare, and less than 60 authentic cases have been reported up to 1972. The ratio of males to females is 5:1, and the majority of cases submitted to operation are between the ages of 40 and 60. In 1965, Manesis,[62] and Smith and Loe,[65] recognized only 21 and 35 cases, respectively, according to their criteria. The following criteria have generally been accepted, as a prerequisite for the diagnosis of primary sclerosing cholangitis:

1. Progressive jaundice of the obstructive type.
2. Absence of biliary calculi.
3. No prior biliary surgery.
4. Generalized thickening and sclerosis of the walls of the biliary ductal system.
5. Absence of biliary tract malignancy, as determined by a reasonably long postoperative follow-up.
6. No evidence of primary biliary cirrhosis as determined by liver biopsy.
7. Absence of associated disease, such as ulcerative colitis, regional enteritis or retroperitoneal fibrosis, in which the biliary tract pathology may be simply secondary, more generalized, or systemic disease process.

In spite of considerable research work, the cause of the *primary* type remains obscure. Glenn and Whitsell (1966) reported 7 patients in whom the diagnosis of *primary* sclerosis cholangitis was clearly established. Holubitsky and McKenzie (1964) reported 4 cases of their own. Miller[63] described, in considerable detail, the clinical picture and operative findings in a 40-year-old doctor who presented what we would now consider a typical example of primary sclerosing cholangitis.

Diagnosis

In the early stages, the signs and symptoms are similar to those of chronic calculous cholecystitis, then of choledocholithiasis, while, later on, cholangitis and jaundice herald the onset of extrahepatic ductal obstruction.

The laboratory investigations suggest a diagnosis of obstructive jaundice, but, when there is marked parenchymal damage, the liver function tests may be misleading.

Intravenous cholangiography, percutaneous intrahepatic cholangiography, and barium-meal intestinal studies are, as a rule, unrewarding. For full details relating to the investigation and management of the jaundiced patient see Chapter 45.

Operation

The operative diagnosis of primary sclerosing cholangitis is made by palpation and visualisation of the fibrotic common bile duct, which feels like a firm cord or the vas deferens. Operative cholangiography is helpful in evaluating the extent of the disease. The gallbadder should not be removed, as it may be required at a later date for a bypass procedure.

T tube choledochostomy, if it is capable of being performed, is the operation of choice.

"It is difficult to explain how drainage through a very small T tube from the middle of the thickened duct with a tiny lumen relieves the signs and symptoms, but its effect at times is dramatic. The T tube should not be removed until it is no longer needed." [65]

All writers have emphasised the effectiveness of steroids and antibiotics in the treatment of primary sclerosing cholangitis.

To sum up: the treatment consists of prolonged T tube choledochostomy (if possible), and of corticosteroid therapy combined with the use of antibiotics and antihistamines for a long period.

FIBROSIS OF THE SPHINCTER OF ODDI

Fibrosis and stenosis of the sphincter of Oddi and/or of the papilla of Vater is a clinical entity and is often responsible for intermittent or continuous attacks of pain in the right hypochondrium, the epigastrium, the back and the scapular regions, with or without associated jaundice or dilatation of the biliary passages. Stenosis of the sphincter of Oddi may be defined as a sphincter that will not allow the passage of a dilator larger than a 3-mm Bakes' (Claude Welch, 1972).

Stenosis of the distal portion of the common bile duct was first described by Flörcken.[70] Fourteen years later Del Valle and Donovan [68] presented a clinicopathological analysis of patients with total or partial obstruction of the common bile duct resulting from chronic cicatricial inflammation of the papilla of Vater and termed the process *sclerosing choledocho-odditis.*

Acosta et al.[66] stated that the concept of biliary dysfunction as a result of spasm of the sphincter of Oddi in the absence of such organic changes in the ampulla was developed by many others. Olivier et al.,[75] and Partington,[76] have reported a number of cases and discussed the treatment of this condition by sphincterotomy.

According to Cattell et al.,[67] exploration of the common bile duct should be considered incomplete unless the surgeon has ruled out obstruction of the papilla or ampulla of Vater. In a few cases, stenosis of the terminal end of the duct may be present without any obvious pathological changes in the entire biliary tree. Hand [72] discussed this subject in his excellent paper An Anatomical Study of the Choledochoduodenal Area.

It is difficult to differentiate fibrosis of the sphincter of Oddi from stone impacted in the ampulla or papilla of Vater, calculus entrapped in the terminal portion of the choledochus, chronic pancreatitis, or cancer of the periampullary region. An impacted stone in the ampullary area is capable of producing a fibrous stricture from intraductal inflammatory reaction, and partial obstruction of the terminal portion of the duct may be a cause of choledocholithiasis. A mucosal stricture may be the only lesion demonstrated at operation. It is of course possible that oedematous papillitis associated with acute duodenitis may lead to "pin-point ampullary opening," "tight ampulla," and "fibrotic ampullary cuff." Previous trauma owing to injudicious dilatation of the bile passages with sounds, Desjardins forceps, etc., may be held responsible at least for a few cases.

Doubilet and Mulholland [69] maintained that fibrosis takes place only when inflammatory reaction has been associated with an impacted calculus in the ampulla or papilla, or when the end of the common bile duct

has been injured during dilatation with probes, sounds, scoops, and the like. They considered that any other obstruction in this region is caused by *spasm.*

Although spasm undoubtedly can occur at this point, the obstruction in many of our patients appeared to be a definite fibrotic stenosis, and it occurred when no common duct stones were present and when there had been no previous surgical treatment.[67]

McPhedran et al.,[73] in an autopsy study, and Gage et al.,[71] in a correlation of specimens obtained at operation and autopsy, concluded that there was no constant histological basis for clinically apparent obstruction of the choledochoduodenal junction. Paulino and Cavalcanti [77] examined 23 surgical biopsy specimens of the papilla of Vater and noted dense fibrosis in 3, glandular alterations in 12, and muscular hypertrophy in 20. Acosta et al.[66] stated that of 38 surgical specimens, 22 (57 percent) showed histological abnormalities consisting of fibrosis of the papilla in 10 instances, acute or chronic inflammatory infiltration in 9, and pseudopolyps composed of granulation tissue in 3. Muscular hypertrophy and cystic glandular dilatation accompanied the fibrosis or chronic inflammation. Fibrosis was the predominant pathological change in 10 instances (16 percent).

Stenosis of the sphincter of Oddi is more common in females than in males, the ratio being 3:1. The condition may reveal itself at any age, but it is most frequently observed between the ages of 50 and 70, the peak incidence being at about age 56.

Diagnosis

Signs and Symptoms

Pain, which is usually severe, is the most important symptom and is present in about 90 percent of patients. It may be continuous or intermittent and is localised to the right hypochondrium—although it may be referred to the back or right scapular region. In some instances pain is felt most acutely below the left subcostal margin.

Symptoms of *gallstone colic* are observed in about 15 to 20 percent of patients.

Approximately 50 percent of patients are

jaundiced or give a past history of jaundice, while about 10 percent suffer from *subclinical jaundice,* that is, the serum bilirubin estimations are above normal values but there is no yellow staining of the conjunctivae.

Other symptoms include *nausea, anorexia, indigestion, epigastric distress* after fatty meals, *vomiting,* and *pruritus.*

In one of my series, of 31 patients, the duration of symptoms ranged from a few months to over 30 years.

Some 80 percent of patients have had a previous cholecystectomy or an exploration of the biliary passages, and these procedures had failed to relieve their symptoms.

BLOOD EXAMINATION

Anaemia and/or leucocytosis may be present; the serum bilirubin estimations are elevated in some 50 percent of the patients; the transaminase estimations show a steep rise in 30 percent, while the alkaline phosphatase is elevated in 50 to 60 percent. (See Chapter 45.)

RADIOLOGICAL INVESTIGATIONS

These include (1) intravenous cholangiography; (2) percutaneous intrahepatic cholangiography (when jaundice is present); and (3) barium-meal or Gastrografin x-ray examination of the stomach and duodenum.

(Operative cholangiography is discussed in Chapter 43, Part A, and Retrograde Pancreatography and Cholangiography by Fibreduodenoscopy in Chapter 34, Part B.)

Operative Procedures

The abdomen is best explored through a right epigastric muscle-splitting incision, and a vertical scar (or scars) of a previous operation should be excised.

In the Lahey Clinic series [67] of 100 consecutive patients with partial or complete stenosis of the sphincter of Oddi—operated upon between October 1952 and January 1956—81 had had a previous cholecystectomy and 40 had also had an exploration of the common duct; 21 had had two previous operations and 1 had had four. In approxi-

mately 70 percent of cases, the common duct was obviously dilated, while in the remainder the duct was not dilated or only moderately so. Stones or biliary sand were found in nearly half of the cases, and cystic duct remnant in 20 percent.

Olivier et al.[75] reported on 92 patients with stenosing sphincteritis with an operative mortality rate of 6.5 percent. Acute pancreatitis was responsible for 4 of the 7 postoperative deaths.

Associated pancreatitis is present in about 15 percent of cases, and concomitant lesions —such as hiatal hernia, duodenal ulcer, and diverticulitis of the colon—are by no means infrequent.[78]

After freeing existing adhesions, the common bile duct is displayed in the manner already described and operative cholangiography carried out, provided this investigation is not considered to be superfluous under the circumstances.

Two stay sutures of fine chromic catgut are introduced into the anterior wall of the duct, about 3 mm apart, and then elevated by an assistant while the surgeon makes a small longitudinal incision through the wall of the duct and between the sutures. Escaping bile and detritus (when present) are immediately aspirated, after which the ducts are explored by means of probes, sounds, dilators, scoops, and the like.

A diagnosis of impacted stone, fibrous stricture of the lower end of the choledochus, or stenosis of the sphincter of Oddi or papilla of Vater is made if a 3-mm dilator cannot be passed through the ampulla and then onward into the duodenum.

It is sometimes difficult to ascertain whether the end of the dilator lies within the lumen of the duodenum or is trapped in the ampulla. It is, of course, possible to force the stenosed and fibrotic ampullary region farther downward in the gut or upward against the anterior wall of the duodenum where it can be palpated—and even mistaken for the bulbous end of the dilator.

The anterior duodenal wall should be incised *obliquely* and at a point opposite to where the end of the probe or sound can be felt through the bowel wall. Duodenal contents are aspirated, small retractors are inserted, the papilla is visualised, Babcock forceps are placed on either side of the

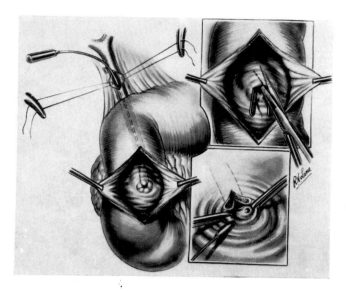

FIG. 10.   Fibrosis of the sphincter of Oddi. Transduodenal sphincterotomy. (Maingot's technique.)

papilla to elevate the posterior wall of the duodenum, and the end of the dilator is gently forced upward in order to deliver the implicated ampulla through the duodenotomy incision.

In a few instances, a small stone is found impacted in the papilla or a mucosal stricture is present, causing obstruction at this site. Papillotomy—simple longitudinal division of the papilla of Vater—followed by sphincterotomy should be performed for such lesions, in spite of the fact that in some cases the ampulla may be normal.

Microscopic examination of a small portion of the papilla and ampulla should be carried out when the sphincter is densely hard, grossly hypertrophied, or the possibility of carcinoma cannot be excluded. When biopsy had been performed on specimens from a number of personal cases, the patho-

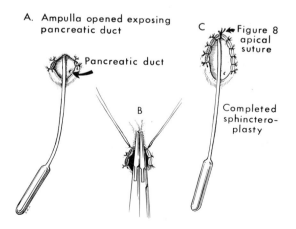

A. Ampulla opened exposing pancreatic duct

Pancreatic duct

B

C   Figure 8 apical suture

Completed sphincteroplasty

FIG. 11.   Sphincteroplasty. (Courtesy of Dr. S. Austin Jones.) (See also Chap. 43B.)

logical findings invariably showed "inflammatory tissue and fibrotic reaction."

The operation of sphincterotomy is described in Chapters 38A, 43A and 44. A simple method of performing transduodenal sphincterotomy is illustrated in Figure 10. The surgeon may elect to perform *sphincteroplasty* (instead of sphincterotomy) by the technique advocated by Austin Jones in Chapter 43, Part B. (See Fig. 11.)

A significant statement by Hand [72] is worthy of emphasis. He writes:

The arrangement of the musculature of the lower duct system is of significance in relation to sphincterotomy, whether performed as part of a duct exploration for calculus or for pancreatic disease. The present studies show that the extent of the usual operation will destroy the common channel and narrowest part of the common bile duct, but will not cut by any means all of the muscle surrounding and controlling the lower end of the common bile and pancreatic ducts, although it will leave a common bile duct whose minimal bore is greater than it was preoperatively.

Following sphincterotomy, or sphincteroplasty, a short-guttered T tube for drainage of the ductal system should be used. Cattell's long-armed T tube is not suitable for choledochostomy, as the lower limb may, on its way through the ampulla into the duodenum, occlude the mouth of the duct of Wirsung and initiate an attack of acute pancreatitis.

The sphincterotomy incision through the papilla and ampulla should be about 1.5 cm long, and in the direction of ten o'clock.

In order to control any bleeding points, a few interrupted sutures of fine catgut may be introduced through each splayed-out margin and tied lightly.

During recent years *lateral choledochoduodenostomy* is being performed on an increasing number of cases of stenosis of the sphincter of Oddi and of recurrent stones in the bile ducts. The results have been gratifying, especially *when a large stoma has been constructed* between the common duct and duodenum. The complication of "ascending" cholangitis is caused by obstruction of the anastomosis and not by the reflux of gastric and duodenal contents. It is, as Madden puts it, a "descending" rather than an "ascending" infection.

Postoperative Complications

The operative mortality rate of sphincterotomy for fibrosis of the sphincter of Oddi is about 2 to 3 percent. In the Lahey Clinic series of 100 cases,[67] there were 2 hospital deaths. Riddell and Kirtley [78] reported on 31 patients with no postoperative fatalities. In my series of 31 cases, 1 death from acute pancreatitis occurred on the fortieth postoperative day.

The *most common complications* are: (1) haemorrhage, (2) duodenal fistula, (3) leakage of bile and duodenal contents around and about the T tube, (4) gastric stasis resulting from partial duodenal obstruction due to excessive inversion of the duodenotomy incision, (5) cholangitis, (6) acute pancreatitis, and (7) subphrenic abscess. Nardi [74] gives an interesting and instructive account of acute cholangitis due to fibrosis of the sphincter of Oddi.

REFERENCES

Choledochus cyst

1. Alonso-Lej et al., Int. Abst. Surg. 108:1, 1959.
2. Arthur and Stewart, Br. J. Surg. 51:671, 1964.
3. Blocker et al., Arch. Surg. 34:695, 1937.
4. Chesterman, J. Obstet. Gynaecol. Br. Emp. 51: 512, 1944.
5. Dexter, Br. J. Cancer 11:18, 1957.
6. Douglas, Monthly J. Med. Sci. London 14:97, 1852.
7. Engle and Salmon, Arch. Surg. 88:345, 1964.
8. Farris and Yadeau, Proc. Mayo Clin. 39:332, 1964.
9. Fischer, Zentralbl. Chir. 83:1234, 1958.
10. Fonkalsrud and Boles, Surg. Gynecol. Obstet. 121:733, 1965.
11. Friend, Br. J. Surg. 46:155, 1958.
12. George and Maingot, Br. J. Surg. 50:339, 1962.
13. Gross, J. Pediat. 3:730, 1933.
14. Gross, The Surgery of Infancy and Childhood, Philadelphia, Saunders, 1953.
15. Irwin and Morison, Br. J. Surg. 32:319, 1944.
16. Jones et al., Ann. Surg. 180:190, 1958.
17. Jones, P., et al., J. Pediat. Surg. 6:112, 1971.
18. Kasi and Asakura, Ann. Surg. 172:844, 1970.
19. Lees et al., Arch. Surg. 99:19, 1969.
20. Lorenzo et al., Am. J. Surg. 121:510, 1971.
21. McLaughlin, Ann. Surg. 123:1047, 1946.
22. O'Neill and Clatworthy, Am. Surg. 37:230, 1971.
23. Rogers and Priestley, Proc. Mayo Clin. 24:568, 1949.
24. Shallow, Eger, and Wagner, Ann. Surg. 123:119, 1946.

25. Shields, Am. J. Surg. 108:142, 1964.
26. Shocket et al., Proc. Mayo Clin. 30:83, 1955.
27. Smith, B., Arch. Surg. 44:963, 1942.
28. Sterry Asby, Br. J. Surg. 51:493, 1964.
29. Swartley, Ann. Surg. 118:91, 1943.
30. Swartley and Weeder, Ann. Surg. 101:912, 1935.
31. Trout and Longmire, Am. J. Surg. 121:68, 1971.
32. Tsardakas and Robnett, Arch. Surg. 72:311, 1956.
33. Tsuchida and Ishida, Surgery 69:776, 1971.
34. Warren et al., Surg. Clin. North Am. 48:567, 1968.
35. Yotuyanagi, Gann 30:601, 1936.

Congenital atresia of bile ducts

36. Beaven and Duncan, Br. J. Surg. 33:378, 1946.
37. Cameron and Brunton, Br. Med. J. 2:1253, 1960.
38. Chesterman, Br. J. Surg. 29:52, 1941.
39. Durell and Halliwell, Lancet 2:1203, 1952.
40. Editorial comment, Congenital Atresia of the Bile Ducts Lancet 2:179, 1963.
41. Foukalsrud et al., Am. Surg. 37:389, 1971.
42. Ghadimi and Sass-Kortsak, New Engl. J. Med. 265:351, 1961.
43. Gray et al., Proc. Mayo Clin. 23:473, 1948.
44. Greaney et al., Am. J. Surg. 88:17, 1954.
45. Ladd and Gross, The Surgery of Infancy and Childhood, Philadelphia, Saunders, 1941.
46. Holder, Am. J. Surg. 107:458, 1964.
47. Holmes, Am. J. Dis. Child. 11:405, 1961.
48. Kove et al., Am. J. Dis. Child. 100:47, 1960.
49. Krovetz, Surgery 47:453, 1960.
50. Ladd, J.A.M.A. 91:1082, 1928.
51. Ladd, Ann. Surg. 102:742, 1935.
52. Longmire, Ann. Surg. 159:335, 1964.
53. Maingot, Br. Med. J. 1:1256, 1955.
54. Moore, Surg. Gynecol. Obstet. 96:215, 1953.
55. Schnug, Ann. Surg. 148:931, 1958.

56. Starzl et al., Ann. Surg. 160:411, 1964.
57. Starzl et al., Surgery 63:549, 1968.
58. Thomson, J., Edinburgh Med. J. 37:523, 1892.
59. White et al., Pediatrics 32:239, 1963.

Primary sclerosing cholangitis

60. Cutler and Donaldson, Am. J. Surg. 169:276, 1969.
61. Delbet and Bull, Mem. Soc. Nat. Chir. 50:1144, 1924.
62. Manesis and Sullivan, Arch. Intern. Med. 115:187, 1965.
63. Miller, R., Jr., Ann. Surg. 86:296, 1927.
64. Myers et al., Am. J. Gastroenterol. 53:527, 1970.
65. Smith and Loe, Am. J. Surg. 110:239, 1965.

Fibrosis of the sphincter of Oddi

66. Acosta et al., Surg. Gynecol. Obstet. 124:787, 1967.
67. Cattell et al., The Surgical Practice of the Lahey Clinic, Philadelphia, Saunders, 1962, p. 595.
68. Del Valle and Donovan, Arch. Argent. Enferm. Ap. Digest 4:1, 1926.
69. Doubilet and Mulholland, J.A.M.A. 160:521, 1956.
70. Flörcken, Dtsch. Z. Chir. 123:604, 1912.
71. Gage et al., Surgery 48:304, 1960.
72. Hand, Br. J. Surg. 50:486, 1963.
73. McPhedran et al., Arch. Surg. 83:146, 1961.
74. Nardi, Surg. Clin. North Am. 50:1137, 1970.
75. Olivier et al., J. Clin. Pathol. 89:269, 1965.
76. Partington, Surg. Gynecol. Obstet. 123:282, 1966.
77. Paulino and Cavalcanti, Surgery 48:698, 1960.
78. Riddell and Kirtley, Ann. Surg. 149:773, 1959.

48

A. TRAUMATIC INJURIES OF THE GALLBLADDER AND BILE DUCTS

RODNEY MAINGOT

TRAUMATIC RUPTURE OF THE GALLBLADDER

Traumatic rupture of the gallbladder without any associated injuries to the other abdominal organs is a rare condition. Nevertheless, cases have been reported wherein the gallbladder alone has been amputated [44] or has been torn—e.g., in automobile accidents, by a kick or direct blow to the right hypochondrium, or when the right lower ribs have been crushed inward by some external violence.

Penn [46] stated that in large series of penetrating and nonpenetrating abdominal injuries the gallbladder injuries constituted only 2 percent. He reviewed the literature and added five cases of his own. To the usual classification of gallbladder injuries—contusion, avulsion, laceration—Penn adds a fourth group: traumatic cholecystitis.

In stabs, gunshot wounds, and other types of penetrating lesions, the liver and adjacent structures are nearly always implicated.

The mortality rates recorded appear to be greatly influenced by the extent of frequently *associated intraperitoneal injuries,* and they vary from 15 to 40 percent.

According to Penn, the following organs are also commonly injured when the gallbladder is contused, avulsed from its bed, or torn as the result of external violence: liver, 72 percent; small intestine, 36 percent; and colon, 32 percent. Diethrich et al. [10] reviewed the case records of three hospitals for 25 years ending in 1965 and found only 61 cases of traumatic wounds of the extrahepatic biliary tract.

Thirteen patients were females and 48 were males; the average age was 26 years. Gunshot wounds accounted for 35 of the injuries; 29 were stab wounds; and 6 were blunt injuries.

The gallbladder was lacerated in 54 cases (88 percent) and the common bile duct was involved in 7 (12 percent). Associated visceral injuries occurred in all but 6 cases. The liver was injured in 15 cases and the liver plus one other organ in 16. About 50 percent of patients with gunshot injuries were admitted to hospital in severe shock.

Suture closure of a perforation or a laceration of the gallbladder was performed only once in 29 patients. Cholecystectomy was carried out in the other cases. One stab wound transecting the common bile duct was treated with end-to-end anastomosis followed by T tube splintage. A laceration of the common hepatic duct and division of the cystic duct were treated by direct repair and excision of the gallbladder, respectively.

Perforation of the duodenum associated with laceration of the choledochus occurred in two cases. Drainage of a bile duct pseudocyst resulted in a satisfactory outcome. The right upper quadrant was drained with a corrugated latex tube in all cases of biliary tract injury. Most patients were given antibiotics. In all 7 patients who died, at least two organs had been injured in addition to the extrahepatic biliary tract. No patients with stab wounds died. Missile injuries involving several organ systems accounted for most deaths.

With *nonpenetrating injuries,* the gallbladder injury may be *solitary,* as is usually the case in some 30 percent of gallbladder injuries caused by blunt trauma.

Manlove et al. [38] stated that blunt-trauma injuries to the gallbladder are rare, only 50 cases being reported up to 1959. Watkins [69] reported that the cystic artery or duct alone may be torn and will necessitate cholecystectomy. Again, instances of rupture of the cystic artery alone have been reported in which, in addition to brisk haemorrhage, thrombosis and gangrene of the gallbladder occurred (Hoffman, 1956).

Nonpenetrating injuries of the gallbladder present a clinical picture that is quite characteristic. Following the receipt of the injury, there is always a marked degree of shock, with recovery from shock within a few hours. The patient will complain that he has a constant dull pain in the right upper quadrant of the abdomen, which may be specially severe below the right costal margin. From the first to the tenth day, the abdomen slowly but increasingly distends with bile, and within 4 to 5 days, the tinge of jaundice will be noticed. The jaundice becomes progressively more intense, the stools become clay-colored, the urine is laden with bile, and wasting is soon evident. By the end of the third week there is progressive loss of strength, with rapidly rising pulse rate, pyrexia, and marked exhaustion. Paracentesis will disclose that there is free bile in the peritoneal cavity and thus clinch the diagnosis.[55]

Treatment. The treatment consists of simple suture of the laceration, cholecystostomy, or cholecystectomy. The treatment employed depends upon the general condition of the patient and the extent of the injury. The majority of cases of perforation or laceration of the gallbladder are best treated by cholecystectomy.

TRAUMATIC RUPTURE OF THE BILE DUCTS

Hart[17] reported eight cases of *spontaneous perforation of the common bile duct* and two cases of spontaneous perforation of the hepatic duct; he also recorded an additional case of gangrene of the common duct with perforation. Snyder,[54] in reporting a case of spontaneous rupture of the hepatic duct, states that a careful review of the literature reveals that this condition is rare, only four such cases having been reported.

Rupture of the bile ducts is another rare complication of trauma to the right upper quadrant of the abdomen. Rudberg[47] reviewed the subject and collected 40 cases.

Lewis[23] found 6 additional cases in the literature (including the one reported by Edlington,[14] and gave an illuminating account of his own patient in whom two operations proved necessary. Lysaght[27] reported a case of complete rupture of the common duct, and Grimault[16] recorded a case of injury to the choledochus associated with transection of the pyloric part of the stomach. Salgado,[48] in reporting a case of traumatic rupture of the common hepatic duct, stated that only 52 similar cases have been described in the literature. Hicken and Stevenson[19] have recorded the successful handling of a case of traumatic rupture of the choledochus associated with acute haemorrhagic pancreatitis and bile peritonitis. In the case reported by Milnes Walker,[59] a successful result was achieved by anastomosing a small rent at the bifurcation of the hepatic duct to a loop of proximal jejunum. Baty[1] reported on a patient with traumatic rupture of the hepatic duct (caused by a buffer accident) who was successfully treated following two operations. Mason et al.[39] were able to trace about 100 cases of bile duct injuries caused by violent trauma. Hinshaw et al.[20] could find only 14 instances of *complete transection of the choledochus;* they also presented an account of a patient they treated successfully. Dobbie and Stormo[4] reviewed 14 cases in 1968; J. Stewart reported a case in 1961, and Parkinson[45] (1970) gave an interesting account of his patient who sustained complete severance of the common bile duct due to blunt trauma and was successfully treated by end-to-end repair of the duct plus T tube choledochostomy. In the period from 1954 through 1963, Hartman and Greaney[18] encountered 5 cases of blunt-trauma *injury to the biliary tract in children.* The most striking feature of the clinical course in their patients was the delay in diagnosis and treatment of the bile peritonitis. As much as 6 weeks elapsed before the free escape of bile into the peritoneal cavity was corrected. Despite the presence of prolonged bile peritonitis in several cases, successful repair of the varied biliary-tract injuries was rewarded with a high recovery rate.

A common cause of rupture of the bile passages is crushing trauma to the right hypochondriac region, and especially the right costal margin. Why the ducts should be torn

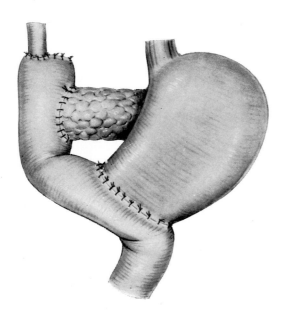

FIG. 1. Pancreatoduodenectomy performed for pulping of the lower end of the bile duct, the second portion of the duodenum, and a localised part of the head of the pancreas.

without there being any associated laceration of the liver, as in the case in many of the reports, is very difficult to understand. The explanation that seems most logical to Lewis is that the force is applied in such a direction as to crush the duct between the liver and the bodies of the vertebrae at that level. The reason for the absence of fractures of the ribs or injury to any of the hollow abdominal viscera in some cases is also difficult to explain. In a number of the reported cases, the trauma resulted from the patients' being crushed between two motorcars.

The *clinical picture* is identical with that of rupture of the gallbladder without associated injuries to the liver and other viscera, i.e., shock, recovery from shock, constant pain over the right costal margin, a slowly filling abdomen, the appearance of jaundice, rising temperature and pulse rate, and the onset of toxaemia.

On tapping the abdomen, large quantities of bile-stained fluid are immediately withdrawn. The bile apparently remains uninfected for a considerable period. Relatively few cases of suppurative "bile" peritonitis

have been reported in the literature. With some *steeringwheel, buffer,* or *"crushing" accidents,* the injuries sustained by the liver, gallbladder, bile ducts, head of the pancreas, and second portion of the duodenum may be very severe and extensive. About 3 years ago I performed *pancreatoduodenectomy* upon a man, aged 42, who was involved in a motorcar accident that caused extensive *pulping* of the lower end of the common duct, the head of the pancreas, and the second part of the duodenum. Following a protracted and stormy convalescence he made a satisfactory recovery (Fig. 1).

Treatment. Access to the biliary passages is obtained through a right paramedian or oblique subcostal incision. As soon as the peritoneum is opened, large quantities of bile will pour through the wound. A suction tube should be inserted into the abdominal cavity and all the pent-up fluid aspirated. It will be noted that all the abdominal organs are deeply bile-stained and that there is, as a rule, no evidence of localised or generalised peritonitis.

Adhesions that are glued to the gallbladder or portal fissure should be gently separated, after which the operative field should be carefully packed off with a long strip of gauze to permit good retraction and exposure of the gallbladder and biliary passages.

Most of these patients are jaundiced, dehydrated, and very ill; thus any prolonged operation is usually out of the question. Nevertheless, a most careful search must be made for a rent in the duct. The most common situation for the laceration is high up in the common hepatic duct close to the junction of the right and left hepatic ducts. It is very difficult to identify and more difficult still to repair. The ideal treatment is closure of the rent in the bile duct with interrupted sutures of 000 medium chromic catgut, making a small opening in the anterior wall of the choledochus for the insertion of a Y tube or a T tube, the upper limb of which acts as an efficient splint for the traumatised area of the duct. The procedure includes aspiration of the bile-stained fluid in the peritoneal cavity and draining the subhepatic region with a sheet of soft corrugated rubber or latex. In desperate cases, however, the insertion of the cigarette drain or a large rubber catheter down to the rent in the hepatic

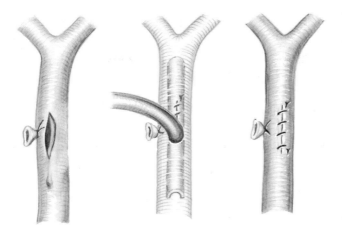

FIG. 2. A small laceration in the anterior wall of the choledochus. The incision in the duct may be closed by the insertion of a few interrupted sutures of 000 chromic catgut or by performing T tube choledochostomy.

duct suffices, as this provides a means of continuous decompression.

Lacerations of the common bile duct are more easily dealt with than those of the hepatic duct, as the majority of them are situated in the anterior wall of the duct. They may be longitudinal or transverse, or again there may be a complete transverse rupture of the duct. When the tear involves only the anterior wall, it is an easy matter to insert a T tube and close the walls of the duct around the issuing limb (Figs. 2 and 3). When, however, the duct is completely torn across, one of two plans may be adopted. If the patient is in good condition, after mobilisation of the duodenum and head of the pancreas, the ends of the duct should be picked up, freshened, and sutured together with a single layer of 000 catgut or Dexon sutures. A T tube is then above the suture line, but never brought out through the line of anastomosis itself.

John and James Donald,[12] in reporting on a patient who had a completely severed common bile duct owing to nonpenetrating

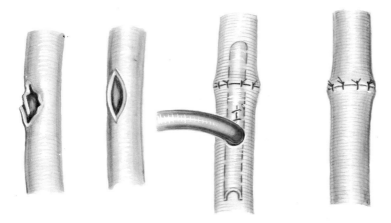

FIG. 3. Avulsion of the gallbladder and cystic duct caused by blunt trauma. The methods of repair are illustrated. Note that the T tube does not emerge through the line of anastomosis.

trauma ("an iron bar struck him across the upper abdomen"), stated that the patient was successfully treated by end-to-end anastomosis of the severed duct combined with T tube choledochostomy. *T tube drainage, however, is unnecessary when the newly fashioned stoma is judged to be "amply capacious."*

If the lower end of the common bile duct is badly lacerated, pulped, or impossible to isolate, it is better to tie and to invaginate the proximal end of the duct and to anastomose the gallbladder to the duodenum or to the proximal jejunum, whichever seems easier and safer in the circumstances.[18] Before proceeding with the anastomosis, the surgeon must be certain that the cystic duct is patent, and is in no way traumatised.

In some instances, it may be possible to anastomose the freshenèd end of the proximal portion of the common bile duct to the duodenum, or, preferably, to a loop of proximal jejunum combined with Braun's jejunojejunostomy. When the right or left hepatic ducts are transected, the surgeon should perform axial anastomoses and splint the union with an inlaying T tube or Maingot's long Y tube, which can be withdrawn after a few weeks. A careful and methodical search should always be conducted for the presence of lacerations and perforations of other abdominal viscera, and these, when found, should be treated *secundum artem*. (See Chaps. 8, 35, 51, and 84.)

The *preoperative diagnosis* is based on the clinical features of the case, a study of plain x-ray films of the abdomen, and paracentesis. *Operative cholangiography* affords considerable help in the diagnosis of some of these complicated lesions of the bile ducts.

B. POSTOPERATIVE STRICTURES OF THE BILE DUCTS: CAUSES AND PREVENTION; DIAGNOSIS: RECONSTRUCTION OPERATIONS

RODNEY MAINGOT

This section deals with man-made strictures of the extrahepatic bile ducts, which account for 90 to 95 percent of all the so-called benign or simple strictures of these ducts.

We are not here concerned with the remaining 5 to 10 percent of benign strictures, which include congenital atresia of the biliary passages, choledochal cyst, fibrosis of the sphincter of Oddi, primary or acquired schlerosing cholangitis, recurrent pancreatitis, hydatid cyst of the liver, pericholedochal abscess, external blunt trauma, stricture due to erosion of a gallstone into the common hepatic duct, or fistulas between the lower end of the common bile duct and the duodenum caused by stone or penetrating posterior-wall duodenal ulcer.

To be more precise, *benign strictures of the bile ducts most frequently follow cholecystectomy* for acute or chronic cholecystitis, exploration of the biliary passages for stone, sphincterotomy, excision of a diverticulum of the second portion of the duodenum, radical pancreatic surgery, partial gastrectomy for a large penetrating duodenal ulcer, and resection of the hepatic flexure of the colon for carcinoma in which the growth has become attached to the liver, gallbladder, and duodenum.

Analyses of numerous cases have proved that the culpable operations were: cholecystectomy, 90 percent; choledochostomy and exploration of the biliary passages, 5 percent; and partial gastrectomy, 3 percent. The remaining 2 percent were caused by other procedures on the choledochus, duodenum, or pancreas.

There is no more distressing situation in abdominal surgery than the responsibility of treating a patient who has developed a stricture of the bile ducts following an operation on the biliary apparatus. The occurrence of such a stricture is a catastrophe not only to the patient but to the surgeon who performs the operation. The tragedy of such an event can be gauged by remembering that the majority of the patients are women under the age of 50, and that only 70 to 75 percent of them are *permanently cured* by a reconstructive procedure.

According to Warren, Mountain, and Midell,[67] the average age of the 987 patients treated for postoperative strictures of the bile ducts at the Lahey Clinic Foundation was 42 years, and the female-to-male ratio was 3:1.

Cattell and Braasch[3] state that in their experience there is approximately a 30 percent chance that the patient will eventually die from attempts made to repair the stricture or from the effects of intermittent or complete biliary obstruction. Many of these unfortunate patients have had several unsuccessful operations for relief of obstruction before being referred to a specialist in this field. I have had patients sent to me who were deeply jaundiced and cirrhotic and who had had as many as six or more previous operations for the correction of strictured ducts. From economic considerations alone, this disability is staggering. The seriousness of these mishaps is so great that minute attention to the details of operative procedures upon the biliary tract should be constantly stressed.

INCIDENCE

Owing to the dearth of statistical material on the subject, except from large institutions such as the Mayo Clinic and the Lahey Clinic Foundations, it is difficult to determine the true incidence of the development of postoperative stricture of the bile ducts following operations upon the gallbladder and biliary passages. At the Mayo Clinic, the yearly average number of reconstructive operations on the bile ducts exceeds 100. For obvious reasons, these statistics are not truly representative of the general experience. Howard Gray believed that postoperative lesions of the bile ducts were increasing in frequency. He reported [11] a series of 700 cases from the Mayo Clinic. Waugh and his colleagues [70] recorded 180 operations in 1951 for benign strictures of the bile ducts, with a mortality rate of 4.4 percent.

Walters and Kelly [63] have recorded their experiences of the operative management of 254 patients with postoperative strictures of the extrahepatic bile ducts. Walters et al.[60] submitted a study of more than 400 cases of strictures of the common and hepatic ducts, to which I will refer presently. Lahey and Pyrtek [22] reported a consecutive series of 314 cases of postoperative stricture of the bile ducts. This comprehensive, authoritative, and profusely illustrated article contains a wealth of important information on the subject. Cosman and Porter [9] recorded a series of 80 common duct strictures and estimate that their hospital incidence of bile duct injury is 0.2 percent, or two cases per 1,000 cholecystectomies. The articles by Cattell and Braasch,[2, 3, 4] and by Warren and Braasch,[66] have proved of immense value to surgeons who are called upon to undertake reconstruction procedures on the bile ducts. These papers contain a number of excellent illustrations, detailed descriptions of operative procedures, and relevant statistical data. Cattell stated that from 1919 to May 1958, 690 patients with benign biliary stricture were treated at the Lahey Clinic, with 1,006 operative procedures.

Michie and Gunn,[42] in an able article, write on the *incidence of bile duct injuries* as follows;

Surgical mishap is not readily publicized and, as reconstructive surgery is not infrequently undertaken in a different hospital from that in which the injury occurred, it may be difficult to obtain an accurate estimate of the number of bile-duct injuries. In the inter-war years, Berner and Norrlin (1931) reported an incidence of 1 injury per 450 cholecystectomies. Rosenqvist and Myrin (1960) quoted 43 in the 21,530 gallstone operations in Sweden in 1956, and concluded that if all total and partial injuries could be calculated, the frequency in Swedish hospitals would be 1 bile duct injury per 300–400 gallstone operations. Madsen, Sorensen, and Trailsen (1960) gave an incidence of 1 case per 327 cholecystectomies in Denmark, and Viikari (1960) 1 per 508 in Finland.

In the hospital complex in Aberdeen, 8 duct injuries were dealt with during the years 1951–1960 inclusive, 2 of which were referred from other hospitals. During these years 2,322 cholecystectomies were performed, giving an incidence of 1 accidental injury per 387 operations. In Scotland, during 1961, which is the first year for which Scottish morbidity statistics are available, 2,532 cholecystectomies were carried out, with (on the basis of 1 injury per 400 cholecystectomies) potential duct injury to 6–7 cases. Assuming gallbladder pathology and surgical competence to be the same for the United Kingdom generally as for Scotland, it can be estimated that approximately 60–65 cases of common duct injury may occur in the United Kingdom annually.

The ratio of women to men is 3:1, and the peak age incidence is about 42.

Few reports on injuries to the bile ducts are available from the British Isles. At a meeting of the Association of Surgeons of Great Britain and Ireland (May 1953), I discussed my experience with 28 cases of my own. Since then a number of my contributions have appeared.[28-30, 34]

This section is based mainly on information collected from the writings of Cattell, Kenneth Warren, Waltman Walters, Waugh, Priestley, Frank Glenn, Rodney Smith, and Warren Cole, and from personal experience gained in performing 131 operations on 109 patients with bile-duct strictures.

I have been fortunate in having had many opportunities of witnessing the courage, endurance, craftsmanship, and skill displayed by various surgeons in the management of these difficult cases in various clinics in the United States. I have been present at no fewer than 35 operations for the repair of strictures of the bile ducts, and such success as I have obtained in this field is due largely to the painstaking tuition and encouragement which I received from Dr. R. B. Cattell and Dr. K. W. Warren.

PREVENTION

The most important aspect of strictures of the bile ducts is *prevention*.

The value of good anaesthesia with complete muscular relaxation, exposure of the operative field through adequate incisions, the best possible illumination, wide retraction with Deaver or Harrington retractors, the putting of the common bile duct on the stretch, and the careful anatomical dissection of the cystic artery and the bile ducts in Calot's triangle has already been stressed. During the performance of cholecystectomy, the cystic artery must be isolated, dissected free, and its point of entry into the neck of the gallbladder must be clearly demonstrated before it is underrun with an aneurysm needle, doubly ligated, and divided. The

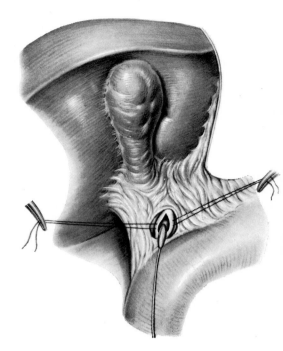

FIG. 4. Preliminary choledochotomy with insertion of a sound into the right hepatic duct to facilitate dissection of Calot's triangle in a difficult cholecystectomy. The sound acts as a useful guide to the lateral borders of the main ducts. (Lahey Clinic.)

cystic artery should in the majority of cases be securely tied and cut *before* the cystic duct is fully straightened out and a ligature applied to it near—very near—to the point where it enters the junction of the common hepatic and common bile ducts.

In those cases in which the hepatoduodenal ligament is laden with fat, fibrotic, and Colot's triangle is obscured with adhesions, it is often advisable to perform a preliminary choledochotomy and insert a sound or a Bakes' dilator into the right hepatic duct. The sound acts as a useful guide during the dissection of the cystic artery and cystic duct (Fig. 4). Again, during the performance of partial gastrectomy for a penetrating duodenal ulcer, the insertion of the arm of a long T tube *into the duodenum* serves as a useful "marker" during a perilous dissection.

These three ducts must be demonstrated to a "critical" assistant before the ligature is applied to the cystic duct (Fig. 5).

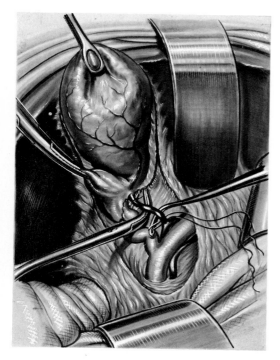

FIG. 5. The cystic artery should be isolated, ligatured, and divided *before* ligating and dividing the cystic duct.

CAUSES

The causes of injuries to the bile ducts during operation and of postoperative strictures of the common and hepatic ducts may be listed as follows:

1. Haemorrhage from the cystic artery, an anomalous cystic artery, an accessory cystic artery, the right hepatic artery, or an aberrant right hepatic artery.
2. Poor exposure; poor assistance; inadequate illumination of the operative field; unsatisfactory anaesthesia.
3. A lack of anatomical knowledge and of the appreciation of anomalies, e.g., accessory bile ducts; aberrant cystic arteries.
4. The easy cholecystectomy.
5. The difficult cholecystectomy.
6. Mutilation or perforation of the duct in the process of exploring it for stones. The formation of a false passage between the choledochus and duodenum by means of dilators in cases of fibrosis of the sphincter of Oddi.

7. Suturing the free margin of the gastro-hepatic omentum too tightly over the bile ducts at the completion of cholecystectomy.
8. Slipping of the ligature which had been applied to the cystic duct; the inadvertent early withdrawal or displacement of a T tube; the profuse discharge of bile from the bared gallbladder fossa; the unrecognised severance of an accessory hepatic duct. In these cases, a subhepatic abscess may form, or the continuous bathing or immersion of the bile ducts with irritating, sclerosing, and cytolytic constituents of the bile may lead to fibrotic contraction of the extrahepatic biliary passages.
9. Angulation of, or injury to (by knife, clamp or suture) the lower end of the choledochus during the process of excising a large penetrating duodenal ulcer, or excessive inturning of the distal end of the duodenum during the performance of the Billroth II types of partial gastrectomy.
10. The lower reaches of the bile duct may be injured during excision of a diverticulum of the second part of the duodenum.
11. A segment of the bile ducts may be excised or incised during a block resection of a mass involving the hepatic flexure of the colon, the great omentum, the gallbladder, and (possibly) a portion of the right lobe of the liver. Such a mass may be caused by an adherent cancer of the large bowel or by calculous cholecystitis, in which the gallbladder had been the seat of repeated attacks of acute cholecystitis.
12. Acute angulation of the common bile duct caused by excessive and persistent traction on a T tube.
13. Excessive devascularization of the bile ducts.

See Table 1.

Table 1. **PROCEDURES RESPONSIBLE FOR BILIARY STRICTURE IN 958 PATIENTS (1940-65)***

Procedure	Number of Patients	
Surgical Trauma		
Biliary tract surgery	918	
Gastric surgery	9	
Pancreatic surgery	2	929 (97 percent)
Nonsurgical Causes		
Inflammatory obstruction	15	
Congenital	5	
Erosion of gallstones	3	
External blunt trauma	2	
Other	4	29 (3 percent)

*I am indebted to Warren, Mountain, and Midell, The Surgical Clinics of North America 51:711, 1971, and to W. B. Saunders Company, for kind permission to tabulate the valuable recent statistical data pertaining to postoperative strictures of the bile ducts, submitted by the Lahey Clinic Foundation.

It is often stated that *abnormalities* in the course, length, and termination of the cystic duct, and variations in the course, origin, and distribution of the cystic artery are important predisposing causes. It is the surgeon's duty, however, to be familiar with these variations and to recognise them at operation when they are present. *He should work by sight and not by faith!* During the performance of a cholecystectomy it should be a rule that the three ducts—the cystic, the common hepatic, and the common bile duct —be displayed and the cystic artery clearly identified before being ligatured and the cystic duct severed.

When access proves difficult or the parts concerned in the operation have not been clearly visualised, excision of the gallbladder is always a hazardous undertaking (Fig. 5).

One of the most common causes of injury to the common hepatic duct is *haemorrhage (occurring from the cystic artery, an anomalous cystic artery, or the right hepatic artery)* during a dissection which aims at displaying the cystic duct and the cystic artery itself. In clearing the fatty tissue away from the neck of the gallbladder, the artery may be torn by dissecting forceps (Fig. 6). The artery may snap and retract under the common hepatic duct, where it is free to hiss and bleed copiously in its hidden retreat if the divided cystic duct is drawn too forcibly upward. Likewise, when cholecystectomy is being performed from the fundus end (retrograde cho-

lecystectomy), if the gallbladder is too firmly pulled downward and outward, *the main force of traction will be applied to the cystic artery* rather than to the cystic duct. In such circumstances, if the gallbladder is tugged upon with a heavy, clumsy hand, the taut cystic artery may snap and give rise to a profuse haemorrhage. It may, too, when picked up with artery forceps, slip through wide and clumsy blades or it may be avulsed when the haemostat which grasps it is used as a tractor by a thoughtless assistant. Artery forceps with their sharp serrations may actually bite through the artery and thus produce a troublesome haemorrhage.

The cystic artery is best tied twice with catgut or Dexon in continuity. This small artery should not be clipped with angulated or other haemostats; after it is displayed it should be underrun with an aneurysm needle and ligated with catgut.

The cystic or even the right hepatic artery may be torn when the peritoneum overlying the anterior surface of the ducts is being dissected to display the structures in the vicinity of the cystic duct. The haemorrhage is always brisk, and blood soon floods the area of operation—obscuring everything. The surgeon in his excitement and hurry to arrest the bleeding makes a blind grab with a haemostat for the bleeding point, and the jaws of the instrument may crush an appreciable portion of the duct in securing the vessel. If a ligature is applied, as shown in Figure 7, a

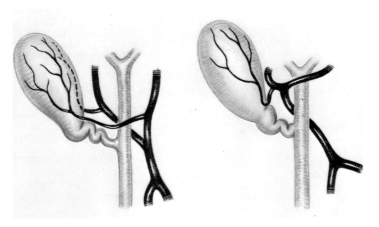

FIG. 6.   Aberrant cystic artery arising from the left hepatic artery. An abnormal left hepatic artery and a short cystic artery are shown.

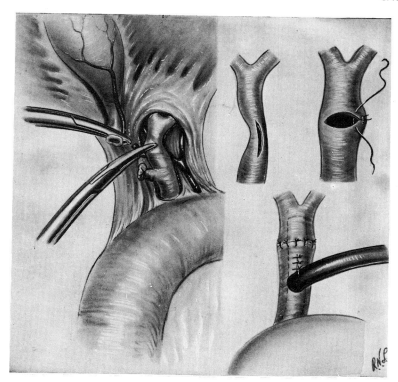

FIG. 7. Stricture of the common hepatic duct—plastic repair. Bleeding from the end of the cystic artery and blind application of a haemostat. The partial stricture of duct which results may be repaired after the Heineke-Mikulicz method. Note that the T tube is introduced into the duct *below* the reconstructed duct. The short arm of the T tube acts as an efficient splint. (From Maingot, *Management of Abdominal Operations,* 2d ed., 1957. Courtesy of H. R. Lewis & Co., Ltd., London.)

considerable portion of the circumference of the duct will be included and blood clot obscuring all traces of the tragedy may prevent the mishap from being realised at the time of its occurrence.

Bleeding from the cystic artery, a pool of blood, and a blind plunge with a haemostat for the spurting point will frequently lead to a number of tragic events!

The method of applying two Moynihan gallbladder forceps or other clamps (the two-clamp method) to the cystic duct so as to include the cystic artery during the performance of retrograde cholecystectomy is to be deprecated. Not infrequently, as the surgeon pulls upon the gallbladder, traction upon the cystic artery will so acutely angulate the right hepatic artery that, as the clamp is applied to the "cystic duct," it will include the angulated V-shaped right hepatic artery.

This places the artery under tension so that as the ligature is tightened about the knuckle of artery there is a tendency for the upper end of the right hepatic artery to retract out of the ligature and result in a serious haemorrhage in the depths of the portal fissure. *Haemorrhage is the most common cause of injury to the hepatic ducts* (Figs. 8 and 9).

When haemorrhage from the cystic artery, an accessory cystic artery, or the right hepatic artery occurs during the performance of a cholecystectomy, it is an easy matter (as Seton Pringle pointed out many years ago) to control the bleeding and to visualise the culpable artery by compressing with the fingers all the structures in the free margin of the hepatoduodenal ligament. The assistant should introduce the index finger of his left hand into the foramen of Winslow and compress the common hepatic artery between

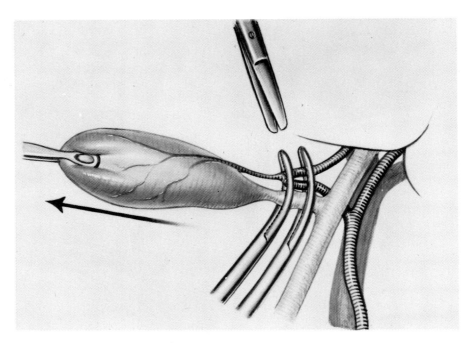

FIG. 8. Two-clamp method of cholecystectomy. Possible cause of massive haemorrhage and stricture of common hepatic duct. (After Dr. Frank Lahey. Courtesy of Butterworths, London.)

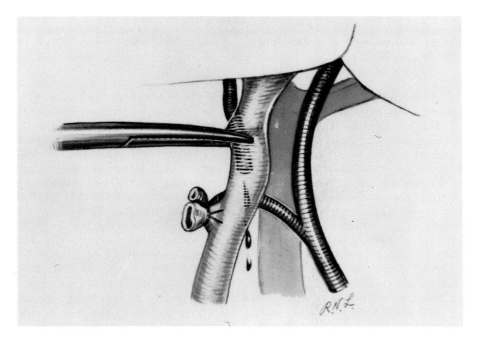

FIG. 9. Blind clamping of the distal end of the right hepatic artery may lead to stricture of the common hepatic duct or its proximal tributaries. (Adapted from Dr. Frank Lahey. Courtesy of Butterworths, London.)

this finger and the thumb. The bleeding point is then visualised, seized with a slender fine-pointed haemostat, and carefully ligatured by the surgeon, after which the pressure is released (Fig. 10).

The subjects of *hepatic artery injury* and the management of patients after hepatic artery ligation are discussed by Karasewich and Bowden [21] and by Truman Mays. [41] (See Fig. 11.)

In examining the records of many cases of benign strictures of the bile duct which have followed operative procedures upon the biliary passages and gallbladder, I have been struck by two things: while haemorrhage has accounted for most of the accidents, it would appear that *overconfidence* has been the cause of not a few. In the overconfidence group, a gallbladder has been unduly mobile and the operation has, to all intents and appearances, been one of great simplicity in a thin and visceroptotic patient. *The easy cholecystectomy and the overconfident "manic" surgeon lacking in technical skill constitute a sinister combination!*

In firmly retracting an unduly mobile gallbladder, a clamp may be applied too close to the junction of the cystic duct and common ducts; in fact, the clamp may even grasp a portion of the common duct, and when the ligature is tightened, it drags up a still greater portion of the duct—thus producing partial stricture.

Figure 12 shows how, during a retrograde cholecystectomy (i.e., commencing the dissection of the gallbladder from the fundus end rather than from the cystic duct end), firm traction upon the gallbladder may angulate and approximate the two common ducts with the result that forceps may inadvertently be applied in such a way as to embrace both *main ducts* instead of the taut and attenuated cystic duct. Kehr was the first to draw attention to the mechanics of this accident.

If the gallbladder is examined after it has been excised, the cystic duct can be traced into the tell-tale segment of the main duct.

This finding should lead the surgeon to examine the common ducts and remove the stuture that binds them together. It is an easy matter *at this stage* to perform an end-to-end anastomosis between the cut ends of the duct. Nevertheless, about 10 percent of injuries to the bile ducts are not recognised during the performance of the primary operation.

Stricture of the common bile duct may be caused by approximating the edges of the

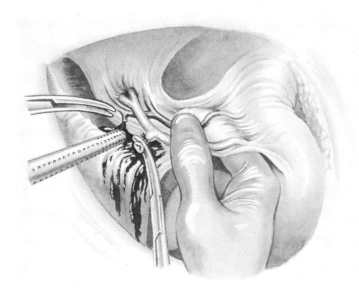

FIG. 10.   Seton Pringle's method of controlling bleeding from a divided cystic artery.

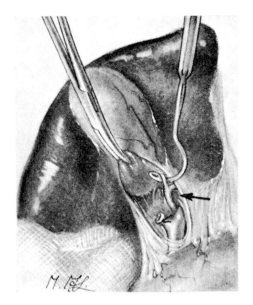

FIG. 11.   Inadvertent ligation of an anomalous right hepatic artery.

peritoneum of the hepatoduodenal ligament over the duct too tightly at the completion of a well-conducted cholecystectomy or a cholecystectomy combined with choledochostomy.

Cholecystectomy is indeed a most difficult undertaking in cases where the gallbladder is small, fibrotic, shrunken and partly calcified, and it lies high up close to the hilus of the liver. It often abuts against the common or right hepatic duct; the planes of cleavage are difficult to identify, the arteries are distorted and are encased in a sheaf of dense fibrous tissue, and in some instances there may even be a fistula between the gallbladder and the duct.

In such difficult cases, it is advisable to open the common bile duct below the cystic duct, where it is readily accessible, and to insert a Bakes' dilator into the right hepatic duct—this sound serving as a useful guide to the surgeon during his dissection. This manoeuvre is likewise advocated in those cases in which *the cystic duct enters the right hepatic duct,* and where the structures in Calot's triangle are involved in an intense inflammatory reaction (Figs. 12B and 13).

In some cases of acute cholecystitis in which the ducts are obscured by dense felt-like adhesions, the surgeon would be well advised to perform cholecystostomy.

The surgeon must not consider this decision as a reflection of his inadequate ability but rather as an indication of his sound surgical judgment.[5]

Caution is also enjoined when the cystic duct is unusually long, emptying its contents into the retroduodenal portion of the choledochus; when the cystic duct is united to the right hepatic duct; when no cystic duct is present, i.e., when the neck of the gallbladder opens directly into the main ducts; when the right and left hepatic ducts separately join the body or fundus of the gallbladder or an ovoid thin-walled cystic structure; and when the cystic and common bile ducts are enveloped by a sheet of fibro-areolar tissue (Figs. 13, 14).

It is difficult to account for some cases in which there has been no injury to the ducts and cholecystectomy has been conducted successfully but in which at a second operation a cartilaginous mass of scar tissue is found somewhere along the course of the main duct, compressing it at one point and giving rise to partial stricture. It is possible that the peritoneal scarring may be caused by an organising haematoma, pericholedochitis, perhaps by a circumscribed patch of localised chronic peritonitis at the margins of the gastrohepatic omentum, or by stripping the blood vessels off the common duct too thoroughly during choledochostomy. Such peritonitis may have been induced by contamination of the operative field at the time of the original cholecystectomy, by leakage from a severed accessory hepatic duct, or by the oozing of bile around the T tube that had been implanted in the common duct.

I believe that any condition which gives rise to the leakage and the pocketing or imprisonment of bile during the early postoperative phase is a potent cause of stricture of the ducts.

Bile salts, infected bile, and other products may excite a low-grade inflammatory process which, in turn, may compress and strangle the ducts. This is especially the case when bile seeps into the retroperitoneal space and cannot escape, when it pools in the subhepatic area and is not efficiently drained, and when, perhaps as the result of a slipped cystic duct ligature, the ductal system is con-

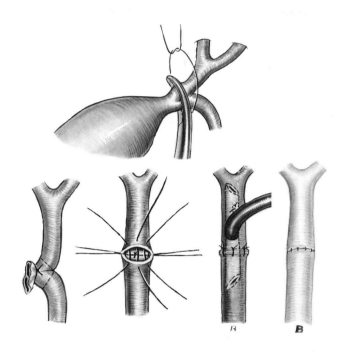

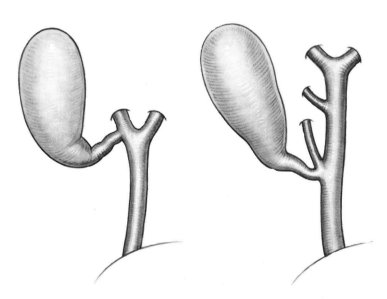

FIG. 12.   (A) The inadvertent excision of a segment of the common ducts during the performance of retrograde cholecystectomy for gallstones. The techniques of primary repair are illustrated. (After Kehr.) (B) In this anomaly, the cystic duct enters the right hepatic duct. Two anomalous or accessory right hepatic ducts are shown on the right side.

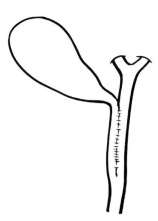

FIG. 13.   In this anomaly, the cystic duct is firmly adherent to a large segment of the common hepatic duct. It joins the choledochus at a rather low point.

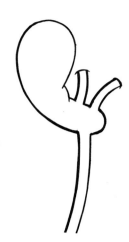

FIG. 14.   No cystic ducts. Hepatic ducts enter the gallbladder above and the common bile duct drains viscus from its inferior margin.

tinuously bathed with this irritating sclerosant fluid. This view has the support of Dragstedt and Woodward,[13] who write as follows:

It seems probable to us that many of these cases of postoperative strictures of the bile passages are due to destruction of the bile ducts by the necrotizing effect of bile that has collected in the peritoneal cavity and pooled in the region of the ducts. The necrotizing and cytolytic action of bile salts was demonstrated by Flexner and others many years ago and has been amply confirmed. Damage to the ducts is often due to some agent acting from without, rather than to some process acting within the duct system or to impairment of the blood supply.

This subject has been discussed by Maingot[33] and by Michie and Gunn.[42]

It is difficult to account for those cases in which a segment of the common hepatic or the right hepatic duct has been removed en masse with the gallbladder. It can only be inferred that the accident occurred because the surgeon thought at the time he was dealing with a long cystic duct!

A rare type of injury to the common duct which can result in stricture is *mutilation of the duct* during the process of exploring it for calculi. The walls of the duct may be torn or partially destroyed by too forcibly applying Allis or other forceps that have teeth, or by the tearing out of stay sutures when they are dragged upon to aid in the retraction of

the margins of the duct. Babcock forceps are often satisfactorily employed in common duct surgery. I prefer stay sutures for retracting the margins of the duct, but only gentle traction is applied to them.

In my opinion, it is a mistake to carry out reconstructive biliary-tract surgery—which may be difficult, exacting, and prolonged—toward the end of a long session of operations when the surgeon may be fatigued or under some tension.

DIAGNOSIS

The most frequent symptom of stricture of the bile ducts is *obstructive jaundice,* which, following blockage, becomes manifest in at least 70 percent of patients within 2 to 3 days after cholecystectomy—provided there is no external biliary fistula. Some patients show no evidence of jaundice until the second or third postoperative week, and a small number may not become jaundiced for several months or even years after injury has been inflicted on the bile duct.

The sequence of (1) biliary fistula, (2) closure of the fistula, and (3) jaundice is characteristic of stricture, but retained stone in the common bile duct may produce the same symptom complex (Fig. 15). The history of a biliary fistula following cholecystectomy for even a few days, with the subsequent

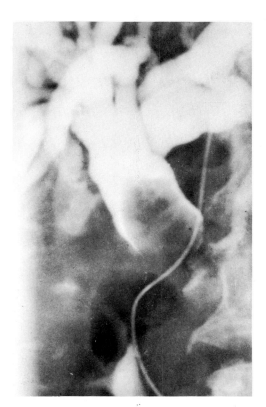

FIG. 15. Percutaneous intrahepatic cholangiography. The patient had had cholecystectomy and choledochostomy for gallstones 5 years previously. Marked jaundice is present. Percutaneous intrahepatic cholangiography shows a large stone in the common bile duct.

development of persistent or intermittent jaundice, is sufficient evidence upon which to make a presumptive diagnosis of stricture with the hopeful realisation that a calculus within the duct may produce an identical clinical picture.

Such symptoms as pain, nausea, anorexia, loss of weight, vomiting, chills, fever, jaundice, dark urine, steatorrhoea with light stools, and pruritus are noted very frequently in this group of patients.

If an external fistula persists, hypoprothrombinaemia develops, which may lead to purpura or frank bleeding.

According to Norcross and Dadey,[43] *remote complications* after injury to the biliary tree are numerous and include: (1) hepatic complications, such as biliary cirrhosis, with portal hypertension (20 percent), and congestive splenomegaly with or without hyper-

splenism; (2) anaemia; (3) hypoprothrombinaemia; (4) hyperphosphatasaemia, and avitaminosis; (5) loss of potassium salts; (6) pancreatitis; and (7) biliary–intestinal fistula formation.

Signs and Symptoms

Following operative injuries to the extrahepatic bile passages, the symptoms and signs are found to vary considerably in individual cases, but actually there are *three* well-defined groups:

In the first, the patient makes an uninterrupted recovery and all appears to be progressing satisfactorily for many months or even years. Then cholangitis ensues and with this are associated recurrent attacks of mild jaundice. This history would suggest an incomplete type of stricture due to choledocholithiasis. The longer intervals which occur between cholecystectomy and the beginning of obstructive jaundice may indicate that sclerosing choledochitis plays a part in the stricturing process; whether this inflammation is a residual of the original cholecystitis or whether it follows the initial stricturing no one can say.

In the second group, the patient has a stormy convalescence and there is a persistent discharge of bile through the wound. This leads to rapid emaciation and digestive disturbances. There is also loss of appetite and of spirit, well-known accompaniments of loss of bile. A profound electrolyte imbalance, with hypochloraemia, may occur from the loss of large quantities of bile externally. At times, the bile ceases to discharge through the fistulous tract, and when this occurs the patient will suffer from pain, backache, chills, fever, jaundice, and a tender epigastric mass —subhepatic abscess.

In the third group, the signs and symptoms are those of frank obstruction of the bile duct. Pain is slight, but when present it is confined to the right upper quadrant of the abdomen and an area just above the right twelfth rib. There is a persistent fluctuating jaundice, and the intermittent hepatic fever of Charcot is in evidence. With this is associated pylorospasm, flatulence, occasional bouts of vomiting and cramp-like sensations in the epigastrium. After a few weeks, the jaundice deepens, the skin becomes tinted a

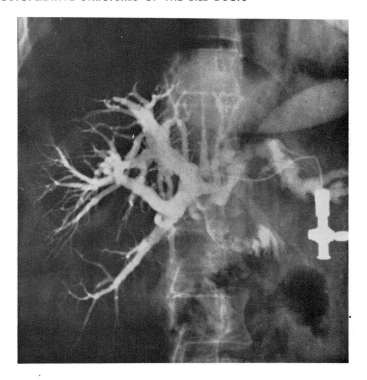

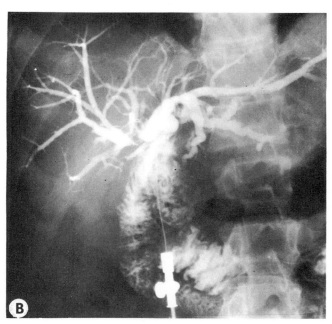

FIG. 16. (A) Postoperative stricture of the common hepatic duct. Percutaneous intrahepatic cholangiography showing slightly dilated common hepatic duct containing sediment and small stones. A previous operation had been hepaticojejunostomy on the Roux-en-Y plan. Note that a small amount of dye is entering the jejunum through the constricted stoma. At the next operation, the patient was successfully treated by the jejunal mucosal graft procedure. (B) Percutaneous intrahepatic cholangiography. A previous operation for postoperative bile duct stricture was hepaticojejunostomy with entero-anastomosis.

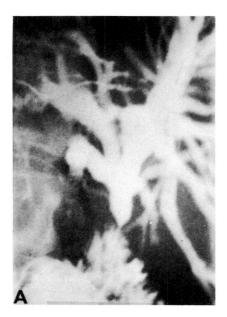 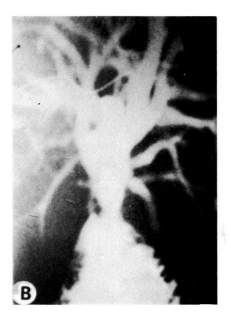

FIG. 17.   Gastrografin-meal x-ray examination. (A) Before operation. (B) Three years after operation. Shows good stoma following Roux-en-Y hepaticojejunostomy.

dark yellow green, and the cirrhotic liver slowly enlarges. Gastrointestinal haemorrhage is a common complication.

As previously stated, the usual history characterising a benign ductal stricture is that of the postoperative development of jaundice or an external biliary fistula or both. A history of haemorrhage from the cystic or the right hepatic artery during the previous operation should fortify the suspicion that the fistula or the jaundice is the result of injury to the common hepatic duct or choledochus.

The main differential diagnostic considerations are: (1) carcinoma of the common bile duct or periampullary region, (2) retained or "residual" stone, or (3) acute sclerosing cholangitis.

All possible causes of obstructive jaundice must be considered. (Laboratory investigations and the management of the jaundiced patient are discussed in Chap. 45.)

Oral or intravenous cholangiography is rarely helpful because of the presence of jaundice. If the serum bilirubin estimation is less than 3 mg per 100 ml and the stricture has only recently developed, visualisation of the biliary tree may be obtained. *Intravenous cholangiography* affords no help in diagnosis when jaundice or an external biliary fistula is present, but *delayed cholangiography,* carried out later by the injection of one of the radiopaque solutions, such as Hypaque, Diodone, or Thorotrast, into catheters or T tubes placed in the ducts at the original operation, has frequently proved of diagnostic value in strictures of the main bile passages. Again, the injection of Hypaque into sinus tracts, followed by x-ray pictures, may prove rewarding.

Percutaneous transhepatic cholangiography is performed, almost as a routine measure in cases of postoperative strictures of the bile ducts, as it so frequently displays the exact site of the obstruction (Figs. 16A and B).

Exploratory laparotomy should be carried out within 3 to 6 hours after the performance of this valuable method of inquiry, as leakage of bile and/or blood into the peritoneal cavity is a common sequel and, if these fluids are not promptly evacuated, peritonitis or "haemorrhagic" shock may ensue, sometimes with grave consequences. (Percutaneous transhepatic cholangiography is described in Chap. 46.)

A *gastrografin-meal x-ray examination* may prove of diagnostic value in certain cases (Figs. 17A and B).

Operative cholangiography is useful in defining the anatomy of the intrahepatic ducts. A small Foley catheter is inserted into the common bile duct or the common hepatic duct, and the balloon is then inflated sufficiently to prevent leakage following the injection of the dye (usually Hypaque).

PREOPERATIVE CARE

All patients require an intensive course of preoperative treatment. A high-carbohydrate, high-protein, low-fat diet is given; liver function tests are carried out on several occasions to determine the degree of hepatic damage present, as well as the response to the treatment prescribed; prothrombin times are investigated in an effort to evaluate bleeding tendencies and vitamin K deficiencies; the routine blood and renal function tests are undertaken to aid in ascertaining and computing the operative risks; water and electrolyte imbalance is corrected by intravenous infusions of glucose and saline; and blood transfusions by the slow-drip method, before, during, and after operation, are given to correct anaemia and hypoproteinaemia. Massive blood transfusions should, however, be avoided. Antibiotic therapy is indicated when cholangitis or liver damage is present (see Chap. 107).

A fistulous tract will demand good drainage, and if there is a profuse discharge of bile, continuous suction applied to an indwelling catheter will diminish the daily dressings and add to the comfort of the patient. In some cases, a temporary ileostomy bag made of cellophane or plastic material may be affixed to the sinus to reduce the number of dressings.

Sedgwick and Hume [49] state that *portal hypertension* occurs in about 20 percent of patients, and if haemorrhage from oesophageal piles occurs, it is advisable to delay the repair of the stricture until after a splenorenal shunt has been carried out.

OPERATIVE TREATMENT

Prognosis

The *prognosis* following reconstructive procedures for postoperative bile duct strictures depends mainly on the following factors:

1. The anatomical site of the stricture and the length and caliber of the remaining proximal portion of the duct.
2. The degree of scarring, cholangitis, and pericholedochitis present, i.e., the quality of the proximal duct.
3. The number of previous repair procedures and the interval between injury and surgical reconstruction or reconstructions.
4. Hepatic function; the presence or absence of cirrhosis of the liver; and the general condition of the patient.
5. The judgement and experience of the surgeon in selecting and carrying out the most suitable corrective operation for a particular type of stricture.
6. The efficiency of the anaesthetist and the assistants; the management of the patient before and after operation; and the operating room facilities.

The most propitious time to obtain a satisfactory result or permanent cure is at the *first time at repair,* more especially when the proximal portion of the duct is of sizeable proportions in length and caliber, and when cholangitis and pericholedochitis are minimal.

On the other hand, the prognosis is poor with intrahepatic and hilar strictures because of the difficulty of access and also in obtaining a satisfactory mucosa-to-mucosa anastomosis.

The general experience is that the final result is governed, in large measure, by the quality of the proximal duct and also by the number of previous attempts to correct recurrent ductal obstruction. (See also further remarks on Prognosis, in Part D of this chapter.)

Types of Repair Procedures

1. Immediate repair of *minor injuries,* such as inadvertent incisions or small lacerations of the ducts inflicted during the performance of cholecystectomy, choledochostomy, partial gastrectomy by the Billroth methods for penetrating posterior-wall duodenal ulcers (see Figs. 2 and 3).

2. Plastic repair for a minimal stricture of the choledochus, followed by T tube choledochostomy.
3. End-to-end ductal anastomosis, with or without T tube choledochostomy.
4. Dragstedt and Woodward's technique.
5. Biliary-intestinal anastomosis:
   a. Choledochoduodenostomy or hepaticoduodenostomy (end-to-side).
   b. Choledochojejunostomy or hepaticojejunostomy by Roux-en-Y method or by employing proximal jejunal loop plus entero-anastomosis—with or without splinting the anastomosis with a T, a Y, or a straight-latex tube.
6. Side-to-side choledochoduodenostomy.
7. Longmire's operation.
8. Cattell's technique for high strictures at the porta hepatis. (See Figs. 40 and 41.)
9. Rodney Smith's techniques:
   a. Hepaticojejunostomy: a method of intrajejunal anastomosis.
   b. Hepaticoenterostomy with *transpatic* intubation.
   c. Mucosal graft operation for hilar or intrahepatic strictures of the hepatic ducts. (See Figs. 64 to 67.)
10. Two-stage procedures.

Principles of Repair

1. If the surgeon recognises that the bile duct has received a minor injury such as a small cut or laceration during the course of an operation such as cholecystectomy, he should carry out an immediate repair with a few interrupted sutures of fine catgut. T tube drainage is rarely called for (see Figs. 2 and 3).
2. If it is possible to perform an axial or an end-to-end ductal anastomosis and thus preserve the sphincteric mechanism, e.g., choledochocholedochostomy or hepaticocholedochostomy, this should be the procedure of choice (Figs. 18 and 19).
3. In those strictures in which it is impossible or hazardous to utilise the distal end of the common duct, it is better to implant the common or hepatic duct into the apex of a moder- ately long loop of proximal jejunum rather than into the duodenum. If a loop of jejunum is used, an entero-anastomosis should be fashioned about 6 to 8 inches (15 to 20 cm) below the biliary-enteric stoma to divert food from the biliary tree. Cole et al.[8] advocate the *Roux-en-Y principle* with the single arm of jejunum. Hepaticoduodenostomy is the procedure of choice when a previous Billroth II partial gastrectomy has been performed.
4. The mucosa should be approximated accurately to the mucosa. This may be the mucosa to mucosa of the approximated duct portion (axial union), or may be the mucosa of the duct to the mucosa of the jejunum or duodenum.

Accurate approximation without tension is important.

Only one row of fine 000 Dexon or chromic catgut sutures employing no more than 8 to 10 through-and-through all-coats sutures should be used for fashioning the anastomoses. However, the insertion of an outer layer of interrupted sutures of fine silk is advocated by many surgeons.

5. When an *end-to-end ductal union* is performed, the suture line should be splinted by a T tube, unless, of course, the stoma is large or of adequate diameter. The long or vertical limb of the T tube must not emerge through the suture line in the duct but at a point above or below it. Re-formation of stricture almost invariably follows if the vertical limb of the T tube is led to the exterior through the newly fashioned suture line. Likewise, withdrawal of a T tube through the healing suture line in the duct in the convalescent period or shortly afterwards is a common source of recurrence of stricture.

If a T tube is used in duct reconstruction, it should be left in situ for about 3 months. It acts as a mould at the line of repair and should remain in place not only until healing is advanced but also until late fibrosis is no longer a possibility.

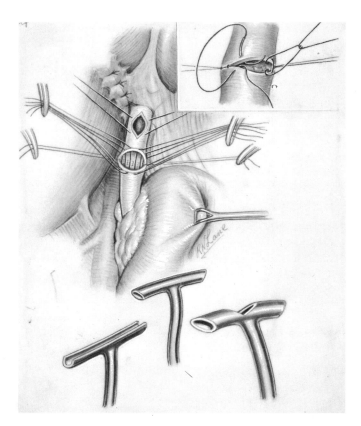

FIG. 18.   Immediate choledochocholedochostomy following cholecystectomy and division of the
common bile duct. Two methods of end-to-end anastomosis are depicted. Note the Maingot
guttered latex T tube. (Courtesy of Butterworths, London.)

6.   Some type of barium-impregnated rubber or latex prosthesis—such as those manufactured by Davol or William Warne, and of the following types: straight tube, Y tube, T tube, Maingot's guttered T tube—will be required for many anastomoses, as these devices serve to splint and mould the anastomoses during the healing period and prevent subsequent contracture. Straight tubes and T tubes are readily removed, and so are the long-limbed latex Y tubes. Under no condition should any plastic tubes such as polyethylene T tubes be used in bile duct surgery, as they are very prone to damage the duct when they are withdrawn.

The best results in operative treatment are obtained when a partial obstruction is present, when after excision of the stricture a direct end-to-end anastomosis of the two ends of the ducts is possible, when the common hepatic or common bile duct can be anastomosed to the jejunum or duodenum without any tension, *when operation can be carried out early in the course of the biliary obstruction* (before the liver has been injured by cirrhosis or infection), and when adequate measures have been adopted to render the patient as fit as possible to withstand operation. It must, once again, be emphasised that it is imperative to achieve a sound mucosa-to-mucosa approximation without tension and that the resulting stoma must be of ample or of generous proportions. Stents should only be employed when the stoma appears to be small.

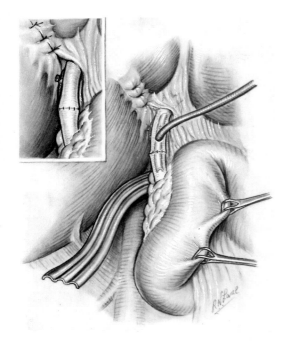

FIG. 19. Immediate choledochocholedochostomy following cholecystectomy and division of the common bile duct. Note the satisfactory axial anastomosis with and without T tube choledochostomy. (From Maingot, in Rob, Smith, and Morgan, 1969. Operative Surgery, 2d ed. Courtesy of Butterworths, London.)

No one operation can be employed for all cases, and each case must be considered individually according to the situation and extent of the lesion.

Repair procedures are best discussed under the following groupings:

One-stage repairs. Choledochocholedochostomy; hepaticocholedochostomy; hepaticojejunostomy; hepaticoduodenostomy; dilatation of partial ductal strictures followed by T tube splintage and drainage of the duct; side-to-side choledochoduodenostomy; Longmire's operation; hepaticojejunostomy with transhepatic intubation; and mucosal graft operation for hilar strictures and for intrahepatic strictures of the hepatic ducts. (See Chap. 48C.)

Two-stage repairs. This category includes those patients in whom an external biliary fistula (*hepaticostomy*) was deliber-

ately produced at a first-stage operation owing to the poor general condition of the patient. Some 2 or 3 weeks later, when the patient's condition has considerably improved, a definitive repair procedure should be performed.

Special repairs. Repair of biliary strictures in which the bifurcation of the hepatic duct has been destroyed or in which only one hepatic duct is involved.

Miscellaneous operations. Those aimed at restoring the flow of bile into the intestinal tract, including: Longmire's operation; Dragstedt's method; and prolonged catheter drainage of the porta hepatis for cases in which no hilar or intrahepatic ducts can be found following careful dissection, and for which Longmire's procedure is not applicable.

Finally, a discussion of Rodney Smith's techniques for postoperative strictures of the bile ducts will be presented.

Types of Definitive Operation

The operative approach to the problem of biliary stricture is the same as that used for all secondary operations on the biliary tract.

The *incision of choice* is a right vertical rectus muscle-splitting one or a long paramedian incision which extends from the right border of the xiphisternum to 2 or 3 inches below and to the right of the umbilicus (Fig. 20).

The preliminary steps consist in freeing omental or other adhesions from the anterior abdominal wall and from the free margin and undersurface of the liver. The ascending colon and the hepatic flexure of the colon is next liberated, displaced downward and medially, well away from the operative field (Fig. 21). The second and third portions of the duodenum now come into view and the peritoneum and fascia propria are incised at their outer margins in order to effect a liberal mobilisation of the head of the pancreas together with these portions of the duodenum. The mobilisation of these structures should extend almost to the middle line so that the ureter, spermatic or ovarian vein, the inferior vena cava, and the lateral margin of the aorta can be clearly visualised (Figs. 21, 22, and 23).

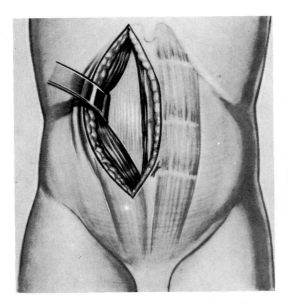

FIG. 20.   Right vertical epigastric rectus muscle-splitting incision. This approach to the biliary system in patients suffering from postoperative strictures of bile ducts cannot be bettered.

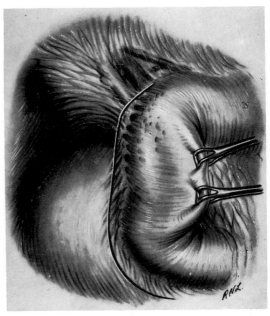

FIG. 22.   Kocher's method of mobilisation of the duodenum and head of the pancreas. Incision of the peritoneum lateral to the duodenum prior to mobilisation of the head of the pancreas and duodenum.

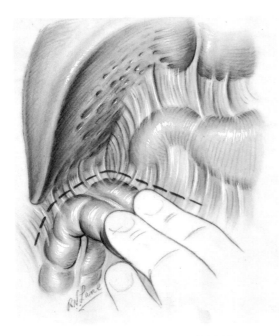

FIG. 21.   Exposure of the operative field. The ascending colon and hepatic flexure should be liberated, displaced downward and medially, well away from the field of operation. During the process of dissection, the phrenocolic ligament will be divided.

The stomach and pylorus are cautiously detached from the undersurface of the liver, after which the first portion of the duodenum is carefully dissected and liberated from the hilus of the liver and the gallbladder or its fossa.

When a fistula is encountered—which is not an unusual finding—its short tract should be cut across and the opening which remains in the duodenum should be closed by a purse-string suture of fine silk. The most common site for such spontaneous internal biliary fistulous tracts is the first portion of the duodenum on the one hand and the upper end of the hepatic duct on the other hand. These fistulas may, in the occasional case, pass unrecognised during the dissection which frees the pylorus and dudenum from the portal fissure. The surgeon on spotting the small hole in the duodenum imagines that he has injured the bowel or has perhaps torn or punctured it at one spot. The opening into the bile duct is usually so small that it is frequently unnoticed until a later stage in the operation.

The next step of the exposure is to find

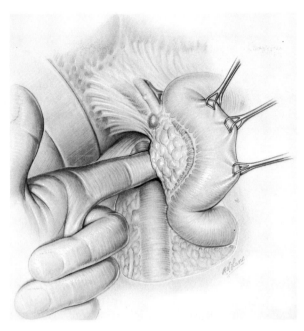

FIG. 23.   Kocher's method of mobilisation of the duodenum and head of the pancreas. Note the inferior vena cava, right ureter, and the common duct lymph node.

and demonstrate the lower end of the bile duct and the common duct gland. Cattell and Braasch [4] write:

The common duct gland is a large lymph node, often about 2 centimeters in diameter, which lies on the posteroinferior aspect of the gastrohepatic ligament and serves as an accurate guide to the lower end of the common duct. The lower end of the common bile duct is almost always located superior and medial to this gland in the anterior aspect of the gastrohepatic ligament. A core of tissue is then dissected out of the hepatico-duodenal ligament anterior to the common duct node and sectioned vertically until a lumen is found. Probes and scoops must then be inserted into the distal end of the duct and into the duodenum to ascertain that no calculi or other forms of obstruction are present. Then a catheter of moderate size is inserted temporarily through the duct and into the duodenum.

Attention is next directed to the hilus of the liver to locate the upper end of the common hepatic duct. Orientation for this dissection is afforded by the location of the hepatic artery, since the duct is usually found *anterior and lateral* to this pulsating vessel. In some instances the duct is evident because of a bulge in the hilus of the liver at this location. Should extensive dissection be necessary, it is usually advisable to accomplish this within the substance of the liver.

The capsule of the liver is incised with a knife, and dissection proceeds within the liver capsule. This dissecton may be accomplished with the electrosurgical unit. If the upper ducts cannot be readily found, they can sometimes be located by needling the hilus of the liver for either white or normal bile. After the lumen of the upper ducts has been encountered and opened, probes and scoops should be passed into the common and right and left hepatic ducts to establish their patency and freedom from calculi. Further dissection can then be accomplished (most readily on the anterior and lateral aspects of the ducts) to outline these ducts more discretely, with probes and scoops defining their course. The ends of both the upper and lower ducts must be free of neuromatous or excessive scar tissue before suture is attempted. We believe that regrowth of neuromatous tissue is a factor in stricture recurrence.

Warren et al.[67] state:

An analysis of the site of the stricture revealed that the common hepatic duct and the right and left hepatic ducts are the commonest areas to be injured. (See Table 2.) This injury is particularly liable to occur when the cystic duct is in firm apposition to the right lateral margin of the common hepatic duct and is prematurely clamped before full delineation of the junction of the cystic and common hepatic ducts has been ob-

Table 2.   SITE OF STRICTURES IN 958 PATIENTS

Site	Number of Patients
Common hepatic ducts	379
Common hepatic and common bile duct	265
Common bile duct, including 14 in distal common bile duct	217
Bifurcation of hepatic ducts	59
Individual hepatic ducts only	38
Right 27	
Left 11	
Total	958

Source: From Warren, et al. Surg. Clin. N. Am. 51:711, 1971.

tained or when the hepatic ducts did not unite until some distance below the liver. The common hepatic duct is also more likely to be injured when uncontrolled haemorrhage from the cystic artery occurs. . . .

Operative cholangiography is useful to confirm the anatomy of the intrahepatic ducts following dissection of a common hepatic or right or left hepatic duct stricture before insertion of the stent. It is best performed using a Foley catheter inserted into the duct with the balloon inflated sufficiently to prevent leakage.

When this stage is reached, the surgeon will have to decide what type of reconstructive operation should be employed in the circumstances. Cattell's operation of choice was an end-to-end anastomosis of the two ends of the bile duct combined with T tube choledochostomy and with the vertical limb of the T tube emerging either above or below the anastomotic junction. Few surgeons possessed the experience or skill of so neatly dissecting out and displaying the lower reaches of a strictured choledochus (when it was embedded and shrouded in adhesions in the head of the pancreas) as the late Richard Cattell. He was in a class by himself; and the excellent results he obtained by his technique of axial union and T tube choledochostomy were unsurpassed by his contemporaries.

Plastic repair. This operation is rarely performed today. It is only possible when there is a minimal stricture of the common bile duct. The stricture area is incised vertically and closed horizontally with a series of interrupted sutures. A T tube stent is usually inserted, with the external

arm being brought out either above or below the repair.

End-to-End Anastomosis

Choledochocholedochostomy or hepaticocholedochostomy is advised when the two ends of the bile duct can be approximated without any tension on the suture line, and when the *"recovered" retroduodenal portion of the common duct has about the same calibre as the stump of the common bile duct.* Conversely, this operation should not be performed if there is a noticeable discrepancy in size between the two ends of the bile ducts, if the lower end is too short, or if the tissues are not suitable for an axial anastomosis.

The chief advantages of choledochocholedochostomy or hepaticocholedochostomy are that the sphincteric mechanism is preserved and the patient is protected against ascending infection (see Figs. 18 and 19).

In this operation, the posterior margins of the opposing ends of the bile ducts are sutured together with 6 to 8 all-coats interrupted sutures of fine chromic catgut, then the horizontal limb of a small T tube is passed into the ducts through an opening made above or below the anastomotic line to act as a splint or mould to the suture line, after which the anterior margins of the ducts are approximated with interrupted sutures of 000 chromic catgut.

It should be noted that, as a rule, not more than ten interrupted catgut sutures are used in fashioning the axial union and that these sutures are placed through all layers of tissue. The vertical limb of the T tube is drawn through the top end of the abdominal incision or through a small stab incision situated to the right of the sutured abdominal incision, where it is securely anchored to the skin by encircling sutures of silk and by means of strips of Micropore, after which it is connected to a segment of rubber tubing that is inserted into a baby's feeding bottle affixed to the left side of the bed, or a URI-BAG (Stille) may be employed.

Biliary-Intestinal Anastomosis

Hepaticojejunostomy should be performed when an axial union between the

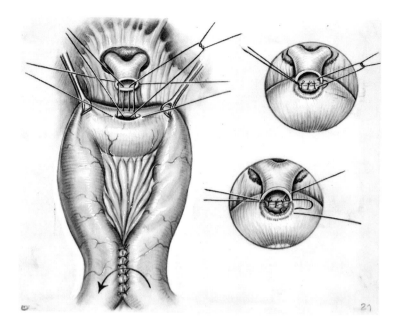

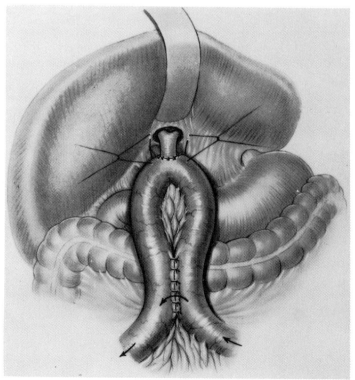

FIG. 24. (A) Hepaticojejunostomy. The jejunal loop method with entero-anastomosis. As the biliary-enteric stoma is of ample proportions, no T tube or Y tube prosthesis is required. (B) Operation completed. This, in my opinion, is the ideal type of reconstructive operation. Note the position of the entero-anastomosis and also the method of anchoring the jejunal loop to the liver to prevent any downward traction of the stoma. (Courtesy of Butterworths, London.)

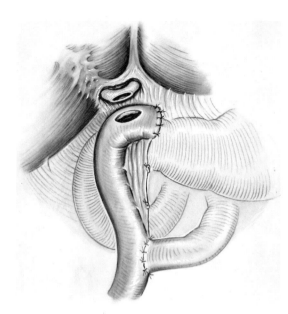

FIG. 25. Hepaticojejunostomy. The Roux-en-Y method. (Courtesy of Butterworths, London.)

ends of the bile ducts is not a feasible or safe undertaking owing to a discrepancy in the size of the proximal and distal ducts or when the distance is considerable between the two ends, which would result in tension if an end-to-end anastomosis were fashioned. This is a highly satisfactory procedure, particularly when the remaining segment of common bile duct is of ample length. I use a *long loop of proximal jejunum* (16 in.), which is drawn upward anterior to the greater omentum and transverse colon (Fig. 24). A point on the antimesenteric border of the jejunum selected for anastomosis to the "freshened" stump of the hepatic duct is steadied with two Babcock forceps and drawn upward and affixed to the porta hepatis to ensure that there will be no tension on the suture line when the union is complete.

It is advisable to adopt the *Roux-en-Y plan* when the mesojejunum proves to be unduly stunted. A small opening corresponding to the calibre of the bile duct is made in the jejunum, and four to six interrupted sutures of 000 chromic catgut are passed through all the layers of the jejunum and the posterior margin of the common hepatic duct. The ends of these sutures are held

together while the apposing posterior margins of the duct and jejunal wall are brought into apposition, after which the sutures are securely tied and divided near—but not too near—to the knots. The anterior edges of the duct and jejunum are likewise united with four or six fine chromic catgut sutures. Eight to 10 sutures in all are ample in constructing this type of anastomosis; more would be superfluous or even harmful.

This anastomosis is often made over some type of prosthesis. The surgeon may elect to use (1) a straight rubber or latex tube (2) a Y tube, or (3) a T tube or the Maingot guttered T tube, depending on the circumstances of the case. The distal end or *long arm* of the tubes should be led to the exterior, anchored to the skin, and then directed into a plastic URI-BAG. The amount of bile discharged each day can be measured accurately and specimens taken for chemical and microscopical investigations. Again, x-ray films can be obtained, after injection of Hypaque or diodone to ascertain the condition of the intrahepatic biliary tree and the biliary-intestinal stoma. In my opinion, *inlaying stents* should not be used to act as splints or supports of anastomotic junctions, as, with

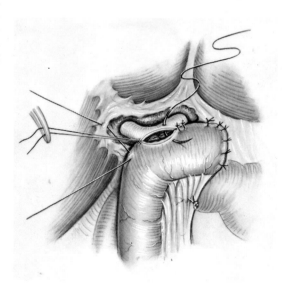

FIG. 26. Hepaticojejunostomy. The Roux-en-Y method of anastomosis. (From Maingot, in Rob and Smith, and Morgan, *Operative Surgery*, 2d ed., 1969. Courtesy of Butterworths, London.)

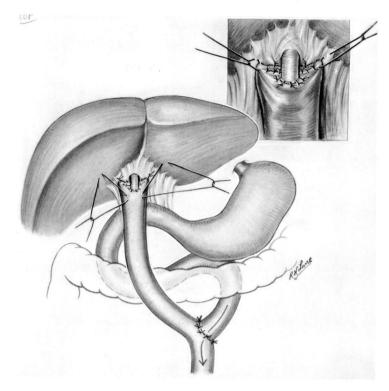

FIG. 27.   Hepaticojejunostomy employing the Roux-en-Y loop.

the passage of time, they frequently become occluded with biliary mud or calculi, thus demanding immediate extraction to circumvent cholangitis, pericholedochitis, and the symptoms associated with obstructive jaundice.

All prostheses—straight rubber tube, T tube, Maingot's guttered T tube and Y tubes which *splint the biliary-intestinal stoma* and drain bile to the exterior—should be left in situ for variable periods depending on the pathologic lesion present and the general condition of the patient, the average time being about 3 months. As has been stated before, tubes (straight, T, or Y) made of any variety of *plastic material,* e.g., polyethylene, should never be employed in biliary tract surgery. Such tubes tend to undergo a process of hardening and discoloration, and while being immersed in bile and they tend to lacerate the duct or adjoining stoma or withdrawal. *If the hepatoenteric stoma is of adequate calibre, the use of such tubes or any other type of tube is, of course, superfluous.* When a T tube is employed as a prosthesis,

it should be inserted either through the anterior wall of the bile duct or through a small puncture hole made in the efferent limb of the jejunal loop. The ascending arm of the T tube is directed through the stoma into the right or left hepatic duct, while the descending arm is led into the efferent limb of the jejunum. The long vertical portion of the T tube is brought to the exterior for drainage purposes.

The final step of the operation consists in performing an entero-anastomosis 5 to 6 inches (102. to 15.3 cm) below the biliary anastomosis, in order to divert gastrointestinal juices and food particles away from the biliary tree (Figs. 24, 30, and 31).

When the Roux-en-Y plan is adopted, the end-to-side anastomosis is fashioned first, after which the long ascending limb of defunctioned jejunum is drawn upward to the hilus of the liver and anastomosed to the open mouth of the bile duct, as is well depicted in Figures 25 to 27.

At the completion of any type of biliary-

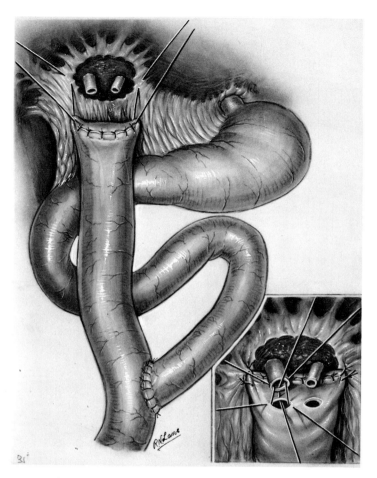

FIG. 28.   Roux-en-Y plan for stricture involving the hepatic ducts. Anastomosis of the right and left hepatic ducts to a Roux-en-Y loop of proximal jejunum. At the prior operation (the fifth), external biliary drainage was established. The artist's impression of the second-stage procedure, which was carried out by Maingot, is depicted.

intestinal anastomosis, it is essential to anchor the adjacent intestine to the hepatoduodenal ligament or to the capsule of the liver, close to the porta hepatis, in order to avoid any downward drag on the newly fashioned stoma. This step in the operation is depicted in Figures 24, 27, and 30.

Hepaticoduodenostomy had the powerful support of Whitman Walters.[60, 61] In this reconstructive procedure, he and others have generally favoured the principle of anastomosing the upper end of the bile duct to the side of the adjacent duodenum. (Good results have been obtained in about 70 percent of patients.) This operation has been accu-

rately and superbly illustrated in the numerous contributions on this subject by Walters during the last 40 years (Fig. 33).

At the Lahey Clinic, hepaticoduodenostomy has been used most frequently for postoperative strictures in patients who had previously undergone partial gastrectomy by the Billroth II method because of peptic ulceration.

Statistical data suggest that the end-results of hepaticoduodenostomy and hepaticojejunostomy are almost identical and that they are both excellent procedures when an ample portion of common hepatic duct is available for anastomosis. Nevertheless, personal experience has biased me in favour of the latter method of reconstruction. Thus, when an axial union between the ends of the bile ducts is not possible I select "jejunal loop" hepaticojejunostomy with entero-anastomoses with confidence. It should be emphasized, once again, that whenever the anastomotic stoma is judged to be large, or, indeed, adequate in diameter, T tube or Y tube splintage is an unnecessary procedure.

Diltatation of ductal strictures. In certain cases, incision of the duct to permit of dilatation of the stricture by means of graduated Bakes' sounds may be undertaken. I refer to *minor strictures* situated relatively low in the ductal system and those which involve the right or left hepatic duct. Following an adequate dilatation, the affected area of the duct should be splinted and discour-

aged from further contraction by means of an inlying guttered T tube.

Excision of a Small Localized Stricture

When a localised fibrous stricture involves the readily accessible middle portion of the ductal system, excision of the fibrotic area, followed by end-to-end anastomosis, is the operation of choice rather than a plastic procedure on the Heineke-Mikulicz plan, which is illustrated in Figure 34.

Lateral choledochoduodenostomy. This operation may be indicated in certain cases of *impassable fibrous stricture of the lower end of the common bile duct* when the patient is ill, wasted, and jaundiced; it is also indicated in some cases of irremovable mul-

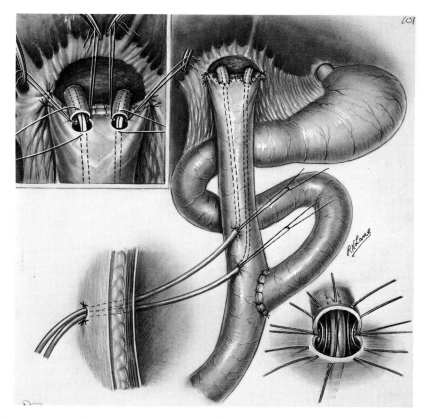

FIG. 29. Roux-en-Y plan for stricture involving the hepatic ducts. Second-stage repair of extensive stricture involving the hepatic ducts. The segment of jejunum through which the rubber tubes emerged was anchored to the peritoneum. The tubes were withdrawn 4 months after the operation. The patient has remained symptom-free for 4½ years.

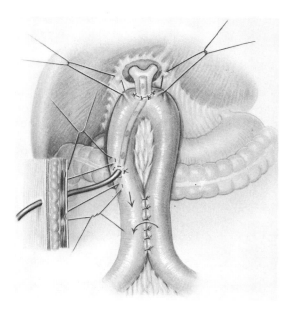

FIG. 30.   Hepaticojejunostomy.   The   straight-tube method.

tiple calculi lodged in the intrahepatic ducts (Figs. 35 and 36).

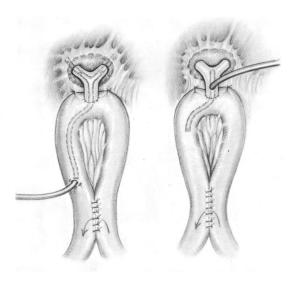

FIG. 31.   Hepaticojejunostomy. The T tube and the Y tube methods of splintage and drainage of the biliary tree.

Two-stage repairs and special procedures. In this group are included those cases in which at the first-stage operation: (a) an external biliary fistula was produced, e.g., *hepaticostomy;* or (b) *an inlying Y tube was used in fashioning a duct-to-duct anastomosis* or for splinting a biliary-intestinal anastomosis. *When the Y tube becomes obstructed with biliary sediment, it is removed at the secondary operation.* The results of this two-stage operation are gratifying, as shown by Warren et al. (1966) in his analyses of 225 patients who were treated by this two-stage Y tube method. Excellent or good results were obtained in 183 (82 percent) of the patients. *Nevertheless, the majority of surgeons prefer to use a Y tube with a long limb that can be brought out through the jejunal wall and abdominal wall and used for irrigation of the ductal system and postoperative cholangiography.* It can be readily and safely removed at a time when it is judged to have performed its functions satisfactorily. The subsequent discharge of bile or intestinal contents is minimal and is rarely prolonged for more than 2 or 3 days.

See also Figures 37, 38, and 39.

According to Cattell and Braasch,[4] *hepaticostomy* is recommended in patients who show the following defects:

1. Severe liver damage as obtains in certain cases of cirrhosis.
2. High serum bilirubin levels, i.e., usually above 30 mg per 100 ml.
3. Portal hypertension (with operative bleeding impeding dissection).
4. General condition deteriorating during the conduct of attempted repair of the duct or ducts.
5. Operative evidence of sepsis in the subhepatic space.

After hepaticostomy, the *second-stage procedure* will consist of anastomosing the remaining stump of the common hepatic duct to the proximal jejunum or to the first portion of the duodenum. This second-stage procedure is carried out some weeks or months after the establishment of the external biliary drainage or when it is deemed that the optimum improvement in the patient's general condition has been achieved.

In cases of stricture of *one hepatic duct,* it is customary to dilate the duct adequately

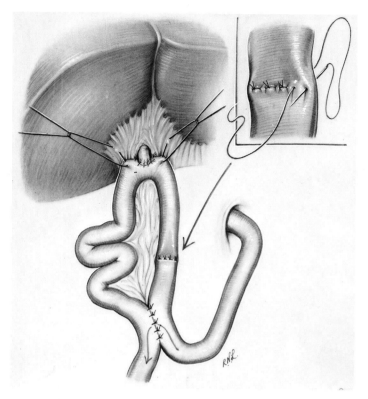

FIG. 32. Hepaticojejunostomy with entero-anastomosis. (K. W. Warren's technique.)

with Bakes' dilators, after which it should be splinted with a long-arm T tube. Should there be any subsequent recurrence following this procedure, at a second stage a biliary-intestinal anastomosis (hepaticojejunostomy) becomes mandatory (Figs. 40, 41).

When at the primary operation no extrahepatic bile duct is found, the surgeon may be tempted to perform *Longmire's operation: intrahepatic cholangiojejunostomy.* Before undertaking Longmire's operation an *operative transhepatic cholangiogram* should be performed to delineate the ducts and to ascertain whether or not there is a free communication between the right and left ductal systems. This ingenious operation may be worthy of a trial when there is no constriction or obstruction at the carina. (Figures 42 and 43).

For hilar and intrahepatic bile duct strictures, Rodney Smith has devised an operation entitled "mucosal graft operation" which is

described and well illustrated later in this chapter.

The surgical treatment of strictures in which *the bifurcation of the common hepatic duct has been ablated or is replaced by dense scar tissue, or in which one or both hepatic ducts are stenosed and fibrotic,* presents many problems. The majority of patients thus afflicted suffer from cholangitis and its effects, i.e., hepatomegaly, cirrhosis, congestive splenomegaly, hypoprothrombinaemia, hypoproteinaemia, hypersplenism, and anaemia. They are indeed serious operative risks, as jaundice is present, the liver enlarged and damaged, and bleeding from the operative site is brisk and difficult to control. The painstaking dissection entailed in the hilar structures and the intrahepatic course of these ducts demands the optimal surgical skill and experience in biliary tract surgery as well as patience and determination—backed by a knowledge of the previous suc-

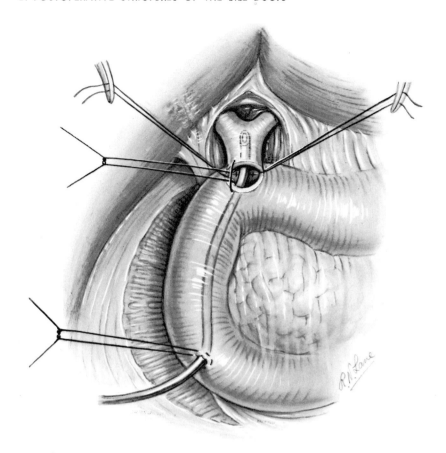

FIG. 33.   Hepaticoduodenostomy.   (Courtesy of Butterworths, London.)

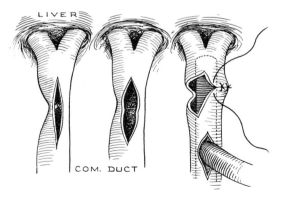

FIG. 34.   Plastic repair of a low, localised stricture of the common bile duct. (Courtesy of Dr. K. W. Warren and W. B. Saunders, Philadelphia.)

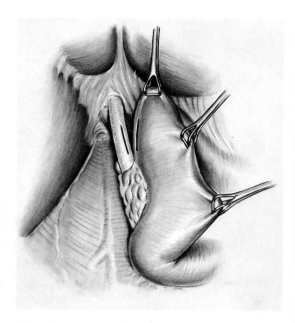

FIG. 35.   Lateral choledochoduodenostomy. (Courtesy of Butterworths, London.)

cesses and failures entailed in such work.

The surgeon should remember that: (1) the pulsating common hepatic artery or the right

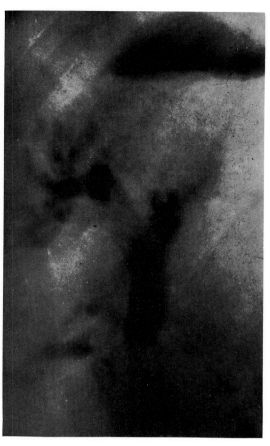

FIG. 37.   Radiograph showing gas in biliary tree following choledochojejunostomy for benign stricture of common bile duct. Picture was taken 3 years after the repair procedure. There has been no recurrence of symptoms, although ducts appear somewhat dilated.

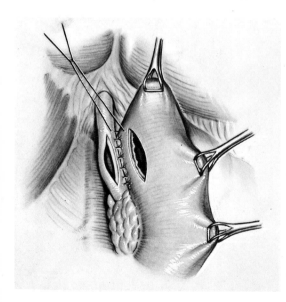

FIG. 36.   Lateral choledochoduodenostomy for stricture of the lower end of the common bile duct. The anastomotic stoma should be fashioned as large as possible. (Courtesy of Butterworths, London.)

usually lies medial to the duct remnant; (2) the portal vein is posterior; (3) a fistula between the nubbin of duct and duodenum is not infrequent, and suitable probing will often outline the proximal ducts; (4) needling the hilus of the liver may be rewarded by the aspiration of white or yellow bile; and (5) operative cholangiography may, at times, illuminate the ductal system and facilitate operative procedures.

These cases present an almost insurmountable problem when the hepatic artery or its main branches course to the liver in a plane which is definitely *anterior* to the damaged ducts in the hilus of the liver.

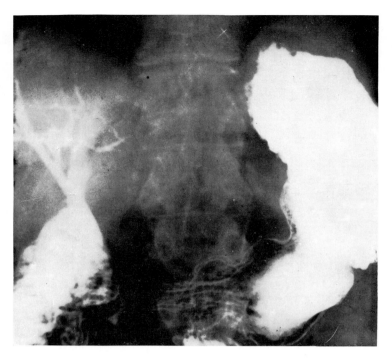

FIG. 38. Hepaticojejunostomy for bile-duct stricture. Barium-meal x-ray examination was carried out 4 years after operation was undertaken by the writer. Note ample stoma.

The dissection of the structures in the porta hepatis proceeds on the lines already described: The hepatic flexure is dropped; the duodenum and head of the pancreas are mobilised; the common duct gland is identified; when possible, the lower end of the common bile duct is recovered, dissected free, and probed; the position of the hepatic artery and of the portal vein is verified, and a search is made in the hilus of the liver (in the right margin of the hepatoduodenal ligament) for the remnant of common hepatic duct and its two main branches.

The treatment recommended will depend upon the *position and extent of the stricture.* For instance:

1. When the common hepatic duct and common bile duct appear to be normal but a stricture of the *right or left hepatic duct* is found, after fulgurating (with a diathermy needle or wire loop) sufficient liver substance in the hilus to demonstrate the ducts, the main bile duct is opened, and the ductal stricture is fully dilated with graduated Bakes' dilators, after which a T tube is placed through the dilated segment. The T tube is left in situ for a period of 6 to 12 months. During convalescence the tube is "spigotted" to allow all the bile to flow freely into the duodenum. Before being discharged from hospital, the patient is instructed to irrigate the tube with sterile warm normale saline, once or twice daily, to take tablets containing bile salts (such as dehydrocholine succinate) twice daily, and to allow the vertical arm of the T tube to drain the bile into a bottle for short periods in each day. The T tube eventually becomes silted up with depositions of bile salts and detritus, and has to be removed.

2. When the bifurcation of the common hepatic duct is destroyed, the involved scarred area will have to be excised with a knife. If, perchance, the "carina" is intact, the fringe of surrounding ductal tissue may be anastomosed over an indwelling *long-armed Y tube.*

Cholangiograms performed through this special radiopaque Y tube may show that the intrahepatic ductal system is well decompressed.

When, however, after excising the bifurcation of the common hepatic duct together with the "carina" the right and left hepatic ducts are seen to lie close to one another, these two ducts should be sutured together and the septum between them should be divided in order to create a new common hepatic duct as practiced by Cattell. (Fig. 41).

The decision whether to employ the proximal freshened end of the common hepatic duct for anastomosis to the jejunum or duodenum depends upon the condition of the lower end of the choledochus. If, after it has been "recovered" following a meticulous dissection, it appears fibrotic and attentuated, it would be foolhardy to attempt a duct-to-duct anastomosis. Again, in those instances in which speed is essential owing to the poor condition of the patient, before and during operation, the surgeon would be well advised to select an expeditious hepaticoduodenostomy rather than hepaticojejunostomy which entails two procedures or anastomoses.

3. When, following excision of a hilar stricture of the ducts, the ends of the right and left hepatic ducts are seen to be too widely separated from each other, it is advisable to bring up the Roux-en-Y limb of proximal jejunum (anterior to the hepatic flexure of the colon) to the hilus and to perform two

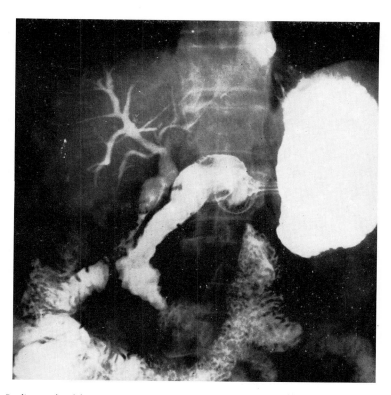

FIG. 39. Radiograph of barium-meal x-ray examination carried out because of repeated attacks of melaena. Hepaticojejunostomy had been performed 5 years previously by the writer for postoperative bile-duct stricture. At operation large leiomyosarcoma was found occupying upper portion of stomach. Subtotal gastrectomy was performed and patient made good recovery. Note satisfactory hepaticocenteric stoma.

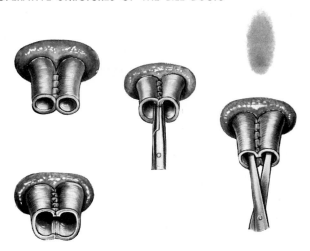

FIG. 40. Cattell's method of performing hepaticojejunostomy for intrahepatic strictures. (From Maingot, in Rob, Smith, and Morgan, 1969. *Operative Surgery*, 2d ed. Courtesy of Butterworths, London.)

separate end-to-side anastomoses. The two minute hepatojejunal stomas should be splinted with rubber tubing. (See Figs. 28 and 29.)

Miscellaneous Procedures

Further special operative techniques are described below.

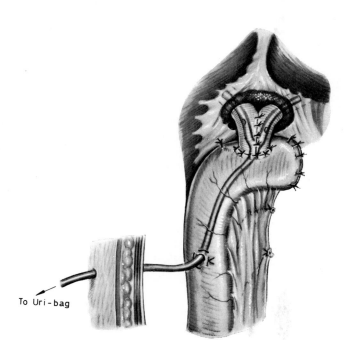

To Uri-bag

FIG. 41. Cattell's method employing a long Y tube. (From Maingot, in Rob, Smith, and Morgan, 1969. *Operative Surgery*, 2d ed. Courtesy of Butterworths, London.)

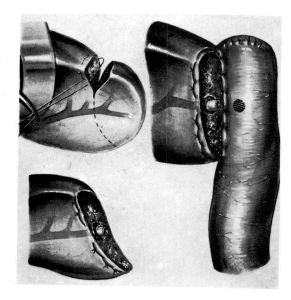

FIG. 42. Longmire's operation of intrahepatic cholangiojejunostomy. (Courtesy of Butterworths, London.)

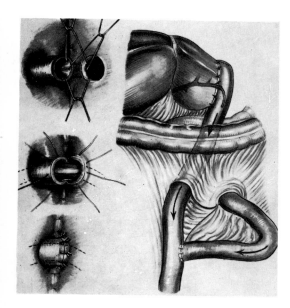

FIG. 43. Longmire's operation of intrahepatic cholangiojejunostomy. (Courtesy of Butterworths, London.)

LONGMIRE'S OPERATION

The operation described by Longmire and Sandford,[25] and as practised by Massie [40] and other surgeons, has been used with a measure of success in the treatment of certain types of intractable postoperative stricture of the extrahepatic bile ducts. Longmire and Sandford reported four successful cases in which *intrahepatic cholangiojejunostomy* was performed, at the Johns Hopkins Hospital, for traumatic stricture of the common hepatic duct. The case reported by Massie (1950) was also a gratifying success.

Preoperative percutaneous intrahepatic cholangiography should be carried out to ascertain whether there is *a free communication* between the intrahepatic ducts of the right lobe of the liver and those of the left lobe. Unless there is a generous communication between these two groups of biliary passages, Longmire's operation is doomed to failure.

The operation is performed as follows: the left lobe of the liver is mobilised and its lateral two-thirds are removed. The largest branch of the left hepatic duct is isolated and then anastomosed to a *Roux-en-Y jejunal loop.* An indwelling latex tube splints the anastomosis (Figs. 42 and 43). The jejunum is then anchored in front and behind to the liver capsule, and a jejunojejunostomy is constructed as close as possible to the duodenojejunal flexure. This procedure offers the last hope in cases in which it is impossible to find any ductal structures after a sedulous search and extensive coring out of hepatic tissue with a diathermy knife or wire curettes in the porta hepatis. As I have noted, the operation has no chance of success if the right and left intrahepatic ductal systems are not in direct communication with each other. An operative cholangiogram, employing the left hepatic duct, may illuminate the ducts and engender a measure of confidence in some instances. Today, this operation has been superseded by the *mucosal graft operation* for hilar strictures. (See Part C.)

* I should like to express my thanks and appreciation to Dr. Dragstedt and to Dr. Woodward for the loan of the illustrations depicting their method of reconstructing the extrahepatic biliary passages, and also for allowing me to quote freely from their instructive article from Surgery, Gynecology and Obstetrics.

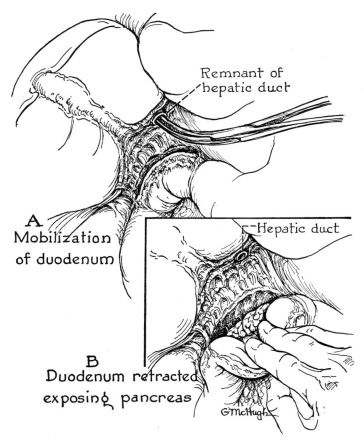

FIG. 44.   Dragstedt's technique. (From Dragstedt and Woodward, *Surg. Gynecol. Obstet.* 94: 53, 1952. Courtesy of *Surgery, Gynecology, and Obstetrics.*)

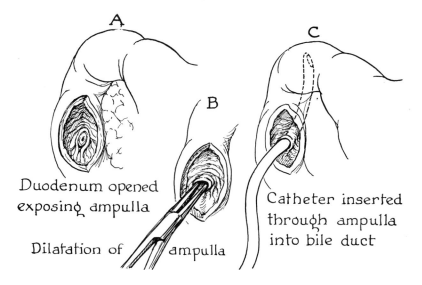

FIG. 45.   Dragstedt's technique. (From Dragstedt and Woodward, *Surg. Gynecol. Obstet.* 94: 53, 1952. Courtesy of *Surgery, Gynecology, and Obstetrics.*)

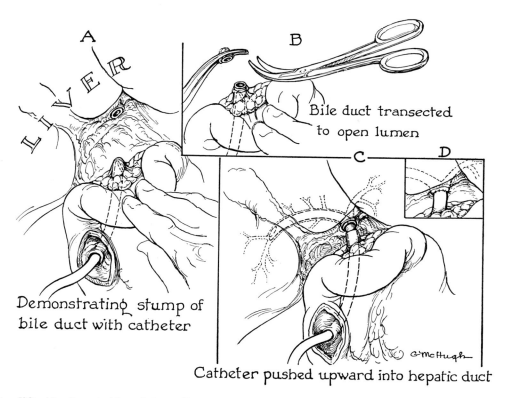

FIG. 46.   Dragstedt's technique. (From Dragstedt and Woodward, Surg. Gynecol. Obstet. 94: 53, 1952. Courtesy of *Surgery, Gynecology, and Obstetrics*.)

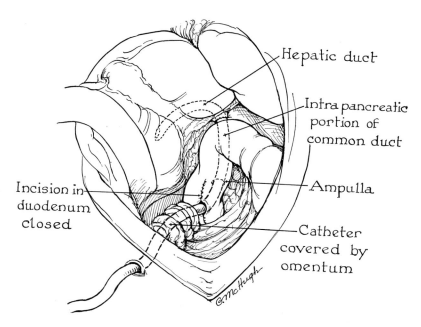

FIG. 47.   Dragstedt's technique. From Dragstedt and Woodward, Surg. Gynecol. Obstet. 94: 53, 1952. Courtesy of *Surgery, Gynecology, and Obstetrics*.)

Dragstedt's Technique

Dragstedt and Woodward [13] have given an account of *transduodenal reconstruction of the bile ducts*. The operation is best described in their own words:

It is the purpose of the present communication to describe a method for reconstruction of the bile ducts, making use of the intrapancreatic portion of the duct and its normal ostium at the ampulla of Vater. The details of technique are best appreciated by inspection of the drawings. The duodenum is mobilized, as indicated in Figure 44, and the remnant of hepatic duct exposed. This is often flush with the surface of the liver. The duodenum should be fully mobilized so that the pancreatic portion of the duct can reach the hepatic remnant without tension. The duodenum is then opened, as in Figure 45, and the ampulla exposed. It is wise for the surgeon to familiarize himself both with the appearance and location of the ampulla so that it may be readily recognized. It is usually necessary to mobilize and displace the transverse colon downward to expose this portion of the duodenum. The ampulla is dilated with a graduated sound or, more simply, with a hemostatic forceps, until it is large enough to admit the rubber catheter. The size of the catheter employed is determined by the diameter of the hepatic duct remnant and is large enough to fit this duct snugly. The catheter is inserted through the ampulla, as in Figure 45C, and passes upward into the pancreatic portion of the common duct which is usually present. As the catheter is pushed upward through the intrapancreatic portion of the common duct, the obstructed end is readily appreciated and can be exposed, as illustrated in Figure 46 A and B. The catheter is then pushed upward until it enters the remnant of hepatic duct, as illustrated in Figure 46 C, and fixed in place with a series of interrupted fine silk sutures, Figure 46 D. This incision in the duodenum is closed, as illustrated in Figure 47, or the catheter may be led outward through a separate stab wound. It is usually wise to fasten the catheter to the duodenum at this point with a suture of chromic catgut. Omentum is then brought up and wrapped about the catheter and sutured so as to cover the incision in the duodenum. The catheter is finally led to the exterior through a stab wound lateral to the incision by the method of Wilson. A Penrose drain is placed in the region of the anastomosis with the hepatic duct and removed after two or three days. It is our practice to leave these catheters in place for at least a year to minimize the tendency for subsequent stricture at the site of the anastomosis. Ill effects from the long continued presence of the tube extending through the ampulla of Vater into the duodenum have not been seen. After a period of several weeks, the catheter may be clamped off, in which case bile escapes around the cannula through the ampulla into the duodenum. In one case an attempt was made to facilitate the passage of bile into the duodenum by making a small opening in the catheter shortly after its exit from the ampulla. This proved to be a mistake because the catheter became displaced outward in the immediate postoperative period and permitted bile to flow into the free peritoneal cavity, and thus a fatal biliary peritonitis was produced.

This method of reconstruction of the bile duct has been employed in three patients in whom the bile duct was more or less completely obliterated, and it has also been used in three patients with chronic relapsing pancreatitis as a method for preventing bile from getting access to the pancreatic duct. The procedure appears to be well tolerated and makes the anatomical reconstruction of the biliary duct system feasible and relatively easy.

Coning-out of External Fistula and Duodenal Implantation

The first successful transplantation of an external biliary fistula into the duodenum was performed by Hugh Williams at the Massachusetts General Hospital, Boston, in 1914. His patient was alive and well many years afterwards. Successful cases have been reported by Williams and Smithwick,[71] Lilienthal,[24] and Waltman Walters.[62] Eliot (1936) recorded that there have been some 41 cases of fistula transplantation, 29 of these having been performed in America. On 18 occasions, the fistula was implanted into the stomach, in one case into the jejunum, and in the remainder into the duodenum. Lahey performed this operation in 14 patients, but in only two was relief obtained. He attributed the failures to the tract's contracting as the result of fibrosis and to obstruction of its lumen with inflammatory debris or biliary sand.

It is the general opinion that this operation is almost invariably doomed to failure and should not in any circumstances be entertained.

"Bridging the Gap"

"Bridging the gap" with a rubber tube or by a heterogenous or autogenous graft (saphenous vein) is an interesting lesson in biliary-tract surgery which will always be linked with the name of Sullivan.[56, 57] In my opinion, it has no place in the modern treatment of postoperative strictures of the bile ducts.

Intrahepatic Biliary-Intestinal Anastomosis

Templeton and Dodd [58] gave an interesting account of the *anatomical separation of the right and left lobes of the liver for intrahepatic anastomosis of the biliary ducts.* They described a case which was successfully treated by this technique. They wrote as follows:

By splitting the liver with blunt dissection along the fissure between the lobes, a most satisfactory exposure of the junction of the right and left hepatic ducts within the liver was rather easily secured.

The liver opened in this fashion very much like the pages of a book and it was quite simple to excise the fibrotic portion of the common hepatic duct and to make a good duct-to-duct, mucosa-to-mucosa union over an indwelling Y tube.

No more difficulty was encountered than in establishing the same type of anastomosis below the liver. The operation was well tolerated by the patient and was followed by a prompt and significant fall in serum bilirubin. The separation of the lobes of the liver did not appear to significantly derange their blood supply. An interlobar hepatic vein encountered during the dissection served as a guide to the proper plane. Bleeders from this vein were controlled readily with ligatures and the coagulating current and mattress sutures were not necessary to control bleeding from the hepatic parenchyma. In this patient the complete interruption of portal venous inflow may have helped diminish the bleeding during the division of the liver. Under other circumstances temporary occlusion of portal vein and hepatic artery with the protection of moderate hypothermia might prove helpful.

Rodney Smith's Techniques

Since 1964, this ingenious and skillful surgeon has devised three original reconstructive procedures for postoperative bile duct strictures:

1. Hepaticojejunostomy: Choledochojejunostomy: a Method of Intrajejunal Anastomosis.[51]
2. Hepaticojejunostomy with Transhepatic Intubation.[52]
3. Mucosal Graft Operation for Hilar or Intrahepatic Strictures of the Hepatic Ducts (Personal communications, 1970, 1973). (See Figs. 64 to 67, Part C of this chapter.)

Hepaticojejunostomy: Choledochojejunostomy: A Method of Intrajejunal Anastomosis

The following important steps should be observed: (1) the biliary-intestinal anastomosis must start by being as large as possible; (2) there must be complete apposition of the bile duct mucosa to the jejunal mucosa; and (3) there must be no tension on the suture line. The stages of the operation are as follows:

The bile duct to be anastomosed is dissected out and in cases of stricture particular care is taken in inspecting the open end to make sure that this is lined with mucosa and not scar tissue. A jejunal Roux loop some 20 cm long is constructed.

The open end of this loop is lifted into the porta hepatis. The hepaticojejunal anastomosis will be sited some 5 to 7 cm from this open end, as shown in Figure 48.

The jejunum is opened at the site chosen and, working through the open end of the

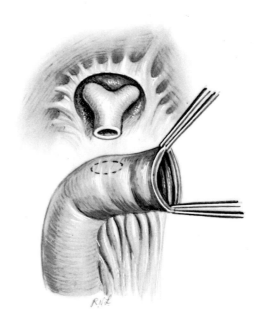

FIG. 48. Hepaticojejunostomy: a method of intrajejunal anastomosis as originally practised by Rodney Smith. (Courtesy of R. Smith and *The British Journal of Surgery.*)

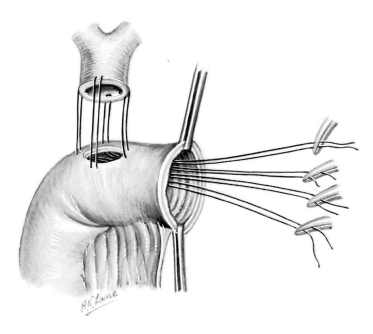

FIG. 49. Hepaticojejunostomy by Rodney Smith's technique. (Courtesy of R. Smith and *The British Journal of Surgery.*)

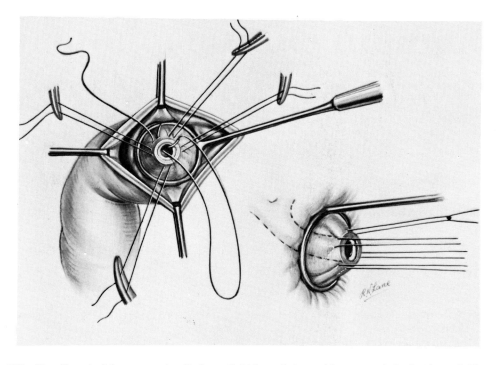

FIG. 50. Hepaticojejunostomy by Rodney Smith's technique. (Courtesy of R. Smith and *The British Journal of Surgery.*)

Roux loop, four stay sutures of fine catgut are inserted—as shown in Figure 49.

The ends of these sutures are threaded through a metal ring with a handle at right angles (Fig. 50), and, by opening up the end of the Roux loop, applying traction to the stay sutures, and pressing back the folds of jejunal mucosa with the metal ring, the end of the bile duct presenting within the jejunal incision is drawn into view.

Anastomosis in one layer is to be constructed with a series of transverse mattress sutures of fine catgut, each inserted as shown in Figure 50 and inset.

The number of sutures depends upon the size of the bile duct and will usually be between six and ten.

With the intrajejunal anastomosis completed, the open end of the Roux loop is closed and the loop itself suspended from the peritoneum or the capsule of the liver so that there is no tension on the anastomosis (Figs. 51 and 52).

The abdomen is then closed, with provision for drainage.

When a sizeable portion of the common hepatic duct can be dissected free from the portal fissure and anastomosed to a Roux-Y jejunal loop (by the plan here described and illustrated), convalescence is smooth and rapid, there is no leakage of bile, and the immediate results are excellent, as demonstrated by Rodney Smith and other surgeons who have adopted this method of reconstruction.

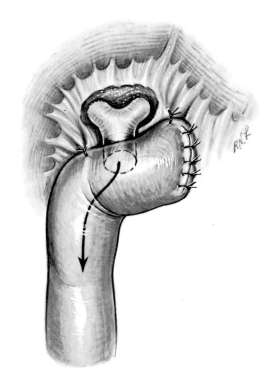

FIG. 51. Hepaticojejunostomy by Rodney Smith's technique. (Courtesy of R. Smith and *The British Journal of Surgery.*)

Hepaticojejunostomy with Transheptic Intubation

If the stricture is located high in the porta hepatis, and *particularly in those cases in which many attempts at reconstruction have already failed,* repair is performed over an indwelling transhepatic tube, as is illustrated in Figures 53 and 54.

The main steps in this operation (regarding which a good critique appeared in *Lancet 1*:597, 1964) include:

1. The fashioning of the *posterior suture line* of the hepaticojejunostomy.
2. The passage of a moderate-sized rubber tube (which has several large holes in its lower portion) through the "uncompleted" stoma upward into one of the main intrahepatic ducts, toward the anterior convex surface of the liver —where a small incision is made in Glisson's capsule precisely over the spot where the end of the tube can be palpated. The anterior or top end of the tube is next projected through the incision in the liver, grasped with a haemostat, and then brought through a laterally placed *subcostal* stab incision. The lower end of the tube is now picked up and directed downward into the lumen of the ascending Roux-en-Y jejunal limb for a distance of 5 to 10 cm. When the surgeon has satisfied himself that there is no kinking of the tube and that it can be made to ride readily up and down in its tunnel, the anterior row of sutures is introduced to complete the biliary-intestinal anastomosis. Care should be taken to avoid "picking-up" the tube with one or

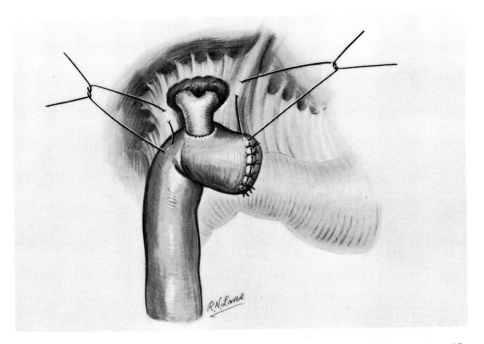

FIG. 52. Hepaticojejunostomy by Rodney Smith's technique. Completion of the operation. (Courtesy of R. Smith and *The British Journal of Surgery*.)

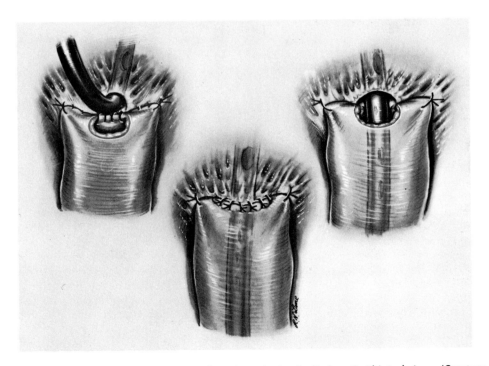

FIG. 53. Hepaticojejunostomy with transhepatic intubation by Rodney Smith's technique. (Courtesy of R. Smith and *The British Journal of Surgery*.)

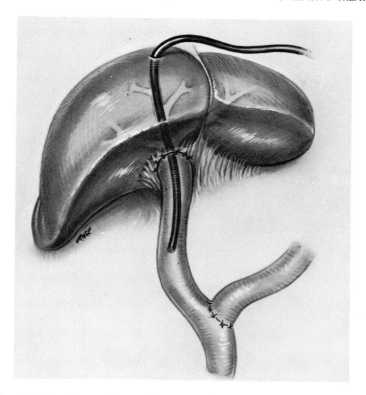

FIG. 54. Hepaticojejunostomy with transhepatic intubation. Roux-en-Y loop. Note position of transhepatic tube, which is eventually led through the abdominal wall for drainage. (Courtesy of R. Smith and *The British Journal of Surgery*.)

more of the interrupted all-coats sutures.

3. The draining of the subhepatic space with a Penrose tube. After closing the abdominal incision, the tube is anchored to the abdominal wall and connected to a polyethylene tube which is introduced into a URI-BAG for drainage purposes. As soon as the patient has recovered from the anaesthetic, suction is applied to this tube for about 1 week in order to divert bile from the healing anastomosis; later the tube is "spigotted" off but washed through daily with sterile normal saline solution. It is left in situ for 6 to 12 months. This long-splinting of the stoma encourages a slow but progressive epithelialization of the anastomotic junction.

In one of my patients, a woman aged 50, the tube remained undisturbed for 18 months without causing any symptoms. When the tube was removed there was no leakage of bile. The removal of the tube was a painless affair, and she has remained in good health. (The operation—hepaticojejunostomy with transhepatic intubation—was performed in May, 1964. When examined in May, 1973, she was enjoying good health.)

MUCOSAL GRAFT OPERATION FOR HILAR AND INTRAHEPATIC STRICTURES OF THE HEPATIC DUCTS

The first account of this operation was given by Rodney Smith at the Meeting of the Association of Surgeons of Great Britain and Ireland, which was held in Dublin, 1967. Figures 55 to 63, clearly depict the essential technical steps and the principles involved in the reconstructions.

A fistulous tract, lined with granulation tissue, when anastomosed to the proximal jejunal loop leads to one thing and one thing only: fibrosis of the stoma and a chain of grave complications, e.g., jaundice, acute cholangitis, etc. When the fistulous tract, together with its surrounding and accompanying hepatic fibrotic tissue, is coned-out and widely excised, a dome-shaped cavity in the liver substance will result. Further dissection in the apex of this dome-shaped space will expose the carina of the hepatic ducts or the right and left hepatic ducts. The terminal portion (or portions) of the fibrosed duct is excised with a knife in order to ensure that the distal end of the duct (or ducts) is healthy and suitable for the mucosal graft approximation. A Roux-en-Y loop is now fashioned, and a circular seromuscular cuff of jejunum is excised. The jejunal mucosa bulges through the defect in the gut wall as illustrated in Figure 57. Smith's special Y tube is next introduced through the open mouth of the jejunum and the splayed-out arms of the tube are led to the exterior through two puncture holes in the mucosa (Fig. 58). The terminal end of the jejunum is securely closed, and the Y tube—together with its clinging tent of jejunal mucosa—is guided upward into the capacious intrahepatic bile ducts (Fig. 59). A finger invaginates the wall of the jejunum into the open end of the Y tube and then forces the mucosal cuff firmly into position before completing the circumferential suturing which completes the anastomosis.

At times, the arms of the Y tube stubbornly "refuse" to be guided and to be snugly placed into the intrahepatic ducts. In such instances, a long flexible silver probe (which has an "eye" in its distal or bulbous end) is guided upward into the right hepatic duct and forced through the curving liver substance and Glisson's capsule, after which 6 inches (15 cm) of 000 chromic catgut is threaded through the eye of the probe and its ends are tied together. The loop of catgut is held while the knotted ends are withdrawn into the operative field. The knot is untied and the strand of the catgut is passed through the distal end of the Y tube and ligated. The loop of catgut on the anterior surface of the liver is next gently pulled upward, drawing the recalcitrant tube with it, and, when it is judged to be lying snugly within the duct, the loop of catgut is cut and then threaded through the eye of a small half-circle needle, and is finally affixed to Glisson's capsule and cut short.

The same procedure is next applied when guiding the left arm of the Y tube up the left hepatic duct.

C. MUCOSAL GRAFT OPERATIONS FOR HILAR STRICTURES AND FOR STRICTURES OF THE HEPATIC DUCTS

RODNEY SMITH

During the past few years, further experience with the *mucosal graft* technique has suggested that the simplest method is to combine it with the method of transhepatic intubation described by me in 1964. After the transhepatic tube has been drawn down through the duct system and out of the widely opened common hepatic duct remnant, the mucosal pocket is constructed and through a snugly fitting stab incision in its apex the end of the tube is inserted and guided well down into the Roux loop. Just below the mucosal graft the tube is anchored by means of two catgut sutures transfixing part of the jejunal wall and the intraluminal tube. Several lateral holes are cut in the tube just above the graft. Traction is now applied to the end of the tube issuing from the dome of the liver, and the graft is thereby pulled firmly into place inside the common hepatic duct, the lateral holes lying in the intrahepatic portion of the duct. If the duct in-

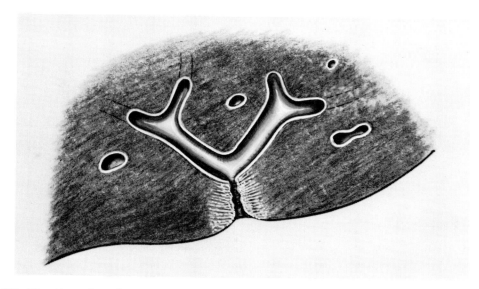

FIG. 55. Mucosal graft operation for hilar and intrahepatic strictures of the hepatic ducts. (R. Smith's technique.) (Courtesy of Butterworths, London.)

jury is so high that no common hepatic duct remains, two transhepatic tubes are used, one through the left hepatic duct system, the other through the right. The Roux loop is anchored firmly in place underneath the liver by means of sutures placed between the edge of the divided seromuscular coat and the scar tissue around the opening into the duct system.

The advantages of combining transhepatic

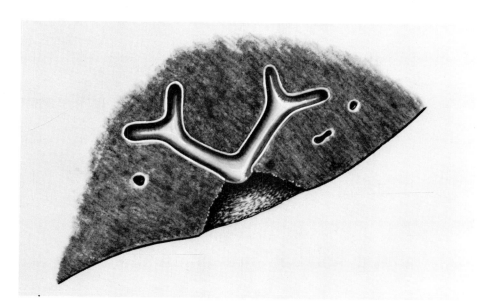

FIG. 56. Mucosal graft operation for hilar and intrahepatic strictures of the hepatic ducts. (R. Smith's technique.)

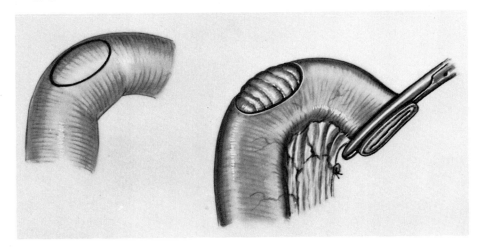

FIG. 57. Mucosal graft operations for hilar and intrahepatic strictures of the hepatic ducts. (R. Smith's technique.)

intubation with the mucosal graft principle are:

1. The ease and simplicity in the placing of the mucosal graft.
2. Bile is diverted by the use of suction applied to the transhepatic tube while the newly made junction is healing.

3. The junction of bile duct epithelium to jejunal epithelium is made by a sutureless technique. No foreign material, absorbable or unabsorbable, lies bathed in bile on the mucosal junction.
4. If the intrahepatic duct system is full of small stones and debris, as not infre-

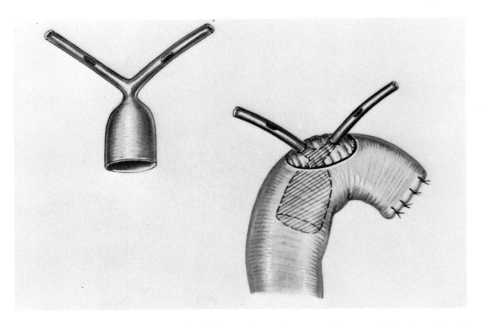

FIG. 58. Mucosal graft operation for hilar and intrahepatic strictures of the hepatic ducts. (R. Smith's technique.) Note R. Smith's special Y tube.

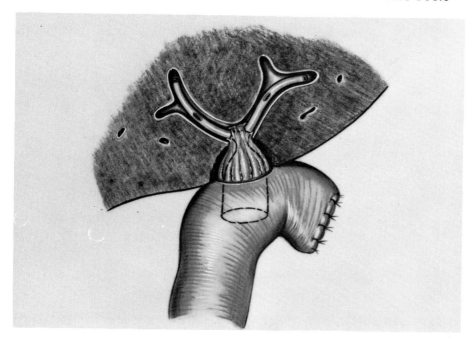

FIG. 59. Mucosal graft operation for hilar and intrahepatic strictures of the hepatic ducts. (R. Smith's technique.) (Courtesy of Butterworths, London.)

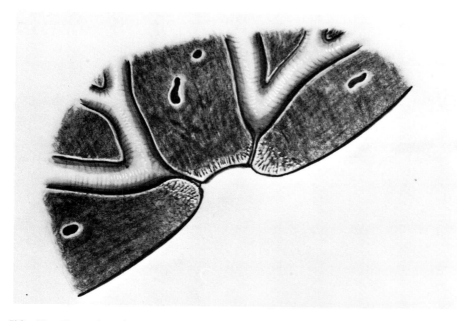

FIG. 60. Mucosal graft operation for hilar and intrahepatic strictures of the hepatic ducts.

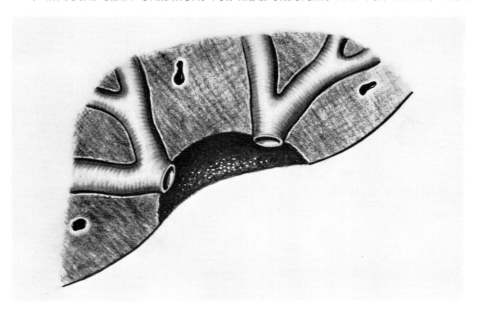

FIG. 61. Mucosal graft operation for hilar and intrahepatic strictures of the hepatic ducts. (R. Smith's technique.) (Courtesy of Butterworths, London.)

quently is the case, washing-out of the duct system can continue postoperatively and this can be most valuable, for the degree to which the duct system can be properly washed out during operation is limited.

5. Postoperative radiological control is easy. Figure 67 shows a postoperative transhepatic cholangiogram, demonstrating well how the transhepatic tube is sited and also the *extremely accurate apposition of the common hepatic duct*

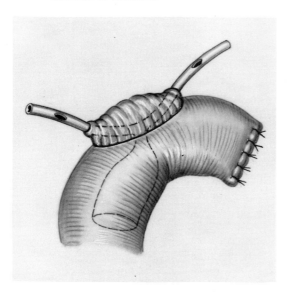

FIG. 62. Mucosal graft operation for hilar and intrahepatic strictures of the hepatic ducts.

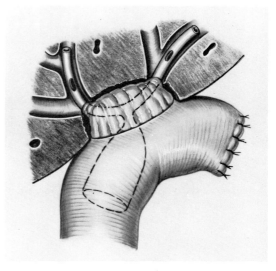

FIG. 63. Mucosal graft operation for hilar and intrahepatic strictures of the hepatic ducts.

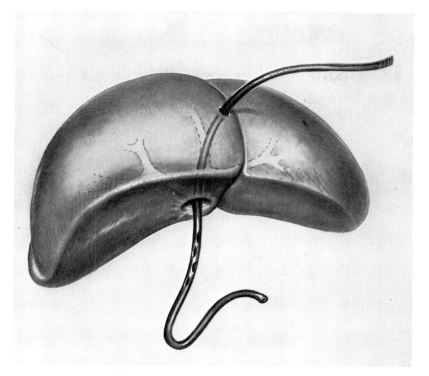

FIG. 64. Mucosal graft technique (R. Smith's new method.) (Courtesy of J. Badenoch and B. Brooke, eds. From Smith, Strictures of the Bile Ducts, Chap. 15, in *Recent Advances in Gastro-enterology*, 2d ed., 1972. Courtesy of Churchill Livingstone, London.)

to the jejunal mucosal graft.

6. Postoperative bacteriological control is easy. Bile is available at any time for culture by applying suction to the transhepatic tube.

7. The deposition of bile pigment within the tube is prevented by a daily wash-out of the tube, the patient being taught before leaving hospital to carry this out for himself. Apart from the daily washing-out, the tube is kept spigoted and does not interfere with normal activities.

8. Support for the anastomosis with the transhepatic tube is continued as long as is desired. Usually 4 months will suffice, the tube being simply removed after a final cholangiogram.

Results

Some 150 patients with high ductal strictures have so far been operated upon em-ploying some form of mucosal graft technique. There have been two deaths. One patient died of bacteraemic shock, having had her very deep obstructive jaundice with severe attacks of cholangitis treated for over a year with a variety of antibiotics (instead of surgery). A variety of resistant organisms were identified on culturing bile taken at operation (an essential step in the surgery of bile duct strictures), but the existence of two resistant strains was not demonstrated until a fatal septicaemia and cardiac arrest had resulted in death 36 hours postoperatively.

A second patient with severe secondary biliary cirrhosis and poor liver function, including clotting deficits, was apparently progressing normally 10 days postoperatively but then suddenly developed gastrointestinal haemorrhage, haemorrhage into the pericardium, and haemorrhage into the pleural cavities, from which she died.

In those patients so far available for one year follow-up, the incidence of restenosis is

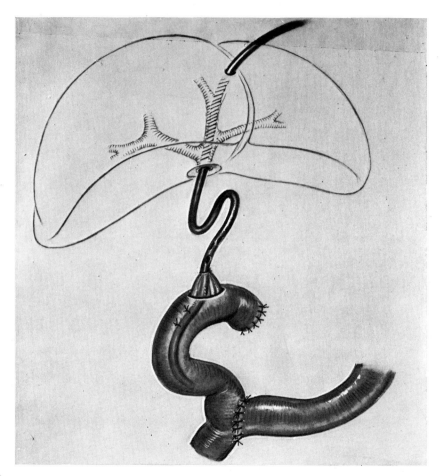

FIG. 65.   Mucosal graft technique (R. Smith's new method.) (Courtesy of J. Badenoch and B. Brooke, eds. From Smith, Strictures of the Bile Ducts, Chap. 15, in *Recent Advances in Gastro-enterology*, 2d ed., 1972. Courtesy of Churchill Livingstone, London.)

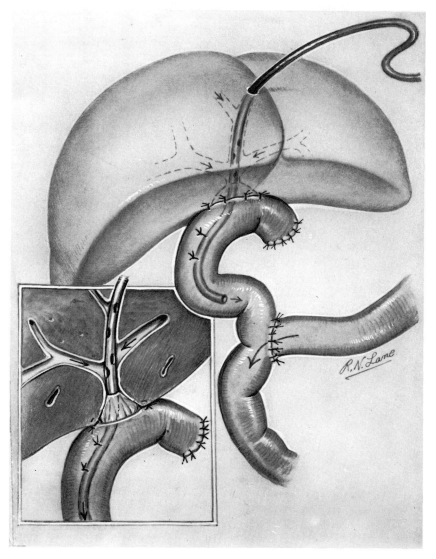

FIG. 66.   Mucosal graft technique (R. Smith's new method.) (Courtesy of J. Badenoch and B. Brooke, eds. From Smith, Strictures of the Bile Ducts, Chap. 15, in *Recent Advances in Gastro-enterology*, 2d ed., 1972. Courtesy of Churchill Livingstone, London.)

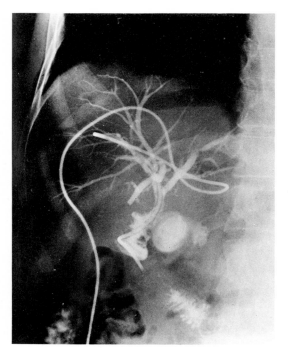

FIG. 67. Postoperative cholangiogram following repair of a high ductal stricture by means of transhepatic intubation combined with a mucosal graft. The extremely accurate apposition of the common hepatic duct to the mucosal graft is clearly visible.

between 7 to 8 percent. There should be a much longer trial than there has been to date before any firm conclusions are put forward, but at the present time it does appear that this technique is not only simpler and easier in terms of the operation itself but also one that is likely to give better results than other techniques so far employed.

Postoperative Complications

Postoperative complications may be summarised as follows: haemorrhage, "shock," external biliary fistula, subphrenic abscess, suppurative cholangitis, hepatic failure, "hepatorenal syndrome," atelectasis, pneumonia, pulmonary embolism, and cardiac infarction. By far the most common causes of death following these reconstructive operations are postoperative "shock," liver failure, and peritonitis.

D. PROGNOSIS
Results Following Various Reconstructive Procedures

RODNEY MAINGOT

A patient who has sustained an injury to the bile duct will have the best chance if the initial repair is done at the time of injury or as soon after the injury as possible, and if the operation reestablishes the continuity of the bile ducts and preserves the sphincter of Oddi. If there is a recurrence of the stricture, the patient is faced with one or more operations, and the chance of a good result will diminish with each additional surgical procedure. In Lahey's entire group of cases (1950), there were 24 postoperative deaths in the total of 344 operative proce-

dures, or a procedure mortality rate of 7 percent. In the period from 1940 to 1948, there were 273 operative procedures in 185 patients, with 12 deaths, or a procedure mortality rate of 4.4 percent; the patient mortality rate was 6.3 percent. Good results were obtained in 81.7 percent and unsatisfactory results were recorded in 18.3 percent. Of 73 patients, 63 (87.2 percent) had a good result when the initial procedure was an end-to-end anastomosis. In those cases in which the proximal duct was anastomosed to a long antecolic loop of jejunum, and an entero-anastomosis was placed below the biliary-enteric stoma, the late results were nearly as good as those obtained with an end-to-end suture (73.1 percent cures).

Walters and Kelly [63] reported that 82 percent of the patients on whom choledocho-duodenostomy had been performed were living and well.

With present-day methods of prevention of bleeding and the control of infection and with accurate anastomosis of the ends of the ducts or of the duct and the intestine, the mortality rate in my last 86 operations has been 2.3 percent. When all cases in which operation was performed are considered, including that unfavourable group in which *no extrahepatic duct could be found* or insufficient duct was present to effect any anastomosis, good results were found in well over 50 percent of cases.

Warren Cole [6] wrote on this subject as follows:

Good results can be expected following repair of strictures in 70 to 80 percent of patients, although the experience of the operator is a very important factor in results. In general, results are jeopardised by numerous previous operations, since scar tissue around the bile duct will be increased by successive operations. When enough proximal and distal duct can be found to do an end-to-end anastomosis, the results should undoubtedly be better than in the other type of lesion. In our series of 63 operations on 49 patients we had 4 postoperative deaths, or a mortality rate of 6.0 percent. Eighty percent of the series had results classified as good to excellent. On a few occasions chills and fever were present for a year or two after operation, but later disappeared.

Cole, Ireneus, and Reynolds [7] later reported a study of 122 cases:

We prefer the use of a defunctionalised loop of jejunum, the open end of which is anastomosed as a so-called Roux-Y to the hepatic end of the bile duct. . . . We have not been reluctant to do without the distal duct because we have found the operation of Roux-Y to be very satisfactory. Each patient who develops recurring symptoms of stricture should be subjected to another attempt to reconstruct the duct. This attitude has resulted in a survival of 102 of our 122 cases, and in satisfactory results in 93 of 122 cases.

Walters et al.[61] have carefully reviewed more than 400 operations for strictures of the common and hepatic bile ducts. Walters states that he has operated upon 429 patients with benign stricture of the bile ducts. Follow-up studies have shown that 70 to 75 percent of these patients have had continuing relief from biliary obstruction without recurrence of intrahepatic infection—unless contraction of the anastomosis occurred. In a long-term group of 191 patients who had had 217 operations, excellent or good results followed in 61 percent, and an additional 7 percent were classified as fair results. The results of choledochocholedochostomy and of choledochoduodenostomy were practically the same, being 68 to 69 percent, respectively, for the long-term (follow-up) group as from 83 to 82 percent, respectively, in the short-term group. Cattell and Braasch [5] state that about 30 percent of the patients died because of operative complications or of the complications of biliary obstruction. About 10 percent of the surviving patients have recurrence of biliary obstruction, and in about 65 percent a good or excellent result is obtained. If a patient is symptom-free after a period of 3 years following a reconstructive procedure on the bile duct for benign stricture, it can be said with a measure of confidence that the chances of permanent cure are extremely good. The patients should, of course, be under close observation during this 3-year postoperative period. If it becomes evident that further obstruction to the biliary outflow is present, prompt operative intervention should be undertaken regardless of the number of previous repairs. Cattell said that under no circumstances should this operation be delayed in the presence of recurrent attacks of cholangitis, persisting jaundice, or increasing hepatic enlargement.

Cattell and Braasch [2] reported the indications for and the results following the use of *primary repair* for benign strictures of the bile ducts. These cases were taken from a series of 501 patients first seen at the Lahey Clinic during the years 1940 to 1955, inclusive; 802 operations were carried out in this group. These procedures included 207 end-to-end ductal repairs, 142 hepatojejunostomies, 46 plastic procedures, 37 dilatations of the stricture, and 15 hepaticoduodenostomies. The postoperative mortality rate ranged from 2 to 5 percent, and a satisfactory result was observed in 43 to 68 percent of the patients 3 years or more after operation. Approximately one-third of the patients in whom Y tubes were used experienced no further trouble related to the biliary stricture and of 36 patients in whom the Y tube became occluded (requiring removal), 31 are still symptom-free—17 for more than 3 years. Cosman and Porter [9] reported that excellent or good results were obtained in 78.5 percent of the patients operated upon by them.

I have performed 131 operations upon 109 patients suffering from postoperative strictures of the bile ducts, with a hospital death rate of about 3 percent. The results of reconstructive procedures on the *extrahepatic or extrahilar* strictures have been gratifying as 75 to 80 percent were judged to be symptom-free during a follow-up period of 5 years or more. The results following operation for intrahepatic or *high hilar strictures* have been disappointing, as less than 35 percent of the patients referred to me could be regarded as being cured after one or more attempts at repair. Nevertheless, I feel confident that the chances of success have been greatly enhanced by performing Rodney Smith's new ingenious method of the so-called *jejunal mucosal graft operation for these hilar strictures.*

Because of the possibility of an eventual good result, each patient who develops recurrent signs and symptoms of bile duct stricture should be subjected to yet another attempt to repair the condition.

Warren et al.[67] of the Lahey Clinic Foundation supplies recent data in Table 3.

Table 3.   OUTCOME FOLLOWING SURGICAL REPAIR OF BILIARY STRICTURE; 1553 OPERATIONS IN 987 PATIENTS (1940-67)

Result	Number of Patients	Percent	
Excellent	513	52	78 percent satisfactory
Good	258	26	
Poor	43	4	
Died	132	13	17 percent unsatisfactory
Lost to follow-up	41	4	

REFERENCES

1. Baty, Br. J. Surg. 43:553, 1956.
2. Cattell and Braasch, Lahey Clin. Bull. 10:194, 1958.
2a. Cattell and Braasch, Surg. Gynecol. Obstet. 109: 691, 1959; 110:88, 1960.
3. Cattell and Braasch, New Engl. J. Med. 261: 929, 1959.
4. Cattell and Braasch, Surg. Gynecol. Obstet. 109: 531, 1959.
5. Cattell and Braasch, Lahey Clin. Bull. 50:147, 1958.
6. Cole, W., Postgrad. Med. 9:349, 1951.
7. Cole, W., Ireneus and Reynolds, Ann. Surg. 142:537, 1955.
8. Cole, W. et al., Ann. Surg. 128:332, 1948.
9. Cosman and Porter, Ann. Surg. 152:730, 1960.
10. Diethrich et al., Am. J. Surg. 112:756, 1966.
11. Dobbie and Stormo, J. Trauma 8:9, 1968.
12. Donald, John, and Donald James, Ann. Surg. 148:855, 1958.
13. Dragstedt and Woodward, Surg. Gynecol. Obstet. 94:53, 1952.
14. Edlington, Br. J. Surg. 20:679, 1933.
15. Gray, Howard, Proc. R. Soc. Med. 44:1005, 1951.
16. Grimault, Mem. Acad. Chir. 73:205, 1947.
17. Hart, Ann. Surg. 133:280, 1951.
18. Hartman and Greaney, Am. J. Surg. 108:150, 1964.
19. Hicken and Stevenson, Ann. Surg. 128:1178, 1948.
20. Hinshaw et al., Am. J. Surg. 104:104, 1962.
21. Karasewich and Bowden, Surg. Gynecol. Obstet. 124:1057, 1967.
22. Lahey and Pyrtek, Surg. Gynecol. Obstet. 91:25, 1950.
23. Lewis, Ann. Surg. 108:237, 1938.
24. Lilienthal, Ann. Surg. 77:865, 1923.
25. Longmire and Sandford, Ann. Surg. 129:264, 1948.
26. Longmire and Sandford, Ann. Surg. 130:455, 1949.
27. Lysaght, Br. J. Surg. 26:646, 1939.
28. Maingot, R., Br. Surg. Prog. 1:1, 1954.
29. Maingot, R., J. Ir. Med. Assoc. 39:41, 1956.
30. Maingot, R., Ann. R. Coll. Surg. Engl. 24:186, 1959
31. Maingot, R., Proc. R. Soc. Med. 53:545, 1960.
32. Maingot, R., London Clin. Med. J. 2:11, 1961.
33. Maingot, R., Proc. R. Soc. Med. 55:587, 1962.
34. Maingot, R., Ann. R. Coll. Surg. Engl. 32:42, 1963
35. Maingot, R., in Smith and Sherlock, eds., Surgery of the Gall Bladder and Bile Ducts, London, Butterworths, 1964, Chaps. 2 and 14.
36. Maingot, R., in Rob and Smith, eds., Operative Surgery, 2d ed., London, Butterworths, 1969, pp. 421–447.
37. Maingot, R., Br. J. Clin. Pract. 26:15, 1972.
38. Manlove et al., Am. J. Surg. 97:113, 1959.
39. Mason et al., Ann. Surg. 140:234, 1954.
40. Massie, Ann. Surg. 131:838, 1950.
41. Mays, Truman, Surg. Gynecol. Obstet. 124:801, 1967.

42. Michie and Gunn, Br. J. Surg. 51:96, 1964.
43. Norcross and Dadey, New Engl. J. Med. 257: 1216, 1957.
44. Parker and Robbins, Ann. Surg. 138:915, 1953.
45. Parkinson, Aust. N.Z. J. Surg. 30:253, 1970.
46. Penn, Br. J. Surg. 49:636, 1962.
46a. Remine, Personal communication, June, 1972.
47. Rudberg, Munch. Med. Wochenschr. 68:1680, 1921.
48. Salgado, Rev. Brasil Gastroenterol. 1:229, 1949.
49. Sedgwick and Hume, Surg. Gynecol. Obstet. 108:627, 1959.
50. Smith, Rodney, Br. J. Surg. 51:25, 1964.
50a. Smith, Rodney, Proc. R. Soc. Med. 62:131, 1969.
51. Smith, Rodney, Br. J. Surg. 51:183, 1964.
52. Smith, Rodney, Br. J. Surg. 51:186, 1964.
53. Smith, Rodney, Personal communications, June, 1970 and April, 1973.
54. Snyder, Ann. Surg. 146:246, 1951.
55. Spencer, Br. J. Surg. 40:283, 1952.
56. Sullivan, J.A.M.A. 53:774, 1909.
57. Sullivan, J.A.M.A. 58:206, 1912.
58. Templeton and Dodd, Ann. Surg. 157:287, 1963.
59. Walker, Milnes, Lancet 2:969, 1953.
60. Walters, W., et al., Proceedings of the World Congress of Gastroenterology, 1958.
61. Walters, W., et al., Proc. Mayo Clin. 50:147, 1958.
62. Walters, W., Surg. Gynecol. Obstet. 48:305, 1929.
63. Walters, W., and Kelly, Arch. Surg. 66:417, 1953.
64. Warren, K. W., Surg. Clin. North Am. 46:611, 1965.
65. Warren, K. W., Personal communications, 1972.
66. Warren, K., and Braasch, Surg. Clin. North Am. 44:717, 1964.
67. Warren, K., Mountain, and Midell, Surg. Clin. North Am. 51:711, 1971.
68. Warren, K., Poulantzas, and Kune, Surg. Gynecol. Obstet. 122:785, 1966.
69. Watkins, Arch. Surg. 80:187, 1961.
70. Waugh et al., Proc. Mayo Clin. 27:578, 1952.
71. Williams and Smithwick, Ann. Surg. 89:942, 1929.

49

ORIENTAL CHOLANGIOHEPATITIS

FRANCIS E. STOCK

Cholangitis means infection of the bile ducts. As is the case in other hollow viscera, it is rarely seen when there is no obstruction to the outflow of fluid from the system. Cholangitis is seen most commonly in association with stones or stricture of the bile ducts and occasionally with ulcerating lesions of the ampulla of Vater that produce partial obstruction. In few of these cases is the liver parenchyma seriously involved.

Oriental cholangiohepatitis (recurrent pyogenic cholangitis) is a recognisable syndrome with a clear geographical and racial distribution. It is found almost exclusively amongst people of the Chinese race, and it occurs most commonly along the coastline of southeast Asia, extending inland around the river deltas (Fig. 1). In Hong Kong, cholangiohepatitis is the disease of the biliary system most commonly seen in the surgical wards. Isolated cases have been found in other parts of the world amongst migrant Chinese.

AETIOLOGY

Age and Sex Incidence

The disease occurs at all ages above infancy, although it is most common in patients between 20 and 40 years. Sex incidence is equal. It is a disease seen much more frequently among the poor than among the well to do.

Infection

The disease is undoubtedly infective in nature, and positive cultures of *E. coli* and *Streptococcus faecalis* can be obtained from the bile and from the portal blood in almost all patients. These organisms come from the bowel. The bowel infections with diarrhoea are certainly no more common amongst the Chinese than in other races in the tropics. Neither is chronic constipation

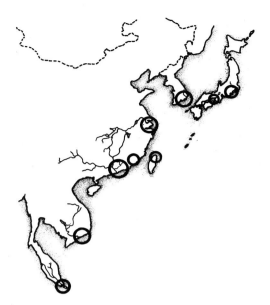

FIG. 1. Southeast Asia: reported endemic areas of *Clonorchis sinensis* infestation and distribution of cholangiohepatitis around major seaports and river estuaries. Actual incidence may be more widespread.

particularly common. There must, therefore, be some other factors which permit the infection to take hold in the biliary system. Many such factors have been implicated. Metabolic causes and especially haemolysis with intraduct stone formation may be important, although the disease is never seen in association with pure cholesterol stones or with pure bilirubin stones in congenital

spherocytosis. Inflammatory oedema or spasm of the sphincter of Oddi has been postulated (Harrison-Levy) but no cause for this condition is known. Furthermore, the narrowed lower end of the common bile duct—sometimes seen in cholangiography and thought to be characteristic—is evidence of underfilling of the ducts and rapidly disappears in most patients if more fluid is introduced.

Infestation of the biliary tree with *Ascaris, Fasciola,* or *Clonorchis* has also been suggested; in some cases the first two worms are found in the duct, dead or alive. Dead worms tend to be encrusted with bile salts and debris. In the Hong Kong series, *Clonorchis* infestation was present in more than 90 percent of patients with the disease compared with a general infestation rate of only 45 percent in the surgical wards; however, this is not true in other places. In Singapore, *Clonorchis* was demonstrated in only 1 of 30 cases.

There is no doubt that infestation with *C. sinensis* produces an intense inflammatory change in the biliary epithelium, with hyperplasia and desquamation and on occasion proceeding to a malignant cholangioma. *Clonorchis* can die out in the biliary tree, particularly in the presence of infection, and there is much to suggest that it plays an important part in the pathogenesis of this disease (Fig. 2). Once established however, other factors may make the disease self-perpetuating.

PATHOLOGY

The changes seen depend both on the acuteness of the individual attack and the chronicity of the disease. In most cases, the gallbladder is not acutely inflamed but is distended with dark, viscous bile and the wall may be thickened. During an acute exacerbation, however, distention and inflammation may combine to produce a gangrenous patch near the fundus—leading to rupture and biliary peritonitis. *Stones are rarely present within the gallbladder.*

The common bile duct is usually grossly distended—often to 2 cm or more in diameter —and contains many stones. These calculi may form a cast of part of the biliary tree. They are found well up into the liver and

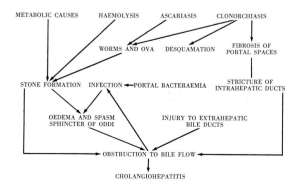

FIG. 2. The aetiological circle.

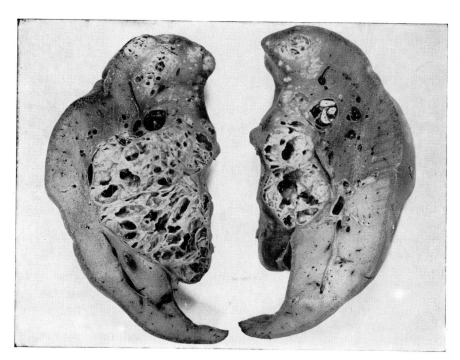

FIG. 3.   Section of liver showing honeycomb abscesses and intrahepatic stones in grossly dilated ducts. (From Smith and Sherlock, eds., *Surgery of the Gallbladder and Bile Ducts,* 1964. Courtesy of Butterworths, London.)

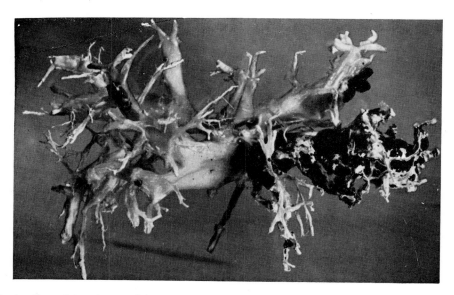

FIG. 4.   Cast of intrahepatic bile ducts showing considerable dilatation of all ducts with many stones in the left lobe and a few on the right side. (From Smith and Sherlock, eds., *Surgery of the Gallbladder and Bile Ducts,* 1964. Courtesy of Butterworths, London.)

on occasion are found only within the liver. Pathological changes in the liver are usually more severe on the left side than on the right. The duct walls are thickened and oedematous and, apart from the stones, may contain epithelial debris, ova, worms, and sometimes pus.

The intrahepatic ducts show changes similar to those outside the liver, but the inflammatory changes in the wall are often more extensive—progressing to fibrosis and stricture formation. The infection passes through the duct wall into the liver parenchyma with the formation of multiple honeycombed hepatic abscesses (Figs. 3 and 4). Stones may be held up behind strictures, and occasionally a lesion on the surface may be found adherent to adjacent viscera.

Sometimes carcinomatous changes occur in the ducts around these stones.

Stones are characteristically *mixed,* containing all biliary elements; however, they are usually soft rather than hard, and are rarely faceted. Thus, they are unlike those found in ordinary cholelithiasis. The nucleus of the stone is frequently an ovum or even a dead *Clonorchis* worm.

Acute pancreatitis is rare in association with the disease, but chronic pancreatitis with fibrosis of the body and head is found quite frequently. It does not seem to be sufficiently severe to produce recognisable symptoms.

CLINICAL PICTURE

Symptoms

Pain is present in almost all cases but not at all stages of the disease. Indeed, the grossest pathological changes may be found in patients with little or no pain. When present, such pain is felt in the epigastrium and the right hypochondrium. It may be colicky at first, perhaps owing to the irritation of the sphincter of Oddi, but rapidly it becomes constant with distention of the biliary tree. The pain rarely radiates to the back.

Pyrexia is present in all acute cases and may be accompanied by rigors. Often, however, there are long periods of this disease when there is no fever.

Jaundice is present clinically in 50 percent of the patients and in almost all there is some elevation of the serum bilirubin levels. Jaundice may progress or disappear. Despite the absence of jaundice, the common bile duct may be filled with stones; in the presence of jaundice this is invariably the case.

Nausea and vomiting are common but perhaps the most characteristic feature of the history is that of recurrence of symptoms often over many years with spontaneous resolution between the attacks.

Physical Signs

The patients are obviously ill when seen in the acute phase. The temperature is elevated to 102 to 103° F. There is often evidence of dehydration due to vomiting. Jaundice is usually obvious.

Examination of the abdomen reveals tenderness in the right hypochondrium, accompanied by guarding or even rigidity and spreading toward the umbilicus. The gallbladder is distended and usually readily palpable unless masked by muscular rigidity. It becomes quite evident under anaesthesia when the abdominal wall is relaxed.

Cholangiohepatitis is thus a unique lesion in producing a palpable gallbladder in a patient with obstructive jaundice caused by the presence of stones.

Laboratory Findings

A low haemoglobin and a low serum protein are frequently present, although not directly related to the disease. Cholangiohepatitis is seen almost exclusively among the poorer classes in whom nutritional defect is common. In the acute phase, leucocytosis up to 15,000 per cubic millimeter is present in most patients. The serum bilirubin is increased up to a level between 2 and 10 mg per 100 ml, and bile is present in the urine. Urobilinogen is also present, as the obstruction is rarely complete. Liver function tests show some evidence of cellular damage.

Radiological Findings

A straight x-ray film may rarely show stones, but occasionally gas is seen in the biliary tree. This radiographic sign is usually regarded as characteristic of gallstone ileus,

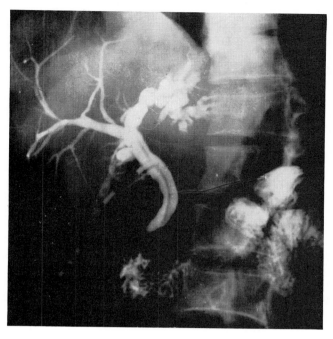

FIG. 5. T tube operative cholangiogram showing relatively normal ducts in the right lobe with gross dilatation and multiple abscess cavities in the left lobe. (From Smith and Sherlock, eds., *Surgery of the Gallbladder and Bile Ducts,* 1964. Courtesy of Butterworths, London.)

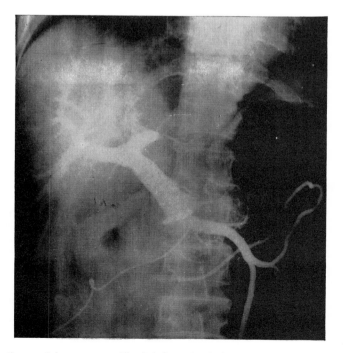

FIG. 6. Operative portal venogram. The left branch of the portal vein is abruptly interrupted by an abscess around which small vessels are displaced. (From Smith and Sherlock, eds., *Surgery of the Gallbladder and Bile Ducts,* 1964. Courtesy of Butterworths, London.)

but in areas where cholangiohepatitis is endemic it occurs quite frequently. This may be due to fistula formation between the common bile duct and duodenum, to a patulous sphincter, or occasionally to gas infection in the biliary tree. (This latter is quite rare.)

Cholecystography and cholangiography are of little value, as jaundice prevents satisfactory excretion. Percutaneous cholangiography, which is such a valuable investigation in patients with obstructive jaundice, is potentially dangerous in these patients and should be avoided if possible. It may release infected bile into blood vessels opened up by the needle and thus produce pyrexia or even bacteraemic shock. Operative cholangiography, however, may show intrahepatic stones and strictures and occasionally large abscess cavities, while portal venography will sometimes show a distortion of the veins around intrahepatic abscesses (Figs. 5 and 6).

Differential Factors

Because of the restricted geographical and racial incidence, this disease will rarely be recognised by those unfamiliar with it. In an endemic area, however, it is almost unmistakable. Nevertheless, in some patients pain is very slight, and the condition can be confused with infective hepatitis. Carcinoma of the head of the pancreas, of the bile ducts, or of the liver itself is not uncommon in Chinese patients and this may cause confusion.

In the absence of jaundice, diagnosis is much more difficult. The recurrent attacks of pain, fever, and right hypochondrial tenderness, however, are suggestive, and in these patients intravenous cholangiography may often show stones.

Clonorchis ova in the stool, although frequently present, are so commonly found in patients in endemic areas that they are of no value in establishing a diagnosis.

TREATMENT

Conservative treatment has no place at all in the jaundiced patient except as a preoperative measure. If the diagnosis is in doubt, e.g., when pain is absent, conservative measures may be adopted for a short time— but unless there is a rapid improvement, continued delay is likely to do greater harm to a patient with cholangiohepatitis than would a negative laparotomy in a patient with infective hepatitis.

Antibiotics, chloramphenicol, tetracycline, or ampicillin should be given preoperatively, together with vitamin K. Dehydration and anaemia should also be corrected as an emergency measure by transfusion. (See Chaps. 106 and 107.)

Surgical Procedure

Surgical intervention is always advised for patients who have jaundice, pain, and pyrexia. The object is to produce adequate permanent drainage of the biliary tree and to effect as complete a debridement as possible.

Any standard operative approach to the biliary tree is acceptable, although the author prefers a vertical transrectus incision. Special care must be taken to protect the wound edges, as the bile is always heavily infected and contamination can readily occur. Antiseptic packs tucked around the peritoneal opening or skin towels stitched to the peritoneum are useful protective measures.

Cholecystostomy. This is reserved for the acutely ill patient in whom there is an immediate risk of perforation and biliary peritonitis. It produces very satisfactory drainage for a short time with minimum risk and allows for further investigation for definitive operation by means of a postoperative cholangiogram.

Evacuation of debris from biliary tree. The main ducts are usually filled with soft stones and a great deal of epithelial debris. If the common bile duct is markedly dilated, it is best opened by a low longitudinal incision made on the front of the duct, just above the duodenum. This will facilitate subsequent procedures. Stones, worms, and other debris are evacuated with forceps and later with irrigation. The ducts are often so large that digital palpation within them is feasible and helpful. A bougie is passed down toward the duodenum and the sphincter is usually easily negotiated, being only rarely constricted.

Choledochostomy. The insertion of a Maingot guttered T tube after debridement allows for continued drainage and, if necessary, for irrigation. It is not recommended by itself, however, because stones usually recur unless steps are taken to improve the drainage from the ducts.

Choledochoduodenostomy. In patients with a common bile duct dilated 2 cm or more in diameter, choledochoduodenostomy provides one form of dependent drainage. A large longitudinal incision in the common bile duct is anastomosed to a similar parallel incision in the front of the first part of the duodenum, and catgut sutures are used to avoid a nidus for recurrent stones. There is a theoretical objection to this procedure in that reflux of duodenal contents into the biliary tree can occur. Provided the anastomosis is *wide* and not stenosed, reflux rarely causes permanent harm. It is reflux with obstruction and impaired drainage that is harmful, and for this reason in the unusual patient in whom there is only slight dilatation, some alternative procedure may be more advantageous.

Choledochojejunostomy, Roux-en-Y. Because of the theoretical risk that choledochoduodenostomy may be followed by reflux, further stone formation, and continued injection, and that stones may also collect in the blind segment of common bile duct below the anastomosis, some surgeons prefer choledochojejunostomy by the Roux-en-Y procedure. In such cases, the common bile duct should be divided completely just above the duodenum and anastomosed to the jejunal loop. This may be done as a primary procedure or as a corrective operation if any of the above-mentioned complications follow choledochoduodenostomy. The latter procedure, however, is simpler and adequate for the majority of patients.

Transduodenal sphincterotomy. This is the procedure favoured in those cases in which the common bile duct is not grossly dilated. It provides completely dependent drainage and, if thought desirable, a *sphincteroplasty* can be done by excising a small wedge of tissue on each side of the sphincterotomy to avoid subsequent stenosis. Full debridement must be carried out through a choledochostomy and not through the sphincterotomy. In all cases, it is best to drain the duct system with a Maingot guttered T tube.

Sphincterotomy avoids the theoretical danger of a short blind loop of common bile duct

behind the duodenum which fails to drain. (In practice, this has rarely been a problem.) In the patient with quite dilated ducts, sphincterotomy can never provide an anastomosis of the same width as the supraduodenal choledochoduodenostomy.

Cholecystectomy. Although the gallbladder is rarely acutely inflamed, if it is left behind after either a choledochoduodenostomy or a transduodenal sphincterotomy, it becomes a stagnant diverticulum which may sometimes cause trouble. Cholecystectomy is not difficult save in the acute phase, and it should be done at the same time as the anastomosis or sphincterotomy.

Drainage and irrigation of dilated intrahepatic ducts. In some cases, the intrahepatic changes are so extensive that it may be desirable to provide for prolonged drainage and irrigation—especially of ducts in the left lobe. This is most readily achieved by the introduction of a soft flexible rubber or latex (plastic tubes should not be used.) tube (1) through the common bile duct, (2) into the left hepatic duct, and (3) out through the superior surface of the liver and an overlying stab wound. The liver may then be irrigated with fluid or antibiotics can be instilled. The measure is of particular value in patients in whom strictures are beginning to develop.

Drainage of abscess and hepatectomy. After the treatment outlined above, occasionally an intrahepatic duct becomes stenosed and abscesses that have formed around the duct enlarge and reach the surface. These must be drained—but, unfortunately, drainage tends to be persistent. Therefore, in patients in whom abscesses form and are localised to the left lobe, a left hepatic lobectomy may be carried out. It should be emphasised that this situation is rarely encountered in the early phases; it is a late complication which may occur several years after the establishment of satisfactory drainage.

PROGNOSIS

The prognosis in this condition should be very guarded. The disease has often been in existence for months or years before treatment is undertaken and changes have occurred in the liver which are slowly progressive. If jaundice is unrelieved, death occurs from hepatic failure; occasionally a small intrahepatic abscess will rupture into an hepatic vein radicle, causing bacteraemia and sometimes sudden death. In a few cases, a cholangiocarcinoma occurs.

Nevertheless, provided the patient is seen early and adequate drainage is established, there is some hope of success. Although the connection between clonorchiasis and cholangiohepatitis is difficult to establish with certainty, continued *Clonorchis* infestation can only do harm, and patients should be warned against the dangers of eating undercooked freshwater fish that are possibly contaminated by the worms.

50

CARCINOMA OF THE GALLBLADDER AND EXTRAHEPATIC BILE DUCTS: OPERATIVE PROCEDURES

RODNEY SMITH

In cases of carcinoma of the gallbladder it is unusual for radical resection to be undertaken with the possibility of a useful long-term survival. More commonly all that can be achieved is *palliation,* e.g., the relief of obstructive jaundice.

The abdomen is usually explored for one of two reasons. (1) Symptoms suggest cholelithiasis and cholecystitis, and x-ray pictures confirm the diagnosis. Carcinoma of the gallbladder may be suspected on account of persistent pain, the presence of a palpable mass, or marked recent weight loss—but it may also be a totally unexpected finding. (2) Laparotomy may be undertaken for obstructive jaundice—perhaps with a mass to be felt in the gallbladder area. Percutaneous transhepatic cholangiography immediately before exploration will suggest malignant obstruction at the level of the porta hepatis.

EXPLORATION: SELECTION OF TECHNIQUE

The presence of a carcinoma may not be immediately obvious. A thick-walled oedematous gallbladder containing stones may be thought to be the site of inflammatory changes only. If there is doubt, frozen-section biopsy studies should be made. The diagnosis of carcinoma being established, the liver, lymphatic fields, and peritoneal cavity are examined for metastases. *Simple cholecystomy alone gives very poor results,* few patients living for more than a year or 18 months. In most cases, therefore, the choice of procedure to be adopted lies between: (a) extended cholecystectomy and (b) extended right hepatic lobectomy—depending upon the age and fitness of the patient and the surgeon's familiarity with hepatic resections.

In extended cholecystectomy, the aim is to remove with the gallbladder a generous margin of continuous liver and all accessible lymphatics draining the gallbladder area.

The procedure starts with division of the peritoneum covering the common bile duct below and the common hepatic duct above. This dissection is carried into the porta hepatis and the right and left hepatic ducts are identified. These ducts are cleared and the loose cellular tissue is stripped from them in a downward direction, using Lahey swabs. To the right of the common hepatic duct the cystic artery is identified and divided between ligatures, the fat around it being similarly stripped away from the liver and hepatic ducts in a downward direction, together with the cystic lymph node (Fig. 1).

The common hepatic duct being well displayed, the cystic duct is put on the stretch

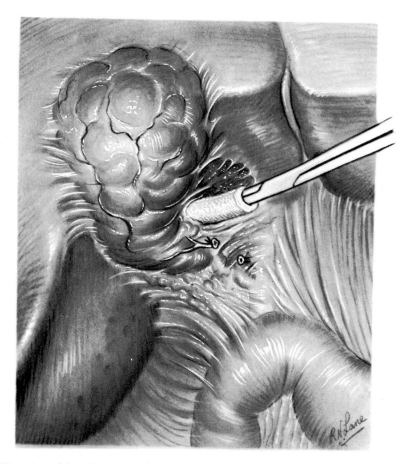

FIG. 1.   Dissection of fat, fascia, and lymphatics covering the common hepatic and cystic ducts.

by traction on Hartmann's pouch and carefully dissected until its junction with the common bile duct is identified. This stage of the operation is so carried out that the loose cellular tissue around the common bile duct, right down to its disappearance into the groove between the pancreas and duodenum —including the "common duct lymph node," is dissected up to be removed en bloc with the gallbladder. Mobilisation of the duodenum by Kocher's method is necessary in order to carry out this fascial clearance adequately.

The cystic duct is ligated and divided as close as possible to the common bile duct (Fig. 2).

The gallbladder is then attached solely to the liver. Whereas in simple cholecystectomy the aim is to identify and stay in the plane between the gallbladder and the liver, the reverse is now the case. Using the diathermy, a wedge of liver substance is removed with the gallbladder so that the hepatic surface of the gallbladder is not approached at any point.

The liver substance is carefully examined and any visible blood vessel or peripheral bile duct is individually ligated. A few mattress sutures may be used to complete haemostasis, and the great omentum may be used to cover the raw surface remaining. The abdomen is closed with drainage.

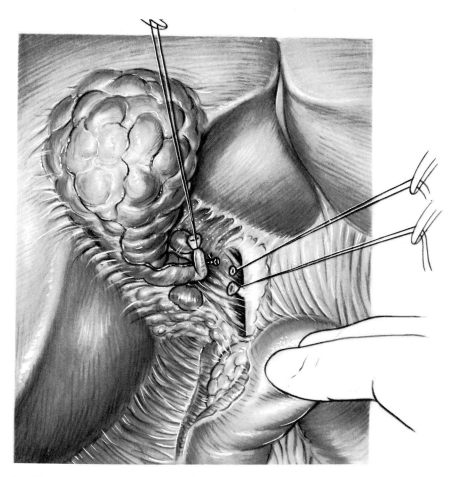

FIG. 2.   The cystic artery and cystic duct have been tied. The fat, fascia, and lymphatics covering the common hepatic, common bile, and cystic ducts are removed with the gallbladder.

EXTENDED RIGHT HEPATIC LOBECTOMY

This radical approach to the problem of carcinoma of the gallbladder is justified by the poor results following performance of lesser procedures. Such poor results are probably due, at least in part, to the early dissemination into the liver of the carcinoma—by direct extension and via blood and lymphatic vessels. Nevertheless it is quite possible [3] for the right lobe to be involved on quite a massive scale while the left lobe remains free of disease.

Extended right hepatic lobectomy [2] means removal of the whole of the liver to the right of the falciform plane. It is thus a more extensive resection than a right hepatic lobectomy (right hemihepatectomy) when the line of division is through the principal plane of the liver and therefore through the gallbladder fossa. The procedure known as "middle lobe hepatectomy" [1]—the central portion of the liver including the gallbladder fossa being removed and the lobus dexter and lobus sinister proper being retained—should not, in the writer's view, be considered. It is rather more difficult technically than an extended right hepatic lobectomy, its risk is at least as great (probably greater), and it is a less effective operation for cancer.

A right thoracoabdominal approach is essential, the incision being extended across the costal margin, which is divided, into the eighth intercostal space. A rib-spreader is inserted and the diaphragm is split from the periphery to the inferior vena caval hiatus.

The peritoneal reflection between the right lobe of the liver and diaphragm is divided and the liver is rotated upward so that dissection in the porta hepatis is facilitated.

The structures in the porta hepatis are dissected out and carefully displayed. The cystic artery is identified and divided between ligatures. The cystic duct is ligated and divided as close as possible to its junction with the common bile duct. This stage of the operation is carried out exactly as it is for extended

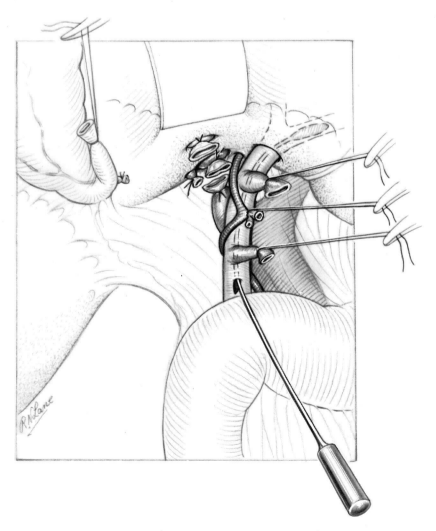

FIG. 3.   Extended right hepatic lobectomy: the right hepatic duct, right hepatic artery, and the right branch of the portal vein have all been tied and divided. A Bakes' dilator in the common bile duct and inserted from this into the left hepatic duct helps in identifying these structures.

cholecystectomy, and it includes clearing all the loose cellular tissue off the hepatic and common bile ducts right down to the duodenum.

The next structure to be divided is the right hepatic duct. In order to make clear the anatomy of the duct system, it is a good plan first to open the common bile duct and to pass a 3-mm Bakes' dilator into the left hepatic duct, leaving it there while the right hepatic duct is ligated and divided. (The opening in the common bile duct is later used for postoperative T tube drainage).

The right hepatic artery and the right branch of the portal vein are identified and divided between ligatures (Fig. 3).

When dissection in the porta hepatis is completed, the table is tilted to the left, the liver is elevated, and dissection proceeds along the inferior vena cava. Several small inconstant veins between the liver and the vena cava in the lower part of its course are secured. Just below the diaphragm the large right hepatic vein is carefully isolated and

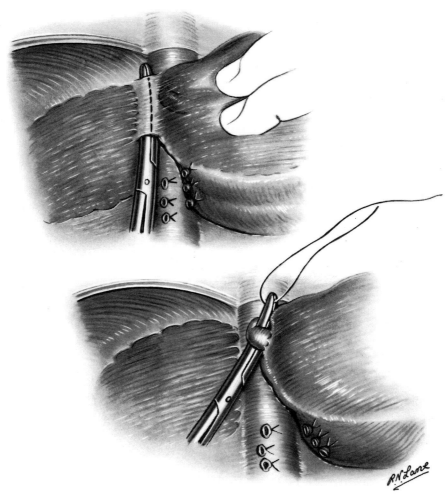

FIG. 4. Extended right hepatic lobectomy: technique for securing and ligating the right hepatic vein behind the liver. (From Smith and Sherlock, eds., *Surgery of the Gallbladder and Bile Ducts,* 1964. Courtesy of Butterworths, London.)

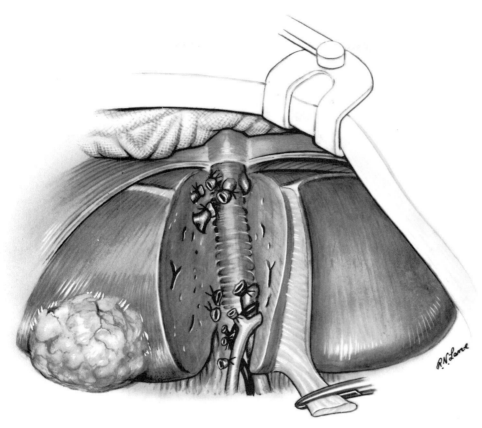

FIG. 5.   Extended right hepatic lobectomy: ligation of the middle hepatic vein. (From Smith and Sherlock, eds., *Surgery of the Gallbladder and Bile Ducts*, 1964. Courtesy of Butterworths, London.)

divided between ligatures (Fig. 4).

For ligation of the middle hepatic vein, the table is tilted back again and the liver is split along the falciform plane. Immediately below the diaphragm, the entry into the vena cava of the left and middle hepatic veins must be identified and the latter divided between ligatures (Fig. 5). These two large veins often enter the vena cava via a common short trunk. The liver substance is split by blunt dissection with the point of a haemostat, the few individual vessels encountered being picked up and ligated. Inferiorly, the left hepatic duct, left hepatic artery, and left branch of the portal vein (already displayed) are carefully preserved as the division of the liver is completed.

The divided liver substance is inspected and complete haemostasis is secured by ligation, diathermy, and one or two interrupted catgut sutures. A T tube is placed in the common bile duct. The diaphragm and costal margin are repaired. The thoracic and abdominal walls are closed, with drainage. The right pleural cavity should be drained with an intercostal catheter connected to an underwater seal drain. The subdiaphragmatic space can usually safely be drained with a corrugated rubber drain, but as air might pass through an unnoticed defect in the repaired diaphragm it is probably better to drain the subdiaphragmatic space also with a catheter (through a separate stab incision) connected to an underwater seal drain.

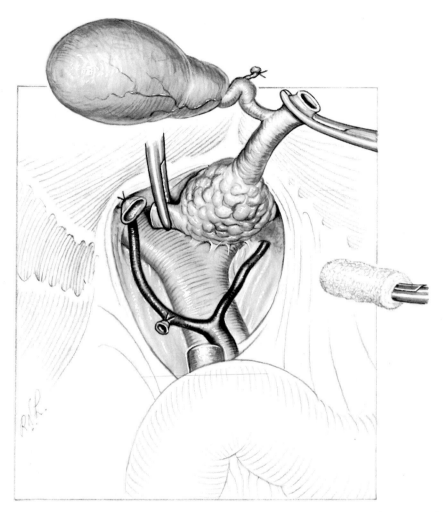

FIG. 6. Resection of carcinoma of the common hepatic duct: the common bile duct and the right hepatic duct have been divided; the left hepatic duct is about to be displayed and divided.

POSTOPERATIVE CARE

The postoperative care after a major hepatectomy is described in Chapter 53. The T tube monitors the bile production by the liver and is removed about 10 to 14 days postoperatively, provided there is no leakage of bile and a cholangiogram shows no extravasation of contrast medium.

CARCINOMA OF THE GALLBLADDER INFILTRATING INTO THE PORTA HEPATIS

Although in theory an extended right hepatic lobectomy might still be possible, the writer has yet to encounter a case in this group in which resection proved practicable.

Palliative T tube intubation is usually the only means of helping the patient. The contracted empty common bile duct is opened and probes of various sizes are used to find a way through the obstructed common hepatic duct into the dilated intrahepatic duct system beyond. When retained bile begins to escape, some is taken for culture (as pyogenic cholangitis is common) and the malignant stricture is dilated with Bakes' dilators to the maximum size possible. A Cattell T tube of the largest possible size is introduced with the upper limb well beyond the stricture, into the dilated ducts above, and the abdomen is then closed.

CARCINOMA OF THE COMMON HEPATIC DUCT

Painless obstructive jaundice in an elderly patient who does not have a palpable gallbladder should arouse suspicion of a carcinoma of the common hepatic duct—a lesion not so rare as is sometimes supposed. Patients presenting in this way should have a percutaneous transhepatic cholangiogram immediately before laparotomy; the site of the biliary obstruction will probably be clearly demonstrable.

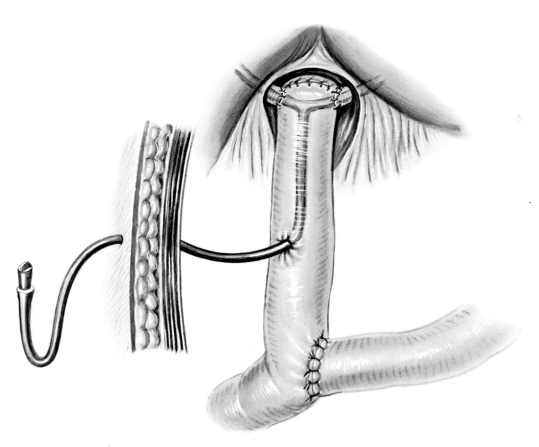

FIG. 7.   Resection of carcinoma of the common hepatic duct; anastomosis of the divided right and left hepatic ducts to the Roux loop of jejunum. (From Smith and Sherlock, eds., *Surgery of the Gallbladder and Bile Ducts*, 1964. Courtesy of Butterworths, London.)

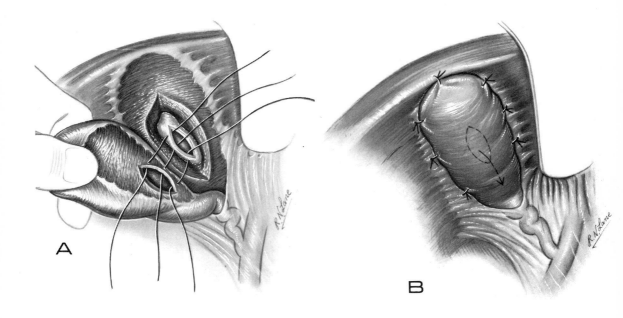

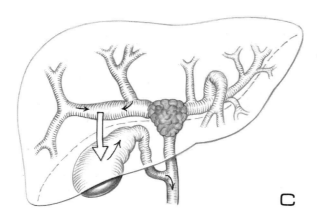

FIG. 8. Inoperable carcinoma of the common hepatic duct: technique for anastomosis of the intrahepatic duct to the gallbladder. (A) The liver has been incised, the duct found, and the anastomosis begun. (B) Completed anastomosis. (C) Short-circuiting procedure. (From Smith and Sherlock, eds., *Surgery of the Gallbladder and Bile Ducts, 1964.* Courtesy of Butterworths, London.)

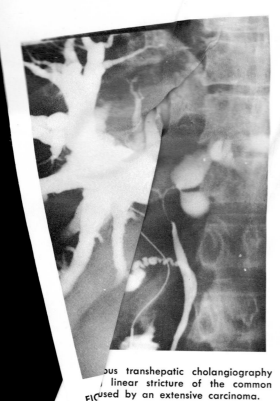

ous transhepatic cholangiography
linear stricture of the common
FICused by an extensive carcinoma.

ir may be small and identifiable
me difficulty. The empty com-
uct is contracted and a misdiag-
sclerosing cholangitis" is sometimes
There should, however, not be any
ulty if an operative cholangiogram is
ded to the already performed percutaneous
transhepatic cholangiogram. The dilated
ducts in the liver and the small but otherwise
normal ducts below the porta hepatis contrast strongly with the generalised irregular
stenosis seen in sclerosing cholangitis.

Resection is rarely possible; palliation of
the obstructive jaundice is usually the aim. If
the tumour is small and considered resectable, the empty common bile duct is divided
just above the duodenum and dissected up
toward the liver together with the surrounding loose cellular tissue and the common duct
lymph node. The cystic artery is ligated and
divided and the gallbladder with the cellular
tissue around its neck, including the cystic
node, is mobilised with the common bile

duct. The common hepatic duct and the
carcinoma are dissected free from the
branches of the hepatic artery and portal
vein with Lahey swabs; the right and left
hepatic ducts are then identified and divided,
allowing removal of the tumour (Fig. 6).

A Roux loop is constructed, the end is
closed, and brought up into the porta hepatis. Each hepatic duct is anastomosed individually to the side (right and left) of the
Roux loop, using a single layer of fine catgut
sutures. Each of these two anastomoses is
splinted with an indwelling latex rubber
tube brought out *transhepatically,* through
the Roux loop or left free in the jejunal
lumen to be passed later. The loop itself is
then sutured to the capsule of the liver for
support (Figs. 7, 8, 9, and 10). The abdomen

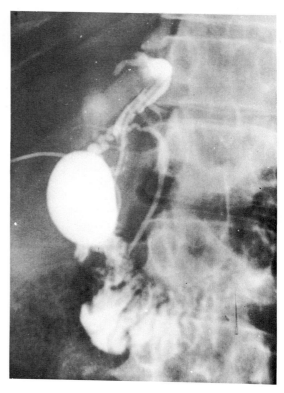

FIG. 10.   Inoperable carcinoma of the common hepatic duct treated by anastomosing the gallbladder
to a large branch of the right hepatic duct. There
was good drainage of the right hepatic duct system with immediate relief of jaundice. (R. Smith's
patient.)

is closed with drainage. An alternative method of effecting a large, stable, epithelium-lined junction between the right and left hepatic ducts and the jejunal loop is to employ *the "mucosal graft" technique* recently described [4] and illustrated in Figures 64, 65, and 66 in Chapter 48C, each duct, of course, being anastomosed independently.

PALLIATIVE T TUBE INTUBATION AND SHORT-CIRCUITING

If, as is usual, the tumour is not considered resectable, the malignant stricture is dilated as described earlier in this chapter and a Cattell T tube is inserted with the upper end well into the dilated intrahepatic duct system. It is important that bile released by the dilatation should be taken for culture so that postoperative antibiotic cover can be related to the drug sensitivity of the organisms. Forcible dilatation of a malignant stricture in the presence of pyogenic cholangitis, which is not uncommon in malignant obstruction, carries a small but distinct hazard of producing a gram-negative septicaemia.

A palliative short circuit is rarely applicable to the problem, but occasionally the anatomy of the ducts favours an operation of this kind. It is indicated if: (a) preoperative percutaneous cholangiography has shown very large dilated ducts in the liver; (b) the tumour is high in the porta hepatis (in fact, mostly intrahepatic); (c) the common bile duct is normal, though empty, and a long

normal cystic duct joins the common bile duct low down, near the duodenum.

CHOLANGIOCHOLECYSTOSTOMY

In these circumstances, the empty gallbladder is detached from the liver after dividing its peritoneal attachment. With use of a needle and syringe inserted through the bare hepatic surface that has been exposed, a dilated intrahepatic duct is sought as near the surface as possible. Aspiration through the liver substance with the point of a haemostat exposes this duct. It is then opened for a distance of ½ in (1.3 to 2.5 cm). Bile pours out and there is no difficulty in confirming that a duct of sufficient size has been entered. An incision of the same length is made in the hepatic end of the gallbladder and the bile duct and gallbladder are anastomosed with a single layer of fine catgut sutures. The gallbladder is reattached to the liver by suturing its peritoneal attachment (Fig. 8).

REFERENCES

1. Pack, G. T., Northwest. Med. 57:881, 1958.
2. Smith, R., in Rob, C. G., and Smith, R., Operative Surgery, London, Butterworths, 1958.
3. Smith, R., Br. J. Surg. 51:886, 1964.
4. Smith, R., Strictures of the Bile Ducts, in J. Badenoch and B. Brooke, Recent Advances in Gastroenterology, 2d ed., London, Churchill Livingstone, 1972, Chap. 15.

INDEX